Nutritional Support of Medical Practice

Editors

Howard A. Schneider, PH.D.
Editor-in-Chief
Director (Retired), Institute of Nutrition
University of North Carolina, Chapel Hill, North Carolina

Carl E. Anderson, PH.D.
Emeritus Professor, Department of Biochemistry and Nutrition
School of Medicine, University of North Carolina,
Chapel Hill, North Carolina

David B. Coursin, M.D.
Clinical Professor of Pediatrics
Georgetown University Medical Center, Washington, D.C.

With 46 Contributors

Nutritional
Support
of
Medical
Practice *Second Edition*

Harper & Row, Publishers

Philadelphia

London São Paulo
Mexico City St. Louis
New York Sydney

1817

Acquisitions Editor: John deCarville
Sponsoring Editor: Richard Winters
Manuscript Editor: Mary K. Smith
Indexer: Ruth Elwell
Art Director: Maria S. Karkucinski
Designer: Arlene Putterman
Production Coordinator: Charles W. Field
Compositor: Waldman Graphics, Inc.
Printer/Binder: The Murray Printing Company

The authors and publisher have exerted every effort to
ensure that drug selection and dosage set forth in this text
are in accord with current recommendations and practice
at the time of publication. However, in view of ongoing
research, changes in government regulations, and the
constant flow of information relating to drug therapy and
drug reactions, the reader is urged to check the package
insert for each drug for any change in indications and
dosage and for added warnings and precautions. This is
particularly important when the recommended agent is a
new or infrequently employed drug.

Library of Congress Cataloging in Publication Data
Main entry under title:

Nutritional support of medical practice.

  Includes bibliographies and index.
  1. Diet therapy. 2. Nutrition. I. Schneider, Howard A.
II. Anderson, Carl E., Date. III. Coursin, David
Baird. [DNLM: 1. Diet therapy. 2. Nutrition. 3. Nutri-
tion disorders. WB 400 N977]
RM216.N864 1983   615.8′54   82-23279
ISBN 0-06-142382-3

To John L. Dusseau, leader and wise counselor in American medical publishing

Contributors

Lilla Aftergood, Ph.D.
Research Biochemist Emeritus, Department of Biochemistry, School of Medicine, University of California, Los Angeles, California

Roslyn B. Alfin-Slater, Ph.D.
Professor of Nutrition, School of Public Health, University of California Los Angeles; Professor of Biological Chemistry, School of Medicine UCLA, Los Angeles, California

Lewis A. Barness, M.D.
Professor and Chairman, Dept. of Pediatrics, University of South Florida College of Medicine, Tampa, Florida

William R. Beisel, M.D.
Deputy for Science, United States Army Medical Research Institute of Infectious Diseases, Frederick, Maryland

Bruce R. Bistrian, M.D., Ph.D.
Associate Professor of Medicine, Harvard Medical School; Lecturer, Massachusetts Institute of Technology; Co-Director, Nutrition Support Service, New England Deaconess Hospital, Boston, Massachusetts

George L. Blackburn, M.D., Ph.D.
Director, Nutrition Support Service, New England Deaconcss Hospital, Cancer Research Institute, Boston, Massachusetts

George A. Bray, M.D.
Professor of Medicine, University of Southern California; Chief, Diabetes, and Clinical Nutrition LAC/USC Medical Center, Los Angeles, California

Robert A. Briggaman, M.D.
Professor of Dermatology and Medicine, Department of Dermatology, School of Medicine, University of North Carolina at Chapel Hill, Chapel Hill, North Carolina

John F. Burke, M.D.
Helen Andrus Benedict Professor of Surgery, Harvard Medical School; Chief of the Trauma Services, Massachusetts General Hospital, Boston Massachusetts

Ronald Cape, M.D., F.R.C.P.
Professor of Medicine, Co-ordinator of Geriatric Medicine, University of Western Ontario, London, Ontario, Canada

Ronni Chernoff, Ph.D., R.D.
Philadelphia, Pennsylvania

Edward M. Copeland, III, M.D.

Professor of Surgery, University of Texas Medical School at Houston, Houston, Texas

Robert G. Crounse, M.D.

Dept. of Surgery, School of Medicine, East Carolina University, Greenville, North Carolina

William T. Dahms, M.D.

Assistant Professor of Pediatrics, Case Western Reserve University School of Medicine, Cleveland, Ohio

Pierre M. Dreyfus, M.D.

Professor and Chairman, Department of Neurology, School of Medicine, University of California, Davis, California; Attending Neurologist, University of California at Davis, Sacramento Medical Center, Sacramento, California

Stanley J. Dudrick, M.D.

Director of Nutrition Support Services, St. Luke's Episcopal Hospital, Houston, Texas

Dianne M. Frazier, Ph.D.

Adjunct Assistant Professor of Biochemistry, University of North Carolina at Chapel Hill, School of Medicine, Chapel Hill, North Carolina

Grace A. Goldsmith, M.D.†

Scott M. Grundy, M.D., Ph.D.

Professor, Internal Medicine and Biochemistry, Director, Center for Human Nutrition, The University of Texas Health Science Center at Dallas, Dallas, Texas

William C. Heird, M.D.

Associate Professor of Pediatrics, Columbia University College of Physicians & Surgeons, New York, New York

Victor Herbert, M.D., J.D.

Chief, Hematology and Nutrition Laboratory, Bronx Veterans Administration Medical Center, Bronx, New York

Malcolm A. Holliday, M.D.

Director, Children's Renal Center, Professor of Pediatrics, University of California, San Francisco, California

B. Smith Hopkins, M.D.

Director of Parenteral Nutrition for the Surgical Services, The Roosevelt Hospital, St. Luke's Roosevelt Hospital Center, New York, New York

---

†Deceased

Francis J. Kane, M.D.

Clinical Professor of Psychiatry, Baylor College of Medicine, Houston, Texas

Irving H. Leopold, M.D., D.Sc. in Medicine

Professor and Chairman, Department of Ophthalmology, California College of Medicine, University of California, Irvine, California

Charles S. Lieber, M.D.

Director, GI-Liver-Nutrition Training Program and Alcohol Research and Treatment Center, Bronx Veterans Administration Medical Center; Professor of Medicine and Pathology, Mt. Sinai School of Medicine of the City University of New York, New York, New York

Morris A. Lipton, Ph.D., M.D.

Department of Psychiatry, School of Medicine, University of North Carolina, Chapel Hill, North Carolina

Bruce V. MacFadyen, Jr., M.D.

Associate Professor, The University of Texas Medical School at Houston, Houston, Texas

H.C. Meng, M.D., Ph.D.

Professor of Physiology and Surgery, Vanderbilt University, School of Medicine, Nashville, Tennessee

Marcia A. Mills, M.A., R.D.

Consulting Nutritionist in Private Practice, President of Profile Associates, Chapel Hill, North Carolina

Mark E. Molitch, M.D.

Associate Professor of Medicine, Tufts University School of Medicine, Boston; Associate Director, Clinical Study Unit and Physician, Division of Endocrinology, Department of Medicine, New England Medical Center, Boston, Massachusetts

Joseph A. Molnar, M.D.

Department of Surgery, Harvard Medical School, Massachusetts General Hospital, Boston, Massachusetts

Michael T. Nakamura, Pharm.D.

Daniel Freeman Memorial Hospital, Inglewood, California

Anita Louise Owen, R.D., M.A.

Nutrition Consultant, President of Owen Associates, Westport, Connecticut

Roy M. Pitkin, M.D.

Professor and Head, Department of Obstetrics and Gynecology, College of Medicine, The University of Iowa, Iowa City, Iowa

Daphne A. Roe, M.D.

Professor of Nutrition, Division of Nutritional Sciences, Cornell University, Ithaca, New York

James H. Shaw, Ph.D.

Professor of Nutrition, Harvard School of Dental Medicine, Boston, Massachusetts

Spencer Shaw, M.D.

Staff Physician, Section of Liver Diseases and Nutrition, Veterans Administration Medical Center, Bronx, New York; Assistant Professor of Medicine, Mt. Sinai School of Medicine of the City of New York, New York

George K. Summer, M.D.

Professor of Biochemistry and Nutrition, Department of Biochemistry and Nutrition, School of Medicine, University of North Carolina at Chapel Hill, Chapel Hill, North Carolina

Robert M. Suskind, M.D.

Professor and Chairman, Department of Pediatrics, University of South Alabama, College of Medicine, Mobile, Alabama

Edward A. Sweeney, D.M.D.

Associate Professor of Pedodontics and Acting Chairman, Department of Orthodontics and Pedodontics, University of Pennsylvania School of Dental Medicine, Philadelphia, Pennsylvania

Keith B. Taylor, M.D.

George DeForest Barnett Professor of Medicine, Stanford University, California

Robert W. Winters, M.D.

Executive Vice-President and Medical Director, Home Nutritional Support, Inc., Fairfield, New Jersey; Formerly Professor of Pediatrics, College of Physicians and Surgeons, Columbia University, New York, New York

Kelly M. West, M.D.†

Robert R. Wolfe, Ph.D.

Associate Physiologist, Massachusetts General Hospital, Associate Professor of Surgery (Physiology), Harvard Medical School, Boston, Massachusetts

Edward K. Wong, M.D.

Assistant Professor, Chief of Ophthalmology, University of California at Irvine, College of Medicine, Irvine, California

†Deceased

Preface

The first edition of The Nutritional Support of Medical Practice has had a gratifying acceptance in the professional community, but with that satisfaction has come responsibility: to remain aware of progress in clinical nutrition, while guarding and retaining what is useful and tested by time; to be receptive to increments to present practical knowledge; and to welcome, although with skeptical restraint, extensions into new areas.

In the first edition we fastened our *raison d'être* to the idea that in addition to the missions of curing and preventing the deficiency diseases, the science of nutrition had a mission in the support of the clinical specialties. We had remarked then, and it is no less true now, that the demand was increasing for the application of nutrition to those diseases which are frequently encountered in practice. We prefer to take a cautious view of the expectations raised by these demands, which, by repetition, continue to escalate.

With the cooperation of our contributing authors we have approached this second edition, then, by sifting and updating the chapter contents of the first edition. Further, we have been successful in obtaining new and important contributions from recognized leaders in some nutritional fields that are identifiable now as meriting a fuller treatment on their own. Here, for the first time anywhere, the reader will find a meshing of the expertise of the dietitian with the needs of the physician-surgeon. This is set forth by dietitian-leaders for settings in the hospital, in private practice referrals, and in the community. The useful structuring of nutrition support services in the hospital has been expanded to include more pointed information on nutritional assessment.

New chapters under the rubric of applications of nutrition to the clinical specialties include the following: geriatrics, hematology, inborn errors of metabolism, and oncology. And following a policy of rotation among our contributors, so that we may hear from new voices, chapters on burns, cardiology, drug and nutrient interactions, endocrinology, immunology, obesity, oral health, and renal disease, have been completely rewritten by authors that we have newly welcomed. Finally, we have expanded the appendix into a new orientation by the inclusion of tables of special use to the practicing physician. Some of these tables are presented here for the first time in the field. Special mention should be made of the newer stance that these tables indicate, on what is "normal" in human populations in the modern industrial society.

A book once launched must strive to breast the current of its time or be swept away. Our boat now is larger but has many more hands at the oars. We look forward not only to staying afloat, but we hope to see what lies around the next bend in the river.

Howard A. Schneider, PH.D.
Carl E. Anderson, PH.D.
David B. Coursin, M.D.

Preface to the First Edition

NUTRITIONAL SUPPORT OF MEDICAL PRACTICE has many authors, but a single idea: to assemble for the medical practitioner in the developed countries those features of nutritional science which are clearly useful and clinically applicable in day-to-day medical practice. We have elected to focus on medical practice in the developed countries because the similarities of their infrastructure of national systems of food supply, transportation, resource use, and industrialization make a unified treatment meaningful, and their historic roles of leadership in medicine recommends our attention. We are not blind to the nutritional problems of the rest of the globe, but these are set in other societal frameworks which seemingly demand systems of medical care delivery adapted to cultures with presuppositions different from those in the West. Further, we are not engaged in probing the tantalizing regions lying beyond the horizons of research, nor are we proposing to revolutionize medicine by some sweeping new paradigms derived from the nutritional sciences. Rather, given the necessarily pragmatic aim of today's medical schools to train practitioners to cope with the preponderance of medical problems they are most likely to encounter, we have come to ask, "How can knowledge of human nutrition help?"

To answer that question the editors sought the expert assistance of their colleagues assembled here. These authorities responded to our appeal to set forward in terms of their own clinical specialty just those aspects of applied nutrition that they had found useful. A broad spectrum emerges in terms of these specific applications, ranging from modalities of a clear and directly curative role, to aspects of prevention, to the more-numerous roles supportive of other modalities which the practitioner may elect as his prime means of intervention. This adds up to an increased effectiveness of the physician–surgeon in practice.

The book itself is structured into three main parts. After a brief description from the viewpoint of human biology, the setting of modern nutritional science, the first main section sets forward a concise review of the basics of the nutritional sciences, that is, energetics, physiology, and the biochemistry and metabolism of the nutrients. Then the various modes of applied human nutrition available to the physician in a variety of settings are described. This particularization of the relationship of human nutrition to the clinical specialties, one by one, is the heart of this book. The scientific advance of medicine inevitably generated the specialties, a process of speciation, if you will, in the evolution of medical practice, and any useful analysis of the role of nutrition in modern medicine, it seems to us, must accommodate this process and this reality.

An appendix provides in tabular form some of the basic reference materials for which the authors of the clinical sections have had general need and which may be of ready use to the reader.

Howard A. Schneider, PH.D.
Carl E. Anderson, PH.D.
David B. Coursin, M.D.

Introduction

Interest in human nutrition as one of the new health sciences of the last half-century has both waxed and waned among practitioners of medicine in the Western world. Indeed we are now at what must be a rather low point in medical interest in the subject, if one is to judge from the short shrift given to identifiable teaching of nutrition in the crowded curricula of the medical schools of the United States. Committees of professional nutrition societies, for their part, wring their hands over their low estate; conferences on nutrition education in medicine are convened; nutrition professors cry havoc before Senate Committees; and harassed curriculum committees in medical schools frown on the importunings of nutrition "enthusiasts."

It was not always thus. Time was when nutritional discoveries brought crowded rooms at medical meetings and pellagra and rickets were not the rare curiosities of today.

The basic thesis of this book is that the waxing and waning of interest in human nutrition in the practice of medicine in the developed world is an inevitable and understandable phenomenon that has its historic–cultural roots in the continuing development both of the health sciences on which medical practice now rests and of the changing societies in which Western medicine is embedded. If this thesis is correct, nutritional science itself can be seen not as a monolithic but ineffectual competitor among the therapeutic modalities of modern medicine, but more appropriately as providing a wide spectrum of usefulness to medicine, ranging from directly curative intervention to aspects of prevention, and further, and most important, to means of supporting therapeutic choices with their own prior claims on the attention of medical practitioners.

This analysis has been confined to Western medicine and especially to the medicine of the developed countries. This view was taken not in a spirit of chauvinism but because of a conviction, generally shared, that modern medicine is led by the West, and by such others who are Western themselves in medical thought and training. This medical tradition is heavily dominated by a preoccupation with curing, and medical interest is indeed first stirred by the presentation of the patient's disease or trauma. The economic base of medicine itself rests on delivery of a healing service that is operationally identifiable with, in one way or another, the hand and thought of the physician or surgeon.

These presuppositions are, of course, reflected in medical education. In a broad sense, all of medical education is directed toward this first concern of how to cure the patient who presses to claim the attention of the medical practitioner.

About a half-century ago a class of diseases of significant proportions in human populations, which could be clearly distinguished through research, became understandable as nutritional deficiency diseases. This set of deficiency diseases was the well-known group of scurvy, rickets, pellagra, and beriberi. Medical practitioners and medical educators showed a high degree of interest when nutritional research revealed the chemical identity of the *curative* vitamins involved and placed them in the practitioner's hand. As long as these clearly identifiable nutritional diseases presented themselves for cure, curative Western medicine was fully interested and busied itself learning to use the newly available vitamins.

But, in these very instances, nutritional knowledge also showed that the same vitamins, if regularly supplied, would *prevent* these diseases. On this knowledge, several events followed which lowered the interest of curative medicine and thereby that of its practitioners. Nutrition education proceeded to inform the general population, and attentive public health authorities, that the almost magic vitamins were available not only on prescription, but also, by proper choice of foods, at the grocery. Two further events ensured that the human dietary in the developed countries came to include preventive levels of the missing nutrients: (1) food fortification and enrichment programs improved supplies of the preventive nutrient and (2) with rising affluence, an expanding food technology and a distribution-marketing system brought a more varied diet within reach of all who could enter the marketplace. And the deficiency diseases went away.

With the monovalent deficiency diseases no longer pressing for attention in medical practice, it is small wonder that nutrition began to fade from the attention of medical educators to its present low visibility.

Nutrition research, of course, has not been idle but, apparently in the very biologic nature of things, has been lead inevitably to recognize the multiple causality of the intractable medical problems that remain to claim attention. As in ischemic heart disease, for example, nutritional parameters are several and of uncertain standing in the hierarchy of multiple causation which includes other nonnutritional parameters. Most importantly, even as they are being elucidated the identifiable nutritional factors are recognized as features of prevention strategies in terms of life styles, income levels, and cultural influences. The medical practitioner, although he is aware of these, no longer identifies them as medical problems amenable to his skills in practice. To the extent that all these matters are preventive, there is the strong inclination to leave them to others and concentrate on those modalities that can be employed in the office, at the bedside, or in the hospital.

If we are not completely wrong in this synopsis, then it is understandable that medical interest was highest when the vitamins cured diseases occurring frequently enough to be seen in practice, that it declined when the diseases disappeared for the socioeconomic reasons just discussed, and that it was relegated to the public health arena to which the responsibility has been assigned for the continuing dynamics of a varied and adequate, but increasingly sophisticated, food supply. Western curative medicine has only modest room for preventive medicine. As we have noted, it has no broadly accepted economic base in this domain, aside from the public health sector. Solutions to this particular problem must be left to the future.

Returning to the medical practitioner, however, we believe that the foregoing discussion does not exhaust the possible relationships of nutritional knowledge to medical practice. This book asserts there is at least one more important but hitherto unarticulated relationship. If medical practice in the West today no longer holds nutrition to be important in its original *curative* sense, and if in a *preventive* sense, nutrition has become the proper concern of other professionals, then nutrition can still be seen as an important claimant to the attention of the practitioner and his educators in a *supportive* sense. What do we mean by this?

We believe that the use of nutritional knowledge in medical practice is not mutually exclusive with the present modalities of therapy that are the proper preoccupation of medical thought and practice. Let the physician and surgeon, in all of the medical specialties, elect their therapies as their special knowledge dictates. And, then, to improve the outcome, to shorten convalescence, to extend the time frame for therapies, and to increase the patient's capability of favorable response, let the practitioner nutritionally support his patient as the hours lengthen into days, weeks, months, and years—as healing is truly achieved.

Nutrition, on its own, can still clearly be curative of certain, now rather rare, diseases. Further, nutrition, as part of the underlying multiple causality, can be an important factor in the prevention of some other and more-common diseases. But in the widest perspective, nutrition can be used *to support* the finest efforts of medical practice to cope with disease in all of its aspects.

Howard A. Schneider, PH.D.

Acknowledgments

As this edition was going to press, editor Carl Anderson died in Chapel Hill on March 26, 1983, after a short illness. Carl was a participant in this book from the earliest discussions concerning its possible publication. As a Professor of Nutrition in a medical school, he saw the need for a textual resource and took personal satisfaction in drafting the three chapters on the fundamentals of nutritional sciences. It is a significant part of his memorial.

All editors are debtors, and the book you now hold in your hands is the visible token of our debt. Our intellectual and scientific creditors are many, indeed a goodly company, but there is a certain pleasure in bringing especially to mind those who helped us on our way.

That this book was ever first begun, and that it was revised and expanded into this second edition, is easily traced to the prescience of David P. Miller, the retired vice president and publisher of the medical department of Harper and Row. It was he who set us on our course and helped us by his experienced advice to hoist the sails and get under way. It is a pleasure as well to record that, with the assumption of corporate responsibilities for publishing in the health professions by the J.B. Lippincott Company, for Harper and Row, we had the continuity and the sustaining help of their leadership and staff.

Another institution deserves explicit mention in these matters. It was the Institute of Nutrition of the University of North Carolina and its Board of Scientific Directors that affirmed the merit of providing some of the resources of the Institute for the endeavor in medical and nutritional education that culminated in our first edition.

Among the many colleagues who made suggestions and offered criticisms to us and to our contributors, several individuals must be granted special mention for giving generously of their time and knowledge when we turned to them for help. We recall with particular gratitude the counsel of Edward H. Ahrens, Jr., M.D.; Edwin L. Bierman, M.D.; D. H. Hornig, Ph.D.; Robert E. Olson, M.D., Ph.D.; and Fred Selzer, Metropolitan Insurance Company.

Finally, we salute our contributing authors. In a very real sense this is their book. It was an honor to serve them.

The Editors

Contents

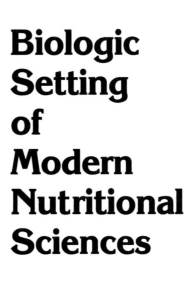

**Biologic
Setting
of
Modern
Nutritional
Sciences**

1
Biologic Setting of Modern Nutritional Sciences

Howard A. Schneider

Natural History of the Planet and *Homo Sapiens*

What a piece of work is a man! how noble in reason! how infinite in faculties! in form and moving how express and admirable! in action how like an angel! in apprehension how like a god! the beauty of the world, the paragon of animals. ("The Tragedy of Hamlet, Prince of Denmark," Act II, Scene 2, pp 307–312)

"The paragon of animals!" So wrote the famous playwright and, as in so many things, so precisely touched the heart of the matter. For although modern biology, studiously eschewing anthropocentricity, still places *Homo sapiens* in a very special place at the terminus of the evolutionary progression, the fact remains that when viewed in an environmental perspective man's nature is incomprehensible if we neglect his animal origins and his animal needs. The unique possession of a mind may set him apart from all other species, but our concern here is with human nutrition, and we must reckon with man as an *eating* animal—as are indeed all the animals. This concern with eating is central to all that will follow, but before we deal with it further it seems profitable to step back in time and view very briefly the whole enterprise of life on the planet Earth and how we came to where we are.

PHYSICAL ENVIRONMENT AND CHEMICAL CONSEQUENCES

Modern estimates of the age of our solar system are now hovering around 4.7 billion years. Our planet, Earth, the third innermost of a group of nine, is orbiting 93,000,000 miles from the sun, a star named Sol, with all ostensibly having "begun" from some grand cosmic explosion. The cardinal feature of this relationship of our planet to the sun as concerns the support of life is that the sun bathes Earth in a flood of energy in the form of electromagnetic waves, some of which is invisible as ultraviolet and infrared radiation, but most of which is visible light. The 93,000,000 miles of empty space between Sol and Earth is traversed in about 8 minutes, but of all the sun's energy thus sent out in all directions, Earth intercepts less than one billionth.

As the sun's radiation enters Earth's film of atmosphere, much of the ultraviolet radiation is absorbed by the ozone layer. This simple fact provides a shield for living things on the Earth's surface, which protects them from what would otherwise be damaging effects, such as skin cancer in humans. Further in, on the path through the atmosphere, water and carbon dioxide absorb infrared radiation. This absorption raises their temperature and thereby that of the total atmosphere. Some solar radiation never reaches Earth but is reflected back into space by dust particles or by the condensed moisture of clouds. Since these processes are selective for ultraviolet and infrared radiation, most of the solar radiation reaching Earth's surface is in the visible part of the light spectrum. The absorption of this visible light is, of course, a function of color. Black is almost totally absorbing, for example, whereas white is almost totally reflecting. It turns out that for life as we know it on our planet, the color green is all important. The absorption of red and blue light, and the reflection of green, is the important feature of chlorophyll, the green substance of plants, that signals the terrestrial trapping of the sun's energy. The physical–chemical consequence of the absorption of energy by a molecule is an increase in chemical reactivity. In a crude way this can be done by merely heating a mixture of the chemical substances one wishes to react with one another, but in a more subtle way the consequences of the absorption of red and blue light by chlorophyll result in a series of chemical reactions, all driven by the push of light, with the end result being a production of organic chemical substances that contain the trapped energy. It is worth pondering that, on Earth, the only significant chemical reaction that can trap the energy of the sun is photosynthesis, wherein the green leaf converts some of the absorbed energy into the potential energy of organic end products. We are not concerned here with the consequences of such organic products as wood or cotton, which serve humans in many ways, but with the central fact that all foods, the metabolizable sources of energy for all life, have this common origin in photosynthesis (see Chap. 2).

EVOLUTION OF THE HUMAN SPECIES

The origin of man and the necessarily antecedent origin of life are problems of great philosophic import, both worthy of volumes in themselves. It is not impertinence, therefore, but sheer necessity that restricts us to a statement, regrettably brief and sketchy, concerning these two great issues. For if we are to place human nutrition in an understandable and logical relationship to the planet and ourselves, we shall need to provide the framework of the origin and elaboration of the life processes and the origin, by evolution, of the species we know as man.

Earlier we alluded to the sheer necessity of remaining sensitive to the animal component of the human species if we are to understand the relationships connecting the species and the nutritional environment. Our emphasis on humans as eating animals may seem brutish to some, but at this cross-section in time of our understanding, incomplete though that be, it is the best stance we can assume. The evolution of those aspects that, in the minds of some, draw a gulf between us and the animals, remains for the future to clarify.

The birth of the solar system about 4.7 billion years ago was in itself followed by a cosmic evolution and a settling down, so to speak, into a system of a sun and nine orbiting planets and their satellites. Then, as Dobzhansky has characterized it, cosmic evolution transcended itself when it produced life:[2]

Life on earth is reckoned to be two billion or more years old. It first arose under environmental conditions quite different from those which exist today; these conditions can be reconstructed only with difficulty. As the earth cooled sufficiently for the water vapor to condense and to form the oceans, the atmosphere consisted of such gases as hydrogen, methane, ammonia, carbon dioxide, and lesser quantities of nitrogen and little free oxygen. Chemical reactions that can take place in such mixtures have been extensively studied in laboratories. Formaldehyde, acetic acid, succinic acid, and as many as ten different amino acids can all be formed. These, and other even more complex substances, now made chiefly or only in living bodies, could arise and accumulate in solution in the then lifeless oceans, making the latter a kind of dilute "soup" of organic compounds.

And he further elaborates:

Much ingenuity has been used to construct models of processes that might conceivably have led to combining the smaller molecular constituents into large molecules, such as DNA, which can facilitate the synthesis of their copies. The best that one can say about these models is that some of the processes which they postulate might conceivably have happened, but not that they did actually happen in the real history of the earth. It is also not quite generally agreed that self-reproduction is both the necessary and sufficient condition for regarding a chemical system as living, though it is agreed that it is at least a necessary condition. The reason for this is as follows: Self-replication means not only that a system engulfs suitable materials from its environment (food) and transforms them into its own likeness (reproduction), but also that any changes that may occur in the self-replicating process (mutation) may be reflected in the relative frequencies of the changed and unchanged systems in the course of time (natural selection). In other words, the origin of self-replication opens up the possibility of biological evolution. This evolution may, although it need not necessarily, be progressive. The evolution of a self-replicating system may be cut short by exhaustion of the environment or by changes in the system which make it less efficient (extinction). It is possible that, if self-replicating systems arose repeatedly, most of them were lost without issue. The point is, however, that at least one system was preserved and "inherited the earth," by becoming the starting point of biological evolution.*

In fact, then, we really do not know how life originated on the planet and transcended the inorganic world. But it surely has not escaped the reader interested in nutrition that Dobzhansky, in discussing self-reproduction as a necessary condition for regarding a system as living, identified the fundamental nature of those "suitable materials from its environment" as "food" when they were capable of being transformed into the very substance of the entity deemed as "living."

This is not the place to discuss the adaptive radiation through evolution into a myriad of living forms, first in the seas and then on land and into the very air. But, remembering our ultimate focus

---

*From *The Biology of Ultimate Concern* by Theodosius Dobzhansky. Copyright © 1967 by Theodosius Dobzhansky. By arrangement with The New American Library Inc., New York, N.Y.

on the human species, we must consider that other fateful transcendence, the appearance of humans among living things. Once again we can do no better than to repeat Dobzhansky's skillful synopsis:

While the origin of life on earth is an event of a very remote past, man is a relative newcomer (even though the estimates of his antiquity have been almost doubled by recent discoveries). The record is still fragmentary, but the general outlines of at least the outward aspects of man's emergence are recognizable. During the early part of the Pleistocene age (the Villafranchian time, perhaps two million to one million years ago), there lived in the east-central and in the southern parts of the African continent at least two species of *Australopithecus*, a genus of Hominidae, the family of man. One of these, larger in body size (*Australopithecus robustus,* and its race *boisei*), apparently represented an evolutionary blind alley, and eventually died out. The other species, of a more supple build (*Australopithecus africanus*), may have been one of our ancestors.

There is good evidence in the structure of their pelvic bones that both species walked erect; their teeth were, if anything, more like ours than like those of the now-living anthropoid apes. The brain case capacity, though large in relation to the body size, was well within the ape range. Perhaps both species of *Australopithecus,* or at any rate one of them, made and used primitive stone tools. The remains of a most interesting creature have recently been found in the Villafranchian deposits in east-central Africa, and given the name *Homo habilis.* The name connotes the opinion of its discoverers that this creature had already passed from the genus *Australopithecus* to the genus *Homo,* to which we also belong. On the other hand, it is closely related to *Australopithecus africanus,* and may even have been only a race of that species. Regardless of the name by which it is classified, this is rather clearly one of the "missing links," which are no longer missing.

Later, during the mid-Pleistocene, there lived several races of the species *Homo erectus,* clearly ancestral to the modern *Homo sapiens.* Remains of *Homo erectus* have been found in Java, in China, in Africa, and probably also in Europe. Roughly 100,000 years ago, during the last, Würm–Wisconsin, glaciation, the territory extending from western Europe to Turkestan and to Iraq and Palestine was inhabited by variants of the Neanderthal race of *Homo sapiens.*

Rough stone tools have been found in association with australopithecine remains both in east-central and South Africa. *Homo erectus* in China is the oldest known user of fire. The Neanderthalians buried their dead. These are evidences of humanization. All animals die, but man alone knows that he will die. . . . A burial is a sign of a death awareness, and probably of the existence of ultimate concern. The ancestors of man had begun to transcend their animality perhaps as long as 1,700,000 years ago. The process is under way in ourselves.*

Several speculations of interest to a science of human nutrition can be drawn from the evolutionary relationships of the Hominòides, which includes apes and humans. From the human viewpoint, for example, considerable interest attaches to the determinants that account for our ancestors' divergence from the rest of the primates. In discussing this issue, Jolly advances certain proposals that rest on features recognized in *Ramapithecus,* the earliest fossil hominoid.[5] These features, which are anatomic, are adaptive for "small object feeding": dental adaptations and the adaptations for feeding while sitting on the ground. The dental evolution, then, of small front teeth and large molars in a small-brained primate could have taken place long before the invention of tools or weapons. The grinding action of molars seems appropriate for the eating of small, hard seeds, and perhaps grass seeds of various kinds. This, in turn, would explain the terrestriality of *Ramapithecus* and the finding of these early hominoid fossils in deposits on the forest fringe and in treeless areas within forests. The functional connection between seed eating and our early ancestors' nutritional and adaptive dependencies is, of course, obvious.

The hominoid adaptation to seed eating resulted in some divergence from the primates in the habits of eating fruit, leaves, insects, and—rarely—meat. Indeed, even among the tool-using and hunting *Australopithecines* the huge grinding molars became the climax of this adaptation to seed eating. From such pathways came eventually our own species, *Homo,* and it seems reasonable that modern man's reliance on starchy grains had its beginnings in the grassy areas of the forest's edge and the search for seeds.

To return, for the moment, to the diet of primates as observed in the wild, three major categories can be distinguished: (1) leaf eating, (2) fruit eating, and (3) insect eating. Intestinal anatomy and stomach contents of specimens give general indications of the predilections of a species. Man is classified as omnivorous, but he is ill-adapted to leaf eating, an accomplishment of certain specialized folivores. Insect and fruit eating are common, however, throughout the order of primates. In general, humans have dropped insects from their diet (quantitatively surely, although there are various exceptions noted in some cultures even today) and taken up meat eating. No other primate except the chimpanzee has so exerted himself, or been so inventive, in the hunt for meat as has been *Homo.* This generalization in turn has led to the error that, aside from humans, the primates are vegetarians. The crucial omission in this erroneous judgment is the neglect of the dietary role of insects among the primates. All primates are in need of vitamin B_{12}, which is obtainable only from animal sources (see Chap. 3). Insects are, of course, invertebrate animals, and as such a source of vitamin B_{12}, as are meat, milk, and other animal products. This dependency on vitamin B_{12} sources, coupled with the erroneous notion that primates are pure vegetarians, has resulted in some captive primates in zoos being deprived of the vitamin and suffering, as a consequence, the nerve degeneration that is a feature of the deficiency. It should be remarked further that capturing the small insect as an important item in the diet probably favored, through natural selection among the primates, the attributes of manipulative skills and manual dexterity that from our vantage point in time we can identify as necessary conditions for the tool-inventing and weapon-wielding *Homo* who was to come.

In this brief sketch of the evolution of man we have emphasized the relationships to food, to its qualitative distinctions, and to its ingathering from the environment. In this complex interplay of evolving organisms and their environment the focus on food has many consequences. One of the most astonishing—another transcendent leap—which that astonishing species *Homo sapiens* now essayed, was to master the very nature of his food supply and embark on a new evolution of a faster pace, his cultural evolution.

Man's Mastery of Food—
The Agricultural Revolution

In dealing with those aspects of the evolution of our species that reflect the necessary adaptations to the securing and use of food we have had occasion to comment on the interactions that led to more and more success in the perpetuation of the species. Tool making from stone was probably widespread throughout the Eurasian and African land mass by ancient types of *Homo* 250,000 years ago. Bladed tools and modern physical man appear in the archaeological record about 50,000 years ago. This modern form of man, the supreme adapter, successfully sought and found food in environmental niches ranging from the frozen tundra to tropical jungles. By about 25,000 years ago a previously man-empty New World was colonized from the Old World by way of the entry at Alaska and diffusion southward and eastward. Man was slowly increasing in numbers and, the archaeological evidence suggests, was penetrating his environment—living into his niche—to a high degree and learning the nature of "the fine structure" of the environment. This was especially true of the processes of food collection. The archaeological record of the era (European Mesolithic, North American Archaic) gives testimony to the vigor and intensity of this preoccupation. Fish, snails, mussels, water birds, and even small, swift animals have left their re-

mains. And in recent years, with the development of the field of paleoethnobotany, it is apparent that plants and seeds were also being brought into familiarity.

And then, about 10,000 years ago, the agricultural revolution was born, not once, but probably three times, in separate, widely separated sites. The first achievement of a food-producing technology occurred in the Near East, on the hills of the fertile crescent, running north along the eastern Mediterranean shore and arching eastward through Turkey down along the eastern banks of the Tigris river to the Persian Gulf. The question naturally arises, Why there? and Why then? The answer, from the archaeological record, is that the agricultural revolution did not take place only there and only then. The same events occurred at slightly later times in Central America (perhaps in the Andes, too) and in southeastern Asia and in China. From all this we can be persuaded that the food-producing revolution came as a cultural climax to an historic process in which, as a consequence of that heightened "living into the environment," there had been accumulated an array of experiences necessary for agriculture, so that, in total, it became a sufficient experience. As Braidwood reminds us, "Here in a climate that provided generous winter and spring rainfall, the intensified food-collectors had been accumulating a rich lore of experience with wild wheat, barley and other food plants, as well as with wild dogs, goats, sheep, pigs, cattle and horses. It was here that man first began to control the production of his food."[1]

The process of domestication of wild species has been defined as one that results in reproductive processes under control by man. A detailed analysis of the various means of husbandry and cultivation is beyond our province here, but in view of the continuing interest in man in earlier "states of nature" it may be of use to view the agricultural revolution in its stages as revealed by the archaeological excavations at Jarmo in Iraq. Approximately 150 people lived in Jarmo about 7000 to 6500 B.C., a permanent year-round settlement. Among the foods identified here were primitive barley, two forms of domesticated wheat, domesticated goats and dogs, and possibly domesticated sheep. Bones of wild animals and the remains of sea foods, acorns, and pistachio nuts indicate that hunting and collection of food had not been abandoned. This total array indicates that the people of Jarmo had a varied, well-balanced diet that was probably an adequate one. The teeth of the Jarmo people showed even wear, the happy outcome of the use of stone mortars and pestles and rubbing stones in food preparation. Food production and food technology had now assumed dimensions and features that make us feel a kinship to the people of Jarmo and others like them. The agricultural revolution was now irrevocably on its way. Man had domesticated his food supply and was himself the servant of his agriculture, with his life settling into the rhythms of the seasons, the planting and the reaping. The dog was the first domesticated animal and was seen on the paths of Jarmo as on the concrete and asphalt of our cities. Certain patterns of life were now set, certain foods becoming favored choices. These choices had consequences which needed to be understood, and the road to this understanding is our next logical concern.

Emergence of the Nutritional Sciences

THE NATURALISTIC ERA (400 B.C.–1750 A.D.)

Thus far, in sketching the biologic origins of man, his food supply, and the increasingly intricate and elaborate nature of the interrelationships of these domains, we have made no mention of medicine and the healing art. This is not to say that efforts by man to cope with disease did not exist or were not attempted. Our problem stems from the fact that we have been dealing with events in prehistory and only the archaeological and paleontological evidence has made our speculations possible. Speculation on the actual intervention by man with the idea of coping with illness is almost profitless until the birth of writing, about 3300 B.C. by the Sumerians of the Fertile Crescent. The art of the scribes diffused from Mesopotamia, and the Babylonians became the inheritors of greatness as the first disciples of the Sumerians; the peoples of the Mediterranean, in turn, learned from the Babylonians. The secret of Mesopotamian cultural dominance lay in the cuneiform script, for now there were records of matters (for our interest here) such as drugs and their corresponding ailments, and medical instructions systematized according to parts of the body or the location of symptoms. Medicine, magic, and the priesthood were, however, all intertwined, as was the case in the Egyptian civilization, which, it so happens, in its isolation on the Nile invented its own writing system of hieroglyphics only a bit later than the Sumerians.

It was in Ionia, on the island of Cos in the 4th century B.C., that what we can now discern as scientific medicine began. It was Hippocrates who advanced the idea that sickness could be understood only if one considered the whole patient and his environment. Successful treatment could be expected only if one used the beneficial experience of similar cases. Clearly, all this has a modern ring

across almost 25 centuries, but aside from some lip-service to "the Father of Medicine," and in spite of the well-known fact that Hippocrates was very much concerned with the diet of his patients, there has been little attention paid by nutrition writers to this remarkable connection. One must except from this stricture, however, E. V. McCollum. His "A History of Nutrition" contains a digest from the Hippocratic writings of the early Greeks' views of special properties and uses of food in medical treatment.[8] The compilation has historic interest, and there is an astonishing prescience of Hippocrates' recommendation that pulses should be eaten along with cereals. But set alongside this, for example, is his listing of "remedial foods," like myrtle, apples, dates, water from crab apples, and milk of asses (taken hot), and foods to be used in the treatment of dysentery, that is, linseed, wheat flour, beans, millet, eggs, and milk, not forgetting barley mush. From this compendium one comes to realize that foods were to Hippocrates what we would now categorize as items of pharmacology, but of an unclear kind. The neglect of Hippocrates by modern nutrition writers is therefore understandable, and McCollum, a lover and student of history, had to yield as much when he concluded "it is clear that Hippocrates had little understanding of the nature of nutrition, and held some groundless opinions about quality in foods."[8]

There is no denying that Hippocrates began the first formulations of a scientific approach to medicine, but we are probably over-zealous to read too much into the ancient words, as was written in *Ancient Medicine:*

For the art of medicine would never have been discovered to begin with, nor would any medical research have been conducted—for there would have been no need for medicine—if sick men had profited by the same mode of living and regimen as the food, drink and mode of living of men in health. . . .[6]

From our vantage point in time we can sense the struggle toward understanding, but for that understanding a new science had to be born, a science of chemistry. Only then could only one hope to untangle the mixture present in a grain of wheat and discern in what way that mixture was similar, and in what way different, from that of a grain of maize. For a chemistry adequate for the task, the world waited two millenia.

THE CHEMICOANALYTIC ERA (1750–1900 A.D.)

Out of the mists of alchemy there gradually coalesced a subject matter and a discipline that we know as chemistry. The recognition of the central and necessary role of quantitation by Lavoisier placed chemistry on its proper foundation, and by the middle of the 18th century, with the added genius of men such as Black and Priestly, chemical investigations of all kinds were well under way. In the domain of what we now name as organic chemistry, the German Liebig began exploring the chemical nature of foods. It was soon evident that foods were complicated mixtures of many various chemical compounds. But what was the nutritional meaning of this complicated and extended array?

The view of Hippocrates, which had prevailed into the 18th century, was that there was but a single essential in all foodstuffs, with foods varying only in the amount of this single aliment that they might contain. But the new chemistry raised obvious difficulties. Among all the chemically definable entities in the mixtures known as foods, which was the aliment of Hippocrates? This, of course, turned out to be a nonquestion; the single "aliment" of Hippocrates never existed except in the conceptual framework of the prechemical era. The new chemistry now forced a revision in concepts, and with the forceful ideas of Liebig and Mulder (who forwarded the notion that the nitrogenous constituents of foods were all one "protein") there gradually emerged by the middle of the 19th century a chemicoanalytic view of the basis of nutrition which rested not on one mysterious aliment, but on four chemically defined categories of substances: (1) protein, (2) carbohydrate, (3) fat, and (4) the minerals left as an ash when the food sample was totally combusted. Chemists then began to develop standardized analytic procedures to measure the agreed-upon four nutrient entities. This important step in the history of nutrition epitomized a significant commitment: the important essentials for animal nutrition were now known; these were four in number, and they were capable of analysis by the procedures of chemists. What is also worth noting is that these developments took place in an economically important field, the scientifically advancing field of agricultural chemistry, and the same advances were being applied in many countries in rapidly increasing numbers of agricultural experiment stations.

For a while enthusiasm ran high that the analysts at the agricultural experiment stations at long last had a methodology that made possible rational advice to the farmer concerning profitable husbandry of his animals and crops to help him achieve the best possible results in the animal industries and place farming on a solid economic footing. It all made a lot of sense, but was in the end brought down by the very test that had been held up as the measure of the advance in the understanding of animal nutrition, that is, the prediction of the equivalence of nutritive value based on equivalent chemicoanalytic data, and the prediction of superior nutritive value based on analytic data being used to achieve the hypothetically ideal composition of rations. All collapsed in the tests of practical use. Farmers who followed the chemists' advice were sometimes successful, but sometimes the animals failed in their response, failed to thrive, and sometimes lay down and died.

By the end of the 19th century the disillusion with the chemicoanalytic approach to a nutritional science was growing. The agricultural chemists, sensing their failure, cast about to patch up matters. A massive effort was made, for example, to mesh the chemical analyses of foods with the calorimetry and respiratory exchanges of the animals consuming these foods. There resulted a marked advance in knowledge of animal energy requirements and the respiratory quotients associated with the catabolism of fats, carbohydrates, and protein, but no new solutions appeared for the overriding problem of the nature and the number of the essential nutrients. The agricultural chemists appointed committees to study the matter, and some refinements in analysis were made, but the ability to predict the nutritive value of a ration based on chemical analysis of the constituents remained impressively erratic and inadequate. The closing years of the century saw an increasing sense of crisis and frustration. Something was wrong, or missing. But what?

THE BIOLOGIC ERA (1900 A.D. TO THE PRESENT)[9]

The resolution of the crisis in nutritional understanding had its roots, as is so often the case, in preceding events whose relationships and usefulness were not appreciated at the time of their original occurrence. The new burst of understanding which launched the present, biologic era came from two sources. One line of research which proved illuminating, but which was pursued so sporadically as to leave but a handful of papers in the scientific literature before 1906, was to give animals food that consisted of mixtures of relatively pure protein, carbohydrate, fat, and those minerals thought to be important. This was, of course, experimentation by means of assembly of the very same four categories that had been the target of chemical analyses and their endless refinement. Sparse though the published record was, it was unanimous in the observations that in all such experiments with chemically simplified diets the animals showed signs of malnutrition, survived for a short time, and died. The conclusion was inescapable that one or more unknown nutrients had not been included and must be sought as the clue to the support of animal health and life. This early record is one of failure, but from its methodology (the use of simplified diets of some chemical definition, which could test the effectiveness of added supplements) investigators gradually fashioned a new and powerful paradigm, which in a Kuhnian sense provided a revolutionary tool for resolving the crisis.[7]

The second line of thought that contributed to the resolution of the crisis in nutritional understanding was the promulgation and investigation of the idea that certain human diseases were due to a dietary deficiency of certain specific chemical substances, which, it was proposed, could be isolated and identified. This second line of research is important because any link between nutrition and human disease is an obvious and legitimate concern of medicine. What was focused upon was no mundane concern with the economics of animal husbandry, important though that might be; rather, nutrition was suddenly seen to touch human life and disease in a very direct way. It was at this point that, spanning the millenia from Hippocrates, the medicine of the West was diminishing its reliance on empiricism and expanding its scientific base and outlook. In an amazingly short time medicine embraced the idea of the deficiency diseases, an idea, it must be remarked, which in its univalent concept of etiology (one dietary deficiency, one disease) was harmonious with the similarly accepted univalent etiology of infectious disease (one pathogenic microorganism, one disease). The idea that disease could be caused by a lack of something, as well as by the noxious and pathogenic presence of something, was a revolutionary idea. First clearly demonstrated for human beriberi, the idea was given a broader generalization by Funk, who in 1912 proposed that not only beriberi but also scurvy, pellagra, and rickets were caused by a lack in the diet of "special substances which are of the nature of organic bases, which we will call vitamines."[3,4] As the chemistry of these "special substances" was gradually mastered, it became clear that they were not uniformly organic bases, but the term has obviously survived, although the "e" has been dropped (see Chap. 3).

The search for the life-sustaining missing dietary ingredient to be added to the chemically simplified diet and the quest for the deficiency disease-curing "vitamines" now were perceived as but one grand and unified agenda for nutrition research. A new era had begun, which has not yet been replaced by any more productive paradigm, although signs of strain have begun to appear. This new era in nutrition, which began in 1900 and continues to the present day, we have designated as the "bio-logic" era, in contrast to the "chemicoanalytic" era which preceded it. All this is to emphasize the fundamental nature in the changeover from the way in which nutritional research was conducted. Instead of presupposing that there were but four important categories of nutrients and that chemical analysis would reveal ideal relations between these, the new and revolutionary presupposition was made that still other important nutrients existed in the natural world of foodstuffs that would expand the list of necessary nutrients. These, it turned out, were so small in their quantitative amounts as to escape the analyst. Instead of turning to analysts, experimenters turned to the experimental animals, in the biologic assay, to signal the presence of the missing and sought-for items. The four categories were now built upon as a basis for the burst of new knowledge, and as of the present about 50 chemically specified compounds are identified as necessary for the nutritional needs of animals, including humans. We will not detail these items here further except to record that since about 1950 no new vitamins have been added to that category, whereas the list of essential trace elements has slowly grown, although the practical significance of many of these remains unspecified (see Chaps. 2, 3, and 4).

THE FUTURE OUTLOOK

The dazzling success of the univalent dietary deficiency hypothesis has placed the classic deficiency diseases under control, and they now occur, when they occur at all in developed countries, because of failures in health delivery systems, or—more usually—because of economic and social distortions of the dietary. But mankind is still left with a burden of diseases with unexplained and complicated etiologies. What, for example, can we say of the relationship of nutrition to coronary heart disease? If univalent etiology does not serve as a suitable framework for understanding causation, even hypothetically, then single entities are not likely to emerge as dominant controlling agencies to be grasped and mastered. Where will nutrition fit now? Although we have raised coronary heart disease as an important medical problem and disease burden in human populations, we have done so only to pose a more general question; in the instance wherein we perceive (and our investigations identify) multicausal sets of parameters, we are faced with the necessity of using a different grammar of biologic science, of abandoning the satisfying imagery of univalent concepts of causation and adopting the apparently necessary conventions and grammar of multivariate statistics. For some this is dismaying. The question seems to have changed from what is true to a recognition that many things are true, but we must decide what is true and important versus what is true but trivial. We now need methodologies for structuring hierarchies of the parameters we have identified. Sometimes, for a given disease, nutrition is but one parameter of many. It is inappropriate then to ask whether nutrition is *a* cause. We must learn to ask not questions but what can only be called a questionnaire. When our education in biology, in science, and in medicine has taught us that, we will be ready to begin. Perhaps, if we look about us, we have begun.

References

1. Braidwood RJ: The agricultural revolution. Sci Am 203: 1–10, 1960
2. Dobzhansky T: The Biology of Ultimate Concern, pp 46–47, 50–52. New York, New American Library, 1967
3. Funk C: Discussion. In McCollum EV: A History of Nutrition, p 217. Boston, Houghton Mifflin, 1957
4. Grijns G: Discussion. In McCollum EV: A History of Nutrition, pp 216–217. Boston, Houghton Mifflin, 1957
5. Jolly A: The Evolution of Primate Behavior, pp 55–69. New York, Macmillan, 1972
6. Jones WHS: Hippocrates, Vol I, p 17. New York, Loeb Classical Library, Putnam's Sons, 1923
7. Kuhn TS: The Structure of Scientific Revolutions. Chicago, University of Chicago Press, 1962
8. McCollum EV: A History of Nutrition. Boston, Houghton Mifflin, 1957
9. Schneider HA: What has happened to nutrition. Perspect Biol Med 1:278–292, 1958

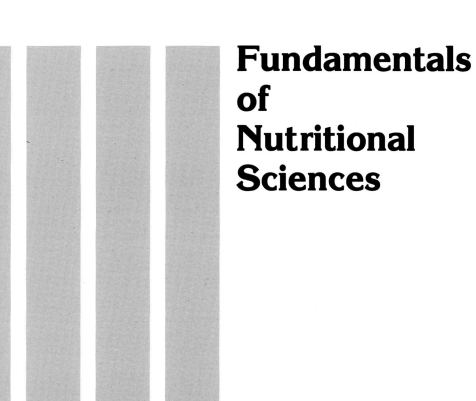

Fundamentals
of
Nutritional
Sciences

2
Energy and Metabolism
Carl E. Anderson

The main purpose of this chapter and the following two chapters is to provide the reader with a brief recall and review of those major sections of biochemistry and physiology that illuminate nutrition. The subject matter of each such chapter is in itself a large one containing much detail, the scope of which would be beyond the practical confines of this book. For the reader wishing to probe more deeply into such detail, the suggested references at the end of this chapter provide an excellent resource.[1,3–8,11,12]

Energy

In the United States, in recent years, consumers have become startingly conscious of shortages in fossil fuel energy, particularly gasoline, so essential to move the automobile and other fuel-propelled machinery. Energy is similarly required to propel humans through their daily tasks, whether active or sedentary. Although the fuels may be different, gasoline in one instance and food in the other, the basic requirement is the same—the need for energy. The dramatic realities of shortages of energy become startingly real when one considers a useless, nonrunning automobile or broken down piece of machinery on one hand, and malnutrition and starvation in humans on the other hand.

The human body needs energy for the metabolic work of the life processes, for example, the action of the heart in circulating blood; the movement of the diaphragm in breathing; osmotic work; to support physical activity, such as running, jumping, and working; for growth, as in the maintenance

and biosynthesis of new tissue; for lactation; and to maintain body temperature, to name but a few of the body's living activities.

In humans, energy is provided by the carbohydrates, fats, and proteins of the diet. In some dietaries alcohol also must be considered because of the significant caloric value (7 Cal/g) of ethanol. Ethyl alcohol, of course, is toxic in high amounts. A typical American diet provides 50% to 60% of its energy from carbohydrate, 10% to 15% from protein, and 35% to 45% from fat. The remaining components of the diet, for instance, water, cellulose, minerals, and vitamins, do not contribute energy. Although carbohydrate has been the chief source of energy in the past, at the present time in the United States some people consume diets in which carbohydrate and fat make nearly equal contributions, approaching 46% and 42% respectively. The total protein consumed has remained nearly constant at 11% to 12% of the dietary energy.[10]

The energy value of food is expressed in terms of a unit of heat, the kilocalorie (kcal). This represents the amount of heat required to raise the temperature of 1 kg (1000 g) water 1°C at the temperature range from 15°C to 16°C. The large calorie (Cal) used by nutritionists is equivalent to the kilocalorie and should not be confused with the small calorie (cal), which is 0.001 Cal. A proposal that the joule (1 Cal = 4.184 kilojoules) be adopted has been endorsed by a number of nutrition groups as a heat measurement unit, but is not as yet widely used.

Much of our information on the energy value of

food is obtained by combustion methods or direct calorimetry using an oxygen bomb calorimeter.[9] This instrument is a highly insulated boxlike container about 1 cubic foot in size. The bomb chamber itself consists of a thick-walled metal vessel equipped with sample dish, electrodes for igniting the sample in an oxygen atmosphere, and a valve for introducing oxygen. This combustion chamber is surrounded with an outer chamber containing a measured quantity of water, a stirrer, and a thermometer. When a dried sample of food is completely burned in the oxygen-rich environment of the combustion chamber, the heat produced is absorbed by the weighed amount of water surrounding the chamber. The change in temperature of the surrounding water is measured by an accurate thermometer. By definition, a kilocalorie is the amount of heat required to change the temperature of the measured weight of water. Because the bomb is well insulated and no heat is exchanged with the environment, the amount of heat resulting from the complete burning of the measured sample can be calculated directly as Cal/g. The energy value of a sample of food thus obtained is known as the heat of combustion.

The first line of Table 2-1 presents the heat of combustion obtained from burning or oxidation of 1 g carbohydrate, fat, protein, or alcohol, respectively. The heat of combustion represents the total energy produced by the oxidation of the carbon of the food in the bomb calorimeter to carbon dioxide, the hydrogen to water, and the nitrogen of the protein to nitrous oxide. In the tissue cells the digested food products are also oxidized. However, unlike the bomb calorimeter, the heat lability of tissue cells prohibits as wasteful and destructive to the cell the direct oxidation of food. Rather, oxidation is accomplished by decarboxylations and by the gradual removal of the hydrogen and electrons of food by a respiratory cycle until the hydrogen and electrons can be united at the end of the cycle with molecular oxygen to form water. During this process the bond energies of the food molecule are released and captured in forming high-energy

adenosine triphosphate (ATP) from adenosine diphosphate (ADP) present in the cell fluid. The combined process of the respiratory cycle and the capture of food bond energies as high-energy ATP is called *coupled oxidative phosphorylation*. The high energy of ATP can be transferred to creatine phosphate for temporary storage or used directly to drive the physiologic processes of the living cell. However, the animal cell cannot release or use the complete energy potential of nitrogen in protein. Therefore, a deduction must be made in the case of proteins because these are not as completely oxidized in the body as in the bomb calorimeter. It is the nitrogen-containing product of protein, urea, that is not oxidized but excreted in the urine. The latent heat of this excreted nitrogen, which amounts to 1.3 Cal for each gram of protein burned in the tissue cell, must be subtracted from the heat of combustion of the protein, yielding a net heat of combustion of 4.35 Cal/g (see line 3 of Table 2-1).

Since the human body is not 100% efficient in digesting and absorbing or metabolizing the major nutrients, it is necessary in determining the amount of energy available to the body from the ingested nutrient to calculate the coefficient of digestibility for each nutrient. This coefficient expresses the percentage of the nutrient ultimately available to the body as fuel value. Carbohydrates are 98% digested, fat 95% digested, and protein 92% digested; the coefficients of digestibility are 0.98, 0.95, and 0.92, respectively. However, it must be recognized that these factors may vary somewhat for any one food. Furthermore, although these coefficients apply generally in the United States, other coefficients may be more appropriate in other countries, reflecting the digestibilities of the predominant foods. The physiologic fuel-value for the major energy-yielding groups are shown in the last line of Table 2-1.

The use and application of these factors can be given in illustration. A sample of milk was found to contain 4.85 g carbohydrate, 3.68 g protein, and 3.80 g fat for every 100-g sample. Using the physiologic fuel values from the last line of Table 2-1,

TABLE 2-1
Physiologic Fuel Value of Major Nutrients

	Carbohydrate (Cal/g)	Fat (Cal/g)	Protein (Cal/g)	Ethanol (Cal/g)
Heat of combustion	4.1	9.45	5.65	7.1
Energy from combustion of nitrogen unavailable to the body			1.3	
Net heat of combustion	4.1	9.45	4.35	7.1
Coefficient of digestibility	0.98	0.95	0.92	Small loss in urine and breath
Physiologic fuel value	4.0	9.0	4.0	7.0

or 4.0 for carbohydrate, 4.0 for protein, and 9.0 for fat, the 100-g sample of milk will have the following caloric value:

Carbo-hydrate	4.85 g × 4.0 Cal/g	= 19.40 Cal
Protein	3.68 g × 4.0 Cal/g	= 14.72 Cal
Fat	3.80 g × 9.0 Cal/g	= 34.20 Cal
	Total	= 68.32 Cal

An 8-oz glass of milk is reported to weigh 244 g and therefore has a caloric value of 68.32 × 2.44, or 166.71 Cal.

ENERGY REQUIREMENT OF ADULTS

The National Academy of Sciences' recommendations of allowances for energy in the United States (see Appendix) are given for two age categories for average mature adults engaged in various occupations.[10] The two age categories are those 23 to 50 years of age and those over 50. The recommendations are made for energy allowances established at the "lowest intake to be consonant with good health in each age group." Since a large number of persons in the American population are overweight, it is quite possible they may need less energy than is recommended because of their sedentary living patterns. Adults and children with excessive amounts of body fat and yet consuming energy-containing diets consistent with their body weight, sex, and age should increase their physical activity until a desired balance is achieved. Adjustments for various degrees of physical activity for body size, and sometimes for climatic changes, are made in the recommendations. When these factors are taken into consideration and allowances for hours of sleep at 90% of the basal metabolic rate are made, as well as adjustments for height, the energy recommendations for various activity periods are as shown in Table 2-2.

AGE

Energy requirements decline progressively after early adulthood because the resting metabolic rate declines and physical activity is slowed. For this reason the energy allowances for persons above 50 years of age should be reduced to 90% of the amount required as mature adults.

PREGNANCY

Additional energy is needed during pregnancy to build new tissues in the placenta and fetus and to accommodate the increased work load of the mother associated with movement. An extra allowance of 300 Cal/day throughout the pregnancy is recommended.[10]

LACTATION

Energy allowances should be increased by 500 Cal/day during the first 3 months of lactation. Allowances should be increased if lactation continues beyond this period.[10]

ENERGY REQUIREMENTS FOR INFANTS, CHILDREN, AND ADOLESCENTS

During the first year of life it is recommended that allowances be reduced in steps from a level of 120 Cal/kg at birth to 100 Cal/kg by the end of the first year.[10]

Energy allowances for children of both sexes de-

TABLE 2-2
Daily Energy Needs for Various Activities*

Activity	Men (Cal/kg/hr)	Women (Cal/kg/hr)
Very light Seated and standing activities, painting, trades, auto and truck driving, laboratory work, typing, sewing	1.5	1.3
Light Walking (2.5–3 mph), electric trades, carpentry, restaurant trades, washing clothes, golf, tennis, volleyball	2.9	2.6
Moderate Walking (3.5–4 mph), weeding, hoeing, scrubbing floors, cycling, tennis, dancing	4.3	4.1
Heavy Walking with load up hill, tree cutting, working with pick and shovel, swimming, climbing, football	8.4	8.0

*Adapted from RDA, National Research Council. For adjustments for heights and example calculations see p. 29 of the RDA.[10]

cline gradually to about 80 Cal/kg through 10 years of age. After the age of 10 there is a gradual further decline to 45 Cal/kg for adolescent males and 38 Cal/kg for adolescent females.

Carbohydrates

Carbohydrates, especially glucose and glycogen, serve as the chief source of readily available energy for the human body. As a class, the carbohydrates are among the most abundant compounds found in nature and the largest component, aside from water, of most diets. They provide 50% to 60% of the energy of the typical American diet. In poorer nations they may reach as high as 90% of the energy of the diet. Because plant life is quite abundant in carbohydrate, plant foods serve as the least expensive form of energy for the diet. In developing nations this reliance on plant foods may reduce the intake of more expensive proteins and fats to critically low levels with prejudice to health.

CHEMICAL CONSTITUTION AND FUNCTION

As a class the carbohydrates are composed of carbon, hydrogen, and oxygen. As a rule they contain two atoms of hydrogen for each atom of oxygen. Since this is the same proportion as in water, they are termed *carbohydrates.*

Of the many compounds classed as carbohydrates, a few are of special importance and interest in human nutrition and metabolism. Among these are the polysaccharides amylose, amylopectin, components of starch, and the animal starch glycogen. These large molecules are all polymers of glucose. Cellulose, also a polymer of glucose, forms a large part of the diet but cannot be used because of the lack of a cellulose-splitting enzyme in the human gastrointestinal (GI) tract.

The disaccharides in many common foods, for instance, sucrose or ordinary table sugar, lactose (found in milk), and maltose (a key component of many polysaccharides), are important in carbohydrate metabolism primarily as sources of energy.

Of prime interest in human metabolism is the monosaccharide glucose, which in phosphorylated form is the chief sugar of carbohydrate metabolism and energy production (Fig. 2-1). Two other monosaccharides, fructose, a component of the disaccharide sucrose, and galactose, a component with glucose of the milk sugar lactose, are of interest (Fig. 2-1). The three monosaccharides are

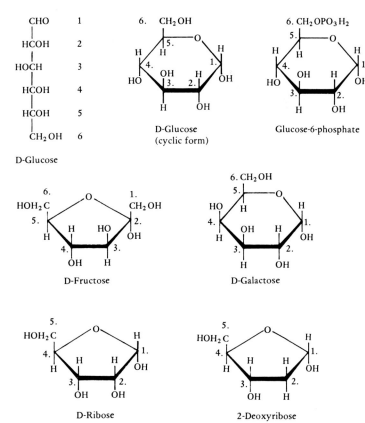

FIG. 2-1 Chemical structures of important monosaccharides.

also known as hexoses since each has 6 linear C atoms in their respective molecules.

Sometimes overlooked are two pentoses (5 carbons) of vital importance, ribose and deoxyribose (see Fig. 2-1). These pentoses are components of nucleic acids and the nucleotides important in cellular biosynthesis and energy production.

The trisaccharide raffinose and the tetrasaccharide stachyose have been suggested as causing the flatulence that occurs after a meal rich in beans. The human small intestine does not produce an enzyme to hydrolyze these sugars.

STARCH

This important food component contains two polysaccharides: (1) amylose, a long unbranched chain of several hundred glucose units comprising about 15% to 20% of starchy foods, and (2) amylopectin, a major component of starch. The latter is a highly branched polymer with many glucose units. The animal starch of human liver and muscle, glycogen, resembles amylopectin but is more highly branched. Cellulose, like starch, is a polymer of glucose units in straight chains. However, the gly-

FIG. 2-2 Chemical structures of important disaccharides.

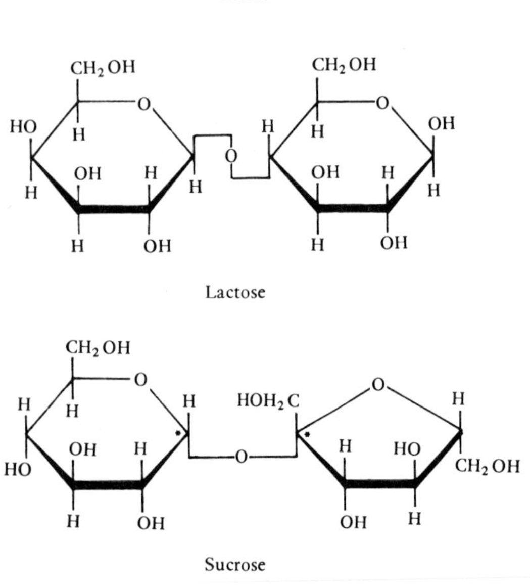

Maltose

Lactose

Sucrose

cosidic linkage between successive glucose units in cellulose is a β-1, 4-linkage instead of the α-1, 4-linkage in starch. The human digestive system does not contain an enzyme that can hydrolyze the β-1, 4-linkage of cellulose. For this reason cellulose is not absorbable as a nutrient, but it does play a role in digestion by aiding in the maintenance of the tone of the intestine because of its bulk. Ruminants can digest cellulose because bacteria in the rumen contain cellulase, a β-1, 4-splitting enzyme.

DISACCHARIDES

Sucrose, or cane sugar, is composed of two monosaccharides: glucose and fructose. Lactose, a milk sugar, contains glucose and galactose, whereas maltose contains two glucose molecules joined by an α-1, 4-glucosidic linkage (see Fig. 2-2).

MONOSACCHARIDES

D-glucose or dextrose, also called grape sugar, is the chief sugar of human metabolism (see Fig. 2-1). It is the only hexose sugar known to exist in the free state in the human body. Blood glucose normally ranges from a concentration of 70 mg/dl to 120 mg/dl, depending on the method of analysis used. Normal fasting blood sugar is about 90 mg/dl to 100 mg/dl. When glucose levels rise to 160 mg/dl, the condition is known as hyperglycemia. Blood sugar levels below 60 mg/dl are characteristic of hypoglycemia. D-glucose contains an aldehyde group and is, therefore, an aldohexose.

Fructose or fruit sugar, also known as levulose, is a component of common table sugar sucrose and is found in many fruits, honey, and plant saps. It is a ketohexose (see Fig. 2-1).

Galactose along with glucose is a constituent of the milk sugar lactose. It is an aldohexose (see Fig. 2-1).

The pentoses ribose and deoxyribose are aldopentoses important in the structure of nucleic acids. D-xylose is also an aldopentose (see Fig. 2-1).

DIGESTION AND ABSORPTION

The major nutrients—carbohydrates, proteins, and lipids—are present in foods either as macromolecules or as other nonabsorbable forms and must be reduced in size before they can be absorbed into the blood and lymph and used by the human body. Until this takes place, all food in the intestinal "tube" remains outside the body.

The first stage in the digestion of carbohydrates takes place in the mouth. Here starches and other polysaccharides are prepared for the catalytic activity of digestive juices by being chewed, mixed, and lubricated with saliva and formed into a bolus that can be swallowed. Some foods if not chewed fail to be digested properly and may cause intestinal flatulence. Other substances, the pith of the orange for example, if not broken up by chewing may coalesce in the stomach and form a ball, or bezoar, which can cause intestinal obstruction.[2]

The digestion of starch begins almost at once when the stimulus of masticated food causes the secretion from salivary glands of a powerful starch-splitting enzyme, α-salivary amylase (called *ptyalin* in the older literature). This enzyme has the capacity to catalyze the hydrolysis of starch into the disaccharide maltose. The limited time food remains in the mouth before being swallowed does not permit extensive digestion. Nevertheless, the salivary enzyme mixed in the interior of the bolus can continue its starch-splitting activity until denatured by the strong acid of the stomach. Furthermore, the acidity of the gastric contents can also cause some hydrolysis of starches and simple sugars. There is no further enzymatic digestion of starches in the stomach.

The digestion of starches and carbohydrates in the lumen of the small intestine is accomplished by an α-amylase secreted in the pancreatic juice. The flow of pancreatic juice containing the amylase is stimulated by the intestinal hormones secretin and cholecystokinin–pancreozymin, produced when acid chyme is introduced into the duodenum. The optimal *p*H in the duodenum for pancreatic amylase is slightly on the alkaline side of neutrality, so its action is enhanced by the alkaline secretions of the pancreas and small intestine.

In the small intestine the amylose and amylopectin of food starches and the animal starch glycogen are broken down to their component disaccharides and glucose. These, along with the table sugar sucrose and the milk sugar lactose and other simple dietary sugars, are absorbed into the mucosal cells of the small intestine. In the microvilli of the brush border of the columnar cells of the intestinal epithelium they are further hydrolyzed to simple monosaccharides by the disaccharidases maltase, sucrase, and lactase. The end product of carbohydrate digestion—the monosaccharides glucose, fructose, and galactose—are absorbed by the portal blood.

If the function of the intestinal mucosa is impaired by disease, as in the malabsorption syndrome or for genetic reasons, patients may become intolerant of dietary sugars, which then can be lost in a watery diarrhea. Lactase deficiency of the small intestine is an example of such a condition.

Cellulose constitutes the great bulk of carbohydrates in nature and cannot be digested in the human GI tract. The human intestine does not produce a cellulase essential for the hydrolysis of cellulose. However, cellulose does contribute to mechanics of the digestive process by the stimulatory action of its fiber and bulk.

The monosaccharides are absorbed through the membranes of the mucosal cells at a rate greater than can be accounted for by such physical processes as diffusion. They are further absorbed against an increased concentration gradient. It is clear that the physiologically important sugars are absorbed by an active process requiring energy and an actively metabolizing intestinal cell as well as by a specific transport system. The various monosaccharides compete for this transport system so that individual absorptions take place at different rates. Galactose and glucose are absorbed most rapidly, followed by fructose, mannose, xylose, and arabinose, in diminishing order. Xylose and arabinose are probably absorbed primarily by diffusion.

METABOLISM

Glucose can be used by all tissues of the body. Some tissues such as the brain use glucose exclusively as an energy source, whereas cardiac muscle uses proportionately more fatty acids for this purpose. Although glucose is the energy source normally used by the nervous system, in total starvation and after periods of adaptation, the brain can use ketone bodies formed from fatty acids and amino acids.

An obligatory reaction in the use of glucose by tissue cells is the phosphorylation of glucose as it passes into the tissue cell from the blood. In so doing the phosphorylated glucose (as glucose-6-phosphate) is locked into the tissue cell and committed to catabolic purposes. It is only with great difficulty, if at all, that it can diffuse back into the blood.

The phosphorylation of blood glucose by the enzyme hexokinase and the energy source ATP is an irreversible reaction because of the large amounts of energy driving the biosynthesis of glucose-6-phosphate. This irreversibility has a number of important consequences in metabolism. It illustrates the fundamental rule that biosynthetic and degradative steps in biologic systems are always separate and distinct. Such a separation affords the body a degree of metabolic control that would not be present if both synthesis and degradation were conducted at the same time along similar pathways.

Liver glycogen is a storage form of glucose energy in the mammal. An important function of liver glycogen is to release glucose to the blood at a rate to maintain a minimal level of 90 mg to 100 mg glucose/100 ml blood. Since the hexokinase reaction described above is an irreversible reaction, this function of glucose release would not be possible were it not for an alternate pathway catalyzed by the liver enzyme glucose-6-phosphatase. This enzyme removes the phosphate moiety, enabling glucose to pass back into the blood and the tissues for oxidative purposes.

In glycogen storage disease there is a characteristic enlargement of the abdomen caused by a massive enlargement of the liver. A pronounced hypoglycemia between meals is also a characteristic symptom of this disease. This disease was first described by von Gierke in 1929. It is caused by a deficiency of glucose-6-phosphatase in the liver. In the absence of the enzyme, phosphate is not removed from glucose-6-phosphate and the liver is unable to contribute glucose to the blood, resulting in an enlarged glycogen-engorged liver and hypoglycemia. This was the first of several glycogen-storage diseases to be described and is one of an increasing number of diseases recognized and designated as *inborn errors of metabolism* that are genetically determined. In muscle tissue there is no glucose-6-phosphatase, so glycogen serves its primary purpose of furnishing glucose as energy for the energy-demanding muscles.

Since the capacity to store glycogen is limited, when carbohydrate is plentiful in the diet excess glucose is converted to fat. The body has a virtually unlimited capacity to store fat and in the dietarily over-indulgent individual reveals the process in corpulence.

Once phosphorylated, glucose-6-phosphate has a number of metabolic options other than storage as glycogen, conversion to fat, or to maintain the blood glucose concentration. Its primary purpose in metabolism is to furnish an energy source for the energy-demanding and metabolizing cells. Once glucose is in the bloodstream, the individual cells take it up and oxidize it at first to pyruvic acid by a process known as glycolysis and ultimately to CO_2 and water with the production of utilizable energy in the form of ATP. This latter oxidative phase takes place in the Krebs citric acid cycle located in the mitochondrion. This oxidation of glucose for energy purposes is the main thrust of carbohydrate metabolism.

Glucose can also furnish the metabolizing cells pentose sugars (ribose and deoxyribose) for nucleic acid and nucleotide synthesis and a source of reduced nicotinamide adenine dinucleotide phosphate (NADPH) for biosynthetic purposes. This takes place in the pentose or hexose monophosphate shunt or cycle.

Glucogenic amino acids can also contribute to the supply of glucose for energy purpose through the process known as gluconeogenesis.

FUNCTION AND REQUIREMENTS

The primary function of carbohydrate in the animal body is to provide a source of energy. Fat also contributes to this function to a significant degree, but carbohydrate, as glucose, is more readily available for use by the tissue cells.

Since carbohydrate, as glucose, can be made in the body from amino acids and the glycerol of fat, there is no specific requirement for this nutrient in the diet. Nevertheless, some preformed carbohydrate is beneficial in the diet to avoid ketosis, excessive breakdown of body protein, loss of cations, especially of sodium, and resulting dehydration.[10]

The undigestible portion of carbohydrate in the diet furnishes fibrous matter to the intestine. Although there is no demonstrated requirement for fiber or bulk, the possible physiologic significance of this has not been adequately explored.[10]

The undigestible portion of carbohydrate in the diet furnishes fibrous matter to the intestine. Although there is no demonstrated requirement for fiber or bulk, the possible physiologic significance of this has not been adequate explored.[10]

Lipids and Fats

Dietary fat provides the human body with a highly concentrated form of energy. Gram for gram fat, or more precisely lipid, contains more than twice the energy (9.0 Cal/g) of either carbohydrate or protein (each 4.0 Cal/g). Ethyl alcohol more nearly approaches the energy value of fat with 7.0 Cal/g.

Lipids, like carbohydrates, contain the three elements carbon, hydrogen, and oxygen; complex lipids also contain phosphorus and nitrogen. However, unlike the carbohydrates, lipids contain much less oxygen per mole in proportion to the amount of carbon and hydrogen. In neutral fat (triacylglycerols), for example, oxygen is confined to the ester linkages formed by the union of long hydrocarbon chain fatty acids with glycerol. Because they are anhydrous and reduced, triacylglycerols are a highly concentrated store of potential energy, and when metabolized by the tissue cell, they can combine with more oxygen and release more energy than either carbohydrate or amino acids. Since triacylglycerols are nonpolar they can be stored in a compact, nearly anhydrous form, whereas protein and carbohydrate, being much more hydrated, require much more tissue space.

There is, unfortunately, some inconsistency in the use of the terms *fat* and *lipid*. These terms are often considered synonymous by many people and are often used loosely by lipid specialists. The biochemist uses the term *fat*, or more properly *true fat*, more precisely to refer to the esters of fatty acids, with glycerol traditionally designated as neutral fat, triglyceride, or more recently, triacylglycerols. This is the fat referred to as *visible fat,* meaning butter, margarine, lard, vegetable oils, and the fat of the animal body depots. The term *lipid* is broader and includes the true fats, the source of energy in fat metabolism, as well as the structural and functional lipids named phospholipids, sphingolipids, cerebrosides, and the sterols.

Chemically, the lipids are a rather heterogeneous group of food substances with no common structural feature other than the presence of fatty acids, either actually or potentially, in the molecule. They are mostly insoluble in water but soluble in such organic solvents as ether, petroleum ether, chloroform, benzene, and hot alcohol.

In the United States the fat content of the average diet has steadily increased from 32% of calories in 1910 to over 41%, or about 160 g/person/day, at present. Most of these dietary lipids, about two thirds, come from animal sources and the remaining one third from vegetables, mostly as vegetable oils.

CHEMICAL CONSTITUTION AND FUNCTION

Functionally, the various classes of lipids can be divided as follows: (1) lipids that serve on oxidation as a source of metabolic energy and (2) lipids that form part of the structure of membranes, are concerned with the transport of fat, or serve as lipid precursors for the biosynthesis of key lipid hormones or catalysts. Cholesterol, for example, acts as a precursor for the biosynthesis of such important compounds as the bile acids, the steroid sex hormones, the adrenal cortical hormones, and vitamin D.

The simple lipid triacylglycerol, also called neutral fat and triglyceride, is the chief example of the group that is oxidized for energy (Fig. 2-3). This molecule of fat consists of glycerol, a trihydroxylic alcohol, esterified with three usually long-chain fatty acids. Naturally occurring fats in the adipose tissue are generally of the mixed type, meaning that the fatty acids represented by R_1, R_2, and R_3 are different. If the three fatty acids in the molecule were oleic, palmitic, and stearic acids, the name of the fat would be oleopalmitostearin. If all three fatty acids were palmitic acid, the compound would be tripalmitin. Triacylglycerols are the chief source of fat energy in the animal body.

The characteristic component of both simple and complex lipids is the fatty acid. Of the fatty acids found in nature, almost all are of the straight-chain type and have an even number of carbon atoms. Of these palmitic (16 C), stearic (18 C), and oleic (18 C:1) are the most commonly occurring. Hu-

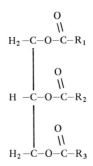

FIG. 2-3 Chemical structure of triacylglycerol.

man depot fat, for example, contains approximately 25% palmitic acid, 6% stearic acid, and 50% oleic acid. The fatty acids can be saturated ($-\overset{|}{C}-$) or unsaturated ($-\overset{|}{C}=\overset{|}{C}-$). The formulas of these typical fatty acids are shown in Table 2-3.

The structural and functional lipids include the phospholipids (also called phosphatides), the sphingolipids (sphingomyelin), glycolipids (cerebrosides), and the sterols.

The phospholipids are composed of glycerol, fatty acids, phosphoric acid, and a basic nitrogen compound. They contain, therefore, hydrogen, oxygen, carbon, phosphorus, and nitrogen. These differ from the triacylglycerols in that R_3 in the above structure for triacylglycerol is an inorganic acid, phosphoric acid, instead of a long-chain fatty acid. In addition these compounds contain nitrogenous bases esterified to the phosphoric acid. In lecithin, or more strictly phosphatidyl choline, the nitrogenous base is choline; in the cephalins (phosphatidyl ethanolamine and phosphatidyl serine) the nitrogenous base is, respectively, ethanolamine and serine. The phospholipids are key components of cellular membranes. The structures of phosphatidyl choline, a sphingomyelin, and cholesterol are illustrated in Figure 2-4.

The sphingomyelins are composed of a complex basic amino alcohol, sphingosine, with a fatty acid in amide linkage on the amino group and a phosphorylcholine group attached by way of the terminal alcohol group. Sphingomyelins are present in brain and nervous tissue.

TABLE 2-3
Composition of Typical Fatty Acids

Acid	Structure	Carbon Molecules	Double Bonds
Palmitic	$CH_3(CH_2)_{14}COOH$	16	None
Stearic	$CH_3(CH_2)_{16}COOH$	18	None
Oleic	$CH_3(CH_2)_7CH{=}CH(CH_2)_7COOH$	18	one

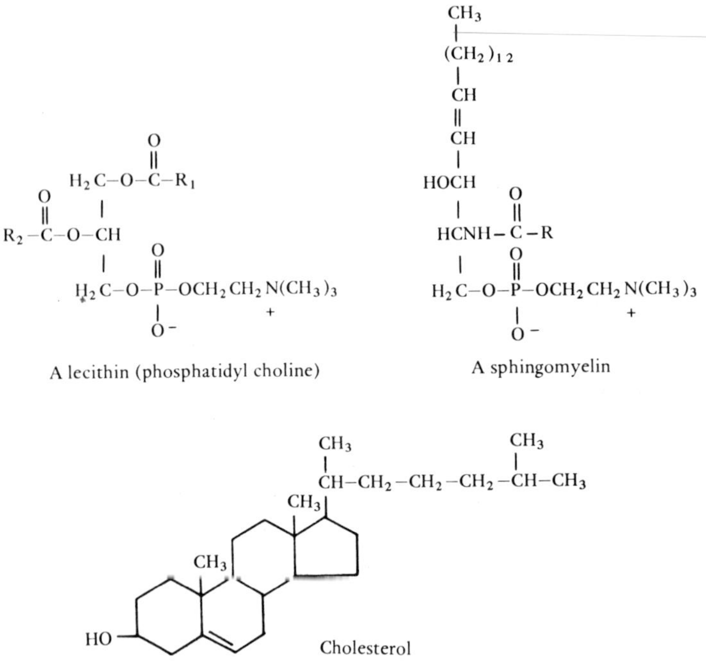

$$CH_3$$
$$|$$
$$(CH_2)_{12}$$
$$|$$
$$CH$$
$$||$$
$$CH$$
$$|$$

A lecithin (phosphatidyl choline)

$$O$$
$$||$$
$$H_2C-O-C-R_1$$
$$O \quad |$$
$$||$$
$$R_2-C-O-CH$$
$$| \quad O$$
$$||$$
$$H_2C-O-P-OCH_2CH_2N(CH_3)_3$$
$$| \quad +$$
$$O^-$$

A sphingomyelin

$$HOCH \quad O$$
$$| \quad ||$$
$$HCNH-C-R$$
$$| \quad O$$
$$||$$
$$H_2C-O-P-OCH_2CH_2N(CH_3)_3$$
$$| \quad +$$
$$O^-$$

Cholesterol

$$CH_3 \qquad CH_3$$
$$| \qquad |$$
$$CH-CH_2-CH_2-CH_2-CH-CH_3$$
$$CH_3|$$

FIG. 2-4 Chemical structures of phospholipids.

Because of its much discussed relationship to atherosclerosis, cholesterol is the best known of the sterols. It is also a constituent of gallstones. Cholesterol is a precursor of the bile acids, the steroid sex hormones, the adrenal cortical hormones, and vitamin D. Less is known of the metabolic origins and fates of glycolipids and the cerebrosides. The latter are found in relatively large concentrations in white matter of brain and in the myelin sheaths of nerves.

DIGESTION AND ABSORPTION

There is very little digestion of lipid in the stomach other than such small hydrolysis of lipid ester bonds that may be catalyzed by the acidity of the stomach chyme. A gastric lipase capable of mild fat-splitting is present in the stomach but does not appear to be important. A polypeptide hormone, enterogastrone, present in the duodenal mucosa, is activated by the discharge of food containing fat from the stomach. It inhibits gastric mobility and retards the discharge of food from the stomach. A meal rich in fat may therefore contribute to the feeling of satiety by delaying the emptying of the stomach, presumably by way of enterogastrone.

The introduction of acid chyme into the duodenum liberates two hormones of importance in intestinal digestion. Secretin, a polypeptide, is liberated from the duodenal mucosal cells by the hydrochloric acid in the chyme and is carried by the blood to the pancreas, where it stimulates the flow of a pancreatic juice rich in bicarbonate. A polypeptide hormone, cholecystokinin–pancreozymin, is produced by the mucosa of the upper small intestine. It stimulates the pancreas to produce a juice rich in enzymes (as inactive zymogens), as well as bicarbonate. The cholecystokinin function of the hormone is to stimulate the contraction of the gallbladder and dilate the sphincter of Oddi.

In the small intestine, bile secreted by the gallbladder acts on the larger fat particles. Such fatty particles divide into smaller particles with greatly increased surface area, enabling the water-soluble pancreatic lipase to hydrolyze them with greater rapidity and ease. Bile salts, small quantities of fatty acids, and monoglycerides liberated by the pancreatic lipase are then able to further emulsify the fat in the alkaline medium of the small intestine (pH 6.0–8.5) with the formation of fine droplets or micelles. Once the fat molecules are reduced to a finely divided form, they are further acted on by pancreatic lipase, which hydrolyzes the triacylglycerols into fatty acids, diglycerides, monoglycerides, and glycerol. Hydrolysis is rapid at first but is slowed at the 2-monoglyceride stage. Pancreatic juice also contains phospholipases and cholesterol esterases that catalyze the hydrolysis of phospholipids and cholesterol esters.

The end product of the digestive phase is a clear emulsion of lipids, which is then absorbed into the microvilli of the mucous membrane of the small intestine. The bile salts are not absorbed into the microvilli at this point but continue down the lumen of the small intestine, where in the ileum they are reabsorbed into the blood and carried back to the liver and gallbladder for reuse. This cycle of bile acids is called the enterohepatic circulation of bile salts. Most fats are 95% to 100% digestible, depending on the length of the fatty acid chain. Fats with melting points below 50°C are more rapidly and completely digested and absorbed than those with higher melting points.

The small fat particles, or micelles, pass into the intestinal mucosal cells, where further hydrolysis may take place and reesterification into new triacylglycerol molecules can take place. During this process new triacylglycerols are formed so that the neutral fat of the food loses its identity and new triacylglycerols characteristic of the human species are formed. These small new fat particles, called *chylomicrons,* are aggregates of triacylglycerols (80%), phospholipid (7%), and cholesterol (9%) coated with lipoproteins to produce very small particles (1 μ in diameter). The formation of chylomicrons renders the water-insoluble fat more soluble and transportable in the aqueous medium of the blood. The chylomicrons are secreted from the mucosal cell into the lacteals and lymphatics and finally into the systemic blood. Triacylglycerols that follow the lymphatic route are predominately the long-chain fatty acids. Medium-chain fatty acids (10 carbons or less) because of their greater water solubility are absorbed directly into the portal blood as free fatty acids bound to albumin.

Absence of bile in the small intestine as the result of disease or the malabsorption syndrome decreases the absorption of fat and results in an increase of undigested fat in the feces, a condition called *steatorrhea.*

METABOLISM

Blood lipids arising from the intestinal absorption of food fat are removed from the blood as it passes through the liver and other tissues. The triacylglycerols are hydrolyzed to fatty acids and glycerol by cellular lipases. Glycerol can be metabolized by entering carbohydrate pathways and is oxidized to CO_2 and water with the transfer of glycerol bond energy to high-energy phosphate bonds in ATP. The fatty acids arising from the adipose and other tissues reappear in the blood as components of lipoproteins. These lipoproteins facilitate the transport of water-insoluble fatty acids to various tissues where they can be oxidized by way of acetyl coenzyme A by removing 2 carbons at a time (β-oxidation) from the long-chain fatty acid molecule. The acetyl coenzyme A so formed can then be condensed with oxalacetate to form citric acid and oxidized in the Krebs aerobic citric acid cycle to CO_2 and water with release and capture of the large amount of potential energy in the fatty acid molecule as high-energy phosphate bond energy in ATP. Subsequently, this high-energy phosphate bond energy (ATP) may be used to cause molecular contractions and movement, to energize the flow and conduction of nerve impulses, to support the biosynthesis of tissues and vital metabolites, and to produce heat. When there is a diminished demand for fatty acids to be oxidized for energy purposes, the fatty acids may be stored in the fat depots for future use.

KETOSIS

The oxidation of fatty acids in the liver by β-oxidation normally produces acetoacetic acid (CH_3COCH_2COOH). At the *p*H of cellular fluids this acid exists as acetoacetate in its coenzyme A form (see Chap. 3). As a parent substance, acetoacetic acid can be degraded to form acetone (CH_3COCH_3) and by reduction, β-hydroxybutyric acid ($CH_3CHOHCH_2COOH$). Although this hydroxyacid is not strictly a ketone, all three substances are called *ketone* or *acetone bodies.*

Ketone bodies serve a very useful purpose in metabolism in that they can diffuse from the liver into the blood where they, especially acetoacetate, can be used by the muscles as a source of energy. Normally, small amounts of ketone bodies are present in the blood and urine.

Under abnormal circumstances (as in diabetes mellitus) ketone bodies can be produced in large quantities (ketosis) by the excessive production of acetoacetate by the liver. When acetoacetate, as acetoacetyl coenzyme A, is formed in the liver it has three possible options: (1) it can condense with oxalacetate and so form citric acid and be used as a source of energy; (2) it can be employed for the biosynthesis of fatty acids; or (3) it can be hydrolyzed to form acetoacetic acid and escape into the blood. When this latter strong acid is produced in large amounts, it causes a condition called ketosis. Unless corrected, this can overwhelm the blood's buffer systems, causing ketonemia and acidosis, and in the urine ketonuria. The oxidation of some glucose seems necessary to prevent ketosis. One possible reason seems to be the need to maintain the level of oxalacetate in the citric acid cycle, a needed intermediate in the oxidation of acetoacetate to CO_2 and water through the Krebs citric acid cycle.

ESSENTIAL FATTY ACIDS

When weanling rats are placed on a fat-free diet, they grow poorly and show signs of deficiency, including dermatitis, poor reproduction, lowered caloric efficiency, decreased resistance to stress, and impairment of lipid transport. If linoleic acid is present in the diet, these deficiency symptoms do not develop. Linolenic acid and arachidonic acid also prevent these symptoms. It is concluded that although mammals can synthesize saturated and monounsaturated (oleic) acids, they are unable to synthesize linoleic acid and α-linolenic acid, which contain respectively two and three unsaturated double bonds. Since linoleic acid and α-linolenic acid cannot be synthesized in mammalian tissues and are required in the diet, they are called *essential fatty acids.*

In tissue metabolism, the essential fatty acids have been shown to be precursors for a group of hormonelike compounds called *prostaglandins.* The name prostaglandin was given by the Swedish physiologist von Euler to those substances that are found in seminal plasma, the prostate gland, and the seminal vesicles. At least 14 prostaglandins occur in human seminal plasma. All the naturally occurring prostaglandins are derived biologically by cyclization of 20-carbon unsaturated fatty acids, such as arachidonic acid, which in turn is formed

FIG. 2-5 Chemical structures of amino acids.

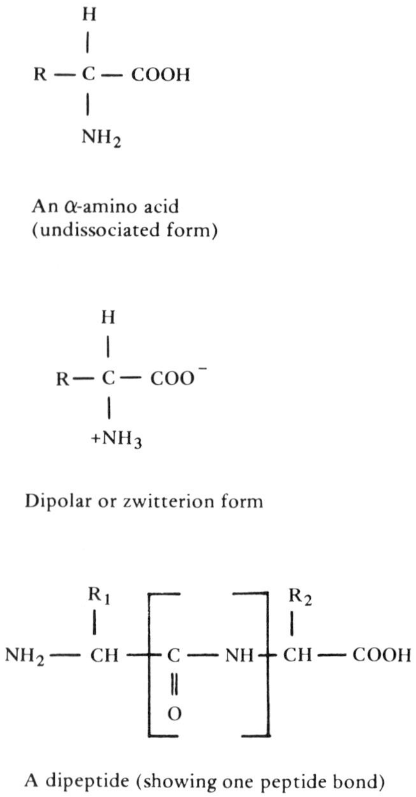

$$R - C - COOH$$

with H above and NH$_2$ below the central C.

An α-amino acid
(undissociated form)

$$R - C - COO^-$$

with H above and $^+$NH$_3$ below.

Dipolar or zwitterion form

$$NH_2 - CH - C - NH - CH - COOH$$

with R$_1$, R$_2$ above and O below (C=O).

A dipeptide (showing one peptide bond)

from the essential fatty acid linoleic acid. Therefore, the essential fatty acids can be considered necessary in the biosynthesis of the prostaglandins. The different prostaglandins have biologic activities that include lowering of blood pressure and causing smooth muscles to contract. The prostaglandins are among the most potent biologically active substances yet discovered. As little as 1 ng/ml causes contraction of smooth muscle. They have been suggested for use in prevention of conception, induction of labor at term, termination of pregnancy, the prevention or alleviation of gastric ulcers, control of inflammation and of blood pressure, and relief of asthma and nasal congestion.

REQUIREMENTS

In addition to serving as an important energy source, dietary fat serves as a carrier for fat-soluble vitamins and provides certain fatty acids that are essential nutrients. These needs can be met by a diet containing 15 g to 25 g food fats. Therefore, except for these needs, there is no specific requirement for fat as a nutrient.[10]

Proteins

The proteins were well named by the Dutch chemist Mulder in 1838 when he named them after the Greek *prōtos,* meaning "primary" or "holding first place." They are the most abundant organic molecule in cells and are fundamental to cell structure and function. The versatile structures of proteins enable them to act as enzyme catalysts that control the rate of biologic reactions, as carriers of essential metabolites within the organism, as regulators (hormones), and as building blocks for subcellular and cellular membranes and tissue structures. The enormous number of permutations possible from the 20-odd α-amino acids that make up protein structures forms the basis for the large number of proteins in nature.

CHEMICAL CONSTITUTION AND STRUCTURE

All proteins contain carbon, hydrogen, oxygen, and nitrogen. Some contain sulfur and others phosphorus, iron, zinc, and copper. All pure proteins on hydrolysis yield α-amino acids, which are the building blocks of protein structure. An examination of the α-amino acid structure in Figure 2-5 reveals that the molecule contains an amino group (—NH$_2$), a carboxyl group (—COOH), and an R group that can be aliphatic (hydrocarbon chain), aromatic as in phenylalanine, heterocyclic (tryptophan), or sulfur containing, as in methionine.

A simple amino acid such as glycine ($CH_2(NH_2)COOH$) in a solution of approximately neutral *p*H is doubly charged. In this doubly charged molecule the carboxyl group is negatively charged and the amino group is positively charged, giving the molecule a net charge of zero. Dipolar ions of this type are known as *zwitterions* (see Fig. 2-5). Because of their zwitterion structure, amino acids can react both as weak acids and as weak bases, that is, they are amphoteric. Most naturally occurring amino acids are L-α-amino acids. The simple properties briefly described above help in the understanding of protein structure.

Proteins are formed from amino acids united by peptide bonds (see Fig. 2-5). There may be many amino acids assembled from the 20-odd amino acids, and those selected determine the particular protein being synthesized. In this manner polypeptides and proteins are formed ranging in molecular size from a molecular weight of several thousand to as high as 40,000,000 as for the tobacco mosaic virus molecule.

DIGESTION AND ABSORPTION

There are no protein-hydrolyzing enzymes in the saliva, and therefore no protein digestion occurs in the mouth. The entrance of the bolus of food into the stomach stimulates the flow from the gastric glands of a strong acid juice containing hydrochloric acid and a powerful protein-splitting enzyme, pepsin. Hydrochloric acid is formed in the parietal cells of the stomach; the chief cells form pepsin in an inactive or zymogen form called *pepsinogen.* The formation of proteolytic enzymes in a precursor or zymogen form protects the protein structure of the enzyme-forming cells from self-digestion or auto-digestion. The zymogen is activated normally, as in the case of pepsinogen, by the acid of the gastric juice. In this acid medium, pepsinogen loses a small masking section of its structure and becomes the active enzyme, pepsin.

Pepsin attacks specific peptide bonds in the food protein molecule, preferably those formed from aromatic amino acids, although peptide bonds formed by other amino acids can be hydrolyzed, but more slowly.

The entrance of the digestive mixture or acid chyme into the duodenum stimulates the hormones, secretin and pancreozymin–cholecystokinin, to cause the flow into the duodenum of a pancreatic juice rich in bicarbonate and enzymes. In the duodenum the food digest is neutralized and made slightly alkaline, producing a *p*H optimal range suitable for the activity of the pancreatic enzymes. In the upper small intestine digestion of the dietary protein continues with pancreatic enzymes, such as trypsin, chymotrypsin, the carboxypeptidases, and dipeptidases. Again, as in the case of pepsin, these enzymes are made in the pancreas as zymogens and become active in the small intestine.

The final result of the action of proteolytic enzymes in the lumen of the small intestine is to hydrolyze proteins to peptides and amino acids. These are absorbed into the microvilli, where further hydrolysis catalyzed by peptidases in the microvilli converts them to the constituent amino acids.

The ultimate amino acids so formed in the process of digestion pass from the intestinal cell into the blood either by diffusion or by the energy-requiring process of active transport. From the intestine, the amino acids are transported by the blood of the portal vein to the liver, where they are released into the general circulation and carried to various tissues and cells for use in repair and synthesis.

METABOLISM

Food proteins provide amino acids for the biosynthesis of body proteins and nitrogenous constituents for the synthesis of other tissue constituents. Since the body is in dynamic equilibrium, proteins themselves are constantly degraded and resynthesized. Some amino acids are reused for the synthesis of new tissue. However, the normal process of catabolism of amino acids removes the amino group. This can be converted to urea in the liver and excreted through the kidney into the urine. The keto acid remaining after removal of the amino group can enter the Krebs aerobic cycle and be oxidized to CO_2 and water with the release of bond energy, which can be stored as ATP.

Amino acids cannot be stored as such and when consumed in excess of the amount needed are rapidly degraded and secreted.

NITROGEN BALANCE

Nitrogen balance implies the balance between intake and output of nitrogen in the body. Here it should be pointed out that nitrogen is found also in other compounds than amino acids. Non-protein nitrogen is present, for example, in urea, uric acid, ammonia, creatine, creatinine, and in other body tissues and fluids. A subject is said to be in N balance when the nitrogen intake in the diet equals the nitrogen output in the urine, feces, and skin. The term *negative nitrogen balance* is used when the output of nitrogen exceeds the intake. *Positive nitrogen balance* refers to that state in which the intake of nitrogen exceeds its output.

ESSENTIAL AND NONESSENTIAL AMINO ACIDS

The human body can synthesize some amino acids. However, there are nine amino acids—histidine, isoleucine, leucine, lysine, methionine, phenylalanine, threonine, tryptophan, and valine—that either cannot be synthesized in mammalian tissues or in certain periods of life cannot be synthesized rapidly enough to fully supply the needs of the human. For example, histidine is required in the diet to maintain growth during childhood. These indispensable amino acids are called *essential amino acids*. They are essential in the diet in adequate amounts to maintain nitrogen balance.

PROTEIN QUALITY

The nutritive value of a protein depends on the relation of its amino acids to those required for the building of new tissue. A diet that is deficient in one or more of the essential amino acids cannot maintain nitrogen equilibrium. If, however, the missing amino acid is provided by another protein added to the diet, nitrogen equilibrium and normal nutrition can be established. It is clear therefore that the quality of a protein depends on the balance of amino acids, especially the essential amino acids, that are present in the protein in question. In humans, the protein requirement must be considered on the basis of the quality and not merely on the quantity of the protein. It is not just a matter of the total amount of protein needed but of the specific amino acids needed. Since the nonessential amino acids can be synthesized in the human body, it is the essential amino acids that are critical to the diet. All the amino acids necessary for the biosynthesis of a protein must be present at the same time, or the protein will not be formed.

PROTEIN ALLOWANCES

The National Academy of Sciences recommended dietary allowances are based on an average requirement of 0.47 g protein/kg body weight/day.[10] This value has been obtained by nitrogen balance studies and has been increased further by 30% to take into account individual variability, giving allowances of 0.6 g/kg/day of high-quality protein. This value has been further increased by allowing for a 75% efficiency of use. The total recommended allowance, therefore, for mixed proteins in the United States diet is 0.8 g/kg body weight/day. The allowance for a 70-kg man is 56 g protein/day, and for a 58-kg woman, 46 g.

The allowance for children is based on the amount of milk consumed and on the amount known to ensure a satisfactory rate of growth. For ages up to one half year the allowance is kilograms weight × 2.2; for one half year to one year it is kilograms weight × 2.0 (see Table A-1).[10]

An additional 30 g protein/day is recommended for the pregnant woman, from the second month until the end of gestation, as a supplement to the 1.3 g protein/kg body weight recommended for a mature woman. For pregnant adolescents and for younger girls see the Tables of Allowances in the Appendix.

Lactation requires an additional 20 g protein/day above the maintenance allowance to cover the requirement for milk production and to allow for 70% efficiency of protein use.

References

1. Bogert J, Briggs GM, Calloway DH: Nutrition and Physical Fitness, 9th ed. Philadelphia, WB Saunders, 1973
2. Davidson S, Passmore R, Brock JF, Truswell AS: Human Nutrition and Dietetics, 7th ed. New York, Churchill Livingstone, 1979
3. Guthrie HA: Introductory Nutrition, 3rd ed. St Louis, CV Mosby, 1975
4. Handbook on Nutritional Requirements. Food and Agriculture Organization of the United Nations, FAO Nutritional Studies No. 28, WHO Monograph Series 61, Rome, 1974
5. Harper's Review of Biochemistry, 18th ed. Los Altos, Lange Medical Publications, 1981
6. Lehninger AL: Biochemistry, 2nd ed. New York, Worth Publishing, 1975
7. Mountcastle VB (ed): Medical Physiology, Vols I and II, 13th ed. St Louis, CV Mosby, 1974
8. Orten JM, Neuhaus O: Human Biochemistry, 9th ed. St Louis, CV Mosby, 1975
9. Oxygen Bomb Calorimetry and Combustion Methods. Technical Manual No. 130, Parr Instrument Co, Moline, Illinois, revised 1968
10. Recommended Dietary Allowances, 9th ed. Washington DC, National Academy of Sciences, 1980
11. Stryer L: Biochemistry, 2nd ed. San Francisco, WF Freeman, 1981
12. Vander AJ, Sherman JH, Luciano DS: Human Physiology. The Mechanisms of Body Function, 2nd ed. New York, McGraw-Hill, 1975

3
Vitamins

Carl E. Anderson

It is not possible to sustain life in animals fed and maintained on a chemically defined diet containing only purified proteins, carbohydrates, fats, and the essential minerals and water. Additional "accessory food factors" called *vitamins* are necessary, although often they are required in only minute amounts. The amount required daily may be as low as a few micrograms to as high as 30 mg.

The first successful preparation of an essential food factor was obtained by Casimir Funk, a Polish biochemist working in the Lister Institute in London. He obtained a potent antiberiberi substance from rice polishings. Since the active factor was an amine and necessary for life, he called it a *vitamine*. As work by many others progressed and other "vitamines" were discovered, it was found that only a few were *amine* in nature, and so the final *e* was dropped to give the now general term *vitamin*. Although a strict definition describing vitamins may be of only modest value, it does help jog the memory.

The vitamins are organic substances that the body requires in small amounts for its metabolism, yet cannot make for itself at least in sufficient quantity. For the most part they are not related chemically and differ in their physiologic role.

This definition holds reasonably true, yet in the light of the most recent work it may not be strictly so. Niacin and vitamin K can be made in the body, but perhaps not in sufficient amounts to allow the neglect of dietary sources. Niacin can be synthesized from the amino acid tryptophan. Vitamin K is a product of intestinal bacterial synthesis, is absorbed, and is, therefore, a nondietary source of

the vitamin. In addition to being present as a dietary source, vitamin D can be produced in one human organ, the skin, and can affect such distant target organs as the intestine and bone, and therefore resembles a hormone in its activity.

During 1913 to 1914, McCollum and Davis extracted a factor from butter fat that they called *fat-soluble A* to distinguish it from the water-soluble unidentified dietary essential called the antiberiberi substance. These two dietary essentials became vitamin A and vitamin B.[25] As one by one the vitamins were discovered, each was assigned a letter. The antiscorbutic factor became vitamin C, the antirachitic factor vitamin D, the antihemorrhagic factor, vitamin K, and so on. When through isolation and synthesis the chemical structure of the vitamin became known, it was given a specific chemical name. Vitamin B_1 (other members of the B-complex vitamins were discovered, such as B_2 and so on) became thiamin, and the antiscorbutic vitamin C became L-ascorbic acid. It was assumed the chemical name assigned the vitamin applied to a single chemical substance of definite activity. It is now clear that some vitamins consist of several closely related compounds. The term *vitamin A* is now used to refer collectively to all active and synthesized forms of the vitamin, vitamin A alcohol is now retinol, vitamin A aldehyde, retinal, and vitamin A acid, retinoic acid.

There are 13 or 14 vitamins that are essential in the human diet (Fig. 3-1). The higher figure is used if the person involved considers one or more of the vitamins in the diet not in conformity with the definition of a vitamin. Some, for example, do not

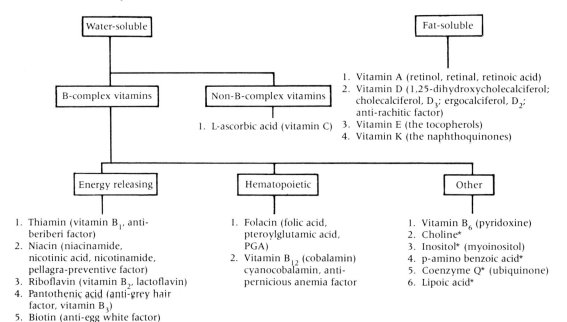

*Dietary substances sometimes given vitamin status but not established as vitamins.

FIG. 3-1 The vitamins.

consider choline a vitamin, although it is of importance in metabolism. The need for this substance for humans has not been proved, and it is retained in the classification as a vitaminlike substance.

The division into fat-soluble and water-soluble vitamins is retained because the four fat-soluble vitamins have some properties in common, although physiologically and structurally, they are quite different. For example, the lipid-soluble vitamins are absorbed from the intestine with dietary lipids. In the malabsorption syndrome (involving the failure of absorption of fat, resulting in steatorrhea) all the fat-soluble vitamins may be excreted, whereas the water-soluble vitamins may not be affected. Also, as a consequence of their lipid solubility significant quantities of the lipid-soluble vitamins are stored in the liver, but the storage of water-soluble vitamins is not significant. Therefore, although it is possible to administer a several weeks' supply of the lipid-soluble vitamins in a single dose, the water-soluble vitamins must be supplied frequently.

The B-complex vitamins are further separated into the group of energy-releasing vitamins, the vitamins concerned with blood formation (the hematopoietic group), and "others," a catch-all group with miscellaneous functions but still essential or important in metabolism.

There are similar properties and functions among the energy-releasing group of vitamins in that they are all components of enzyme systems as components of coenzymes. They have the ever-vital function in living cells of assisting in the release of energy. The remaining non-B-complex vitamin is ascorbic acid, which is important in the synthesis of connective tissue.

Although at present there is a vast body of information on the vitamins, there are only the most meager clues to the mechanism connecting, in the vitamin deficiency, the tissue lesion with the biochemical defect. Much good research remains to be done.

The Water-Soluble Vitamins

THE ENERGY-RELEASING VITAMINS

THIAMIN (VITAMIN B₁)

Function. The principal role of thiamin, the antiberiberi vitamin, is as part of the coenzyme thiamin pyrophosphate in the oxidative decarboxylation of alpha-keto acids. In animal cells this coenzyme plays a critical role in the attainment of energy. The decarboxylation of pyruvate to "active acetate," or acetyl coenzyme A, connects the glycolytic cycle of carbohydrate metabolism with the high energy-producing Krebs or citric acid cycle. Similarly, the decarboxylation of α-ketoglutaric acid to succinyl coenzyme A is a key step in the energy-producing Krebs cycle itself. In these steps other energy-connected vitamins and vitaminlike substances, for instance, lipoic acid, pantothenic acid, nicotinic acid, and riboflavin, also are involved. Thiamin also has a role in the conversion of the amino acid tryptophan to nicotinic acid and nicotinamide. It has been shown that tryptophan normally contributes to the niacin supply of the body.

Deficiency. A thiamin deficiency in animals, including the human, is called beriberi (Singhalese *beri*, weakness or "I can't"). It is characterized biochemically by an accumulation of pyruvic and lactic acids, particularly in the blood and brain. There is impairment of cardiovascular, nervous, and gastrointestinal (GI) systems. The neurologic changes are believed by some to be due to other concomitant vitamin deficiencies. However, neurologic lesions have been induced by thiamin deficiency in pigeons and rats, and some evidence indicates that neurologic lesions in man can result from a thiamin deficiency.

The deficiency disease beriberi has been known since earliest time. In rice-eating people, it is endemic because of the still widespread consumption of decorticated or polished rice. In the Western world, particularly in the United States and Europe, where the diet contains more thiamin, the disease is rarely seen except in alcoholism, food faddism, and sometimes in the malabsorption syndrome. In the alcoholic, the deficiency may lead to Wernicke's disease and Korsokoff's syndrome (see Chap. 15). Here it is of importance to differentiate whether the Wernicke–Korsokoff syndrome is due to the alcohol consumed or to other causes of a thiamin deficiency. Irreversible brain damage may occur unless the disorder is recognized early and treatment properly instituted.

Beriberi can be separated into three forms: (1) wet beriberi, (2) dry beriberi, and (3) infantile beriberi. There are early clinical features common to both wet and dry beriberi. The deficient person tires easily, his limbs feel heavy and weak, and mild degrees of swelling may appear around the ankles. The legs may become numb, and a feeling of "pins and needles" in the leg may appear. Palpitation of the heart may occur. At this stage a close examination may reveal reduced motor power, alterations in gait, and patchy anesthesia over the skin of the lower legs. A better diet or thiamin administration can improve the condition. If left untreated the disease will progress to either the wet or dry beriberi.

In wet beriberi the main feature of the disease is the accumulation of edema fluid in the legs and often in the scrotum, face, and trunk. Cardiac palpitations, chest pains, and dyspnea may develop. The pulse is rapid and often irregular. The neck veins are distended with visible pulsations, and the heart becomes enlarged. In spite of the edema the urine contains no albumin—an important diagnostic feature. Wet beriberi must be distinguished from renal edema and congestive cardiac failure. In both of the aforementioned conditions there is albuminuria; in beriberi there is none. A person with wet beriberi is in danger of rapid deterioration, acute circulatory failure, and death.

Dry beriberi is so called because edema is not a feature of the disease. The condition is similar to peripheral neuritis. A common feature is anesthesia and paraesthesia of the feet followed by difficulty in walking, a peculiar ataxic gait, foot drop, and wrist drop. Muscular wasting may occur, and anesthetic patches (especially over the tibia) occur. Tenderness of the calves and other muscles when pressure is applied may be present. The person may have great difficulty in rising from the squatting position. The disease may be chronic, and a better diet or thiamin supplementation improves the disease in most instances. Untreated the disease progresses; the person becomes bedridden and often dies of some chronic infection.

Infantile beriberi may occur in otherwise normal infants under 6 months of age receiving inadequate thiamin in the milk of a lactating mother, particularly if her diet is deficient in thiamin. The mother may not present overt signs of beriberi. Infantile beriberi often occurs between 2 to 6 months of age. In the acute form the infant develops dyspnea and cyanosis and dies rapidly of cardiac failure. Aphonia may be present, and the infant may appear to be crying without emitting much sound. Diarrhea, wasting, and vomiting may occur. Edema is sometimes seen, and convulsions may occur at the terminal stage. Measurement of thiamin in the blood is of limited value. Most useful are determinations of lactate and blood pyruvate, especially if performed after glucose administration and exercise.

Chemical Properties and Structure. Thiamin hydrochloride is a compound consisting of a pyrimidine ring joined by a methylene bridge to a thiazole nucleus. The bond between the two rings is weak with the result the compound is easily destroyed in an alkaline medium. The active coenzyme form is thiamin pyrophosphate.

Thiamin is highly soluble in water and will resist destruction at temperatures up to 100°C. Since it can be destroyed if heated above 100°C, it will be destroyed in food fried in a hot pan or cooked too long under pressure. Because of its insolubility thiamin is easily leached out of food being washed or boiled.

Absorption and Metabolism. Thiamin and its salts are easily, under normal conditions, absorbed from the small intestine. As with most of the water-soluble vitamins, the body is unable to store thiamin in any great quantity.

Liver, heart, and brain have higher concentrations of the active vitamin than muscle tissue or other organs. A person on a high-thiamin intake becomes saturated and begins to excrete increased quantities in the urine.

Sources. Thiamin is found in foods of both animal and vegetable origin. The richest sources among commonly eaten foods are pork, whole grains, enriched cereal grains, and legumes. Green vegetables, fish, meat, fruits, and milk all contain useful quantities. In cereals the vitamin is present mainly in the germ and in the outer coat of the seed. Much of the vitamin is lost if cereals are milled and refined.

Requirement. The activity of thiamin hydrochloride is expressed in milligrams of the chemically pure and synthesized substance. From 1.2 mg to 1.5 mg daily is recommended for men. Similar amounts are recommended for women. For allowances in pregnancy and lactation and in children, see Appendix Table A-1.

Toxicity. Taken in excessive amounts thiamin is excreted in the urine and hence has no known toxicity. The kidney has no known threshold. Intolerance to thiamin is rare; daily doses of 500 mg have been administered for as long as a month without ill effects. A few cases of sensitization have been described following repeated parenteral injections.

NIACIN

The discovery of niacin (nicotinic acid, nicotinamide, pellagra-preventive factor) and its association with the disease pellagra are closely linked. Pellagra was first described by Casals, a physician in Spain in 1730, soon after the introduction of corn (maize) into Europe. It was given its name (It. *pelle*, skin, + *agra*, rough) in 1771 by an Italian physician, F. Frapolli. The disease seems to have spread with the cultivation of corn, but it was not until 1917 that Goldberger, studying the disease among the poor and those in prisons in southern United States, confirmed his theory that the incidence of the disease is closely related to the quality of the diet and that certain foods (*e.g.*, yeast, milk, and meat) are pellagra preventive and can be used to treat the disease.

In 1916 Spencer, a veterinarian of Concord, North Carolina, first called attention to the similarity between the symptoms of a spontaneous canine disease known to veterinarians as "blacktongue," and those of human pellagra.[49] He diagnosed blacktongue as pellagra in dogs, and from his successes in curing the animals by giving them milk, eggs, and meat, he concluded that it was caused by a diet low in nitrogen.

In 1937 Elvehjem and co-workers working at the University of Wisconsin found that nicotinic acid was effective in curing blacktongue in dogs and pellagra in man.[10,38] Shortly thereafter the use of nicotinic acid in treating human pellagra brought dramatic curative results.

Function. Niacin (nicotinic acid) is an essential part of the enzyme system concerned with hydrogen transport (oxidation) in living cells. It is the functional group of two coenzymes: (1) nicotinamide adenine dinucleotide (NAD) and (2) nicotinamide adenine dinucleotide phosphate (NADP). As coenzyme components of dehydrogenase enzyme systems they assist in removing hydrogen from (oxidation of) the food substrate and then passing the hydrogens on to other components of the respiratory chain. At the end of the chain hydrogen is united to oxygen to form water. The energy released during the oxidation of the food substrate is captured as high-energy adenine triphosphate. This energy can then be released and transformed into other forms of energy (*e.g.*, mechanical, heat, the energy required for synthesis, and nervous energy) and used in other energy-requiring cellular functions.

Deficiency. The specific disease caused by a deficiency of niacin is pellagra. The disease involves the skin, GI tract, and central nervous system. It progresses through dermatitis, diarrhea, dementia, and, unless corrected, death. These are the four Ds well known to medical students. The typical features of the disease are increasing weakness and a characteristic rash found only on the surfaces of the body exposed to the sun or heat. Early symptoms include glossitis, stomatitis, insomnia, anorexia, weakness, irritability, abdominal pain, burning sensations in various parts of the body, numbness, forgetfulness, marked fears, and vertigo. There are ill-defined disturbances of the alimentary tract with changes of bowel function. Patients debilitated and weakened by diarrhea often die of infection or become subjected to mental disorder.

Chemical Properties and Structure. Niacin is a simple derivative of pyridine and is very stable.

It is a water-soluble, white compound that is moderately resistant to heat and to both acid and alkali.

The human body has the ability to convert the amino acid tryptophan to niacin. It is believed that about 60 mg dietary tryptophan is equivalent to 1 mg niacin. Diets in the United States often contain 600 mg or more tryptophan, and this provides a substantial contribution to the niacin pool.

Sources. Niacin is widely distributed in plants and in animal foods, but in most cases in small amounts. Particularly rich sources of niacin are lean meats (especially liver), peanuts, yeast, and cereal bran and germ. The main source in the diet is frequently the cereal staple consumed. Whole grain or lightly milled cereals contain more niacin than refined cereal grains and flours. Niacin is now often added to many manufactured food products, especially those made from cereals.

Corn is poor in niacin, and its principal protein, zein, is very low in tryptophan, a biosynthetic source of the vitamin. There is evidence that some of the niacin in corn is present in a bound form that may not be available.

Requirement. Estimations of niacin requirements are complicated by the fact that tryptophan is converted to niacin in humans and by the paucity of studies of diets and of people at different ages. The allowance recommended for adults, expressed as niacin, is 6.6 mg/1000 Cal, and not less than 13 mg at caloric intakes of less than 2000 Cal. There is no data on the niacin requirements of children from infancy through adolescence. However, for recommendation, see Appendix Table A-1. There is no information on the niacin requirements of pregnant and lactating women.

Toxicity. Niacin is related chemically to nicotine but has quite different physiologic properties. It is essentially nontoxic. Niacin (but not niacinamide) acts as a vasodilator and, therefore, may cause flushing of the skin, dizziness, and nausea. These symptoms are temporary and not harmful but may be disturbing to those not aware of this physiologic effect.

RIBOFLAVIN

Riboflavin functions as a coenzyme or active prosthetic group in a group of flavoproteins concerned with tissue oxidation and respiration. Despite its fundamental role in the respiratory cycle as a hydrogen acceptor in energy and protein metabolism, no recognized disease is associated with an exclusive deficiency of riboflavin.

Riboflavin was discovered during the search for a hypothetical heat-stable vitamin B_2. Using its growth-promoting properties in the rat, Kuhn and his colleagues in 1933 finally isolated from 5400 liters milk 1 g active crystalline riboflavin. Unfortunately, it did not have the properties previously ascribed to vitamin B_2, such as curing blacktongue in dogs. It was clear, therefore, that riboflavin was just another of several factors present in the heat-stable fraction of the vitamin B complex.

An important clue to the nature of Kuhn's crystals was that they had a yellow color. A year earlier Warburg and Christian described a "yellow enzyme," a respiratory catalyst capable of acting as a hydrogen acceptor and donor. Riboflavin and Warburg's yellow enzyme were found to be related. The yellow enzyme proved to be a flavoprotein comprising a flavin pigment linked to a protein carrier. In 1935 riboflavin was synthesized by two independent groups, Kuhn and his colleagues in Heidelberg and Karrers' group in Basel.

Function. Combinations of riboflavin and various proteins form enzymes that function in tissue respiration as components of the electron-transport system. These include L-amino and D-amino oxidases, xanthine oxidase, cytochrome-c reductase, and a number of dehydrogenases. The flavin coenzyme or prosthetic group is usually flavin adenine dinucleotide (FAD), or in some instances it can be flavin mononucleotide (FMN). The flavoproteins, therefore, are an important group of enzymes involved in oxidation–reduction reactions.

Deficiency. Characteristic lesions of the lips, the most common of which are angular stomatitis and cheilosis, occur in the deficiency. Localized seborrheic dermatitis of the face, a particular type of glossitis (magenta tongue), and certain functional and organic disorders of the eyes may result from riboflavin deficiency. Many of these symptoms are not due to riboflavin deficiency alone but result from other deficiencies of the B-complex group.

Chemical Properties and Structure. The riboflavin molecule consists of an isoalloxazine nucleus with a ribityl side chain attached to the middle ring. It is an orange yellow crystalline compound. It is water soluble and heat stable, especially in acid solution, but is easily decomposed by light. It exhibits a yellow green fluorescence in water solution.

Absorption and Metabolism. Riboflavin is readily absorbed from the small intestine. It is phosphorylated in the intestine, liver, and other tissues. The bulk of riboflavin in the body is stored to a limited extent in the liver, heart, and kidney. In man, riboflavin is excreted predominantly in the feces. Fecal riboflavin arises both from the intestinal wall and bacterial synthesis. It is excreted in the urine to some extent as riboflavin or riboflavin phosphate.

Sources.   Riboflavin is widely distributed in plant and animal tissues. The best food sources include milk, eggs, liver, kidney, heart, and green leafy vegetables.

Riboflavin is lost in appreciable quantities in food preparation if the food is cooked while exposed to light. Losses also occur in dehydrated vegetables. Considerable quantities of riboflavin can be destroyed in milk if it is bottled and exposed to sun or bright daylight for any length of time.

Requirements.   Recommended allowances are 0.4 mg to 0.6 mg for infants, 0.8 mg to 1.2 mg for children, 1.3 mg to 1.8 mg for men depending on age, and 1.1 mg to 1.3 mg for women. Increases as shown in the Appendix Table A-1 are made for pregnant and lactating women.

Toxicity.   There is no evidence of toxicity in the human when large amounts are consumed.

PANTOTHENIC ACID

Pantothenic acid is an essential vitamin in the nutrition of man, many species of animals, plants, bacteria, and yeast. Because of its widespread occurrence in food, it was named from the Greek word *pantos,* meaning everywhere. It had been called vitamin B₃ and was given its present name by its discoverer, R. J. Williams, in 1938. It occupies a central and basic role in the metabolism of carbohydrate, fat, and protein because of its posi-

tion and role as a part of the structure of a key enzyme in metabolism, coenzyme A (Fig. 3-2).

Function.   As a constituent of coenzyme A, pantothenic acid is essential to a number of fundamental reactions in metabolism. It participates in this way in the release of energy from the catabolism of all three energy-yielding nutrients, that is, carbohydrate, fat, and protein. The acetyl coenzyme A that is formed from the three major nutrients combines with oxaloacetic acid to form citric acid, which initiates the citric acid or Krebs oxidative cycle, with the liberation and capture of the bond energies involved as high-energy adenosine triphosphate.

Pantothenic acid is involved in providing acetyl groups in the formation of acetylcholine and with the sulfonamide drugs, which are acetylated prior to excretions.

Although a major function of pantothenic acid is in conjunction with its role as a constituent of coenzyme A, a protein-bound pantothenic acid is contained in a compound known as *acyl carrier protein.*[36] Acyl carrier protein is a coenzyme required in the biosynthesis of fatty acids.

Pantothenic acid as a component of coenzyme A is also concerned with the biosynthesis of cholesterol and other sterols and of porphyrin, a component of hemoglobin.

Because of its role in energy metabolism, it can be considered to be vital to all energy-requiring processes within the cell.

Deficiency.   In humans, pantothenic acid deficiency has been produced in volunteers by the use of a purified diet and a specific antagonist. Evidence of dietary deficiency has not been clinically recognized in humans, and the administration of a metabolic antagonist appears to be necessary to

FIG. 3-2   Coenzyme A (CoA).

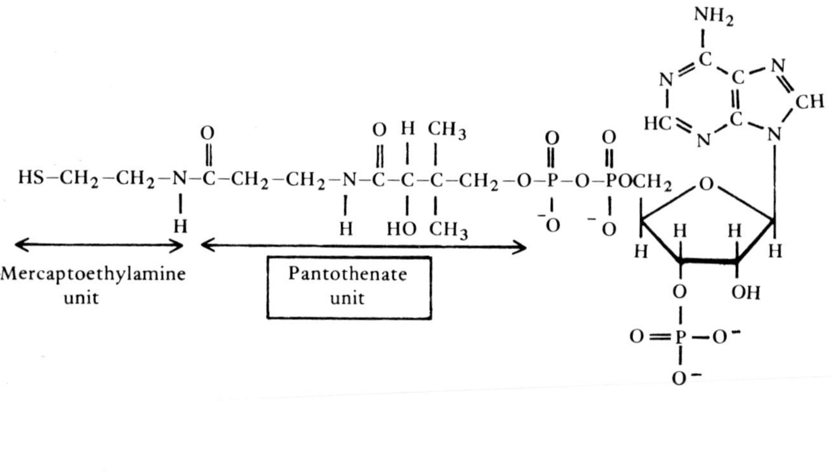

produce clinical symptoms.[17] The symptoms noted include fatigue, sleep disturbances, personality changes, nausea, abdominal distress, numbness and tingling of hands and feet, muscle cramps, impaired coordination, and loss of antibody production. All symptoms were cured by the administration of the vitamin. A well-defined pantothenic acid deficiency has not been observed in humans under normal conditions, but it is an essential nutrient for all animal species that have been investigated.

In the rat, pantothenic acid deficiency is characterized by retardation of growth, impaired reproduction, graying of the hair of black rats, and hemorrhagic adrenal cortical hypofunction. This may be related to reports that indicate that the synthesis of coenzyme A from free pantothenic acid can take place in the zona fasciculata of the adrenal cortex. Pantothenic acid neither prevents nor cures graying of hair in the human, contrary to claims so made.

Calcium pantothenate has been used successfully in treating paralysis of the GI tract after surgery, which causes the accumulation of gas and severe abdominal pain. It may act by stimulating GI motility. High levels of the acid (10 g–20 g) cause diarrhea. Intestinal bacteria synthesize considerable amounts of pantothenic acid. This, together with its widespread natural occurrence, makes a deficiency unlikely.

Chemical Properties and Structure. Pantothenic acid is a pale yellow oily liquid that has never been crystallized, although its calcium salt crystallizes readily. It is generally available in this latter form. Though stable in neutral solution, it is easily destroyed both on the acid and alkaline side of neutrality. It is readily soluble in water, somewhat soluble in ether, and practically insoluble in benzene and chloroform.

The acid is a β-alanine derivative with a peptide bond linkage. It is a component of coenzyme A, the critically essential cofactor for acylation reactions in the animal body (see coenzyme A, Fig. 3-2). As a component of coenzyme A, pantothenic acid is involved in the intermediary metabolism of carbohydrate, fat, and protein, leading to energy release, synthesis of fatty acids and sterols, gluconeogenesis, and many other essential reactions.[22]

Sources. Pantothenic acid is widely distributed in food, especially in foods from animal sources. The best sources are liver, kidney, egg yolk, yeast, wheat bran, and fresh vegetables (100 μg/g–200 μg/g dry material); broccoli, lean beef, skimmed milk, sweet potatoes, and molasses are fair sources (35 μg/g–100 μg/g dry material). It is probably synthesized by intestinal bacteria.

In most cooking and baking procedures there is little loss of the vitamin, but temperature above the boiling point may cause considerable loss. Frozen meat may lose much of its original content in the drip that occurs with thawing.

Requirement. Pantothenic acid is readily available in most foods, and isolated dietary deficiencies are unlikely. Some subclinical deficiencies may be found in individuals who are greatly malnourished.

There is not yet adequate evidence on which to base recommended allowance for pantothenic acid. Dietary intake in the adult population is 5 mg to 20 mg/day. Diets that meet nutritional needs of children contain 4 mg to 5 mg/day of the vitamin. A daily intake of 5 mg to 10 mg is thought to be adequate for adults, with the upper level suggested for pregnant and lactating women.[37]

Toxicity. Toxicity from large intakes of pantothenic acid is not known to occur in humans.

BIOTIN

Biotin is a water-soluble vitamin that is widely distributed in nature and is essential for many animal species including man.[57] The addition of 15% to 30% raw, dried egg white as a source of protein to a diet low in biotin will induce symptoms of biotin deficiency. Raw egg white contains a glycoprotein, avidin, which binds biotin into a large biotin–avidin complex that cannot be absorbed from the GI tract.

Biotin was crystallized in 1936. It was given the name biotin because it is part of the *bios* factor needed for yeast growth, but early in the research of biotin deficiency it was also called the "anti-egg-white injury factor." Cooking denatures avidin so that it loses its ability to bind biotin and prevent absorption.

Ordinarily, biotin deficiency does not occur in man except when induced experimentally. In the human, a diet must provide 30% of its calories from egg white to induce a biotin deficiency. Since this represents the egg whites from more than two dozen eggs it is obvious that a reasonable intake of egg white will not precipitate a deficiency state.

Function. Biotin is one of the most active biologic substances known. As little as 0.005 μg stimulates the growth of yeast and certain bacteria. In foods and tissues, biotin occurs bound to protein as part of an enzyme system.[28]

Biotin functions primarily as a coenzyme for enzymatic reactions involving the addition of carbon dioxide to other units. Termed *carbon dioxide fixa-*

tion, this process is a means of lengthening carbon chains.

Biotin is of prime importance in the carboxylation that occurs in the conversion of pyruvic acid in mitochondria to oxaloacetate. This bypass of the pyruvate dehydrogenase system serves to replenish oxalacetate under metabolic conditions where there is a strain on the supply of α-keto acids, as in gluconeogenesis.

Biotin as a coenzyme carrier of carbon dioxide is essential for the carboxylation that occurs in the conversion of acetyl coenzyme A to malonyl coenzyme A in the biosynthesis of fatty acids. In a similar manner it functions in the conversion of propionyl coenzyme A to methylmalonyl coenzyme A in reactions involving the oxidation of odd-numbered carbon chains.

There are studies indicating that biotin may be involved in carbohydrate and protein metabolism. However, evidence for its role in these reactions is either meager or indirect.[6]

Deficiency. The effects of a biotin-deficient diet in animals are varied but seem to be characterized by early changes in the skin. Rats fed large amounts of egg white develop a eczemalike dermatitis characterized by either scaliness or hardening of the affected area and often starting as a characteristic alopecia in the region of the eye. This is sometimes called "spectacle eye." Loss of hair and muscular atrophy follow these signs.

Although no evidence exists of a natural biotin deficiency in human adults, evidence has suggested that two types of dermatitis, Leiner's disease and seborrheic dermatitis (which occurs in infants), may be caused by a lack of the vitamin. Both of these conditions respond rather dramatically to biotin therapy, although a similar condition in adults is not responsive (see Chap. 35).

Yeast and bacteria of many species either make or retain biotin. Conditions that reduce the number of microorganisms in the diet may reduce the amount of biotin synthesized. Sulfonamides and oxytetracycline are known to reduce the number of biotin-synthesizing organisms. It is possible, therefore, that some of the symptoms that develop with the use of sulfonamides may be evidence of biotin deficiency, since biotin administration seems to counteract these antibiotics.

In a study of four human subjects, Sydenstricker and colleagues showed that biotin is a dietary essential for humans.[55] They produced a biotin deficiency by feeding four volunteers a diet very poor in all vitamins of the B complex except riboflavin supplied by the egg white. The diet was supplemented with dried uncooked egg white, which is high in avidin. The symptoms that developed were similar to those of thiamin deficiency, including dermatitis, glossitis, loss of appetite, nausea, loss of sleep and depression, muscle pains, and a high blood cholesterol. An injection of a concentrated preparation containing 150 µg to 300 µg biotin daily brought about a marked improvement of symptoms in 3 to 4 days.

A spontaneous case of biotin deficiency was reported by Scott in a boy with bulbar poliomyelitis who had received 6 raw eggs daily by gastric tube for 18 months.[45] He developed scaly dermatitis.

Baugh and colleagues reported a deficiency in a man with cirrhosis of the liver who consumed raw eggs.[2]

A biotin deficiency has been described by Williams in a man whose diet consisted mainly of six dozen raw egg whites daily, washed down by 4 quarts of red wine.[61] He developed a severe dermatitis that responded to injections of the methyl ester of biotin.

Chemical Properties and Structure. Biotin is a white compound stable to heat in cooking, processing, and storage. However, being a somewhat water-soluble vitamin, losses will occur during cooking. It is relatively insoluble in chloroform, ether, and petroleum ether. In 1942 biotin was synthesized and its structure determined. Like thiamin it contains sulfur in its molecule. It is labile to alkali and oxidation.

Biotin has been isolated in at least five active forms. One of these, biocytin, is a combination of biotin with the amino acid lysine, which may represent a fragment of the protein–coenzyme complex. Other important forms are biotin sulfone, a potent antagonist, and biotinal, which can be oxidized to an active form.

Protein-bound biotin in animal tissues is fat soluble, and the active substance in plants is water soluble. The bound form is liberated by the action of proteolytic enzymes, and therefore the linkage is believed to be peptide in nature.

Sources. Biotin is present in almost all foods, particularly those known to be good sources of the B-complex vitamins. Human milk contains an average of 0.16 µg/100 ml and seems little affected by variations in diet.[31] Human milk has only one tenth as much biotin as does cow's milk. Liver, kidney, milk, egg yolk, and yeast have been shown by biologic assay to be the richest sources. Pulses, nuts, chocolate, and some vegetables, such as cauliflower, are fair sources. Animal meats (except for those listed above), dairy products, and cereals (unless fortified) are relatively poor sources. Except for cauliflower, nuts, and legumes, most vegetables are poorer in content than the meats. Most diets contain 150 μg to 300 μg biotin, which is supplemented by bacterial intestinal synthesis that is stimulated by sucrose in the diet.

Requirement. It is believed that the body uses approximately 150 μg/day, an amount that appears to be adequately provided for in most diets, even without the amount of biotin provided by intestinal microorganism synthesis. Dietary intake of biotin is believed to be 100 μg to 300 μg daily.

Three to six times more biotin is excreted in the urine than is ingested, reflecting a major contribution of the active substance by the intestinal microflora.[1] It seems probable, therefore, that humans can obtain all the required biotin from the numerous microorganism present in the intestines.

Although biotin is recognized as being essential for humans, because of the uncertainty as to the amount contributed by intestinal microorganisms, a precise recommended daily allowance cannot be established at this time.[37]

Toxicity. Biotin has little or no toxicity. It is well tolerated by animals given large doses over prolonged periods.

THE HEMATOPOIETIC VITAMINS

FOLACIN

The discovery of folacin (or folic acid, or pteroylglutamic acid) began with the studies of Dr. Lucy Wills in Bombay, India, in 1931, when she called attention to a megaloblastic anemia found in pregnant women. Wills produced the anemia in monkeys by feeding them a diet similar to that eaten by her patients—primarily polished rice and white bread. She was unable to prevent or cure the anemia by using any of the vitamins known at that time or by feeding purified liver extract. Good responses were obtained, however, by feeding autolyzed yeast that had been found ineffective in cases of pernicious anemia.[62] Therefore, it appeared yeast contained an antianemic factor (Will's factor) that was different from the factor present in purified liver extract so effective in preventing pernicious anemia.

In 1941, Mitchell and coworkers in the United States obtained from spinach a factor that was a growth factor for *Lactobacillus casei*. They called the material folic acid because it came from foliage plants such as spinach. The pure synthetic substance, pteroylglutamic acid (folic acid), contained a complex component called pterin. This substance had been studied by Hopkins in England as early as 1885 during an investigation of the pigments of butterfly wings. Because of the similarity of his preparation to purine of nucleic acids, Hopkins suggested they might be important in the metabolism of mammals.

Folic acid was found to be effective in curing the dietary anemia of chicks and also monkeys. In 1945, Spies found folic acid, or folacin, effective in the treatment of the macrocytic anemias of pregnancy and also of tropical sprue.

Function and Deficiency. Tetrahydrofolic acid plays an essential role in one-carbon transfers in metabolism. In this role it receives one-carbon radicals from such amino acids as serine, glycine, histidine, and tryptophan and transfers them at two steps in purine synthesis. In pyrimidine synthesis it is essential in the insertion of the methyl group in deoxyuridylic acid to form thymidylic acid, the characteristic nucleotide of DNA. Failure in this synthetic step is responsible for the megaloblastosis seen in folate deficiency and in vitamin B_{12} deficiency.

Folic acid is needed for thymidylate synthesis as 5,10-methylene-tetrahydrofolate. This molecule is made from tetrahydrofolate by methyl-tetrahydrofolate, the principal form of folate in the human liver. The distinction between a folic acid deficiency and vitamin B_{12} deficiency appears to lie in that when vitamin B_{12} is deficient, most of the folate is trapped in the methyl-tetrahydrofolate, which cannot then be used in the subsequent necessary reactions for the formation of thymidylate for DNA synthesis.

Chemical Properties and Structure. Folacin is a yellow crystalline substance consisting of a pterin ring attached to a *p*-aminobenzoic acid and conjugated with glutamic acid. It is sparingly soluble in water and stable in acid solution. When heated in neutral or alkaline solution it is rapidly destroyed. Consequently, it may be destroyed by some methods of cooking.

Up to seven additional molecules of glutamic acid may be attached through the α-carboxyl moiety to pteroylmonoglutamic acid.

Absorption. The small intestine has a conjugase (γ-L-glutamyl carboxypeptidase) in the intestinal epithelium that hydrolyzes polyglutamyl forms of folic acid to free folic acid. Free folic acid is then absorbed from the upper part of the small intestine. During absorption it is believed that folic acid is reduced and methylated to methyl-tetrahydrofolic acid. This form is the principal form of folate present in the liver as well as the plasma.

Sources. Good sources of folic acid are green leafy vegetables, liver, kidney, lima beans, asparagus, whole grain cereals, nuts, legumes, and yeast. The folacin content of many foods has not yet been established.

Requirement. The minimum need for adults is believed to be approximately 50 μg, or 0.05 mg. This allows a wide degree of difference that may be due to differences in the availability in various foods. For further recommendations in pregnancy and lactation and for children see Appendix Table A-1.

Toxicity. No toxic reactions to folacin have been seen when doses up to 15 mg have been taken daily for 1 month. Certain synthetic analogues are toxic, such as methotrexate, which is used as an antimetabolite in the treatment of leukemia.

VITAMIN B$_{12}$ (COBALAMIN, CYANOCOBALAMIN)

Thomas Addison, a physician working in Guy's hospital, London, discovered in 1849 an anemia that occurred mostly in middle-aged and elderly patients and that led to the death of the patient in 2 to 5 years. So inevitable was death that the disease became known as pernicious anemia. Later, in 1926, Minot and Murphy in Boston found that a remission in pernicious anemia occurred when patients were fed large amounts of whole liver.

At this time, W. B. Castle, also in Boston, observed that pernicious anemia patients had an abnormal gastric secretion. From his observations of gastric secretion and the knowledge that the anti-pernicious-anemia factor was present in liver and meat, Castle concluded that the disease was not dietary in origin but a failure of the stomach to secrete an "intrinsic factor" essential for the absorption of the dietary "extrinsic factor" from the small intestine. Progress in the search for the liver anti-pernicious-anemia factor was impeded by the necessity for using the human being as a test animal. Fortunately, it was found that the microorganism *Lactobacillus lactis* also needed the factor. This finding greatly facilitated the search for the factor.

In the human an injection of a protein-free extract of liver is far more potent in preventing pernicious anemia than the equivalent amount of ingested liver. This cast doubt on Castle's theory that the extrinsic and intrinsic factors combined to form the anti-pernicious-anemia factor, but it is now known that the favorable result obtained by feeding massive amounts of liver enabled the absorption by diffusion of a small amount of the liver factor (1%–3%) rather than by active transport. It is now believed Castle's extrinsic factor in food is

the anti-pernicious-anemia factor, which is aided in its transport into the mucosal cell by the "intrinsic factor" secreted by the parietal cells of the gastric mucosa.

The observation that concentrated liver extract has a characteristic red color led rapidly to the isolation of the crystalline vitamin by Smith and Parker[48] in England and simultaneously in the United States by Rickes[41] and others. Proof was soon obtained of the effectiveness of vitamin B$_{12}$ treatment by the alleviation of both the hematologic and neurologic manifestation of pernicious anemia.

Function and Deficiency. Vitamin B$_{12}$ is essential to the proper functioning of all mammalian cells. A lack of the vitamin is most severely felt in tissue where the cells are normally dividing such as the blood-forming tissues of the bone marrow, and in the GI tract. In the nervous system a deficiency may lead to degeneration of nerve fibers in the spinal cord and peripheral nerves. In the bone marrow abnormal cells, megaloblasts, can be seen. When these are present in the bone marrow the circulating red cells derived from them are bigger than normal (macrocytes) but usually carry a normal hemoglobin concentration (normochromic).

The formation of megaloblasts, or megaloblastosis, occurs because the formation of DNA is inhibited. Synthesis of RNA does not appear to be affected. Vitamin B$_{12}$ has been shown to be necessary as a coenzyme in the synthesis of thymidylate, the nucleotide of thymidine which is the characteristic base of DNA. Folate is also necessary in the synthesis of thymidylate.

The manner in which vitamin B$_{12}$ affects the nervous system is not clear. Carbohydrate metabolism may be involved since vitamin B$_{12}$ helps keep glutathione, a part of several enzymes involved in carbohydrate metabolism, in its biologically active reduced state. Since the nervous system relies almost entirely on glucose as a source of fuel, any interference in the energy supply to the nervous system unquestionably has a profound effect.

Vitamin B$_{12}$ also appears to be necessary for myelin formation since a deficiency gives rise to myelin damage. Here it is possible the mechanism may involve propionate or odd-chain fatty acid metabolism. In this pathway L-methylmalonyl coenzyme A is converted to succinyl coenzyme A by means of methylmalonyl CoA-mutase, which requires adenosyl B$_{12}$ as a coenzyme. This pathway is important whenever fatty acids with odd numbers of carbon atoms are catabolized. The reaction requires biotin as well as vitamin B$_{12}$. Patients suffering from pernicious anemia who are deficient in vitamin B$_{12}$, usually because of a lack of the intrinsic factor, excrete large amounts of methylmalonic acid and its precursor propionic acid in the urine.

Vitamin B_{12} is also involved in the metabolism of single carbon units.

Chemical Properties and Structure. Vitamin B_{12} is present in the body in several forms. The coenzyme form is 5-deoxyadenosyl cobalamin. The originally isolated vitamin B_{12} was a cyanocobalamin. This form has not been found in natural materials. In the isolation of the vitamin cyanide was added to promote the crystallization of the red crystals. The natural form appears to be hydroxycobalamin.

Crystalline vitamin B_{12} is freely soluble in water and is resistant to boiling in neutral solutions. It is unstable in solutions in the presence of alkali.

Absorption. Vitamin B_{12} requires for intestinal absorption a heat-labile glycoprotein called by Castle the intrinsic factor. This substance is secreted from the parietal cells of the stomach during the normal secretion of gastric juice. Food vitamin B_{12} released from a protein complex binds to the intrinsic factor, which it is believed helps attach the vitamin to a receptor in the intestinal mucosa of the lower ileum. Calcium seems to be required in this process. In the intestinal cell membrane, vitamin B_{12} is released from the intrinsic factor and absorbed into the blood.

If the gastric juice secreted by the stomach lacks intrinsic factor, absorption does not take place. Under these conditions massive intakes of vitamin B_{12} may be given on the assumption that some diffusion into the blood will take place.

The plasma concentration of the vitamin in healthy persons normally lies between 200 pg/ml to 960 pg/ml. The capacity of the intestine to absorb cyanocobalamin is a valuable test (Shillings test) of absorptive capacity. Normal subjects usually absorb 30% of the test dose and excrete most of it in the urine. Persons with pernicious anemia absorb and excrete only 2% of the test dose.

Sources. Since plants are unable to synthesize vitamin B_{12} it can be found only in food of animal origin. Microorganisms in the human GI tract can synthesize the vitamin, but the site of synthesis in the colon does not permit absorption. In ruminants, microorganisms synthesize vitamin B_{12} from the plants eaten, and this can then be absorbed from the GI tract. Therefore, domestic animals are a good food source.

Best sources of the vitamin are beef liver, kidney, whole milk, eggs, oysters, fresh shrimp, pork, and chicken.

Requirement. The human needs very small amounts of B_{12}. The recommended amount in the diet is 3 µg/day, of which 1 µg to 1.5 µg are absorbed. A range of 0.5 µg to 2.5 µg appears desirable (Appendix Table A-1). The average American diet contains 7 µg to 30 µg of the vitamin. The requirement is increased if the body metabolic rate is raised, as in fever or hyperthyroidism.

OTHER WATER-SOLUBLE VITAMINS

PYRIDOXINE (VITAMIN B_6)

Vitamin B_6 was first identified as essential in the nutrition of the rat for preventing a dermatitis called *acrodynia*. Acrodynia is characterized by a dermatitis that appears on the tail, ears, mouth, and paws of the rat and is accompanied by edema and scaliness of these tissues. A crystalline compound, pyridoxine, was isolated and when included in the diet of the rat prevented the dermatitis.

Pyridoxine owes its name to its structural resemblance to the pyridine ring. Originally, pyridoxine was used synonymously with vitamin B_6. From the work of Snell and colleagues it is now clear that pyridoxine (or pyridoxol, an alcohol) is biologically converted into two other compounds:(1) pyridoxal (an aldehyde) and (2) pyridoxamine (an amine). All three of these compounds are active biologically as the vitamin, and pyridoxine is often used as the collective term for all three. The active coenzyme forms of pyridoxine are pyridoxal phosphate and pyridoxamine phosphate.

It should be pointed out that other nutritional deficiencies can lead to dermatologic lesions similar to those described above for the rat. Only edema distinguishes acrodynia from the dermatitis of rats seen in a deficiency of essential fatty acids. It is possible, therefore, that acrodynia may reflect a deficiency in polyunsaturated fatty acids because of a failure of arachidonic acid synthesis, from linoleic acid, in the deficient rat.

Function. Unlike thiamin, niacin, and riboflavin, which act primarily as coenzymes for energy metabolism, vitamin B_6 plays no role in energy production. Instead the vitamin is involved primarily with reactions involving the synthesis and catabolism of amino acids and is therefore critical to protein synthesis.

Pyridoxal phosphate and pyridoxamine phosphate are very versatile coenzymes functioning in a large number of different enzymatic reactions in which amino acids or amino groups are transformed or transferred. For example, pyridoxal phosphate is required as a coenzyme in transamination reactions in which the α-amino acid groups of an amino acid are transferred to the α-carbon of an α-keto acid. In this manner the amino group of L-alanine in the presence of alanine transaminase transfers its amino group to α-ketoglutaric acid to form L-glutamate and pyruvate.

During the metabolic conversion of tryptophan to acetyl coenzyme A, the enzyme kynureninase catalyzes the conversion of 3-hydroxykynurenine to 3-hydroxyanthranilic acid. This step requires pyridoxal phosphate. In the deficiency, large amounts of L-kynurenine are excreted in the urine. This step is critical in the biosynthesis of the vitamin nicotinic acid, which will not be synthesized in a deficiency of pyridoxal phosphate.

Pyridoxal phosphate plays a role in hemoglobin synthesis as a cofactor in the formation of a precursor to porphyrin, an essential part of the hemoglobin molecule.

Pyridoxine appears to be involved in the metabolism of the central nervous system. Changes in electroencephalograms used to evaluate the function of the nervous system occur in pyridoxine deficiency. In a severe deficiency convulsive seizures take place; vitamin B_6 appears to be necessary to prevent uncontrolled excitation of the central nervous system, and eventual uncontrolled muscle seizures.

Deficiency. In adults the only symptom that can be ascribed to a lack of pyridoxine is a microcytic hypochromic anemia. This occurs with a high serum iron level. Other symptoms are weakness, nervousness, irritability, insomnia, and difficulty in walking.

Efforts to produce a dietary deficiency have not been successful unless the antagonist deoxypyridoxine was fed. Glossitis, cheilosis, and stomatitis occurred; these were different from those seen in a niacin or riboflavin deficiency.

Since citrate favors the solubility of oxalates, it is possible that the formation of kidney stones, which occurs in pyridoxine deficiency, may be due to low levels or the lack of citrate found in the deficiency.

Absorption and Metabolism. Pyridoxine is water-soluble and heat-stable, but sensitive to light and alkalis. As with the other B vitamins it is absorbed in the upper part of the small intestine, where a lower pH facilitates passage. Once absorbed, all three forms are converted to pyridoxal phosphate, the coenzyme form.

Following absorption the vitamin phosphate is distributed throughout the body tissues, emphasizing its essential role in metabolism.

It is excreted in the urine chiefly as 4-pyridoxic acid along with small amounts of pyridoxal and pyridoxamine.

Sources. Pyridoxine is widespread in nature but frequently occurs in very small amounts. Good sources of the vitamin are yeast, wheat and corn, egg yolk, liver, kidney, and muscle meats. Limited amounts are present in milk and vegetables. Vegetables that are frozen may lose as much as 20% of their original activity. Milling of cereals can lead to losses as high as 90%.

Requirement. Since there are no areas in the world in which pyridoxine deficiency has been defined as a problem resulting from poor nutrition, establishing a firm requirement is difficult. The Food and Nutrition Board has recommended 2 mg/day for adults. Data are not sufficient to permit an evaluation of the requirement for pyridoxine or vitamin B_6 for children and adolescents. The allowances recommended range up to 2.2 g/day (see Appendix Table A-1).

Toxicity. Toxicity has been described in humans receiving 300 mg/day. Since this dose far exceeds any recommended for drug treatment and is impossible to obtain from food in the diet, one would expect that pyridoxine has little if any toxicity from normal daily required dietary amounts.

Rats can tolerate doses of pyridoxine up to 1 g/kg body weight. Above this amount convulsions appear, and with oral doses of 4 g/kg to 6 g/kg death occurs.

When pyridoxine is given intramuscularly to humans it causes some pain, probably due to the acidity of the solution.

ASCORBIC ACID (VITAMIN C)

The disease scurvy has been known to man for centuries. Before the substance necessary for its prevention and cure was found, it was known as the scourge of sailors and soldiers because of the scorbutic diets they were fed. In 1753 Lind, a Scottish naval surgeon and outstanding investigator of the prevention and cure of scurvy, published his first edition of *A Treatise on the Scurvy*. In this treatise he related the experience of the explorer of the St. Lawrence waterway, Jacques Cartier, when 110 men in his command were disabled by scurvy. Forced to spend the winter of 1535 in Canada, Cartier's men were saved because they learned from friendly Indians, who were familiar with the disorder, that an infusion of the needles of some evergreen trees was a remedy. In a second edition of his treatise in 1757, Lind described in vivid language the symptoms of scurvy he had seen in sailor patients on board the British ship Salisbury; all men suffered from putrid gums, spots caused by hemorrhage in the skin, lassitude, and weakness of the knees. Lind found that the symptoms disappeared when their diet was supplemented with oranges and lemons.[25]

In 1907 Holst and Fröhlich found that although guinea pigs remained healthy on a diet of cereal grains and cabbage, when restricted to cereal grains alone they developed scorbutic lesions.[18] Supplements of fruits, fresh vegetables, and juices protected the animals. An important aspect of this work was that it provided an experimental animal, the guinea pig, effective in the study of scurvy. Somewhat later (1928) while studying oxidation–reduction factors, Szent–Györgyi isolated a very active hydrogen carrier in cell respiration from the adrenal gland, cabbages, and oranges and named it *hexuronic acid.*[56] He was concerned chiefly with the reducing properties of the acid and did not recognize it as vitamin C.

Waugh and King isolated the active substance from lemon juice and found that the crystalline material had antiscorbutic properties.[60] They called the substance *ascorbic acid,* a shortened form of "antiscorbutic factor" effective in preventing scurvy (L. *scorbutus*). Svirbely and Szent–Györgyi found ascorbic acid to be identical with hexuronic acid.[54]

Synthesis of ascorbic acid was first accomplished in 1933 by Reichstein, Grussner, and Oppenauer.[40]

Function. Although it was assumed at one time that the metabolic role of ascorbic acid was related to its reversible oxidation and reduction properties, no role in biologic oxidation systems has been described in which ascorbic acid serves as a specific coenzyme.

However, there is no question but that ascorbic acid is essential in the daily diet of humans. Many species of animals are able to synthesize ascorbic acid in their tissues and therefore do not require it in their diet. Humans, however, and other primates and the guinea pig, by consuming food deficient in ascorbic acid will soon develop scurvy, a potentially fatal disease characterized by a deterioration of collagenous connective tissues and structures.

Connective tissue consists of a system of insoluble protein fibers embedded in a continuous matrix called *ground substance.* Its chief function is supportive, and this is performed by fibrils of insoluble protein, such as collagen and elastin. Collagen is the most abundant protein in mammals, constituting one quarter of the protein of tissues and providing the major fibrous structure of skin, cartilage, tendons, ligaments, blood vessels, bone, and teeth. The intercellular cement, collagen, functions to hold the tissue cells together in discrete organized systems.

The amino acid composition of collagen is unique among mammalian tissues. Glycine represents about one third of the amino acids present. Amounts of proline are higher, and amounts of lysine slightly less, than those found in most proteins. Hydroxyproline and hydroxylysine, which are present in collagen, are found in only a few other proteins. They are vital in maintaining the tertiary structure of collagen. Neither hydroxyproline nor hydroxylysine is incorporated directly into the growing protein chains. There are no codons for these two amino acids. Rather hydroxylation of proline and lysine occurs after the peptide bond is formed in the growing polypeptide chain. Hydroxylation requires a proline hydroxylase and a lysine hydroxylase, molecular oxygen, ferrous ions, α-ketoglutaric acid, and a reducing substance in the reaction. Ascorbic acid appears to play a key role in the synthesis of collagen as the reducing substance.[34]

In scurvy, the hydroxylation of collagen is impaired. The collagen synthesized in the absence of ascorbic acid cannot properly form fibers, thereby resulting in the skin lesions and blood vessel fragility prominent in scurvy. Without vitamin C to provide a firm wall, capillaries are easily ruptured with consequent diffuse tissue bleeding. Similar clinical conditions include easy bruising, pinpoint peripheral hemorrhages, easy bone fracture and joint hemorrhage, poor wound healing, and friable bleeding gums with loosened teeth (gingivitis).

Bone consists of an organic phase that is nearly all collagen and an inorganic phase that is calcium phosphate essentially. Collagen is necessary for the deposition of the calcium phosphate crystals and the formation of bone. Ascorbic acid appears essential in this process.

The participation of ascorbic acid in the synthesis of corticosterone and 17-hydroxycorticosterone may account for the high concentration of vitamin C in adrenal tissue as well as for its rapid disappearance following stress when cortical hormone activity is high.

Staudinger and co-workers report ascorbic acid in the electron transport chain of mammalian microsomes and have suggested that this reaction is coupled with hydroxylation.[51]

Ascorbic acid can function as a reducing agent for iron in the GI tract and thereby enhance its absorption into the intestinal mucosal cell.

Deficiency. With knowledge of preventive measures, scurvy is not a common disease today. It can be observed in infants, food faddists or cranks, alcoholics, and in older people. Individuals with frank scurvy can be readily recognized, but borderline cases require experience in diagnosis. The gums are swollen, particularly between the teeth, and they bleed easily. Bleeding may occur in all parts of the body, and numerous small hemorrhages or petechiae may be seen under the skin. Trivial injuries may give rise to large bruises. Large joints, such as in the knee or hip, may appear swollen owing to bleeding into the joint cavity. Severe internal hemorrhages may lead to sudden death and heart failure. And adequate intake of ascorbic acid rapidly reverses these signs or symptoms.

The increased use of artificial milk products as a sole source of food for infants soon after birth produced an increase in the number of cases of infantile scurvy. In the older person, declining appetite, immobility, and reduced income tend to reduce the intake of ascorbic acid and produce borderline cases of ascorbic acid deficiency. In both of the above deficiencies the symptoms can be reversed and prevented by fruit juice or supplements of ascorbic acid.

Chemical Properties and Structure. L-ascorbic acid is a simple 6-carbon organic compound ($C_6H_8O_6$) closely related to glucose. It is an enediol lactone of an acid whose chemical configuration is analogous to L-glucose. The D-form of ascorbic acid and many such closely related compounds show very little antiscorbutic activity. To avoid confusion, it has been proposed that D-ascorbic acid (inactive) be called erythrobic acid.

Ascorbic acid is a white crystalline substance that is stable, when dry, in air and light. It is stable to acid but easily destroyed by oxidation, alkali, and heat. It is soluble in water (1 g/3 ml water), moderately soluble in alcohol, and practically insoluble in petroleum ether. In aqueous solution and in the presence of copper (but not aluminum) it is readily destroyed. This property is of interest in connection with cooking utensils.

The most prominent chemical properties of L-ascorbic acid are its acidity, due to the dissociation of the enolic hydroxyl groups, and its ready oxidation (—2H) to dehydroascorbic acid. This oxidation product has about 80% the activity of the vitamin itself. Further oxidation produces diketogulonic acid, which is inactive. This reaction is irreversible. In mammalian tissues the reversible reduction of dehydroascorbic acid to ascorbic acid appears to be aided by reducing agents, such as the sulfhydryl group of glutathione. In fact, it has been postulated that glutathione may be involved in maintaining the vitamin in the reduced form under physiologic conditions. Ascorbic acid itself is the most active reducing agent known to occur naturally in living tissues.

D-araboascorbic acid (isoascorbic acid) has antiscorbutic properties but cannot support growth.

Most animals have the ability to synthesize ascorbic acid and therefore need no dietary supply.

However, a few species (man, monkeys, and the guinea pig) lack the necessary enzyme to complete the conversion of glucose or galactose to L-ascorbic acid. A dietary supply of the vitamin is therefore essential to prevent scurvy.

Absorption. Ascorbic acid is easily absorbed in the normal human from the upper part of the small intestine. The exact mechanism is not clear, but there is evidence that in some cases it may be absorbed by simple diffusion and in others by an active sodium-dependent transport. Following absorption into the portal blood it passes into the tissues. There is no extensive storage of vitamin C, but certain tissues, such as the adrenal cortex, have relatively large amounts of the acid.

Sources. Fruits, especially citrus fruits, and tomatoes, are rich sources of vitamin C. Green vegetables are also good sources, but much of the vitamin C activity may be lost in preparation and cooking.

Although rather low in ascorbic acid, potatoes and the root vegetables are consumed in such large quantities that they become a good source. Storage lowers the content of ascorbic acid in potatoes, and excessive cooking completely destroys the vitamin. Animal products, such as meat, fish, eggs, and milk, are not a good source. The vitamin C contained in meat is easily destroyed by heating.

The loss of ascorbic acid by oxidation in foods is hastened by the action of ascorbic acid oxidase, which is present in raw fruits and vegetables. This enzyme becomes active when leaves or fruits are damaged by drying, bruising, or cutting.

Requirement. An intake of 30 mg/day is sufficient to replenish the quantity of ascorbic acid metabolized daily. An intake of 45 mg/day will maintain an adequate body pool. Although not known precisely, the infant's need for ascorbic acid seems to be met satisfactorily by the amount provided by the milk of the adequately fed mother, 40 mg/liter to 55 mg/liter. For children up to 11 years of age, 40 mg/day is recommended. For the adult man and woman 45 mg/day is recommended. Pregnant women should receive 60 mg/day, with an increase to 80 mg/day for lactating women.[37]

Large doses of ascorbic acid (0.5 g–5 g/day) have been reported as reducing the frequency of the common cold, but these claims have not been sufficiently substantiated.

Toxicity. Ingestion by mouth of massive amounts of ascorbic acid have not produced toxicity. This may be due to its rapid excretion in the urine and limited storage in the human body.

The Fat-Soluble Vitamins

VITAMIN A

Although vitamin A was the first vitamin to be discovered and has been known chemically since Karrer determined its structure in 1931, the chief metabolic role or function of the vitamin is still puzzling and unclear. Active preformed vitamin A is found only in foods of animal origin. However, the carotenoid pigments of plants contain inactive precursor substances, or provitamin A, which can be converted to the active vitamin when eaten and digested by animals. There are therefore two sources of the vitamin: (1) the vitamin present in animal foods and (2) the inactive provitamins present in foods of plant origin.

Vitamin A is a collective term now used to refer to all forms of the vitamin that are biologically active. Vitamin A alcohol is called *retinol,* vitamin A aldehyde *retinal,* and vitamin A acid *retinoic acid.*

Function. Even though at present it is not possible to relate the symptoms of vitamin A deficiency to a specific biochemical defect, except perhaps for the pigments of the eye, it is possible to identify five distinct metabolic roles for the vitamin: (1) visual purple and vision in dim light, (2) growth, (3) reproduction, (4) health of epithelial cells, and (5) a role involving the stability of membranes.

MAINTENANCE OF VISUAL PURPLE. The specific role of vitamin A in biochemical and physiologic mechanisms of vision has been worked out largely by Wald and Morton (see Chap. 30).[29,59] During the light reaction rhodopsin, a photoreceptor pigment or visual purple occurring in the rod cells of the retina, is split into a protein component, opsin, and vitamin A aldehyde or retinal. This reaction occurs during the light-bleaching reaction. As light strikes the retina, visual purple is bleached to visual yellow and retinal is separated from opsin. The light stimulus causes a reaction to excite the optic nerve, which in turn transfers the stimulus to the brain. During this process some retinal is reduced to retinol. Most of this retinol in the presence of a dehydrogenase is oxidized to retinal, which then can recombine with opsin to regenerate visual purple. Small losses occur through excretion, probably as retinoic acid, which must be replaced from the blood. The amount of retinal in the blood determines the rate at which rhodopsin is regenerated and made available to act as a receptor substance in the retina.

In vitamin A deficiency there may be a long lag in the ability of the visual mechanism to regenerate rhodopsin. This results in night blindness or nyctalopia. Examples of this phenomenon can be seen in the lag in adaptation to dim light of a person entering a dimly lit theater from a brightly lit street, or in the temporary blindness experienced by a driver at night meeting the headlights of an oncoming car.

The biochemical mechanism underlying color vision in the cones of the retina is analogous to that of rod vision. Here again retinal combines with a specific protein that in this case differs from opsin.

GROWTH. An animal deprived of vitamin A will cease to grow and will die when its tissue reserves of vitamin A are depleted. A possible initial reason may be loss of appetite. This in turn can be attributed to loss of the sense of taste that may result from keratinization of taste bud spores.

One of the earliest symptoms to appear in a vitamin A deficiency, growth failure is due to a lack of retinoic acid, which normally promotes growth. It should be pointed out that growth failure is not peculiar to a lack of vitamin A, since deficiencies of other vitamins and nutrients can produce similar results.

In young animals, experimentally produced vitamin A deficiency is accompanied by a cessation of bone growth. Bones fail to grow in length, and although there appears to be normal intramembranous bone formation, the remodeling sequences become abnormal and stop. The defect in bone growth is thought to result from a failure in the normal conversion of osteoblasts (cells responsible for an increase in the number of bone cells) to osteoclasts, which failure causes a breakdown of bone during the process of remodeling. The bones of young vitamin A–deficient animals may be short and thick. Bone disorders have not been observed in the adult during induced vitamin A deficiency.

Nerve lesions observed in experimental vitamin A deficiency are the result of disproportionate growth between nerve tissues and bone. Under conditions of bone growth failure, undue pressure may occur in the brain and other nervous tissues as the protective bony framework fails to grow fast enough to accommodate these tissues. Bone growth is stimulated when vitamin A again is made available.

A defective formation of nervous tissue independent of the effect of a deficiency of vitamin A on bone growth may occur. It is believed that in the absence of vitamin A the protective layer of tissue surrounding nerve fibers does not form satisfactorily.

REPRODUCTION. Vitamin A, either as retinol or retinal, is essential for normal reproduction. Retinoic acid does not appear to be involved in reproduction. In the absence of vitamin A, failure of spermatogenesis occurs in the male, and fetal resorption occurs in the female. The biochemical defect is unknown. A decrease in estrogen synthesis where there is a failure to convert cholesterol to the hormone may be related to the reproductive abnormality in the female. In the male, vitamin A acts directly on the testes in some unknown manner which is diminished in the deficiency.

MAINTENANCE OF EPITHELIAL CELLS. A major function of vitamin A is to maintain the health of the epithelial tissues. Epithelial cells are found in the linings of all openings into the interior of the body, for instance, the alimentary tract, respiratory tract, and the genitourinary tract, as well as the glands and their ducts. They form the outer protective layer of the skin. It is clear, therefore, that these cells form an important "first line of defense" against invading bacteria and other microorganisms. The presence of degenerative changes when vitamin A is lacking is evidence that vitamin A is essential to the normal biochemical reactions underlying the health of these cells. Epithelial cells are characterized by continuous replacement and differentiation. They produce protective mucopolysaccharides as secretory products.

When deprived of an adequate supply of vitamin A, epithelial tissues undergo changes that lead to a horny degeneration called keratinization. Drying of the cells of the cornea and skin occurs. The mucous membranes lining the mouth, throat, nose, and respiratory passages are damaged. This is one of the earlier signs of vitamin A deficiency. In addition to a general deterioration of the epithelial cells and membranes, the cells lack normal secretions, and there is a loss of cilia, which by constant movement aid in keeping the membrane surface clean. Susceptibility to infections, such as sinus trouble, sore throat, and abscesses in ears, mouth, or salivary glands, is a common finding when vitamin A is lacking in the diet.

STABILITY OF CELL MEMBRANES. Vitamin A participates in some unknown manner in reactions involving the stability of the membranes of subcellular particles of the lysosomes and mitochondria as well as the cell membranes. The association between many of the changes just described and vitamin A cannot be explained with certainty. It is possible that vitamin A may play a role in cell differentiation through an influence on RNA and DNA.

Deficiency. The liver reserves of vitamin A must be depleted before symptoms of a deficiency appear. Growth ceases when the reserves are de-

pleted. Most deficiency symptoms seen are directly or indirectly a reflection of the health of epithelial cells. A deficiency can result from (1) a low dietary intake of vitamin A for various causes, (2) interference with absorption from the small intestine due to diseases of the pancreas, liver, gallbladder, or mucosal cells, as in malabsorption, (3) interference with the conversion of carotene to vitamin A, and (4) rapid loss of vitamin A.

In a vitamin deficiency the concentration of vitamin A in the plasma is usually below 20 µg/100 ml, but may be so low as to be undetectable. It must be low for a prolonged period to produce clinical signs of vitamin A deficiency. Normal levels are 30 µg to 50 µg/100 ml.

NIGHT BLINDNESS. An early symptom of vitamin A deficiency is night blindness, or nyctalopia. The visual purple pigment rhodopsin in the receptor cells or cones of the retina is necessary for vision in dim light. These receptor cells require a constant replenishment of the small amounts of vitamin A lost in the visual cycle during which a nerve impulse is transmitted to the optic nerve and rhodopsin is regenerated. A low or depleted liver reserve of vitamin A is reflected in the blood level and slower rate of regeneration of vitamin A. If continued, this will show up as slow dark-adaptation time and eventually night blindness.

XEROPHTHALMIA. This disease usually begins with a drying of the conjunctiva, which loses its shining luster. The condition may then spread to the cornea, which also becomes dull and loses its power to reflect. The lacrimal gland fails to secrete tears due to a blocking of the duct or a reduced ability to synthesize mucopolysaccharide. This pathologic dryness of the eye, which robs it of its normal epithelial protection, is called xerophthalmia and is a precursor to keratomalacia. If the condition remains untreated, ulceration leading to perforation, loss of intraocular fluid, and severe secondary infection may occur. Pus is exudated, and the eye will hemorrhage. This condition is known as Bitot's spots in its mildest form, as xerosis conjunctivae in moderately severe form, and as xerophthalmia in advanced stages. At this last stage, the patient is seriously ill with pyrexia and a grossly inflamed eye. Blindness in the infected eye is the inevitable result.

Severe cases of xerophthalmia should be treated at once as the sight and life of the individual, usually a child, are at stake.

Many children probably succumb to other forms of vitamin deficiency or an infection before xerophthalmia develops. Xerophthalmia occurs frequently in children in developing tropical countries where a low protein intake may be a contributive factor.

CHANGES IN THE EPITHELIAL CELLS OF TISSUES.   One of the chief functions of vitamin A is to maintain the health of epithelial tissues (see above).

FAILURE OF TOOTH ENAMEL.   In the enamel organ of rats there is an atrophy and degeneration of ameloblasts (which ultimately change to keratin) when the animals are fed a vitamin A–deficient diet. Such a deficiency can slow down and even completely stop the growth of incisor teeth in rats. The deficiency is characterized by a disturbance in enamel formation which produces a hypoplastic and chalky white incisor as the result of a loss of orange pigment.

OTHER ABNORMALITIES.   Vitamin A deficiency can lead to a loss of taste and smell. This may be partially responsible for growth failure because of the decreased appetite and food intake.

The formation of thick bones in a vitamin A deficiency may cause an increase in cerebral spinal fluid pressure because of failure of absorption of fluid from the deficient membrane or because of the decrease in space resulting from the thickening of the bones.

Chemical Properties and Structure.   Only foods of animal origin contain preformed vitamin A. The active vitamin is a complex primary alcohol containing a β-ionone ring with an unsaturated side chain terminating in an alcohol group. The β-ionone ring is essential for vitamin activity, and when it is absent or altered structurally, the compound may become inactive. The compound is pale yellow, almost colorless, soluble in fat or fat solvents, and insoluble in water. It can be destroyed by oxidation when exposed to air at high temperatures or to ultraviolet light. The vitamin A content of fats and oils can be destroyed by oxidation as they become rancid unless protected by antioxidants or stored in a cool, dark place.

The ultimate source of vitamin A is plants. Here the provitamin form occurs as highly colored yellow or orange carotenoid pigments or carotenes. These give color to carrots, sweet potatoes, peaches, and other colored vegetables and fruits. The green color of vegetables often masks the yellow orange color of the carotenes because of the green pigment chlorophyll, which does not have vitamin A activity. There are a number of carotenoid pigments in plants, but the three known as alpha (α), beta (β), and gamma (γ) carotene and a fourth, cryptoxanthine, the yellow pigment of corn, are of importance in human nutrition. Their ability to re-

place vitamin A in the diet depends on the integrity of the β-ionone ring. Of these forms β-carotene is the provitamin member that when eaten and digested is theoretically cleaved in the intestinal mucosal cell into two molecules of vitamin A. Unfortunately, the ability of the human mucosal cell to split β-carotene into the two active forms of vitamin A does not approach this degree of efficiency.

Absorption and Metabolism.   Both vitamin A and the carotenes are fat soluble. Their absorption from the intestine and utilization in tissues may therefore be decreased in the malabsorptive state. Such diseases as celiac disease and sprue, and liver disease which interferes with bile production or flow, may induce a vitamin A deficiency. Diarrhea and excessive intakes of mineral oil may also interfere with the absorption of vitamin A and the carotenes.

Preformed vitamin A in food, usually esterified with palmitic acid as retinyl palmitate, must be hydrolyzed by pancreatic enzymes before being absorbed by the mucosal cell as retinol. The carotenes and cryptoxanthine are absorbed intact in the presence of bile salts and are converted to retinol by a cleavage enzyme in the intestinal mucosal cell.

Retinol, either from dietary sources or the result of hydrolysis, is esterified inside the mucosal cell, preferentially with palmitic acid. Retinyl palmitate incorporated in chylomicrons is introduced to the bloodstream through the lymphatic system and thoracic duct; it is stored in the liver.[32,43]

Sources.   Preformed vitamin A is available only in animal products in which the animal has converted the carotene of food into active vitamin A. Food sources of preformed vitamin, therefore, include liver, kidney, cream, butter, and egg yolk. The major dietary sources of active vitamin A are the provitamins in yellow and green vegetables and fruits, for example, carrots, sweet potatoes, squash, apricots, spinach, collards, broccoli, cabbage, and dark leafy greens. In some defects of the intestinal tract, such as the malabsorption syndrome, because of lack of bile salts, defects in the epithelial cells of the intestinal mucosa, or conditions leading to diarrhea, the provitamins are not absorbed or converted to the active enzyme and are often excreted in the stools.

Requirements.   In the current National Academy of Sciences' Table of Allowances, requirements are given in retinol equivalents.[37] By definition, 1 retinol equivalent is equal to 1 μg of retinol or 6 μg of β-carotene or 12 μg of other provitamin A carotenoids. In terms of international units, 1 retinol equivalent is equal to 3.33 IU retinol or 10

IU β-carotene. The vitamin A values of diets, expressed as retinol equivalents, can be calculated by following the example presented in the recommended daily dietary allowance (RDA).[37] The recommended allowances for infants, children, men, women, and pregnant and lactating women are presented in Appendix Table A-1.

Toxicity. High intakes of vitamin A are toxic. Smith and Goodman have reported three cases of human vitamin A toxicity.[47] A 4-year-old girl for 2 years before admission to a hospital had been given daily doses of 25,000 IU vitamin A by her anxious, compulsive mother. Three weeks before admission she developed increasingly severe pain in the ankles and feet, followed by transient loss of vision. On the day of admission she was found to have papilledema by her pediatrician. In addition, she had a faint yellow tint to the skin over her palms, a faint, erythematous eruption over her wrists, hands, and buttocks, and widespread excoriated areas over her entire body. Vitamin A supplement was discontinued, and she was given a diet low in vitamin A and carotene. By the time of her discharge 9 days after admission she no longer had visual difficulties, the dermatitis was improved, and the papilledema had disappeared. One month later she was asymptomatic except for continued scalp–hair loss.

A 9-year-old boy was admitted after a period of daily treatment with 50,000 IU vitamin A. Prior to admission to a hospital a generalized erythematous eruption—"like sunburn"—developed. He complained of pain in all four extremities and became lethargic. On hospital admission he had dry, scaling skin; a maculopapular eruption, most pronounced over the extensor surfaces of the arms; and dried, fissured lips. The liver edge was palpable and nontender 4 cm below the right costal margin, and there was tenderness and soft-tissue swelling over his ankles and feet. After a hospital diet low in vitamin A and carotene, his papilledema, dermatitis, and bone pain improved, and he was discharged. When seen 33 days later, he was asymptomatic.

A 20-year-old female college student who voluntarily had gradually decreased her weight from 56 kg to 41 kg was admitted to the hospital for evaluation of a possible cerebral neoplasm. On repeated questioning she indicated that a dermatologist had recommended vitamin A supplementation in doses of 50,000 IU/day for acne and that she had increased her daily intake to a maximum of 400,000 IU in addition to eating six carrots each day in hopes of improving her complexion. After being placed on a diet low in vitamin A and car-

otene she was discharged and 22 days later was found to be asymptomatic.

Smith and Goodman report that their limited clinical data support conclusions from detailed studies in hypervitaminotic rats that suggest that vitamin A toxicity occurs when excessive amounts of vitamin A are presented to cell membranes in association with plasma lipoproteins, rather than specifically bound to retinol-binding protein.[47] Retinol-binding protein may not only regulate the supply of retinol to tissues but also protect surface-active properties of the vitamin.

The early explorers of the Arctic learned from the Eskimos that eating the liver of the polar bear caused drowsiness, headache with increased cerebrospinal fluid pressure, vomiting, and extensive peeling of the skin. Rodahl and Moore found that polar bear liver may contain nearly 600 mg retinol/100 g liver.[42]

Muenter and colleagues have reported on 17 cases, mostly women, who had taken 14 mg to 19 mg retinol/day for over 8 years for chronic skin diseases.[30] The clinical findings were skin changes, headache, muscular stiffness, and enlarged liver. Plasma retinol concentrations were 0.8 mg to 20 mg/liter.

The symptoms of vitamin A toxicity are many: headache, drowsiness, nausea, dry skin and loss of hair, diarrhea in adults, scaly dermatitis, weight loss, anorexia, and in infants skeletal pain. Carotenoid deposits may cause a yellow dyspigmentation of the soles of the feet, palms of the hands, and nasolabial folds. Increased intracranial pressure and edema may develop. In young women, following periods of excessive intake of vitamin A there is loss of hemoglobin and potassium from the red blood cells and cessation of menstruation.

Wide individual differences in sensitivity to high levels of vitamin A appear to exist. Infants have shown bulging on the head, hydrocephalus, hyperirritability, and increased intracranial pressure after doses of 25,000 IU/day for 30 days. At least one death has occurred in a food faddist.[47]

Recovery from hypervitaminosis A is rapid and complete on withdrawal of the excessive intake. In some instances symptoms subside within 72 hr. Although permanent effects of vitamin A toxicity may be rare, high intakes by the mother can produce harmful effects in the fetus. Single injections of vitamin A to pregnant female animals have produced cleft palate in the young.

Excessive intake of carotenes does not appear to be harmful even though it may result in deposition of yellow pigments in the skin since the pigments disappear after reduction in the excessive intakes of the carotenoids, but toxic reactions do occur after the consumption of high doses of preformed vitamin A.

A high blood concentration of vitamin A can result in decreased stability of membrane structures. It is possible this may account for the increase in fragile bones when excess intake is provided, since the resultant release of enzymes leads to degeneration or resorption of bone tissue. This may explain the simultaneous increase in calcium in both urine and blood.

Because of the toxicity that can be induced by high concentrations of vitamin A, the FDA has imposed a ceiling of 10,000 IU on the amount of vitamin A that can be included in a multivitamin preparation available without prescription.

VITAMIN D

In 1918 Mellanby first clearly showed by his classic studies in puppies that rickets, a crippling bone deformity in children, is a nutritional disease responding to a fat-soluble vitamin present in cod-liver oil.[27] If an infant lacks the vitamin, the growing portion of his bones are affected so that they do not harden. If the deficiency persists as the child grows, the bones are unable to support the weight of the body and this results in bowlegs, knock-knees, and enlarged joints. Other deformities of the chest, spine, and pelvis develop. The disease is known as rickets. The preventive or antirachitic substance in cod-liver oil is known as vitamin D.

Vitamin D is actually a group of closely related steroid alcohols with vitamin D activity that promotes the absorption of calcium from the small intestine and is also involved in an essential way in the mineralization of bone. From the point of nutritional importance, vitamin D exists in two forms: (1) vitamin D_2 (ergocalciferol) and (2) vitamin D_3 (cholecalciferol). Vitamin D_1 is now known as an impure mixture of sterols.

Function. Vitamin E has been aptly described as "the vitamin in search of a disease." In a like spirit, vitamin D can be described as a vitamin with a split personality. It is present in foods and therefore functions as a vitamin in the diet of man. Since in the human, cholecalciferol is formed in one organ of the body (the skin) and acts on distant target organs (the intestine and bone), it also can be considered to function as a hormone.[23] A recent thorough description of the chemistry and metabolism of vitamin D is contained in DeLuca and Schnoes.[10]

Vitamin D is necessary for the formation of normal bone. In this role it acts on the small intestine, where it promotes the absorption of calcium and phosphorus from the intestinal lumen. It is not certain, but it also may act directly on the bone, kidneys, and other tissues. These functions of vitamin D depend on the conversion of cholecalciferol in the body into two more active substances.[15,33] Dietary vitamin D is absorbed from the intestinal lumen and carried from the intestinal cell in chylomicrons. In the blood, vitamin D of both dietary and cutaneous origin is carried on an α-globulin to the liver. In the liver it is converted into 25-hydroxycholecalciferol (25-HCC). A summary of the metabolism of vitamin D is shown in Figure 3-3. Carried in the blood from the liver to the kidney, 25-HCC is further hydroxylated to 1,25-dihydroxycholecalciferol (1,25-DCC), which is secreted by the kidney into the blood and carried to the target tissues.[21]

In the small intestine, 1,25-DCC enters the intestinal epithelial cell, where it functions apparently through DNA in the nucleus of the intestinal cell to initiate the synthesis in the cytoplasm of a specific calcium-binding protein. This calcium-binding protein serves to actively transport calcium from the brush border into the blood. The increased concentration of calcium in the blood promotes bone deposition. This may be regulated by calcitonin and parathyroid hormone, but the vitamin may have a direct action on bone by initiating a cellular transport system for calcium.

Vitamin D also promotes tubular absorption by the kidney of phosphate. An increased urinary excretion of phosphate and a fall in plasma phosphate may interfere with the mineralization of bone.

Deficiency. Vitamin D deficiency in children is called rickets. In adults, vitamin D deficiency is known as osteomalacia.

Rickets is essentially a disease of defective bone formation caused by an inadequate deposition of calcium and phosphorus in bone. The bones are normally incompletely calcified at birth and in the deficiency remain soft and pliable. When these poorly calcified bones are called on to perform weight-bearing functions for which they are not properly prepared, they yield, and bowing of legs occurs when the child starts to walk or to support on the incompletely mineralized bone a weight of any kind. The ends of the large bones become enlarged, causing great difficulty in movement. At this stage, knock-knees can be seen. Deformities of the ribs results in a concave breast that causes crowding in the breast cavity. The ribs also develop irregularly spaced areas of swelling that take on the appearance of beading. The term rachitic rosary is applied to this condition. The failure of the fontanel of the skull to close, allowing rapid enlargement of the head, is also a condition of the devel-

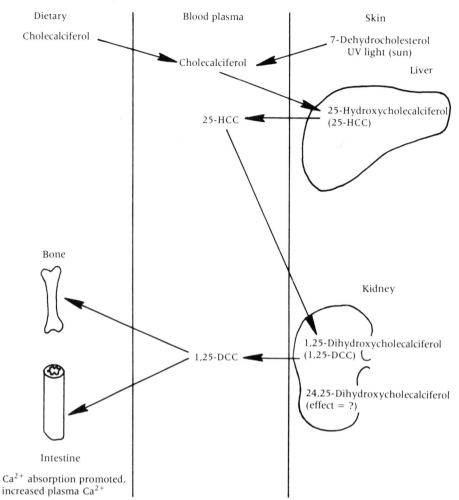

Dietary
Blood plasma
Skin

Cholecalciferol

7-Dehydrocholesterol
UV light (sun)

Cholecalciferol

Liver

25-Hydroxycholecalciferol
(25-HCC)

25-HCC

Bone

Kidney

1,25-Dihydroxycholecalciferol
(1,25-DCC)

1,25-DCC

24,25-Dihydroxycholecalciferol
(effect = ?)

Intestine

Ca^{2+} absorption promoted,
increased plasma Ca^{2+}

FIG. 3-3 Vitamin D metabolism.

oping deficiency. The eruption of teeth is delayed; they are poorly formed and subject to earlier decay. Growth is frequently retarded.

Rickets is primarily a deficiency of children. Unless effective measures are employed early in the disease, permanent malformation of bone may persist.

Osteomalacia, sometimes called adult rickets, is characterized by an accumulation of uncalcified osteoid tissue in the costochondral joints. It is prevalent in women, frequently in the Orient, whose bodies have been depleted of calcium by numerous pregnancies, prolonged nursing, and long periods of protection from the sun, and who receive diets low in calcium and vitamin D.

Chemical Properties and Structure. Because vitamins D_2 and D_3 and some of their related me-

tabolites produce similar effects in the body, vitamin D is used as a collective term to describe the effect of this group of antirachitic vitamins. Vitamin D_3, or cholecalciferol, is the natural form of vitamin D. Humans can synthesize the vitamin by the ultraviolet irradiation of 7-dehydrocholesterol in the skin. Vitamin D_2, or ergocalciferol, is produced by exposing ergosterol, a sterol found in ergot or black fungus, and yeast, to the action of ultraviolet light. Irradiation of ergosterol gives rise to a number of related substances, some toxic, of which only ergocalciferol has marked antirachitic properties. Ergocalciferol (D_2) has the same chemical structure as cholecalciferol (D_3) with the exception of the side chain, which has an unsaturated double bond and an extra methyl group. Ergosterol, from which it is derived, occurs only in plants. Although ergocalciferol is used as a therapeutic agent, it rarely occurs in nature.

Sources. Vitamin D occurs naturally in such animal foods as fatty fish, eggs, liver, and butter. Milk is a poor source of vitamin D unless fortified. Much of the milk now available has vitamin D added to provide a concentration of 400 IU (10 µg vitamin D_3) per quart. Cod-liver oil and other fish-liver oils are excellent natural sources of the vitamin. It is present in very small quantities in green plants and mushrooms.

Although the vitamin is not widely distributed in nature, consumption of the vitamin as it occurs naturally in food or by enriched foods, the irradiation of foods containing precursors of the vitamin, and irradiation of the skin with ultraviolet light or sunlight, all ensure an adequate daily supply.

Vitamin D is stable in foods; storage, processing, and cooking do not affect its activity.

Requirement. Because there are two sources of vitamin D, the naturally occurring form (D_3) and the synthetic (D_2), the evaluation of minimum requirement is difficult. It is only when exposure to sunlight is inadequate, dietary intake restricted, and needs high, that deficiency symptoms develop. The amount of vitamin D needed, therefore, is determined by the degree of exposure to sunlight. A person living and working indoors, primarily, would need more vitamin D than a person working outdoors all day.

One international unit vitamin D equals 0.025 µg vitamin D, or cholecalciferol. The minimum requirement for vitamin D has not yet been established.[37] The amount of vitamin D formed by the action of sunlight on the skin is dependent on a number of variables, including length and intensity of exposure and color of skin. Heavily pigmented skin can prevent up to 95% of ultraviolet radiation from reaching the deeper layers of the skin, where vitamin D is synthesized.[23]

An intake of 2.5 µg (100 IU) vitamin D/day prevents rickets and ensures adequate absorption of calcium from the intestine, a satisfactory growth rate, and normal mineralization of the bone in infants. However, the ingestion of 7.5 µg to 10 µg (300 IU–400 IU) vitamin D seems to promote better calcium absorption and some increase in growth. Therefore, this higher level is recommended as the daily allowance (RDA). For infants the allowance should be provided in the diet or as a supplement since exposure to sunlight may be insufficient.

The precise requirement for vitamin D in older children and adults is not known. Normally, the requirement can be met by exposure to sunlight, but if exposure to sunlight is insufficient, a dietary source must be provided. An intake of 400 IU vitamin D/day is advisable for pregnant and lactating women, infants, children, and adolescents. Since the requirement for the normal healthy adult seems to be satisfied by nondietary sources, no dietary recommendation is necessary. However, a dietary intake of 400 IU for normal individuals of all ages incurs no risk of toxicity.

Toxicity. The ingestion of vitamin D in excess of the recommended amounts (hypervitaminosis) provides no benefit, and large doses can be harmful. It should be emphasized that the fat-soluble vitamins, such as vitamin D, can be stored in the body for considerable lengths of time and that, since they metabolize slowly, they therefore may produce toxic symptoms. The reason for this toxicity involves the difficulty of excretion rather than its storage. Excretion is gradual by way of the bile. In contrast, the water-soluble vitamins are not stored to any great extent but when consumed in excess of needs are rapidly excreted in the urine.

There is evidence that infants are especially sensitive to the toxic effect of vitamin D. Infants need only 400 IU daily, whereas intakes such as 3000 IU to 4000 IU daily may produce toxic symptoms as shown by abnormally high calcium levels in the blood, loss of appetite, and retarded growth.[35,39] With daily doses of 20,000 IU to 40,000 IU in infants, or 75,000 IU to 100,000 IU for adults, toxic symptoms usually develop. These symptoms include sudden loss of appetite, nausea, vomiting, intense thirst, and resulting polyuria. There may be diarrhea, and the child may become thin, irritable, depressed, and stuporous. Fatal cases have been reported in which the arteries, renal tubules, heart, and lungs have shown evidence of considerable calcification.

Vitamin D is probably the most toxic of all vitamins. Very high doses, for instance, 100,000 IU, for weeks or months may, in addition to deposition of calcium in many of the organs such as the arteries and kidneys, induce characteristic dense calcification of the bone along the metaphysis. Such toxic symptoms may arise when the vitamin is given in massive amounts for the treatment of bone disease caused by malabsorption of chronic renal disease.

The quantities of vitamin D necessary to induce toxic symptoms cannot be obtained from natural sources.

VITAMIN E (THE TOCOPHEROLS)

Current popular interest in vitamin E has probably come about through a hoped for, but unwarranted, expectation that results obtained and reproducible in experimental animals are without question directly applicable to humans. Among conditions for which vitamin E is supposedly effective are sexual impotence, sterility, habitual abortion, muscular dystrophy, arthritis, aging, and acne, to name only a few. Fortunately, much confirmed biochemical and metabolic information rigorously obtained by experimentation in animals can be, with reason, applied to humans. Unfortunately, this is sometimes not true. At present there is no satisfactory evidence that any of the human ailments noted above are correctable by eating, injecting, or any other means of taking vitamin E into the human body.

Vitamin E has been known as the antisterility vitamin since its discovery in 1922. In that year, Evans and Bishop found a third, unknown fat-soluble factor in lettuce, wheat germ, and dried alfalfa essential for successful reproduction in rats.[13] A deficiency of their unknown "factor X" caused resorption of the fetus in the female and in the male atrophy of spermatogenic tissue and permanent sterility. Sure in 1924 independently came to the same conclusion, and because the then four known vitamins were called A, B, C, and D, he suggested that this "fertility vitamin" be called vitamin E.[52] Evans in 1936 isolated crystalline vitamin E from the unsaponifiable fraction of wheat germ oil and named it tocopherol, an alcohol which helps in the bearing of young (Greek *tokos*, childbirth + *phero*, to bear + *ol*, an alcohol).[14]

In some animals, such as the rat, guinea pig, rabbit, and dog, the lack of vitamin E produces a condition resembling muscular dystrophy. The dystrophic muscles exhibit increased oxygen uptake. This may be due to increased oxidation of polyunsaturated fats, which appears to occur chiefly in the muscles. The degeneration is reported to resemble Zenker's necrosis observed in severe infections such as typhoid fever and epidemic influenzal pneumonia. Muscle fibers may be replaced by fat and connective tissue. Increased urinary excretion of creatine may reflect the inability of skeletal muscle to use creatine. A brown discoloration occurs in the voluntary muscles of these vitamin E–deficient animals, and similar pigmentation can be seen in the uterus, ovaries, and seminal vesicles. The increased oxygen consumption of the dystrophic muscles and other abnormal findings can be decreased, sometimes dramatically as in the rabbit, by adding the vitamin to the diet. The use of vitamin E as a curative agent in the treatment of muscular dystrophy in the human subject has without exception met with failure.

Function. It is reasonable to suspect from evidence that is now available that vitamin E may function in tissues as an antioxidant. In the tissues vitamin E may prevent the destructive nonenzymatic oxidation of polyunsaturated fatty acids by molecular oxygen. Some products that result from oxidation of fat may appear in tissues as pigments. These may be associated with cell damage, and they are found in tissues of older animals as well as animals on diets lacking in vitamin E. A role for vitamin E in tissues as an agent for preventing degenerative disorders therefore cannot be discounted. It is also possible that vitamin E may function either as a coenzyme or in some other manner in enzymatic reactions. The many questions that can be raised in regard to the functional role of vitamin E offer great opportunities for investigative work.

Deficiency. At present, investigations conducted in laboratory animals have contributed to our knowledge of vitamin E. Data obtained from such animal experiments vary substantially when examined in such species as the rat, guinea pig, rabbit, dog, and chicken. Equally puzzling and seemingly unrelated is the variety of symptoms involving the reproductive, muscular, vascular, nervous, and glandular systems. Only recently have vitamin E deficiencies been observed in human beings, and the results are too incomplete to support firm conclusions or to verify the applicability of results obtained in animal experimentation to human beings.

DEFICIENCY IN ANIMALS. *Reproduction.* As pointed out earlier in this section, vitamin E deficiency results in infertility and reproductive failure in the rat. The female rat conceives normally, but the fetuses die during gestation and are reabsorbed. The deficiency in the female rat is not permanent, and if vitamin E is administered prior to the fifth or sixth day, resorption of the fetus can be prevented, allowing the female rat to continue to reproduce normally. If vitamin E restitution to the diet is delayed, many congenital abnormalities may occur. In the male rat, vitamin E deficiency produces permanent degeneration of testicular germinal epithelium and sterility. Liver degeneration may occur along with reproductive failure. The male mouse, however, does not show signs of testicular damage when made vitamin E deficient. In addition to α-tocopherol, the administration of selenium, cystine, and ubichromenol may be effective in relieving the reproductive symptoms. The element selenium either replaces vitamin E as an antioxidant or spares it.[44] The sulfur-containing amino acid cystine also may influence the antioxidative effectiveness of vitamin E. Ubichromenol and DPPD (N,N'-diphenyl-p-phenylenediamine) can replace vitamin E in preventing fetal resorption in rats.

In Muscles. A frequent finding in vitamin E deficiency in the guinea pig, rabbit, and monkey is muscular dystrophy. This is characterized by degenerative changes in skeletal muscle fibers followed by atrophy and replacement by connective tissue and fat. The weakened muscles, fatty degeneration, and fibrotic changes resemble the signs seen in muscular dystrophies in humans. The muscular changes are accompanied by a large increase in urinary creatine, a decrease in muscle creatine, and an increase in the oxygen consumption of the muscle. Changes in EKG have been reported for cardiac muscles, and death may be caused by cardiac failure. No relationship has been established between human muscular dystrophy and the similar condition seen in experimental animals. Vitamin E supplementation does not appear to relieve the symptoms of human muscular dystrophy.

Encephalomalacia and Exudative Diathesis. In chicks vitamin E deficiency causes central nervous system changes known as encephalomalacia and exudative diathesis. In this latter condition, areas of fluid accumulation appear beneath the skin, on the breast, legs, abdomen, and neck. Hemorrhage and leakage of plasma from the capillaries are seen, particularly those under the skin. Encephalomalacia in chickens is characterized by convulsions, paralysis, ataxia, head retraction, and sudden death.

Hepatic Necrosis. Hepatic necrosis in rats has been observed to be aggravated by a vitamin E deficiency. The condition was induced by a low-protein diet that was very low in cystine, a sulfur-containing amino acid. The condition was much improved when the diet was supplemented with cystine, vitamin E, and a selenium preparation. It was prevented, or did not occur, when the substances described above were included in the initial diet fed. It is possible selenium may replace or spare vitamin E in a mixed diet.

It is of interest that hepatic necrosis in the rat occurs only if the diet contains appreciable quantities of unsaturated lipids. Diets in which casein, rigorously purified, served as the sole source of protein resulted in 1 month or more in sudden death owing to hepatic necrosis. A constituent found in food, which has not been completely characterized but contains a selenite, when added to the diet afforded complete protection.

Hemolysis of Red Blood Cells. In the presence of peroxide or dialuric acid (an alloxan derivative) the red blood cells of vitamin E–deficient animals are more easily hemolyzed than red blood cells not subjected to the influence of peroxide and acid. A macrocytic anemia has been observed in vitamin E–deficient monkeys.

Steatitis. In some animals the feeding of vitamin E–deficient diets containing large amounts of polyunsaturated fatty acids results in yellow fat disease or steatitis. Peroxidation and polymerization of the polyunsaturated fatty acids result in the production of acid-fast ceroid pigments, which deposited in the fat give it a brown or yellow orange appearance.

DEFICIENCY IN THE HUMAN. A vitamin E deficiency is rarely seen except in persons suffering from some form of the malabsorption deficiency. It may be that in normal individuals on a Western-style diet a vitamin E deficiency is not an important problem in human nutrition.

Studies conducted in newborn infants and in children with steatorrhea have shown increased red blood cell hemolysis that has been related to low serum tocopherol levels.

Creatinuria, ceroid pigment deposition, increased hemolysis rates, and muscle lesions have been reported in individuals with cystic fibrosis of the pancreas, which reduces vitamin E absorption.

It is difficult to find a single theory to explain all the varied physiologic abnormalities cited above. It is possible that the ability of vitamin E to act as an antioxidant may underlie much of the pathology. Death of the rat fetus may result from the toxic effects of peroxides formed because of an absence of the vitamin, or the increased oxygen consumption in dystrophic muscles in vitamin E–deficient animals may result from the low stores of vitamin E. The possibility of α-tocopherol participating in a specific enzyme system cannot be discounted.

Chemical Properties and Structure. Like vitamins A and D, vitamin E exists in more than one form. Of these, eight substances of plant origin (four tocopherols and four tocotrienols) are of interest (Fig. 3-4). All are derivatives of 6-hydroxychroman and contain a 16-carbon isoprenoid side chain. They differ structurally in the number and position of methyl groups in the ring structure, and in the case of the tocotrienols the side chain is unsaturated. All have the same physiologic properties, but α-tocopherol is the most active of the group as a vitamin. The remaining compounds have lower biologic activities estimated to be 1% to 50% of the activity of α-tocopherol. Synthesized in 1938 by Karrer in Switzerland and Smith in the United States, this is the form in which the vitamin is produced commercially. In accordance with a recommendation by the International Union of Nutritional Sciences (IUNS) Committee on Nomenclature, the term vitamin E should be used as the general description for all tocol and tocotrienol derivatives exhibiting qualitatively the biologic activity of α-tocopherol.[19]

Vitamin E compounds are light yellow, viscous oils, insoluble in water but freely soluble in fat solvents. They are stable to heat but readily destroyed

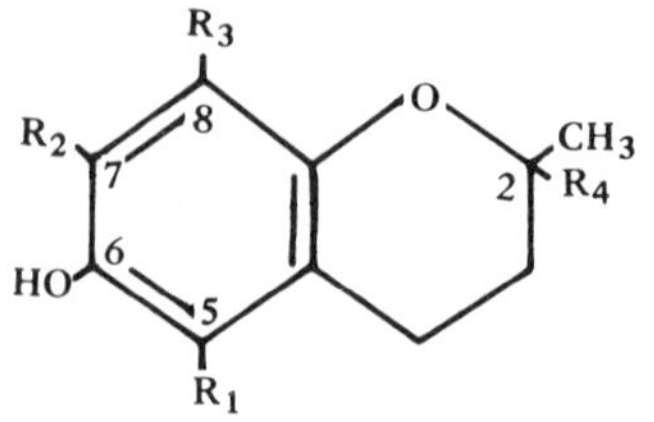

Tocols

$R4 = (CH_2\ CH_2\ CH_2\ CH)_3\ CH_3$ with CH_3 substituent

Tocotrienols

$R4 = (CH_2\ CH_2\ CH = C)_3\ CH_3$ with CH_3 substituent

Tocol	Tocotrienol	Methyl positions
α -(alpha)	ζ-(zeta)	5, 7, 8
β-(beta)	ϵ-(epsilon)	5, 8
γ-(gamma)	η-(eta)	7, 8
δ-(delta)	8-methyl-tocotrienol	8

FIG. 3-4 Naturally occurring tocopherols.

by oxidation and ultraviolet light and are not destroyed to any extent by temperatures used in cooking, though some loss occurs in frozen foods and processing.

Because vitamin E is capable of taking up oxygen and oxidizing slowly, it can function in the body as a potent antioxidant to protect other vital metabolites such as vitamin A, the carotenes, and unsaturated fatty acids, from destructive oxidation. The tocopherols are the chief antioxidants in natural fats and act to prevent fats from becoming rancid.

The tocopherols are themselves easily oxidized, and this property presents difficulties in analytic procedures devised to estimate this vitamin.[20]

Absorption and Metabolism. As a fat-soluble substance, vitamin E requires the presence of bile for absorption from the small intestine. It is absorbed best in the presence of fat. Any abnormal or disease state that interferes with the absorption of fat, such as pancreatic, liver, and biliary disease, or diseases of the intestinal mucosal cell and transport, will interfere with the absorption of vitamin E. Although some vitamin E may be absorbed into the portal blood, the bulk of the vitamin enters unchanged into the lymph system and is transported to the bloodstream as tocopherol attached to lipoproteins. It is stored largely in adipose tissue, muscle, liver, and in somewhat smaller amounts in heart, uterus, testes, and adrenals.

Sources. The richest sources of vitamin E are the vegetable oils. Wheat germ oil, from which α-tocopherol was first isolated, is a good source, as are salad oils and mayonnaise, beef liver, milk, eggs, butter, leafy vegetables, and cereals (particularly if fortified). Many of these foods are also excellent sources of polyunsaturated fatty acids.

Fish-liver oils are rich in vitamins A and D but are low or devoid of vitamin E.

Requirement. As pointed out previously in this section the exact mechanism by which vitamin E functions in the body is unknown. Foods contain significant amounts of nearly all the eight tocopherols. For this reason the milligram of α-tocopherol equivalent has been recommended as a summation term for all vitamin E activity.[46] Vitamin E is an essential nutrient. The National Research Council's revised statement of 1980 recommends about 3 mg vitamin E for infants, increasing to 10 mg for men and 8 mg for women (see Appendix Table A-1).

Toxicity. Vitamin E appears to be relatively nontoxic. Human adults have been reported to consume as much as 1 g/day for months without developing signs of toxicity.

VITAMIN K (THE NAPHTHOQUINONES)

McFarlane and co-workers in 1931 reported on experiments conducted to determine the needs of chickens for fat-soluble vitamins.[26] In their work they employed a diet consisting of 70% polished rice, 15% yeast as a hydrolysate, together with protein from fish meal and casein. When their fish meal was ether-extracted before being fed, they sustained heavy losses of birds from hemorrhage. No losses or hemorrhage were noted when the fish meal was not ether-extracted. Also, they observed that when blood from their hemorrhagic chickens was kept overnight in the laboratory, it failed to clot. This latter observation appears to be the first relating blood-clotting time with an ether-soluble substance in fish meal.[26]

In 1935 Henrick Dam at the University of Copenhagen, studying hemorrhagic disease in chicks fed a fat-free diet, reported that bleeding could be prevented by giving a variety of foodstuffs, especially alfalfa and decayed fish.[9] The active material could be extracted by ether. The bleeding was not due to a lack of vitamin C (ascorbic acid). He succeeded in isolating the substance from alfalfa and showed that the antihemorrhagic substance was fat soluble but not identified with vitamins A, D, or E. He called the active substance *koagulations-vitamin* (after the Danish word for coagulation), which then became vitamin K.

Function. The primary function of vitamin K is to catalyze the synthesis of prothrombin by the liver. Without this step, the normal process of blood clotting could not take place. In addition, the synthesis of other factors necessary in the clotting process, such as factors IV (proconvertin), IX (Christmas factor), and X (Stuart factor), depends on vitamin K. In the absence of vitamin K, hypoprothrombinemia develops and blood clotting is greatly prolonged. In fact, defective blood coagulation is the only well-established sign of vitamin K deficiency in animals. It should be pointed out that the ability of vitamin K to alleviate hypoprothrombinemia is dependent on the capacity of liver cells to produce prothrombin. Advanced liver damage, as in cirrhosis or carcinoma, may be accompanied by a prothrombin deficiency that cannot be reversed by vitamin K—a normal liver is required.

The major defense of the human body against blood loss is the formation of a blood clot. Normal human blood when shed will clot in 5 min to 8 min at 37°C. The process of forming a clot is a complex cascade of enzyme activations in which a very small amount of the first factor initiates a series of catalytic reactions until the amplified response to the injury results in the formation of the clot. Prothrombin, a precursor enzyme, is in some way not yet clear formed as the result of the presence of vitamin K, which in the presence of thromboplastin and calcium ions is converted to the enzyme thrombin. This in turn catalyzes the conversion of the soluble protein dimer fibrinogen into the insoluble monomer fibrin, the basis of the clot.

The only generally accepted function of vitamin K in higher animals is that of regulating the synthesis of prothrombin and other plasma-clotting factors. The vitamin regulates the rate of synthesis of prothrombin after transcription, but the nature of the control site is still undetermined. Some investigators believe that protein synthesis is not required for the step sensitive to vitamin K in the production of prothrombin. Suttie has found data consistent with the formation of a precursor protein in the liver which is converted to prothrombin in a step requiring vitamin K.[53]

Certain snake venoms as well as strains of Staphylococci contain vitamin K–like proteolytic enzymes that can cause clotting.

Deficiency. A dietary deficiency of vitamin K is unlikely because of the intestinal synthesis of the vitamin by microorganisms and because it is quite widely distributed in foods. As pointed out previously, a vitamin K deficiency may occur in biliary obstruction and in any defect in the intestinal absorption of fat, such as may occur in malabsorption syndromes, for example, sprue and celiac disease, and in conditions giving rise to steatorrhea.

In severe liver disease the destruction of liver cells may cause a failure in the synthesis of prothrombin, and bleeding may result. Normal liver cells are necessary for vitamin K to participate in the synthesis of prothrombin.

The newborn infant has a sterile intestinal tract and is often fed on foods relatively free from bacterial contamination. Breast milk and cow's milk are very poor sources of the vitamin. As a result, the neonate may have a low prothrombin level and prolonged coagulation time. Usually, there is a spontaneous improvement in the prothrombin levels and clotting time, but where this does not occur, supplementation of the infant's diet with vitamin K is necessary. Treatment with antibiotics may give rise to a prothrombin deficiency.

Surgical procedures involving the biliary tract, such as operations on the common bile duct or removal of the gallbladder (cholecystectomy), usually necessitate vitamin K therapy to prevent excessive postsurgical hemorrhage.

Dicoumarol, which is used as an anticoagulant, resembles vitamin K in structure and can act as an antagonist to vitamin K, thereby giving rise to a hemorrhagic condition.[50] An important therapeutic use of vitamin K is as an antidote to the anticoagulant drug. The prothrombin time, which is lengthened by the use of dicoumarol, will usually return to normal within 12 hr to 36 hr after the administration of the vitamin, provided the liver function is adequate to synthesize prothrombin.

Chemical Properties and Structure. The term *vitamin K* is used to include a group of antihemorrhagic substances with similar biologic activity. There are two naturally occurring vitamins in the group, vitamin K_1 and vitamin K_2, required for the biosynthesis of prothrombin essential in the blood-clotting process. Vitamin K_1 is present in green leaves and other plant tissues that are eaten in the diet. Vitamin K_2 is present in putrefying fish meal and is synthesized by intestinal bacteria. Chemically, they are quinones and related to the parent compound α-methyl-1,4-naphthoquinone (Fig. 3-5).

Following the IUNS Committee on Nomenclature, vitamin K_1 is *phytylmenaquinone* (formerly phylloquinone or phylonadione), and vitamin K_2 *multiprenylmenaquinone* (formerly farnoquinone), of which there are several active forms in bacteria and in the animal body. Vitamin K_3 is *menaquinone* (formerly menadione), which is produced syn-

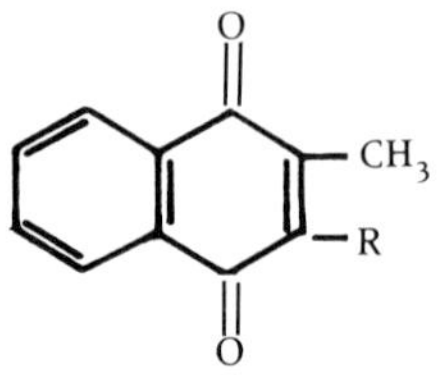

2-Methyl-1,4-Naphthoquinone

K_3, or menaquinone ——————— R = H

K_1, or phytylmenaquinone ——————— R = 3-Phytyl-1,4-Naphthoquinone

$$—CH_2—CH = \overset{\overset{\displaystyle CH_3}{|}}{C}—[CH_2\ CH_2\ CH_2\ \overset{\overset{\displaystyle CH_3}{|}}{CH}]_3—CH_3$$

K_2, or multiprenylmenaquinone ——————— R = 3-Polyprenyl-1,4-Naphthoquinone

$$—(CH_2—CH = \overset{\overset{\displaystyle CH_3}{|}}{C}—CH_2)_n—H \quad (n = 7, 8, \text{or } 9)$$

FIG. 3-5 Chemical structure of some vitamin K compounds.

thetically, is fat soluble, and has about twice the biologic activity of the natural forms of the vitamin. Vitamin K_2 has approximately 75% of the activity of vitamin K_1. It is believed that phytylmenaquinone is the biologically active form of the vitamin and that animal cells are able to convert the other forms into this active form.

When fat absorption is impaired, as in the malabsorption syndrome, several water-soluble and water-miscible preparations are available for the treatment of vitamin K deficiency. Menadione sodium bisulfite (Hykinone) and sodium menadiol diphosphate (Synkayvite) are water soluble; Mephyton, Konakin, and Mono-kay are water miscible.

All forms of the natural vitamin K are yellow oils. They are quite stable to heat, air, and moisture, but not to light. They are unstable in ultraviolet light and destroyed by oxidation. Cooking destroys very little of the activity because the natural forms are insoluble in water.

It has been known for some time that cattle develop a tendency to bleed if fed on spoiled sweet clover. The substance responsible for this bleeding tendency was isolated and synthesized by Link and his students as dicoumarol.[50] Dicoumarol prolongs the prothrombin time of blood and so aids as an anticoagulant in the treatment of arterial and venous thromboses. Other synthetic analogues, such as warfarin (a rat poison which prevents the rat's blood from clotting) and phenindione, are antag-onistic to the action of vitamin K and inhibit synthesis of prothrombin and blood-clotting factors (IV, IX, and X) in the liver.

The biochemical function of vitamin K has been clarified considerably in recent years. The vitamin catalyzes the gamma carboxylation of glutamic acid residues in precursor prothrombin protein, and in other vitamin K–dependent proteins. Calcium binding properties are a consequence.[37]

Absorption. Like vitamins A, D, and E, vitamin K is fat soluble and requires a normal supply of bile for intestinal absorption. It is absorbed in the duodenum and jejunum of the small intestine. A deficiency of vitamin K can appear as a result of the malabsorption syndrome as for example, in biliary tract obstruction or if there is a defect in fat absorption, such as in sprue and celiac disease.

Normally, vitamin K is absorbed and enters the metabolic system by way of the lacteals, lymph, and blood. It is transported from the intestine in chylomicrons and subsequently transported by the blood in β-lipoproteins.

Sources. The synthesis of vitamin K by intestinal bacteria and the levels obtained in a diet from vegetables, especially green leafy vegetables, normally supply sufficient vitamin K. However, in the neonate before the establishment of intestinal bacteria, in malabsorption syndromes such as cystic fibrosis, diarrhea, and failure of bile secretion, and in patients requiring antibiotics, the amount of vitamin K in the body is reduced and supplements of the vitamin are recommended.

Lettuce, spinach, kale, cauliflower, and cabbage are excellent sources of vitamin K. Very little vitamin K is present in most cereals, fruits, carrots, peas, meats, and highly refined foods. Breast milk and cow's milk, although the latter is better than human milk, are very poor sources of the vitamin.

A primary deficiency of vitamin K in adults has never been clearly demonstrated. It must be assumed therefore that even a poor diet contains enough vitamin K to sustain normal human needs.

Requirement. Vitamin K is synthesized by intestinal bacteria. Although the role of the intestinal flora in synthesizing the vitamins is not fully known, absorption of synthesized vitamin K from the small intestine and of that supplied in the diet appears in the normal individual to be efficient. Therefore, because of the above observations and the abundance of vitamin K in the diet, no daily recommendation of intake is made. The American Academy of Pediatrics estimates that the neonate requires 0.15 µg to 0.25 µg/kg/day.[58] If about 10% of orally administered vitamin K is assumed, a daily intake of 0.2 mg (200 µg) appears adequate for the newborn infant. Adults are believed to require 0.3 µg to 15 µg/kg/day.[34]

Toxicity. The natural vitamins K_1 and K_2 are nontoxic in large doses. Excessive doses (over 5 mg) of menaquinone (formerly menadione) and its derivatives have led to hemolytic anemia in rats and kernicterus in low-birth-weight infants, owing probably to an increased breakdown of red blood cells. Vitamin K_1 seems to be free from these side-effects.[37]

Vitaminlike Compounds

The essential nutrients described in the previous sections of this chapter are definitely established as vitamins. In addition to these, there are vitaminlike substances that presently do not meet the necessary criteria to be classified as vitamins. These are choline, inositol, coenzyme Q, lipoic acid, p-aminobenzoic acid, and the bioflavonoids. All of these vitaminlike substances fail to meet one or more of the following established criteria for a vitamin: (1) they do not on the basis of present knowledge have an essential biological role; (2) the animal body can synthesize sufficient amounts to meet metabolic needs; (3) they are present in the diet and tissues in larger amounts than the catalytically involved and established vitamins.

As knowledge increases, it is possible that some of these compounds may become accepted as "vitamins." For this reason descriptions of these substances are presented here.

CHOLINE

Choline is not a vitamin for humans because it is synthesized in the body from the amino acid glycine, provided there is present another source of methyl groups, such as the methyl group in methionine. Furthermore, the amount of choline utilized by the human organism is much larger than the catalytic amounts expected in metabolic reactions involving vitamins. Choline probably cannot be considered a vitamin since the human is not dependent on a dietary source of either choline or a choline precursor. In addition, there is little evidence to suggest that in man the administration of choline alleviates fatty liver, cirrhosis, chronic liver disease, or other defects that resemble those associated with a choline deficiency.[5] (For discussion of choline in liver cirrhosis in alcoholism, see Chap. 15.)

Choline is a simple molecule containing three methyl groups. It is strongly alkaline in its free form. It is water soluble and takes up water (*i.e.*, it is hygroscopic) on exposure to air. Choline is more stable in the form of the chloride. It serves as a source of labile methyl groups. In many organic compounds the methyl group is fixed and not detachable. However, in choline the labile methyl groups can be transferred from one compound to another in a process called transmethylation. In this way, choline provides methyl groups, for example, for the synthesis of creatine and epinephrine and for methylating certain substances for excretion in the urine.

In the young growing rat on a low-protein diet, fatty livers develop in 4 to 6 weeks on a diet deficient in choline. Depending on the composition of the deficient diet and the length of time fed, there is poor growth, edema, and an impaired cardiovascular system, which in turn may result in hemorrhagic lesions in the kidney, heart muscle, and adrenal glands. Older animals and the young that survive may develop cirrhosis. Best and co-workers have shown that choline, and less efficiently betaine (another methyl group donor), prevents the occurrence of fatty livers in rats fed diets low in protein and high in fat, cholesterol, and sucrose.[3,4] Betaine, which is formed by the oxidation of choline, has choline activity and resembles choline in that it has a nitrogenous base and three methyl groups.

Chickens and turkeys are quite immune to fatty livers but develop slipped tendon (a bowing of the legs), which makes walking so difficult that death usually results in 6 to 8 weeks. Best and co-workers found that lecithin (phosphatidyl choline) prevented fatty livers in dogs.

Choline is essential in the synthesis of phosphatidyl choline, a component of cell membranes and lipoproteins involved in the transport of fat-soluble substances. It is a constituent of sphingomyelin (a sphingolipid present in high concentrations in the brain) and acetyl choline, which functions in the transmission of nerve impulses.

Choline is present in foods in which phospholipids occur, such as egg yolk (a very rich source), whole grains, legumes such as soybeans, peas and beans, meats of all types, and wheat germ. Vegetables and milk have small amounts. Fruits have low or no choline content.

The Food and Nutrition Board of the National Academy of Sciences does not suggest a human allowance of choline because of lack of evidence for a recommendation.

MYOINOSITOL

The inositols are cyclic alcohols (cyclohexanols). Chemically, inositol is hexahydroxycyclohexane. Because of the presence of hydroxyl groups in the molecule, inositols can be considered as related to the sugars. There are nine isomers of inositol (seven optically inactive forms and one pair of optically active isomers), but only the *myo*-inositol (also called *meso*-inositol or i-inositol) is biologically active and of importance in animal and plant metabolism. Inositol is found in nature in at least four forms: (1) free inositol, (2) phytin, a mixed calcium and magnesium salt of inositol hexaphosphate (phytic acid), (3) the phospholipid, phosphatidyl-inositol, and (4) a nondialysable, water-soluble complex. Large amounts of phytic acid in cereals and grains when taken into the GI tract can combine with calcium and prevent the absorption of this essential mineral by the excretion of the insoluble complex into the feces.

In mice a dietary deficiency causes alopecia and a failure of lactation and growth. It has sometimes been classified as a vitamin because mice require traces of *myo*-inositol in the diet. In rats a deficiency causes a "spectacled-eye" condition due to denudation about the eyes.

In inositol-deficient chicks an encephalomalacia and an exudative diathesis have been reported. There is no evidence for a requirement in humans.

Eagle, studying the nutrient requirements of cells in tissue culture, found that 18 different human cell strains maintained on a semisynthetic medium failed to grow without the addition of *myo*-inositol.[11] None of the other isomers of inositol was effective. A similar finding was true of experiments in animals.

Like choline, inositol has a lipotropic effect in preventing certain types of fatty livers in experimental animals. This lipotropic activity may be associated with the formation of inositol-containing lipids such as phosphatidyl inositol.

In plants, monophosphoric, diphosphoric, and triphosphoric esters of inositol are found in large quantities. The hexaphosphatic phytic acid is present in high concentrations in grains. In nucleated erythrocytes of birds, phytic acid tends to bind hemoglobin in the same manner as 2,3-diphosphoglycerate in mammalian erythrocytes. It is of interest that McClure has found a beneficial effect of phosphates, primarily in the form of phytates of whole grain cereals, in preventing dental caries.[24] However, dietary phytic acid is rachitogenic because formation of the insoluble salt, calcium phytate, in the GI tract prevents normal absorption of dietary calcium, and possibly of iron as well.

Inositols occur widely in the plant kingdom in whole grains and nuts and in fruits and vegetables. Considerable concentrations are present in yeast and milk.

COENZYME Q (UBIQUINONE)

The biologically active and ubiquitous coenzyme Q is so widely distributed in nature that it is appropriately called "ubiquinone." It is the collective name for a group of chemical compounds that differ from one another merely by the number of isoprenoid units in a side chain. Thus far five crystalline homologues that differ from one another by the number of isoprenoid units have been obtained from natural sources. Coenzyme Q obtained from beef heart has 10 isoprenoid units in the side chain (Q_{10}); yeast (*Saccaromyces cerevisia*) has 6 units (Q_6) and the active material from *Torula* 9 units (Q_9). Coenzyme Q is quite similar in structure to vitamin K and vitamin E.

In recent years it has become clear that an additional electron carrier is present in the respiratory chain linking the flavoproteins to cytochrome b, the member of the cytochrome chain of lowest redox potential. Crane has demonstrated such a function for coenzyme Q as an electron carrier in terminal electron transport and oxidative phosphorylation.[7]

Coenzyme Q is a constituent of the phospholipids of the mitochondrial membrane. It exists in the mitochondria in the oxidized or quinone form under aerobic conditions and in the reduced or quinol form under anaerobic conditions.

Coenzyme Q is synthesized in the cell and therefore is not a true vitamin.

α-LIPOIC ACID

Also called thioctic acid, α-lipoic acid is a sulfur-containing fatty acid. Both thiamin pyrophosphate and α-lipoic acid are required for the oxidative decarboxylation of α-keto acids, such as pyruvic acid to acetate or more properly to acetyl coenzyme A. This is a key step in the production of energy from carbohydrate, linking the oxidation of glucose in the mammalian glycolytic cycle with the complete oxidation of glucose to carbon dioxide and water in the citric acid or Krebs cycle. In this process the bond energy of the glucose molecule is captured as high-energy phosphate bonds in adenosine triphosphate (ATP).

The complete system for the oxidative decarboxylation of pyruvic acid involves not only thiamin and α-lipoic acid but also pantothenic acid (as coenzyme A), riboflavin (as FAD), and nicotinamide derivatives (as NAD). This step is considered in detail in the previous section on the function of thiamin as a coenzyme.

α-Lipoic acid occurs in a wide variety of foods and is active in extremely minute amounts. It has not been demonstrated to be required in the diet of higher animals. No attempt to induce a dietary deficiency of lipoic acid has been successful.

α-Lipoic acid is not considered a vitamin for mammals because it can be synthesized in adequate amounts in the mammalian cell.

p-AMINOBENZOIC ACID

p-Aminobenzoic acid (PABA) is a growth factor for bacteria and lower animals. It is synthesized by bacteria and is essential to the growth of the bacterial cell. It is antagonistic to the bacteriostatic action of sulfonamide drugs. It also acts as an anti-grey hair factor in black rats and mice and as a growth-promoting agent in chicks. These properties are considered the basis of PABA's putative status as a vitamin, but no role has been elucidated for humans. Cruikshank has reported that an autopsy of two cases of acute rheumatic fever and one of arthritis treated with large doses of PABA showed fatty changes in the liver, kidneys, and heart of these persons.[8]

A portion of the folic acid molecule is formed by PABA, and its suggested role is to provide this chemical component for the synthesis of folic acid by those organisms that do not require a preformed source of folic acid. In chemical structure PABA resembles sulfanilamide; this fact may underlie its activity as an antagonist to the bacteriostatic action of sulfa drugs.

When fed to deficient animals in which the intestinal synthesis of folic acid takes place, PABA has considerable folic acid activity. In the rat and the mouse it can completely replace the need for dietary folic acid. This may explain why it was once considered to be a vitamin. At the moment it is not certain whether PABA has a role in metabolism independent of folic acid.

The best food sources of PABA are yeast, liver, rice, bran, and whole wheat. Since PABA does exist in a free form in food, it can be considered a dietary precursor of folic acid. It is not regarded as a vitamin for animals.

References

1. Appel TW: Studies of biotin metabolism in man. J Med Sci 204:856–875, 1942
2. Baugh CM, Malone JM, Butterworth CE: Human biotin deficiency. A case history of biotin deficiency induced by raw egg consumption in a cirrhotic patient. Am J Clin Nutr 21:173, 1968
3. Best CH, Channon HJ: The action of choline and other substances in the prevention and cures of fatty livers. Biochem J 29:2651–2658, 1935
4. Best CH, Hershey JM, Huntsman ME: The control of the deposition of fat. Am J Physiol 101:7, 1932
5. Best CH, Lucase CC: Choline malnutrition. In Jolliffe N (ed): Clinical Nutrition, 2nd ed, pp 227–260. New York, Harper & Row, 1962
6. Bridgens WF: Present knowledge of biotins. Nutr Rev 25:65–68, 1967
7. Crane FL, Hatefi Y, Lester RL, Widmer C: Isolation of a quinone from beef heart mitochondria. Biochim Biophys Acta 25:220–221, 1952
8. Cruikshank AH, Mitchell GW Jr: Myocardial, hepatic and renal damage resulting from para-aminobenzoic acid therapy. Bull Johns Hopkins Hosp 88:211, 1951
9. Dam H: Antihaemorrhagic vitamin of chicks: Occurrence and chemical nature. Nature 135:652–653, 1935
10. DeLuca HF, Schnoes HK: Metabolism and mechanism of action of vitamin D. Ann Rev Biochem 45:631–666, 1976
11. Eagle H, Oyama VI, Levy M, Freeman AE: Myoinositol as an essential growth factor for normal and malignant human cells in tissue culture. J Biol Chem 226:191–205, 1957
12. Elvehjem CA, Madden RJ, Strong FM, Woolley DW: The isolation and identification of the anti-black tongue factor. J Biol Chem 123:137–149, 1938
13. Evans HM, Bishop KS: On the existence of a hitherto unrecognized dietary factor essential for reproduction. Science 56:650–651, 1922
14. Evans HM, Emerson HP, Emerson GA: The isolation from wheat germ oil of an alcohol α-tocopherol, having the properties of vitamin E. J Biol Chem 113:319–322, 1936
15. Fraser DR, Kodicek E: Unique biosynthesis by kidney of a biologically active vitamin D metabolite. Nature 228:764–766, 1970
16. Griffith WH, Nye JF, Hartroft WS, Porta EA: Choline. In Sebrell WH, Harris RS (eds): The Vitamins, Vol III, 2nd ed, pp 1–154. New York, Academic Press, 1971
17. Hodges RE, Bean WB, Ohlson MA, Bleiler R: Human

pantothenic acid deficiency produced by omega-methyl pantothenic acid. J Clin Invest 38:1421–1425, 1959

18. Holst A, Fröhlich T: Experimental studies relating to ship-beriberi and scurvy. II. On the etiology of scurvy. J Hyg (Camb) 7:634–671, 1907
19. IUNS committee on nomenclature. J Nutr 101:133–140, 1971
20. Köfler M, Sommer PF, Bolleger HR, Schmidli B, Veccki M: Physiochemical properties and assay of the tocopherols. Vitam Horm 20:407–439, 1962
21. Lawson DEM, Fraser DR, Kodicek E, Morris HR, Williams DH: Identification of 1,25-dihydroxycholecalciferol, a new kidney hormone controlling calcium metabolism. Nature 230:228–230, 1971
22. Lipmann F, Kaplan NO, Novelli GD, Tuttle LC, Guirard BM: Coenzyme for acetylation of a pantothenic acid derivative. J Biol Chem 167:869–870, 1953
23. Loomis WF: Skin pigment regulation of vitamin D biosynthesis in man. Science 157:501–506, 1967
24. McClure FJ: Cariostatic effect of phosphates. Science 144:1337–1338, 1964
25. McCollum EV: A History of Nutrition. Boston, Houghton Mifflin, 1957
26. McFarlane WD, Graham WR, Richardson F: The fat soluble vitamin requirement of the chick. 1. The vitamin A and vitamin D content of fish meal and meat meal. Biochem J 25:358–366, 1931
27. Mellanby Sir E: A story of nutritional research: The Abraham Flexner Lectures, Vanderbilt Univ. Baltimore, Williams & Wilkins, 1950
28. Mistry SP, Dakshinamutri K: Biochemistry of biotin. Vitamins and Hormones: Advances in Research and Applications 22:1–55, 1964
29. Morton RA: Vitamin A and vision. Br J Nutr 5:100–104, 1951
30. Muenter MD, Perry HO, Ludwig J: Chronic vitamin A intoxication in adults. Am J Med 50:129–136, 1971
31. Neuweiter W, Ritter W: Über den biotingehalt den frauenmilk. Intern Z Vitaminforsch 21:239–245, 1949
32. Olson JA: Metabolism and function of vitamin A. Fed Proc 28:1670–1677, 1969
33. Omdahl JL, DeLuca HF: Regulation of vitamin D metabolism and function. Physiol Rev 53:327–372, 1973
34. Peterkotsky B, Undenfriend S: Enzymatic hydroxylation of proline in microsomal polypeptide leading to formation of collagen. Proc Natl Acad Sci USA 53:335–342, 1965
35. Prophylactic requirement and the toxicity of vitamin D. Committee on Nutrition, American Academy of Pediatrics. Pediatrics 31:512–525, 1963
36. Pugh EL, Wakil SJ: Studies on the mechanism of fatty acid synthesis. XIV. The prosthetic group of acyl carrier protein and the mode of its attachment to proteins. J Biol Chem 240:4727–4733, 1965
37. Recommended Dietary Allowances, National Academy of Sciences, 9th ed. Washington DC, National Academy of Sciences, 1980
38. Relation of nicotinic acid and nicotinic acid amide to canine black tongue. J Am Chem Soc 59:1767–1768, 1937
39. Relation between infantile hypercalcemia and vitamin. Committee on Nutrition, American Academy of Pediatrics. Pediatrics 40:1050–1061, 1967
40. Reichstein T, Grussner A, Oppenauer R: Synthesis of d- and l-ascorbic acid (vitamin C). Helv Chim Acta 16:1019–1033, 1933

41. Rickes EL, Brink NG, Konuiszy FR, Wood TR, Folkers K: Crystalline vitamin B_{12}. Science 107:396–397, 1948
42. Rodahl K, Moore T: The vitamin A content and toxicity of bear and seal liver. Biochem J 37:166–168, 1943
43. Roels OA: Vitamin A physiology. JAMA 214:1097–1102, 1970
44. Schwarz K, Foltz CM: Selenium as an integral part of factor 3 against dietary necrotic liver degeneration. J Am Chem Soc 79:3292–3293, 1957
45. Scott D: Clinical biotin deficiency (egg white injury). Acta Med Scand 162:69, 1958
46. Slover HT: Tocopherols in food and fats. Lipids 6:291–296, 1971
47. Smith FR, Goodman DS: Vitamin A transport and toxicity. N Eng J Med 394:805–806, 1976
48. Smith EL, Parker LF: Purification of antipernicious anemia factor. Biochem J 43:viii, 1948
49. Spencer TN: "Black tongue" in dogs pellagra? Am J Vet Med 11:325, 1916
50. Stahmann MA, Huebner CF, Link KP: Studies on the hemorrhagic agent. J Biol Chem 138:513–526, 1941
51. Staudinger H, Krisch K, Leonhäuser S: Ascorbic acid in microsomal electron transport and the possible relationship to hydroxylation reactions. Ann NY Acad Sci 92:195–207, 1961
52. Sure B: Dietary requirement for reproduction. II. The existence of a specific vitamin for reproduction. J Biol Chem 58:693–709, 1924
53. Suttie JW: Mechanism of action of vitamin K. Demonstration of a liver precursor of prothrombin. Science 179:192–194, 1973
54. Svirbely JL, Szent-Györgyi A: The chemical nature of vitamin C. Biochem J 26:865–870, 1932
55. Syndenstricker VP, Singal SA, Briggs AP, deVaughn NM, Isbell H: Observations of the "egg-white injury" in man and its cure with biotin concentrate. J Am Med Assoc 118:1199–1200, 1942
56. Szent-Györgyi A: Observations on the function of peroxidase systems and the chemistry of the adrenal cortex: Description of a new carbohydrate derivative. Biochem J 22:1387–1409, 1928
57. Terroine T: Physiology and biochemistry of biotin. Vitam Horm 18:1–42, 1960
58. Vitamin K compounds and the water-soluble analogues. Committee on Nutrition, American Academy of Pediatrics. Pediatrics 28:501–507, 1961
59. Wald G: The biochemistry of vision. Ann Rev Biochem 23:497–526, 1973
60. Waugh WA, King CG: Isolation and identification of vitamin C. J Biol Chem 97:325–331, 1932
61. Williams RH: Clinical biotin deficiency. N Eng J Med 288:247–252, 1943
62. Wills L, Camb MA, Lond MB: The nature of the haemopoietic factor in Marmite. Lancet 224:1283–1286, 1933

Suggested Reading

Bogert LJ, Briggs GM, Calloway DH: Nutrition and Physical Fitness, 9th ed. Philadelphia, WB Saunders, 1973

Davidson S, Passmore R, Brock JF, Truswell AS: Human Nutrition and Dietetics, 7th ed. London, Churchill Livingstone, 1979

Guthrie HA: Introductory Nutrition, 3rd ed. St. Louis, CV Mosby, 1975

Handbook on Human Nutritional Requirements. (Monograph 61). Food and Agriculture Organization of the United Nations. Rome, WHO, 1974

Harper's Review of Biochemistry, 18th ed. Los Altos, Lange, 1981

Mahler HR, Cordes EH: Biological Chemistry, 2nd ed. New York, Harper & Row, 1971

Nizel AE: Nutrition in Preventive Dentistry: Science and Practice. Philadelphia, WB Saunders, 1972

Orten JM, Neuhaus OW: Human Biochemistry, 9th ed. St Louis, CV Mosby, 1975

Pike RL, Brown ML: Nutrition: An Integrated Approach. New York, John Wiley & Sons, 1967

Williams SR: Review of Nutrition and Diet Therapy. St Louis, CV Mosby, 1973

4
Minerals
Carl E. Anderson

Nomenclature

There are 92 natural chemical elements, with 50 or more of these being found in human body tissues and fluids. The four elements, oxygen, hydrogen, carbon, and nitrogen, form and make up 96% of the weight of the human body. Over one half of this is oxygen, and oxygen and hydrogen together constitute three fourths of the human body by weight, largely as vital body water. The remaining 4% of the body weight is composed of the essential and nonessential minerals and the mineral contaminants.

The term *inorganic element* or *mineral* is not entirely satisfactory as a true description for these nutrients. For example, although essential in the diet and an element, chlorine is not a mineral. Carbon, a major element in the organic matter of tissues, is neither inorganic nor a mineral. However, custom has established this terminology, and because of the lack of a better designation and to avoid confusion with the preexisting literature, these terms will be used in this chapter.

In accordance with present knowledge and the National Academy of Science's description and dietary recommendations, the inorganic elements or minerals will be treated in this chapter under four headings: (1) the essential *macro*nutrients, that is, those minerals needed in the diet at levels of 100 mg/day or more; (2) the essential *micro*nutrients, that is, those minerals needed in amounts no higher than a few milligrams per day; (3) trace minerals that may be essential but for which human requirements have not been established although there

is some evidence that they may be essential in animal metabolism; and (4) the trace contaminants.[14,23] Many trace elements that have no essential function gain entrance to the human body through food, water, and air. Strontium, for example, is probably not an element essential for life, but small amounts often are associated with calcium in bone. In this way strontium-90 in the atmosphere from atomic bomb explosions may create a hazard by contaminating food and water.

It is possible that what is now regarded as mineral contaminants may be found in the future to be vital in man's metabolic processes. With the development of highly sensitive analytic tools such as atomic absorption spectrometry, flame photometry, purified diets, and the "isolator" technique for handling laboratory animals in a contamination-free atmosphere developed by Schwarz, such investigative work is possible.[27] It is unfortunate that more work in this area is not vigorously pursued, since detection and proof of essentiality may become increasingly difficult with increasing contamination of the air, sea, and earth by expanding populations, industrial wastes, and the application and use of radioactive substances.

The four groups of minerals may be listed as follows:

A. Essential *macro*nutrients (needed in amounts of 100 mg/day or more)
   1. Calcium
   2. Phosphorus
   3. Sodium
   4. Potassium

5. Chlorine
6. Magnesium
7. Sulfur
B. Essential *micro*nutrients (trace elements needed in amounts no more than a few mg/day)
   1. Iron
   2. Copper
   3. Cobalt
   4. Zinc
   5. Manganese
   6. Iodine
   7. Molybdenum
   8. Selenium
   9. Fluorine
   10. Chromium
C. *Micro*nutrients that may be essential for the human
   1. Tin
   2. Nickel
   3. Silicon
   4. Vanadium
D. Trace contaminants
   1. Lead
   2. Cadmium
   3. Mercury
   4. Arsenic
   5. Barium
   6. Strontium
   7. Boron
   8. Aluminum
   9. Lithium
   10. Beryllium
   11. Rubidium
   12. Silver
   13. Antimony
   14. Others

No free element, metal, or nonmetal, is present in the body. They exist as simple ions, polyatomic ions or in covalently bonded molecules.

The essentiality of a mineral in animal and human metabolism is determined if (1) altered or diminished physiologic function is observed in a diet adequate in all respects except for the mineral under study, (2) a growth response is demonstrated after repeated supplementation by the mineral in question, or (3) the deficiency state can be correlated with lower than normal levels of the mineral in blood or tissues of the body.

Although the essential mineral nutrients are present in only a small fraction of the total body tissue, they nevertheless are required for a large number of varied and essential purposes in body metabolism. They are interrelated to each other so that a deficiency of one inorganic element may affect the functioning of another. Additionally, the quantity of an essential mineral may not indicate

its importance in body function. A very small amount of one mineral can be as essential as large quantities of another.

In general, the function of minerals in metabolism can be considered under two headings: (1) structural components of body tissues, such as the insoluble portions of the skeleton and other softer tissues, and indispensable components of important metabolites, for example, phosphates and (2) solutes and electrolytes in solution as free ions in body fluids.

STRUCTURAL COMPONENTS

Calcium, phosphorus, and magnesium provide hardness and rigidity to bones and teeth. The sulfur of the amino acids cystine and methionine is present in such protein-containing tissues as hair, nails, and skin. Iron is a vital component of hemoglobin, myoglobin, and—with copper—a component of metalloenzyme complexes, such as cytochrome oxidase, essential in the respiratory chain. Cobalt is an essential component of vitamin B_{12}, and iodine of thyroxine, the hormone of the thyroid.

SOLUTES AND ELECTROLYTES IN SOLUTION AS FREE IONS

Sodium, potassium, chlorine, and phosphorus are vital in the regulation of acid–base balance and normal metabolism. Sodium and potassium play a primary role in osmotic regulation and in the flow of tissue fluids, absorption and secretion. Calcium is important in cell permeability and with sodium and potassium and magnesium, and manganese ions function as enzyme activators. These are only a few illustrative roles for minerals in body metabolism.

Essential Macronutrients (100 mg/day or more)

CALCIUM

FUNCTION AND DISTRIBUTION

The body of a healthy (70 kg) human adult contains about 1250 g calcium, 99% (about 1.2 kg) of which is in the bones and teeth as deposits of calcium phosphates. The small amount of calcium not present in the hard tissues is in the body fluids, partly ionized. In blood serum, calcium is present in small amounts, usually about 10 mg/100 ml (9 mg/dl–11 mg/dl). Approximately 60% of serum calcium is ionized; the remainder is bound to serum proteins. Tetany develops when serum calcium is reduced substantially. Such a reduction can lead to respiratory or cardiac failure because of impaired muscle function.

Calcium is necessary for blood coagulation, for the integrity of intracellular cement substances, and membranes, and for myocardial function.

Calcium is deposited in an organic matrix in bone that is essential to normal calcification. The inorganic portion of bone is largely a crystalline form of calcium phosphate, which resembles the mineral hydroxyapatite $[Ca_{10}(PO_4)_6(OH)_2]$. Additionally, bone contains a noncrystalline and amorphous calcium phosphate. This amorphous material is predominant in early life but is replaced in later life by the crystalline apatite.[14]

Although it would appear that the mineral deposits in bone are permanent, bone is constantly being formed and resorbed. This occurs at a rapid rate during the early developmental period of life and at a declining rate during adult life. In older people and with advancing age the bones become fragile and may break easily. When accelerated this process gives rise to the frequently painful and debilitating disease known as osteoporosis. About 700 mg of calcium enters and leaves the bones each day.

SOURCES

A large variety of foods such as leafy vegetables, legumes and nuts, and whole grain cereal products contain calcium. Among common foods, milk and cheese are the richest source of calcium. Cow's milk contains 120 mg/100 ml, considerably more than human breast milk (30 mg/100 ml). Sardines and other small fish in which the bones are eaten can be important sources of calcium.[17]

ABSORPTION AND METABOLISM

The absorption of calcium from the human intestine is influenced by a number of factors, including the *p*H, the calcium to phosphorus ratio, the presence of free fatty acids, and—importantly—vitamin D, which promotes the absorption of calcium. Even if the intake of calcium is adequate, calcium absorption is reduced and calcium balance may be negative if the individual is deficient in vitamin D.

Citric acid, lactose, and some amino acids enhance the absorption of calcium. On the other hand, phosphates, oxalates, and phytates inhibit calcium absorption. In the past the above factors weighed heavily in considering calcium absorption, however, it is doubtful if any of the above factors ordinarily affect the calcium requirement to any marked degree.

The average person has a high degree of adapt-ability to high or low amounts of calcium in the diet. Those eating low-calcium diets appear to have a more efficient absorption of calcium than those consuming a diet high in calcium. Thus, as the intake of calcium is lowered, intestinal efficiency and the ability to absorb and retain calcium increases, whereas raising calcium intake reduces utilization.

Calcium is present in the feces, urine, and sweat of humans. Fecal calcium is chiefly dietary calcium that for various reasons, such as the insolubility of some salts, has not been absorbed. Urinary calcium is variable and reflects the calcium that has been absorbed but not retained by the skeleton or soft tissues. Individuals working under conditions of high temperature may lose significant amounts of calcium.

There is very little calcium in blood cells. Most of the calcium is in the plasma. Here it exists both as ionized (also called diffusible calcium) and as un-ionized calcium largely bound to protein, including a small amount bound as a calcium–citrate complex. About one half the calcium is in the ionized form, and the rest is un-ionized calcium. The calcium of blood, extracellular fluid, and soft tissues has important roles in metabolism, such as in determining the excitability of peripheral nerves and muscle and in the clotting of blood. As noted previously, a decrease in the ionized fraction of serum calcium causes tetany.

Although a great deal of publicity has been given to the importance of a high calcium intake, there is no convincing evidence to show that a deficiency of calcium even at low levels of 250 mg to 300 mg daily is harmful. Apparently the adult can achieve a balance at the level of intake supplied by the usual diet, and has the ability to adapt to the dietary intake.

Women on a habitually low-calcium intake can, as the result of repeated pregnancies and prolonged lactation, deplete their body stores of calcium. This can lead to the development of osteomalacia. However, evidence indicates that vitamin D deficiency probably plays a greater role in this condition.

Rickets is a disease characterized by faulty calcification of bones due to a low vitamin D content of the body, a deficiency of dietary calcium and phosphorus, or both. An increase of alkaline phosphatase activity is characteristic of rickets.

Osteoporosis is a common disease of aging in many parts of the world. There is some evidence that a high protein intake is associated with low calcium intake and may play a role in the pathogenesis of osteoporosis. Calcium losses can be large when protein intake is high. Also, there is evidence to show that a high intake of fluoride benefits calcium retention in osteoporosis.[17] The effect of fluoride in calcium retention needs confirmation.

Appreciable losses or gains in calcium are often reflected in similar changes in phosphorus content.

REQUIREMENTS

The recommended allowance for adults in the United States is put at 800 mg calcium daily (see Appendix Table A-1). This value is well above theoretic estimate of needs. For recommended allowances for infants, children, and during periods of increasing growth see RDA in the Appendix Table A-1.

The Food and Agriculture Organization of the United Nations has stated that high intakes of calcium are unnecessary and that requirements can be met with one half of the customary intakes and recommendations, or 400 mg to 500 mg daily for adults.[13]

Additional calcium is needed during pregnancy and lactation to meet the needs of the growing fetus and mother. The full-term infant body contains about 25 g calcium. Most of this is deposited during the last 2 to 3 months of pregnancy. The RDA therefore recommends that 1200 mg calcium be given daily during lactation and pregnancy.

Because children are constantly rapidly increasing their skeleton in size, they have an especially high calcium requirement. The 1980 RDA (see Appendix Table A-1) recommends 360 mg to 540 mg calcium/day for infants, 800 mg/day for children, and up to 1200 mg/day for the teen-age pubertal growth period.

TOXICITY

There are conditions in which excessive calcium is found in the serum, urine, or soft tissue. Idiopathic hypercalcemia is one such condition; others are the "milk alkali syndrome" (alkalosis along with hypercalcemia and renal tubular calcification), renal stone formation, hypercalciuria, and fluorosis. At the present time there is no epidemiologic data to prove that a high calcium intake *per se* is responsible for these conditions.

PHOSPHORUS

FUNCTION AND DISTRIBUTION

Phosphorus constitutes 1% (0.8%–1.2%) of the human body weight. Along with calcium it has a chief role in the formation of bones and teeth. Because of its more obvious role in the growth of the skeleton, an essential and perhaps more vital role in the production and transfer of high-energy phosphates is often overlooked.

The human adult body contains approximately 12 g phosphorus/kg fat-free tissue, or about 670 g in the adult man and 630 g in the adult woman. About 80% of the phosphorus is combined with calcium in the form of insoluble calcium phosphate (apatite) in the bones and teeth.

Calcification of Bones and Teeth. The start of the calcification process involves the concomitant precipitation and fixation of phosphate to the matrix of bone and teeth. It should be pointed out that the term calcification has led to the belief by some that a lack of calcium is a major cause of failure of this process. On the contrary, failure of bone calcification results from a lack of phosphorus as often as from a lack of calcium. Where there is poor bone calcification, there is an increase in the enzyme phosphatase, and this facilitates the hydrolysis of tissue metabolites into the blood to yield a proper calcium to phosphorus ratio, which is of importance in proper bone growth. Low phosphorus blood levels are more likely to be a reflection of excessive excretion of phosphorus in the urine than of inadequate dietary phosphorus.

Regulation of Release and Transfer of Energy. The controlled release of energy resulting from the oxidation of carbohydrate, lipid (fat), and protein is accomplished through phosphorus-containing intermediates as phosphates. Prominent among these phosphates is adenosine triphosphate (ATP). Of the three phosphate bonds in ATP, two contain higher bond energies than the usual ester bond and are known as high energy phosphate bonds (A-O-P-O~P-O~P; the symbol ~ indicates a high-energy bond). In a sense, ATP stores the bond energy released in the oxidation of foodstuffs.

As energy is needed by the body, ATP is hydrolyzed to ADP (sometimes to AMP) and orthophosphate. The energy so released is used to drive many energy-consuming reactions of metabolism. In animals, including the human, a prime and essential function of living cells is the capture and transfer of food energy as high-energy phosphate bonds (ATP). This provides the energy to drive living processes.

Absorption and Transportation of Nutrients. Many metabolites, as for example the monosaccharide glucose, are metabolized in the form of phosphorylated intermediates. The phosphorylation of glucose to glucose-6-phosphate is an obligatory process that must be accomplished before it can be metabolized properly. Fats are insoluble in the aqueous solution of the bloodstream, but by packaging or coating them with phospholipids and protein into fat droplets called chylomicrons, they are rendered transportable in the bloodstream. When glycogen is degraded in the liver and muscles, it appears as metabolizable phosphorylated glucose (glucose-6-phosphate) and is rapidly oxidized in the tissue cells.

Components of Essential Metabolites. The energy-releasing and vitamin-containing coenzymes, such as thiamin pyrophosphate, nicotinamide adenine dinucleotide (NAD), and pyridoxal phosphate, are active only in a phosphorylated form. Even more critical is the role of phosphate as part of the nucleic acids, such as DNA and RNA, both of which are essential for cell protein synthesis.

Regulation of Acid–Base Balance. Because of an ability to combine with hydrogen ions, phosphorus-containing compounds are important as blood and tissue buffers. In this role they help prevent changes in the acidity of body fluids as protons are released in metabolism.

SOURCES

Animal foods rich in protein are also rich in phosphorus. Meat, fish, poultry, eggs, and cereal products are good sources of phosphorus for the average diet.

Whole grain cereals contain phytic acid, a phosphorus-containing organic acid (hexaphosphate of inositol). This acid many combine with calcium as an insoluble complex so that neither nutrient will be absorbed.[2]

The high phosphorus content of carbonated beverages (up to 500 mg/bottle) can contribute, when taken in excess, to an imbalance of the calcium to phosphorus ratio and can cause abnormal intestinal absorption of these elements. A large excess of either element (unbalanced Ca:P ratio) seems to hinder absorption from the intestine.[2]

ABSORPTION AND METABOLISM

The organic phosphorus of food particles must be hydrolyzed or removed from the food before phosphorus can be absorbed as phosphate. This is accomplished in the gastrointestinal (GI) tract. The amount of phosphorus absorbed will be conditioned by the amount made available during the process of digestion. Some phosphorus will be made unavailable for absorption by forming insoluble complexes with magnesium, iron, and other elements. Under these conditions phosphorus is excreted in the feces. Fecal phosphate will also include organic and inorganic phosphates secreted into the intestine along with desquamated epithelial cells of the intestinal lining.

Unabsorbed phosphorus can account for as much as 30% of dietary phosphorus. The control of the amount of phosphorus in the body is exercised through excretion in the urine rather than by control of absorption. Urinary phosphorus increases during the catabolism of body tissues and represents the phosphorus released from the tissues. It is temporarily decreased after the ingestion of those carbohydrate foods that require phosphorus for metabolism.

In addition to being associated in bone and tooth structures, calcium and phosphorus are influenced by the same metabolic and hormonal factors. The parathyroid, which regulates the level of blood calcium, also affects the level of blood phosphorus and its rate of resorption from the kidneys. Vitamin D (dihydroxycholecalciferol) facilitates absorption of calcium and phosphorus from the gut and also increases the rate of resorption of phosphorus from the kidney. In this way the level of both calcium and phosphorus needed for calcification of bone is raised simultaneously. Blood levels of total phosphorus may be 35 mg to 45 mg/100 ml, of which 3 mg to 5 mg is in the form of orthophosphate. Like calcium, phosphorus is in dynamic equilibrium between fluids and cells and is constantly being released and rebuilt into bone structure. Evidence exists to indicate that the phosphorus of tooth enamel is exchanged with that of the saliva and the phosphorus of dentin with that of the blood supply.[11]

REQUIREMENTS

The widespread distribution of phosphorus in food renders a phosphorus deficiency, except in the malabsorptive state and starvation, quite unlikely.

SODIUM

FUNCTION AND DISTRIBUTION

Sodium is the principal cation of extracellular fluid, and potassium is the principal cation of intracellular fluid. Sodium is associated in the extracellular fluid with chloride and bicarbonate in the regulation of acid–base equilibrium. Another important function for sodium is maintenance of the osmotic pressure of body fluids, which thereby protects against excessive fluid loss in the body. In addition, sodium has an important role in the preservation of normal muscle irritability and contractibility and the permeability of the cells. It has a vital role in maintaining the *p*H of blood.

Most of the sodium in the body is found in the extracellular fluid, but the inorganic portion of the skeleton contains about one third of the total sodium content of the body.

SOURCES

Foods of both animal and plant origin contain sodium. As a rule, animal foods contain more than plant foods. In the United States, the chief source is common table salt.

ABSORPTION AND METABOLISM

The metabolism of sodium is influenced by the adrenocortical steroids. In a deficiency of these steroids a decrease of serum sodium and an increase of sodium excretion occur. Excessive and prolonged periods of sweating may lead to signs and symptoms of salt depletion if only water and not salt is replaced. Under such conditions nausea, giddiness, apathy, exhaustion, cramps, and vomiting occur. Respiratory failure may be a consequence. These symptoms can be prevented by adding a little more salt to food or if necessary adding 1 g salt/liter to the water consumed.

REQUIREMENTS

The Food and Nutrition Board has not established dietary allowances for sodium.[23] Intakes of sodium in the United States average about 5 g/person/day. This is about five times more than the physiologic requirement. A maximum sodium chloride intake of about 5 g/day may be permitted for adults who have no history of hypertension. This is about one half the daily amount ordinarily consumed.[14] For persons with a family history of hypertension Dahl recommends a diet containing not more than 1 g sodium chloride/day.[5] (See Chap. 17.)

POTASSIUM

FUNCTION AND DISTRIBUTION

As stated in the section on sodium, potassium is the chief cation of the intracellular fluid. Its concentration in this fluid is much greater than in the extracellular. Nevertheless, potassium does have a very important role in extracellular fluid in that it influences muscle activity, notably cardiac muscle. Within the cells it functions, like sodium in the extracellular fluid, by influencing acid–base balance and osmotic pressure, including water retention.

The concentration of potassium in tissue cells is about 440 mg/100 g. Blood contains 200 mg/100 ml, whereas plasma has 20 mg/100 ml. Muscle tissue contains 250 mg to 400 mg/100 g and nerve tissue 350 mg/100 g.

SOURCES

Potassium is present in most commonly eaten foods.

ABSORPTION AND METABOLISM

Potassium deficiency usually occurs as a result of inadequate intake coupled with excessive loss due to diarrhea, diabetic acidosis, or to the use of diuretic drugs or purgatives. The deficiency is associated with general muscle weakness. This may lead to reduced intestinal tone and distention, to cardiac abnormalities, and to respiratory failure. Common causes of potassium depletion are infectious and nutritional diarrheas of infancy.[6]

REQUIREMENTS

The normal dietary intake of this element is about 4 g/day.[14] It is so widely distributed that a deficiency is unlikely to occur under normal dietary circumstances.

CHLORINE

FUNCTION AND DISTRIBUTION

Chlorine as chloride is present in body tissues and fluids. In extracellular fluids it is closely associated with sodium. It is essential in a number of vital body processes, including water balance, osmotic pressure regulation, and acid–base equilibria. In connection with this latter function, it should be noted that human life is possible only if blood is kept within a narrow range of neutrality, in health, between a range of pH of 7.35 to 7.45. As a component of gastric juice, the strong mineral acid hydrochloric acid is especially important in initiating the digestion of protein.

The chloride concentration is lowest in muscle (40 mg/100 g tissue) and highest in spinal fluid (440 mg/100 ml). Intermediate values are found in whole blood (250 mg/100 ml), plasma or serum (365 mg/100 ml), and nerve tissue (171 mg/100 g tissue).[14]

SOURCES

Chloride usually occurs in the diet as sodium chloride. For this reason an intake of chloride can be considered as satisfactory as long as the sodium intake is adequate.

ABSORPTION AND METABOLISM

During the loss of gastric juice by vomiting, or in pyloric or duodenal obstruction, there is often a loss of chloride in excess of sodium. This leads to a decrease in plasma chloride and is compensated for by an increase in bicarbonate which results in a state of hypochloremic alkalosis. In Cushing's disease, or after the administration of an excess of corticotropin (ACTH) or cortisone, hypokalemia with an accompanying hypochloremic alkalosis may be observed.[14] In diarrhea due to an impairment of intestinal secretions and absorption there is often a loss of chloride.

Abnormalities of chloride metabolism are generally accompanied by abnormalities in sodium metabolism. Chloride disturbances can accompany excessive losses of sodium, as in diarrhea, profuse sweating, and endocrine disturbances.

REQUIREMENTS

Dietary chloride occurs almost entirely as sodium chloride. It has been known since the time of ancient man that the best available food preservative is salt. Salted meats and fish were an important part of the diet of hunting man. Yet, interestingly, a separate supply of salt in addition to that present in the food is not essential to humans. Most people suffering from congestive heart failure or hypertension benefit if the salt in their diet is restricted.[7] (See Chap. 17.)

MAGNESIUM

FUNCTION AND DISTRIBUTION

Magnesium is an essential constituent of all soft tissues and bone in the human. The adult body contains 20 g to 25 g, of which 70% is combined with calcium and phosphate in bone, the rest being in the soft tissues and body fluids. This mineral is an important metallic cation and is required for the activity of a large number of enzymes concerned with oxidative-phosphorylation and the transfer in cells of phosphate bond energy.

Magnesium is essential in nerve impulse transmission and muscle contraction. A deficiency of magnesium causes muscle tremors, twitches, and convulsions.

It seems the skeleton provides a reserve supply of magnesium, as it does for calcium and sodium, which becomes available when there is a shortage elsewhere in the body.[7] Like the iron in hemoglobin, magnesium occupies a central role in the plant pigment chlorophyll. Whole blood contains 2 mg to 4 mg/100 ml, whereas serum contains less than one half that amount.

SOURCES

Most foods, especially those of vegetable origin, contain useful amounts of magnesium. Whole grains and raw dried beans and peas contain about 100 mg to 200 mg/100 g. Cocoa, various nuts, soybeans, and some seafoods are rich in magnesium (100 mg to 400 mg/100 g). Human milk contains approximately 4 mg/100 ml; cow's milk has about 12 mg/100 ml.[14] Meat and viscera are sources of the element. Fortunately, most foods contain useful amounts of magnesium, particularly those of vegetable origin, partly due to the magnesium-containing chlorophyll.

ABSORPTION AND METABOLISM

In contrast to calcium, vitamin D does not aid in the absorption of magnesium. Failure of absorption is not known to be a problem. Magnesium deficiency in humans occurs in such conditions as chronic malabsorption syndromes, acute diarrhea, chronic renal failure, chronic alcoholism, and protein–calorie malnutrition.

Magnesium deficiency in man has been described.[9] Symptoms include emotional lability and irritability, tetany, hyperreflexia, and occasionally hyporeflexia. Alcoholics have low serum magnesium levels, but the condition responds dramatically to magnesium administration.[32] Magnesium deficiency has been described in kwashiorkor.[20] In the United States, many diets are marginal in their content of magnesium.[17]

REQUIREMENTS

The recommended intake for adults is 350 mg/day. An intake of 300 mg/day has been found to maintain a positive balance in women.[23] Estimates of magnesium requirements are based on very limited information regarding the absorption, metabolism, and excretion of this nutrient (see Appendix Table A-1).

SULFUR

FUNCTION AND DISTRIBUTION

Sulfur is an essential macronutrient, present in the proteins of all cells, that represents about 0.25% of body weight. A large part of the sulfur in the human body is present in the amino acids methionine, cysteine, and cystine. It is present also in such physiologically important substances as the vitamins, thiamin, pantothenic acid, and biotin, hormones such as insulin and the anterior pituitary hormones, sulfhydryl-containing compounds of which glutathione is an example, and the bile acid taurocholic acid. Several enzyme systems, such as those containing coenzyme A and glutathione, depend for their activity on free sulfhydryl (—SH) groups. Sulfur serves an important role in the body's detoxication mechanisms and as high-energy sulfur bonds, similar to the phosphate bonds in ATP and so important in the body's energy producing and transferring mechanisms.

SOURCES

Sulfur is ingested in the food as inorganic sulfates and as sulfur bound in organic form. The latter group contains (1) the complex sulfur-containing lipids, such as the sulfolipids and sulfatides, and (2) protein sulfur, derived from the sulfur-containing amino acids methionine, cysteine, and cystine and from glycoproteins, such as mucin, ovomucoid, and the chondroitin sulfuric acid in cartilage and tendons. The most important source of sulfur is the cystine and methionine of ingested proteins, both animal and vegetable. A diet containing 100 g protein will provide 0.6 g to 1.6 g sulfur, depending on the quality of the protein.

ABSORPTION AND METABOLISM

Inorganic sulfur as sulfate is absorbed from the intestine into the portal circulation. It is believed not to be used. The sulfur-containing amino acids liberated by the digestion of protein are absorbed into the portal circulation and used for the synthesis of tissue protein and other amino acid-containing metabolites.

The highest concentration of sulfur is found in hair, skin, and nails. As far as is known, there is no reliable metabolic balance of sulfur intake and output in man.[11] The urinary output of sulfur ranges up to 2 g daily, most of which is sulfate, with a small amount of organic sulfur. The bulk of the organic sulfur is oxidized in the liver to inorganic sulfur and is excreted in the urine. Some inorganic sulfate is combined in the liver with bilirubin and some phenol compounds, such as indole formed in the bowel through bacterial activity to form ethereal sulfates, which are excreted in the urine. Sulfur is excreted in the urine in the three forms found in the blood: (1) inorganic sulfate, (2) ethereal sulfate, and (3) neutral sulfur (organic sulfur-containing compounds).[18]

Essential Micronutrients

IRON

FUNCTION AND DISTRIBUTION

Although the total amount of iron in the adult human body is small (4 g–5 g, or 0.004%), it is one of the most important elements in nutrition and is of fundamental importance to life. Iron-deficiency anemia is a major public health problem especially in young girls and women in their child-bearing years. Its role in the human is almost exclusively confined to oxygen transport and cellular respiration.

Iron is a component of such important macromolecules as hemoglobin (60%–70% of the total adult body iron, or about 3 g); muscle myoglobin (3%–5%, or about 0.13 g); the iron porphyrin enzymes, catalase, and peroxidase (0.2%, or 0.008 g); ferritin, the storage form of iron (15%, or 0.4 g–0.8 g); and transferrin, the transport form of iron (0.004%, or 0.1 g).

SOURCES

The recommended allowances of 10 mg/day for adult men is readily obtainable from a normal diet; obtaining the greater recommended allowances for women from dietary sources is difficult without including fortified foods.

The best dietary sources of iron are such organ meats as liver, heart, kidney, and spleen. Egg yolk, fish, oysters, clams, whole wheat, beans, figs, dates, molasses, and green vegetables are other good sources.

Meat extenders or meat analogs may not contain iron and other nutrients present in the meat they replace. When these extenders replace meat, additional sources of iron as from meat extracts or the addition of ferrous sulfate USP should be considered.

ABSORPTION AND METABOLISM

Absorption of iron can take place from the stomach and the entire small intestine, but the greatest absorption occurs in the upper part of the small intestine. Normally, very little iron is absorbed, and the amounts excreted in the urine are exceedingly small (0.1 mg or less/day). In the man excretion from the body is less than 1 mg/day and in the woman during the child-bearing years 1.5 mg to 2 mg/day. Because there is no way to excrete excess iron, its absorption from the intestine must be controlled if iron is not to accumulate in the tissues in toxic amounts. In the ordinary diet, 10 mg to 20 mg iron are taken in each day, but less than 10% is absorbed. Only 10% of the iron present in cereals, vegetables, and pulses, excluding soybeans, is absorbed. Absorption from other foods, particularly meats and fish, is higher, for example, 20% from meat, 20% from soybean, and 15% from fish.

Food iron occurs in the ionic (Fe^{3+}) state, either as ferric hydroxide or as ferric organic compounds.

During digestion the food-bound iron is broken down into free ferric ions. Ascorbic acid, sulfhydryl groups, and other reducing substances in the intestinal lumen reduce the ferric iron to the ferrous (Fe^{2+}) state, in which form iron seems to be more readily absorbable.

There appears to be some control of absorption by the intestine, but the exact mechanism still is not clear. Recent work has shown evidence for the presence of a ferritin-independent active transport system for iron.[14] The state of the body stores of iron appears to regulate the absorption of iron. Iron absorption increases when there is increased hemoglobin synthesis, as for example, following hemorrhage or as the result of anemia. Absorption increases during growth and pregnancy. Phytic acid and phosphates in excess may impair iron absorption.

Iron released from storage in the mucosal cell as ferritin is transferred to the plasma or tissues as transferrin. In the plasma the Fe^{2+} iron is rapidly oxidized to the ferric (Fe^{3+}) state and then incorporated into the transport form transferrin. Normally, almost all the iron-bound transferrin is rapidly taken up by the bone marrow cells actively synthesizing hemoglobin.

The storage form of iron, ferritin, is found in the intestine, liver, spleen, and bone marrow. If iron is taken into the body, as for example parenterally, in amounts exceeding the capacity of the body to store ferritin, it accumulates in the liver as microscopically visible hemosiderin.

Iron-deficiency anemias are of the hypochromic microcytic type. A deficiency of iron may result from inadequate intake of food iron or as the result of GI disturbances, such as diarrhea, steatorrhea, malabsorption syndromes, and surgery, as well as from excessive loss of blood.

Because of the absence of an excretory pathway for iron, patients receiving many blood transfusions over a period of years, or with an excessive capacity for iron absorption, accumulate iron in the liver in a condition known as hemochromatosis.

Iron intake is often inadequate (1) in infancy, because of the low iron content of milk and the low amount of iron in the infant at birth; (2) during the female reproductive period because of menstrual iron losses; and (3) in pregnancy, owing to the demands of the fetus and losses in childbirth from hemorrhage at labor. A woman, therefore, during her reproductive life has a loss of iron at least double that of man.[7] The intake of iron in the diet may often be insufficient to meet the demand, with the result that anemia is very common in women in all countries of the world. Fortunately, there are simple automated methods for the determination of serum iron and total iron-binding capacity based in the color developed using 2,4,6-tripyridyl-1,3,5-triazine.[34] Rapid determinations of blood and serum iron are therefore available to the physician from hospital or commercial laboratories for the assessment of the iron status of a patient.

REQUIREMENTS

Only very small amounts of iron are lost daily from the body. This loss occurs mostly in the cells or is shed from the skin and epithelial surfaces lining the alimentary and urinary tracts. The average loss of iron in the healthy adult is estimated to be only about 1 mg/day. During growth, pregnancy, and lactation additional iron is required. Pregnancy and lactation increase the iron requirement (see Appendix Table A-1). In addition to the physiologic losses, women who are menstruating normally also lose about 0.5 mg/day. This is the amount in menstrual blood averaged over a period of 1 month. In pregnant women iron is required in addition to basal physiologic losses to allow for expansion of the red cell mass and to provide for the needs of the fetus and placenta.

The need for iron in the human diet varies greatly with different ages. The recommended intakes of iron for different age groups, including increases to accommodate for growth, pregnancy, and lactation, are given in detail in Appendix Table A-1. Briefly, these daily allowances are for infants and children, depending on age, 10 mg to 15 mg/day; adult men, 10 mg to 18 mg; adult women, 10 mg to 18 mg, with increases to 18 and more mg/day during pregnancy and lactation.

Infants of low birth weight have relatively high iron needs because of their rapid growth. In the premature of low-birth-weight infant iron reserves are often low, whereas reserves of the full-term infant are rapidly depleted. It should be noted that milk, the usual food during the first months of life, contains negligible amounts of iron. Therefore, supplementary iron furnished, for example, by iron-fortified formulas, iron-enriched infant cereals, and by strained meats should be made available.

COPPER

FUNCTION AND DISTRIBUTION

Copper is an essential nutrient for all mammals.[8] It is a component of, or essential to the activity of, such enzymes as cytochrome oxidase, tyrosinase, catalase, monoamine oxidase, ascorbic acid oxidase, and uricase. Copper has a role in the biochemical reactions whereby iron is inserted into the hemoglobin and cytochrome molecules and is also believed to facilitate the absorption of iron. The exact mechanism or role of copper in these enzyme systems has not been established.

A copper deficiency has not been reported in human adults, although moderate to severe degrees of anemia have been reported in infants. These infants manifest pallor, retarded growth, edema, and suffer from anorexia. They are responsive to copper and iron therapy. Low serum levels of iron and copper are among the diagnostic signs.

In Wilson's disease, or hepatolenticular degeneration, there is accumulation of excessive copper in the body tissues, probably due to a genetic absence of a liver enzyme. This disease is characterized by neurological degeneration and cirrhotic liver changes. A reduction in dietary copper may be useful in the treatment of this disease, particularly the use of chelating agents to bind free copper.[7]

SOURCES

Copper is widely distributed in foods and a diet containing 2 mg to 3 mg/day seems sufficient to meet human requirements. The richest sources of dietary copper are liver, kidney, shellfish, nuts, raisins, and dried legumes. Milk is a poor source of copper. Homogenized cow's milk may contain 0.015 mg to 0.18 mg copper/liter. This is much less than human milk, which can range from 1.05 mg/liter at the beginning of lactation to 0.15 mg/liter at the end.[14]

REQUIREMENTS

A daily allowance of 2.5 mg copper has been suggested for adults, with about 0.05 mg/kg body weight being suggested for infants and children.

COBALT

This mineral is an integral part of vitamin B_{12}.[29] As such it is an essential nutrient for man. There is no evidence that cobalt has a function in normal human nutrition other than as a component of the vitamin B_{12} molecule.

Cobalt is readily absorbed from the human intestinal tract, but most of the absorbed mineral is excreted in the urine. Retained cobalt appears to serve no physiologic function since human tissues cannot synthesize vitamin B_{12}.

A deficiency of cobalt in ruminants results in impaired growth, listlessness, emaciation, and varying degrees of anorexia.[13]

ZINC

FUNCTION AND DISTRIBUTION

Zinc is a component of a number of enzyme systems. These include carbonic anhydrase, alcohol dehydrogenase, alkaline phosphatase, and enzyme systems concerned with nucleic acids and protein and carbohydrate metabolism.[29] It is a structural and functional component of the digestive enzyme carboxypeptidase and participates directly in the catalytic activity of this enzyme.[30] Zinc is also found in the insulin molecule. Here two zinc atoms are apparently involved in the spatial organization of the insulin molecule. For the above reasons, it is generally accepted that humans have a requirement for zinc.

SOURCES

In the United States an average mixed diet contains about 10 mg to 15 mg zinc. An intake of 15 mg/day is recommended for adults.[23] A breast-fed infant consumes 0.7 mg to 5 mg zinc/day. An additional allowance for lactation is therefore indicated for breast-feeding women. Recommended allowances for all ages and for growth, pregnancy, and lactation are given in the RDA included in the Appendix Table A-1.

Meat, liver, eggs, and seafoods, especially oysters, are good sources of zinc. Milk and whole grains are also good sources. Fruits and leafy vegetables appear to be poor sources of zinc.

ABSORPTION AND METABOLISM

The highest concentration of zinc in human tissues are reportedly found in the prostate gland, spermatozoa, and in parts of the eye.[7]

Halsted, Reinhold, and coworkers have reported a clinical syndrome characterized by small stature, hypogonadism, a mild anemia, and low plasma zinc in older children and adolescents in villages near Shiraz, Iran.[12] The major constituent of the diet of these communities is unleavened bread prepared from low extraction flour. Zinc-chelating substances such as phytates probably are present in these breads and other nonabsorbable complexes. After giving supplements of 120 mg zinc sulfate daily for several months, puberty developed and growth rates were accelerated. It should be pointed out that Caughey has suggested that the clinical features might be due to a dietary deficiency of protein since plasma albumin was also low in these cases.[3]

Zinc appears to be necessary to maintain the

normal concentration of vitamin A in the plasma. Here it seems to be involved in the mobilization of vitamin A from the liver.[14] The occurrence of a marginal deficiency of zinc in apparently healthy children who show impaired taste acuity has been reported.[14] Those children were found responsive to additional zinc in their diet. Accelerated rates of wound healing also have been observed with increased zinc intakes.

MANGANESE

This element is known to be needed for normal bone structure, reproduction, and the normal functioning of the central nervous system and is therefore an essential element in the diet.[4,23] Manganese deficiency has not been described in the human, but it can be produced in laboratory animals and may occur in cattle grazing on pastures poor in manganese. Under these circumstances the cattle exhibit poor growth and reproduction, bone changes, and disturbances of the nervous system.

The average adult daily dietary intake of 2.5 mg to 5 mg appears to be adequate. A recommended daily allowance cannot be made with the knowledge presently available.

The total body content of manganese is about 10 mg, with the kidney and liver being chief storage organs.

The functions in the human body of manganese are not known, although *in vitro* manganese activates several enzymes including blood and bone phosphatases, liver and intestine phosphatases, arginase, carboxylase, and cholinesterase; therefore, an essential function may exist in man.[14,23]

IODINE

FUNCTION AND DISTRIBUTION

Iodine is an essential nutrient for the human because it is an integral component of the thyroid hormones thyroxine and triiodothyronine. In an iodine deficiency, or if the availability of iodine is very low for a prolonged period of time, the gland attempts to compensate for the deficiency by increasing its secretory activity. This activity causes the thyroid to enlarge or hypertrophy, a condition known as simple or endemic goiter. The lack of hormones causes an accumulation of mucinous material under the skin and other areas, which presents a coarseness of features giving the patient the characteristic appearance of myxedema.

SOURCES

Iodine is obtained from food and water. Since some soils have little or no iodide, vegetables and other plant foods grown in these soils are low or lacking in iodide. Seafoods are a rich source of iodide; products such as eggs may be low in iodine, depending on the iodine content of the poultry ration. In the United States and a number of other nations, a ready source of iodine is iodized salt. The current level of enrichment furnishes 76 μg iodine/g salt. The use of iodized salt has caused a marked reduction in goiter in iodine-deficient areas.

ABSORPTION AND METABOLISM

Iodine is readily absorbed from the intestinal tract. About 30% is removed by the thyroid gland, and the remaining iodine is excreted in the urine. In the thyroid gland the iodide is oxidized to and bound to tyrosine with the formation of monoiodotyrosines and diiodotyrosines. These are converted into the thyroid hormones in the epithelial cells of the thyroid and bound to a globulin to form thyroglobulin, in which form the hormones are stored.

REQUIREMENTS

The body of an average adult contains 20 mg to 50 mg iodine. The suggested RDA intake of iodine for adults is 150 μg/day.[23] This is quite adequate for the adult. Women during pregnancy and lactation have increased needs (see Appendix Table A-1).

MOLYBDENUM

Evidence that molybdenum is an essential trace element for humans is based on the fact that it is a part of the molecular structure of two enzymes, xanthine oxidase and aldehyde oxidase; deficiencies have been produced in animals.[14,24]

The molybdenum content of foods is variable. Beef kidney, some cereals, and some legumes seem to be good sources. The amount of the mineral in plant foods depends on the amount in the soil.

Molybdenum has been reported to have a cariostatic effect in animals, and dental caries rates are lower than average in children brought up in areas where the soil is high in this element.[7]

There is no evidence suggesting that a low-molybdenum diet produces clinical deficiency signs in the human. A dietary intake of 2 μg molybdenum/kg body weight has been suggested.[7]

SELENIUM

Selenium appears to be a dietary essential for many animal species, but direct evidence of a role for selenium in human nutrition is lacking.[14] The element is essential in the diet of a number of domestic and laboratory animals (*e.g.*, sheep, cattle, pigs, poultry, rabbits, horses, mice, and rats). Its presence can be detected because certain weeds and grasses grow well in soils containing selenium. Horses grazing in these areas (central United States) develop an acute disease called "blind staggers" and a chronic disease called "alkali disease." Both of these diseases have been attributable to selenium.[7] In New Zealand and in parts of the United States the addition of selenium to diets of lambs and calves markedly improves their health and reduces the incidence of "white muscle disease."

Schwarz has evidence to indicate selenium may be an essential factor in tissue respiration.[14] Hepatic necrosis produced in the rat by dietary means can be protected against by a "factor 3," which is an organic compound containing selenium as the active agent. Factor 3 and sodium selenite apparently not only prevent dietary liver necrosis in the rat but also multiple necrosis in mice, muscular dystrophy and heart necrosis in minks, and exudative diathesis in chicks, among other deficiency diseases. In some of these fatal diseases, factor 3 seems to act synergistically with vitamin E and cystine.[14] There is now evidence that selenium is an essential component of the enzyme glutathione peroxidase.[25] This enzyme catalyzes the destruction of peroxides by glutathione, which in turn protects tissues and membranes from oxidative damage.

There is insufficient evidence at this time for the establishment of a human requirement, but daily intakes of 50 μg to 200 μg occur on varied diets.

FLUORINE

FUNCTION AND DISTRIBUTION

Fluorine, as fluoride, is present in small and variable concentrations in nearly all soils, water supplies, plants, and animals. Because of its widespread distribution, it can be found as a constituent of most diets. In the human, fluoride deposition is found mainly in the teeth and skeleton, but the total quantity is small. Nevertheless, the presence of traces of this mineral in the teeth helps to protect them against dental caries. Fluorine is therefore essential to optimal health (see Chap. 31).

The protective effect of fluoride occurs primarily during infancy and early childhood when the teeth are developing. However, its caries-preventive action appears to be carried over into adulthood as long as fluoridated water is available.

Bernstein has reported that an adequate intake of fluoride is important in the elderly as a protection against osteoporosis, although the issue remains in doubt.[1]

SOURCES

The main source of fluorine for humans is the drinking water. If this contains approximately 1 part per million (1 ppm) fluoride, it will supply adequate amounts of fluorine for the prevention of dental caries.

Where water supplies contain quantities of fluorine less than 1 ppm, the addition of fluoride (fluoridation) to reach a level considered optimal is an important public health measure. Such an addition of fluoride to drinking water has been shown to reduce the incidence of caries by 60% to 70%. Many medical and public health measures have clearly demonstrated the safety and nutritional advantage that results from fluoridation of water supplies.[10]

Tea and sardines are two good sources of dietary fluoride, the latter because of the bones consumed.

REQUIREMENTS

A deficiency of fluoride during infancy and childhood leaves the teeth unprotected from dental caries. There is evidence to suggest that in areas where the fluoride content of the water is high there is less osteoporosis than in comparable areas where the fluoride content of the water is low.

Bernstein has obtained evidence to suggest that arterial calcification may be less marked in high than in low fluoride areas.[1]

Because of the widely varying fluoride concentration of diets consumed in the United States, a total intake (from food and drinking water) of 1.5 mg to 4 mg/day is tentatively recommended as safe and adequate for adults. For younger age groups, the range is reduced to a maximal level of 2.5 mg in order to avoid the mottling of teeth.[23]

In those areas where the daily fluoride intake is not sufficient to afford optimal protection against dental caries, standardization of water supplies by addition of fluoride to bring the concentration to 1 mg/liter has proved to be safe, economical, and an efficient way to reduce the incidence of tooth decay.[23]

TOXICITY

An excessively high intake of fluoride during childhood causes a condition known as dental fluorosis in which the teeth become mottled and discolored. Very large intakes of fluoride may also cause bone changes that increase bone density, calcification of muscle insertions, and exostoses. This can be diagnosed by radiography.

Dental and skeletal fluorosis do not occur in communities with a properly controlled fluoridated water supply of 1 ppm.

CHROMIUM

Chromium is present in most organic matter. Only the trivalent form is biologically active. Mertz has reported that trivalent chromium is required for maintaining normal glucose metabolism in experimental animals, and it may act as a cofactor for insulin.[19] In some patients with impaired glucose tolerance, especially children with protein–calorie malnutrition, tolerance has improved after giving a chromium supplement.

Schroeder found that the levels of chromium in tissues declined with age.[26] A precise recommendation for chromium intake cannot presently be given. A chromium intake of 50 μg to 200 μg/day is tentatively recommended for adults.[23] Brewer's yeast, meat products, cheeses, whole grains, and condiments are good sources of available chromium. Leafy vegetables, polished rice, and table sugar are poor sources.

Micronutrients That May Be Essential

TIN

At the present time naturally occurring tin deficiency is unknown either in animals or man. Schwarz however, has presented evidence indicating that rats raised in an all-plastic "isolator" system to prevent trace element contamination and fed a highly purified basal diet do not grow normally until they receive a supplement of 8.5 μmol to 17 μmol (1 mg–2 mg)/kg body weight.[27] The weanling rats maintained on the basal diet showed signs of a deficiency within 1 to 2 weeks from the beginning of basal diet feeding. They grew poorly, lost hair, developed a seborrhea-like condition, and were lacking in energy and tonicity. Schwarz has proposed this work identifies tin as an element essential for the growth of rats maintained at first under trace element sterile conditions in the isolator system and later, similarly, in plastic cages instead of the isolator.

Human diets have been reported to contain 30 μmol to 140 μmol (3.5 mg–17 mg) tin/day.[7] Since the toxic dose for man is about 40 μmol to 60 μmol/kg body weight, such intakes have a high safety margin. The formerly widespread use of tin and tinfoil in cans and packages of food presents potential hazards to man. However, in most countries now, plastic containers or lacquer-coated containers greatly reduce the hazard of food contamination by tin.

The upper limit permissible in canned food is usually taken as 250 mg/kg.[7]

Dietary tin is poorly absorbed and is mainly excreted in the feces. At this time there is a lack of information regarding the metabolic or dietary need for tin.

NICKEL

Traces of nickel are present in human tissues, and there is evidence suggesting that it is an essential nutrient for rats and chicks.[7] Nielsen has concluded from work presently in the literature and from his own work with chicks that nickel might have an essential role in animals.[21] In Nielsen's work, low levels of nickel in the diet of chicks caused changes including "a different shade of yellow in the shank skin, slightly swollen hocks, slightly thickened legs, a dermatitis on the shank skin, a change in the texture and color of the liver, a reduction in ether-extractable lipid in the liver, heart, aorta, and kidneys."[21]

Nickel may play a role as an activator of liver arginase and in maintaining the conformation of membranes.[22] The average intake of normal adults is 0.3 mg to 0.6 mg/day.[22]

The occurrence of nickel in human tissues and the fact that a nickel deficiency has been produced in chickens and rats, both suggest some possibility of a human need for this trace element.

An essential role in the human cannot be established at this time.

SILICON

Although deficiencies of silicon reportedly have been produced in laboratory animals, suggesting a possible human requirement, positive data implicating silicon in human nutrition are lacking. Carlisle in 1972 reported that silicon is needed by the chick in microgram amounts for normal growth and bone development.[7] There is some suggestion that silicon enhances calcification, especially when calcium is limited.

Silicon, as silicates, is ingested chiefly in vegetable foods. Human blood serum ordinarily carries about 1 mg/100 ml.[7] Among stone workers the lungs are highest in silicon concentration because of inhalation of dust particles in stone-cutting and stone-working industries. Workmen inhaling this dust often develop silicosis.

The amount of silicon in both plant and animal foodstuffs appears to be effective for normal growth and development. Therefore, a deficiency in the human appears to be remote. Milk is a good source of silicon for mammals.

VANADIUM

The essentiality of an element can be determined by reducing the level of the nutrient in a diet below the requirement of the organism. If fed under these conditions for an adequate length of time, deficiency symptoms will appear when contrasted to a control group receiving a supplement of the same nutrient in greater amount. In 1970, Hopkins and Mohr presented evidence that indicated the essentiality of vanadium in the diet of chicks studied under strict conditions of housing and diet.[15] These investigators showed that when chicks were consuming a diet containing 10 parts per billion vanadium there was significantly slower growth in both the chicks' wings and tail feathers. Blood cholesterol levels, interestingly, in these chicks were significantly lower than those in control animals. In 1971, Schwarz and Milne showed that the growth of rats raised on carefully controlled and deficient diets under "ultraclean" conditions increased their growth 40% in 21 to 28 days after the addition of 0.25 mg to 0.5 mg sodium orthovanadate/kg diet.[28]

Vanadium is present in human body tissues. In view of this fact and the findings reported above for the chick and rat, there appears reason to believe that vanadium may be necessary for the human dietary.[2] No figure can be given for the vanadium requirement of the human at present, but it may be in the range of 0.1 mg to 0.3 mg/day. Normal diets contain about 10 times this amount.

Trace Contaminants

There are many elements present in trace amounts in human body tissues and fluids. Some of these are described briefly here, and others are merely listed as being present. As far as is known, all of these are foreign to the human and animal body function and metabolism and are present as trace contaminants. It is possible that as analytic tools become sharpened and refined more will be learned of these "incidental" tissue substances, including possibly their toxic qualities.

LEAD

Lead does not appear to have an essential role in animal metabolism. In fact, no biologic role in plants or animals is known. Rather, interest in lead is due its toxicity. In industrial societies people are at risk of absorbing toxic amounts in their drinking water, in their food, and from the air they breathe. Lead has been found in high concentrations in plants and soils in areas in the vicinity of major highways owing to discharges of lead from automobile engines.[2] In children, lead toxicity has occurred through chewing toys or other surfaces painted with lead paints. Some dishes with lead glazes can be toxic, particularly if used in cooking. The burning of refuse containing lead paints, old lead batteries,

or other lead-containing materials is a possible source of toxicity.

Lead is stored in the bones and, to a lesser extent, in the liver. Enzymes that depend on sulfhydryl groups (—SH) for their activity are inhibited by lead, for example, δ-aminolevulinic acid dehydratase, which is involved in the biosynthesis of heme. For this reason patients with lead poisoning causing an anemia will excrete coproporphyrin III in the urine. This is such a constant finding that the examination of urine is one of the best screening tests for suspected lead poisoning or toxicity.[33]

In industrial areas, 1 μmol to 2 μmol (200 μg–400 μg) may be ingested daily. A blood concentration above 2 μmol/liter suggests more than usual exposure to lead, and higher amounts invite the risk of developing lead poisoning. A stool sample containing more than 4 μmol, or a urine sample with more than 400 μmol/liter is indicative of excess lead contamination of food.[7]

CADMIUM

Although cadmium exists in tissues in trace amounts, it does not appear to be an essential nutrient. It is absent or extremely low in concentration in the body at birth. However, by age 50 the amount present in tissues has accumulated slowly to 200 μmol to 300 μmol (20 mg–30 mg).[7]

Cadmium poisoning is recognized as an industrial hazard. In Japan, cadmium has been shown to be the cause of a severe and often fatal osteomalacia with aminoaciduria called Itai-itai disease. This disease affected over 200 people living on rice grown on land irrigated by waste water from a zinc mine upstream from the area.[7]

In 1960 Kagi and Vallee isolated from equine renal cortex a metalloprotein containing cadmium.[16] It contained 2.9% cadmium, 0.6% zinc, and 4.1% sulfur. Because of its high metal and sulfur content, it was named metallothionein. Although the metabolic function of this metalloprotein has not been explained, it may suggest a role for cadmium in biologic systems.

MERCURY

Compounds of mercury have a number of industrial uses, and the toxicity of the metal is therefore a hazard. Poisoning produces tremors and stomatitis, but the symptoms appear to be reversible when the patient is removed from further exposure to the metal. The dangerous forms of mercury are the alkyl derivatives, methylmercury and ethylmercury.[7] When absorbed or ingested, these compounds produce an apparently irreversible encephalopathy. Mercury poisoning can be produced by eating fish from polluted waters containing these and other mercury–organo compounds or seed grains treated with mercurial fungicides to prevent fungal disease. Following a latent period of 2 to 5 weeks, ataxia and visual disturbances develop which may lead to permanent paralysis or death.[7]

Blood or hair can be examined when mercury poisoning is suspected. Concentrations below 100 μmol (20 μg/liter) of whole blood are desirable.

ARSENIC

Although arsenic is present in soil, water, and in many plant and animal foods, it does not seem to have an essential role in biology. In the form of organic arsenicals it is sometimes added to animal feeds to stimulate growth.[7] Such animals may have higher than normal amounts of arsenic in their liver and muscles.

Reduction of growth and reproduction and pathological changes in various organs are described in some animals fed diets deficient in this element.[23]

The diet of an adult man normally contains 6 μmol to 50 μmol (0.4 mg–3.9 mg)/day. It has been suggested that 43 μmol/day is an acceptable upper limit of intake.[7]

STRONTIUM

As mentioned in the introduction to this chapter, the radioactive isotope of strontium (strontium-90) attracted attention first as fall-out from atomic explosions. Like calcium and magnesium it is a divalent ion, and its biologic behavior is somewhat similar to calcium. In general, strontium is present in foods rich in calcium, such as milk and to a lesser degree vegetables. It is stored in bone.[7]

BORON

This element has been shown to be essential for plants, but there is no evidence that it plays a role as an essential nutrient in animal metabolism. The growth of laboratory animals (rats) maintained on diets very low in boron is not impaired.[14]

ALUMINUM

Aluminum is the third most abundant element in the earth's crust, and the human body contains 50 mg to 150 mg. There is no evidence that it is essential. The hydroxide, however, has value as an antacid and appears to be effective in patients with chronic renal failure to help reduce phosphate absorption. The daily intake of aluminum in the human diet varies from 10 mg to over 100 mg, and in addition small amounts may be derived from aluminum cooking utensils or added to the diet as sodium aluminum sulfate in baking powder. Absorption of aluminum from the intestine is poor.[14]

LITHIUM

This element is not an essential nutrient for animals or man. According to Voors the concentration of lithium in drinking water appears to be inversely related to the prevalence of coronary heart disease.[31] Lithium salts have been found to be effective in the treatment of mania and related mental disorders in which there is a disturbance of amine metabolism. It seems to have a place in psychiatry and is used in the prevention of recurrent attacks of mania and depression.[7] This element inhibits the release of norepinephrine and serotonin from brain slices stimulated by an electric current.

References

1. Bernstein DS, Sandowsky N, Hegsted M, Guri CD, Stare FJ: Prevalence of osteoporosis in high- and low-fluoride areas in North Dakota. JAMA 198:85–87, 1966
2. Bogert J, Briggs GM, Calloway CH: Nutrition and Physical Fitness, 9th ed. Philadelphia, WB Saunders, 1973
3. Caughey JE: Etiological factors in adolescent malnutrition in Iran. NZ Med J 77:90–95, 1973
4. Cotzias GC: Manganese in health and disease. Physiol Rev 38:503–532, 1958
5. Dahl LK: Salt intake and salt need. N Engl J Med 258:1152–1158, 1205–1208, 1958
6. Darrow DC, Pratt DL, Flett J, Gamble AH, Weise HF: Disturbance of water and electrolytes in infantile diarrhea. Pediatrics 3:129–156, 1949
7. Davidson S, Passmore R, Brock JF, Truswell AS: Human Nutrition and Dietetics, 6th ed. New York, Churchill Livingstone, 1975
8. Elvehjem CA: The biological significance of copper and its relation to iron metabolism. Physiol Rev 15:471–507, 1935
9. Flink EB: Magnesium deficiency syndrome in man. JAMA 160:1406–1409, 1956
10. Fluoride as a nutrient. Committee on Nutrition, American Academy of Pediatrics, Pediatrics 49:456–460, 1972
11. Guthrie HA: Introductory Nutrition, 3rd ed. St Louis, CV Mosby, 1975
12. Halsted JA, Ronaghy HA, Abadi P, Haghshenass M, Amirhakemi GH, Barakat RM, Reinhold JC: Zinc deficiency in man. Am J Med 53:277–284, 1972
13. Handbook on Human Nutritional Requirements. Food and Agriculture Organization of the United Nations, FAO Nutritional Studies No. 28. Rome, WHO Monograph Series 61, 1974
14. Martin DW, Mayes P, Rodwell VW: Harper's Review of Biochemistry, 18th ed. Los Altos, Lange Medical Publications, 1981
15. Hopkins LL, Mohr HE: The biological essentiality of vanadium. In Mertz W, Cornatzer WE (eds): Newer Trace Elements in Nutrition. New York, M Dekker, 1971

16. Kagi JHR, Vallee BL: Metallothionein: a cadmium- and zinc-containing protein from equine renal cortex. J Bio Chem 235:3460–3465, 1960

17. Latham MC, McGandy RB, McCann MB, Stare FJ: Scope Manual on Nutrition, Kalamazoo, MI, Upjohn Co, 1970

18. Latner A: Clinical Biochemistry, 7th ed. Philadelphia, WB Saunders, 1975

19. Mertz W: Chromium occurrence and function in biological systems. Physiol Rev 49:163–239, 1969

20. Montgomery RD: Magnesium metabolism in infantile protein malnutrition. Lancet II:74–75, 1960

21. Nielsen FH: Studies on the essentiality of nickel. In Mertz W, Cornatzer WE (eds): Newer Trace Elements in Nutrition. New York, M Dekker, 1971

22. Orten JM, Neuhaus OW: Human Biochemistry, 9th ed. St Louis, CV Mosby, 1975, p 551

23. Recommended Dietary Allowances, National Academy of Sciences, 9th ed, Washington DC, 1980

24. Rickert DA, Westerfeld WW: Isolation and identification of xanthine oxidase factor as molybdenum. J Biol Chem 203:915–923, 1953

25. Rotruck JI, Pope AL, Ganther HE, Swanson AB, Hafeman DG, Hoekstra WG: Selenium: biochemical role as a component of glutathione peroxidase. Science 179:588–590, 1973

26. Schroeder HA, Balassa JJ, Tipton IH: Abnormal trace metals in man—chromium. J Chron Dis 15:941–964, 1962

27. Schwarz K: Tin as an essential growth factor for rats. In Mertz W, Cornatzer WE (eds): Newer Trace Elements in Nutrition, p 314. New York, M Dekker, 1971

28. Schwarz K, Milne DB: Growth effects of vanadium in the rat. Science 174:426–428, 1971

29. Underwood EJ: Trace Elements in Human and Animal Nutrition, 3rd ed. New York, Academic Press, 1971

30. Vallee BL, Neurath H: Carboxypeptidase, a zinc metalloenzyme. J Biol Chem 217:253–261, 1975

31. Voors AW: Does lithium depletion cause artherosclerotic heart disease? Lancet II:1337–1339, 1969

32. Wacker WEC, Moore FD, Ulmer DDD, Vallee BEJ: Normocalcemic magnesium deficiency tetany. JAMA 180:161–163, 1962

33. Wintrobe MM, et al (eds): Harrison's Principals of Internal Medicine, 6th ed, p 665. New York, McGraw–Hill, 1970

34. Young DS, Hicks JM: Method for the automatic determination of serum iron. J Clin Path 18:98, 1965

Modalities
of
Applied
Nutrition

5
The Dietitian in the Hospital Setting

Ronni Chernoff

The term *dietitian* was first used in 1899 to describe a person working in a hospital who provided nutritious meals to patients.[22] Since then the duties of the hospital dietitian have continued to grow, especially in providing nutritional services to hospital patients. The first dietitians were primarily home economists until 1917, when, in recognition of the professional nature of their work, the American Dietetic Association was founded. Dietitians then had a professional organization and the beginning of a means of communicating with each other, sharing experiences, and developing professional goals.[22] The first dietitians' conference was concerned with nutritional standards and standards for hospital food service.[7] This regard for the quality of food service has continued.

Dietitians' Education

From the beginning, there was concern among the members of the American Dietetic Association for the establishment and maintenance of educational standards for dietitians. As early as 1926, a bachelor of science degree was required for membership in the Association. Undergraduate programs in food, nutrition, and dietetics included training in both the natural sciences (biology, chemistry, biochemistry, bacteriology, and physiology) and the social sciences (psychology, sociology, and philosophy), as well as in languages and management skills. By 1930 an apprenticeship system was established to provide postbaccalaureate on-the-job training. By 1940, there were 60 internship programs functioning as formal apprenticeship training programs.

These programs provided a multifaceted practical experience for student dietitians. The continued desire to raise professional standards for practicing dietitians eventually led to the institution of dietetic registration.

To be eligible to take the registration examination, a dietitian must have completed a bachelor's degree program, served in a practical experience program, and performed at minimal competency levels. Registration was officially sanctioned in 1969 by a vote of the membership of the American Dietetic Association. Because of the limited number of internship programs, other routes to registration examination eligibility were opened. Traineeship programs were developed to allow hospitals to provide practical experience in a variety of settings (patient care areas, administration, out-patient facilities, research units) for one or two students at a time. Because of the unevenness of these experiences, traineeship programs have since been phased out. However, so many students have become interested in pursuing dietetics as a career that more training programs have had to be developed.

A relatively new program design, called *coordinated undergraduate programs* (CUP), is available to interested students. These programs provide academic and applied experiences during the usual four-year undergraduate program. Work experiences are interspersed with classroom experiences. A student graduating from such a program is eligible to take the registration examination.

Still another route to registration examination eligibility is that of the student with a bachelor's degree in a discipline other than nutrition who then earns a masters' level degree in nutrition. (Graduate degrees in nutrition and dietetics were evident by 1940.) After a six-month apprenticeship under a registered dietitian who provides the student with a variety of experiences in a broad area of dietetics, the student can apply for registration eligibility. After review by a committee of the Commission on Dietetic Registration, eligibility can be awarded and the student can take the examination. The purpose of these standards is to ensure that a professional dietitian possesses a certain body of knowledge and experience common to everyone with the title "dietitian."

The registration examination covers the area of relevant information for the sciences, administration skills, and clinical dietetics. A registered dietitian thus has met a minimum standard of knowledge in the very broad spectrum of content areas that constitute dietetics.

In a hospital setting, the shared areas of knowledge serve to provide a common basis of professionalism between the dietitians who are responsible for food preparation, storage, and delivery and those who are responsible for providing modified diets and nutritional care to the patients. As in any other profession, a mutual understanding between those performing different job functions enables both parties to better fulfill their assigned responsibilities. Dietitians who have successfully completed the requirements to be eligible for registration, and have then attained registered status by passing the examination, share experiences and knowledge that will serve them well in whatever job they seek in dietetics.

As with other professions, the training of dietitians has changed with time. The practice of medicine and the delivery of health care have become more sophisticated, specialized, and individualized, and so has the delivery of nutritional care. The role of the dietitian in the hospital setting has changed and expanded considerably in recent years. Over half the dietitians in the United States work in hospitals serving in one of two capacities, as administrative dietitians or as clinical dietitians.

Administrative Dietitians

Administrative dietitians are concerned with the standardization of food and services in order to provide the best food in a quality-controlled setting. Administrative dietitians are part of the hospital management team in that they develop budgetary programs and manage their fiscal resources in accord with institutional policies. Hospital and nursing-home food services are not income-generating cost centers; usually overall financial re-

sources are drawn as a percentage of the daily room and board charge. From that single resource, equipment must be purchased and maintained, overhead paid, salaries and benefits accounted for, and food costs covered.

The administrative dietitian is responsible for food production and quality control in the delivery of hospital meal service. This often extends beyond patient food service to include staff meal service as well. This may mean the production of thousands of meals per day, depending on the size of the institution. Not only is the administrative dietitian responsible for the procurement, storage, and deployment of material goods, but often is also responsible for dietary department staffing and the assignment of professional time.

One of the major budget items in many dietary departments is labor, including both professional and support staff. Many patients and hospital staff members are often unaware of the number of people who work in hospital dietary departments. Both the number of meals produced per day and the number of menu items required to provide acceptable alternatives for the many modified and special diets are impressive. To simplify the planning of food purchase orders and daily work flow in the kitchen, cycle menus are often used.

Cycling of menus allows for a three- or four-week pattern of food purchase orders and employee scheduling to be written and repeated without major change. This approach to menu writing allows administrative dietitians to anticipate work flow and also to take advantage of seasonal foods, such as fruits and vegetables, to ensure variety on the menu, and yet to retain control over costs.[19]

Administrative dietitians often relate to hospital managers and administrators but rarely have direct contact with the medical staff. The clinical dietitian is the person who has direct contact with the medical and paramedical staff concerned with the delivery of care to the patient.

Clinical Dietitians

The clinical dietitian's role in the hospital setting has changed a great deal in recent years. Traditionally, the primary role of the clinical dietitian in the hospital was to ensure compliance of patients placed on modified diets by the managing physician. Patients on regular or "house" diets were visited by the dietitian, but attention was focused on patients on diets with one or more nutrients modified from the standard diet. (A hospital menu is planned to provide the recommended dietary allowances for each patient each day.) One of the reasons for this has been the number of patients for whom each dietitian is responsible. The patient:dietitian ratio ranges from 400:1 to 45:1, with the average range at 100:1 to 150:1.[4] This ratio is not conducive to seeing every patient every day, or even taking time to visit patients on regular diets. This problem has persisted for many years with no impetus for change.

Although clinical dietitians recognized the need for more visibility and participation in the health delivery system, change was slow until the mid-1970s when the extent of hospital malnutrition that existed in certain medical centers was documented.[1-3] A parallel development in the sophisticated area of intravenous nutritional support contributed to the rapid changes that have taken place in the definition of the role of the dietitian in the hospital setting.

The recognition of the need for nutritional support of patients who did not seem to need modified diets, by investigators working with problems of surgical sepsis, preceded the identification of generalized malnutrition in both medical and surgical patients.[20] However, the development of the sophisticated technology for assessing nutritional status by physical measures coincided with the ability to deliver nutrients to the very sick or severely malnourished patient directly into the blood in a form to be immediately metabolized or used for tissue repletion. The hospital dietitian has had to learn quickly and apply this knowledge to keep up with the rapid changes brought about by this interest in nutrition by physicians and other paramedical personnel.

Although the use of nutrition-care plans has been supported for many years, the scientific basis for making judgments of nutritional status was not commonly used. With the suggestions made by Drs. Blackburn and Butterworth for standard nutritional assessment programs in hospitals (see Chap. 9), many dietitians have been able to take on this responsibility and incorporate it into their roles.[3] Continuing education programs have promoted training and understanding of this new technique. In the clinical setting, the cooperative support of the physician is essential for the dietitian to break new ground and perform functions beyond the traditional ones, such as modifying menus and teaching discharge diets. The dietitian must be more assertive and recognize that active participation at rounds and conferences is necessary to perform adequately some of these responsibilities. The dietitian is now a recognized member of the health-care team.

NUTRITION ASSESSMENT RESPONSIBILITIES

Aside from the traditional expectation of translating orders for modified diets into practice (in some institutions the dietitian writes the diet orders with the physician's approval), dietitians are prepared to take on additional responsibilities and assume a more active role in patient care. The introduction of nutritional assessment programs in many hospitals during the past five years has created challenges. Although encouraged to read patients' charts, the dietitian, overwhelmed with paperwork, found it difficult to find time. With some reorganization of duties and the use of dietetic technicians, the clinical dietitian has been able to create time in which to perform these responsibilities effectively.[13] A review of the patient's chart will give the dietitian an overview of the medical and nutritional problems of each patient; the medical care plan or differential diagnosis plan may indicate procedures that could have some deleterious effects on the patient's ability to ingest adequate nutrients for nutritional status maintenance. Subsequent stress related to surgery or other treatment modalities may lead to additional nutritional problems. Many diagnostic tests require that the patient not eat for twelve hours prior to the procedure; this is not a hardship, but when patients are kept on clear-liquid diets for several days and miss even those meals because they are waiting for tests, a toll will be taken. For a sick patient who has reduced food intake prior to entering the hospital, the added stress of hospitalization and a "starvation" diet of clear liquids will serve to deplete whatever nutritional stores the patient had upon admission. If it is known that a patient will not be eating for more than three days, and the patient has some indication of nutritional compromise (weight loss, dehydration, nausea, vomiting, diarrhea) prior to admission, intervention with some kind of nutritional support is indicated. The dietitian, as well as the responsible physician, should be aware of the feeding alternatives.

It has been suggested that all patients be assessed for nutritional status within a few days of admission.[15] The tools that the dietitian requires to perform this function are not difficult to obtain. As indicated, the first step should be to review the patient's past medical history and admission laboratory data, including serum electrolytes and hematologic values. Urinary tests should be reviewed, especially for renal patients or diabetics. Temperature, respiration and pulse, blood pressure, and fluid intake and output should be noted in this review. At this time, a quick perusal of the medication cardex may be appropriate. There are many drugs that may have an effect on nutritional status by affecting nutrient intake or by interfering with nutrient absorption or use. Medications such as steroids, insulin, chemotherapy agents, or antibiotics, for example, will have some type of effect on nutritional status. Even the fact that a patient has a fever will impact on nutritional requirements, if only by necessitating additional fluids.

Although in the past recording heights and weights in the patient chart was a rare occurrence, this is becoming more common. Having weights recorded at periodic intervals (at least two times per week) will help monitor the patient's response to, or need for, nutritional therapy throughout a hospitalization. It is a desirable routine to establish and maintain in any hospital.

Once the dietitian knows the chief complaint and probable diagnosis, additional pertinent information can be elicited from the patient during interview. The dietitian should visit every patient within 48 hours of admission to the hospital.[15] During the process of taking a diet history, information about impaired intake, appetite changes, nausea, vomiting, diarrhea, weight history, meal patterns, unusual food cravings, changes in food consumption, and vitamin pill and drug history can be gathered by the dietitian. This is an appropriate time to establish a relationship with the patient as a foundation for later diet instruction and teaching, if necessary.

During this first visit, the dietitian can take anthropometric measurements to contribute to an overall nutritional evaluation and to serve as baseline data for future assessments. The most common measurements taken are triceps skinfold and upper arm circumference at the midpoint between shoulder and elbow. Some dietitians may also measure suprailiac and subclavicular skinfolds.

It is important to note, however, that anthropometric standards are poor and have questionable value as a criterion of nutritional status in much of the adult American population.[6,8] The Metropolitan Life Insurance Company height and weight tables, for instance, were compiled over 20 years ago on a middle-class population of life insurance purchasers.

The dietitian can be responsible for estimation of energy requirements for patients and can be expected to extrapolate requirements for additional needs related to surgery, trauma, sepsis, and other metabolic problems. Research on energy expenditure under unusual metabolic conditions is beginning to appear in the literature, and it is the dietitian's responsibility to stay abreast of new developments in the field.[14] The reference material concerning nutritional assessment has expanded greatly in just a few years. Newer techniques are being used experimentally and, when perfected, may come into general use. Arm radiography, neutron stimulation, ultrasound, ^{40}K counting and radial immunodiffusion for retinol-binding protein and prealbumin are among these techniques.

For several years, the dietitian has been encouraged to write relevant observations in the medical chart. A technique called *SOAPING* has been advocated. The acronym SOAP refers to a *S*ubjective observation of the patient's status and possible related concerns, *O*bjective measurement supporting these subjective observations, an *A*ssessment of the situation, and a *P*lan to either avoid or solve potential difficulties. By following such a format, problems may be anticipated before they interfere with the delivery of necessary medical care. There was some initial resistance to the dietitian adding to the progress notes, but it is now an acceptable practice that affords the dietitian an opportunity to share relevant information with other health-care team members.

SPECIALIZATION—THE COUNCIL ON PRACTICE, AMERICAN DIETETIC ASSOCIATION

The practice of medicine has become highly specialized, as is reflected in the delivery of health care in American hospitals. As the other members of the medical team (physicians, nurse clinicians, clinical pharmacists) specialized, so did dietitians. Although the dietitian has long been considered a generalist whose function has been to deliver attractive, healthful food and to provide dietary counseling after taking a dietary history, the dietitian's role is perforce becoming more specialized.[24] While there are still generalists in small community hospitals and nursing homes, dietitian specialists have appeared in more identifiable, specific areas of practice.

In 1978, the American Dietetic Association Council on Practice was established. The Council is made up of five divisions of areas of dietetic practice: clinical dietetics and research, management practice, consultation and private practice, dietetic educators, and community dietetics practice. Each division is further subdivided into more specialized units known as dietetic practice groups. When the Council was organized in 1978, there were nine dietetic practice groups; since then more groups have been identified and formed every year.[10]

The Division of Clinical Dietetics and Research is the division with which clinical hospital dietitians will opt to align themselves, even those hospital dietitians who do not consider themselves specialists in a specific practice area. Administrative dietitians can join a dietetic practice group under the Division of Management Practice.

CLINICAL RESEARCH DIETITIANS

The first clinical dietetic practitioners to be identified in a specialty area were the clinical research dietitians, who organized as an informal group under the auspices of the Section on Diet Therapy of the American Dietetic Association (since replaced by the Council on Practice) in the early 1960s. Their group became the forerunner of other dietetic practice groups. The research dietitian's responsibilities often include participation in metabolic research studies. Many metabolic research studies require very specialized, highly controlled dietary intakes, since diet is often one of the dependent variables. Some clinical research units specialize in one or two areas of research, while others have broad-based research projects related to a variety of protocols and investigators. A thorough understanding of metabolism and biochemistry is required in order to participate in these research activities.

Sometimes new techniques for clinical care are tested under grant-supported research before becoming part of standard medical practice. Organ transplantation was first done on metabolic research units, as are many drug clinical trials. Depending upon the sophistication of the investigations in any particular research center, the dietitian has the opportunity to become familiar with the newest approaches to medical care.

Recently, more research dietitians are conducting their own research in cooperation with experienced investigators. The opportunity for dietitians to initiate clinical research is new and exciting, and perhaps indicative of the future direction of research dietetics.

Aside from the original group, the Division of Clinical Dietetics and Research has dietetic practice groups for diabetes education and care dietitians, renal dietitians, dietitians in pediatric practice, and dietitians in critical care. It is possible that more special-interest groups will be formed and become members of this division. A group can formally petition to become a dietetic practice group when it has identified 50 members. This new structure in the organization of the American Dietetic Association serves to better meet the interests and educational needs of the practitioner.

DIABETES CARE AND EDUCATION DIETITIANS

Dietitians in the Diabetes Care and Education Group have a growing role in clinical care that extends to both an inpatient and an outpatient setting. Teaching a newly diagnosed diabetic how to control his or her blood sugar has been left to the dietitian. With the increasing importance of diet control, the dietitian has become more pivotal in the care of the diabetic. Knowledge of insulin action and oral hypoglycemic agent functions must be integrated with knowledge of metabolism in order for the dietitian to provide the most appropriate diet plan for the medical care plan. Flexibility and creativity are

necessary for the dietitian in diabetes care and education because juvenile, insulin-dependent, diabetics require a different approach than do adult, non-insulin-dependent, diabetics (see Chap. 18).

The dietitian reviews diet orders to see that caloric requirements are appropriate to attain or maintain normal body weight. The dietitian's job is to begin patient education in the hospital and to follow the patient after discharge (see Chap. 6). When patients resume a more normal activity pattern, caloric requirements, insulin requirements, medications, and meal times may change. Group teaching has not proved very successful for some diabetics, and more individualized instruction and care plans are necessary, especially when the patient has diabetes secondary to another disease process or when the diabetic develops complications.

The dietitian in diabetes care and education also serves as an educator for other health professionals. There are many new devices being tested and advances being made in this clinical specialty. The dietitian can participate in research as well as in clinical care.[23]

RENAL DIETITIANS

The Dietetic Practice Group for Renal Dietitians is comprised of dietitians who work with patients suffering from varying degrees and types of renal disease. For dietitians who work in dialysis or kidney transplantation units, the status of their specialty derives from specific funding legislation. In 1976, regulations supporting the law for Medicare reimbursement of patients with end-stage renal disease required that a "qualified dietitian" must be part of the professional team that develops long-term and short-term patient care plans for renal patients. The dietitian, along with a nephrologist, has the responsibility for nutritional assessment, therapeutic diet recommendations and counseling, and monitoring dietary adherence and response (see Chap. 34).

The renal dietitian must be able to understand and interpret laboratory data that reflect changes in renal function status, stage of disease, or form of treatment.

As with the dietitian who works in diabetes care and education, the renal dietitian is often faced with the problems of other ongoing disease processes and must have the ability to design individualized nutritional care plans for each patient. In many instances, the dietitian has patients with various stages and types of renal disease and may care for patients who are being treated with medical-management predialysis; patients on chronic hemodialysis, peritoneal dialysis, or continuous ambulatory peritoneal dialysis; or patients undergoing transplantation. All of these modalities affect nutritional needs differently. A thorough understanding of renal physiology, treatment courses, and medication interactions is required for the renal dietitian to perform effectively.[11]

PEDIATRIC DIETITIANS

A more recently formed Dietetic Practice Group is Dietitians in Pediatric Practice. The dietitian's role in pediatrics is also a multifaceted one, similar to those already discussed, yet unique. The pediatric dietitian is responsible for the assessment of the nutritional requirements related to the growth and development of pediatric patients. Caring for healthy children may be straightforward, but caring for sick children requires knowledge of the metabolic requirements of the disease process as well as the normal nutritional needs for growth and development. The dietitian working in pediatrics may specialize in more specific areas: neonatology, infancy, childhood, or adolescence. The dietitian is responsible for modifying the diet when necessary to accommodate food preferences, altered requirements, or feeding problems that may be mechanical or physiological. A nutritional care plan must be developed that can be adapted as the child grows and changes. Nutritional requirements change with the age of the child, with improving or deteriorating disease states, or with developmental changes, and the dietitian has to anticipate and be prepared for future modifications.

The dietitian in pediatric practice has an unusual role as an educator. The dietitian may teach the patient in certain circumstances and the parent or caretaker in others. For the mother who is trying to manage unusual dietary requirements for her child (*i.e.,* inborn errors of metabolism, diabetes, renal disease, cystic fibrosis) and feed the rest of the family too, the dietitian must be an accessible resource. The pediatric dietitian has access to resource material on many dietary products made especially for formula feeding or diet modifications that are frequently difficult for a parent to locate.

The dietitian becomes part of a support system for the parents of a sick child. Whether the child has cancer, phenylketonuria, or allergies, the dietitian must act as a stimulus for the parents to be creative and comfortable with the restrictions imposed upon the child. As with other dietitian specialists, the pediatric dietitian can help direct the patient or parent to appropriate and quality resource material and, sometimes, to support groups where the knowledge of an experienced patient can ease adjustments for the newly diagnosed patient.[17]

DIETITIANS IN CRITICAL CARE

Until recently, the clinical dietitian specialist has functioned in a clearly defined specialty. Research dietitians have had their activities confined to the metabolic research centers, renal dietitians to dialysis centers and transplantation units, and pediatric dietitians to isolated areas of the hospital or hospitals where the sole medical practice is pediatrics. Diabetes specialists seem to be primarily located in outpatient clinics and work more closely with the ambulatory patient who is followed on a chronic basis at home. Dietitians in critical care are becoming more visible because their area of practice extends beyond the critical care units to touch on many other patients in the hospital. The reason is that many of these dietitians serve as members of nutritional support teams. Dietitians specializing in the care of the critically ill patient may be involved with burn, trauma, or cancer patients as well as with surgical or medical patients who are deemed to be at risk nutritionally because of admission nutritional status or plans for treatment.

Dietitians who work and specialize in the area of critical care must have a thorough knowledge of the metabolic changes that occur with critical illness. They must understand the altered requirements of patients who have been severely injured and adjust nutritional care plans accordingly. The dietitian in critical care must also have a working knowledge of the nutritional support modalities frequently used to nourish critically ill patients: enteral feeding by tube (nasoenteric, gastrostomy, jejunostomy, needle catheter jejunostomy, and so forth), by peripheral vein, or by central vein. The dietitian must be familiar with the myriad products and hardware used for these feedings, be able to make suggestions for nutritional modification when the patient's condition changes, and be involved in the transitional process of changing feeding modalities and monitoring laboratory values during this time. The dietitian in critical care must also have knowledge of drug–nutrient interactions related to many pharmaceutical products and be aware of side-effects that may affect nutritional status (*i.e.,* drugs that may cause diarrhea, chemotherapeutic agents, and the like). The dietitian working with critically ill patients must be able to change approaches to nutritional support as rapidly as the patient's condition changes and often does not have time to establish relationships with patients because of the short-term contact with many of them.

NUTRITION-SUPPORT-TEAM DIETITIANS

Nutrition-support-team dietitians have helped to make the other members of the health-care team aware of the contribution that the dietitian can make to the overall care of the patient.

The dietitian's role in the clinical setting has been to translate the physician's order for dietary modification into the practical terms of food or nutritional products. With the rapid advances in the development of supplemental and tube-feeding products, the dietitian should serve as the resource person for the team. The dietitian should also be familiar with the tube-feeding access routes and the appropriate use and composition of commercially available products. The monitoring of tube-feeding administration may be shared with a nurse, but the dietitian should be aware of the intake and tolerance for these products by the patients for whom the nutrition-support team is responsible.[5]

In addition to the nutritional assessment responsibilities previously described, the dietitian serves as the nutritional resource person for both the nutrition-support team and the extended medical-care team. Dietitians are specific members of the health-care team who have been formally trained in nutrition. Too few medical schools offer courses in nutrition for physician instruction in a systematic curriculum.[18]

DIETITIANS AS EDUCATORS

The dietitian's role as an educator in the clinical setting is a multilevel one. The relationship between attending staff and dietitians is usually dependent on the individual physician's interest in the nutritional care of his or her patients. The members of the house staff are generally interested in and receptive to learning abut the nutritional problems of the patients under their care. An interesting technique that may be used to familiarize young physicians with the realities of a therapeutic diet is to provide free, modified-diet meals to the house staff. It is quite instructive for a medical student, intern, or resident to eat a low-sodium or low-fat diet. This also holds true for formula feedings. A managing physician, for example, may order two liters of an oral defined-formula diet and expect a sick patient to drink it. The physician may not know what it tastes like or whether his expectation of what the patient will ingest is reasonable. The dietitian can take an educational role with the other members of the health-care team as well. An effective method is to participate in daily rounds and to focus on problems that patients may be having. For example, a patient starting on antibiotic therapy may have problems with diarrhea, or a patient receiving chemotherapy may have nausea and vomiting and should be supported nutritionally by an alternate route.

The dietitian has a prime role as an educator of the patient. Teaching a modified diet should begin while the patient is still in the hospital. Teaching discharge diets an hour before a patient is to leave the hospital is ineffective because at that time patients are overwhelmed with details of health insurance and bill paying, medication instructions, follow-up appointment arrangements, and simply getting home. Effective teaching should be gradual and planned. It is of highest priority that the patient understand dietary restrictions and the rationale for the restrictions. It is also helpful if the physician has explained that there will be a dietary modification, so the patient is not taken by surprise when the dietitian starts the diet instruction.

The dietitian should have access to information relating to discharge; whether the patient is going home, to an extended-care facility, or to a nursing home will be important to the discharge planning. Knowledge of meal-preparation facilities and the person responsible for the meal preparation is also crucial in order for the dietitian to successfully teach a diet. If someone else in the family does the meal preparation, that person should be present during the instruction. The dietitian should be available to the patient and family to answer questions that may not arise until the patient is settled at home and has to start planning meals and purchasing food. The dietitian should provide for some follow-up after discharge, be it a phone number or an appointment with the clinic or outpatient dietitian. If the patient is being transferred to an extended-care facility or nursing home, the diet instruction should go with him. Sometimes it is helpful for the clinical dietitian to call ahead and speak with the dietitian who will be responsible for the patient's care at the transfer facility. Any unusual orders can be explained, and problems or requests unique to the patient can be discussed in more detail than a written note may allow.

PHYSICIAN–DIETITIAN RELATIONSHIP

Studies indicate that there is a discrepancy between the way dietitians see their role and the way physicians see it.[21] Dietitians frequently have not had the opportunity to make a contribution to decision making. Physicians must concur if the dietitian is to assume responsibility. Many physicians think that dietitians are only concerned with food, and they tend to overlook dietitians' backgrounds in biochemistry, physiology, and diet therapy.[18] However, the physician and the dietitian need to work together to provide the best nutritional care for the patient.

To best effect quality patient care, the physician and the dietitian must communicate openly and frequently. The physician has a responsibility to keep the dietitian apprised of changing plans concerning the patient's care; this can be accomplished easily if the dietitian attends daily rounds with the other members of the primary-care team. The dietitian has a responsibility to keep the physician apprised of the patient's compliance with dietary restrictions, his intake of certain nutrients where appropriate, and the progress he makes with necessary modifications. A fair portion of the communication between physician and dietitian is done in writing, so written orders must be clear and comply with the hospital diet manual. Members of the house staff often rotate among various institutions, and the diets and the names given to diets may differ. It takes only a few moments for the physician to locate the diet manual and check the diets available. Every nurses' station has a hospital diet manual accessible for reference. Some institutions provide pocket manuals with available modified diets listed. If a diet is ordered that is not reasonable, the dietitian has an obligation to make the physician aware of the discrepancy between what was ordered and its ability to be translated into food. Diet manuals are revised at periodic intervals, some continuously, and staff should be alerted as a matter of course.

Changes may even be initiated in diet manuals by the physician. There is generally a representative of the dietary or nutritional services department on the formulary committee. Many hospitals have diet-manual committees, sometimes chaired by a physician. When diet manuals are being revised, physicians are often asked to review changes related to their specialities. There is a sharing of responsibility in keeping diet manuals as up to date as possible. The opportunity to work together should be a positive experience for both professionals.

DISCHARGE PLANNING

When planning for patient discharge, the resources available to the patient in the community should be explored. As previously mentioned, communication with the nursing home dietitian can be invaluable for continuing nutritional care for the patient. Most dietary prescriptions can be met within the nursing home and its resources. In some cases, adjustments can be made prior to discharge, such as allowing the patient time to control his medications while still in the hospital or changing a commercial tube-feeding product and providing adequate time for adaptation before transferring the patient to another facility. A preparatory phone call is always a good idea, but is not always possible; written orders should be as explicit as possible. The hospital dietitian should have knowledge of, and attempt contact with, the resources in the community. The contact between the hospital dietitian and the patient is often the patient's first contact with a nutrition professional.

The dietitian will be viewed as a source of basic information and will often receive calls from members of the lay public who are seeking reasonable answers to nutrition questions. Having a reference list of community health professionals and resources will often be useful (see Chap. 7). A new resource is the dietitian in private practice (see Chap. 6). Because of the lack of accessible resources in some communities, the private practice dietitian can provide a valuable service both to physicians in private practice who have patients who require dietary counseling but cannot take time from work to attend hospital outpatient clinics, and to the patient who requires more time and individualized attention.

Hospital dietitians can also serve to follow-up patient care in out-patient clinics. An effort must be made to pass information from the clinical dietitian to the outpatient dietitian if the patient is to be followed in the clinic. More progressive institutions have clinical dietitian specialists who provide inpatient service, then follow their patients in clinics after discharge. This procedure offers a tremendous advantage in continuity of care.

Future Directions

Dietitians have been challenged to exercise their expertise and make a visible contribution to their profession.[24] They have had a need to show individual creativity, initiative, and adaptability.[7] More dietitians are acquiring higher academic degrees and feel competent to accept additional responsibilities and to take a more active role as members of the health-care team. They have a need to continue to upgrade their scientific and medical knowledge and to extend their study of behavioral sciences. Continuing education becomes a lifelong responsibility.[16] Dietitians are beginning to take leadership roles in many areas of clinical nutrition and to make an impact in research, clinical care, administrative positions, and legislative activities. Minimal competencies defined by the peer-review process are raising the quality of the entry-level professional. Inclusion of dietetics in patient-care audits has had an impact on the quality of care by increasing awareness of patient needs.[9]

More challenging positions are opening to dietitians who have proven clinical competency and expertise. In the hospital setting, the increasing support of physicians and the burgeoning interest in nutrition of other health professionals have stimulated the clinical dietitian to rise to the challenge. The changes yet to come will provide stimulation for both the dietitian and health-care colleagues for the future. In the process, the nutritional care for the hospitalized patient will continue to improve.

References

1. Bistrian BR, Blackburn GL, Vitale J et al: Prevalence of protein calorie malnutrition in general medical patients. JAMA 235:1567, 1976
2. Bistrian BR, Blackburn GL, Hallowell E et al: Protein status of general surgical patients. JAMA 230:858, 1974
3. Butterworth CE Jr, Blackburn GL: Hospital malnutrition. Nutrition Today 10:8, 1975
4. Casey T: How to determine dietitian staffing requirements. Hospitals 51:82, 1977
5. Chernoff R: The team concept: The dietitian's responsibility. JPEN 3:89, 1979
6. Collins JP, McCarthy ID, Hill GL: Assessment of protein nutrition in surgical patients—the value of anthropometrics. Am J Clin Nutr 32:1527, 1979
7. David BD: Quality and standards—the dietitian's heritage. J Am Diet Assoc 75:408, 1980
8. Dugdale AE, Griffiths M: Estimating body mass from anthropometric data. Am J Clin Nutr 32:2400, 1979
9. El–Beheri BB: Dietetic audit—a giant step for nutritional care. J Am Diet Assoc 74:321, 1979
10. Henderson PR: The president's page. J Am Diet Assoc 73:66, 1978
11. Henry RR: Personal communication, 1980
12. Inglebleek Y, De Visscher M, De Nayer P: Measurement of prealbumin as index of protein-calorie malnutrition. Lancet 2:106, 1972
13. Jensen TG: Roles of the Dietetic Technician in Nutritional Assessment Programs. ASPEN monograph, American Society for Parenteral and Enteral Nutrition, Washington, D.C., 1980
14. Long CL, Schaffel N, Geiger JW, Schiller WR, Blakemore WS: Metabolic response to injury and illness: Estimation of energy needs from indirect calorimetry and nitrogen balance. JPEN 3:452, 1979
15. Malnutrition in the hospital. Dialogues in Nutrition, Health Learning Systems, Volume 2, No. 2, 1977
16. McLeish J: The challenge of professional and personal renewal. Journal of the Canadian Dietetic Association 39:274, 1978
17. Murray CA: Personal communication, 1980
18. Nutrition training of health professionals, Hearing before the Subcommittee on Nutrition of the Committee on Agriculture, Nutrition and Forestry, United States Senate, November 8, 1979
19. Position paper on recommended salaries and employment practices for members of the American Dietetic Association. J Am Diet Assoc 69:412, 1976
20. Rhoads JE: Development of surgical nutrition at the University of Pennsylvania. JPEN 4:464, 1980
21. Schiller MR, Vivian VM: Role of the clinical dietitian: I. Ideal role perceived by dietitians and physicians, II. Ideal role vs. actual role. J Am Diet Assoc 65:284, 1974
22. Weigley ES: Professionalization and the dietitian. J Am Diet Assoc 74:317, 1979
23. Wylie–Rosett JA: Personal communication, 1980
24. Young CM: The therapeutic dietitian—a challenge for cooperation. J Am Diet Assoc 21:424, 1965

6
Private Practice of Dietetics
Marcia A. Mills

Role of the Dietitian

The conventional portrait of the trained dietitian places the professional in a variety of institutional settings. It is probable that the most prominent among these, and the most familiar to the practicing physician, is the hospital (see Chap. 5). But this portrayal neglects a growing development in the application of the nutritional knowledge of the trained dietitian, a development indeed under way for at least 25 years in the United States.[11] This is the private practice of dietetics by registered dietitians, separate from hospitals and clinics or in independent association with them as will be further described below. The American Dietetic Association (ADA) has defined several terms to specify these relationships, new and old, of the application of the dietitian's expertise.[1]

Nutritional care describes the application of the science of nutrition to the health care of people.

Dietary counseling is the process of providing individualized, professional guidance to assist people in adjusting their daily food consumption to meet their health needs. The objective of dietary counseling is to modify the client's behavior so that he chooses appropriate foods.

Team approach to nutritional care is a concept combining the expertise of physicians and dietitians in addition to other allied health professionals to improve the health of a patient. The team approach is now used in various hospitals, which presently use over half of the practicing dietitians.[13]

With these terms in mind it is possible to sketch and categorize the current systems of nutritional care with a view toward delineating the role of the privately practicing dietitian.

CURRENT SYSTEMS OF NUTRITIONAL CARE

The nutritional care available at the present time in the United States is delivered predominantly in hospitals, nursing homes, or large clinics by registered dietitians and occasionally by dietetic technicians. The ADA registered dietitian has successfully completed a comprehensive examination and fulfills continuing education requirements in addition to having a Bachelor of Science or Arts degree in Dietetics. One can recognize a registered dietitian's title by the R.D. following the name. The registered dietitian provides nutritional care by applying science as well as the art of human nutrition to help people select food for the purpose of nourishing their bodies during health and disease throughout the life cycle.[13,15]

The dietetic technician is a technically skilled person who has successfully completed an associate degree program that meets the educational standards established by the ADA. The dietetic technician works under the direct guidance of a registered dietitian and has specifically assigned responsibilities in food service management and in teaching food and nutrition principles or dietary counseling.

The practicing physician is likely to find access to professional dietetic assistance in the person of the registered dietitian in several settings: the hospital, the nursing home (see Chap. 5), the public health agency (see Chap. 7), and—as a relatively new development—in private practice, relating to the medical community through referrals.

APPLIED NUTRITION
AND THE PRIVATE PHYSICIAN

The rapid increase in expectation of health-care delivery and the equally rapid expansion of scientific knowledge has forced the physician in private practice to carefully evaluate his priorities for patient health care. Since the physician has been charged with the major responsibility of medical care in his community, he feels an increased pressure to decide which facet of health care each patient will receive. However, the private practitioner is well aware that a number of resources are available that will benefit both his patients and his practice. In other words, he is usually interested in building an effective health-care team.

The private physician is hampered by the amount of time he can spend with patients. The average physician sees each patient for perhaps 15 minutes, during which he must evaluate the specific problem presented. In the past, when the general practitioner dealt with a patient who needed dietary counseling, the favored tool was a diet sheet, with allowed and prohibited foods printed in columns. Another common patient-teaching device has been the 1000-Cal or 1200-Cal menu plan given to a patient for a quick solution to a weight problem coupled with his own professional awareness of the complexities of losing weight.[14] Therefore, the time-limited practitioner often leaves the dietary changes necessary to lose weight to the patient's "will power." Since specific instructions are not given, this generally guarantees that the patient will do nothing more than he is already doing. The patient has probably used his will power, ineffectively, before he arrived at the doctor's office.

If the private medical practitioner did have the time to work individually with patients on dietary behavior changes, the cost to the patient would be extremely high. For example, health insurance companies generally do not provide third-party payment for "simple" exogenous obesity. The discussion time necessary to discount misinformation on which the patient has based his food-intake behavior would double the time required to provide factual information regarding a dietary change. The physician rarely has the required time to teach patients to the extent demanded.

The science of nutrition has grown tremendously in the past 50 years, and progress continues, but national food supplies continue to change qualitatively and quantitatively. The registered dietitian, having an educational background focusing on food composition as well as on the role of food itself in the maintenance of health, is a logical source of continuing dietary information.[7]

THE TEAM APPROACH
IN THE MEDICAL COMMUNITY

The expanding advances of science have brought an increasing complexity to health care. The cooperation of a team of specialists who share their respective knowledge for the welfare of the patient is now required. A wide range of facilities is essential, but they must also be available to the people whom the health care team seeks to serve.

Nutrition is an integral part of total health and life. All efforts in nutrition education, either normal or therapeutic, need to be multidisciplinary in approach. Registered dietitians are the most numerous professionally educated group whose primary concern is the application of nutrition science to health care. Dietitians must be involved in the planning and execution of health-care programs.

There has been a trend in recent years for the medical-team approach, as applied in hospitals, to move outward to the community and to function as a cooperative group. Physical therapists, nurse practitioners, and social workers, in addition to dietitians, have initiated private practices to serve the community in this manner.

The Privately Practicing Dietitian as a Resource

Therapeutic dietary objectives can be specified following a medical diagnosis by the private physician. The privately practicing dietitian is identified by referral, and the dietitian–physician team then determines the therapeutic dietary means that need to be implemented.

The dietitian works with the patient to evaluate dietary recollections, or records, and then can suggest and plan with the patient the course of action to change dietary habits to meet objectives agreed upon by the physician–dietitian team. Follow-up with the patient is usually necessary so that new questions and situations can be handled appropriately. Dietitians work in their own offices, in the physician's office, or in the patient's immediate food environment. Dietitian and physician interaction at appropriate intervals is necessary after changes have taken place. This communication can take place by telephone, letter, or personal discussion.[9]

Patient self-referrals are also made to dietitians in private practice. The client may want to have his normal dietary intake evaluated to determine if his eating pattern meets the recommended dietary allowances.[12] He may want to lose weight, having failed in the past. The self-referred client may want to improve the family's eating habits.

Food-habit change may be desired to reduce the cost of a well-balanced meal pattern or to switch to a lower animal-protein dietary plan.

Consulting dietitians, in addition to working with physicians and patients, provide educational services for allied health professionals in the form of workshops, classes, or individual training in a specialized area of therapeutic dietetics.

Dietitians often set up consulting services within large clinics, or with groups of physicians, sharing office and waiting-room space and secretarial help. This practice enables convenient referral by the physicians within the same day, at a relatively low overhead cost to the dietitian. The disadvantage of having the dietitian's office within a medical complex is that other physicians in the community may be reluctant to send their patients to a different medical complex.[2]

Private practices are established throughout the country in a variety of settings. Some registered dietitians have offices within their homes, in allied health buildings, in office buildings, or in physicians' offices, or they may exist solely through house calls. Practices are designed as solo practices, partnerships, and corporations.

A special dietetic practice group, in the Council on Practice within the ADA, is the "Consulting Nutritionists in Private Practice." Members of this group are Registered Dietitians who have established or plan to establish independent counseling practices throughout the United States, Canada, and Mexico. Through unity and communication the specialty group promotes consistency of quality among its members. Almost every state has a state coordinator for the group who can contact other dietitians in private practice within the state quickly and efficiently.

By combining individuals into a unified force, this professional group is expected to improve medical insurance coverage for physician-referred therapeutic dietary instructions and to create a professional unity visible to the allied health professional and the general public. The group will also provide the opportunity for improvement and growth in each dietitian's practice through planned meetings for continuing education credit.

To contact dietitians in private practice, one may consult the yellow pages of the telephone directory under "Dietitian" or "Nutritionists." Contact may also be made by inquiry to the state or local dietetic association or a major hospital director of dietetics.

DIETARY COUNSELING—PREVENTIVE MEDICINE

Preventive medicine is a well-accepted concept in the effort to improve the health of the nation. Many medical problems are best dealt with before they become medical crises, and proper nutrition is a modality *par excellence.*[16]

The consulting dietitian or nutritionist can assist in evaluating present dietary habits. Some clients, in the absence of illness, are concerned about the quality of their diet for promoting optimal health. Other persons may look for assistance with making deliberate food changes, such as becoming a partial vegetarian.

Weight gain is one aspect of preventive medicine in which the consulting dietitian nutritionist can assist the physician or client. Young children, adolescents, and adults may desire and need to gain weight. Senior citizens sometimes lower their weight to such an extent that preventive dietary counseling may be desirable.

A physician may order some type of surgery which necessitates his patient being in optimal nutritional status before the stress and tissue injury of the surgery. Patients may need to lose weight before surgery can be contemplated owing to the increased risk for obese surgery patients.

Postsurgical care ideally keeps the dietary intake at optimal levels within the restrictions of any necessary therapeutic changes. Home follow-up by the consulting dietitian or nutritionist after surgery can help to maintain appropriate levels of protein and calories, while providing vitamins and minerals necessary for optimal healing to take place.

Consulting dietitians or nutritionists in several areas of the country consult within home environments as well. Close follow-up work enables patients to gain control of diseases that require dietary changes within their own homes.

Dietitians in private practice are equipped to obtain and evaluate nutritional histories, perform dietary assessment, and teach patients to adapt prescribed dietary modifications to their life style. This service is particularly advantageous when multiple dietary restrictions are involved or when a patient needs to be followed over a period of time for dietary intervention. The consulting dietitian or nutritionist can assist the family to adapt special dietary combinations when several family members need dietary modifications.[3] The registered dietitian also reinforces and offers more detailed explanations to patients who are unable to follow a prescribed diet following a hospital diet instruction.

Chronic diseases or poor dietary habits require lifetime dietary modifications. These changes are difficult to comprehend by the patients or families who refuse to "go on a diet," when in reality their dietary habits are already one kind of a "diet." Most people consider diets to be painful or a form of deprivation and thus view food-habit changes in a negative sense.

Dietitians see food habits and therapeutic dietary changes as goal-oriented, with readily measurable objectives to be achieved. The dietitian ideally takes time to explain the benefits of changing dietary habits and how these changes can be measured. The patient then knows where he is going and how he is going to get there, and thus can adopt a more positive attitude toward taking responsibility for directing his behavior toward the new dietary goals. The patient and his family must participate in the dietary management that will eventually develop into permanent appropriate dietary habits for his particular disease or health. The privately practicing registered dietitian is well-positioned to support this effort.

Dietary instruction by a consulting dietitian nutritionist can be seen as four distinct steps: (1) assessing current dietary habits, (2) creating the new therapeutic dietary habits with revisions for better patient acceptance, (3) assistance with implementing the changes, and (4) evaluating the changes made.[2]

Individual likes and dislikes, allergies, and family composition must be considered during the creation of a therapeutic diet. If nutrient supplementation is necessary, the dietitian is in a position to suggest a supplementation to both the patient and the referring physician.

Several methods are available to help the family implement a dietary change. The technique chosen depends on the family's interests. Some techniques could include shopping ideas or practice, menu planning, recipe modification, appropriate use of specially developed products or seasonings, food economy, or ways to incorporate new food habits while entertaining or dining in a restaurant. Other methods include behavior-modification techniques in small group settings.[4]

Evaluations of changes made are assessed by designing suitable records for clients to keep with corresponding weight changes. Discussion of attitude changes is helpful to determine if the new habits will remain long term.

ECONOMICS OF PRIVATE DIETARY COUNSELING

The registered dietitian in private practice in the community may be viewed as economical, in view of historic costs of dietary counseling within institutions. Patients and physicians are well-advised to ask how to obtain economically the best dietary management counsel.

The physician–dietitian team can reduce the frequency of hospitalization and provide necessary management for patients with diabetes, hyperlipidemia, and weight control problems who are screened through physical examinations and routine laboratory procedure in the physician's office.

The patient benefits by avoiding the negative effect of fears associated with hospitalization, and significant savings result for the health insurers.

The patient receives better follow-up and more time for learning with a consulting dietitian or nutritionist at a lower cost than with a heavily scheduled physician. Flexible scheduling is more readily available with a dietitian in private practice.

Individual physicians or small groups of physicians can make referrals to a consulting dietitian or nutritionist from all parts of the community they serve and thereby save themselves the cost of retaining dietitians. They may also wish to subcontract consulting nutritionist services on a fee-for-service basis in their own office.

The insurance industry is now considering third-party payment for therapeutic dietary counseling. In the past, health insurers paid only for crisis and disease-related treatment.[2] This may be extended to preventive medicine and already has begun to provide payments for mental health.[6]

Reimbursement of dietary counseling fees rarely occurs at the present time, although some labor union policies reimburse clients for such outpatient services. The majority of clients personally pay the charges for dietary counseling, which are considered medical expenses by the Internal Revenue Service. When the insurance industry does move toward dietary coverage, professional qualifications will be closely related to the fee reimbursement. Dietetic registration as a requirement separate from membership in the ADA will probably be necessary for the inclusion of nutritional services under this third-party payment scheme.

QUALITY OF CARE

In the opinion of many, the patient obtains improved care from a team approach. Physician and allied health professionals together use their expertise in an expedient manner, thus saving valuable time and money for the patient. The dietitian in this team personalizes dietary instruction and is capable of expending the effort necessary to use the best teaching and behavioral tools available for each patient's individual needs and desires. The dietitian, as a consulting nutritionist, is particularly able to keep abreast of the expanding body of knowledge from nutrition scientists as well as the medical research dealing with nutrition. The communication feedback system between physician, dietitian, and patient allows consistent treatment, leading to greater progress and satisfaction for the client.

Hospital dietitians can refer patients for outpatient care and follow-up to the privately practicing consulting dietitian nutritionist. This continuation of health care outside the hospital increases the probability of dietary compliance and attitude changes necessary for long-term improved health.

Conclusion

There is a well-documented relationship between adequate nutrition and health, vigor, and achievement. Poor nutrition can lead to poor health, reduced work output, and low morale. Good nutritional status is regarded as a desirable health-related goal. It is necessary to recognize that eating behaviors are learned. When nutritional care services are recognizably a part of the community health team, the opportunity is available for the individual to learn new more appropriate behaviors based on medical evaluations.

Nutrition care availability in the community will become a resource for the public to obtain reliable nutrition information. Privately practicing dietitians as consulting nutritionists can provide better information to people in the community than earlier sources, often misinformed, have in the past.

Preventive nutritional care is indeed a concrete way of decreasing the effect of poor nutrition and poor eating habits as major contributing factors in several expensive health problems, such as birth defects, anemia, diabetes, coronary heart disease, hypertension, diverticulitis, obesity, and dental disease. In certain of these cases, diet becomes the basic means of managing the disease or maintaining health. Therapeutic nutrition education will probably shorten the time necessary for a person to reach certain health goals and therefore lessen the total amount of service needed, thereby reducing the cost of health care.

Health insurance coverage for dietary counseling and any national health insurance program adopted to provide both preventive and restorative nutritional care will solve numerous costly nutritional problems of the past. The current public interest in nutrition, the recognition of the significance of nutritional care to the maintenance and improvement of health, and the rising concern of government for making quality health care available to all people, all point to the greater use of registered dietitians and nutritionists in the community.

The health-care team already has used registered dietitian nutritionists in health maintenance organizations, day care programs, and programs for the aging.[5] Now it is time to include the privately practicing dietitian and nutritionist, outside the hospital or special program, working with the physician, as part of the community's health-care team.

References

1. The American Dietetic Association Fact Sheet Nutritional Care—Dietary Counseling, Chicago, October 1974
2. Donahoe CT: Realities in Private Practice, 3rd ed, Pasadena, Nutrition Plus, 1982
3. Dresser CV, Roth JH: Private practice: Nutritional counseling, perspectives in practice. J Am Diet Assoc 69:475, 1975
4. Ferguson J: Dietitians as behavior–change agents. J Am Diet Assoc 73:231, 1978
5. Light I: Challenging perceptions of the health team members. J Am Diet Assoc 59:13, 1971
6. Myers ES: Insurance lowers the barriers to mental health care. Med Insight 3:42, 1971
7. Ohlson MA: The philosophy of dietary counseling. J Am Diet Assoc 63:13, 1973
8. Oller JA: The dietitian in community home programs. J Am Diet Assoc 76:267, 1980
9. Parant D: Starting a Private Practice—One Dietitian's Experience. New Haven, D Parant, 1974
10. Peck EB: The public health nutritionist–dietitian: An historical perspective. J Am Diet Assoc 64:642, 1974
11. Perspective 1974: Unusual positions and newer dietetic specialties: Perspectives in practice. J Am Diet Assoc 64:649, 1974
12. Recommended Dietary Allowances. Washington DC, National Academy of Sciences, 1980
13. Titles, definitions and responsibilities for the profession of dietetics. J Am Diet Assoc 64:661, 1974
14. Tobias AL, Gordon JB: Social consequences of obesity. J Am Diet Assoc 76:338, 1980
15. Trithart ES, Noel MB: New dimensions: The dietitian in private practice. J Am Diet Assoc 73:60, 1978
16. Winterfeldt EA: The president's page. J Am Diet Assoc 76:490, 1980

7
Community Nutrition Resources

Anita L. Owen
David Baird Coursin

The nutritional well-being of the nation is a central concern of the dietetics and nutrition profession and, to some, predates medicine itself. H. M. Sinclair made this observation: "Medicine arose from dietetics; the Pythagoreans, including Hippocrates, used diet to prevent and cure diseases, and drugs only if these failed."[3]

In the past decade, the physician has effectively applied the science of nutrition to improved management of the hospitalized patient, but prevention of disease and the promotion of health are of increasing interest to physicians, dietitians and nutritionists. As expenditures for curative care escalate, understanding of diet and life style, considered to play a major role in the promotion of "wellness," must be encouraged by health-care providers, including dietitians and nutritionists. In earlier chapters (see Chaps. 5 and 6), the role of the dietitian has been described in relation to the physician in the hospital and in private practice. In this chapter, this is expanded to the community, narrowly or broadly defined, from which the patient emerges and to which he returns. The community can thus be considered as a public part of the environment, and its nutritional features naturally compel attention. The fact that this environment has public features has opened the door to governmental attention and policy formation. Community dietitians and nutritionists are the visible mentors and purveyors of these community-wide influences, and the alert physician will be aware of these.

The Patient in the Nutrition Landscape

Available evidence indicates that current dietary habits and certain food elements may be linked with health problems as diverse as heart disease, tooth decay, obesity, and some types of cancer, yet consumers often find it difficult to make informed choices about food.[7] The consumer is bombarded with confusing and even conflicting information from books, newspapers, magazine articles, and advertising, thus making the wise selection of food even more complex.

Today one out of two American families is cutting back in some essential health area in order to cope with inflation. The figures are higher for low income families, minorities, and single parents.

There is a backlash against the constant barrage of information about products hazardous to health. And, despite all of the material on health released by the government and available in the media, only about one in four families feels well-informed about good health practices.

Sedentary jobs are only partly responsible for physical inactivity. Women working outside the home and increased leisure-time alternatives have placed time constraints on many families. Most families are more interested in relaxing, watching television, or going out to a restaurant or the movies than they are in exercising regularly.

Two recent reports provide some useful insights into the consumers' views of health and nutrition. The General Mills reports concluded that the majority of American families are ready to accept in principle a new and more active approach to health and health care—one that would require supplementing traditional means of health care with new approaches aimed primarily at preventing health problems before they arise.[10,22] Yet only a small minority are even beginning to put these new beliefs into action, with many obstacles still to be overcome before families are prepared to make the life style changes necessary to improve their health.[22] These are some of the major barriers, presented in the reports, that need to be dealt with if the preventive health message is to be understood and if the health practices of Americans are to be significantly and appropriately changed.[22]

At the same time, there are some optimistic trends in health attitudes and behavior:

1. Health is a subject of growing interest and concern and is given a high priority by families.
2. A new set of personal values, emphasizing self-realization, has helped to create an emphasis on physical well-being.
3. Americans show signs of concern about cholesterol, fats, and additives in the diet, which were not matters of concern in the past.
4. Overweight is recognized as a serious health hazard.
5. Crash diets are regarded by many persons as a serious health hazard.
6. In many areas of health care, there is evidence that extensive education has been accomplished, although more effective means of motivating family members to better practices must be found.
7. American family members feel confident about the medical profession and their own physicians. For most, the problem is not the quality of medical care, but the cost.
8. The knowledge of how a nutritious, healthful diet can be selected has no influence on an individual's health status unless it is translated into positive attitudes and behavior—good dietary habits.
9. When consumers are well informed and motivated about nutrition, it is reflected in their eating behavior. Consumers, who relate excessive ingestion of calories, fat, and cholesterol to an increased risk of heart disease, have cut down on their consumption of calories, cholesterol, and saturated fats.

Analysis of 32 recent surveys on nutrition, knowledge, attitudes and practices of consumers revealed the following information:[10]

1. While consumers have traditionally considered cost, convenience, and family taste preferences in their food choices, in recent years increasing concern about the overall "healthfulness" of the food supply, nutritional quality, and food safety has developed.
2. The traditional "Basic Four" concept is understood in general terms by most consumers. However, some consider certain of the food groups to contribute to the nutritional quality of the diet and others to detract from it. For example, the meat group is perceived by some to be more important nutritionally than the bread–cereal group.
3. Consumers appear to have negative attitudes toward certain nutrients and ingredients in food. This is especially evident in the area of food processing and calorie control.

Two thirds of American adults believe that they would be healthier if they made some changes in their diet. Changes that the largest number of people see as desirable include increased consumption of fruits, fish or poultry, whole grain bread, and fresh or frozen vegetables and decreased intake of fried foods, sugar, soft drinks, salt, coffee, pretzels and potato chips, and white bread.[12]

The role of the dietitian and nutritionist in providing quality nutrition services in the community, outside the hospital, will be discussed in the sections to follow (see Chaps. 5 and 6).

The Nutrition Component of the Health-Care System

Since adequate food and sound nutrition are essential to good health, every effort must be made to counsel patients and clients about sound nutrition practices.

The American Medical Association's definition of nutrition describes the broad scope of this subject:

> Nutrition is the science of food, the nutrients and other substances therein, their action, interaction and balance in relation to health and disease, and the process by which the organism ingests, digests, absorbs, transports, utilizes and excretes food substances. In addition, nutrition must be concerned with social, economic, cultural and psychological implications of food and eating.[7]

The role of environmental factors in nutritional diseases is the result of their effect on the availability of nutrients, nutrition requirements, and the intake of nutrients. The environment includes not only the important physical and ecological environment but also the social or cultural environment. As our nation looks for ways to prevent disease and to improve health delivery systems and the quality of care for our citizens, the science of nutrition becomes important.

Physicians, dietitians or nutritionists, nurses, and other health-care providers are often prone to think in terms of pathology and therapy when considering the subject of nutrition, but the majority of Americans are basically healthy. Therefore, attention may well be drawn to normal nutrition in its most positive aspects, to the preventive role of nutrition, and to the changing life style of the population.[18]

Nutrition services, integrated with medical and social services, ideally should be included at all levels of the health-care delivery system. The primary level of community care focuses on the welfare of the whole individual and provides an assessment of people's needs. At the secondary and tertiary levels, health care becomes increasingly specialized, but nutrition services may constitute either a major part of the treatment plan or a part of the ancillary life-support system (see Chap. 5).

Community-Oriented Nutrition Services

Quality nutrition services can be achieved best by providing continuity of care from the hospital setting to the community and to the home setting. Intensive care units are at one end of the spectrum and community health centers at the other; nutrition services have a major role throughout the entire spectrum.

The five basic elements required to deliver quality nutrition care in community settings include the following:

1. Screening and assessment
2. Intervention, including nutrition education, nutrition counseling, and referral
3. Assessing quality of nutrition services
4. Data collection and recording
5. Monitoring and evaluation

NUTRITION SCREENING AND ASSESSMENT

In order to identify nutrition problems in individuals or groups, nutrition screening and assessment must occur. Screening is the process by which various parameters are evaluated in groups or individuals for the purpose of identifying those persons likely to be at greatest risk. Once these individuals have been identified through the screening process, a more detailed evaluation and assessment of nutrition status is undertaken.

Assessment of the nutrition status of individuals includes the following components:

1. Dietary assessment, which includes review of food availability and dietary practices, which in turn may reflect socioeconomic, cultural, and other factors.
2. Biochemical measurements of body fluids and tissue
3. Clinical examination by a physician
4. Anthropometric examination; assessment of growth

The American Public Health Association has published a useful guide to nutritional assessment to assist the physician, dietitian or nutritionist, and other health workers in completing various levels of assessment in specific age groups.[4] The guide includes minimal, mid-level, and in-depth approaches. These levels have been designed for infants and children from birth to 24 months of age, 2 to 5 years old, and 6 to 12 years old; for adolescents; for pregnant women; for adults, and for the elderly. The dietary, medical, socioeconomic, clinical, and laboratory assessments are covered. (For further discussion of nutritional assessment see Chap. 10.)

INTERVENTION—PREVENTION, TREATMENT, AND FOLLOW-UP SERVICES

The three major elements of community nutrition intervention are nutrition counseling, nutrition education, and referral for additional services, including food assistance programs.

NUTRITION COUNSELING

Nutrition counseling is the process by which clients are most effectively helped to acquire more healthful behaviors.[15] In attempting to counsel, consideration should be given to understanding the client's problems and concerns and those of other persons such as family, peers, and colleagues who interact with the client and the health team.

The screening and assessment results are the first tools to be used in determining a client's care plan for nutrition counseling. Counseling may be carried out to obtain more information about the individual and his family, to teach new information so as to review and strengthen acquired knowledge and desirable habits, or to help the individual set goals and make decisions.

The composite roles of the counselor in client-centered nutrition counseling are those of communicator, facilitator, and manager. These roles are supported by the nutrition knowledge base, understanding of human behavior, and those skills that are essential to the varying roles.[15] The term *nutrition counseling* is often used in conjunction with clinical practice, but this may include community modalities as well.

A recent report by the American Dietetic Association addressed the potential health outcomes and economic benefits from sound nutrition counseling.[6] Potential health and economic benefits include reduction in mortality, disability, and debility, and use of crisis medical care.

NUTRITION EDUCATION

Nutrition education, including community nutrition education, promotes beliefs, attitudes, environmental influences, and an understanding about food that lead to practices that are scientifically sound, practical, and consistent with individual needs and available food resources.[2] Nutrition education should be addressed to an individual or group at a suitable level, including appropriate cultural adaptations. Because of its preventive aspects, nutrition education is profitably included at all levels of the health delivery system.

For efforts in nutrition to be successful they should do the following:

1. Assess the needs of the individual or group
2. State objectives that are measurable, feasible, or able to be accomplished in a stated period of time
3. Determine content based on the assessment of needs and statement of objectives
4. Select techniques that are appropriate to the ages, educational and cultural backgrounds, and problems of the individual or group
5. Evaluate progress at stated periods of time in order to review, continue, and make changes in program design

The dietitian or nutritionist must be knowledgeable about behavioral-change strategies. The difficulties in motivating changes in eating behavior and other health behaviors are well known to the health community.

Some concepts that nutrition educators should keep in mind in obtaining behavioral change include the following:[11]

1. Information alone is often not enough to cause or enable a person to improve his eating habits and nutritional status.
2. The benefits of improved nutrition habits may be delayed, as in the case of weight reduction, or not directly experienced, as in the case of averted illness.
3. It is difficult to offer a sound nutritional alternative to combat the conflicting and often highly emotional claims that immediate benefits can be achieved through the use of specific foods or food patterns.
4. The goal is to promote variety in food selection and to be sensitive to the range of acceptable choices associated with ethnic, economic, geographic, and age variations in our society.

Evans and Hall stress the importance of the patient's assuming responsibility for his own behavior.[8] Zifferblatt and Wilbur indicate that there are a number of illusions that hinder nutrition counselors in their efforts.[23] One such illusion is that dietary counseling forcefully guides the patient in assuming responsibility and in learning skills for managing his own dietary habits.

Vickstrom and Fox addressed nurses' knowledge and attitudes about nutrition.[20] In general, nurses had favorable attitudes toward nutrition. Although their knowledge was adequate, they lacked confidence in their ability to impart the information. Older nurses had more favorable attitudes, but were less knowledgeable than younger ones. More knowledgeable nurses had more positive attitudes toward their own role in nutrition education and toward the team approach to health care.

General practitioners, pediatricians, and obstetricians in British Columbia were surveyed concerning their opinions and practices regarding maternal and infant nutrition.[14] Scores were significantly higher for physicians who (1) were female, (2) consulted with a dietitian or nutritionist, (3) had additional training, (4) attended continuing education training, and (5) had studied nutrition in medical school. Pediatricians' and obstetricians' practice scores were significantly higher than those of general practitioners.

REFERRAL SYSTEMS

Referral procedures provide an opportunity for individuals and groups to take advantage of services available from various sources. A properly coordinated health-service delivery system can contribute to a consumer's sense of continuity and to the consistency of care and advice.[9]

Physicians should be aware of existing food assistance programs in their communities, since they are an important part of nutrition services available to high-risk groups. Indigent patients in the community may be eligible for these services. Most of the major food assistance programs are administered by the United States Department of Agriculture (USDA), including the following: School Lunch, School Breakfast, Supplemental Food Service, Child Care Food Program, Special Milk Program, Food

Stamps, Commodity Distribution, and the Special Supplemental Food Program for Women, Infants and Children (WIC).

The Department of Health and Human Services administers the Title III Program, which is the National Nutrition Program for the Elderly.

Table 7-1 provides a list of these federally financed food assistance programs available in most counties throughout the country, with information on the purposes and objectives of these programs.

ASSESSING QUALITY-OF-NUTRITION SERVICES

Quality-of-nutrition services can be considered in three categories: structure, process, and outcome. *Structure* is related to the environmental and personnel factors in delivery of services, such as the adequacy of the facility, availability of equipment, and availability of skilled personnel. *Process* deals with the interaction between providers and patients and with follow-up of problems over time. The main focus of this element has traditionally been the medical record. In nutritional assessment, the pertinent medical record is generated by determining the biochemical, clinical, dietary, and anthropometric indices. This information provides the data base for implementing a plan to correct a problem and for measuring the *outcome.*

DATA COLLECTION AND RECORDING

On an individual client basis, the problem-oriented medical record (POMR) is an acceptable method for recording data. The POMR is particularly adaptable to nutrition services and is based on four essential elements of health care: (1) a data base, (2) problem identification, (3) plan formulation, and (4) progress notes.

Nutrition *surveillance* involves frequent and continuous watching over a specific population. It provides for the early detection of community nutrition problems so that they can be quickly corrected. A good surveillance system not only gathers and analyzes data but also quickly presents the data to those who make administrative decisions that will affect the health and nutrition of the community.

On a population basis, the Center for Disease Control Nutrition Surveillance System has the greatest potential for developing data sources on local nutrition problems.[16] In 1980, 25 state public health departments were involved in nutrition surveillance of pediatric populations in the United States.

MONITORING AND EVALUATION

Evaluation may be described as the process of determining the value of, or amount of success in achieving, a predetermined objective. Evaluation is a two-step process that includes measurement and comparison.

James has listed several major rules of evaluation for the health-care provider that can be applied to nutrition programs:[13]

1. The practical objective of each program to be evaluated should be clearly stated.
2. The underlying assumption of validity associated with these objectives should be meticulously identified.
3. Evaluations should always be done according to effort. Evaluation by performance, adequacy of performance, and efficiency should be done whenever possible.
4. The entire program should be reexamined in light of the findings.
5. The status of all significant conditions associated with the use of the standard must be specified.

Community Nutrition Resources

Table 7-2 provides guidelines for delivery of nutrition services in a community. These guidelines cover the elements of quality nutrition services, including nutritional assessment, intervention strategies, and referral sources. The guidelines are presented for pregnant women, infants and children, adolescents, adults, and the elderly.

With a growing awareness that more attention should be given to nutrition considerations in the practice of medicine, the New York Academy of Medicine Committee on Public Health recently took official action by issuing a statement entitled "Recommendations Concerning Consulting Dietitians in Private Practice."[17] These recommendations clarify for the physician the selection of qualified dietitians or nutritionists to provide nutrition counseling for patients. It describes the qualifications and professional responsibilities for both the dietitian or nutritionist and the physician (see Chap. 6).

At the White House Conference on Food, Nutrition and Health in 1969, dietitians and nutritionists were identified as the only health professionals whose education and training have been directed toward the application of food and nutrition science to the health care of people.[21] As a "specialist educated for a profession responsible for the nutritional care of individuals and groups," the registered dietitian (RD) not only has completed

TABLE 7-1
Federally Financed Food Assistance Programs

Agency, Program— Administering Agencies	Purpose of Program	Objective of Program
Department of Agriculture: Food Stamp Program—USDA, Food and Nutrition Service (FNS), and state welfare agencies	Assist families in providing nutritious meals	Permit eligible households to buy food stamps at less than face value for purchase of food at authorized retail stores
Special Supplemental Food Program for Women, Infants, and Children (WIC)—USDA, FNS, and state health agencies	Assist mothers in obtaining specified nutritious foods for herself, infants, and children	Provide vouchers for purchase of foods to qualifying pregnant and lactating women, new mothers up to 1 year postpartum, and children up to 5 years old
National School Lunch Program—FNS and state educational agencies	Safeguard the health and well-being of the nation's children and educate children about proper food habits	Provide meals free or at reduced prices to children attending participating schools (high school, grade school, or under)
School Breakfast Program—FNS and state educational agencies	Serve nutritious breakfasts to needy children or those who travel distances	Provide meals free or at reduced prices to children attending participating schools (high school, grade school, or under)
Special Milk Program—FNS, state educational agencies, and public or private nonprofit day care centers and summer camps	Encourage the consumption of fluid whole milk by children	Provide subsidy for milk served to children in participating schools, child care centers, and summer camps; free milk to needy
Summer Food Program—FNS, state educational agencies, and public or private nonprofit summer camps	Initiate, maintain, or expand foodservice programs to children in summer camps	Provide meals or snacks to children at participating institutions
Child Care Food Program—FNS, state educational agencies, and public or private nonprofit day care centers	Initiate, maintain, or expand foodservice programs to children in child care centers	Provide free meals or supplemental snacks to children in participating institutions
Food Donation, Commodity Distribution Programs	Encourage and maintain the domestic consumption of commodities; prevent the waste of commodities	Use foods donated by USDA to needy persons and institutions
Title III Nutrition Services—HHS, Office of Human Development for aging, and state agencies on aging	Provide low-cost nutritious meals to the elderly who are needy, lack meal preparation skills, have limited mobility, or are lonely	Provide at least one hot meal per day 5 days a week as well as social contact for the elderly
Community Services Administration, Community Food and Nutrition—Community Services Administration Office of Operations and local sponsoring organizations	Reduce the incidence of hunger and malnutrition and improve the nutritional status of the poor	Improve participation in federal food programs; provide food directly to target population; supplement and fill gaps in existing food programs; mobilize other resources toward local feeding problems

(Owen AL, Owen GM, Lanna G: Health and Nutritional Benefits of Federal Food Assistance Programs in Costs and Benefits of Nutritional Care Phase I, Chicago, The American Dietetic Association, October 1979.

basic academic and experience requirements and has passed the qualifying examination for registration, but is also required to update her knowledge with continuing education activities[5] (see Chap. 5).

The physician may obtain further assistance in nutrition information from the following areas:

STATE AND LOCAL LEVELS

1. Public health nutritionists in the state and local health departments
2. Dietitians or nutritionists in voluntary agencies such as local Diabetes Associations, local Heart Associations, or Visiting Nurse Associations

(Text continues on p. 96)

TABLE 7-2
Guidelines for Population Groups in Community Nutrition

Pregnant Women

Determining Risk	Standard Criteria (Technique/Equipment/Standards)	Problem	General Guidelines	Sample Client Behavioral Objectives	Referral Sources
				Intervention	
Anthropometric					
Height Prepregnant weight	Steel tape measure Balance scales	Short stature Underweight	Promote adequate weight gain and nutrient intake	Client will identify difference between nutrient needs during pregnant and nonpregnant states	Maternal and Infant Care Project Prenatal care
Weight gain	Follow pattern of National Academy of Balances weight gain grid	Weight loss or inadequate weight gain		Participant will plot and determine the components of her weight gain during pregnancy	WIC Program Food stamps
Biochemical					
Hemoglobin Hematocrit	Center for Disease Control Standards adjusted for altitude	Anemia Diabetes Toxemia	Promote regular and early use of prenatal services	Participant will identify reasons for early use of prenatal services and relationship to outcome of pregnancy	Regional perinatal programs
Urine	Stick test for sugar, ketones, protein				
Clinical					
Obstetric history Blood pressure	Questionnaire Sphygmomanometer	Repeated pregnancy and lactation at intervals of less than 1 year	Encourage decision on breast or bottle feeding during last trimester	Participant will identify reasons to *breast feed* or *bottle feed* an infant	Title XIX
Smoking, alcohol, and drug intake questionnaire		Previous problem pregnancies High parity Mothers 19 or 35 years old Smoking, alcohol, and drug use increase risk of low birth weight or birth defects Pica and allergies			Maternal and Child Health Services
Dietary					
24-hour recall or food frequency	24-hour recall or food frequency form				

Measure	Method	Finding	Intervention	Objective	Resources/Referral
Anthropometric					
Height Weight Head circumference (to 2 years of age)	Balance scales, steel measuring tape, infant measuring board, calipers; National Center for Health Statistics (NCHS) growth grids	Poor growth (ht/age <5th percentile, wt/ht <5th percentile, head circumference <5th percentile)	Rule out child abuse or neglect Check diet for energy and nutrient adequacy	Parent will plot and interpret screening values for height, weight, and head circumference on growth grids	Private physician WIC Program Children and Youth Crippled Children's Services Regional center for high-risk newborns Title XIX (Early Periodic Screening, Diagnosis, and Treatment Program) Head Start
Skinfold thickness (over 5 years of age)	Triceps skinfold according to Seltzer and Mayer, Postgrad. Med. 38: A-101, 1965	Failure to thrive (drop in position on growth grid)	Check feeding environment	Parent will explain relationship between weight/height and health problems	
		Obesity (wt/ht >95th percentile)	Aim for child to "grow into" ideal weight range rather than lose weight	Parent will identify ideal weight for his/her infant	
Biochemical					
Hemoglobin Hematocrit Serum cholesterol	Center for Disease Control Standards; adjusted for altitude Cyanmethemoglobin method for hemoglobin Wybenga method on microsample	Anemia	Identify cause of anemia (malabsorption, dietary, bleeding)	Parent/participant will identify causes, symptoms, and consequences of anemia	Child Abuse and Neglect Center Food Stamps Commodity foods
		Elevated serum cholesterol (>160 mg/dl)	Investigate other cardiovascular disease risk factors	Client/parent will identify cardiovascular disease risk factors and state those which can be modified	
Clinical					
Birth weight Blood pressure Dental caries	Sphygmomanometer with child-size cuff; quiet environment	Birth weight <5½ lb.	Monitor low birth weight infant to determine catch-up growth rate	Parent explains meaning of systolic and diastolic readings	
		Diastolic blood pressure for 3- to 12-year-olds greater than 90 mm/Hg	Caution should be exercised in labeling children as hypertensive because of psychosocial and economic implications; use of term "high normal blood pressure" is appropriate during evaluation and follow-up*	Parent explains factors that contribute to hypertension	

*Report of the Task Force on Blood Pressure Control in Children, Pediatrics Supplement, vol. 59, May, 1977.
(Frankle R, Owen A: Nutrition in the Community: The Art of Delivering Services. CV Mosby, St. Louis, 1978.)

TABLE 7-2 (cont.)
Guidelines for Population Groups in Community Nutrition

Determining Risk	Standard Criteria (Technique/ Equipment/Standards)	Problem	Intervention		
			General Guidelines	Sample Client Behavioral Objectives	Referral Source
Dietary 24-hour recall or food frequency Feeding development	24-hour recall or food frequency form	At risk of nutrient and energy intake inappropriate to age according to RDA	Identify key nutrients, function, and food sources Describe introduction of foods and food preparation Discuss weaning	Parent will explain factors affecting weight gain during infancy Parent will identify eating problems occurring during infancy leading to obesity Parent will identify appropriate feeding skills for their infant or child	

		Adolescents			
Anthropometric Height Weight Skinfold thickness	Balance scales, steel measuring tape, calipers NCHS growth grids for ht/age and wt/age and wt/ht before puberty	Teenage pregnancy Obesity (wt/ht >95th percentile in prepuberty)	Concentrate on fact that mother is still physiologically developing, as well as supporting growth of fetus Explain rotation between weight, self-image, and poor acceptance	Client will identify reason for increase of nutrient and energy needs due to (1) her own physiologic development, and (2) her pregnant state Client will explain how obesity relates to social problems in adolescence, hypertension, diabetes, cardiovascular disease risk, and obesity as an adult	Prenatal care WIC Program Maternal and Infant Care Project Weight Watchers International, Inc. Physical fitness programs and recreational facilities

Assessment	Methods/Standards	Risk factor	Intervention	Behavioral objective	Resources
Biochemical Hemoglobin Hematocrit Serum cholesterol	Center for Disease Control Standards; adjusted for altitude Cyanmethemoglobin method for hemoglobin Wybenga method on microsample	Anorexia nervosa	Concentrate on psychological factors and influence of entire family	Client will identify ideal weight for age and sex and identify health risks associated with rapid weight loss	Physician, psychologist, or guidance center
Clinical Blood pressure Dental caries Drug and alcohol abuse and venereal disease questionnaire	Sphygmomanometer; quiet environment	Alcohol and drug abuse	Investigate social environment in terms of peer pressure and peer acceptance	Client will state energy/nutrient requirements and explain how substance abuse affects satisfying these requirements	Drug treatment centers Alcoholics Anonymous Free clinics Neighborhood health centers Nontraditional alternative health centers
Dietary 24-hour recall or food frequency Feeding development	24-hour recall or food frequency form	At risk of nutrient and energy intake inappropriate to age according to RDA	Identify key nutrients, function, and food sources Describe introduction of foods and food preparation Discuss weaning	Parent will explain factors affecting weight gain during infancy Parent will identify eating problems occurring during infancy leading to obesity Parent will identify appropriate feeding skills for their infant or child	
Adults					
Anthropometric Height Weight Skinfold thickness	Balance scales Steel tape measure, calipers	Obesity (>20% over ideal weight for height)	Relate obesity to chronic health problems	Client will explain association between obesity and chronic health problems	Weight Watchers International, Inc. Physical fitness

(Frankle R, Owen A: Nutrition in the Community: The Art of Delivering Services. CV Mosby, St. Louis, 1978)

TABLE 7-2 (cont.)

			Adults		
				Intervention	
Determining Risk	Standard Criteria (Technique/ Equipment/Standards)	Problem	General Guidelines	Sample Client Behavioral Objectives	Referral Source
	Metropolitan Life Insurance Height and Weight tables Triceps skinfold according to Seltzer and Mayer, Postgrad. Med. 38: A-101, 1965		Develop personalized intervention plan on desirable life-style modifications that include diet and exercise	Client will identify which disease risk factors he has and how he can modify them	program and recreational facilities
Biochemical Hemoglobin Hematocrit Serum cholesterol and other lipids Blood glucose	Center for Disease Control Standards, adjusted for altitude	Anemia Diabetes Elevated cholesterol (>200 mg/dl) Hyperlipidemias, Types I to V Hypertension (blood pressure >140/90 mm Hg)	Concentrate on personal diet modifications using diabetes exchange list	Client will describe rotation between insulin, physical activity, and diet intake and importance of reaching and maintaining ideal weight to control diabetes	Food stamps
Clinical Blood pressure Cardiovascular disease risk factor questionnaire; family history, diabetes, smoking, physical activity, stress	Sphygmomanometer Treadmill, lung function test	Risk of heart attack, stroke, and certain cancers (lung, esophagus, bladder) increases with number and severity of risk factors such as overweight, fat intake, hypertension, elevated cholesterol, smoking, inactivity, and stress			Stop smoking clinics Alcoholics Anonymous
Dietary 24-hour recall or food frequency	24-hour recall or food frequency form	Alcoholism and drug abuse	Investigate causal factors in substance abuse and suggest coping mechanisms	Client will state energy/nutrient requirements and explain how substance abuse affects satisfying	

Anthropometric Height Weight Skinfold thickness	Balance scales Steel tape measure, calipers Metropolitan Life Insurance height and weight tables Triceps skinfold according to Seltzer and Mayer, Postgrad. Med. 38: A-101, 1965	Obesity (20% over ideal weight for height)	Increase nutrient density of diet to adjust for decreased energy need Stress importance of food in social environment	Client will identify own decreased energy needs and name specific foods high in nutrients, low in calories Client will identify food/social programs for which he is eligible and which are available in his community	Weight Watchers International, Inc. Title VII Congregate meal site Meals on Wheels Food stamps
Biochemical Hemoglobin Hematocrit Serum cholesterol and other lipids Blood glucose	Center for Disease Control Standards, adjusted for altitude	Anemia Diabetes Elevated cholesterol (with elevated proportion of low density to high density lipoproteins)		
Clinical Blood pressure Cardiovascular disease risk factor questionnaire; family history, diabetes, smoking, physical activity, stress Dental Socioeconomic status	Sphygmomanometer Treadmill; lung function test	Hypertension (blood pressure > 140/90 mm Hg) Risk of heart attack, stroke and certain cancers (lung, esophagus, bladder); increases with number and severity of risk factors such as overweight, fat intake, hypertension, elevated cholesterol, smoking, inactivity, and stress Osteoporosis		
Dietary 24-hour recall or food frequency	24-hour recall or food frequency form	Inadequate food intake due to poor dentures, low income, and deprived social environment		

(Frankle R, Owen A: Nutrition in the Community: The Art of Delivering Services. St. Louis, CV Mosby, 1978.)

[95]

3. Dietitians or nutritionists in clinics, health centers, and hospitals
4. Dietitians or nutritionists in Headstart programs at the regional, state, and local levels
5. Professional organizations such as the American Dietetic Association and the Society for Nutrition Education, with their state or local affiliate chapters
6. University nutrition faculty members
7. State Departments of Education, particularly the Nutrition Education Training Program (NET)
8. Local affiliations of the National Dairy Council
9. State and local welfare agencies

NATIONAL LEVEL

1. U.S. Department of Health and Human Services
   Health Services Administration/Bureau of Community Health Services
   Food and Drug Administration, Rockville, Maryland.
2. U.S. Department of Agriculture
   Agricultural Research Service
   Consumer and Food Economics Research Division
   Food and Nutrition Service
   Federal Extension Service, Washington, D.C.
3. National Academy of Sciences
   Food and Nutrition Board, Division of Biological Sciences, Assembly of Life Sciences, National Research Council, Washington, D.C.
4. U.S. Government Printing Office, Superintendent of Documents
   (mailing list for publications related to food, nutrition, and health), Washington, D.C.
5. American Academy of Pediatrics, Evanston, Illinois.
6. The American College of Obstetricians and Gynecologists, Chicago, Illinois.
7. The American Home Economics Association, Washington, D.C.
8. American Institute of Nutrition, Bethesda, Maryland.
9. The American Medical Association, Chicago, Illinois.
10. American Public Health Association, Food and Nutrition Section, Washington, D.C.
11. Society for Nutrition Education, Berkeley, California.

Community Nutrition Advice— The Case of the Americans

The ethnic, geographic, cultural, and educational diversities of the people of the United States warn against too facile a generalization in any particular. This is true for the American diet and for the putative but, in some instances, unclear role of nutrition in the public health. Recognition of such diversity is not nihilism, but rather honesty in the face of facts.

It must be recognized that in the aggregate of citizens, certain nutritional practices in choosing a dietary are now emerging as a phenomenon in national life. The physician should be aware of these influences on the patient as an important fact in the description of the nutritional environment.

The growing national interest in human nutrition has been reflected recently in governmental advice, and it is probable that this response will continue to be sensitive to political forces. That human nutrition should attract political interest is in itself a tribute to the growing perception that nutrition is a manipulatable determinant in the pursuit of an improved quality of life. In the United States, however, even governmental advice given *ex cathedra* cannot escape criticism. As a result of criticism by professional groups, and in the face of lack of consensus, the most prudent advice is probably the most conservative.[1,19] By this criterion the publication of the Food and Nutrition Board of the National Research Council merits mention here. The final comments on "Conclusions and Recommendations," in "Toward Healthful Diets" are as follows:[19]

Select a nutritionally adequate diet from the foods available, by consuming each day appropriate servings of dairy products, meats or legumes, vegetables and fruits, and cereals and breads.

Select as wide a variety of foods in each of the major food groups as is practicable in order to ensure a high probability of consuming adequate quantities of all essential nutrients.

Adjust dietary energy intake and energy expenditure so as to maintain appropriate weight for height; if overweight, achieve appropriate weight reduction by decreasing a total food and fat intake and by increasing physical activity.

If the requirement for energy is low (*e.g.*, reducing diet) reduce consumption of such foods as alcohol, sugars, fats, and oils, which provide calories but few other essential nutrients.

Use salt in moderation; adequate but safe intakes are considered to range between 3 g and 8 g of sodium chloride daily.

It is probably inevitable that community nutrition, in its trends and in its resources, will continue to reflect nationally perceived goals. Knowledge will bring change. It is the final responsibility of the physician to adapt such broad generalizations to the particulars presented by the patient.

In his larger role as a member of the community, the physician should insist on the maintenance of rigorous scientific standards in the continuing process of formulating community nutrition policies.

References

1. Ahrens EH et al: The evidence relating six dietary factors to the nation's health. Am J Clin Nutr 32:2621–2748, 1979
2. The American Dietetic Association position paper on nutrition education for the public. J Amer Diet Assoc 62:429–430, 1973
3. Birch GG, Green LF, Pasketts LG (eds): Health and Food. New York, John Wiley & Sons, 1972
4. Chritakis G (ed): Nutritional assessment in health programs (Supplement). American Journal of Public Health 63:1, 1973
5. Committee to Develop a Glossary of Terminology for the Association and Profession, American Dietetic Association: Titles, definitions and responsibilities for the profession of dietetics. J Amer Diet Assoc 64:661, 1974
6. Costs and Benefits of Nutritional Care Phase I, The American Dietetic Association, Chicago, October 1979
7. Department of Health, Education, and Welfare: Healthy People, The Surgeon General's Report on Health Promotion and Disease Prevention (DHEW No 79-55071). Washington, DC, US Government Printing Office, 1979
8. Evans RI, Hall Y: Social psychological perspective on motivating change in eating behavior. J Amer Diet Assoc 72(4):378–382, 1978
9. Frankle RT, Owen AY: Nutrition in the Community: The Art of Delivering Services. St Louis, CV Mosby, 1978
10. General Mills, Inc: A summary report on US consumers' knowledge, attitudes and practices about nutrition. Minneapolis, 1979
11. Guthrie HA: Is education enough? J Nutr Education 10:2, June 1978
12. Harris, Louis and Associates, Inc: Health Maintenance, Pacific Mutual Life Insurance Co, November 1978
13. James G: Evaluation in public health practice. Amer J P Health 52:1145–1146, 1962
14. Johnston EM, Schwartz NE: Physician's opinions and counseling practices in maternal and infant nutrition. J Amer Diet Assoc 73(3):246–250, 1978
15. Mason M, Wenberg BG, Welsch PK: The Dynamics of Clinical Dietetics. New York, John Wiley & Sons, 1982
16. Nichaman MZ: Developing a nutritional surveillance system. J Amer Diet Assoc 65:15–17, 1974
17. Nutrition Today: The colors of dietetics are raised on a medical flagship. Sept.–Oct. 1979
18. Owen AY: Community Nutrition in Preventive Health Care Services: A Critical Review of the Literature. Department of Health, Education, and Welfare, Washington, DC, US Government Printing Office, 1978
19. Toward Healthful Diets. Washington, DC, Food and Nutrition Board, National Research Council, National Academy of Sciences, 1980
20. Vichstrom JA, Fox HM: Nutritional knowledge and attitudes of registered nurses. J Amer Diet Assoc 68:453–456, 1976
21. White House Conference on Food, Nutrition and Health: Final Report. Washington, DC, US Government Printing Office, 1970
22. Yankelovich, Skelley and White Inc: Family Health in an Era of Stress. Minneapolis, General Mills Inc, 1979
23. Zifferblatt SM, Wilbur CS: Dietary counseling: Some realistic expectations and guidelines. J Amer Diet Assoc 70:591–595, 1977

8
Food Fads

Roslyn B. Alfin–Slater
Lilla Aftergood

From the earliest days of recorded history humans have been endowing certain foods with properties and qualities above and beyond those benefits derived from nutrient composition. The reasons for this type of food faddism are many and varied, including tales and traditions handed down from parents and grandparents, cultural practices, religious beliefs, and misinformation dispensed freely—but not without cost—through books, magazines, newspapers, radio, and television. The last two decades have been accompanied by an increased interest in foods and nutrition by the general public. In the United States, improved food technology has made possible the distribution and increased the availability of a wide variety of food products. International cooperation, ease of travel, and the subsequent intermingling of peoples of different religious and cultural backgrounds have introduced new types of foods and new methods of preparing existing foods. Furthermore, the need to feed increasing numbers of people has brought about improved agricultural methods and new means of food processing which provide more food for more people with a minimum of contamination and spoilage. Yet, although improved communication serves a nutrition-conscious public by introducing new types of food and food preparation, it also provides an excellent medium for the wide dissemination of misinformation about foods and their role in health and disease.

Knowing what to eat is not instinctive. The selection of food is influenced by many factors, but a knowledge of nutrient requirements seems to be the least available and least considered of these.

Since food faddism thrives on ignorance and superstition, the new awareness of food as a factor in health coupled with a lack of nutrition information provides productive ground for the food faddist movement. Food becomes more than a source of nutrients; it is endowed with glamorous and beneficial properties that appeal to the imagination and hope of both the sick and the healthy.

There are many reasons for this preoccupation with food. First of all, the fear of incapacitating illness and disease, the uncertainty of life, and the innate dread of death make most people susceptible to nutritional quackery. A particularly vulnerable group is the elderly, who are urged to spend money needlessly on useless supplements and special food items. Then, too, people may be exploited due to their ignorance of nutrition. Most lay people have little basis for judgment in the area of nutrition and therefore believe the exalted claims for special diets and foods. They may also believe that the faddist is privy to some discovery of which medical science is still ignorant, that the faddist is too far ahead of his time to be accorded recognition or is a victim of organized medical jealousy or professional monopoly. It is difficult for the average person to distinguish between the respectable scientist and the self-proclaimed expert, and there are too few places where people may seek reliable nutrition information. Also, in some cases, even reputable scientists disagree in their interpretation of research findings.

In many cases, food faddism and self-medication result from dissatisfaction with medical care, particularly the high cost of an office visit, the lack of communication between patient and busy clinician, and the inability of many people to accept reality when faced with an incurable illness. Obviously, in such instances a sympathetic health food proponent will find a very receptive customer for any dietary regimen that promises help.

Also, the appeal of food fads has recently been enhanced by an outgrowth of the ecological movement; people are abandoning food treated with pesticides and various chemical additives and turning to "natural," organically grown foods. The "naturalist" argument against such additives as preservatives, stabilizers, and emulsifiers seems self-evident to the lay person overcome by the complicated chemical names of these substances, and the food faddist exploits this denouncement of processed foods to sell his "natural" product at elevated prices.

Furthermore, the many environmental problems of our industrial society, such as air and water pollution, oxidants in smog, and pesticide residues in foods, have led some people to the feeling that something extra must be done to protect their health. Hence, large amounts of vitamins, especially vitamins C, E, and A, are ingested as a result of newspaper reports of preliminary experiments yet to be evaluated by the scientific community under laboratory conditions.

Finally, the faddist may seek fulfillment of specific desires and needs. Certain foods are supposed to act as aphrodisiacs; others are supposed to increase intelligence and brain function, reproductive ability, strength, beauty, and vision. Still other special foods are associated with religious and ceremonial practices. The Zen macrobiotic diet has been said to make an individual "transcend to a level of consciousness never before experienced by ordinary man."

In a society where people are hungry, obtaining food for survival becomes a goal, and it is difficult to relate to commercial food faddism. But when food is plentiful and time and money are available, the climate is ripe for an increased interest in nutrition. Such interest without knowledge can lead to eating habits that range from a conscious avoidance of certain food items ordinarily considered edible to the ingestion of one food or group of foods at the exclusion of all others in the hope that these new patterns of eating may be the ultimate cure for all physical and mental ills. Although sometimes limited only to a financial drain, the results may lead to suboptimal or frank malnutrition and may be expressed in serious physiologic or pathologic changes, or both.

Food faddism encompasses two general areas. One is the promotion of untested, unbalanced diets or single dietary components to prevent disease; the other involves using single food items and specific nutrients in large amounts for curative purposes. In both instances, the advocates do not consider the fact that both the prevention and the cure of illness by dietary means will depend on the etiology of the condition, for example, whether it was caused by a dietary deficiency, impaired absorption of a particular nutrient or nutrients, or both.

Diet and Prevention of Disease

Many factors in the relationship of disease states and pathologic symptoms to nutritional deficiencies are still unknown. Furthermore, all disease is not nutritionally generated, and nutritional deficiencies or nutrient excesses are usually neither the sole cause nor cure for all pathologic conditions. A drastic departure from a well-balanced diet in an attempt to prevent or treat a disease may result in a potentially health-endangering situation. Most often such dietary changes are based on unfounded theories propagated by not always well-meaning pseudoscientists. In general, one should never depart too far, or for too long a period, from moderation in the choice of a diet.

One of the examples where the importance of nutrition is now being stressed, unfortunately not always to the best advantage, is the so-called holistic medicine.[11] Holistic practitioners profess to treat the whole person, not simply the disease. This is a new concept in health care which emphasizes preventive techniques and integrates physical and spiritual approaches. The holistics who are Eastern-oriented attempt to balance positive forces with the negative (Yin–Yang), whereas the followers of the American Indian concept claim that disease is due to a disharmony with nature. This preventive-medicine approach to disease states may be of some merit as long as it does not impart cure-all properties to specific foods or nutrients, and as long as the medical intervention is available and not delayed if needed.

The two diseases in this country that have the highest mortality rates are heart disease and cancer. A third problem, perhaps not as life-threatening but very widespread and a potential health hazard, is obesity. Although obesity is not the cause of heart disease or cancer, it does predispose to conditions such as diabetes and hypertension that increase the susceptibility to coronary heart disease and enhance the formation of tumors. It is therefore not surprising that these are the areas to which much dietary attention is being directed. Dietary manipulations to prevent or alleviate these diseases involve changes in the intake of dietary fat, vitamins, and minerals, and the omission of specific additives. In the same category are the alleged reducing diets that are used for both the prevention and cure of obesity.

OVERCONSUMPTION OF VITAMINS

The gradual understanding of the role of vitamins in nutritional well-being and the fact that vitamin deficiencies are associated with specific disease conditions have led to overdosing with these potent nutrients as a result of misinterpretation and extrapolation of experiments done with animals. The old, misapplied theory that "more must be better if a little is good" still persists. While curative properties of many vitamins in well-established deficiency states are well-recognized, many claims for the disease-preventing activity of megadoses of all or even a few specific vitamins are unfounded and may even result in disastrous side-effects.

The vitamins for which megadoses are recommended most often include vitamin E, vitamin C, and sometimes niacin.

VITAMIN E

The 1980 recommended dietary allowance (RDA) for vitamin E is 8 IU to 10 IU (RDA 1980). However, it is possible that larger amounts of vitamin E than the RDA may be of value for individuals living in areas seriously affected by smog, since the inherent antioxidative activity of vitamin E may exert some degree of protection for the lungs against oxidizing compounds in smog.[27]

The major sources of vitamin E are the polyunsaturated oils—corn, soybean, cottonseed—and wheat germ. Approximately 64% of our dietary vitamin E comes from fats and oils; fruits and vegetables supply 11%, and cereal and grain products supply 7%. Vitamin E is also present in egg yolk and in very small amounts in meats.

Vitamin E therapy is being practiced by individuals and is prescribed by clinicians as well for a variety of ailments, including heart disease, with no experimental substantiation. A recent statement of the Food and Nutrition Board, Division of Biology and Agriculture, National Research Council, points out that the claims for vitamin E's curative effect on such noninfectious diseases as heart disease, sterility, muscle weakness, cancer, ulcers, skin disorders, burns, and shortness of breath, result from misinterpretations of research on experimental animals or from fertile imaginations.[29] Similarly fallacious are the claims that vitamin E promotes physical endurance, increases sexual potency in men, enhances reproductive performance in women, prevents heart attacks, and delays the aging process. It is true that vitamin E deficiency in animals interferes with reproduction in the female, results in testicular degeneration and the formation of immature sperm in the male, and causes cardiac fibrosis in the ruminant.[2,26] A nutritional muscular dystrophy has been induced in susceptible species of animals by vitamin E deprivation. However, supplementation with the vitamin E requirement for these animals (1 mg dl-α-tocopherol for the rat) prevents and cures these deficiency symptoms.[28]

Studies done over a number of years have not confirmed any of the virtues claimed for large doses of vitamin E. In fact, there is increasing evidence that vitamin E in excess is similar to excesses of the other fat-soluble vitamins A and D and may have some measure of toxicity. In studies with chicks, scientists from the University of British Columbia showed that large doses of vitamin E depressed growth, interfered with the uptake and release of iodine by the thyroid, and increased the requirement for vitamins D and K.[25] The interference of large doses of vitamin E with vitamin K activity has recently been confirmed.[14] Other studies in rats have resulted in fatty livers containing elevated levels of cholesterol and triglycerides after 6 months supplementation with high levels of vitamin E.[1] A report on the development of "flulike" symptoms in humans taking 800 mg vitamin E/day that disappeared when the dose was reduced to half also indicated that excess vitamin E may not be as well tolerated as had been previously believed.[13]

VITAMIN C

When Linus Pauling's *Vitamin C and the Common Cold* was published in 1970, the public rushed to buy every conceivable type of vitamin C preparation available.[31] It was an appealing idea—that an extra amount of a vitamin found in such "anticold" foods as citrus fruits could protect against an affliction that plagues the population at the most inconvenient times. Pauling recommended 1 g to 5 g vitamin C daily to prevent a cold and to treat a cold, a substantial 15 g daily. The maintenance or prophylactic dose was arrived at from extrapolations of calculations of how much vitamin C a gorilla normally consumed from vegetation and how much vitamin C the rat could synthesize per day. The therapeutic dose was derived principally from personal recommendations. Unfortunately, scientific evidence for the efficiency of vitamin C in preventing colds has not been conclusive; the experiments available to date are open to criticism and controversy. Although doses larger than the 1980 RDA (60 mg for adults) may possibly be advantageous in treating respiratory ailments, large amounts of vitamin C are not without toxic effects.[12]

It should be noted that Anderson's report on his studies with massive doses of vitamin C concluded that large doses (250 mg–2000 mg) may under certain circumstances indeed reduce the severity of upper respiratory infections in those individuals whose tissues are not fully saturated with this vitamin.[3] He pointed out, however, that levels above those necessary for tissue saturation could conceivably be harmful, but also indicated that respiratory infections might increase the amount of vitamin C required for tissue saturation. Obviously more research on large numbers of persons is required to resolve this controversy.

Infants born to mothers who take megadoses of vitamin C during their pregnancies are at risk to develop scurvy after birth. The adaptability of the infant's body to high circulating levels of vitamin C results in an accelerated destruction and excretion of this vitamin. Also, there are indications that the resultant acid urines may contribute to the formation of renal calculi in those with a tendency to gout. Furthermore, ascorbic acid is metabolized through the formation of oxalic acid, a substance that also contributes to renal calculi.[5] Large amounts of vitamin C also interfere with the activity of certain drugs (see Chap. 19).[27,34]

Other possible toxic effects as well as beneficial effects await further investigation. For instance, the role of vitamin C in atherosclerosis and cancer still needs clarification. Vitamin C, for example, interferes with the formation of carcinogenic nitrosamines from nitrites.

Most recent claims involve vitamin C in both the prevention and cure of cancer. Well-controlled, double-blind studies, however, have shown that megadoses of vitamin C for cancer patients are of no value.[15]

NIACIN

Large doses of niacin in amounts over and above those recommended by the Committee on Dietary Allowances of the Food and Nutrition Board, National Research Council, have been used to reduce hypercholesterolemia. Although side-effects were noted early in the treatment ("flushing" reactions), changes in the form of niacin used and a decrease in the amount minimized these undesirable effects. However, although niacin is a water-soluble vitamin and, in general, water-soluble vitamins are nontoxic even when consumed in relatively large amounts, studies on humans strongly suggest that large doses of niacin have an undesirable effect on

the metabolism of the heart muscle.[22] In fact, it is suggested that excessive niacin might be especially dangerous if taken by athletes before an event.

When a significant success rate in improvement of schizophrenia with megadoses of niacin was reported, this "orthomolecular" treatment was widely promoted.[41] However, a more detailed study revealed that some of the previous "cures" may have been successful because an actual niacin deficiency disease was being treated.

VITAMIN A

Large quantities of vitamin A (50,000 IU–150,000 IU/day) have been prescribed for adolescents in the treatment of *acne vulgaris*. The benefits of this treatment have not been substantiated, nor is there a valid reason for the use of this treatment. If it is necessary to take vitamin supplements, the vitamin A content of the supplement should approximate the RDA.

It is known that vitamin A is an essential nutrient required for the maintenance of healthy epithelial tissue, for growth, and for vision. Vitamin A deficiency causes impaired dark adaptation and night blindness. The Ten-State Nutrition Survey revealed that a significant proportion of the population had a low vitamin A intake (below the 5000 IU recommended for adults in the 1980 RDA), and methods to increase the vitamin A intake by proper selection of foods and diets should be advised by nutritionists and clinicians.

On the other hand, there is no advantage to be derived from exceeding the recommended level of vitamin A. Excessive intake may result in toxic effects (see Chap. 3). For example, five times the RDA or 25,000 IU vitamin A (which is unfortunately present in some vitamin preparations), when taken daily for extended periods is risky, especially during pregnancy. Ingestion of such amounts by pregnant women may produce in them CNS anomalies, and in the fetus teratologic effects have been observed.[6] In older children or adults, hypervitaminosis A may result in increased intercranial pressure with its accompanying effects on the CNS in as little as 30 days of ingesting 25,000 IU to 50,000 IU/day.[18] Longer usage has been shown to result in optic atrophy and blindness. In general, the toxicity of large doses of vitamin A has been well established.[35]

Since it has been established in animals that chemical carcinogenesis in epithelia can sometimes be prevented by vitamin A derivatives, there has been an upsurge of interest in the possible relationship of vitamin A to cancer.[37] For instance, a regression of papillomas of the urinary bladder and leukoplakia of the mouth has been observed as a result of oral administration of retinoic acid.[8] Similarly, a decreased consumption of vitamin A was shown in patients with lung cancer.[36]

Because of the potential toxicity of the common forms of vitamin A esters, synthetic analogs of retinoids have been developed; they are less toxic and have different patterns of tissue distribution and storage.[37]

Until recently it has been believed that while an overdose of a fat-soluble vitamin may present some danger, the overconsumption of water-soluble vitamins may be simply just wasteful, since excesses are automatically excreted. More expanded knowledge, however, points out that this is not necessarily so. Not only are megadoses of vitamin C harmful, but megadoses of niacin may also have undesirable side-effects.

"VITAMINS" B_{15} AND B_{17}

A discussion of "vitamins" in regard to fad diets would not be complete without mentioning pangamic acid (so-called vitamin B_{15}) and laetrile (so-called vitamin B_{17}).[20,21]

Pangamic acid, isolated from various plant sources, has no clearly defined standard of identity. It is primarily a gluconodimethyl aminoacetic acid. It has been claimed that it detoxifies products formed in human metabolism and is also of value in cancer, alcoholism, hepatitis, and diabetes, among other disease. Spectacular results have been described without substantiating data. According to the FDA this is not an identifiable substance, not even a provitamin, and furthermore, no usefulness for it has been established, nor is there a deficiency disease resulting from its absence.

Laetrile, which is the common name for the compound amygdalin, a cyanogenic glycoside occurring in apricot pits and similar plant material, has been named vitamin B_{17} by its promoters, and along with a so-called antineoplastic diet has been claimed to cure many varieties of cancer. The diet itself is nutritionally inadequate since it excludes meat and dairy products and is based on ingestion of fruit, nuts, and megadoses of vitamins. Such diets tend to further weaken the patients.

The activity of laetrile is theoretically based on the release of hydrocyanic acid, which unfortunately destroys all cells, normal as well as cancer, and may lead to permanent destruction of the host. Another major risk involving laetrile is that its use often delays or replaces conventional treatment during the potentially treatable stage of cancer. Laetrile has been shown to be totally ineffective in controlled studies.[20]

LECITHIN

In recent years, lecithin, a phospholipid present in many foods, especially in egg yolks and meats, has become a favorite supplement in the world of quackery. Commercial preparations are made from soybeans. It can also be synthesized in the body from readily available precursors. When ingested in foods, lecithin is broken down into glycerol, phosphate, choline, and fatty acids. In the body, phospholipids are essential parts of living cells; appearing particularly in cell walls and mitochondria, they are used in transport and utilization of fats and fatty acids.

It has been claimed that lecithin reduces hypercholesterolemia and therefore is effective in prevention and treatment of cardiovascular diseases. However, there is no good evidence available as yet to indicate that lecithin lowers serum cholesterol levels or that it has a role in the treatment of coronary disease. Nor is there any evidence for the miraculous effects attributed to a combination of lecithin, kelp, cider vinegar, and vitamin B_6 in removing fat deposits from special places in obese subjects. In fact, overusage of kelp (dried seaweed) may result in iodine toxicity.

FATS AND HEART DISEASE

An example of potential harm brought about by a lack of moderation and insufficient testing is the use of large amounts of polyunsaturated fat to treat hypercholesterolemia and to reduce the risk of heart disease. It now appears that diets excessively high in polyunsaturates may not be as advisable as originally believed. These diets may result in an increased risk of gallstone disease and an enhancement of certain types of cancer.[39] A moderate substitution of a portion of saturated fat with polyunsaturated fat may perhaps improve plasma lipid profiles, but data showing that reducing serum cholesterol levels reduces the incidence and morbidity of coronary heart disease are sparse and unconvincing.

FIBER

In recent years, mainly as a result of demographic studies, dietary fiber came to prominence. It became the panacea for obesity, cancer of the colon, diabetes, gall-bladder disease, and especially constipation.[10] There is no question that fiber absorbs water, softens the stools, and decreases the fecal transit time. It also changes the type and concentration of the bacterial flora. However, there are many different types of fiber, and not all dietary fiber is identical in its action. Whereas pectin has plasma cholesterol lowering properties, wheat bran alleviates constipation but does not affect hypercholesterolemia. There is also the risk of the indiscriminate use and overuse of fiber. A deficiency of trace elements may result, since high fiber cereals contain phytate, which binds trace minerals making them unavailable. Thus, even though the increased use of fibrous foods may be advisable, they should be used in moderation by eating whole grain wheat products, fruits, and vegetables rather than food supplements.

Organic and Natural Foods— Problems of Processing and Refining

Related to the promotion of megavitamin therapy is the promotion of "natural" foods that retain the nutrients supposedly lost through processing. The need for increased supplies of food to feed a burgeoning population, and the changes in life style that have come about in the last 20 years have led to remarkable advances in food technology, as is reflected by the large numbers and variety of food products with greater visual and taste appeal now available. To circumvent problems involved in food storage and transportation, new ways of treating raw materials were devised to assure the least spoilage and a longer shelf life. Furthermore, there is a great demand for convenience foods that are easily and quickly prepared. No longer does either the housekeeper or family cook devote a large part of the day to meal preparation. In the first place, housekeepers are no longer readily available; the wife and mother has been liberated from the kitchen, and cooking "from scratch" has become the exception rather than the rule.

Food processing is done for a number of reasons, one of which is to increase the shelf life of the product. Wheat is processed to yield white flour because whole grain products have comparatively low keeping qualities, and millers and bakers therefore make use of large amounts of the more stable refined products. Obviously, processing or refining foods results in the loss of several nutrients, but modern processing methods attempt to keep nutrient losses as low as possible. Furthermore, processed foods are enriched to restore some of the nutrients that may be removed in their preparation. For example, white flour is now enriched with thiamin, riboflavin, niacin, and iron. Minor quantities of other nutrients present in small amounts in whole grain which might be lost during processing are widely available in other foodstuffs. Man does not—and should not—live by eating bread alone, even whole wheat bread.

The refining of sugar causes a similar loss of minute amounts of vitamins and some minerals. To the faddist, honey, brown, and raw sugar possess great nutritional value, whereas refined sugar does nothing but cause dental caries, obesity, and heart disease. Actually, sugar in any form essentially provides only calories. Honey, raw sugar, brown sugar, and white sugar are nutritionally practically the same. Honey, raw, and brown sugar possibly have more pleasant flavors, as well as traces of minerals and vitamins due to the presence of small amounts of molasses, but these are of no real significance. Sugars eaten in moderate amounts are not harmful—they add taste, color, and texture to the diet. The danger arises when these are consumed in excess. The possible role of sugar in the genesis of diabetes, heart disease, cancer, and other diseases is a controversial subject still unresolved.

Related to the problem of processed food is the controversy surrounding the question of raw versus pasteurized milk. It is claimed that the pasteurization process destroys important enzymes and vitamins found in raw milk. Actually, the enzymes that are present are of no use to humans; since enzymes are protein in nature, they are denatured and destroyed by the acid of the stomach. Furthermore, the small amount of vitamin C present in milk that is destroyed by heating it to 60°C, as required in the pasteurization process, is of little consequence as far as human diets are concerned. Milk is not considered a source of vitamin C; other foods in a balanced diet provide sufficient amounts of this vitamin to more than satisfy the recommended dietary allowance. Pasteurization was adopted to destroy pathogenic microorganisms that might be present in milk and therefore to provide a safe product for the greatest number of people. Although the standards for the safety and cleanliness of certified raw milk are quite high, there is always a possibility that some pathogens will find a way into the final product. Pasteurization has largely eliminated undulant fever and tuberculosis; the organism that caused them may be found in fresh milk. The preparation of yogurt from milk involves introducing a nonpathogenic bacterial culture that produces an acid taste and changes the consistency of the milk. The same nutrients are present in yogurt that are present in milk except for the partial breakdown of lactose (milk sugar) into its components, glucose and galactose.

Vitamins *per se* have not escaped the controversy of "natural" versus "synthetic," despite the fact that a vitamin has the same chemical formula whether it is extracted from natural sources or has been synthesized in the laboratory. The only possible advantage of preferring the former is the remote possibility that some as yet unidentified but beneficial substance may accompany the "natural" product.

ADDITIVES

Few topics have aroused more heated comment than the practice of adding various substances to food. On one hand, the food industry maintains that food additives enhance the quality, attractiveness, and nutritive value while reducing the perishability and therefore the price of the product. On the other hand, representatives of various consumer groups claim that all kinds of chemical substances are added to food without regard for the consequences. Actually, many allowable food additives are derived directly from food itself, and some that are synthesized are identical to those found in food. All additives are chemicals, and the body does not distinguish between those isolated from food and those synthesized in the laboratory.

Additives are used for specific purposes, namely, to preserve the quality of the food, to improve the nutritive value, and to add or enhance flavor, texture, color, and odor. One of the oldest additives known is salt. Spices have also been used for a long time. Both of these were and are used as preservatives as well as for flavor. Nutritional supplements are also additives. For example, the B vitamins and iron added to bread for "enrichment" are considered to be additives, as is the vitamin D added to milk and the vitamin A added to margarine. The addition of potassium iodide to salt provides iodine in a safe, effective way, especially for those areas where goiter is a prevalent disease.

Probably still one of the most contested issues is the question of adding fluoride to water to bring the level up to 1:1,000,000 in order to decrease the incidence of dental caries, particularly in children. Although many studies have shown that fluoride at this level is safe and effective,[18] the outspoken and vigorous opponents of fluoridation have blocked attempts of government agencies at various levels to adopt a uniform policy on fluoridation. Most of the opposition to fluoride stems from misinterpretation of data concerning people who have been subjected to high fluoride levels. The opponents of fluoridation feel that the line of demarcation between what is safe and what is dangerous is not that well defined. If the fluoride concentration in drinking water exceeds 1.4 ppm to 1.6 ppm, the first signs of dental fluorosis (mottled enamel) may appear.[16] Also, sodium fluoride itself bears the stigma of being a component of rodenticides and some insecticides. In the meantime many children who are not receiving fluoride treatments will needlessly suffer the discomfort and expense of unhealthy teeth.

Other intentional additives include those that are added to enhance flavor. If food lacks flavor, it will not be eaten. Our cultural life style includes living in large cities away from the source of farm crops, including fresh fruits and vegetables, and synthetic flavors are used when natural ones are in short supply. The increased use of quick, easy to prepare, convenience foods has led to the increased use of both natural and synthetic flavoring agents, but synthetic flavors may also be used to give consistently good flavor where the naturally occurring flavors may be destroyed or altered in processing.

Antioxidants are also added to foods to reduce food spoilage. Foods are at their best immediately after they are harvested. As a result of oxidative processes that continue to function in the food until it is used, fresh fruits and vegetables—and processed foods as well—change in color, flavor, texture, and appetite appeal as they age. The enzymatic browning of sliced fresh apples, peaches, and potatoes can be prevented or delayed by the use of such antioxidants as vitamins C or E, and these antioxidants seem to be generally acceptable since they are natural food components. However, butylated hydroxytoluene (BHT) and butylated hydroxyanisole (BHA), commercial antioxidants usually added to polyunsaturated oils to prevent the formation of toxic lipoperoxides, are suspect even though they have been tested and found to be acceptable at the levels used, because they are "chemicals" with unpronounceable names. Antioxidants of all types lengthen the shelf life of a variety of products and therefore help maintain a reasonable price on many foodstuffs.

Potassium nitrate, or "saltpeter," has been used to cure meat for centuries. Nitrites are derivatives of nitrates, approved by the FDA as an additive. Currently they are used to cure processed meat such as bacon, ham, and sausage. They also give these foods their characteristic color and flavor and inhibit the growth of bacteria and botulism.

Nitrites can form nitrosamines on cooking and also during digestion in the intestine. A problem arises because certain nitrosamines were found to be carcinogenic in some animal species when given in very large amounts. But whether or not nitrites actually cause cancer in humans is not known. The dilemma still exists. Is it better to cut out nitrites completely and risk botulism or continue nitrite use and risk cancer?

The Council for Agricultural Science and Technology recently reported that only 2% to 20% of the exposure of humans to nitrites is due to the consumption of cured meats. Part of the nitrite originates in the saliva as a result of eating nitrate-rich leafy green vegetables, such as carrots, beets, radishes, and celery, and even some waters. Nitrites are also produced in the lower intestines where the nitrite can form nitrosamines. Elimination of nitrite from cured meats would only eliminate a small proportion of the total. However, in any event, the FDA and the USDA are reducing the levels of nitrite in bacon, and a general phasing out of nitrites from food is taking place.

Other additives that are suspect are emulsifiers, stabilizers, thickeners, acids, synthetic coloring agents, alkalis, buffers, neutralizing agents, leavening agents, bleaching agents, sequestrants, humectants, foaming agents, foam inhibitors, and many others. Whether all of these are necessary is open to question. The food industry claims that they are safe, nutritious, and essential for satisfying consumers' tastes and convenience, and it feels that meeting the food demands of this country would be impossible without food additives. Critics of food additives contend that some are hazardous to humans, others are suspect, and most are designed to deceive the consumer. The United States government through the FDA protects the food purchaser by the National Pure Food and Drug Law, which requires that chemicals used in food production must be shown to be safe before they may be used commercially. The Food Additives amendment requires that manufacturers of food additives test their substances and then submit evidence for the safety of these substances to the Food and Drug Administration, which examines the tests and evidence and then rules on whether the products are indeed safe. Only after they are given this clearance are they placed on the generally recognized as safe (GRAS) list and cleared for commercial use. It is a fact, however, that some additives now on this list have not been given this rigorous testing but were part of a "grandfather" clause on the basis of experience drawn from their common and safe use in food over many years (prior to 1958).

Sometimes, unrealistic and unscientific constraints are placed on food additives by the Delaney clause (a 1958 Amendment of Pure Food and Drug Act) because several scientists contend that if enough of a substance were ingested, almost anything would be harmful. For example, the cyclamate dose that induced bladder cancer in rats was 50 times the daily maximum recommended for humans by the World Health Organization (WHO). It is also incorrect to assume that results of tests on animals necessarily apply to man.

Testing and retesting of additives are rapidly becoming too expensive for smaller companies to carry out. Evaluating and regulating food safety create research problems that scientists outside the FDA would not understand and in which they would not be interested.

Results on rats fed quantities of cyclamates that would be impossible for humans to consume in presently marketed foods and beverages, cost Abbott a $16 million per year market. The issue is still one of contention.

We probably could get along without additives, but not very well. The variety and quality of foods would be drastically reduced, the nutritional and keeping qualities of foods sharply curtailed, and the price of foods considerably higher. The alternative is to keep the additives and encourage more testing and more vigilance on the part of the FDA, and this would seem to be a partial answer to the growing suspicion of "chemicals" added to foods.

FERTILIZERS VERSUS "ORGANICALLY GROWN" FOODS

Organically grown foods are defined as "foods grown without the use of any agricultural chemical and processed without the use of food chemicals or additives."[40] Unfortunately, no agency of law defines or supervises the label "organic" and certifies that foods so labeled actually fit this description.

Claims have been made that organically grown foods are nutritionally superior to foods grown under more usual agricultural conditions during which chemical fertilizers are used. However, there are no scientific experiments or reports to support these claims. It is known that the nutrient composition of a fruit or vegetable is determined genetically—the seed carries this information. Furthermore, organic fertilizers (*e.g.*, compost, manure) cannot be absorbed *per se* by plants. They must be broken down to inorganic compounds (the same compounds found in chemical fertilizers) by the bacteria in the soil, since plants only absorb inorganic compounds. Moreover, there is the risk that manure and moldy leaves and other organic material used as fertilizers in organic gardening may be infected with any number of mycotoxins (fungal toxins, *e.g.*, aflatoxin, which is an extremely potent carcinogen) that could be transferred to the plant by means of maggots, insects, and other pests that have been shown to concentrate some of these fungal toxins. Also, there is the possibility of *Salmonella* contamination, which can result in food poisoning.

Chemical fertilizers are needed to produce enough food for our population. For the commercial production of food, nutrients that promote good plant growth are added to the soil in these fertilizers, and the food crops that result have the expected nutritional value.

The use of pesticides seems to be a necessary evil in our modern civilization. Although methods of pest control without the use of toxins are now in effect in limited areas, including the use of natural predators, pheromones, and insect hormones, it will be many years before these methods are sufficiently effective and widespread to protect the food supply in the same way as the pesticides now in use. Even the banning of DDT, a "hard" pesticide that was found to be stored in adipose tissue, is not well received in some areas, where it is feared that there will be a reappearance of the malaria-bearing *Anopheles* mosquito.

Pesticide residues on plants are carefully monitored by both the FDA and the Environmental Protection Agency (EPA); if a pesticide is allowed, the amount is set at the lowest level that will accomplish the desired purpose, even when larger amounts would still be safe.

Diets

ZEN MACROBIOTIC DIET

A typically harmful fad which was promoted some years ago is the so-called Zen macrobiotic diet, which if followed religiously results in severe malnutrition. This diet represents the extreme in adherence to a natural diet containing only organic foods. It is supposed to create a spiritual rebirth and to be a cure for all disease, tension, and aging. The prescribed diets (there are ten) are predominantly vegetarian and range from a rather varied diet (Diet − 3) to the final Diet + 7. Diet + 7 is composed of 100% cereals with fluid restriction as well and is said to achieve the ultimate in well-being. True adherents of this mode of eating risk the danger of developing serious nutritional deficiencies. Depending on the length of adherence to this diet, cases of scurvy, anemia, hypoproteinemia, hypocalcemia, emaciation, loss of kidney function, and death have been reported.

VEGETARIANISM

Vegetarianism as such does not constitute faddism unless its advocates profess that it cures illness. Although the number of adherents to vegetarian diets has increased considerably in recent years, especially in the younger populations, vegetarianism is not a new pattern of eating. Large populations of the world have lived for generations on diets almost or completely vegetarian, either because of religious beliefs or because of the unavailability of animal protein. The newer proponents of vegetarianism believe that this type of diet is more conducive to good health and also that it preserves the life of animals—the latter a fact that cannot be argued.

The several different types of vegetarian diets have in common the fact that they do not include meat, poultry, or fish. They do contain vegetables, fruits, enriched or whole grain bread and cereals, dry beans and peas, lentils, nuts, and seeds. A pure vegetarian diet excludes all foods of animal origin; an ovo-lactovegetarian diet allows eggs and dairy products; a lactovegetarian diet includes dairy products but excludes eggs.

Vegetarian diets can be nutritionally adequate if the foods are selected wisely.[33] They should include as much of a variety of foods as is permissible to make sure that all of the nutrients required for good health are present. One of the main concerns in adherence to an all-vegetable diet is the quality of the protein component. It has long been known that animal protein has a higher biologic value than do vegetable and grain proteins, which are often lacking in one or more essential amino acids. However, individual vegetable proteins with low biologic value can be mixed with others to provide an amino acid pattern that is adequate for growth and maintenance of populations. For example, grain–legume combinations provide much better nutrition than either grains or legumes separately. This mixing of two incomplete proteins to provide a complete mixture is known as mutual supplementation.

One difficulty arising during the use of vegetarian diets is the possible lack of vitamin B_{12}, which is found only in foods of animal origin, such as meat, fish, eggs, and dairy products. Although there is no problem for the ovolactovegetarians or lactovegetarians, those whose protein is derived solely from vegetable sources (vegans) must either select foods fortified with vitamin B_{12} or take a vitamin B_{12} supplement. Strict vegetarians who do not ingest a source of vitamin B_{12} may develop nerve damage and blood dyscrasias.

Other nutrients that may be in short supply in persons consuming only vegetable products are calcium, since milk and milk products are the major sources of calcium; vitamin D, which occurs naturally only in foods of animal origin (but this is a problem only for children, since vitamin D can be manufactured in sufficient quantities to satisfy adult requirements by the action of sunlight on the skin); and—possibly—riboflavin and iodine. However, by the proper selection of foods, based on a knowledge of the nutrient composition of foods and of the requirements for health as recommended by the RDA, there is no reason why a vegetarian diet cannot be as nutritious as one that includes animal products. Only when the selection of foods is limited do vegetarians encounter potential dangers of malnutrition.

Reducing Diets

The dictionary defines obesity as "an excessive accumulation of fat in the body." The reasons for this accumulation are now recognized to be of complex etiology, involving genetic, physiologic, psychologic, and socioeconomic factors to various degrees, and perhaps other undefined environmental factors. Once the complexity of this disorder is recognized, it becomes obvious that there is no simple cure and that weight reduction and maintenance requires a variety of treatments, including the motivation of the subject, a diet that is nutritionally adequate except for calories, and a learning process wherein the palate is reeducated to new dietary patterns. This cannot be accomplished overnight (see Chap. 28).

And yet, there are many fad reducing diets available today that promise quick weight loss with no discomfort—no abstinence from high-caloric, high-fat foods, no need to count calories, no need for exercise—a veritable "something for nothing." These diets are dissimilar from the ordinary in that they (1) differ in the proportion of fat, carbohydrate, and protein allowed, (2) make use of a limited number of foods, and (3) are usually deficient in one or more essential nutrients.

It is of course possible to lose weight on these diets, but in most cases the weight is usually quickly regained. The small number of foods allowed results in a diet that becomes monotonous and therefore cannot be followed for long periods of time. Furthermore, no education has been achieved, and a return to the prediet eating pattern is accompanied by a return of the lost pounds. When essential nutrients are missing from a reducing diet, long-term adherence is dangerous and may lead to pathologic deficiency symptoms.

LOW-CARBOHYDRATE DIETS

The more popular fad diets today are based on the low-carbohydrate principle. Since protein in the diet is limited by the fact that most high-protein foods are less than 40% protein, these are actually high-fat diets. These diets have high satiety value and do show an encourging quick weight loss. The proponents of low-carbohydrate diets maintain that they are effective because in the overweight person carbohydrates are rapidly converted to adipose tissue (rather than being used for energy), whereas the calories from fat and protein are used in metabolic processes and do not form fat, nor are they

stored as body fat. This convenient theory has no justification. Actually, the initial weight loss on the low-carbohydrate diet is due to a shift in water balance and a loss in body water.[9,30] The continued weight loss is a result of the self-imposed calorie restriction because of the monotony and high satiety value of the allowable foods.[42]

Restriction of carbohydrate to under 100 g/day results in the synthesis of glucose from protein with an extra load imposed on the kidney to excrete the nitrogen by-products. Furthermore, carbohydrate is required for the complete oxidation of fat. In the absence of sufficient carbohydrate, acetyl-CoA molecules (intermediary products in fat metabolism) accumulate and condense, forming ketone bodies, and these accumulate in the blood, cause ketosis, and disturb the acid–base balance of the body. High-fat diets also may be undesirable in that they may promote or aggravate atherosclerosis. And low-carbohydrate diets are often deficient in fiber, minerals, and vitamin C. These diets are indeed similar to the diets fed to laboratory rats to induce fatty livers, diabetes, and hyperlipidemia.[7]

DR. STILLMAN'S DIET

Dr. Stillman's reducing diet is basically a carbohydrate-restricted, high-protein, high-animal-fat diet.[38] Experimental subjects lost weight in the early period of the diet but showed a 16.3% increase in serum cholesterol levels after 5 days. Most subjects also complained of fatigue, lassitude, nausea, and diarrhea.

DR. ATKINS' DIET

Dr. Atkins' Diet Revolution is another variant of the low-carbohydrate diet.[4] Potential hazards of this diet include the possibility of hyperlipidemia with the risk of accelerating atherosclerosis. Ketogenic diets also may cause elevations in blood uric acid concentration with a possibility of inducing gout in susceptible individuals. Subjects on this diet also complained of fatigue, lack of energy, and other symptoms previously described due to the low-carbohydrate diet. Dr. Atkins' book contains statements that have never been substantiated; for example, he claims that this diet promotes the production of a "fat mobilizing hormone" (FMH), which is why his diet is successful and all others fail. Unfortunately, no such hormone has been positively identified in humans. Among Dr. Atkins' other recommendations are megadoses of the vitamin B complex and vitamins C and E, which are supposed to help keep blood sugar at an even level. This has never been found to be either necessary or efficacious in patients with deranged carbohydrate metabolism. All in all, the rationale given to justify this diet is without scientific merit.

SIMEONS REGIMEN

One of the fad reducing diets to achieve popularity is the use of human chorionic gonadotropin (HCG) obtained from the urine of pregnant women in conjunction with a 500-Cal diet, the so-called Simeons regimen. Patients are given daily intramuscular (IM) injections of 125 IU of HCG six times per week for a total of 40 injections. The 500-Cal diet is given in two daily meals. The weight loss is inevitable if the patient adheres to the low-calorie diet, but whether HCG contributes to this weight reduction is questionable. Here again, there have been no well-designed studies to determine the relative influences of HCG, caloric restriction, and the psychologic effects of daily injections and daily weighings on weight reduction. It is known that HCG stimulates testes to produce androgens and at high doses produces headache, restlessness, depression, pain at the injection site, edema, and fatigue. However, the amount of HCG used for weight reduction is much less than that which has been shown to produce these symptoms. The 500-Cal diet, which is actually semistarvation, probably results in the loss of considerable protein from the body, and malnutrition could be expected. In summary, the efficacy of this regimen has not been confirmed.

THE PRITIKIN DIET

One of the more drastic approaches to dieting in an attempt to treat so-called diseases of affluence— heart disease, diabetes, and obesity—is the Pritikin diet.[32] It is based on a reduction of daily fat intake to less than 10% of the total calories, a very low protein intake, with most of the proteins from vegetable sources, a high complex carbohydrate intake, no sugar, and an extreme limitation of caffeine, cholesterol, and salt. Together with a supervised exercise program, this diet, developed at a "Longevity Institute," has been claimed to result in great improvement in the health of many men and women with dangerously occluded arteries and heart conditions. Since no reports have been published in reputable scientific journals, it is impossible to evaluate these claims or the long-range effects of this imbalanced diet. Furthermore, no follow-up studies have been done to explore adherence to the diet after 26 days of "in-house" treatment, or to evaluate its effectiveness.

This type of diet is difficult to follow for prolonged periods of time. Additionally, the high fiber content may lead to malabsorption of trace minerals and subsequent deficiencies. Long-term effects of adherence to the diet have not been satisfactorily assessed.

LIQUID-PROTEIN DIET

One of the most recent and potentially dangerous attempts at weight reduction is the so-called last chance, or protein-sparing, diet.[24] This is actually a modification of the protein-sparing modified fast.[23] The weight reduction is achieved through the low-calorie, low-carbohydrate diet that is accompanied by ketosis. The heavy protein load (approximately double the RDA) places a heavy burden on the kidney as well as on the individual, who is additionally stressed by the minimal caloric intake. There is the possibility of cholelithiasis and kidney disease. In some cases the administered protein is of low biological value, lacking one or more of the essential amino acids. Electrolyte deficiencies, particularly of potassium, develop; this has resulted in arrhythmias, cardiac failure, and death.

Other more recent entries into the field of weight reduction include the low-carbohydrate "Scarsdale Diet;" the very-low-calorie, protein-insufficient "Cambridge Diet;" the use of glucomannan, a water-absorbing compound that expands in the stomach and ostensibly promotes satiety thereby; and of so-called "starch blockers" that diminish the digestion of some complex carbohydrates. These two latter methods are now classified as drugs and are undergoing extensive testing.

The cure for obesity is not in fad "quick weight loss" diets but rather in the maintenance of correct balance between energy intake and energy expenditure. And prevention is always better than cure. Good habits of food intake and physical activity should be initiated early in childhood.

Conclusions

It has been estimated that the direct economic waste attributable to food faddism reaches approximately $500,000,000 per year. However, the greatest damage lies in the deliberate and distorted misinformation given to the public and in the suspicion that is aroused concerning our food supply, which is probably the most abundant and the most nutritious of any in the world. Furthermore, promises of cures for incurable and terminal diseases have caused much anguish as well as financial ruin to the many people unlucky enough to be deceived by nutritional "confidence artists."

The scientific community is only now beginning to fight back vigorously by countering misinformation and false claims with data based on experimental fact and providing information on nutrition where none has been available before. It is absolutely essential that more valid information on nutrition be provided to the public as simply and as comprehensively as possible. In particular, nutrition education is needed for those who influence the public—physicians, dentists, public health workers, social workers, and teachers at all levels of instruction.

Another answer to the problem lies in governmental regulation. The advent of food labeling has involved setting up stringent new labeling requirements for foods designated for "special dietary use." No longer may foods be said to prevent or treat disease because of nutrients they may or may not contain. No longer can it be claimed that a diet of ordinary foods cannot supply adequate nutrition and that "deficient" soil produces "deficient" food. No longer can suspicion be thrust on the nutrient content of a food because it is "processed." Foods that contain substances for which the need in human nutrition has never been established cannot be claimed to have special health properties. Furthermore, claims that natural vitamins are in any way superior to synthetic vitamins will be prohibited. From now on, a vitamin is a vitamin is a vitamin.

Finally, the public must become more discriminating in the evaluation of nutritional reports made directly available through various mass media channels. In the past, nutritional scientists reported their studies in scientific journals, and their work was reviewed and evaluated by their peers prior to publication. Scientists with divergent opinions were then able to assess critically areas in which there were points of contention. A third or fourth study might be necessary to clarify a confusing situation. Now, unevaluated findings are reported in newspapers, magazines, radio, and television, promising immediate solutions to very complex problems. As a result, pressure is brought to bear on government agencies to rule on issues for which available information may be inadequate and irrelevant. The public must realize that many of these reports are derived from persons with little or no education or training in nutrition and biochemistry who are not recognized as part of the reputable scientific community. The problem is one of informing the public on what is known and what is guesswork; to accomplish this, resource facilities should be designated where valid scientific facts would be freely available to those who seek them.

References

1. Alfin–Slater RB, Aftergood L, Kishineff S: Investigations on hypervitaminosis E in rats (abstr). Ninth International Congress on Nutrition, p 191, Mexico City, 1972
2. Ames SR: Age, parity, and vit A supplementation and the vit E requirement of female rats. Am J Clin Nutr 27:1017, 1974
3. Anderson TW: Vitamin C: Report of trials with massive doses (abstr). Miami Beach, Fourth Western Hemisphere Nutrition Congress, p. 67, 1974
4. Atkins RC: Dr. Atkins' Diet Revolution. New York, David McKay, 1972
5. Baker EM, Saari JC, Tolbert BM: Ascorbic acid metabolism in man. Am J Clin Nutr 19:371, 1966
6. Bernhardt IB, Dorsey DJ: Hypervitaminosis A and congenital renal anomalies in a human infant. Obstet Gynecol 43:750, 1974
7. Blumenfeld A: Low carbohydrate diet debate. Obesity and Bariatric Medicine 3:93, 1974
8. Bollag W: Retinoids and cancer. Cancer Chemotherapy & Pharmacology 3:207, 1979
9. Bortz WM, Howat P, Holmes WL: Fat, carbohydrate, salt and water loss. Am J Clin Nutr 21:1291, 1968
10. Burkitt DP: Relationships between diseases and their etiological significance. Am J Clin Nutr 30:262, 1977
11. Callan JP: Holistic health or holistic hoax? JAMA 241:1156, 1979
12. Chalmers, TC: Effects of ascorbic acid on the common cold: An evaluation of the evidence. Am J Med 58:532, 1975
13. Cohen HM: Fatigue caused by vit E. Calif Med 119:72, 1973
14. Corrigan JJ, Marcus FI: Coagulopathy associated with vit E ingestion. JAMA 230:1300, 1974
15. Creagan ET, Mortel CG, et al: Failure of high doses of vit C to benefit patients with advanced cancer. N Engl J Med 301:687, 1979
16. Dean HT: Fluorine in the control of dental caries. Int Dent J 4:311, 1954
17. Eastwood MA, Kay RM: An hypothesis for the action of fiber along the gastrointestinal tract. Am J Clin Nutr 32:364, 1979
18. Fluorides and Human Health (Monograph 59). Geneva, World Health Organization, 1970
19. Furman, KI: Acute hypervitaminosis A in an adult. Am J Clin Nutr 26:575, 1973
20. Herbert V: Laetrile: The cult of cyanide. Promoting poison for profit. Am J Clin Nutr 32:1121, 1979
21. Herbert V: Pangamic acid ("vit B_{15}"). Am J Clin Nutr 32:1534, 1979
22. Lassers BW, Wahlqvist ML, et al: Effect of nicotinic acid on myocardial metabolism in man at rest and during exercise. J Appl Physiol 33:72, 1972
23. Lindner PG, Blackburn GL: Multidisciplinary approach to obesity, utilizing fasting modified by protein-sparing therapy. Obes Bariat Med 5:198, 1976
24. Linn R, Stuart SL: The Last Chance Diet. Secaucus, NJ, L Stuart, 1976
25. March BE, Wong E: Hypervitaminosis E in the chick. J Nutr 103:371, 1973
26. Mason KE, Horwitt MK: Tocopherols X. Effects of deficiency in animals. In Sebrell WH Jr, Harris RS (eds): The Vitamins, p 272. New York, Academic Press, 1972
27. Mustafa MG: Influence of dietary vit E on lung cellular sensitivity to ozone in rats. Nutr Rep Int 2:473, 1975
28. National Research Council. Nutrient requirement of the laboratory rat. In Nutrient Requirements of Laboratory Animals, Vol 10, p 64. Washington, DC, National Academy of Sciences, 1972
29. Nutrition misinformation and food faddism. Nutr Revs (Suppl) 32:37, 1974
30. Olesen ES, Quaade F: Fatty foods and obesity. Lancet 1:1048, 1960
31. Pauling L: Vitamin C and the Common Cold. San Francisco, WH Freeman, 1970

32. Pritikin N, McGrady P Jr: The Pritikin Program. New York, Grosset and Dunlap, 1978
33. Register UD, Sonnenberg LM: The vegetarian diet. J Am Diet Assoc 62:253, 1973
34. Rosenthal G: Interaction of ascorbic acid and warfarin. JAMA 215:1671, 1971
35. Smith FR, Goodman DS: Vitamin A transport in human vit A toxicity. N Engl J Med 294:805, 1976
36. Smith PG, Jick H: Cancers among users of preparations containing vit A. Cancer 42:808–11, 1978
37. Sporn MB, Newton DL: Chemoprevention of cancer with retinoids. Fed Proc 38:2528, 1979
38. Stillman IM, Baker SS: The Doctor's Quick Weight Loss Diet. New York, Dell Publishing, 1967
39. US Senate, Select Committee on Nutrition and Human Needs: Diet Related to Killer Diseases, p 676. Washington, D.C., G.P.O., 1977
40. White HS: The organic food movement. Food Technol 26:29, 1972
41. Wyatt RJ: Comment. Am J Psychiat 131:1258, 1974
42. Yudkin J, Carey M: The treatment of obesity by the "high fat diet." The inevitability of calories. Lancet 2:939, 1960

Suggested Reading

McBean LD, Speckmann EW: Food faddism: A challenge to nutritionists and dieticians. Am J Clin Nutr 27:1071, 1974

Ellenbogen L (ed): Controversies in Nutrition. New York, Churchill-Livingstone, 1981

Jellife DB, Jelliffe EFP (eds): Adverse Effects of Foods. New York, Plenum Press, 1981

Herbert V, Barrett S: Vitamins and "Health Foods." Philadelphia, Stickley, 1981

9
The Nutrition Support Service in Hospital Practice

George L. Blackburn,
B. Smith Hopkins,
Bruce R. Bistrian

Initial evidence that a significant number of hospitalized patients suffer moderate to severe protein–calorie malnutrition (PCM) came from university municipal hospitals dealing with acute medical and surgical care.[1,2] More recent nutritional surveys confirm the prevalence of PCM or hypoalbuminemic malnutrition in many institutional settings.[16,25,27]

The advent of total parenteral nutrition (TPN) and defined formula diets has made it possible to feed patients in most disease states (Tables 9-1 and 9-2).[15,28] Although there is controversy as to the optimal nutritional support for a variety of clinical situations (see Chaps. 13 and 14), it has been established that adequate nutritional support can maintain the nutritional status of all patients and can replete all malnourished patients except those with advanced age, severe stress such as prolonged sepsis, and possibly some forms of cancer.[3,24]

Preliminary evidence suggests that nutritional maintenance or repletion substantially improves mortality and morbidity of hospitalized patients with nonmalignant disease and may reduce postoperative complications in malnourished patients.[10,21] Further preliminary evidence shows that short-term preoperative nutritional repletion of malnourished patients substantially reduces morbidity and mortality.[19] The nutritional maintenance or repletion of hospitalized patients is becoming part of standard medical care in hospitals of all types. Yet there remains a general lack of knowledge by physicians about nutrition that contrasts with the growing sophistication in nutritional diagnosis and treatment. This disparity, and a concern about the poor nu-

tritional status of hospitalized patients, led to the development of the *nutrition support service* (NSS) concept and the specialty of clinical nutrition to allow for the optimal use of increasingly complex nutritional therapies with a minimum of unnecessary morbidity and mortality.[22]

Assessment of Nutritional Risk

The challenge for an NSS is to establish a team approach to malnutrition appropriate to the individual setting. The NSS should provide surveillance for all patients in order to screen for those patients who require complete nutritional assessment and to further identify those who will benefit from nutritional support therapies. A standard medical examination is often inadequate to evaluate "nutritional risk," specifically in those patients who have deficient visceral organ function and impaired host defense, which can prevent optimal response to medical therapies. In these at-risk patients, who may not have obviously significant deficits in lean body mass, a relatively selective and rapidly occurring deficit in visceral protein status develops during semi-starvation in association with a stress response to acute illness, injury, or medical therapy.[14,19]

Procedures for surveillance, assessment (see Chap. 10), and treatment of malnutrition will vary in different hospital settings (*i.e.,* chronic care, primary care, medical center, or university or tertiary-care hospitals). Surveillance must include a dietary history and at least some simple biometric measurements.

TABLE 9-1
Concentration* Amino Acids and Various Salts of Commercially Available Products

Components	Aminosyn M 3.5% (Abbott)	Aminosyn 5% (Abbott)	Aminosyn 7% (Abbott)	Aminosyn 10% (Abbott)	FreAmine II 8.5% (McGaw)	Travasol 5.5% (Travenol)	Travasol 8.5% with Electrolytes (Travenol)	Travasol 8.5% (Travenol)	Veinamine 8% (Cutter)
Essential Amino Acids (mg)									
L-isoleucine	252	360	510	720	590	263	406	406	490
L-leucine	329	470	660	940	770	340	526	526	350
L-lysine	252	360	510	720	870	318	492	492	670
	(as Ac)	(as Ac)	(as Ac)	(as Ac)	(as Ac)	(as HCl)	(as HCl)	(as HCl)	
L-methionine	140	200	280	400	480	318	492	492	430
L-phenylalanine	154	220	310	440	340	340	526	526	400
L-threonine	182	260	370	520	340	230	356	356	160
L-tryptophan	56	80	120	160	130	99	152	152	80
L-valine	280	400	560	800	560	252	390	390	250
dL-methionine			450						
dL-tryptophan									
Nonessential Amino Acids (mg)									
L-alanine	448	640	900	1280	600	1140	1760	1760	†
L-arginine	343	490	690	980	310	570	880	880	750
L-histidine	105	150	210	300	240	241	372	372	240
L-proline	300	430	610	860	950	230	356	356	110
L-serine	147	210	300	420	500				
Aminoacetic acid (glycine)	448	640	900	1280	1700	1140	1760	1760	3390
L-cysteine HCl									
L-tyrosine	31	44	44	44	20	22	34	34	†
L-glutamic acid									430
L-aspartic acid									400
Electrolytes (mEq)									
Sodium	4.0					7.0	7.0	0.3	4.0
Chloride	4.0					7.0	7.0	3.4	5.0
Potassium	1.84	0.54	0.54	0.54	1.0	6.0	6.0		3.0
Magnesium	0.3					1.0	1.0		6.0
Acetate	2.7					10.0	13.0	5.2	5.0
Phosphate					2.0	6.0	6.0		
Calcium									†

*Per 100 ml

†Reduced by process

(Bistrian B, Bothe A: Management of nutrition: Hyperalimentation. In Lokich, JJ (ed): Clinical Cancer Medicine. Boston, GK Haal Medical Publishers, 1971.)

TABLE 9-2
Enteral Formulas

	Cal/ml	Osmolarity*	% Cal Protein	% Cal CHO	% Cal Fat	N:Cal	Protein Source	CHO Source	Fat Source	mEq Na/l	Function
SUPPLEMENTS											
Carnation Inst. Breakfast + whole milk (Carnation)	1.05	NA	22	51	27	1:85	Whole milk nonfat dry milk, sodium caseinate, soy protein isolate	Sucrose, corn syrup solids, lactose	Whole milk fat	40.4	High-protein supplement, oral or tube feeding
Citrotein (Doyle)	0.66	500	24	73	0.5	1:178	Pasteurized egg white solids	Sucrose, maltodextrins	Vegetable oil	31	Minimal fat, high-protein supplement
Lanolac (Mead–Johnson)	0.67	NA	21	30	49	1:93	Casein	Lactose	Coconut oil	1.1	Low-sodium protein beverage
Lolactene (Doyle)	0.8	670	26	53	21	1:70	Low lactose nonfat dry milk, sodium caseinate	Corn syrup solids, sucrose	Vegetable oil	38	99.6% lactose-free supplement
Meritene liquid (Doyle)	1	560–617	24	46	30	1:79	Concentrated sweet skim milk, sodium caseinate	Corn syrup solids	Vegetable oil	40	High-protein supplement for oral or tube feeding
Meritene Powder plus whole milk (Doyle)	1.06	690	26	45	29	1:71	Processed nonfat dry milk	Corn syrup solids, sucrose	Cow milk fat	41.8	High-protein supplement for oral or tube feeding
Sustacal liquid (Mead–Johnson)	1	625	24	55	21	1:79	Calcium caseinate, soy protein isolate	Sucrose, corn syrup	Partially hydrogenated soy oil	40	Lactose-free high-protein supplement
Sustacal powder + whole milk	1.3	756	24	54	22	1:79	Nonfat dry milk	Sucrose, corn syrup	Cow milk fat	30.7	High-protein supplement when mixed with milk contains 114 g lactose
Sustacal pudding (per 5 oz-37 g can)	1.6/g	NA	11.3	53.2	35.5	1:196	Nonfat milk	Sucrose, starch	Hydrogenated soy oil	5.2	High-calorie supplement offers change in consistency

TABLE 9-2
Enteral Formulas (*Continued*)

	Cal/ml	Osmolarity*	% Cal Protein	% Cal CHO	% Cal Fat	N:Cal	Protein Source	CHO Source	Fat Source	mEq Na/l	Function
Sustagen powder	1.7	721	24	68	8	1:79	Nonfat milk, powdered whole milk, calcium caseinate	Corn syrup solids, dextrose	Cow milk fat	54	High-calorie (mainly from CHO), high-protein, low-fat formula for oral use or tube feeding
MEAL REPLACEMENTS											
Compleat 'B' (Doyle)	1.0	517	16	48	36	1:131	Puree beef, nonfat dry milk	Maltodextrin, vegetable & fruit purees, sucrose	Corn oil, beef fat	55.1	Blenderized house diet for tube feeding
Ensure (Ross)	1.06	450	14	54.5	31.5	1:153	Sodium & calcium caseinats, soy protein isolate	Corn syrup solids, sucrose	Corn oil	32.2	Lactose-free meal; replacement formula for oral or tube
Ensure Plus (Ross)	1.5	600	14.6	53	32	1:146	Sodium & calcium caseinates, soy protein isolate	Corn syrup solids, sucrose	Corn oil	46	Calorically dense formula for oral or tube feeding
Formula 2 (Cutter)	1.0	435–510	15	49	36	1:142	Skim milk, beef, egg yolk	Sucrose, vegetables, orange juice, wheat flour	Corn oil, egg yolk, beef fat	26	Blenderized tube feeding, nutritionally complete
Isocal (Mead–Johnson)	1.06	300	13	50	37	1:168	Calcium & sodium caseinates; soy protein isolate	Glucose oligosaccharides	Soy oil (80%), MCT (20%)	23	Unflavored tube feeding formula, lactose-free
Magnacal (Organon)	2.0	590	14	50	36	1:154	Calcium caseinate, sodium caseinate	Maltodextrin, corn syrup solids, sucrose	Soy oil mono-, diglycerides	43.5	High-calorie formula, nutritionally complete tube or oral feeding

	cal/ml	mOsm				ratio	Protein source	Carbohydrate source	Fat source		
Nutri-1000 LF (Cutter)	1.06	304	15.1	46.7	38.2	1:141	Skim milk	Sucrose, lactose, dextrin-maltose, dextrose	Corn oil	22.9	Lactose-free meal replacement formula for oral or tube feeding
Osmolite (Ross)	1.06	300	14	54.6	31.4	1:157	Sodium & calcium caseinates, soy protein isolate	Corn syrup solids	MCT (20%), corn oil, soy oil	23	Unflavored tube feeding formula; lactose-free
Portagen (Mead–Johnson)	1.0	354	14	46	40	1:154	Sodium caseinate	Corn syrup solids, sucrose	MCT (86%), corn oil (14%)	20.4	Intended for use with those patients who malabsorb long-chain fats, essentially lactose-free (<0.3 g lactose/960 ml)
Precision Isotonic (Doyle)	0.96		12	60	28	1:184	Pasteurized egg white solids	Glucose oligosaccharides, sucrose	Soy oil	33	Isotonic formula for oral or tube feeding
Renu (Organon)	1.01	330	13	51	36	1:166	Sodium & calcium caseinates	Maltodextrin, corn syrup, corn & malt syrup	Soy oil, mono-, diglycerides	21.7	Tube or oral feeding, low sodium
Travasorb whole protein liquid (Travenol)	1.06	450	14	54.5	31.5	1:154	Sodium & calcium caseinates, soy protein isolate	Sucrose, corn syrup solids	Corn oil, soy oil (partially hydrogenated)	32	Lactose-free tube or oral feeding
Vitaneed (Organon)	1.02	400	14	51	35	1:157	Puree beef, calcium caseinate	Corn syrup solids, maltodextrin, puree fruit/vegetables	Soy oil, mono-diglycerides	23.9	Blenderized tube feeding; nutritionally complete
FORMULA DFD† Flexical (Mead–Johnson)	1.0	550	9	61	30	1:253	Hydrolyzed casein, methionine, tyrosine, tryptophane	Corn syrup solids, dextrioligosaccharides	MCT (20%), partially (80%) hydrogenated soy oil	15.2	Protein source is 70% free a.a., 30% small peptides; usually for tube feeding; flavor packs available

TABLE 9-2
Enteral Formulas (Continued)

	Cal/ml	Osmolarity*	% Cal Protein	% Cal CHO	% Cal Fat	N:Cal	Protein Source	CHO Source	Fat Source	mEq Na/l	Function
Precision–LR (Doyle)	1.08	600	9.5	89.9	1.3	1:239	Pasteurized egg white solids	Maltodextrin, sucrose	Soy oil, MCT	30.5	Low-residue minimal fat formula for oral or tube feeding. Protein source requires digestion
Precision–HN (Doyle)	1.1	580	16.6	82.6	1.1	1:125	Pasteurized egg white solids	Maltodextrin, sucrose	Soy oil, MCT	42.6	High-nitrogen, low-residue, minimal fat formula for oral or tube feeding. Protein source requires digestion
Travasorb std. (Travenol)	1.0	450	12	76	12	1:202	Oligopeptides of fortified lactalbumin	Glucose oligosaccharides	MCT (40%), sunflower oil (60%)	40	"Elemental" oligopeptide; protein source of high biological value. Although easily absorbed, some digestive capacity required. Minimal residue. Unflavored packs available (increase osmolarity)

[116]

							Protein source	Carbohydrate source	Fat source		Comments
Travasorb HN (Travenol)	1.0	450	18	70	12	1:126	Oligopeptides of fortified lactalbumin	Glucose oligosaccharides	MCT (40%), sunflower oil (60%)	40	"Elemental" oligopeptide; high nitrogen. Although easily absorbed, some digestive capacity required. Minimal residue, unflavored packs available (increase osmolarity)
Travasorb MCT (Travenol)	1.0	250	20	50	30	1:100	Lactalbumin, potassium caseinate	Corn syrup solids	MCT, sunflower oil	15	Protein source requires digestion; high-protein content. Low osmolarity. Low sodium, 80% of fat calories from MCT, unflavored
Vipep	1	520	10	68	22	1:228	Enzymatically hydrolyzed whole fish protein concentrate	Corn syrup solids, glucose, potassium gluconate, corn starch	MCT oil, corn oil	32.6	19.6% free amino acids; 72.5% di-, teti peptides; 7.9% 4–14% a.a. chain; 18% fat calories as MCT; 4% as corn
Vital (Ross)	1.0	450	16.7	74	9.3	1:125	Enzymatically hydrolyzed soy, whey, meat, free amino acids	Glucose oligo- & polysac-charides, sucrose	Safflower oil, MCT oil	17	Hydrolyzed protein source (due to tetrapeptides) for oral or tube feeding
Vivonex Std. (unflavored) (flavored) (Morton–Norwich)	1.0	550 610–678	8.2	90.5	1.3	1:281	Crystalline amino acids	Glucose oligosaccharides	Safflower oil	20	Minimal fat, low residue formula: easily absorbed protein source

TABLE 9-2
Enteral Formulas (*Continued*)

	Cal/ml	Osmolarity*	% Cal Protein	% Cal CHO	% Cal Fat	N:Cal	Protein Source	CHO Source	Fat Source	mEq Na/l	Function
Vivonex HN (unflavored) (flavored) (Morton–Norwich)	1.0	810 850–920	17.7	81.5	.8	1:125	Crystalline amino acids	Glucose oligosaccharides	Safflower oil	23	Minimal fat, low residue, high protein formula; easily absorbed protein source
Amin–Aid (McGaw)	1.95	850	4	74.8	21.2	1:638	Essential amino acid	Maltodextrins, sugar, citric acid	Partially hydrogenated soy oil, mono- & diglycerides	14.7	Provides high calorie, low protein diet of essential a.a. only; for use in renal failure; contains no vitamins; limited electrolytes
Hepatic–Aid (McGaw)	1.6	900	10.4	69.8	19.8	1:225	Essential & nonessential a.a.; BCAA enriched	Maltodextrins, sucrose	Soybean oil, mono- & diglycerides	None	Provides high calorie BCAA enriched formula; theoretically useful in treatment of hepatic encephalopathy; no vitamins or minerals
FEEDING MODULES											
Casec (powder) (per 100 g) (Mead–Johnson)	3.6/g		95	0	4.8		Calcium caseinate	None	Butter fat	6	Concentrated protein source
Controlyte (powder) (Doyle)	5.0/g		Negligible	57	43		Trace	Polysaccharides of deionized partial hydrolysate of corn starch	Vegetable oil	0.65/100 g	Provides calorie source

Product										Comments
Pro-mix (Nubro)	3.7		0.80	4.2	3.9	Whey	Lactose	Milk fat	6.5/100 g	Concentrated protein source
Polycose (powder) (Ross)	4 cal/min		0	96	0	None	Hydrolyzed corn starch	None	4.7/100 g	Provides calorie source; low osmolarity; tasteless
Polycose (liquid) (Ross)	2.0	570	0	96	0	None	Hydrolyzed corn starch	None	26.2	
MCT oil (per 100 ml) (Mead–Johnson)	7.7		0	0	100		None	MCT	0	Special dietary supplement for patients malabsorbing long-chain fats
Microlipid (Organon)	4.5	32	0	0	100	None	None	Safflower oil; mono-, diglycerides	0	A 50% fat emulsion used to increase caloric density of enteral feedings
Sumacal	2.0	680	100	0	0	None	Maltodextrin; glucose, syrup solids	None	8.7	Liquid carbohydrate source used to increase caloric density of enteral feedings
Sumacal Plus (Organon)	2.5	890	100	0	0	None	Maltodextrin, glucose syrup solids	None	9.1	Liquid carbohydrate source used to increase the caloric density of enteral feedings

NA = Not available
*mOsmol/kg H$_2$O
†Defined Formula Diets
MCT = Medium Chain Triglycerides

NUTRITIONAL RISK AS A PREDICTOR OF PATIENT OUTCOME

Seltzer and colleagues have suggested monitoring the routine admission values of albumin and total lymphocyte count.[26] In a review of 500 consecutive hospital admissions, they found an abnormal serum albumin (<3.5 g/dl) associated with a four-fold increase in complications and a sixfold increase in mortality, while an abnormal lymphocyte count (<1500/mm³) reflected a fourfold increase in the likelihood of mortality. If both serum albumin and total lymphocyte count were abnormal, the risk of complications was again four times that of the "normal" hospital population, and deaths were 20 times as common.

More elaborate predictive models of nutritional assessment and surveillance include the prognostic nutritional index (PNI) developed by Mullen and associates as a linear predictive marker of postoperative mortality and morbidity:[20]

PNI (%) = 158 − 16.6 (ALB) − 0.78 (TSF) − 0.20 (TFN) − 5.8 (DH), where ALB = serum albumin in g/100 ml, TSF = triceps skinfold in mm, TFN = serum transferrin in mg/100 ml, and DH = cutaneous delayed hypersensitivity to any of three recall antigens (candida, mumps, SK/SD) scored as follows: nonreactive = 0, <5 mm = 1, ≥5 mm = 2. Buzby and colleagues have prospectively validated the PNI as a sensitive predictor of risk in surgical patients.[9]

While estimating risk of mortality in a mixed medical surgical population referred for nutrition support consultation at a large university hospital, Harvey and colleagues developed a more elaborate discriminant function, 0.91 (ALB) − 1.00 (DH) − 1.44 (SEPSIS) + 0.98 (DIAGNOSIS) − 1.09, where ALB = serum albumin in g/100 ml, DH = cutaneous delayed hypersensitivity to three standard recall antigens (candida, mumps, SK/SD) with any ≥5 mm induration = 1 and all three <5 mm induration = 2, SEPSIS = no = 1, yes = 2, and DIAGNOSIS = cancer = 1, noncancer = 2. The overall predictive value for subsequent hospital mortality was 72%, with a discriminant function value of ≥ + 2 predicting a 90% survival rate, ≤ − 1 predicting a 25% survival rate, and 0 predicting a 50% survival rate.[14] Of these four factors found to significantly predict outcome, only improvement in DH response was a significant predictor of improved prognosis with nutritional support in this patient population.

The current status of nutritional assessment, the metabolic response to injury, and the role of protein–calorie management in hospitalized patients are reviewed elsewhere (see Chaps. 10 and 11). It is the purpose of this chapter to discuss the safe management of clinical nutrition in the hospital by a nutrition support service, describing some of its essential components and functions. For more detailed discussions, see also the proceedings of a symposium on the establishment and function of an NSS, as well as a variety of available manuals on the subject.[8,12,17]

The Establishment of a Nutrition Support Service

GOALS

The first step in the establishment of an NSS is the creation of a nutrition committee with appropriate representatives from the departments of medicine, surgery, pediatrics, nursing, dietitians, pharmacy, social service, physical therapy, and other interested groups. This committee will begin to develop policy and procedure guidelines with the following goals:

1. To provide the clinical support for the safe delivery of nutritional therapies
2. To establish a mechanism for the surveillance (for clinically significant malnutrition) of all hospital admissions
3. To nutritionally assess all patients found to be at-risk for protein–calorie malnutrition and, where indicated, to institute nutritional support prior to elective therapies and procedures likely to be complicated by malnutrition
4. To evaluate the effectiveness of nutritional therapies in individual patients
5. To ensure quality control in the delivery of nutritional therapies

These goals can best be accomplished by a multidisciplinary approach of a nutrition support group, although the specific design and functioning of an NSS will vary widely within a range of different hospital settings. Without the organized interaction of a number of clinical professionals, safe, effective nutritional therapies cannot be guaranteed, and are in fact unlikely.[22]

NUTRITIONAL MANAGEMENT GOALS IN HOSPITAL PRACTICE

1. Formulation of Hospital Policy
   — Guidelines for nutritional surveillance and assessment
   — Procedures for nutritional support
2. Nutritional Surveillance
   — Mechanism for good nutritional history, especially relating to weight loss, in all hospital admissions

3. Nutritional Assessment
   — Standard techniques (see Chap. 10) in all patients at risk for malnutrition based on nutritional surveillance
   — Triggering a nutrition support consultation in patients whose *prognostic nutritional index* or *hospital prognostic index* documents moderate or severe risk of morbidity on a nutritional basis[9,14,19]
4. Assessment of Nutritional Therapy
   — Periodic monitoring of nitrogen balance and serum, albumin, and transferrin levels; total lymphocyte counts; anthropometrics; grip strength testing; and delayed hypersensitivity reactivity
5. Quality Control
   — Periodic monitoring of liver function tests, catheter infections, metabolic and catheter-related complications, and efficacy of therapies

An NSS should combine the services of nursing, dietetics, pharmacy, and physical therapy with the major clinical disciplines and emphasize the treatment of protein–calorie malnutrition (PCM). There is a high prevalence of this disorder in hospital settings, in large measure caused by disease, but in part resulting from the frequent association of semistarvation with medical treatment.[1,2,16,25,27] A minimum of 5% of the patients in any acute medical/surgical hospital will meet established criteria for severe PCM and require intensive nutritional support. Thus, any hospital caring for patients should have an identifiable nutrition counseling service, even if it consists of only an interested physician, a therapeutic dietitian, and a nurse who functions as an epidemiologist. Education in nutrition has been so limited and poorly organized in most medical schools that most physicians are unable either to recognize nutritional problems or to use available nutritional techniques to reverse PCM.

The smaller hospital dealing with the acutely ill medical and surgical patient and offering total parenteral nutrition (TPN) requires a clinician, a therapeutic dietitian, and a pharmacist under the supervision of an interested, properly trained physician to care for routine nutritional problems that seriously affect response to illness. The hospital nutrition service developed in larger hospitals should expand to include a multidisciplinary team able to use the many scientific and technologic advances in nutrition. Another responsibility that can be assumed by this enlarged service includes clinical evaluation of the safety and efficacy of many meal-replacement items, food supplements, defined formula diets, and parenteral feeding solutions (see Chaps. 13 and 14). Larger contributions to post-graduate training through grand rounds, consultations, supervised therapy, lectures, and formal continuing education courses are useful ancillary activities.

The established NSS in larger hospitals will be able to provide outpatient nutritional support for patients undergoing cancer therapy or those with convalescent nutritional problems secondary to primary disease, for instance, "short gut," inflammatory bowel disease, pancreatic insufficiency, renal disease, or obesity. Major research efforts would be in the areas of metabolism, endocrinology, gastroenterology, nephrology, and cardiology, in addition to clinical nutrition.

An ancillary, important, and entirely appropriate role of all NSSs, large and small, is to correct by lay nutritional education the misinformation and half-truths that exist among the community at large. Through these efforts, NSSs will rapidly attract the lay and professional attention, respect, and support necessary to bring nutrition abreast of the other health-care specialists. The role of the public health nutritionist in community medicine is a separate entity and beyond the scope of this chapter. (See Chap. 7.) Further, the primary function of a nutrition service is in patient treatment, not public health nutrition, which is best served through other agencies. These two specialists can, however, complement each other, and mutual referrals may be an appropriate avenue for exchange of experiences.

PROCEDURE FOR ESTABLISHING A NUTRITION SUPPORT SERVICE

Establishment of an NSS progresses from the formation of a nutrition committee. Representatives on this committee should include administrators as well as interested staff from medicine, surgery, pediatrics, obstetrics, gastroenterology, oncology, and other subspecialties; a senior therapeutic dietitian; a pharmacist; a nurse clinician; and the supervisor of nurses. The purpose of such a committee is to ascertain the needs of the hospital for nutritional support, to provide guidelines for parenteral "hyperalimentation" and nutritional assessment, to prepare standard order sheets and instructions for therapeutic dietitians, and to establish guidelines for the pharmacy. In addition, determination of personnel requirements and job descriptions are appropriate tasks. Preliminary requests for estimated salary requirements, space, equipment and supplies, and solutions should be formulated. Application for status as a reimbursable service from third-party carriers, development of a schedule of charges, and preparation of a budget are prerequisites for viability. It must be remembered during this planning stage that an NSS is an evolving, growing entity.[5,8,12,17] Plans should allow reasonable flexibility and should anticipate a considerable increase in the use of nutritional therapies as the success of the NSS becomes known.

RESPONSIBILITIES OF COMMITTEE PERSONNEL

THE CHAIRMAN

The chairman of the committee would be the anticipated nutrition service director, a physician who must have the time and interest to develop knowledge in clinical nutrition and the metabolism of stress as well as the techniques of nutritional assessment and interpretation, and the techniques of parenteral and enteral hyperalimentation. Within the framework of a hospital nutrition support service, the first priority for this physician is to develop a team that will deliver parenteral hyperalimentation effectively, since this represents the most immediate clinical need. Further expansion of nutritional techniques to include defined-formula diets and other tube feedings in the "fed" state and with various protein-sparing regimens in the semistarved state should follow (see Chap. 11). Programs for nutritional rehabilitation of patients with inadequate digestive function (*e.g.,* short bowel syndrome, jejunoileal bypass, radiation enteritis, Crohn's disease) and of oncology patients, both prior and subsequent to specific therapy, will require protocols for nutritional therapy. As the nutritional aspects of other diseases (renal, cardiac, pulmonary, gastroenterologic, for instance) are explored, associates from other specialties can contribute to the expansion of knowledge in clinical nutrition (see section on Application of Nutrition to Clinical Specialties, beginning with Chap. 15).

Clinical laboratory facilities are necessary to determine parameters of energy and nitrogen metabolism (*i.e.,* urinary urea nitrogen), body composition (*i.e.,* creatinine height index), and assays of micro- and macronutrient components of tissues and blood fluids (*i.e.,* albumin, transferrin, carotene, B_{12}, folic acid). Bacteriologic facilities and infectious disease consultants are essential because of the reduction in host immune function in the malnourished patient and the increase in the hazard of serious infection with TPN (see Chaps. 13 and 14).[13]

THE HYPERALIMENTATION NURSE

In the smaller hospital providing only TPN, total staff may include only the part-time services of a nurse or dietitian, a physician, and a pharmacist.

A full-time nurse clinician will be the key person to ensure safe and optimal delivery of parenteral hyperalimentation. In addition, she or he can serve the hospital as an infectious disease epidemiologist. Responsibilities of the nurse clinician would include in-service teaching, technical help with catheter insertions, the routine management of catheters and dressings, and administration and reading of delayed hypersensitivity skin tests (thus ensuring quality and uniformity). Other duties should include responsibility for integrating the nursing-care plan for the patient in order to ensure that a diagnostic work-up takes place in an efficient manner while not interfering with basic requirements for adequate nutrition and exercise, fully utilizing the expertise of physical therapy. The nurse clinician will frequently develop a close relationship with the seriously ill patient, which in itself can be of therapeutic value, as well as provide more information to the service about the patient's other ongoing problems and an assessment of the patient's ability for self-care. In the setting of a large university hospital, the nurse clinician is also often the coordinator of care, services, and training of home TPN patients.

THE DIETITIAN

The therapeutic dietitian or nutritionist would coordinate his work with a nurse and assume particular responsibility for composition and techniques of oral and tube feedings (see Chap. 5). Either the nurse or the dietitian can gather the data necessary for the nutritional assessment of the patient, specifically doing the anthropometric measurements or an estimate of lean body mass and fat stores. The "hyperal" dietitian serves as a liaison with the dietary department, coordinates the obtaining of a complete admission, the dietary history, including loss of appetite and rate of weight loss, and the gathering of accurate calorie counts, and supervises the program of transitional feedings in patients being weaned from TPN and modular feeding supplementation. Together with the nurse clinician, the dietitian nutritionist also coordinates home enteral feeding programs when required.

THE PHARMACIST

Preparation of parenteral feeding solutions and procurement of many dietary supplements require a pharmacist who specializes in this area to protect against errors in medication orders, to prepare the nutritional products for patient use, and to deal with the manufacturing representatives for these products. This pharmacist's knowledge of the physiochemical properties of macro- and micronutrients in TPN can minimize waste and provide considerably increased flexibility in preparation of TPN solutions to include a variety of other medications. The usual close relationship of the pharmacy to the IV therapy department can also be exploited through the "hyperal" pharmacist to enlist the full understanding and cooperation of IV nurses in the delivery of safe TPN. Again, in the setting of the large university hospital, training home TPN patients in solution preparation and coordinating procurement of home TPN supplies requires a pharmacist specializing in nutritional therapies.

THE ADMINISTRATION

An interested and dedicated administrator is also essential in the large hospital setting. Administrative duties include data collection, fiscal reporting, and the monitoring of productivity and cost effectiveness, as well as education, public relations, and communications. Without such data, maintenance of a viable reimbursable service is impossible.

THE PHYSICIAN

The supervision of these specialists requires an interested and properly trained physician. His primary training need not interfere with the ability to deliver nutrition for all types of patients, since the major nutritional problem in American hospitals is PCM, which transcends specialty lines.

In larger hospitals a team with increased number, types, and time commitment of personnel is desirable. Additional functions can be assumed by this multidisciplinary team, such as clinical investigation to advance nutritional science.[6] Consideration should be given to the establishment of a special area with quasi-metabolic ward characteristics for nutritional care in complicated cases when careful monitoring of intake and output is necessary. Finally, a nutrition outpatient clinic for follow-up care and management will extend the benefits of the service to the ambulatory patient and to the community at large.

EDUCATIONAL TEAM

In both large and small hospitals the NSS personnel should conduct intensive education for house staff and practicing physicians by informal rounds, bedside instruction, and the consultation service. A library of basic nutrition information and recent developments in the treatment of PCM should be provided, and periodic newsletters and memoranda involving techniques of parenteral and enteral feedings should be distributed to the hospital community, including the patient and his family,

to encourage everyone's interest and compliance in nutritional therapies.

The Functioning of the Nutritional Support Service

A description of the functioning of the service at the New England Deaconess Hospital serves as a model. Under the co-directors, the team consists of therapeutic dietitians, nurse clinicians, pharmacists, and a nurse epidemiologist. Several residents from medicine and surgery and a nutritional fellow complete the consulting team, although consultants from several specialty services dealing with infectious disease, renal, pulmonary, and GI disorders, and social work can be employed.

FORMULATION OF A NUTRITIONAL PROGRAM

Patients admitted to the hospital who are in a state of moderate PCM necessitating parenteral or enteral nutrition and hospitalized patients whose nutritional requirements cannot be met by standard nutritional practice are referred to the service. The following data are procured from both categories of patients:

1. Age
2. Sex
3. Height
4. Usual weight
5. Present weight
6. Nutritional assessment and characterization of type of PCM (Fig. 9-1; see Chap. 10).

The data accumulated in Figure 9-2 is derived from a series of nomograms incorporated into a computer program that provides the metabolic data necessary to formulate nutritional programs for treatment when parameters 1 to 6 are provided (Figs. 9-2, 9-3). The basal energy expenditure (BEE) is derived from the Harris–Benedict equation using the first four above parameters to allow for factors not adequately covered by formulas based on weight alone. In states of mild to moderate catabolism, delivery of standard TPN at 1.75 times the BEE should produce positive nitrogen balance. By the oral route 1.3 to 1.5 times the BEE is sufficient for maintenance.[4] After the protein and calorie requirements for maintenance and anabolic therapy have been obtained, selection of parenteral and oral diet may begin; fed versus starved and oral versus IV decisions are determined by the results of nutritional assessment (see Chaps. 10 and 11). Formula diets, supplemental feedings, and parenteral feedings provide a wide variety of techniques to

Anthropometric Measurements	Percent Standard				
	Actual	Severe	Moderate	Mild	Standards
Weight (usual) (kg)					
(present)				—	
Arm circumference (cm)		—	—	—	
Triceps skinfold (mm)				—	
Arm muscle circumference (cm)				—	
Height (cm)					
Biochemical indices					

	Actual	Severe	Moderate	Mild	Standards	
					M	F
Urine Creatinine height index (CHI)				—		
Urine urea nitrogen (UUN)				—	/////	
Nitrogen balance (N$_{bal}$)				—	/////	
Catabolic index (CI)					>5 g = severe, <0 = mild 0–5 = moderate	
Serum: Albumin (Alb)					≥3.5 g/dl	
Transferrin (TFN)				—	≥170 mg/dl	
Total lymphocyte count (TLC)				—	≥1500 cells/mm^3	
Immune function						
Candida			—	—	≥5 mm induration	
Mumps			—	—	≥5 mm erythema/ind.	
Tetanus toxoid			—	—	≥5 mm induration	
Other						

	Actual	High	Moderate	Low	
Prognostic nutritional index (PNI)					High <40% Moderate 40%–49% Low ≥50%
Hospital nutritional index (HNI)					High <−1, Low >+1 Moderate +1−−1

Summary:

☐ Not depleted

☐ Marasmus

☐ Hypoalbuminemia (Kwashiorkor-like)

☐ Mixed marasmus–hypoalbuminemia

Marasmus: Depressed anthropometrics. Maintenance of visceral proteins.

Hypoalbuminemia: Depressed visceral proteins. Depressed cellular immunity. Maintenance of anthropometrics.

Mixed: Depressed anthropometrics. Depressed visceral proteins. Depressed cellular immunity.

Suggested energy requirements:

Basal energy expenditure: (Harris–Benedict)

Males: $66 + (13.7 \times W) + (5 \times H) - (6.8 \times A)$

Females: $665 + (9.6 \times W) + (1.8 \times H) - (4.7 \times A)$

W = actual weight in kg
H = height in cm
A = age in years

Anabolic requirements:

BEE × 1.76 (parenteral)

BEE × 1.54 (enteral)

Maintenance:

BEE × 1.2

FIG. 9-1 Initial assessment of nutritional status (Nutrition Support Service, N.E.D.H., 1981).

overcome the catabolic response to illness, and modification of a fast by oral or IV protein can minimize protein catabolism by maximum utilization of endogenous fat.

INITIATION OF TREATMENT

The group functions in the following manner: after a consultation request is received, the nutritional fellow or resident, the therapeutic dietitian, and the hyperalimentation nurse together provide "on the spot" expertise to the ward team. At this time each member of the group can review and evaluate with the house staff the theoretic and practical aspects of available nutritional therapies. Direct responsibility for nutritional support is often assumed by the service at the responsible physician's request, and this responsibility is invariably assumed with cases requiring TPN. After the course of therapy has been decided, each group member provides guidelines for application of the therapy to the particular patient. The physician discusses medical care and fluid, electrolyte, and nutrition monitoring procedures. The nurse instructs and supervises in special nursing procedures, including a nursing plan that minimizes the immobilization and weakness created by bed rest. The dietitian establishes and monitors all oral and tube feedings and vitamin supplementation and also works with the patient to stress the importance of nutritional therapy. A pharmacist trained in additive techniques under aseptic conditions is essential if complications are to be minimized and good results achieved. Each of these positions requires a mature, empathetic specialist who is able to communicate with these seriously ill patients, gain their confidence and cooperation, and design appropriate plans to optimize care.

MONITORING OF THERAPY

Each consultation is monitored by one of the co-directors, as is the daily follow-up of the patient throughout the course of therapy during which special laboratory data is interpreted and staff education provided. In patients requiring TPN, the nutritional service provides the primary care for this process, writing all orders, inserting catheters, and assuming responsibility on a 24-hour basis. The nurse clinician generally handles the three-times-weekly dressing changes except for special care units or when the IV therapy department substitutes for the off-duty "hyperal" nurse. This approach has minimized the infectious complications generally associated with TPN.[23]

Data fed into computer
1. Height in
2. Weight (usual) lb
3. Frame type (ring) small, medium, large
4. Weight (at Rx) lb
5. Weight (ideal) lb
6. Surface area M^2 (Based on weight at Rx)

Computer feedback
Height cm (in x 2.54)
Weight (usual) kg (lb x 2.2)
Weight (at Rx) kg (lb x 2.2)
Weight (ideal) kg (lb x 2.2)
Usual weight − ideal weight
Weight at Rx − ideal weight
Weight at Rx/ideal weight %
Weight at Rx/usual weight %

Basal energy expenditure (BEE)
Cal/24 hr
Cal/hr/M^2

Anabolic requirements (Cal/24 hr)
IV (BEE x 1.76) Cal
Oral (BEE x 1.54) Cal

Nitrogen anabolic requirements/24 hr
IV (Cals ÷ 150) g
Oral (Cals ÷ 150) g

Protein (amino acid) requirements/24 hr
IV (nitrogen x 6.25) g
Oral (nitrogen x 6.25) g

Maintenance requirements (Cal/24 hr)
Oral (BEE x 1.22) Cal

Nitrogen maintenance requirements/24 hr
Oral (Cals ÷ 300) g

Protein (amino acid) requirements/24 hr
Oral (nitrogen x 6.65) g

FIG. 9-2 Computer/calculator determination of protein and calorie requirement for nutrition maintenance or anabolism either orally or parenterally. Estimates are based on surface area plus age and sex.

Regular meetings of the NSS are attended by the member physicians, therapeutic dietitians, specialized nurses, and supportive members. Patient cases are reviewed, therapies discussed, new products evaluated, and policies and procedures for special therapies established.

GROWTH EXPERIENCE

Since the formation of the NSS in New England Deaconess Hospital in 1973, considerable success in some high-risk patients has increased the patient load of the NSS to its current daily load of greater than 20 (see Table 9-3). During this period, increased efficiency in the preparation and delivery

Derived Clinical Metabolic Rate

Identification data

Name	John Doe
Hospital	New England Deaconess
Record No.	
Building and Room No.	Farr 715

Input

Height (in)	70.0
Body type	Medium
Usual weight (lb)	160.0
Weight at initiation of therapy (lb)	137.0
Ideal weight (in lb from a nomogram)	153.0
Age (years)	55.0
Body surface area (M^2 — from a nomogram)	1.781
Sex	Male

Output

Height (cm)	178	
Ideal weight (kg)	69.5	
Weight on initiation of therapy as % of ideal weight	89.6%	
Weight on initiation of therapy as % of usual weight	85.7%	
Basal energy expenditure (BEE)	1585	Cal/day
Calories required for anabolism in this patient	2908	Cal/day
BEE corrected for BSA and hourly requirements	37.0	$Cal/hr/M^2$

Metabolic maintenance required at two different nitrogen-to-calorie ratios

1. 1-to-150 ratio — nitrogen required	16	
protein required	99	
2. 1 -to-300 ratio — nitrogen required	8	
protein required	50	

FIG. 9-3 Individual patient nutritional requirements to aid Nutrition Support Service (NSS) and staff in developing a nutrition therapy plan.

of TPN solutions has significantly decreased the number of liters of solution per patient (a major cost item). The identification of high-risk patients with serious nutritional deficiencies (approximately 5% of the hospitalized patient population) treated prior to elective or postponable surgery appears to have favorably influenced the demand for intensive-care beds, the incidence of sepsis, and the use of antibiotics.

There has also been a considerable increase in the teaching commitments of the NSS. Course subject matter covers topics including the following:

1. Metabolic basis of optimal nutrition in cachexia
2. TPN—theory, administration, special aseptic techniques, and nursing procedures
3. Elemental diets—rationale and administration
4. Tube feedings—rationale and administration
5. Diet as related to GI dysfunction
6. Protein-sparing therapies
7. Interpretation of biochemical data
8. Nutritional assessment of the hospitalized patient

The Future for Nutritional Support Service in Hospitals Rendering Acute Care

With the recent data by a number of investigators showing the predictive value of nutritional assessment and the positive benefit of nutritional support in a variety of clinical settings, the value of enteral and parenteral nutrition is firmly grounded.[9,14,20,26] Similarly, the value of the team approach outlined above has become increasingly clear, most recently documented by Nehme in a study that showed markedly fewer catheter-insertion complications, catheter-related infections, and metabolic complications from TPN in patients managed by an NSS.[22] The efficacy and safety of TPN in a smaller community hospital also has been documented in the setting of a knowledgeable physician directing a small group of interested professionals.

In an era when nutritional deficiencies, specifically protein–calorie malnutrition and hypoalbuminemic malnutrition are better understood and corrective therapies are now available, the devel-

TABLE 9-3
Growth of the Nutrition Support Service (NSS) Role at the New England Deaconess Hospital

	1973–74	*1974–75*	*1975–76*	*1976–77*	*1977–78*	*1978–79*	*1979–80*
NSS Patient Days	2,228	3,575	5,191	5,269	7,032	7,459	8,356
Total Hospital Patient Days	159,866	160,111	159,409	165,303	166,862	170,639	167,633
NSS % Total Patient Days	1%	2%	3%	3%	4%	4%	5%

(Blackburn GL, Bothe A, Lahey MA: Organization and administration of a nutrition support service. Surg Clin North Am, 61:709–719, 1981)

opment of an NSS to ensure adequate hospital surveillance of possible PCM, nutritional assessment of patients at risk, ongoing assessment of the effectiveness of nutritional therapies as well as quality control through audits, can and should be achieved in any hospital rendering the best possible acute care.

References

1. Bistrian BR, Blackburn GL, Hallowell E, Heddle R: Protein nutritional status of general surgical patients. JAMA 230:858–860, 1974
2. Bistrian BR, Blackburn GL, Vitale J, Cochran D, Naylor J: Prevalence of malnutrition in general medical patients. JAMA 235:1567–1570, 1976
3. Bistrian B, Bothe A: Management of nutrition: Hyperalimentation. In Lokich JJ (ed): Clinical Cancer Medicine, pp 249–272. Boston, GK Haal Medical Publishers, 1971
4. Blackburn GL, Bistrian BR, Maini BS, Schlamon HT, Smith MF: Nutritional and metabolic assessment of the hospitalized patient. JPEN 1:11–22, 1977
5. Blackburn GL, Bothe A, Lahey MA: Organization and administration of a nutrition support service. Surg Clin North Am 61:709–719, 1981
6. Bothe A, Bistrian BR, Blackburn GL: Nutrition support in a University Hospital. In Dudrick SJ (ed): Team Approach to Nutritional Support. New York, Appleton-Century-Crofts (in press)
7. Bothe A, Wade JE, Blackburn GL: Enteral nutrition—an overview. In Hill GL (ed): Nutrition and the Surgical Patient p 76–103. New York, Churchill-Livingston, 1981
8. Burke WA, Burkhart VP, Pierpaoli PG: A guide for a nutritional support service. Travenol Laboratories, 1981
9. Buzby GP, Mullen JL, Matthews DC, Hobbs LL, Rosato EF: Prognostic nutritional index in gastrointestinal surgery. Am J Surg 139:160–167, 1980
10. Collins JP, Oxby CB, Hill GL: Intravenous aminoacids and intravenous hyperalimentation as protein-sparing therapy after major surgery. Lancet 1:788–791, 1978
11. Dudrick SJ, Long JM, Steiger E, Rhoads JE: Intravenous hyperalimentation. Med Clin North Am 54:577–589, 1970
12. Establishing a nutrition support service. Abbott Laboratories, 1980
13. Goldman, DA, Maki DG: Infection control in total parental nutrition. JAMA 223:1360–1364, 1973
14. Harvey KB, Moldawer LL, Bistrian BR, Blackburn GL: Biological measures for the formulation of a hospital prognostic index. Am J Clin Nutr 34:2013–2022, 1981
15. Heymsfield SE, Bether RA, Ansley JD, Nixon DW, Rudman D: Enteral hyperalimentation. Ann Intern Med 90:63–71, 1979
16. Hill GL, Blackett RL, Rickford I, Birkinshaw L, Young GA, Warren JV, Schorah CJ, Morgan DB. Malnutrition in surgical patients: An unrecognized problem. Lancet 1:689–692, 1977
17. Hooley RA: Parenteral nutrition—general concept, part II. Nutritional Support Services 1 (3):41–44, 1981
18. Kaminski MV, Burke WA, Blackburn GL: Intravenous Hyperalimentation in Modern Hospital Practice. USV Pharmaceutical Corp, 1977
19. Mullen JL, Buzby GP, Smalls BF, Rosato EF: Reduction of operative morbidity and mortality by combined preoperative and postoperative nutritional support. Am Surg 192:604–613, 1980
20. Mullen JL, Gertner MH, Buzby GP, Goodhart GL, Rosato EF: Implications of malnutrition in the surgical patient. Arch Surg 114:121–125, 1979
21. Nasrallah SM, Galdubos JT: Amino acid therapy of alcohol hepatitis. Lancet 2:1276–1277, 1980
22. Nehme AE: Nutritional support of the hospitalized patient: The team concept. JAMA 243:1906–1908, 1980
23. Padberg FT, Ruggiero J, Blackburn GL, Bistrian BR: Central venous catheterization for parenteral nutrition. Ann Surg 139:264–270, 1981
24. Popp MB, Morrison SD, Brennan MF: Total parenteral nutrition in a methyl cholanthrene-induced rat sarcoma model. Cancer Treatment Rep (in press)
25. Reinhardt GF, Myscofski JW, Wilkens DB, Dobrin DB, Wangan JE, Stannard RT: Incidence and mortality of hypoalbuminemic patients in hospitalized veterans. JPEN 3:157–159, 1979
26. Seltzer MH, Bastudas JA, Cooper DM, Engler P, Slocum B, Fletcher HS: Instant nutritional assessment. JPEN 3:157–159, 1979
27. Shaver HJ, Loper JA, Lutes RA: Nutritional status of nursing home patients. JPEN 4:367–370, 1980
28. Stephens RV, Randall HT: Use of concentrated, balanced liquid elemental diet for nutritional management of catabolic states. Ann Surg 170:642–667, 1969

10
Assessment of Protein–Calorie Malnutrition in the Hospitalized Patient

Bruce R. Bistrian
George L. Blackburn

Prevalence of Protein–Calorie Malnutrition

Nutrition surveys in the United States and England have documented the existence of protein–calorie malnutrition among hospital patients.[4,7,12,27,36,49] Other studies have suggested that vitamin deficiencies are also common in hospital patients.[36,49] Both conditions have frequently gone unrecognized and untreated. Although many patients are malnourished on admission, the further consequence of a hospital stay of several weeks or longer can include a deterioration of nutritional status.[49]

A sampling of prevalence rates from different studies shows the following: 26% of patients presented hypoalbuminemia in Hill's study of surgical patients in an English teaching hospital; 43% of patients were hypoalbuminemic on admission in Butterworth's study of medical patients at the University of Alabama; and 45% of medical patients and 54% of surgical patients were similarly affected in our studies at a municipal hospital (see Fig. 10-1).[4,7,27,49]

Other measures that reflect protein nutritional status, such as weight related to height, arm muscle circumference, triceps skinfold thickness, total peripheral lymphocyte count, and hematocrit, have yielded similar results, although rates vary widely (see Figs. 10-1 and 10-2).[4,7] The lack of close correlation between different parameters suggests that the degree of sensitivity of the parameters differs, and that there may be different types of protein–calorie malnutrition.

Vitamin status of hospital patients is also severely affected. In one study, Butterworth found abnormal folic acid nutriture in 69% of patients and low Vitamin C levels in 20% of patients.[4] Hill found a low folate somewhat less often (24%), but Vitamin C was low in 24% of the patients.[27] In this latter study, riboflavin and pyridoxine were low in 20% and 6% of patients, respectively.

This amount of malnutrition is alarming, particularly since it is not restricted to people with diseases like cancer but is widely distributed among broad disease categories. If effective therapy to reverse malnutrition were not available, these findings would be of theoretical interest only. However, techniques of nutritional support that are now well established can restore or maintain a satisfactory nutritional status in most disease conditions.

CAUSES OF MALNUTRITION

The primary reason for most malnutrition present on patient admission is the anorexia that is nearly a universal accompaniment of disease. Anorexia may be part of the metabolic response to injury that is effective in mobilizing body energy and protein stores during acute stress. The denial of nutrients to invading microorganisms or to tumor tissue that results from limiting food intake might well have had survival benefit in the past, when there was no specific therapy for the underlying disease. However, with the development of effective treatments for the primary illness, the accompanying malnutrition that results from semistar-

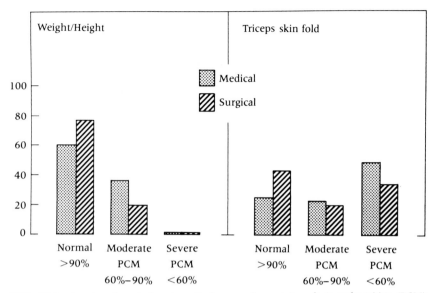

FIG. 10-1 Results of surgical and medical survey for protein–calorie malnutrition (PCM) in a municipal hospital population, in percent of "normal" standards for weight/height and triceps skinfold. (Bistrian BR, Blackburn GL, Vitale J, et al: Prevalence of malnutrition in general medical patients. JAMA 235:1567–1570, 1976)

vation can be detrimental if prolonged, because it can impair the response of the host itself to disease. The reverse is also true. Where there is still no effective therapy for a disease, such as with certain cancers, the goals of nutritional support must often be altered. There is no good evidence, for example, that nutritional support of the malnourished patient with cancer will substantially prolong life in the absence of effective cancer therapy.

A second factor in the development of protein–calorie malnutrition is that many gastrointestinal tract disturbances, such as obstruction, ileus,

FIG. 10-2 Results of surgical and medical survey for protein–calorie malnutrition (PCM) in a municipal hospital population, in percent of "normal" standards for arm muscle circumference and serum albumin. (Bistrian BR, Blackburn GL, Vitale J, et al: Prevalence of malnutrition in general medical patients. JAMA 235:1567–1570, 1976)

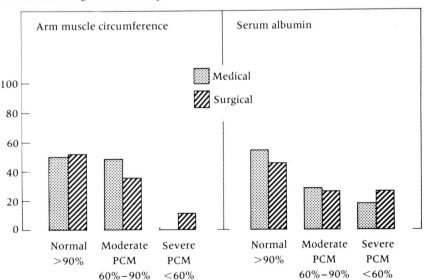

fistulas, and malabsorption syndromes, impair function. After admission, anorexia remains a factor further exacerbated by an environment that is not conducive to eating, the "missed meals" characteristic of hospitalization and the many therapies that reduce appetite. Compounding these problems is the fact that the injury or infection that generally precipitates hospital admission reduces the efficiency of utilization of most nutrients. Protein and calorie needs are increased by the metabolic response to the stress of injury or infection. In the early phase of response to injury, this is beneficial in the well-nourished host, but can be harmful if persistent or if occurring in a previously compromised host.

These two variables, semistarvation and stress, determine the degree and type of resulting malnutrition. Figure 10-3 portrays the body fuel stores available when energy needs are not met by the diet.[3,39] The body's store of carbohydrate as glycogen is extremely limited, representing about 2000 Calories, and is rapidly depleted by several days of starvation or stress.

The *lean body mass* (LBM) is the protein-containing portion of the body and represents about 75% of the body weight (slightly less in women). The LBM is the fat-free mass of the body and thus represents the body weight minus body fat (LBM = total weight − body fat). A portion of the LBM is active metabolizing tissue composed of skeletal muscle and visceral organs, representing about 40% of the body weight. This is called the *body cell mass* (BCM) by Moore.[7]

When the diet is inadequate, deficit calories are provided from three body sites—skeletal muscle, viscera, and fat. Fat tissue is the largest fuel depot, containing in excess of 150,000 stored calories in most normal adults, and can be considered dispensable. Fat represents about 25% of body weight in men and 30% in women. Protein in skeletal muscle is of functional importance but can also serve as a source of amino acids for energy and protein synthesis in visceral organs during injury and semistarvation, without serious consequence as long as losses are not great. There is far less protein in visceral organs, and even mild protein loss from these sites can impair vital functions.

When the cause of malnutrition is primarily semistarvation resulting from anorexia, fat and muscle provide most of the deficit calories, and adult marasmus is produced. This condition is characterized by a reduction in body weight reflecting loss of muscle and fat, a decrease in the triceps skinfold thickness reflecting loss of body fat, and a reduction in the arm muscle circumference reflecting loss of skeletal muscle. Serum albumin and transferrin, along with immune competence, is generally well maintained until marasmus becomes very severe. The stress of injury or infection causes a graded increase in protein loss, with increasing impairment of visceral function manifested by the development of anergy and hypoalbuminemia. This would best be categorized as hypoalbuminemic malnutrition when seen in adults in hospitals of the industrialized nations. The condition superficially resembles the kwashiorkor of children in less developed countries in that the etiologies are similar (*i.e.*, stress), but the settings in which they occur are quite different. However, true kwashiorkor (see Chap. 35) with classic skin changes, edema,

FIG. 10-3 Body composition and energy equivalence in reference man. (Data from Bistrian BR: Nutritional assessment and therapy of protein–calorie malnutrition in the hospital. J Am Diet Assoc. 71:393–397, 1979) In malnourished patients the body compartments are altered. The major energy stores (skeletal muscle protein, visceral protein, fat) can be estimated by anthropometry or appropriate secretory proteins. The sizes of the various body compartments are approximate values based primarily on data from Moore FD, Olsen K, McMurray J, et al: The Body Cell Mass and Its Supporting Environment, Philadelphia, WB Saunders, 1963.

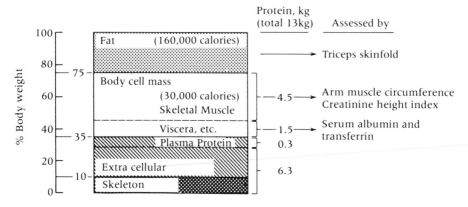

and even hair changes can and does occur in American hospitals.

The major purpose for identifying the marasmic individual is not that this condition itself is particularly life threatening, because, in fact, it is extremely well tolerated as long as there is no catabolic stress from injury, including surgery or infection. However, hypoalbuminemic malnutrition occurs very rapidly in the marasmic patient, much more quickly than in the normally nourished person, when stress is superimposed. Hypoalbuminemic malnutrition *is* a potentially life-threatening condition. A malnourished patient with hypoalbuminemia has a much greater risk of being anergic, becoming septic during hospitalization, and failing to survive hospitalization, than does his normoalbuminemic counterpart.

Figure 10-4 displays the relationship between serum albumin level and the likelihood of anergy, sepsis, and survival in 229 patients who underwent serial nutritional assessment from a representative Nutrition Support Service.[22,23] Anergic patients were 6.4 times more likely to die during hospitalization. Hypoalbuminemic patients (<3 g/dl) were 1.7 times more likely to be anergic, 1.9 times more likely to become septic, and 2 times more likely to die during hospitalization. Are these simply associated phenomena, or can nutrition make a difference? Consider the following: if a patient is anergic due to malnutrition, two weeks of nutritional support with 40 Cal and 1.5 g protein/kilogram body weight will restore immune competence and improve prognosis. In the study quoted above, 43 patients improved their immune status

with nutritional support and had a favorable mortality experience comparable to patients who were originally skin-test positive. Given this fact, and the availability of new techniques of nutritional support, such as total parenteral nutrition and commercial formulas for tube feeding, greater attention to the nutritional care of patients can no longer be ignored.

Although vitamin and mineral deficiencies occur in hospitalized patients, there are distinct differences between these deficiencies and protein malnutrition. Vitamin and mineral deficiencies are relatively easy to treat and do not require central venous access for parenteral administration. Protein–calorie malnutrition (PCM), on the other hand, generally has a profound impact on diverse body functions. In the case of protein, there is essentially no storage form as a reserve that would allow a substantial interval before significant malnutrition ensues. Because of this fact and the consideration of vitamin and mineral deficiencies elsewhere in this volume (Chaps. 4 and 12), this chapter will primarily consider the assessment of PCM and mention only briefly the routine assessment for minerals and vitamin status.

Nutrition Assessment

Three simple tests yielding four pieces of information provide most of the information necessary for assessment and categorization of protein malnutrition. These tests are weight/height, percent weight loss, serum albumin, and delayed hypersensitivity.

FIG. 10-4 Serum albumin levels in 229 patients on admission to a nutrition support service (8,19). Serum albumin levels were significantly lower in anergic patients, those with a septic hospital course, or those who died during hospitalization.

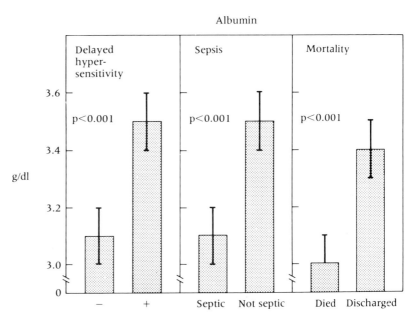

WEIGHT/HEIGHT

The measurement of height and weight is a very useful indicator of nutritional status, particularly because of the ease of assessment and the well-established norms for comparison, which have been recently updated to answer the criticism regarding frame size (see Table 10-1) although other criticisms exist.[30,47] In hospitalized individuals many pathological states lead to water retention in excess of normal (*edema*), which elevates body weight, while body cell mass (BCM) or protein content of the body is unchanged. PCM can also alter (*i.e.,* increase) the normal ratio of water-to-protein intracellularly, leading to underestimation of the severity of body protein loss.[43]

Beam balance scales for weight are preferred due to their greater accuracy. Weights in hospital gowns and bare feet or light-weight slippers are an acceptable compromise between the ease and convenience of the measurement of clothed persons and the greater reliability of nude weights. Height can be measured with a vertical measuring rod, but often in the hospitalized patient a compromise is necessary. Use of a measuring tape to estimate length (height) in the reclining subject or reliance on the patient history may often be necessary. Assessment of weight in hospitalized patients in industrialized societies is concerned both with undernutrition and obesity. The criterion for PCM would be 85% of

standard, since this has been demonstrated to have functional correlates and also approximates the fifth percentile (see later discussion of standards).[9]

PERCENT WEIGHT LOSS

As obesity becomes more prevalent in our society, categorical reliance on the 85% standard weight/height can be misleading in many instances. For example, a patient who initially exceeded 150% standard weight/height would be suffering from significant PCM long before he descended to the 85% standard. This emphasizes the point that several measures to assess PCM are necessary, and percent weight loss is one of the more important. A 10% weight loss from the former weight represents significant PCM, and would have about the same significance as it would in a patient who is at the 85% standard weight/height.[32,34] It is probably more than coincidental that a 10% weight loss from the 95% standard weight/height is approximately the 85% standard. The percent weight loss from usual weight can be considered roughly equivalent to 95% standard weight/height minus the percent weight loss. For example, a 5'5" male weighing 200 lb (150% ideal body weight) who has lost 30 lb (15% weight loss) is similar to a patient at the 80% standard weight/height (95% standard weight/height − 15% weight loss = 80% standard weight/height). Twenty percent weight loss should be considered severe and 30% life threatening. The cause of weight loss is also important, because starvation alone does not lead to high mortality rates until a 40% weight loss has occurred, whereas starvation plus stress leads to high mortality at a 25% weight loss.[19,33,35] However, as we have already discussed, the latter patients have hypoalbuminemic malnutrition; the former, adult marasmus.

TABLE 10-1
Fogarty International Center Conference on Obesity: Recommended Weight in Relation to Height

	Men		Women	
Height	*Average*	*Range*	*Average*	*Range*
METERS	KG	KG	KG	KG
1.47			46.3	41.7–54.0
1.50			47.1	42.6–55.3
1.52			48.5	43.5–56.7
1.55			50.0	44.9–58.1
1.58	55.8	50.8–63.9	51.3	46.3–59.4
1.60	57.6	52.2–65.3	52.6	47.6–60.8
1.63	58.9	53.5–67.1	54.4	49.0–62.6
1.65	60.3	54.9–68.9	55.8	50.3–64.4
1.68	61.7	56.2–70.8	58.1	51.7–66.2
1.70	63.5	58.1–73.0	59.9	53.5–68.0
1.73	65.8	59.9–75.3	61.7	55.3–69.9
1.75	67.6	61.7–77.1	63.5	57.2–71.7
1.78	69.4	63.5–78.9	65.3	59.0–73.9
1.80	71.7	65.3–81.2	67.1	60.8–70.2
1.83	73.5	67.1–83.5	68.9	62.6–78.5
1.85	75.3	68.9–85.7		
1.88	77.6	70.8–88.0		
1.91	79.8	72.6–90.3		
1.93	82.1	74.4–92.5		

Height without shoes, weight without clothes. Adapted from the Table of the Metropolitan Life Insurance Company.

SERUM ALBUMIN

Serum albumin is the major plasma protein that serves to maintain colloid osmotic pressure and to transport metals, ions, hormones, drugs, and metabolites.[45] Albumin is synthesized in the liver and equilibrates between intravascular and extravascular compartments, with about 55% of the exchangeable albumin pool in the plasma. The half-life of albumin is about 20 days. Albumin synthesis falls with fasting or protein deprivation, followed by a fall in catabolism after several days. Refeeding stimulates synthesis rapidly. Serum albumin levels fall with stress from surgery, trauma, and infection, probably owing to increased breakdown and extravasation.

Serum albumin has been considered the primary

index of significant PCM and, although insensitive to early phases of nutritional repletion and reduced in states of stress, still remains the benchmark for other measures of PCM.[5,30] This is particularly true given the evidence of the value of a hypoalbuminemia in predicting anergy, sepsis, and death during hospitalization.[22,40]

Local standards vary, but a serum albumin less than 3 g/dl represents significant PCM, since other changes characteristic of PCM occur at about this level.[50] Serum albumin can be assessed by a standard "salting-out" technique, autoanalyzer (colorimetric), or by radial immunodiffusion.

ANERGY

It is generally recognized that PCM underlies the most common type of acquired immunodeficiency. Although both antibody-producing capacity and cellular immunity are impaired by PCM, cellular immunity is affected earlier and more severely. With adult hypoalbuminemic malnutrition, recall to primary and secondary antigens, total peripheral lymphocyte counts, total thymus-derived cells, and *in vitro* lymphocyte response to mitogens are all reduced.[5,34] Adult marasmus causes little effect on cellular immune function in terms of total and T-lymphocyte counts and *in vitro* lymphocyte tests, although anergy is common if patients are less than 85% standard weight/height and have had recent weight loss.[9] The effects on anergy, at least, in both conditions can be rapidly reversed.[9,23] The above findings further support the general clinical impression of better preservation of vital body functions in marasmus than in hypoalbuminemic malnutrition.

Delayed hypersensitivity skin testing is used to determine anergy in the assessment of nutritional status. The recall antigens used are generally from this group: candida (Hollister-Stier), streptokinase/streptodornase (Lederle), Mumps Skin Test Antigen (Lilly), and occasionally Dermatophyton (Hollister–Stier), although the latter is less helpful in northern climates. At least three antigens are placed intradermally on the forearm and read at 24 and 48 hours. Greater than 5 mm of induration is considered positive. A patient is considered anergic if he does not react positively to any of the three antigens at 24 or 48 hours.

Skin test preparations typically are 0.1 ml of a solution of 20,000 units of streptokinase and 5,000 units of streptodornase (Varidase) diluted to 100 ml with normal saline solution, supplying approximately 10 units of streptokinase and 2.5 units of streptodornase; 0.1 ml of a solution of Candida allergic extract (1:10 w/v in 50% glycerin) diluted 1:100 with normal saline solution; and 0.1 ml of Mumps Skin Test Antigen (Lilly).

SECONDARY ASSESSMENT TECHNIQUES

UPPER ARM ANTHROPOMETRY

Approximately 50% of the body fat is located in the subcutaneous tissue and its measurement reflects total body fat. While there are complex techniques using computed tomography or ultrasound, physical anthropometry using skinfold calipers is most practical for routine clinical use.[26] Lange calipers are most widely used for this purpose. The skinfold consists of a double layer of skin and subcutaneous fat. The most appropriate site for precision in location and accessibility is the triceps skinfold. The left arm should be used, although there are no substantial differences between arms.[14] The technique according to Jelliffe is as follows: the skinfold is grasped by finger and thumb and lifted away from the underlying muscle at a point half way between the tip of the acromion process of the scapula and the olecranon process of the ulna.[30] The calipers are applied 1 cm below the point of grasp. Three measurements should be made and the results averaged. Skinfold measurements are more difficult and less accurate in the obese. Standards from Jelliffe for the United States population are found in Table 10-2. (See later discussion.)

The upper arm circumference is measured with the left arm hanging freely, at the same point that the triceps skinfold is measured.[30] A steel or fiber glass tape is placed firmly without compressing the underlying soft tissues. From the skinfold and the arm circumference the arm muscle circumference can be derived by the following formula: arm muscle circumference (AMC) in cm = arm circumference − π triceps skinfold (in cm). Although the arm circumference is not perfectly circular, a comparison of derived estimates and those determined by tomography are correlated closely. Standards for arm muscle circumference for the United States population are now available in addition to those of Jelliffe.[18,30] (See Table 10-2.) Similar values are obtained whether the 85% of standard or the fifth percentile is used to categorize PCM. The arm muscle circumference is a sensitive measure of protein nutrition and is correlated with other estimates of body protein status such as serum albumin, prealbumin, and percent weight loss.[7,27,51] Its value lies primarily in the edematous states of patients, where weight standards are inaccurate.

CREATININE HEIGHT INDEX[6]

In the hospitalized adult with PCM, gross abnormalities in body composition resulting from disease reduce the reliability of weight as an index of protein depletion. In normal persons, creatinine ex-

TABLE 10-2
Standards for Arm Muscle Circumference and Triceps Skinfold*

Upper Arm Circumference (mm)	Standard†	‡	Lower 5th† Percentile	Percent of Standard Represented by 5th Percentile
Male	270	(253)	220	81
Female	213	(232)	177	83
Triceps Skinfold (mm)				
Male	11	(12.5)	7	36
Female	19	(16.5)	9	47

*Standard is 50th percentile of 30-year-olds.
†From Frisancho AR: Triceps skinfold and upper arm muscle size norms for assessment of nutritional status. Am J Clin Nutr 27:1052–1058, 1974.
‡Jelliffe DB: The Assessment of the Nutritional Status of the Community: WHO Monograph 53, Geneva, 1968.

cretion correlates equally well with LBM, surface area, and body weight.[16,38] In patients with wasting disease, creatinine excretion is reduced and no longer correlates with body weight.[46] Presumably this reflects the distortion of body composition produced by disease, particularly protein loss. Since height is minimally affected in adult malnutrition and creatinine excretion continues to correlate with BCM, a creatinine height index affords a means of assessing the status of the metabolically active tissue by comparing expected and actual body cell mass for height.[6,25,48] Standards for young males and females of various heights are shown in Table 10-3. Creatinine excretion falls with age, and standards have not been developed for those older than 55 years. This technique has not been widely applied, and there is insufficient data to develop percentiles. Only an estimate can be made for the level denoting significant PCM. This is approximately 75% of standard.

OTHER VISCERAL PROTEINS

Other liver secretory proteins with a shorter half-life have been shown to be more sensitive than serum albumin, particularly in assessing response to adequate nutritional support. Transferrin is a globulin and the main iron-binding protein. There is an equal distribution of transferrin in the intravascular and extravascular spaces with an equilibrium time of 4 to 5 days. Transferrin synthesis is less dependent on amino acid supply than albumin and increases in response to iron deficiency. A value less than 150 mg/dl represents significant PCM. There is a good correlation between serum albumin and transferrin levels,[5] but transferrin levels do respond more rapidly and reflect the severity (mortality) of PCM.[31,40,44] Two other liver secretory proteins, prealbumin and retinol binding pro-

tein, continue to be used on a research basis as indicators of visceral protein status.[27,28,29] Because they have even shorter half-lives (Table 10-4), their serum levels respond more rapidly to nutritional repletion. However, standards and their ultimate role as nutritional markers have not been established.

CURRENT CONTROVERSY IN NUTRITIONAL ASSESSMENT

Recent concern has been raised about the appropriateness of current anthropometric standards used in nutritional assessment.[14,18,30] With the increasing recognition of the importance of nutrition in clinical medicine, it is imperative that there be general agreement about standards, for objective assessment has been instrumental in fostering the growth of clinical nutrition. Arm anthropometry to assess hospital protein–calorie malnutrition was first used in a report of a substantial prevalence of PCM among surgical patients.[4] At the time this study was conducted, the only standards available were from Jelliffe.[30] His reference population for triceps skinfold standards was not delineated, and the samples for left arm circumference were from right arm measurements in military personnel from several Mediterranean countries and from volunteer American women in 1941.[24,42]

The standards for left arm muscle circumference were calculated by Jelliffe from the above group standards for both triceps skinfold and arm circumference, and a single standard was developed for adults of each sex.[30] Jelliffe also suggested that a surveyed population should be divided into deciles in terms of percent of standard, with the population median being considered the standard.[30] We used this procedure in both surveys even though, as Burgert and Anderson note, this would not be

TABLE 10-3*
Expected 24-hr. Urine Creatinine Excretion of Normal Adult Men and Women of Different Heights†

	Men‡					Women§			
Height		Ideal Weight	Creatinine Coefficient	24-hr Urine Creatinine	Height		Ideal Weight	Creatinine Coefficient	24-hr Urine Creatinine
IN	CM	KG	MG/KG	GM	IN	CM	KG	MG/KG	GM
62	157.5	56.0	23	1.29	58	147.3	46.0	17	0.782
63	160.0	57.6		1.32	59	149.9	47.2		0.802
64	162.5	59.0		1.36	60	152.4	48.6		0.826
65	165.1	60.3		1.39	61	154.9	49.9		0.848
66	167.6	62.0		1.43	62	157.5	51.3		0.872
67	170.2	63.8		1.47	63	160.0	52.6		0.894
68	172.7	65.8		1.51	64	162.6	54.3		0.923
69	175.3	67.6		1.55	65	165.1	55.9		0.950
70	177.8	69.4		1.60	66	167.6	57.8		0.983
71	180.3	71.4		1.64	67	170.2	59.6		1.01
72	182.9	73.5		1.69	68	172.7	61.5		1.04
73	185.4	75.6		1.74	69	175.3	63.3		1.08
74	188.0	77.6		1.78	70	177.8	65.1		1.11
75	190.5	79.6		1.83	71	180.3	66.9		1.14
76	193.0	82.2		1.89	72	182.9	68.7		1.17

*Bistrian BR: Nutritional assessment and therapy of protein–calorie malnutrition in the hospital. J Am Diet Assoc 71:393–397, 1977.

†Creatinine: height index is defined as the 24-hr creatinine excretion of the patient divided by the expected 24-hr creatinine excretion of a normal adult of the same height.

‡Bistrian BR, Blackburn GL, Sherman M, Scrimshaw NS: Therapeutic index of nutritional depletion in hospitalized patients. Surg Gynecol Obstet 141:512–516, 1973.

§Unpublished observations.

the best alternative were standards available from the population to be measured, with subcategorization according to age and with the fifth percentile identified to define abnormal values.[4,7,14] Recently, Frisancho published American standards for triceps skinfold and arm muscle circumference by age and sex.[24] The 50th percentile values from this survey were within 15% (triceps skinfold) and 10% (arm muscle circumference) of Jelliffe's standards for 30-year-old men and women. These differences are statistically significant, but the clinical significance is unknown.[14] Other than noting that new standards were available, in the interest of comparability with the earlier survey, Jelliffe's standards were again used in the survey of medical patients.[7] A later publication did suggest the use of Ten State Nutrition Survey standards, but reserved the diagnosis of clinically significant protein–calorie malnutrition to those with a weight/height measurement less than 85% standard or an albumin level less than 3 g/dl.[3]

As clinical experience with arm anthropometry increased, it became obvious that using percent of standard (median) values for triceps skinfold overstated the prevalence of malnutrition and that using the fifth percentile from the Ten State Nutrition Survey better identified the truly abnormal. How-

ever, malnutrition defined by percent of standard arm muscle circumference does not differ a great deal from that determined by the fifth percentile (Table 10-2). In a recent publication we recommended the consideration of the fifth percentile of triceps skinfold and arm muscle circumference to define abnormal.[8] However, for clinical purposes we have always been reluctant to use the triceps skinfold to diagnose protein–calorie malnutrition because fat is a dispensable tissue, the lack of which generally does not correlate with function.[32] Nei-

TABLE 10-4
Serum Proteins as Nutritional Markers

	Half-life
Albumin*	20 days
Transferrin†	7–8 days
Prealbumin†	2 days
Retinol-binding protein†	12 hours

*From Rothschild MA, Oratz M, Schreiber S: Albumin synthesis. N Engl J Med 286:748–757, 816–821, 1972.

†From Ingenbleek Y, Van Den Schriek HG, DeNayer P, DeVirscher M: Albumin, transferrin, and the thyroxine binding prealbumin/retinol-binding protein (TBPA–RBP) complex in assessment of malnutrition. Clin Chim Acta 63:61–67, 1975.

ther in Mullen's original study nor in our study were triceps skinfold measurements correlated with subsequent hospital morbidity or mortality.[22,40] More recently, Buzby and colleagues have claimed a prognostic value for triceps skinfold thickness.[40] Our feeling, however, is that the primary value of triceps skinfold measurements is in the calculation of the arm *muscle* circumference, which correlates with serum albumin and with percent weight loss, plasma prealbumin, and hemoglobin.[7,51] Although weight/height is the primary anthropometric index of protein–calorie malnutrition, the arm muscle circumference is of value in patients with fluid retention from cardiac, renal, or hepatic disease, in which weight/height underestimates protein–calorie malnutrition.[3,9]

The situation is somewhat different with proper weight/height standards to be employed in nutritional diagnosis. Gray and Gray have suggested that in addition to the use of HANES and Ten State Nutrition Survey standards for upper arm anthropometry, similar to recommendations of Burgert and Anderson, the HANES weight standards should be used instead of Metropolitan Life Insurance data owing to criticisms of the latter.[13,14,18,20,41] The likely differences in standards based on insured individuals from four decades ago, who were weighed and measured in clothes and shoes, from those of hospitalized patients is apparent. However, there are three very important characteristics that favor their continued use: (1) wide acceptance and use among clinicians and researchers, (2) the concept of an ideal body weight related to optimal mortality experience, and (3) the desirability of using the same standard for the diagnosis of malnutrition and obesity. The HANES standards have not been related to mortality experience and primarily document the increasing prevalence of obesity in our population.

Gray and Gray are also concerned that there may be conflicting results in the diagnosis of protein–calorie malnutrition by the different parameters if the standards are inappropriate.[20] Misapplication of the diagnosis of protein–calorie malnutrition is a legitimate concern, but the use of the fifth percentile does not obviate this problem. There is no assurance that the fifth percentile will define dysfunction. For instance, the fifth percentile for weight in 18- to 34-year-old women who are 5 feet 4 inches tall is 89 lbs.[20] Most surgeons would be concerned about the metabolic response to injury in such a patient without nutritional support some time before weight declined to this point. Any level chosen to indicate an abnormal condition must also be associated with functional consequences if it is to be of clinical value. Some authors have suggested such prognostic levels for triceps skinfold and arm muscle circumference.[11,15] At the present state of knowledge however, in our opinion only the standards of greater than 10% recent weight loss, albumin less than 3 g/dl, weight/height less than 85% of standard, and anergy have been shown to have functional consequences.[3,5,9,17,22,34,37,40,50]

In summary, the points of Burgert and Anderson and Gray and Gray are well taken.[23,34] Present standards for anthropometry are not from the curren U.S. population and are not represented in terms of the fifth percentile. On the other hand, many are now familiar with their use, and consistency among investigators is a valuable asset. Further, the triceps skinfold is of limited clinical value for the diagnosis of protein–calorie malnutrition; changes in standards for arm muscle circumference would lead to statistically significant changes, but the biologic significance of these changes for clinical purposes is uncertain. There are compelling reasons to maintain the present standards of weight/height, at least for clinical use.

DYNAMIC NUTRITIONAL ASSESSMENT

Secretory protein levels and delayed hypersensitivity skin testing can also be used to monitor changes in nutritional status. Weight change is important, although subject to changes from fluid retention. Upper arm anthropometry has been used but is relatively insensitive over brief periods, such as several weeks.[21,27] Serum protein levels and immune competence are the most important and sensitive measures for alteration in nutritional status. Both tests have been shown to correlate with subsequent hospital morbidity and mortality, and improvement in either with therapy improves prognosis.[15,21–23,37,40] Of these two measures, immune competence is a somewhat more valuable indicator because serum albumin levels are slower to respond to nutritional support as long as significant stress persists. This is less true of serum transferrin; immune responsiveness as measured by antigen recall appears to respond to nutritional repletion even in the presence of usual stresses. When anergy persists despite nutritional support, this usually portends a poor prognosis.

Various other methods have evolved for the clinical assessment of nutritional status. Nitrogen balance measurements indicate protein balance, and thus changes in LBM. This is particularly important in hospitalized patients whose response to nutrient intake can not be predicted with certainty owing to the confounding variables of nutritional depletion and stress. However, the nitrogen balance technique has remained essentially one of research because of the cumbersome, time-consuming, and expensive method for measuring total nitrogen in stool and urine. A clinical estimate of total urine nitrogen excretion can be achieved by measuring the 24-hour urine urea nitrogen, which can be simply and inexpensively accomplished in any hospital clinical laboratory.[10] Because urine nitrogen, as urea, changes in response to protein breakdown, whereas the nonurea urine nitrogen and fecal and integumental nitrogen losses are relatively stable, an estimate of 2 g for the former and 2 g for the latter two, added to the measured urine urea nitrogen, gives a useful measure of total urine nitrogen excretion. The equation for clinical nitrogen balance is as follows:

$$\text{Nbal} = \frac{\text{Protein intake (g)}}{6.25*}$$
$$- (24 \text{ urine urea nitrogen (g)} + 4)$$

This technique provides an effective and simple method to assess and to adjust suitably the nutritional therapy in hospitalized patients.

CATABOLIC INDEX

The other important variable in addition to nutritional status is the degree of catabolic stress. The efficiency of the use of dietary protein is reduced by stress, with an increased conversion of dietary and endogenous protein to glucose and urea by gluconeogenesis. When the diet is low in or devoid of protein, such as when hospitalized patients are maintained on dextrose or electrolyte solutions intravenously, the urinary urea nitrogen excretion can be used as an index of protein catabolic rates (see Fig. 10-5).[8,10] However, the presence of dietary protein in excess of 20 g/day will contribute significantly to urinary nitrogen excretion. To compensate, the catabolic index (CI) has been derived:[1]

CI = 24 hr urine urea nitrogen excretion
   − (½ dietary nitrogen (g) intake + 3)

Then, CI < 0 = no significant stress
   CI = 1–5 = mild stress
   CI > 5 = moderate to severe stress

This formula is based on the premise that approximately 50% of dietary protein will be converted to urea in mild to moderately stressed individuals and that 3 g of urea nitrogen would be produced even in the absence of dietary protein.

The combination of degree of stress and degree of malnutrition can be combined to help determine

*Protein intake is divided by 6.25 because the average protein contains 16% nitrogen.

the proper mode of nutritional therapy; that is, whether total enteral or parenteral nutrition or various protein-sparing hypocaloric regimens (see Fig. 10-6) should be employed.

VITAMIN AND MINERAL DEFICIENCIES

Although vitamin and mineral deficiencies secondary to various pathologic conditions occur with distressing regularity in hospitalized patients, as evidenced by reduced blood or urinary values for these nutrients, there is substantially less clinical vitamin or mineral deficiency than PCM, and a lack of correlation with physical findings generally.[12] Unlike protein, vitamins and minerals are needed in small amounts that can be easily and inexpensively provided orally or parenterally to most hospitalized patients as a routine. Finally, vitamin and mineral levels in blood often fall in response to injury and infection; the meaning of this as a true deficiency state is unknown. For these reasons, and because classic vitamin-deficiency syndromes are rarely seen, a brief description of the routine assessment of patients in the Nutrition Support Service is given. The goal is to identify the most common and clinically important conditions that often co-

FIG. 10-5 Rates of hypermetabolism estimated from urinary urea nitrogen excretion. The rate of protein catabolism varies with the degree of stress and can be measured as the 24-hour urinary urea nitrogen excretion. Because the protein contribution to caloric expenditure is relatively constant during stress, urea production can be related to energy consumption. *RME*, resting metabolic expenditure. (Blackburn GL, Bistrian BR: Curative nutrition: Protein calorie management. In Schneider HA et al (eds): Nutritional Support of Medical Practice. Hagerstown, Harper and Row, 1977)

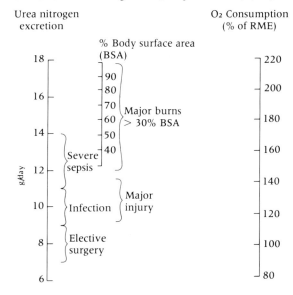

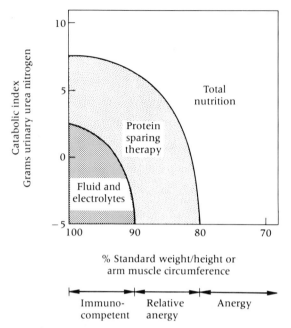

FIG. 10-6 Degree of stress and extent of malnutrition as the prime variables in the design of nutrition support therapy. (Data from Bistrian BR, Bothe A: Nutritional management of the patient with cancer. In Lokich J (ed): Clinical Cancer Medicine, Boston, GK Hall, 1980.) Any patient who is either severely stressed (catabolic index > 7–8) or severely malnourished (anergic) deserves full nutritional support providing adequate calories and protein. Patients who are neither (catabolic index < 2–3, immunocompetent) do not specifically need attempts to minimize protein loss over the short term (7 days). Intermediate states can benefit from active nutritional support by either protein sparing or total nutrition therapy; the particular route and method chosen will be determined by other factors such as the state of the gastrointestinal tract, the familiarity of the medical staff with the various nutritional techniques, and the goals for the patient.

exist with PCM and to rely on the adequate intake of nutrients in the feeding formulas to treat marginal deficiencies. Where specific deficiencies are thought to exist, standard diagnostic measures are employed. The reader is referred to other chapters (Chaps. 4 and 12) for the routine assessment of vitamin and mineral status. The following tests are performed:

1. A Chem 18—which includes sodium, potassium, calcium, phosphorus, alkaline phosphatase
2. Complete bloodcount (CBC)—to identify nutritional anemia
3. Serum folate, B_{12}—(commonly low in hospitalized patients)
4. Magnesium
5. Iron, total iron binding capacity, transferrin—to assess protein and iron status

6. Zinc—the level in serum primarily reflects current intake rather than body status

The total parenteral solutions routinely provided contain all nutrients for which an RDA has been established, as do most commercial enteral formulas (see Chap. 11).

RAPID NUTRITIONAL SURVEYS

One of the first priorities for a hospital aiming to develop a nutrition support team may be to identify the extent of the problems faced. One quick, convenient, and inexpensive way to do this is to determine the prevalence of protein–calorie malnutrition by using simple criteria, such as 85% weight/height, 10% recent weight loss, and serum albumin < 3 g/dl. A random sample of at least 50 patients can be chosen from the total hospital inpatient population. Then the most recent serum albumin, weight, height, and history of weight loss can be gathered from the charts. This can be easily accomplished in a matter of hours by several people, particularly with prior planning. It is often interesting to record other information, such as whether malnutrition has been listed as a diagnosis in the chart. Not only will such a simple survey identify protein–calorie malnutrition, but it can also serve as a reflection of current nutritional assessment practices at the surveyed hospital. It should not be surprising to find no available weights, heights, or serum albumins in a substantial fraction of patients.

In summary, epidemiologic evidence strongly supports the high prevalence of hospital malnutrition and its potentially devastating impact on patient care. The first step in the solution of such a problem is its recognition, since the technique and products to treat this problem, once its importance is accepted, are widely available.

References

1. Bistrian BR: A simple technique to estimate severity of stress. Surg Gynecol Obstet 148:675–678, 1979
2. Bistrian BR: Interaction of nutrition and infection in the hospital setting. Am J Clin Nutr 30:1228–1232, 1977
3. Bistrian BR: Nutritional assessment and therapy of protein–calorie malnutrition in the hospital. J Am Diet Assoc 71:393–397, 1977
4. Bistrian BR, Blackburn GL, Hallowell E, et al: Protein status of general surgical patients. JAMA 230:858–860, 1974
5. Bistrian BR, Blackburn GL, Scrimshaw NS, et al: Cellular immunity in semi-starved states in hospitalized adults. Am J Clin Nutr 28:1148–1155, 1975
6. Bistrian BR, Blackburn GL, Sherman M, et al: Therapeutic index of nutritional depletion in hospitalized patients. Surg Gynecol Obstet 141:512–516, 1973
7. Bistrian BR, Blackburn GL, Vitale J et al: Prevalence of

malnutrition in general medical patients. JAMA 235:1567–1570, 1976

8. Bistrian BR, Bothe A: Nutritional management of the patient with cancer. In Lokich J (ed): Clinical Cancer Medicine, Boston, GK Hall, 1980

9. Bistrian BR, Sherman M, Blackburn GL, et al: Cellular immunity in adult marasmus. Arch Intern Med 137:249–272, 1977

10. Blackburn GL, Bistrian BR: Curative nutrition: Protein–calorie management. In Schneider HA, Anderson CE, Coursin DB (eds): Nutritional Support of Medical Practice, pp 101–123, Hagerstown, Harper & Row, 1977

11. Blackburn GL, Thornton PA: Nutritional assessment of the hospitalized patient. Med Clin North Am 63:1103–1115, 1979

12. Bollet AJ, Owens SO: Evaluation of nutritional status of selected hospitalized patients. Am J Clin Nutr 26:931–938, 1973

13. Build and Blood Pressure Study. Chicago Society of Actuaries, 1959

14. Burgert SL, Anderson CF: An evaluation of upper arm measurements used in nutritional assessment. Am J Clin Nutr 32:2136–2142, 1979

15. Buzby GP, Mullen JL, Matthews DC, et al: Prognostic nutritional index in gastrointestinal surgery. Am J Surg (in press)

16. Edwards KDG, Whyte HM: Creatinine excretion and body composition. Clin Sci 18:361–365, 1959

17. Faintuch J, Faintuch JJ, Machado MCC, et al: Anthropometric assessment of nutritional depletion after surgical injury. JPEN 3:369–371, 1979

18. Frisancho AR: Triceps skinfold and upper arm muscle size norms for assessment of nutritional status. Am J Clin Nutr 27:1052–1058, 1974

19. Garrow JS, Fletcher J, Halliday D: Body composition in severe infantile malnutrition. J Clin Invest 44:417–425, 1965

20. Gray GE, Gray LK: Validity of anthropometric norms used in the assessment of hospitalized patients. JPEN 3:366–368, 1979

21. Harvey KB, Bothe A, Blackburn GL: Nutritional assessment and patient outcome during oncological therapy. Cancer 43:2065–2069, 1979

22. Harvey KB, Moldawer LL, Bistrian BR, et al: Index for identifying and monitoring high risk patients. Clin Res 27:571A, 1979

23. Harvey KB, Ruggiero JA, Regan CS, et al: Hospital morbidity–mortality risk factors using nutritional assessment. Clin Res 26:581A, 1978

24. Hertzberg HTE, Churchill E, Dupertis CN, et al: Anthropometric Survey of Turkey and Italy. New York, Pergamon Press, 1963

25. Heymsfield SB, Bethel RA, Ansley JD, et al: Enteral hyperalimentation: An alternative to central venous hyperalimentation. Ann Intern Med 90:63–71, 1979

26. Heymsfield SB, Olafson RP, Kutner MH, et al: A radiographic method of quantifying protein–calorie undernutrition. Am J Clin Nutr 32:693–702, 1979

27. Hill GL, Blackett RL, Rickford I, et al: Malnutrition in surgical patients: An unrecognized problem. Lancet 1:689–692, 1977

28. Ingenbleek Y, DeVisscher M, DeNayer P: Measurement of prealbumin as index of protein–calorie malnutrition. Lancet 2:106–108, 1972

29. Ingenbleek Y, Van Den Schrieck HG, DeNayer P, et al: The role of retinol-binding protein in protein–calorie malnutrition. Metabolism 24:633–641, 1975

30. Jelliffe DB: The Assessment of the Nutritional Status of

the Community: WHO Monograph 53, Geneva, World Health Organization, 1968

31. Kaminski MV, Fitzgerald MJ, Murphy RJ, et al: Correlation of mortality with serum transferrin and energy. JPEN 1:27A, 1977

32. Keys A, Brozek J, Henschel A, et al: The Biology of Human Starvation. Minneapolis, University of Minnesota Press, 1950

33. Kinney JM, Duke JH, Long CL: Tissue fuel and weight loss after injury. J Clin Pathol [Suppl] 4:65–72, 1978

34. Law DK, Dudrick USJ, Abdou NI: Immunocompetence of patients with protein calorie malnutrition. Ann Intern Med 79:545–550, 1973

35. Lawson LJ: Parenteral nutrition in surgery. Br J Surg 52:795–800, 1965

36. Leevy CM, Cardi L, Frank O, et al: Incidence and significance of hypovitaminemia in a randomly selected municipal hospital population. Am J Clin Nutr 17:259–271, 1965

37. Meakins JL, Pietsch JB, Bubenick D, et al: Delayed hypersensitivity: Indicator of acquired failure of host defenses in sepsis and trauma. Ann Surg 186:241–250, 1977

38. Miller AT, Blyth CS: Estimation of lean body mass and body fat from basal oxygen consumption and creatinine excretion. J Appl Physiol 5:73–78, 1952

39. Moore FD, Olesen K, McMurray J, et al: The Body Cell Mass And Its Supporting Environment, Philadelphia, WB Saunders, 1963

40. Mullen JL, Gertner MH, Buzby, GP, et al: Implications of malnutrition in the surgical patient. Arch Surg 114:121–125, 1979

41. National Center for Health Statistics: Weight by height and age of adults 18–74 years: United States, 1971–1979, Advanced data 14, 1977

42. O'Brien R, Sheldon WC: Women's measurement for garment and pattern construction. USDA Miscellaneous Publication No. 454, Washington, D.C., USDA, 1941

43. Patrick J, Reeds PJ, Jackson AA, et al: Total body water in malnutrition: The possible role of energy intake. Br J Nutr 39:417–424, 1978

44. Reeds PJ, Laditan AAO: Serum albumin and transferrin in protein energy malnutrition. Br J Nutr 36:255–263, 1976

45. Rothschild MA, Oratz M, Schreiber S: Albumin synthesis. N Engl J Med 286:748–757, 816–821, 1972

46. Ryan RJ, Williams SJD, Ansell BM, et al: Relationship of body composition to oxygen consumption and creatinine excretion in healthy and wasted man. Metabolism 6:365–377, 1957

47. Stoudt HW, Damon A, McFarland RA: Weight, height, and selected body dimensions of adults. Vital and Health Statistics, Series II, No. 8, Washington, D.C. United States Public Health Service, 1965

48. Viteri FE, Alvarado J: The creatinine index: Its use in the estimation of the degree of protein depletion and repletion in protein–calorie malnourished children. Pediatrics 46:696–706, 1970

49. Weinsier RL, Hunker EM, Krumdieck CL, et al: Hospital malnutrition: A prospective evaluation of general medical patients during the course of hospitalization. Am J Clin Nutr 32:418–426, 1979

50. Whitehead RG, Coward WA, Lunn PG: Serum albumin and the onset of kwashiorkor. Lancet 1:63–66, 1973

51. Young GA, Hill GL: Assessment of protein–calorie malnutrition in surgical patients from plasma proteins and anthropometric measurements. Am J Clin Nutr 31:429–435, 1978

11
Protein–Calorie Management in the Hospitalized Patient

B. Smith Hopkins,
Bruce R. Bistrian,
George L. Blackburn

Among the essential nutrients required for daily metabolism are amino acids for protein synthesis and nonprotein calories (NPC) to provide the energy for cell work. Since these nutrients have the largest daily requirements and their utilization is uniquely interdependent, they are considered together in this chapter.[74]

Protein–calorie malnutrition (PCM) results in deficiencies that the body is slow to restore because it is rate-limited by a total body protein turnover of approximately 4% per day, with any surplus converted to fat.[95] Restoration of body protein is particularly difficult owing to the priority of energy over protein requirements and the complex interactions of the ten essential amino acids.[74]

To further complicate matters, there are different priorities for net protein synthesis in the various organs in response to partial starvation during recovery from illness, injury, or sepsis. Prolonged starvation in mild chronic illness, representing a balanced deficit of calories and protein, primarily depletes the somatic protein compartment. Except for loss of labile protein mass, visceral organ protein status is conserved at an adequate level, while protein (muscle) and energy (fat) are mobilized in sufficient quantity from the periphery until somatic depletion ultimately becomes severe.

Increased rates of proteolysis during severe stress or sepsis, as well as diminished adaptation to starvation by the provision of protein-free calories, will deplete the visceral protein compartment. An acute hypoalbuminemic syndrome develops because of the normally rapid turnover of liver, gut, bone marrow, and other visceral proteins now accentuated by increased demand. This is a frequent cause of increased morbidity in hospitalized patients. It also represents an opportunity, since effective nutritional support can prevent or reduce the usual clinical consequences of visceral protein losses if it is provided prior to or without stress, even for a relatively short period of time (7–10 days).

Rarely will the clinician see any nutritional deficiency of significant medical importance that is not associated with PCM, in part because nearly all essential nutrients are involved in optimal protein synthesis. A favorable outcome may sometimes result from therapies that selectively replace some nutrients before or without overt treatment of PCM; but given the overriding importance of protein and calories in the common clinical situation, this selective supplementation cannot be the wisest course, and in some instances may even be detrimental.[10] Restoration of iron depletion without proper therapy of PCM may paradoxically support adventitious bacterial growth to the host's detriment.[50,87] Conversely, protein and calorie repletion may precipitate acute vitamin A deficiency in children with kwashiorkor.[56] The point is that protein and calories should not be restored preferentially to other nutrients. Utilization of protein requires an adequate balance of zinc, magnesium, potassium, phosphate, and other vitamins and micronutrients. However, the amounts required are relatively small and easily included.

Successful treatment of PCM is affected by certain key variables, particularly the depth of nutritional depletion and the degree of hypercatabolism.[74] Many secondary conditions, such as the particular disease state (*e.g.,* cancer, diabetes, trauma, or infection) or age group (*e.g.,* pediatric, adult, or geriatric), also influence the type and effectiveness of therapy. Considered first, here, is the metabolic response to illness, second, the nutritional state obtainable (*fed* state versus the *nonfed* or *starved* state), and finally, the various specific patient conditions and organ failures that will affect the nutritional support plan.

Metabolic Response to Illness

Trauma, sepsis, and injury have long been recognized as producing significant alterations in body metabolism.[24,25,60] These insults evoke from the central nervous system a sympathetic-mediated reaction that triggers the release of substrate *mobilizing* hormones.[17,90] Phagocytosis also represents an important mechanism in the metabolic response to illness. During the initial *acute phase,* generous mobilization of metabolic reserves, including skeletal protein, ensures that an adequate supply of substrates is available for energy production and biosynthesis. This is quite different from starvation without injury, in which initial losses occur from the liver and other labile proteins of the viscera, and substantial depletion of skeletal protein begins only after 3 to 4 days.[86]

With the stress of illness, the glucocorticoid-induced peripheral protein catabolism results in an overall negative nitrogen balance that classically has been deplored.[25] Only recently has consideration been given to the possibility that peripheral catabolism might provide amino acids for synthesis of acutely needed blood proteins, structural proteins, and enzymes.[17] The mobilization of body protein from skeletal muscle does provide energy fuels as precursors for gluconeogenesis, but it also enables the synthesis of acute phase globulins, white blood cells, and other protein mediators of immune function, host resistance, and would healing. It is essential that this be recognized when nutritional support therapies are designed.[4,16]

ACUTE PHASE

The hormones released during the initial *acute catabolic phase* of the response to injury include signals to specifically antagonize the action of insulin, the key anabolic hormone for the two major peripheral tissues, skeletal muscle, and adipose tissue. Catecholamines inhibit the release of insulin, and glucocorticoids reduce the sensitivity of peripheral tissues to it. The body cell mass appears to be temporarily sacrificed during the acute phase in favor of maintaining a relative abundance of circulating substrates to meet any particular working cell's requirement.

The major energy reserves in the body are in the form of triglycerides stored in adipose tissue. Because of the high caloric value of fat and the low water content of adipose tissue, this tissue contains some 3500 Cal/pound. During the acute phase of injury, this energy reserve is mobilized to meet the metabolic demands, even in severely calorie-restricted states.[13] Given such fat depots, it is clear that the concerns about the lack of energy fuel substrate during the immediate postoperative period, or during conditions of early starvation, do not appear to be warranted. In contrast, during major stress and sepsis, labile protein reserves can be rapidly depleted, producing hypoalbuminemic malnutrition.

ADAPTIVE PHASE

The acute phase of illness gives way to an *adaptive phase* during which the organism seeks to adapt its metabolism to the changes in nutritional state. The timing of the transition between phases is dependent on the degree of illness, injury, or sepsis, and associated nutritional depletion.[16] Effective nutritional support can occur in this adaptive phase, once the strong catabolic signals resulting from high levels of catecholamines and glucocorticoids have subsided. The hormonal situation is complex and variable, but the adaptive phase can be identified by measurements of blood sugar, blood urea nitrogen, serum and urine ketones, and urinary urea nitrogen excretion. The adaptive phase of injury without dietary carbohydrate is recognized by a falling blood glucose, normal blood urea nitrogen, ketosis, ketonuria, and decreasing excretion of urea nitrogen. A fall in blood glucose level is of major significance in identifying this transition, since high rates of catabolism are associated with increased rates of gluconeogenesis and hyperglycemia. Administration of exogenous glucose, such as the infusion of isotonic 5% dextrose solutions, prevents the recognition of a transition and is of no consistent demonstrable protein-sparing value during the acute phase of injury.[68]

It is important to design nutritional support with an appropriate sense of timing. In the setting of planned metabolic stress, such as during the early postoperative period, providing the patient with protein that will only be metabolized to glucose by gluconeogenesis and ureagenesis, or with calories that will only result in lipogenesis, can be considered detrimental because these processes require work and result in increased hypermetabolism.[74] Optimal nutritional support must be equated with the retention of administered protein (net protein utilization), and this depends on an appropriate hormonal situation.

PROLONGED STRESS

Special conditions exist during prolonged stress, such as that observed in major burns, and in periods of systemic infection or sepsis.[24,91] The ability to develop an effective nutritional support plan is temporarily muted, and most efforts are limited to preserving the present nutritional state until the hypercatabolism and disease state can be treated. One important problem, particularly in conjunction with systemic infection or sepsis, is the increased use of protein as an energy source from muscle tissue, particularly the ketogenic amino acids: leucine, isoleucine, and valine. Logically, effective therapy would be to increase the intake of dietary protein fortified with up to 50% of these branched-chain amino acids in an attempt to render normal the profile of amino acids released from skeletal muscle as a result of selective loss of the branched-chain amino acids. Since injury is often associated with increased amounts of aromatic amino acids that are poorly "cleared" by the liver, their intake should be limited. Protein intakes of 1.5 g/kg to 2 g/kg with 250 g to 300 g carbohydrate, providing approximately 1300 Cal at a nitrogen to calorie ratio of 1:50, appears to be indicated in these states. Additional calories can be provided as exogenous fat to a total energy intake of 40 Cal/kg to 45 Cal/kg, if volume limitations allow. The resulting high rates of ureagenesis are not a problem if renal function is adequate, and this high rate of amino acid infusion appears to preserve protein synthesis in visceral tissues.

In this context, fever is a marker of hypercatabolism that can have potentially beneficial effects such as increasing metabolic rate, fostering protein synthesis in specific tissues, and providing ample glucose calories for certain tissues (e.g., phagocytes of white cells, fibrous tissue). As such, the treatment of fever with antipyretics in patients who are neurologically and hemodynamically stable and are tolerating hypermetabolism may in fact reduce the effectiveness of the metabolic responses to stress and reduce survival.[50]

A contrasting hypothesis condones the feeding of stressed patients with a formula relatively high in glucose calories, providing infusions of hypertonic glucose (400 g/day–600 g/day) with appropriate exogenous insulin and potassium as a means of curtailing the loss of body protein. Indeed, bolus administration of glucose, potassium, and insulin is known to be effective hemodynamic support during "low-flow" septic states. However, the pre-ferential peripheral uptake of amino acids produced by this therapy may not result in effective support of visceral protein synthesis unless adequate protein is also provided. Furthermore, the ability to oxidize glucose directly appears to be limited during stress, with large amounts of glucose merely fostering lipogenesis and excessive carbon dioxide production.[49,94] This latter therapy uses metabolism for a pharmacologic resuscitation, whereas the former uses metabolism to optimize nutrition. These contrasting nutritional therapies reemphasize the sophistication now necessary in this field. The use of standard parenteral hyperalimentation (hypertonic glucose and amino acids) as a combination of the two therapies does improve hemodynamic support by its inotropic effect on cardiac function.[12,24] A separate chapter will consider nutritional care of the burn patient (see Chap. 16).

Restoration of body cell mass, and in particular the visceral compartments, is the prime goal of nutritional support. Maintenance of adequate protein synthesis will support body cell mass and provide optimal organ response to injury. Proper utilization of protein intake is dependent on adequate energy fuel substrate to meet caloric requirements so as to minimize oxidation of amino acids for energy by gluconeogenesis. Factors that will best determine the nitrogen balance and net protein utilization include the metabolic rate, nonprotein caloric intake, nitrogen intake, and a favorable metabolic state as described above.[74,90]

The caloric requirement, although difficult to measure clinically, may be estimated from the equation of Harris and Benedict, that furnishes the basal energy expenditure (BEE):[74]

For men: $BEE = 66 + (13.7 \times W) + (5 \times H) - (6.8 \times A)$

For women: $BEE = 655 + (9.6 \times W) + (1.7 \times H) - (4.7 \times A)$

W = actual weight in kg H = height in cm
A = age in years

This simply calculated basal energy expenditure (BEE), based on age, sex, height, and weight, gives a better estimate of caloric requirements than the standard practice of using weight alone. The degree of increase of metabolic expenditure over BEE can be estimated from the daily urinary urea nitrogen loss.[29,74]

Table 11-1 provides a classification for surgical catabolism and Figure 11-1 relates catabolic rates to energy expenditure. Most medical illnesses will fall in the first or second degree of catabolism. Using regression analysis in a variety of mildly to moderately catabolic surgical patients, it has been

TABLE 11-1
Surgical Catabolism*

Degree of Net Catabolism	N_{obg}† (g urea − N/24 hr)	% Increase of RME over BEE
1° Normal	<5	10–20
2° Mild	5–10	20–50
3° Moderate	10–15	50–80
4° Severe	>15	>80

*Classification of patients is according to the following: (1) obligate nitrogen loss (N_{obg}) expressed in g urea − N/24 hr, (2) energy expenditure expressed as percent increase of the resting metabolic expenditure (RME) over calculated basal energy expenditure (BEE)
†No nitrogen intake and 3 days of at least 100 g carbohydrate

found that the delivery of 1.76 times BEE can be expected to produce positive nitrogen balance with a 95% confidence interval during parenteral feeding, whereas an intake of 1.54 times BEE will be effective for oral intake at the same confidence limit. Net protein utilization is optimal (72% ± 10%) at this level of intake. In rare patients with energy requirements in excess of 1.75 times BEE, attempts to meet those requirements with carbohydrate can become self-defeating. The specific dynamic action of glucose (i.e., the proportion of calories used in the metabolism of glucose and lost as heat) becomes clinically significant (up to 20% of infused glucose) in the higher ranges of carbohydrate feeding as the efficiency of glucose utilization decreases (see Fig. 11-3).[54,93] CO_2 production is also increased as the respiratory quotient (CO_2 production/O_2 consumption) exceeds 1 with lipogenesis. No demonstrable benefit is observed when feeding at or above 2 times BEE. Fourth degree hypercatabolism, as is seen primarily in major burns where energy requirements exceed 2.5 times BEE, may require a nitrogen–calorie ratio of 1:150.[91] Even here, glucose loads in excess of 5 mg/kg/min (500 g/day for a 70-kg man) appear to meet such limitations and suggest the remaining needs should be met by fat. The addition of exogenous insulin to larger glucose loads, while lowering blood glucose by increasing clearance from the serum, does not increase direct glucose oxidation.[92,95]

The optimal protein intake for positive nitrogen balance and restoration of lean body mass (LBM) in depleted, stressed adults is 16% of caloric input. This would appear to reflect the fact that precisely 16% of the caloric expenditure comes from protein sources during injury.[17] Since this value is approximately twice that seen during nonstress maintenance diets, the reutilization of body protein for

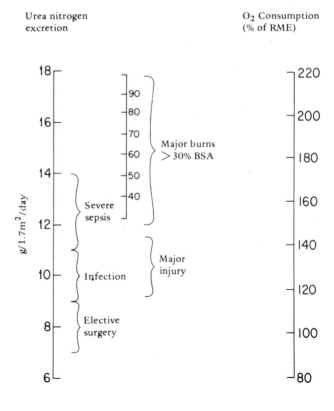

FIG. 11-1 Rate of endogenous protein breakdown rises with increasing degrees of hypermetabolism, reflecting relatively constant (12%–16%) contribution of protein to energy expenditure during periods of catabolic stress in various disease states (*left*). *BSA,* body surface area. Determination of daily urea nitrogen excretion (g/m²/day) can provide a simple and effective clinical estimate of magnitude of hypermetabolism, as percent above resting metabolic expenditure (*RME*), normally obtained by measurement of oxygen consumption (*right*).

synthesis is obviously decreased. Thus, a nitrogen–calorie ratio of 1:150 would appear optimal to meet the protein requirements for anabolism. In the future, alteration of the amino acid profile for enteral and parenteral nutritional support in stressed patients, specifically a crystalline amino acid mixture enriched with branched-chain amino acids, may alter this optimal nitrogen–calorie ratio somewhat. Although therapy with branched-chain enriched formulas in stress is experimental at this time, animal studies suggest a unique role of these amino acids in supporting the synthesis of visceral proteins important to the body's response to stress. This unique role may go beyond the normalization of the serum amino acid profile discussed below.

Special considerations are necessary in the nitrogen accumulation disorders, for instance, renal failure, in which the nitrogen–calorie ratio may range from 1:450 Cal/day to 1:700 Cal/day. Liver failure also has an upper limit of tolerance of protein intake that may be metabolized without creating encephalopathy.[33] In liver and probably also in renal failure, branched-chain enriched protein sources appear to be better tolerated in terms of the level of nitrogen intake possible without excessive urea or ammonia production or encephalopathy.

Maintenance diets in which 8% of the calories are provided as protein result in effective preservation of LBM in convalescent patients, but these diets are slow to restore lean tissue in depleted patients.[44] This 1:300 nitrogen–calorie ratio is an important consideration when *elemental* or chemically defined formula diets are used, because each additional gram of amino acids over the ideal will influence osmolarity, taste, and ultimate acceptibility and utilization of protein intake. The source of the nonprotein calories, such as sugars, starches, dextrins, and medium-chain and long-chain triglycerides, is also important an determination of osmolarity and digestibility and thus of the likelihood of meeting energy and protein requirements.[70] For this reason, tube feeding is often appropriate when elemental diets (*i.e.*, Vivonex, Precision, Vipep, Vital) are used. Tube feeding may also be helpful to meet total volume needs when the more palatable fat-containing formulas are used.

In summary, careful appreciation of the metabolic response to illness is necessary prior to consideration of nutritional support plans. Knowledge as to the phase of response to illness or injury and the degree of hypercatabolism will influence the attainable goals and timing of therapy.[13] These issues are discussed in more detail, as they relate to specific situations of organ failure, later in this chapter.

Modes of Therapy

ENTERAL FEEDING AND DEFINED FORMULA DIETS, NUTRITIONAL SUPPLEMENTS, MEAL REPLACEMENTS

Figure 11-2 provides a general scheme of nutritional products and feeding situations. Major consideration must be given to whether the goal of treatment is the *fed* state or *nonfed* (modified starved) state and to whether the route of administration, will be enteral or parenteral. Combination of the various categories of feeding is implied from this figure, since in many instances both parenteral and enteral feeding are used to obtain fed-state requirements. For example, enteral feeding may require some additional parenteral feeding (*e.g.*, isotonic amino acids) to obtain the appropriate protein–calorie ratio in pancreatitis or malabsorption syndromes.

Classic hyperalimentation using hypertonic glucose and amino acids may be improved, in terms of support of visceral protein synthesis, by enteral feeding of small amounts of protein or by *cyclic* hyperalimentation.[14] In this latter instance hyperalimentation solutions are infused only at night, and a nonfed routine is used during the day to free the patient from some of the constraints of his "lifeline" and to provide a feeding schedule more compatible with normal feeding patterns.[54] During the *nonfed* period, lower insulin levels allow for a relative shift of protein synthesis to favor the visceral compartment.

In general the common nutritional supplements provide 1 Cal/ml in their normal mixtures but differ widely in their protein and calorie sources and nitrogen–calorie ratios. Some newer products now contain up to 2 Cal/ml. In fact, many of the diets exceed the optimal nitrogen–calorie ratio and can therefore serve in a comprehensive nutritional support plan as *modules* to supplement low-protein, high-calorie food that is acceptable to the patient but that is by itself inadequate nutrition.

Since many patients in need of nutritional support have lactose intolerance and the oligosaccharides are less osmotically active than monoforms or diforms, the type of carbohydrate is specified for screening purposes. The complexity of fat digestion and its impairment in many disease conditions make it necessary, when evaluating a product, to consider fat levels beyond the minimal 1% required to prevent essential fatty acid deficiency. The rationale for using medium-chain triglycerides as an energy source is based on their unique metabolism. Medium-chain triglycerides are digested more rapidly than long-chain triglycerides, are not depend-

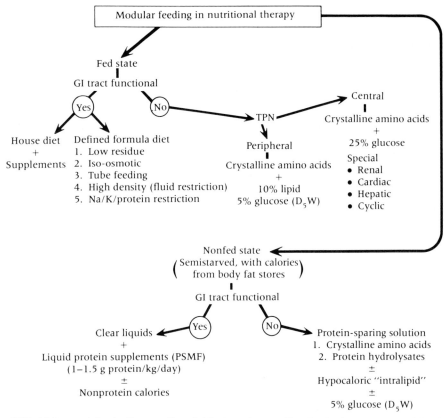

FIG. 11-2 Modular feeding. In all available therapies consideration is given to two nutritional states (fed and semistarved) and two possible means of delivery (enteral and parenteral). The use of this concept is depicted in this algorithm, which allows a systematic approach to nutritional support. *PSMF,* protein-sparing modified fast.

ent on micelle formation, are transported rapidly across the cell, and enter the portal circulation directly where they are oxidized preferentially.[76] Structured lipids, which are triglycerides that may contain one or two medium-chain fatty acids and linoleic acid or other long-chain fatty acids in other positions, also have a unique metabolism intermediate to medium- and long-chain triglycerides. The taste, osmolarity, and viscosity are important, depending respectively on patient cooperation, irritability of bowel, and whether tube feeding will be used. Most preparations are started at half strength with slow feeding rates in order to obtain the best utilization.

Most available preparations contain a high biologic value protein. No important clinical difference has been shown in the digestibility and utilization of egg albumin, hydrolysates, or amino acids that have the egg–protein profile. However, significantly improved taste acceptance and cost differential of whole proteins over hydrolysates or amino acids are a strong recommendation for their preferential use, except in those few instances where protein maldigestion is likely to be clinically significant. Besides the meal supplements available, defined formula diets (DFD), commonly known as elemental diets, originated from a NASA requirement for a low-residue, concentrated food compatible with the conditions on early spacecraft. This first generation of products was adapted for use in the medical field without due consideration of the differences in nutritional status, physical requirements, and activity levels between astronauts and hospitalized patients. Significant long-term comprehensive evaluation on the effect, utilization, efficacy, safety, and metabolism in a variety of patients using these products is not available. A more detailed discussion of protein sources, fat content, carbohydrate content, osmolality, effect on gut flora, indications, and methods of utilization is beyond the scope of this chapter (See refs. 45 and 71, and Chap. 13).

One important criticism of these products is the fixed-compounding of the products, which makes in necessary to stock many products. For this reason the concept of *modular* feeding is useful (see Fig. 11-2). Maintaining one or two basic diets that would provide maintenance nutrition (30 Cal/kg/day–35 Cal/kg/day with a nitrogen–calorie ratio of 1:300) and an anabolic nutrition product (40 Cal/kg/day–45 Cal/kg/day with a nitrogen–calorie ratio of 1:150) appears adequate for most purposes. These products can be supplemented with a variety of single nutrient supplements such as protein, fat, and carbohydrate. Indications for the modified and the standard DFD would come from the assessment of protein utilization, which has been previously described (see Chap. 10) (*e.g.,* nitrogen balance using urinary urea nitrogen excretion).

Since some of these products are relatively expensive compared to the normal hospital food budget, it is important that they be provided in a way that results in optimal therapy. Equally important, however, is the cost in relation to total daily hospital cost. Considered in this way the cost is often small, particularly when compared to the benefit resulting from effective nutritional support. However, it is important that a qualified dietitian (see Chap. 5) monitor the use of these products to ensure that they are acceptable to the patient, are taken in sufficient, but not excessive, quantity, and are integrated into the medical and nursing plan for the care of the patient. Only with further experience in clinical nutrition will proper use of these beneficial products occur, based on careful consideration of objective nutritional assessment and evaluation of nutritional therapy. An appropriate use of these new modular forms is to prepare high-density feedings that contain 2 Cal/ml to 4 Cal/ml rather than the more usual 1 Cal/ml. The resulting small volume is an effective therapy for patients requiring fluid restriction, such as those with renal or cardiac failure. This reduction in volume is also useful in patients with anorexia who still must meet their protein and calorie requirements.

Parenteral Feeding— Total Parenteral Alimentation

The development of total intravenous (IV) feeding by Dudrick and colleagues at the University of Pennsylvania in large part makes possible clinical nutrition as a full-time hospital medical speciality (see Chaps. 13 and 14).[28] The substantial life-saving results of total parenteral nutrition (TPN) require an experienced team to obtain appropriate risk/benefit and cost/benefit results. Available products are by necessity modular in that the Maillard reaction precludes compounding them prior to use. In addition, reports by Freeman and Stegink show significant chelation of zinc and copper by sugar–amine complexes when protein and carbohydrate are autoclaved together.[35]

When protein hydrolysates are compared to amino acid infusions in the same patient the former are found to be deficient by serum amino acid analysis and nitrogen balance techniques. That is, improved net protein utilization occurs with amino acid infusion. Therefore, in computing the relative cost of hydrolysate versus crystalline amino acid one must take into consideration the percent of the product retained in evaluating ratios of cost to benefit. This observation, together with the relative availability of casein, fibrin, and amino acids, has resulted in a substantial shift to amino acids as a source of protein for parenteral feeding. Furthermore, the potential for allergic reaction is minimized by amino acid infusion. A final advantage is the number of versatile patterns possible from amino acids, which can be expected to provide better treatment for renal failure, hepatic failure, and probably sepsis and major injury.[1,18,32] The cost of individual amino acids is variable, and by allowing utilization of cellular pathways for transamination and synthesis of nonessential amino acids, new patterns can be designed that will improve clinical results and reduce the cost of the first and second generation of products currently available. It is possible that single amino acids and their ketoanalogues can also improve parenteral feeding by a pharmacologic effect.[75]

Despite the small contribution that branched-chain amino acids make to the caloric expenditure of muscle, this fraction appears to be important in control of muscle–protein synthesis and in the flux of amino acids to the liver to supply substrate for liver–protein synthesis. Inappropriate amino acid mobilization, in degree and composition, occurs if there is impaired availability of nonprotein calories for muscle metabolism. With the consumption of branched-chain amino acids to meet muscle energy needs, the efflux of amino acids from catabolized protein is relatively devoid of branched-chain amino acids, and this imbalance upsets the amino acid profile for secretory protein synthesis by the liver. This is the usual finding during the acute phase of stress and systemic infection and sepsis, in which a combination of carbohydrate intolerance, impaired free fatty acid oxidation, and lack of ketonemia secondary to hyperinsulinism account for this phenomenon.[16] Branched-chain-amino-acid-enriched formulas appear to improve nutritional therapy during major injury and sepsis.[18]

Although good results may be obtained using

commercially available *hyperalimentation kits,* many ill patients can benefit from individualization of infusate composition. These products are already provided in separate modules, that is, protein, calories (glucose and fat), minerals, electrolytes, vitamins, and minerals, which may be tailored to the patient's requirements. Customizing the formulation, infusion rates, and duration of feeding each day can result in better protein utilization (net protein utilization) with less alteration in blood chemistry and improved organ function as well. Proper concentrations and dilutions of formulas should also allow for fluid and electrolyte management in the presence of renal failure, cardiac failure, or fluid-loss conditions, such as gastric, fistula, or diarrhea drainage, without the need for supplementation by peripheral infusion. By the proper mix with other feeding techniques (oral fed or nonfed schedules) as well as the use of parenteral fat, optimal nutritional support can be obtained.

Some new developments and concepts in parenteral nutrition should be considered in more detail because they portray the increasing sophistication of this field. The consequence of over-feeding by standard hyperalimentation is shown in Figure 11-3. The calculated specific dynamic action is twice that usually considered for glucose metabolism.[11] If calories sufficient to meet this increased energy requirement are not provided, the energy cost incurred in the specific dynamic action of glucose conversion to fat will result in negative nitrogen balance. Increased caloric intakes that allow even or positive nitrogen balance are in themselves partially responsible for the hypermetabolism associated with TPN.[11,74] This is discussed in more detail below with regard to respiratory failure.

An in-depth discussion of the science of hyperalimentation is beyond the scope of this chapter (see Chaps. 13 and 14). Briefly, efforts should be made to maintain normal limits of serum electrolytes, blood urea nitrogen, glucose, near-normal liver function tests, avoidance of fatty liver, hepatomegaly, and impaired secretory protein synthesis usually associated with overfeeding, particularly in stressed or septic patients. Monitoring and provision of cofactors, such as phosphate, magnesium, iron, copper, zinc, and linoleic acid, are also essential.[38,57]

It is now clear that infusions of fresh frozen plasma and impurities in amino acid solutions cannot be relied upon to provide sufficient trace elements to prevent deficiencies, as was previously believed. Zinc deficiency, the most commonly seen trace element deficiency except for iron, presents as diarrhea, hair loss, dementia or irritability, a herpetiform rash in the perioral and peroneal areas, and inability to achieve nitrogen balance or growth. Replacement

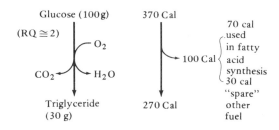

$$\text{"SDA" for amount of Dextrose given in excess of BMR} = \frac{70}{370} \times 100 = 20\%$$

[Estimates based on *in vitro* carbon flow of glucose conversion to triglycerides.]

FIG. 11-3 Energy cost of glucose conversion to fat. (Estimates based on *in vitro* carbon flow of glucose conversion to triglycerides.) Specific dynamic action (SDA) for dextrose given in excess of basal metabolic requirements is $70/370 \times 100$, approximately 20%. This is higher than normally considered.

in the range of 3 mg/day will prevent zinc deficiency during TPN providing there are no abnormal zinc losses. Diarrhea or high ileostomy output needs to be replaced with 10 mg/liter to 15 mg/liter of losses.[94] Copper deficiency presents as a hypochromic, microcytic anemia with neutropenia, and can be avoided with 1 mg/day to 2 mg/day replacement. Chromium replacement of 0.01 mg/day to 0.02 mg/day will prevent a rare deficiency state characterized by glucose intolerance caused by impaired release of insulin and decreased insulin sensitivity.[49] The possibility of manganese deficiency, although ill-defined at present, is felt by most authorities to justify the administration of approximately 0.4 mg/day. Replacement of iodine in the range of 0.05 mg/day is also recommended to maintain normal thyroid function. Adequate maintenance for the non-iron–depleted patient requires 2 mg/day of iron. However, hypoferremia is a consequence of the metabolic response to infection and injury, and cannot be relied upon as an index of iron nutriture in the hyperalimented patient.[80] Furthermore, iron replacement therapy in the septic patient is probably contraindicated.[49,87]

Cyclic hyperalimentation provides for a daily dextrose-free period of 12 to 14 hours during which the standard infusion is discontinued. This can free the patient from "life lines" and so allow better exercise schedules, which prevent the adverse effect of immobilization while providing considerable psychological support of the long-term hospitalized patient. Cyclic techniques are also used for home hyperalimentation, particularly to allow a better life style, but also to resemble more closely the normal feeding pattern. The essential fatty acid (EFA) deficiency produced by standard hyperalimentation is also treated by this technique.[55,88] Most hyperalimentation patients have ample stores of linoleic acid (10%–12%) in their body fat, and feedings designed for mobilization of this body fat can be incorporated into a daily plan (see Fig. 11-4). A discontinuation of glucose infusions with or without substitution by isotonic amino acid solutions (30 g/12 hr–60 g/12 hr) allows insulin levels to decline to a level that permits lipolysis. The composition of the released free fatty acids reflects previous dietary intake stored in adipose tissue.[88] In those patients in whom EFA stores are truly deficient, IV fat (Intralipid or Liposyn, 10% or 20%) can be provided.

Proper delivery of parenteral nutrition requires an experienced team with knowledge of nutritional metabolism. Clearly, this therapy represents a major medical advance that ranks with antibiotics, heart–lung bypass machines, and renal dialysis in its influence on the survival of many patients. However, failure to recognize that the proper use of this therapy is a sophisticated science precludes satisfactory results in many patients. The practitioner responsible for this therapy must have proper training and must check his patients daily in order to avoid unnecessary complications and to provide each patient with optimal care.

FIG. 11-4 Cyclic hyperalimentation. Preceded by a reduction in the infusion rate to 75 ml to 80 ml/hr for 1 hour, the infusion of hypertonic glucose and amino acids is discontinued for 8 to 10 hours of each day. Dextrose-free solutions, saline or isotonic 3% amino acids (*AA*), or oral protein 20 g to 30 g bid or tid are administered in this period.

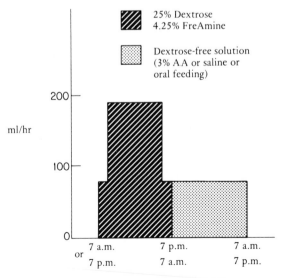

NONFED PARENTERAL

A modified starved state has been relatively ignored as a significant feature of nutritional support. Although the nutrient losses over the short term and adverse findings of nutritional depletion are well documented, most practitioners have been counseled that it is not worthwhile to provide nutritional support during short periods of starvation.[21,24,51,70,72,84] In part, this attitude is justified in the well-nourished individual with losses occurring over a short period, when the hormonal response is strongly catabolic and precludes significant utilization of exogenous nutrients, either as protein or calories.[43,68,74] However, many ill patients are already malnourished. Further, poor utilization of exogenous nutrients does not last as long as the classic catabolic phase of injury. Although net protein catabolism occurs from several days to weeks after injury, the ability to reverse this condition improves daily and justifies early efforts. Failure to minimize continuing losses from body cell mass, particularly in nutritionally depleted patients, affects the quality of recovery as well as morbidity and mortality.[61,82]

The realization that substantial protein sparing could occur in the starved state came when Owen and colleagues at the Joslin Research Laboratories demonstrated that ketones were a major fuel for brain energy requirement.[67] This observation accounted for the reduced requirement for glucose, decreased rates of gluconeogenesis, and amino acid oxidation seen late in fasting. Felig, from the same group, advanced the understanding of peripheral muscle metabolism, particularly the shuttle of gluconeogenic precursors (alanine and glutamine) to the liver for the production of glucose.[31]

Blackburn and Flatt developed the metabolic fuel cycle that provided a first-order approximation of the interrelationship of protein, fat, and carbohydrate and provided a basis for meeting the protein–calorie requirements during a modified starvation state.[17,34] In this state substantial protein sparing could occur by the infusion of amino acids to maintain protein synthesis, particularly in the viscera, while allowing the continued mobilization of the body fat stores.[16] The importance of ketone metabolism in this regard has been confirmed in studies by Felig.[77] This concept runs counter to the inferred interpretation of Gamble's classic studies on the life-raft ration.[38] He noted decreased nitrogen losses in human volunteers without stress who were fed 100 g glucose, and these findings were associated with elimination of ketosis and ketonuria. Others have proposed that this technique represents the most effective protein-sparing therapy during the nonfed starved state.[64] However, an increasing body of evidence indicates that during the early phase of illness, surgery, or major trauma, glucose is not more protein-sparing than is total starvation in a control patient with stress or injury, or both.[16,68] The sympathetic-mediated response to injury increases the mobilization of peripheral stores of fat and improves utilization of the mobilized amino acids to maintain LBM better than starvation alone.[40,89] In contrast, by raising insulin levels the administration of glucose preferentially shunts amino acids into the periphery and may be harmful for the important function of supporting visceral protein synthesis.

Recent studies in animals and humans have demonstrated the major protein-sparing effect of glucose in stress to result from decreased protein breakdown.[58,66] The protein-sparing effect of amino acids, particularly the branched-chain amino acids, however, is based primarily on increased protein synthesis. The efficacy of carbohydrate in small amounts (either orally or intravenously), particularly in the adaptive phase of stress or in prolonged stress, when glucose potentially blocks the mobilization of amino acids for visceral protein synthesis, must now be subject to question.[30,66] A growing body of evidence is accumulating to show that the use of 1 g to 1.5 g protein/kg ideal body weight/day, with appropriate cofactors of vitamins, minerals, fluids, and electrolytes is the optimal modification of the starved state.[15,36,47] This nutritional support is more compatible with the response to injury in preserving homeostasis and electrolyte balance. A characteristic series of changes in fluid and electrolyte status occurs in the acute phase after injury. Insulin secretion is known to decrease after injury and lipolysis to increase in response to increased catecholamine levels. Secretion of adrenocorticotropic hormone (ACTH) produces a glucocorticoid response and is associated with insulin resistance, glucose intolerance, and proteolysis. The free water production by tissue catabolism of muscle and fat and the secretion of antidiuretic hormone (ADH) produce increased free-water retention. In addition, a natriuresis secondary to an obligate cation coverage of the metabolically generated anions for excretion occurs.[78] Further, elevated plasma levels of glucagon and low plasma levels of insulin, characteristic of this natural state of injury, antagonize the action of aldosterone.[79] Thus, given poor utilization of exogenous substrate, initial resuscitation fluid should contain slightly hypertonic balanced electrolyte solutions for optimal preservation of the metabolic response to injury.[68]

Once the acute phase of injury has passed, the judicious incorporation of isotonic amino acid solutions can be expected to best support the patient.

The role of hypocaloric amounts of glucose in addition to protein has not been resolved. Although such therapy does not reduce net nitrogen sparing over an equivalent amount of protein alone, and in some instances has marginally improved nitrogen balance, the usual consequence clinically is to increase the osmolarity beyond the limits of peripheral vein tolerance.[39] Further research may demonstrate that even more vigorous use of oral and parenteral diets using formulas high in branched-chain amino acids and low in aromatic amino acids will benefit the acutely injured and septic patient unable to adapt to starvation by increased use of free fatty acids and ketone bodies.

ORAL PROTEIN SPARING

The provisions of protein orally, when gastrointestinal function permits, contrasts with the current practice of providing clear liquids in the form of fruit juice and gelatin. Not only is nitrogen balance improved, but oral protein may be selectively used by the GI tract, liver, and other key viscera, as reflected by improvements in serum albumin and transferrin levels and by immunocompetence. Currently available liquid protein sources, for instance, casein, whole egg, and soy protein isolate, allow early protein intake as clear liquid diets, although there is not yet a very palatable formula of protein alone.

It is important to remember the primacy of oral protein intake for reversing negative nitrogen balance and stimulating trophic gut hormones and visceral protein synthesis whether in semistarvation or adequate nutrition. The ability of enteral therapies to foster visceral protein synthesis makes them highly important, both for the pure nonfed state and its combination with parenteral nutritional therapies (cyclic hyperalimentation).

Development of a Nutrition Plan

A wide range of protein and nonprotein calorie sources exists. These products allow the nutritionist a versatile armamentarium to meet the many variations that various organ system failures and disease states present. Despite the potential complexity arising in patient care, nutrition support can easily be reduced to an effective plan by consideration of the following criteria:

A. Nutritional assessment (see Chap. 10)
　1. Degree of depletion of LBM (weight for height, creatinine–height index, arm muscle circumference, total body nitrogen by neutron activation analysis, N_{ae}/K_e ratio, or ^{40}K counting)

2. Degree of visceral protein depletion (serum albumin, serum transferrin, cell–mediated immunity)
B. Degree of hypercatabolism[74]
  1. Disease categories and measured or estimated metabolic rates
  2. Inspection of the patient, presence of tachycardia, fever
  3. Rate of weight loss and nitrogen excretion (urea nitrogen, corrected for nitrogen intake)[8]
C. GI function
  1. Dietary history of intake (complete, partial loss of, no effective intestinal function)
  2. Presence of a high intestinal fistula, low intestinal fistula
  3. Use of a nasogastric, transpharyngeal, gastric, enteric, or transfistula feeding tube
D. Appetite
  1. Solid or liquid food preference
  2. Taste preference (bland, fruits, sweet food groups)
E. Category nutritional support
  1. Fed
  2. Modified starved
  3. Combination
  4. Enteral versus parenteral

Consideration of these questions and calculation of the protein–calorie requirements based on age, sex, height, and weight allow development of a comprehensive nutritional support plan.

Nutritional Support in Specific Disease States

INFECTION

Infection is a major stress, producing a greater catabolic response than major elective surgery when viewed in terms of nitrogen loss. Protein kinetic studies have demonstrated that the mechanism of negative nitrogen balance in major, uncomplicated surgery is primarily through increased whole-body protein breakdown and protein flux (turnover). Whole-body protein synthesis may be slightly decreased, depending on the level of protein intake, while the efficiency of protein utilization is diminished by increased rates of amino acid oxidation, primarily from muscle, resting gut, and connective tissue proteins. As the hormonal milieu of stress diminishes with time, the protein synthetic machinery can be manipulated by provision of exogenous substrate (dietary protein or parenteral amino acids) to increase synthesis.[59]

Burns, multiple trauma, and systemic infection represent a higher level of metabolic stress. These prolonged moderate to severe stresses, as recognized by fever, even greater ureagenesis, and protracted lack of keto-adaptation show a somewhat different pattern of protein catabolism. Utilization of protein remains about as efficient as in lesser stresses. However, whole-body protein breakdown is increased, and protein synthesis is also increased but to a lesser degree than breakdown, yielding a greater negative nitrogen balance. While nutritional support is still possible in this setting, this generally means merely maintenance of present nutritional status. Full repletion of LBM deficits and the visceral protein compartment using currently available TPN techniques is not possible until the stress response has abated. The role of nutritional support is in maintaining the high level of visceral protein synthesis needed for survival, while trying to prevent or minimize further whole-body protein losses. A mildly hypocaloric feeding regimen with a high nitrogen–calorie ratio appears optimal to provide this support.

Besides the potential benefits of branched-chain amino acid-enriched solutions and mixed fuel systems of fat and carbohydrate to support protein synthesis in systemic infection, another area of promising work is the study of a possible mechanism underlying many of the phenomena seen in severe stress and infection. A small, as yet not fully characterized protein, produced by leukocytes and fixed tissue phagocytes, may represent a common pathway for major stress response. This leukocyte endogenous mediator (LEM) has been shown to increase somatic protein breakdown while increasing visceral protein synthesis (acute phase protein, white blood cells), to lower serum iron, zinc, and perhaps chromium to acute levels, and to produce fever.[5,70] It has been suggested that the withdrawal of iron from the serum is a protective mechanism, denying this micronutrient to invading microorganisms. Hence, it seems appropriate to withhold iron from TPN solutions in septic patients.[50,70] The ability of leukocytes to produce LEM (and therefore the ability of the patient to mobilize a full functional stress response to severe injury or sepsis) appears to be diminished in patients with hypoalbuminemic malnutrition and visceral protein depletion, and can be restored rapidly by feeding when unstressed. Whether this condition is nutritionally correctable in the setting of established stress is not known, but it does reemphasize the importance of feeding malnourished patients prior to the anticipated stress of surgery.

RENAL FAILURE

By almost any nutritional assessment parameter, patients with chronic renal failure are among the most likely to be malnourished. The introduction of a low-protein diet containing protein of high biologic value and adequate-to-excess calories by Giordano and Giavonetti in 1963 revolutionized the treatment of renal failure.[41] The diet was based on the pioneering work of Rose and colleagues that had established in the 1950s the human requirements for essential amino acids and nonessential nitrogen.[73] Not only does the Giavonetti diet provide adequate essential amino acids, but experience has also shown that endogenous urea nitrogen production is reduced.

The benefit of this diet in the treatment of chronic renal failure has been demonstrated by improvement in the hypoplastic anemia, lower blood urea nitrogen (BUN) levels, achievement of nitrogen balance, and disappearance or improvement of uremic symptoms, such as anorexia, vomiting, muscle twitching, and mental changes. The effectiveness of this diet depends on (1) a low nitrogen–calorie ration, (2) the number of calories delivered as related to the BEE, and (3) provision of adequate essential amino acids. Originally developed as an oral diet for chronic renal failure, it has been adapted to IV use for acute renal impairment, such as frequently occurs owing to tubular necrosis in severely traumatized patients or following major surgery. Since such patients are often unable to use their GI tracts for ingestion of nutrients, IV feeding can offer substantial support during recovery from various disease states and associated renal failure.

It is important to emphasize that this therapy is supportive and not a replacement for hemodialysis or peritoneal dialysis. In 1973 Abel and colleagues published the results of an extensive trial using essential amino acids in hypertonic glucose that confirmed the beneficial effects of renal-failure hyperalimentation as a support therapy.[1] In addition to optimizing wound healing, minimizing the catabolism of tissue proteins, and reducing the frequency of dialysis, metabolic benefits include normalization of serum protein, phosphate, and magnesium levels. In fact, the natural history of acute renal failure was altered with nutritional support, hastening the return of renal function in those patients who recovered.

There are, however, several unanswered questions about renal failure patients. The improvement in survival has not been confirmed in later studies.[53] Some workers have suggested this may be due to failure to maintain net protein synthesis under conditions of high rates of protein catabolism prevailing in acute renal failure.[20] Clinically, the use of solutions with both essential and nonessential amino acids in crossover studies, with the patient receiving essential amino acids alone, has not shown a substantial difference in the results.[19]

Several investigators have demonstrated the semiessential nature of histidine, and indeed improved utilization of protein has occurred with the provision of arginine and some nonessential amino acids.[7] It would appear that provision of the optimal number of calories needed to meet the metabolic expenditure and sufficient protein for optimal protein synthesis and turnover is more important than the amino acid profile. Data would suggest that administration of some protein, 20 g/day to 30 g/day (given with adequate calories) results in the best protein utilization. This suggests an optimal nitrogen–calorie ratio of 1:450. Protein and calorie intake at this level will minimize the BUN, and hence increase the interval between required dialyses. This seems appropriate in patients in renal failure who are only mildly catabolic. (A rise of the BUN of 5 mg/dl/day in a 70-kg man represents approximately the equivalent of 2 g urea–nitrogen production/day). Mild catabolism therefore represents up to 5 g/day to 6 g/day of urea production in the fasting state, either as urine urea output or as an elevation of BUN of 10 mg/dl to 12 mg/dl per day. However, it may be important to increase protein intakes to 50 g/day to 70 g/day in the more catabolic patient despite increased urea production and increase dialysis frequency in order to improve net nitrogen balance, since it is obvious from reported studies that 20 g/day to 30 g/day cannot replete a patient even under optimal conditions of malnutrition without disease.[2,52]

At greater levels of metabolic stress, greater protein intake is clearly required in the long run to preserve visceral protein synthesis and LBM. Although marginal protein utilization will be less, and ureagenesis greater, total protein synthesis will be greater at higher levels of protein intake. It is anticipated that adequate nutritional support to avoid further nutritional depletion in stressed patients with renal failure will have the same value as seen in non-renal-failure patients. Since sepsis is the major cause of death in acute renal failure, the importance of visceral protein support should not be underestimated in this group. Supportive nutritional therapy in moderately to severely catabolic renal-failure patients should be nearly identical in protein and calorie content to similar non-renal-failure patients, so long as effective dialysis to maintain the BUN under 75 mg/dl to 100 mg/dl is available.

Conversely, dialysis must be performed in this patient group as frequently as is required to keep the BUN and other metabolic wastes at an acceptable level, to allow the utilization of carbohydrate, fat, and protein in as normal a way as possible. Some patients on such a regimen will require replacement of intracellular minerals, specifically potassium and phosphate, that are required for ana-bolism. In general, sodium, calcium, and magnesium are not given to patients in renal failure. Trace elements and vitamins are given in normal amounts. Careful metabolic monitoring to determine true mineral requirements is mandatory. Restriction of sodium and fluid in the anuric patient is also important, with requirements being limited to measured and calculated losses once adequate fluid and sodium balance is achieved.[52]

A defined formula diet containing essential amino acids and their ketoanalogues is also a promising variant in the nutritional support of patients with chronic renal failure, although here too, the importance of adequate long-term nutrition must be emphasized.[75] Techniques of amino acid infusion during the latter half of hemodialysis, or intraperitoneal instillation at the end of peritoneal dialysis, although still experimental, also appear promising in aiding the goal of adequate long-term nutrition. On a theoretical basis, branched-chain enriched formulas (Hepatic–Aid) actually may be the best available for renal failure, since renal failure also alters peripheral utilization of the branched-chain amino acids (see Chap. 34).

HEPATIC FAILURE

The failing liver is characterized by a decreased ability to metabolize various amino acids. Patients with liver failure are frequently malnourished and require nutritional support in order to prevent a worsening of their condition. As in renal failure, protein intake of 20 g/day to 30 g/day with adequate calories will maximize nitrogen utilization over the fasting-stressed condition, and will minimize metabolic derangements. However, protein intake above that level often can and should be achieved, if adequate nutrition is to be provided.

The unique metabolism of the branched-chain amino acids and aromatic amino acids suggests that they represent the most critically regulated amino acids in circulation.[62,65,77] For example, tryptophan detoxification is primarily dependent on liver function. Therefore, it is not surprising that the level of tryptophan is elevated together with the other aromatic amino acids during liver failure. Branched-chain amino acids, on the other hand, are not significantly metabolized by the liver and become depleted during limited protein intakes. These observations form the basis for development of a defined-formula diet for liver failure (Hepatic–Aid) that has proved to be beneficial in allowing greater levels of protein intake before encephalopathy occurs, presumably relating to a normalization of the amino acid imbalance.[33] Experimental work with a

branched-chain enriched intravenous crystalline amino acid solution also appears to show a similar benefit in increased protein tolerance in liver failure.[32] The nonprotein calories are also important components of the diet for liver failure and have given rise to alcohol-free products that include medium-chain triglycerides and a judicious distribution of sugars, starches, and dextrins. Use of intravenous fat emulsions (Intralipid, Liposyn) is also helpful, because triglycerides can be utilized for energy by peripheral tissues, while minimizing intrahepatic lipogenesis. In liver failure, large glucose loads alone promote intrahepatic lipogenesis and may worsen liver function.[54] The provision of calories as a mixture of carbohydrate and fat (70%:30%) sufficient to meet energy requirements without causing the extra work of lipogenesis, gluconeogenesis, and ureagenesis will minimize nutrient imbalances resulting from liver failure. Sodium is poorly tolerated due to the hyperaldosteronism associated with liver failure. If given at all, sodium must be carefully restricted. Fluid balance must also be observed, as sodium retention will lead to fluid retention, if excess fluid is provided. The temptation to give sodium to patients with ascites and dilutional hyponatremia must be avoided, as additional sodium will only lead to increased fluid retention.

RESPIRATORY FAILURE

The role of nutritional support in respiratory failure is all too frequently ignored. Maintenance of LBM and repair of protein deficiency in the somatic and visceral compartments are vital not only to patient survival from the frequently accompanying respiratory sepsis, but for support and improvement of respiratory mechanics. Other than in the somewhat unique situation of the Pickwickian syndrome, where ketosis has been shown to increase sensitivity to an elevated pCO_2, maintenance of the fed state (with calorie intakes in excess of 1,000 Cal/day) in respiratory-failure patients is beneficial both in terms of central response to anoxia and in support of the primary and secondary muscles of respiration.[27,37]

The appropriate fuel mix for patients with respiratory failure presents a complicated picture. In patients with problems of adequate oxygenation, reliance primarily on glucose appears to be appropriate. In some studies fat emulsions appear to decrease oxygen diffusion across the alveolar–capillary membrane, but no clinically significant detrimental effect of using fat emulsions in respiratory failure has been demonstrated in adults.[42] Glucose consumes less oxygen per calorie than does fat. However, more CO_2 is produced per calorie when using glucose rather than fat as a fuel source.

In patients with CO_2 retention due to hypoventilation, manipulation of the respiratory quotient ($RQ = CO_2$ production/O_2 consumption) by altering the mix of fuels used for energy can be beneficial in ranges of carbohydrate feeding above 1000 Cals/day. This can be accomplished either by substituting exogenous fat calories for carbohydrate calories or by decreasing caloric intake to allow utilization of endogenous fat. The respiratory quotient when burning triglycerides is in the range of 0.7, for amino acids 0.8, and for glucose oxidation 1. As one approaches and exceeds the patient's metabolic expenditure with glucose feedings, net *de novo* lipogenesis from glucose becomes an important factor, as the RQ of conversion of glucose to long-chain fatty acids is in the range of 9. Hence patients who are overfed glucose in excess of metabolic requirements can have an RQ greater than 1, often as high as 1.25 or more.[48] This can be a cause of continued CO_2 retention and can precipitate respiratory failure in patients previously at borderline compensation.

Metabolic requirements in respiratory failure, in terms of protein and energy needs, should not be neglected. Deitel has shown improved ability to wean respiratory-dependent patients with effective nutritional support.[26] A caloric intake slightly under the estimated resting metabolic expenditure will avoid the possibility of excess CO_2 production owing to overfeeding and will minimize the hypercatabolism caused by the hyperalimentation itself. Both increased CO_2 production and increased hypercatabolism in the severely stressed patient limit carbohydrate feeding to a range below 5 mg/kg/minute in a 70-kg adult.[93]

CARDIAC DISEASE

The role of malnutrition in patients with advanced cardiac decompensation is another relatively ignored area. Cardiac cachexia has long been known as a consequence of disease or chronic congestive heart failure.[69] In its more advanced form, there is evidence to suggest depressed cardiac function both serves as a cause for and can be further depressed by malnutrition. Little data is available on the clinical significance of refeeding large numbers of patients with cardiac cachexia, although some benefit would be anticipated. Studies in preoperative cardiac surgery patients suggest a similarly increased morbidity and mortality in patients with concurrent protein–calorie malnutrition (measured by anthropometry, cell-mediated immunity, and serum albumin) as seen in general surgical patients, in whom the beneficial effect of preoperative refeeding has been shown. The value of preoperative refeeding in cardiac surgical patients is suggested but not yet proven by available data.

Techniques of enteral or parenteral hyperalimentation in patients with cardiac dysfunction rely on marked fluid and sodium restriction, careful clinical and metabolic monitoring, strict avoidance of excessive hypercatabolism from overfeeding, and provision of high-density alimentation solutions. As high glucose loads tend to produce increased salt and fluid retention by an antinatriuretic effect of insulin, a mixed fuel system may be of benefit. Insofar as fluid intake cannot be adequately restricted, increased use of diuretics may be required.

In patients with ischemic cardiac disease and ventricular irritability, an additional benefit of hypertonic glucose infusion can be shown. Mild hyperglycemia (up to the 150 mg/dl–200 mg/dl range) provides by mass action a non-insulin-dependent fuel to ischemic muscle that can be used anaerobically (by degradation to pyruvate and lactate, which are then transported to the liver for resynthesis into glucose). This inefficient fuel recycling obviously does not represent a true anaerobic fuel source on the whole body level but can decrease oxygen requirements of ischemic, irritable cardiac muscle. As discussed with respect to respiratory failure, glucose as a fuel requires less oxygen per calorie than does fat.

CANCER

Cancer is frequently associated with anorexia and semi-starvation. Factors other than anorexia responsible for the weight loss in cancer include disease-related dysfunction of the GI tract, malabsorption, organ failure, and infection. Cancer therapy by surgery, chemotherapy, radiotherapy, and immunotherapy also contributes to cancer cachexia. Finally, alterations in intermediary metabolism produced by cancer can affect the utilization of foodstuffs and the maintenance of the nutritional status of the patient.

These metabolic aspects of cancer and nutrition have been extensively reviewed.[83] The maintenance of a favorable nitrogen economy is dependent on the organism's ability to regulate both the synthetic and catabolic processes of a diverse variety of proteins and still maintain a relative constant whole body protein. Although the mechanisms are not precisely understood, it is felt that wasting in cancer is due primarily to anorexia and to the use of both host and dietary proteins by the tumor. The relatively more active metabolism of tumor tissue allows it to act as a nitrogen and energy trap, resulting in preferential growth at the expense of the host when dietary intake of energy and protein is inadequate. This tumor utilization of nitrogen is comparable to the situation following trauma or stress in which protein wasting rather than protein conservation is seen in spite of reduced protein intake. Although the BMR of cancer patients is rarely elevated more than 20% to 30% by the tumor, if at all, decreased glucose tolerance, increased gluconeogenesis not explicable by energy demands alone, decreased insulin sensitivity, and negative nitrogen balance can frequently be seen. Stein postulates that tumor utilization of specific amino acids leads to an imbalance in the amino acid profile.[82] Hence, increased ureagenesis and gluconeogenesis represent the body's only means of disposal of those amino acids in excess.

As yet unanswered questions arise about the role of branched-chain amino acids in cancer patients, as in stressed patients, and about hypocaloric protein regimens to support visceral protein metabolism in cancer patients. It has been noted that patients with the greatest weight loss also have the highest rates of Cori cycle activity, and this may imply another mechanism of cancer cachexia. However, the energy expenditure for the measured Cori cycle activity amounts to a small fraction of the total daily energy expenditure. This may also represent altered metabolism by a substrate imbalance affecting substrate-regulated pathways, again having an effect much greater than increased energy requirements alone can explain.

Although the mechanism of the nutritional depletion of cancer has remained partially unexplained, recent work demonstrates that weight loss does not necessarily have to result from tumor growth. Although conceptually and metabolically different, the anorexic share the similarity of inadequate dietary protein and calorie intake to meet metabolic requirements. Concepts useful in the treatment of anorexia nervosa, namely using techniques to produce behavior that will encourage the patient to maintain his nutritional status, have been found to be useful in some cancer patients as well. The basic principle underlying behavioral approaches to anorexia involves positive reinforcement of food intake coupled with negative reinforcement of episodes of food rejection. Within a hospital ward, positive reinforcement may consist of increased activity, visiting privileges, and social activities. On an outpatient basis, visits from friends, the interest of professional staff, and special treats can also be supportive. Continued outpatient care consists primarily of behavioral therapies to overcome loss of appetite. Such an approach does not require intensive psychological intervention or the use of psychotherapeutic drugs. The basic principles can be learned and implemented on a medical ward by physicians, nurses, and dietary staff, and at home by family and friends.

There can be little doubt that optimal nutritional support influences the results of new cancer therapies. Forced-feeding programs using enteral and parenteral hyperalimentation serve as acute short-term nutritional support in conjunction with specific tumor therapy. Since the cancer patient with significant weight loss has a poor therapeutic response, it is important to minimize and repair protein–calorie deficiency and support visceral protein synthesis. This enhances destruction of cancer cells and allows optimal function of normal tissue populations, particularly those cells or proteins with high rates of protein turnover, such as the GI mucosa and visceral proteins. Proper nutrition may minimize the ability of tumors to parasitize nutrients from the host and may increase tumor cell mitoses, which is a desired target-increasing effect during radiotherapy and chemotherapy. Conversely, nutrition-induced depression of cell-mediated immunity can be expected to have an adverse effect on certain aspects of cancer therapy, particularly (but not exclusively) immunotherapy, as well as to increase the risk of sepsis in immunosuppressed patients.

Nutritional therapy is now at a high enough level of development to provide support during effective antitumor therapies, and is one area in which the patient can actively participate in efforts to survive. Clearly, the multidisciplinary approach provided by a nutritional support service is essential. Efforts to design diet therapy to satisfy individual taste and to be consistent in the use of solid or liquid foods with adequate amounts of nutrients are important. The frequently altered taste patterns of cancer patients, including an aversion to red meat, strong flavors, and especially sweetness must be taken into account as well. The long-term use of feeding tubes by nasogastric, transpharyngeal, or gastrostomy route, however, and occasionally home hyperalimentation by parenteral-feeding programs, must be increasingly employed in the care of cancer patients. It must be clearly understood that continued weight loss is not a necessary component of advanced cancer, and concentrated efforts at treatment must be pursued simultaneously with specific cancer therapy (see Chap. 36).

At the same time, no evidence exists indicating that nutritional support is in any way beneficial, in terms of survival, in the treatment of tumors for which no effective palliative therapy exists. In this setting, maintenance of weight by provision of maintenance levels of protein and caloric intake can be of psychological benefit and may improve a patient's sense of well-being, while maintaining strength or limiting further loss. Aggressive refeeding of patients with advanced cancer who are undergoing no specific treatment or ineffective treatment will be unsuccessful in repairing lean body mass deficit and may be harmful, since tumor growth will occur at least at the same rate as that of lean tissue repletion.[64] Any moderately to severely malnourished cancer patient who is to undergo surgical treatment should be aggressively fed preoperatively for 7 to 10 days, because the importance of reversing the consequences of visceral protein depletion prior to surgical stress probably outweighs any potentially harmful effect on tumor growth.

DIABETES

In patients with diabetes mellitus, aggressive nutritional support is often avoided, particularly by the parenteral route, owing to the difficulty of managing diabetes on TPN and the fear that prohibitive rates of complications will outweigh the benefits. Under the care of an experienced nutrition support group capable of providing meticulous catheter care, expert preparation of tailor-made TPN solutions, and frequent metabolic monitoring, nutritional therapy can be provided to even brittle insulin-dependent diabetics without unacceptable risks, although metabolic complications and infections are considerably more common.

Insulin-dependent diabetics require a careful history detailing insulin requirements and insulin sensitivity. Parenteral insulin requirements added into the TPN solution for a full-feeding regimen (35 Cal/kg/day–40 Cal/kg/day) without significant stress will be 1.5 to 2 times the usual dosage, when the patient was previously consuming an adequate oral intake (35 Cal/kg/day–40 Cal/kg/day). This is because regular insulin in TPN solutions is about 50% effective due to loss of insulin in the bottle or tubing. The use of plastic bags and of filters for TPN solutions will further decrease the effectiveness of the insulin. Attempts to achieve tight control of blood glucose will lead to hypoglycemia (although this is usually remarkably well tolerated at high levels of glucose infusion). Maintenance of capillary blood sugars in the range of 150 mg/dl to 250 mg/dl, with one blood sugar per day less than 200 mg/dl, represents good control of insulin-dependent diabetes on TPN.

In order to initiate TPN in an insulin-dependent diabetic patient, the initial glucose load should be 150 g/day to 200 g/day, with insulin added to the infusate in an amount proportional to the caloric intake, based on the previous known insulin requirements for the caloric intake of full feeding. For example, a patient requiring 35 units of NPH insulin when eating 2000 Cal/day is being started on 1 liter of 15% glucose per day (150 gm = 600 kcal). Then $35 \times 600/2000$ = approximately 10 units of regular insulin is added to the first TPN bottle. Capillary blood sugars are determined every 6 to 8 hours, and elevated blood sugars are covered with subcutaneous regular insulin on a sliding scale:

5 u for > 200 mg/dl	or if conservative
10 u for > 250 mg/dl	5 u for > 250 mg/dl
15 u for > 300 mg/dl	10 u for > 300 mg/dl
20 u for > 350 mg/dl	15 u for > 350 mg/dl
>400 mg/dl emergency!	>400 mg/dl emergency!

This does require a maximum response time of 1 hr between capillary blood sugar sampling and administration of the insulin. The sliding scale doses are decreased in patients with known increased sensitivity to insulin, as occasionally occurs in association with diabetic nephropathy and renal failure.

If adequate control is achieved with less than twenty units of additional subcutaneous insulin required, the daily glucose load may be advanced toward full-feeding goals with the insulin dose increased proportionally (usually by maintaining the glucose and insulin concentrations and increasing the rate). If greater than 20 units additional insulin coverage is required, two thirds of the additional insulin is added to the TPN solution for the next day, and feeding is not advanced until adequate control is achieved. Usually full-feeding can be achieved by this method in 4 days. Once insulin requirements are established, they will remain stable if there is no new metabolic stress. Patients stabilized on a full feeding regimen must continue to be monitored with capillary blood sugar determinations every 8 hours.

In patients who are also receiving significant enteral calories, subcutaneous insulin (either NPH in the morning or regular insulin as needed) should be used to manage enteral calories. Insulin in the TPN solution is meant only to manage the parenteral glucose load. If the patient receives no additional subcutaneous insulin overnight, the fasting blood sugar each morning will be the sole determinant of the adequacy of the insulin in the TPN solution and should be above 120 mg/dl. The use of fat emulsions is often helpful in improving the control of blood sugars in diabetic patients, and need not be considered in determining insulin requirements. A step-wise tapering of TPN in diabetic patients can also be accomplished. This is done by maintaining the insulin to glucose ratio as carbohydrate is withdrawn until 150 g per day or less of glucose is given. At this point insulin in the infusate can be discontinued and the patient's blood sugars controlled easily with subcutaneous insulin alone.

A unique indication for nutritional support, diabetic gastropathy, exists in the insulin-dependent diabetic group. The development of this complication of diabetes becomes a vicious cycle, since the disease is worsened by poor nutrition. Conversely, full nutritional support is often extremely valuable in reversing this neurogenic gastric atony. In some patients, this can be accomplished by constant drip tube feeding, which is better tolerated than is eating or other bolus feeding. In others, TPN is required. Often a period of three weeks of full feeding with good diabetic control is sufficient to allow gradual resumption of normal oral intake. Whether denial of the oral route aids in the return of function, or whether TPN plays only a supportive role in maintaining acceptable nutrition while the disease pursues its own variable course is not known, since random clinical trials have not been conducted.

The common association of diabetes with renal failure also often requires nutritional intervention. TPN in diabetic patients with chronic renal failure is managed in the manner described above, with additional limitations of fluid, sodium, potassium, phosphate, magnesium, and calcium appropriate in renal failure. Vitamins and trace elements should be given daily, although vitamin D may have to be omitted or limited, because patients with renal impairment may be additionally sensitive to parenteral vitamin D, causing elevation in bone alkaline phosphatase and serum calcium. Patients on peritoneal dialysis absorb large amounts of glucose during their dialyses. Hence, blood sugar control and potassium and phosphate stability may all be easier to maintain by omitting glucose from the TPN solution during the dialysis.[3]

Metabolic complications of TPN in diabetes, besides hyper- and hypoglycemia, include an increased incidence of hyperkalemia, particularly when glucose concentrations are rapidly changing. This requires more frequent monitoring of serum potassium levels in patients not fully stabilized, but can be acceptably controlled. Cyclic hyperalimentation is contraindicated in insulin-dependent patients owing to the excessive risk of hyper- and hypoglycemia and hyperkalemia. Hypophosphatemia, particularly in diabetics with renal failure on chronic phosphate restriction, must be watched for carefully and corrected. There is no obvious increased incidence of mechanical complications with catheter insertion in diabetes, nor any increase in subclavian vein thrombosis. TPN catheter infections appear to be somewhat more common in insulin-dependent diabetic patients, indicating the necessity for increased awareness of this potential problem and an aggressive approach both to proper catheter management and to diagnosis of catheter infection that is present. The increased risks even from properly managed TPN in the insulin-dependent diabetic group are outweighed by the benefits to be derived from nutritional support.

CRITICAL ILLNESS

Many of the specific problems and concerns of providing nutritional support in the intensive care unit (ICU) patient have been discussed under sepsis, organ failure, and diabetes. It is worthwhile to consider briefly the more general problem of nutritional support in the ICU.

Frequently, ICU patients cannot be fully fed because of the inability to tolerate sufficient fluids. Intolerance to large protein loads or glucose loads also limits therapy. Most ICU patients present a variety of limitations to feeding, as well as significant prolonged stress. In this setting, the importance of flexibility in creating widely disparate feeding regimes based on individualized TPN and tube-feeding solutions from modular sources cannot be overemphasized. A 10% crystalline amino acid solution and a 70% hydrous dextrose solution are now commercially available and provide a wide range of nutritional blends for use in the critically ill. Protein and glucose combinations can be prepared in minimal fluid volumes as seen in Table 11-2.

The goals of nutritional support in the intensive care unit are similar to the goals of other invasive therapies, such as pressors, cardiotonics, respiratory support, and acute hemodialysis. Namely, metabolic support is needed until the acute critical decompensation is resolved. Weight gain in pa-

TABLE 11-2
Protein and Glucose Combinations in Minimal Fluid Volumes

Amino Acids (%)	(g/liter)	Glucose (%)	(g/liter)	N:cal ratio
8	80	14	140	1:37
7	70	21	210	1:64
6	60	28	280	1:97
5	50	35	350	1:149
4	40	42	420	1:223
3.5	35	45.5	455	1:276
3	30	49	490	1:347

tients with severe acute illness cannot represent repair of LBM deficit and should be interpreted as fluid accumulation. Maintenance of somatic protein status while maximally supporting and driving the protein synthetic machinery should help optimize survival. Refeeding will then become the goal of convalescence. Nutritional and metabolic support for the critically ill ICU patient, although undoubtedly riskier than nutritional support for a more stable patient, must be viewed as crucial, and must not be neglected.[6]

Summary

Nutritional support has been clearly established as beneficial in patients with long-standing disease in order (1) to prevent or repair malnutrition, (2) to correct moderate to severe PCM prior to elective or postponable surgery, thereby minimizing morbidity and mortality from surgery, and (3) to nourish patients whose gastrointestinal tracts cannot, or for therapeutic reasons should not, be used for a prolonged period. Less widely appreciated, and therefore more often neglected or suboptimally treated, are a variety of conditions in which metabolic stress and catabolism acutely create or compound the problem of visceral protein depletion. Although the effects of nutritional support in these conditions are less easily demonstrable, a rationale and a basis for understanding have been provided for nutritional support in acute illness.

Protein–calorie management is uniquely influenced by disease, and effective nutritional support in the ill must include consideration of nutritional status, particularly the degree of protein depletion. The presence of hypercatabolism must also be considered because the hormonal substrate response is distinctly antagonistic to replacement therapy. Further, enteral feeding regimens are often limited by impaired digestive function associated with disease. Although each patient has a unique response, a systematic approach based on objective measures will more often result in effective nutritional therapy. The accomplished therapist will be aided by the flexible modular approach using the wide variety of products and techniques now available. Certainly it is no longer considered good patient care to ignore the management of the semi-starved state when it is possible to support, either orally or intravenously, protein synthesis and to preserve lean body mass. With proper skill in the techniques of protein–calorie therapy, the morbidity and mortality of most disease states can be expected to be favorably influenced. The science and art of nutritional assessment and therapy now provide the basis for an important clinical advance and specialty.

References

1. Able RM, Beck CH, Abbot WM, et al: Improved survival from acute renal failure after treatment with intravenous essential L-amino acids and glucose. N Engl J Med 288:695, 1973
2. Barac–Nieto M, Spurr GB, Dahners HW, et al: Aerobic work capacity and endurance during nutritional repletion of severely undernourished men. Am J Clin Nutr 33:2268, 1980
3. Batist G, Bistrian BR, Kaldany A, et al: Intravenous total parenteral nutrition in diabetic renal failure. Nephron 28:244, 1981
4. Beisel WR: Interrelated changes in host metabolism during generalized infectious illness. Am J Clin Nutr 25:1254, 1973
5. Beisel WR, Sobocinski PZ: Endogenous mediators of fever-related metabolic and hormonal responses. In Lipton JM (ed): Fever, p 39–48, New York, Raven Press, 1980
6. Benotti PN, Blackburn GL: Protein and calorie or macronutrient metabolic management of the critically ill patient. Crit Care Med 7:520, 1979
7. Bergstrom J, Bucht P, Furst E, et al: Intravenous nutrition with amino acid solutions in patients with chronic uraemia. Acta Med Scand 191:359, 1972
8. Bistrian BR: A simple technique to estimate severity of stress. Surg Gynecol Obstet 148:675, 1979
9. Bistrian BR, Blackburn GL, Scrimshaw NS, et al: Cellular immunity in semi-starved states in hospitalized adults. Am J Clin Nutr 28:1147, 1975
10. Bistrian BR, Blackburn GL, Vitale J, et al: Prevalence of protein–calorie malnutrition in general medical patients. JAMA 235:1567, 1976
11. Blackburn GL: Adipose tissue as a valuable source of essential fatty acids. Proc on Fat Emulsions in Parenteral Nutrition. Chicago, American Medical Association, 1975
12. Blackburn GL: Glucose, potassium and insulin therapy in critical clinical states. Journal of St. Barnabus Medical Center Symposium on Surgical Advances, p 43, December 1975
13. Blackburn GL, Bistrian BR: Nutritional care of the injured and/or septic patient. Surg Clin N Am 56:1195, 1976
14. Blackburn GL, Bistrian BR, Flatt JP, et al: Restoration of the visceral component of protein malnutrition during hypocaloric feeding. Clin Res 23:315A, 1975
15. Blackburn GL, Flatt JP: Metabolic response to illness: Role of protein-sparing therapy. Compr Ther 1:23, 1975
16. Blackburn GL, Flatt JP, Heddle R, et al: The significance of muscle protein and fat mobilization following injury for the design of parenteral fluid, electrolyte and nutritional therapy. Cuthbertson D (ed): Glasgow Injury Symposium, 1975
17. Blackburn GL, Flatt JP, Hensle TE: Peripheral amino acid infusions. In Fischer J (ed): Total Parenteral Nutrition, p 363–394, Boston, Little, Brown & Co, 1975
18. Blackburn GL, Moldawer LL, Usui S, et al: Branched chain amino acid administration and metabolism during starvation, injury, and infection. Surgery 86:307, 1979
19. Blackburn GL, Rutten P, Stone M, et al: Proc Int Conference on Parenteral Nutrition, Montpellier, France, 1974
20. Blumenkrantz MJ, Kopple JD, Koffler A, et al: Total parenteral nutrition in the management of acute renal failure. Am J Clin Nutr 31:1831, 1978

21. Buzby GP, Mullen JL, Matthews DC, et al: Prognostic nutritional index in gastric intestinal surgery. Am J Surg 139:160, 1980

22. Christon NV, Meakins JL, MacLean LD: The predictive role of delayed hypersensitivity in preoperative patients. Surg Gynecol Obstet 152:297, 1981

23. Close JH: The use of amino acid precursors in nitrogen accumulation diseases. N Eng J Med 290:663, 1974

24. Clowes GHA Jr, O'Donnell TF, Ryan NT, et al: Energy metabolism in sepsis: Treatment based on different patterns in shock and high output state. Ann Surg 175:584, 1974

25. Cuthbertson DP: Post-shock metabolic response. Lancet 25:235, 1942

26. Deitel M, Bassili HR: Nutritional support in weaning patients off ventilators (abstr). JPEN 4:584, 1980

27. Doekel RC, Zwillich CW, Sloggin CH, et al: Clinical semistarvation: Depression of hypoxic ventilatory response. N Engl J Med 295:358, 1976

28. Dudrick SJ, MacFayden BV, VanBuren CT: Parenteral hyperalimentation: Metabolic problems and solutions. Ann Surg 176:259, 1972

29. Duke JH, Jorgensen SB, Broel JR, et al: Contribution of protein to caloric expenditure following injury. Surgery 68:168, 1970

30. Elwyn DH, Bryan–Brown CW, Shoemaker WC: Nutritional aspects of body water dislocations in postoperative and depleted patients. Ann Surg 182:76, 1975

31. Felig P, Wahren J: Protein turnover and amino acid metabolism in the regulation of gluconeogenesis. Fed Proc 33:1092, 1974

32. Fischer JE, Freund H, Rosen H, et al: Effects of F080 in clinical hepatic encephalopathy: Result of a phase I study (abstr). Gastroenterology 75:963, 1978

33. Fischer JE, Funovics JM, Aguirre A, et al: The role of plasma amino acids in hepatic encephalopathy. Surgery 78:276, 1975

34. Flatt JP, Blackburn GL: The metabolic fuel regulatory system: Implications for protein sparing therapies during caloric deprivation and disease. Am J Clin Nutr 27:175, 1974

35. Freeman JB, Stegink LK, Meyer PD, et al: Excessive urinary zinc losses during parenteral alimentation. J Surg Res 18:463, 1975

36. Freeman JB, Stegink LD, Meyer PD, et al: Metabolic effects of amino acids vs. dextrose infusion in surgical patients. Arch Surg 110:916, 1975

37. Fried PI, McCleen PA, Phillipson EA, et al: Effect of ketosis in respiratory sensitivity to carbon dioxide in obesity. N Eng J Med 294:1081, 1976

38. Gamble JL: Physiological information gained from studies on the life raft ration. Harvey Lect 42:247, 1946

39. Gazitua R, Wilson K, Bistrian BR, et al: Factors determining peripheral vein tolerance to amino acid infusions. Arch Surg 114:897, 1979

40. Gilder H, Valcre M, DeLeon V, et al: Comparative effect of experimental injury and hydrocortisone injection on liver and plasma composition of rats. Metabolism 19:562, 1970

41. Giordano C: Use of exogenous and endogenous urea for protein synthesis in normal and uremic subjects. J Lab Clin Med 62:231, 1963

42. Greene HL, Hazlett D, Demaree R: Relationship between Intralipid-induced hyperlipemia and pulmonary function. Am J Clin Nutr 29:127, 1976

43. Gump FE, Long CL, Geiger JW, et al: The significance of altered gluconeogenesis in surgical catabolism. J Trauma 15:704, 1975

44. Hallowell E, Sasvary D, Bistrian BR, et al: Factors determining optimal use of defined (elemental) formula diets. Clinical Research 24:500A, 1976

45. Heymsfield SB, Bethai RA, Ansley JD, et al: Enteral hyperalimentation: An alternative to central venous hyperalimentation. Ann Intern Med 90:63, 1979

46. Hoffman–Goetz L, McFarlane D, Bistrian BR, et al: Febrile and plasma iron responses of rabbits injected with endogenous pyrogen from malnourished patients. Am J Clin Nutr 34:1109, 1981

47. Hoover HC, Grant JP, Gorschboth C, et al: Nitrogen-sparing intravenous fluid in postoperative patients. N Engl J Med 293:172, 1975

48. Hunker FD, Bruton CW, Hunker VM, et al: Metabolic and nutritional evaluation of patients supported with mechanical ventilation. Crit Care Med 8:628, 1980

49. Jeejeebhoy KN, Chu RC, Marliss EB, et al: Chromium deficiency, glucose intolerance, and neuropathy reversed by chromium supplementation in a patient receiving long-term parenteral nutrition. Am J Clin Nutr 30:531, 1977

50. Kluger MJ, Rothenburg BA: Fever, trace metals, and disease. In Lipton JM (ed): Fever p 31–38. New York, Raven Press, 1980

51. Law DK, Dudrick SJ, Abdou NI: Immunocompetence of patients with protein calorie malnutrition. Ann Intern Med 79:543, 1973

52. Lee HA: Nutritional support in renal and hepatic failure. In Karran SJ, Alberti KGMM (eds): Practical Nutritional Support p 275–282, New York, John Wiley & Sons, 1980

53. Leonard CD, Luke RG, Siegel RR: Parenteral essential amino acids in acute renal failure. Urology 6:154, 1975

54. Maini BS, Blackburn GL, Bistrian BR, et al: Cyclic hyperalimentation: An optimal technique for preservation of visceral protein. J Surg Res 20:515, 1976

55. Mascioli EA, Smith MF, Trerice MS, et al: Effect of total parenteral nutrition with cycling on essential fatty acid deficiency. JPEN 3:171, 1979

56. McLaren DS: Xerophthalmia: A neglected problem. Nutr Rev 22:289, 1964

57. Mills CB, Kaminski MV: Trace element requirements. In Deitel M (ed): Nutrition in Clinical Surgery p 113–123, Baltimore, Williams & Wilkins, 1980

58. Moldawer LL, O'Keefe SJD, Bothe A, et al: *In vivo* demonstration of nitrogen-sparing mechanisms for glucose and amino acids in the injured rat. Metabolism 29:173, 1980

59. Moldawer LL, Sakamoto A, Blackburn GL et al: Alterations in protein kinetics produced by branched-chain amino acid administered during infection and inflammation. In Walser M, Williamson JR (eds): Metabolism and Clinical Implications of Branched-Chain Amino and Ketoacids, p 533–534. New York, Elsevier/North Holland, 1981

60. Moore FD: Metabolic Care of the Surgical Patient, Philadelphia, WB Saunders, 1959

61. Mullen JL, Buzby GP, Matthews DC, et al: Reduction of operative morbidity and mortality by combined preoperative and postoperative nutritional support. Ann Surg 192:604, 1980

62. Munro HN, Fernstrom JD, Wurtman RJ: Insulin, plasma amino acid imbalance and hepatic coma. Lancet 1:722, 1975

63. Nixon DW, Moffitt S, Lawson DH, et al: Total parenteral

nutrition as an adjunct to chemotherapy of metastatic cancer. Cancer Treat Rep 65:121, 1981

64. O'Connell RC, Morgan AP, Aoki TT, et al: Nitrogen conservation in starvation: Graded responses to intravenous glucose. J Clin Endocrinol Metab 29:555, 1975
65. Odessey R, Khaitallah EA, Goldberg AL: Origin and possible significance of alanine production by skeletal muscle. J Biol Chem 249:7623, 1974
66. O'Keefe SJD, Moldawer LL, Young VR, et al: The influence of intravenous nutrition on protein dynamics following surgery. Metabolism 30:1150, 1981
67. Owen OE, Morgan AP, Kemp HG, et al: Brain metabolism during fasting. J Clin Invest 46:1589, 1967
68. Page G, Blackburn GL, Heddle R, et al: Crystalloid therapy in resuscitation during routine surgery and severe trauma. Surg Forum 26:18, 1975
69. Pittman JG, Cohn P: The pathogenesis of cardiac cachexia. N Engl J Med 271:403, 1964
70. Powanda MC: Changes in body balance of nitrogen and other key nutrients: Description and underlying mechanisms. Am J Clin Nutr 30:1254, 1977
71. Proceedings of AMA Conference on Defined Formula Diets. Washington, D.C. Acton, MA, Publishing Sciences Group, 1975
72. Reinhardt GF, Myscofski JW, Wilkins DB, et al: Incidence and mortality of hypoalbuminemic patients in hospitalized veterans. JPEN 4:357, 1980
73. Rose WC, Wixom RL: The amino acid requirement of man: 16. The role of the nitrogen intake. J Biol Chem 217:997, 1955
74. Rutten P, Blackburn GL, Flatt JP, et al: Determination of optimal hyperalimentation infusion rate. J Surg Res 18:477, 1975
75. Sapir DG, Owen OE, Pozefsky T, et al: Nitrogen sparing induced by a mixture of essential amino acids given chiefly as their keto-analogues during prolonged starvation in obese subjects. J Clin Invest 54:974, 1974
76. Senior JR (ed): Medium Chain Triglycerides, Philadelphia, University of Pennsylvania Press, 1968
77. Sherwin RS, Hendler RG, Felig P: Effect of ketone infusions and amino acid and nitrogen metabolism in man. J Clin Invest 55:1382, 1975
78. Sigler M: The mechanism of the natriuresis of fasting. J Clin Invest 55:377, 1975
79. Sparks RF, Arky RA, Boulter PR, et al: Renin, aldoster-

one, and glucagon in the natriuresis of fasting. N Engl J Med 292:1335, 1975
80. Stead N, Curtas M, Grant J: Changes in ferrokinetics during parenteral nutrition (abstr) JPEN 4:585, 1980
81. Stein TP: Cachexia, gluconeogenesis, and progressive weight loss in cancer patients. J Theor Biol 73:51, 1978
82. Studley HO: Percent of weight loss: A basic indicator of surgical risk. JAMA 106:458, 1936
83. Theologides A: Pathogenesis of cachexia in cancer. Cancer 29:484, 1972
84. Trinkle JK, Fischer LJ, Ketcham AS, et al: The metabolic effects of preoperative intestinal preparation. Surg Gynecol Obstet 118:739, 1964
85. Vitter RW, Bozian RC, Hess EV, et al: Manifestations of copper deficiency in a patient with systemic sclerosis on intravenous hyperalimentation. N Engl J Med 291:188, 1974
86. Waterlow JC, Stephen JM: The measurement of total lysine turnover in the rat by intravenous infusion of L (U^{14}C) lysine. Clin Sci 33:389, 1967
87. Weinberg ED: Nutritional immunity. JAMA 231:39, 1975
88. Wene JD, Connor WE, DenBesten I: The development of essential fatty acid deficiency in healthy men fed fat-free diets intravenously and orally. J Clin Invest 56:127, 1975
89. Whipple GH, Hooper CW, Robscheit FS: Blood regeneration following simple anemia in fasting compared with sugar feeding. AM J Physiol 53:167, 1920
90. Wilmore DW, Long JM, Mason AD, et al: Catecholamines: Mediator of the hypermetabolic responses to thermal injury. Ann Surg 180:653, 1974
91. Wolfe RR, Allsop JR, Burke JF: Glucose metabolism in man: Responses to intravenous glucose infusion. Metabolism 28:210, 1979
92. Wolfe RR, Durkot MJ, Allsop JR, et al: Glucose metabolism in severely burned patients. Metabolism 28:1031, 1979
93. Wolfe RR, O'Donnell TF, Stone MD, et al: Investigation of factors determining the optimal glucose infusion rate in total parenteral nutrition. Metabolism 29:892, 1980
94. Wolman SL, Anderson GH, Marliss EB, et al: Zinc in total parenteral nutrition: Requirements and metabolic effects. Gastroenterology 76:458, 1979
95. Young VR, Steffee W, Pencharz P, et al: Protein turnover in the whole body. Nature 253:157, 1975

12
Curative Nutrition—Vitamins
*Grace A. Goldsmith**

Vitamin-deficiency diseases due primarily to an inadequate dietary supply of specific nutrients are relatively rare in the United States and other developed countries of the world although they remain common in many developing nations. However, these deficiencies are encountered secondary to numerous pathologic conditions both in this country and elsewhere. Each of the vitamin-deficiency diseases will be discussed separately, including prevalence, clinical and laboratory findings, diagnostic features, and treatment.

In addition, there are a number of changing concepts of vitamin requirements and clinical uses that deserve mention. In the functioning organism there must be a sufficient quantity of dietary intake of each vitamin in order to accomodate satisfactorily each of the biochemical systems requiring them. When a number of systems require the same vitamin for their operations, each has its specific capacity to bind the vitamin so that it can function adequately. These genetically-based capabilities are different for each system and, therefore, are rank ordered with respect to this binding capacity. While all are operational in the presence of sufficient quantities of the vitamin, any given magnitude of

*The first edition of the *Nutritional Support of Medical Practice* was fortunate in having this chapter written by Dr. Grace Goldsmith whose professional career had spanned the era when the biochemical and clinical roles of these essential nutrients were being defined. This chapter was so well done, that indeed it is now a classic. Although Dr. Goldsmith died in 1975, its strength is such that the consensus of reviewers recommended that it be republished with but minor changes and such additions as are in keeping with current knowledge in the field. (D.B.C., 1982.)

deficiency will preferentially affect those with the weakest binding kinetics. Under these circumstances, selected metabolic and clinical changes may take place that will be further influenced by other factors such as previous state of health and nutrition, age, degree of severity of the deficiency, its duration, and accompanying deficiencies. With correction of the deficiency and adequate maintenance by administration of the normally required quantities of the vitamin, these changes usually will be reversed.

In providing guidelines for prevention of vitamin deficiencies in the general population, the Food and Nutrition Board of the National Research Council, National Academy of Science, has developed the Recommended (Daily) Dietary Allowances (RDAs). The details of their formulation are presented in Appendix Table A-1, and the recommended values are shown in Appendix Tables A-1 and A-3. As outlined, each of the RDAs has purposely been quantified to contain a large margin of safety that is in excess of what may be adequate as a minimum daily requirement for a particular individual. This assures that the quantities will be sufficient for virtually all of the "normal healthy" population.

It is anticipated that the healthy individual's varied diet of appropriate composition and quantity will meet their requirements. However, some circumstances in health and in disease may dictate the need for vitamin supplementation with quantities that are several times larger than the RDAs. Appendix Table A-4 addresses this issue.

During the past decade, a special situation of

higher "conditioned nutrient requirements" has emerged as a result of the widespread use of parenteral hyperalimentation. The details of this subject are discussed in Chapters 9, 11, 13, 14, 16, and 34, which deal with its use in a variety of disorders and diseases. Appendix Table A-41 outlines suggested amounts to meet the needs under such circumstances.

In addition to their roles as essential nutrients, there are a number of disorders in which very large (pharmacologic) dosages of vitamins may have a therapeutic effect. These quantities far exceed the normal nutritional requirements or the amounts needed to correct deficiencies and appear to effect the mechanisms that are impaired.

The classic example of the successful use of pharmacologic dosages of a vitamin is in cases of inborn errors of metabolism of a specific enzyme system that is dependent on the vitamin for activity (see Chap. 25). In this instance, the genetically abnormal structure of the enzyme will not permit it to bind satisfactorily to its coenzyme (the vitamin) to produce a functional holoenzyme. This occurs despite the fact that the individual's dietary intake and tissue levels of the vitamin are adequate for normal operation of similarly dependent enzyme systems that are genetically sound.

Correction of this abnormality may require the pharmacologic action of administration of hundreds of times the RDA as soon as possible, with long-term continuation—perhaps for a lifetime. In some cases, newer diagnostic techniques can facilitate identification of such cases *in utero*, permitting very early effective treatment and prevention of irreversible damage and possible death.[32]

In an increasing number of other disorders, there is an apparent effectiveness of "pharmacologic" dosages of various vitamins. The results are generally less well defined biochemically but have demonstrable metabolic, functional, and clinical consequences. Examples of such relationships include those between vitamin C and some features of the common cold, vitamin A and skin cancer, vitamin E and retrolental fibroplasia as well as vitamin E and fibrocystic breast disease.[9,56,62,64] Continued research is needed to clarify these dual capabilities of vitamins as nutrients and as pharmacologic agents so that their true potential can be realized.

Vitamin A Deficiency—Xerophthalmia

PREVALENCE

Vitamin A (retinol) deficiency is extremely rare in North America and Western Europe, but it is an important cause of preventable blindness in South-east Asia, certain parts of Africa, and Central and South America. It is frequently associated with protein–calorie malnutrition. Severe deficiency occurs most frequently in infants and young children and is more common in males than in females. In this country, deficiency of vitamin A and its precursor, carotene, is observed as a result of a number of conditions in which fat absorption is defective. These include diets very low in fat, the steatorrheas (*e.g.*, sprue), fibrocystic disease of the pancreas and other pancreatic diseases, intestinal lipodystrophy (Whipple's disease), gluten-induced enteropathy, and intestinal defects following operative procedures. Since bile is necessary for the absorption of carotene and vitamin A, deficiency may occur when bile is absent or when amounts in the intestinal tract are insufficient, such as in obstructive jaundice and biliary fistula. In cirrhosis of the liver, storage of vitamin A may be impaired with resultant deficiency. Infectious diseases associated with massive urinary excretion of vitamin A include tuberculosis, pneumonia, chronic nephritis, urinary tract infections, and prostatic diseases. Increased excretion also occurs in cancer. In children with vitamin A deficiency, there is a high incidence of respiratory infections, gastroenteritis, measles, and other infectious diseases. This is particularly true in areas where marasmus or kwashiorkor are endemic. Whether this susceptibility is due to vitamin A deficiency or whether the infection led to lowered vitamin A reserves is unknown. Vitamin A deficiency has been reported in diabetes mellitus and in myxedema, presumably owing to failure of conversion of carotene to vitamin A.

CLINICAL FINDINGS

The earliest symptom of vitamin A deficiency is night blindness caused by an inadequate supply of vitamin A aldehyde to the retina for the formation of rhodopsin. This lesion is fully reversible with prompt treatment but may be followed rapidly by structural changes in the retina. Night blindness may be difficult to detect in infants and young children. They may be seen to stumble at dusk or be unable to feed themselves when the light is failing.

A second early finding is xerosis (dryness) of the conjuntiva. The bulbar portion exposed in the eye slit is particularly affected. Oomen describes the appearance as fatty dryness, most pronounced at the thickened, wrinkled corners of the eye.[8] Slit lamp examination shows that the transparent structure has become opaque due to fine milky droplets. The white of the eye looks muddy and greasy, like oil paint. The pores of the meibomian glands enlarge and resemble a string of beads along the margin of the eyelids. The skin is thin and dry around the eyes, and fine points of folliculosis may be present. The skin between the eyelashes is often scaly.

Xerosis may progress rapidly to xerophthalmia and keratomalacia. As the disease advances, the cornea is involved, appearing hazy, rough, and dry, and becoming insensitive to touch. Small erosions or punctate superficial infiltrations may be seen on the surface, frequently in the lower nasal quadrant. These develop rapidly into small, dark, berrylike protrusions to which a tiny slip of iris is attached. Following this, perforation occurs, and the iris may collapse or the lens may be expelled. The condition is not painful, but the child keeps his eyes closed in order to avoid light. In late stages, there may be inflammatory symptoms that resemble conjunctivitis and—rarely—panophthalmitis. The end result is a large thick scar that prevents the entrance of light, and consequently blindness results.

Corneal involvement is called keratomalacia by some authors. Oomen, however, considers the latter to be a different process, which he describes as colliquative necrosis, or ''a rather sudden, spongy swelling and melting down of the cornea with subsequent shrinkage of the eyeball without infection. The adjacent structures become irritated and xerosis of the bulbar conjunctiva is difficult to demonstrate.''[8] Keratomalacia is a medical emergency requiring immediate therapy. It usually involves both eyes. Blindness occurs if treatment is not instituted before an advanced stage is reached.

Several other findings are seen in association with vitamin A deficiency. Bitot's spots occur in the equatorial region of the eye on the lateral side. They are triangular in shape with the base lying at the corneoscleral junction. The appearance is similar to patches of paste that have been striated with a pin. The color resembles aluminum paint. Smears made from these areas show Corynebacterium xerose and keratinized epithelium. Bitot's spots are probably nonspecific findings of malnutrition. They are found in areas where vitamin A deficiency is common but are seldom associated with night blindness, keratomalacia, or low concentrations of vitamin A in blood. Administration of vitamin A has not led to disappearance of the lesions. However, Bitot's spots are useful indicators of potential vitamin A deficiency due to their association with xerophthalmia (see Chap. 30).

A number of changes in the skin have been ascribed to vitamin A deficiency, including xeroderma, mosaic or crackled skin, phrynoderma, folliculosis, and follicular hyperkeratosis. All of these conditions are characterized by abnormal keratinization of the epithelium. Folliculosis of the skin around the eye is seen in xerophthalmia, and xeroderma may be present in children with this disease. Phrynoderma (toad skin) has been noted in children of school age with mild xerophthalmia but also in children without eye symptoms. The characteristic findings in phrynoderma are pointed, horny, pigmented spikes in the skin, particularly in the knees and elbows. Follicular hyperkeratosis may be a variant of this condition. Abundant evidence indicates that not all cases of xeroderma, crackled skin, phrynoderma, or follicular hyperkeratosis are due to vitamin A deficiency. Some investigators question whether follicular hyperkeratosis is ever due to deficiency of this vitamin alone. Administration of oils containing polyunsaturated fatty acids, without vitamin A, has resulted in a cure in some instances but not in others. In all likelihood, these abnormalities of the skin are of varied etiology, some due to lack of vitamin A, others to lack of essential fatty acids or ascorbic acid or to multiple deficiency (see Chap. 35).

Within the past several years, these phenomena have been explored further, with extensive research into the role of vitamin A in the development of cancers of the skin and their successful treatment with vitamin A analogues (retinoids).[3] Another interesting observation has emerged from a number of epidemiological studies of cancer in which there has been a significant correlation between low vitamin A levels and an increased risk of cancer in other organs, especially the lung and the gastrointestinal tract.[9] These findings are currently under further study and if such significant relationships can be substantiated, may open yet another area of prophylactic usefulness for the vitamin.

BIOCHEMICAL FINDINGS

The concentration of vitamin A in serum of well-nourished subjects is 40 μg to 80 μg/100 ml. Concentrations less than 30 μg/100 ml are considered low, and a level of less than 10 μg/100 ml is indicative of deficiency if infections have been ruled out.[2] In severe protein deficiency, such as kwashiorkor, vitamin A concentration in serum is very low. The level returns to normal in some subjects, but not in all, as a result of treatment with a high-protein diet. This is dependent on liver stores of vitamin A. When improvement occurs with protein alone, the low serum vitamin A was due probably to an inadequate amount of serum protein for transport of the vitamin. Determination of carotene in serum is useful in evaluating recent dietary intake of this substance. Normal levels are 25 μg to 50 μg/100 ml.

Absorption of vitamin A can be determined by administering a test dose and estimating the concentration in the serum at intervals thereafter. The maximum rise usually occurs in 3 to 6 hours.

The earliest abnormality in experimental vitamin A deficiency was detected by measurement of the visual fields under the condition of dark adaptation, that is, using rod scotometry.

With long-term vitamin A deficiency, changes may occur in iron status, with reductions in serum iron levels, hemoglobin, and hematocrit.[4]

PREVENTION AND TREATMENT

Vitamin A deficiency can be prevented by a diet that furnishes sufficient amounts of this vitamin to meet daily requirements. Administration of 100,000 IU vitamin A, orally or parenterally, every 6 months protects most of the preschool population. In the treatment of mild vitamin A deficiency, oral administration of 30,000 IU vitamin A daily is adequate. In severe xerophthalmia and keratomalacia, treatment consists of large doses that will cause a rapid increase in the level of vitamin A in the blood. The adult liver can absorb at least 500,000 IU. Accordingly, doses should be adjusted to make this amount available during the first few days of therapy. Somewhat smaller doses are used in children. On the first day, 100,000 IU of an aqueous dispersion of vitamin A, such as the palmitate (30,000 μg retinol), should be given parenterally. On the second through the sixth day, 50,000 IU should be given twice daily orally. Subsequently 10,000 IU should be provided daily in the form of cod liver oil to promote storage and prevent relapse; 30 ml cod liver oil provides 25,000 IU vitamin A (7500 μg retinol). Aqueous preparations of vitamin A should be used in conditions in which there are abnormalities in intestinal absorption of fat. Supportive therapy includes a high-protein, high-calorie diet rich in sources of vitamin A and carotene. Antibiotics may also be required.

TOXICITY—HYPERVITAMINOSIS A

A single dose of a million units of vitamin A can cause severe, acute toxicity. Persons have died from eating large amounts of polar bear liver. Acute manifestations include transient hydrocephalus and vomiting. Chronic hypervitaminosis A has been observed with as little as 18,500 IU of the water-dispersed vitamin daily for 1 to 3 months in infants 3 to 6 months of age. In adults, chronic hypervitaminosis A has occurred in patients receiving large doses (20–30 times RDA) as a treatment for dermatologic conditions. It has been reported, also, in food faddists. Symptoms have included anorexia, irritability, loss of weight, low-grade fever, sparseness of hair, and a prurigenous rash. There is tend-

erness over the long bones, and periosteal elevations may be seen on x-ray examination. Hepatomegaly and splenomegaly have been reported. In a few instances, an increase in intracranial pressure has occurred with signs suggestive of brain tumor. Concentrations of vitamin A in serum are greater than 100 μg/100 ml. The only therapy is to stop administration of vitamin A.

Recognizing these inherent dangers from the use of very large doses of vitamin A, there are nevertheless circumstances under which they must be used with appropriate caution in order to combat major medical problems successfully. These include prophylactic use to prevent serious damage caused by hypovitaminosis A in the malnourished pediatric populations of developing countries and theraputic use in skin cancers. The subject of the judicious use of such very large doses of vitamin A is well presented in the Report of the Vitamin A Consultative Group.[1]

Hypercarotenemia may occur as a result of prolonged ingestion of large quantities of green leafy and yellow vegetables, carrot juice (often by food faddists), citrus fruits, and tomato. Hypercarotenemia may occur as a result of disturbed carotenoid metabolism in some cases of hypothyroidism, diabetes, and various hyperlipemic states. Yellow or orange discoloration of the skin may be present when serum carotene levels are above 250 μg/100 ml. Since carotenoids are secreted in sweat and sebum, the skin changes are especially prominent on the nasolabial folds, forehead, axilla, groin, palms of the hands, and soles of the feet. The scleral and buccal mucosa are unaffected, aiding in differential diagnosis from jaundice. Hypercarotenemia, *per se,* appears to be compatible with health and disappears within a few weeks in cases of dietary origin after withdrawal of the cause. Underlying metabolic disturbances require appropriate therapy.

Thiamin Deficiency

PREVALENCE

Thiamin deficiency occurs primarily in countries where polished rice is the staple cereal in the diet. Various preventive measures, including the use of undermilled or parboiled rice, enrichment of rice with thiamin, and distribution of the vitamin itself in health clinics, have decreased the incidence markedly. In the United States, deficiency is seen primarily in association with chronic alcoholism (see Chap. 15). The increasing use of highly refined white flour in many African countries has increased the liability to deficiency, as occured in Newfoundland some years ago. Thiamin deficiency may develop in pathologic states that interfere with ingestion and absorption of food and is characterized by profound anorexia, nausea, vomiting, and diarrhea. Diseases in which the metabolic rate is elevated can lead to deficiency. Thiamin requirement is related to caloric intake, the minimum need being in the neighborhood of 0.3 mg/1000 Cal. Overloading the tissues with glucose may precipitate deficiency if thiamin intake has been borderline. Thiamin may be lost in the urine following the administration of diuretics.

CLINICAL SYNDROMES

The syndromes due to thiamin deficiency in man are beriberi, Wernicke's syndrome, and Korsakoff's syndrome. Manifestations of deficiency depend on the degree and duration of deprivation. Severe deficiency leads to Wernicke's encephalopathy and Korsakoff's syndrome, less severe deficiency to beriberi heart disease, and still milder deficiency to polyneuritis or dry beriberi.

WERNICKE'S ENCEPHALOPATHY AND KORSAKOFF'S SYNDROME

In the United States and Europe, these syndromes, which represent severe acute thiamin deficiency, are found primarily in alcoholics. They occasionally follow prolonged vomiting, such as in pyloric obstruction or toxemia of pregnancy, or they may occur in carcinoma of the stomach or other conditions of severe digestive failure. They have been precipitated by overloading the tissues with glucose when thiamin stores are depleted.

Wernicke's encephalopathy is characterized by mental disturbances, weakness, paralysis of the eye muscles, and an ataxic gait. Early symptoms are anorexia, nausea and vomiting, and also photophobia, diplopia, and failing vision. Eye signs are always present and include nystagmus, paralysis of the extraocular muscles (particularly the external rectus), and paralysis of conjugate gaze. Ptosis of the eyelids and abnormalities of the pupils may occur. Rarely, papilledema and hemorrhages of the retina are noted. Ataxia is a frequent finding both in standing and walking and is probably of cerebellar origin. Occasionally, cranial nerves other than those supplying the eye muscles are involved. The pyramidal tracts may be affected.

The most common mental symptoms are apathy and confusion. Less often, delirium dominates the picture. Following the administration of thiamin, the patient begins to improve, and the features of Korsakoff's syndrome become evident. A defect in memory retention, particularly for recent events, is the most important finding. This is often associated with confabulation. Retrograde amnesia may involve periods of months or years. Events that happened in the past cannot be recalled in proper sequence. Derangement in perception of time occurs. Delusions may be present, and defects in cognitive function may be observed. Some patients have polyneuropathy.

The mortality of Wernicke's syndrome is 90% without therapy, the most common cause of death being sudden heart failure. Early treatment may result in complete recovery. However, some findings of Korsakoff's syndrome may persist, including loss of memory or confabulation. other residues may include nystagmus and slight ataxia (see Chap. 27).

BERIBERI (ADULT)

Symptoms and signs of beriberi and the course of the disease are extremely variable. Thus, it is difficult to describe a characteristic sequence of development. Early writers divided the disease into several types: (1) dry beriberi, characterized by peripheral neuritis; (2) wet beriberi, in which edema was a prominent finding (this was usually associated with some evidence of peripheral neuritis); and (3) acute, pernicious or cardiac beriberi. Any one of these forms may merge into another.

Early symptoms of neutitic beriberi include a sensation of numbness of the feet, heaviness of the legs, and paresthesias (*e.g.*, sensations of pins and needles, numbness, formication, and itching). Pain and tenderness in the calf muscles are common. In early stages, the tendon reflexes may be exaggerated, whereas later they are decreased or disappear. These changes are bilateral. Muscular weakness develops gradually, beginning in the dorsiflexors of the foot and extending to the calf muscles, the extensor muscles of the legs, the gluteal muscles, and the flexors of the leg. The patient has difficulty in rising from a squatting position due to weakness of the quadriceps muscles. The squat test has been widely used in the diagnosis of beriberi in the Orient.

Sensory disturbances occur first on the inner surface of the legs below the knee and on the dorsum of the feet. Anesthesia over the tibia is common, as is delayed response to pain. In extensive polyneuritis, anesthesia may extend upward and involve both legs, the arms, the trunk, and even the face and neck. Factors that appear to influence the affected areas include length of the nerve, the amount of work done by the part, and—possibly—the blood supply.

Foot drop and wrist drop are observed in advanced polyneuritis. Aphonia is often noted due to paralysis of the muscles of the larynx as a result of involvement of the laryngeal nerves. Complete flaccid paralysis of the lower extremities or even of the upper extremities is observed occasionally. Paralysis is associated with marked muscular atrophy and absence of deep tendon reflexes (DTRs).

Cardiac disturbances develop at some stage of beriberi in most subjects. Palpitation and dull precordial or epigastric pain are common complaints. The pulse may be rapid and bounding, although this is not always the case, and pulsations may be visible in the vessels of the neck. The extremities are pale and cold, and edema may be present. Cyanosis occurs when cardiac involvement is severe. The heart is enlarged to both sides, but enlargement is more marked to the right. Heart sounds are often loud, and systolic murmurs may be detected. Edema may occur without obvious cardiac involvement. When heart failure is present, the edema is dependent at first, gradually extending upward. Effusions may develop in all of the serous cavities. Edema of the lungs is a late occurrence. Oliguria is a prominent finding in wet beriberi.

Gastrointestinal (GI) disturbances, including anorexia, nausea, vomiting, and constipation, are usually noted in thiamin deficiency but are nonspecific.

The acute form of cardiac beriberi has been termed *sho-shin* by the Japanese. The patient is severely dyspneic and complains of violent palpitation and intense precordial pain. He is cyanotic and restless, tossing and turning violently from one side of the bed to the other. Hoarseness or aphonia may be present. The patient prefers the lying to the sitting position. Respiration is superficial and rapid, the pulse is weak and regular, and about 120 beats/min to 150 beats/min. Pulsations may be visible in the neck, precordium, and epigastrium. The heart is enlarged in all directions, but more to the right than to the left. The area of aortic dullness may be increased. Systolic murmurs are often present. The liver is enlarged and may pulsate. Pistol shot sounds are heard over the peripheral vessels. A stocking and glove type of peripheral cyanosis has been described. Systolic pressure may be normal and diastolic pressure low. The lungs are clear until just before death, when rales appear at the bases. At this time the pulse becomes thin, and the veins dilate. The patient usually dies intensely dyspneic and fully conscious.

The cardiac failure of beriberi is usually of the high output type. Circulation time is rapid, despite an elevated venous pressure. Serial ECGs show fleeting, variable, and nonspecific changes, such as transient T-wave inversion, S-T segment changes or low voltage of the (QRS) complexes. Roent-genographic examination of the chest shows generalized cardiac enlargement. Following therapy, the heart returns to normal size unless other factors are contributing to the heart failure.

Diagnosis of beriberi heart disease may be very difficult. Blankenhorn suggests that the following criteria are useful: an enlarged heart with normal sinus rhythm, dependent edema, elevated venous pressure and an associated peripheral neuritis or evidence of deficiency of one or more of the B vitamins, nonspecific ECG changes, no other demonstrable etiology, and a history of a grossly deficient diet for three or more months.[10] Improvement following the administration of thiamin rapidly corroborates the diagnosis. Digitalis is not effective in thiamin deficiency heart failure.

INFANTILE BERIBERI

This disease is seen in breast-fed infants, usually between the second and fifth months of life. It is rare in the United States. The mother may have no clinical signs of beriberi, but she will have a history of a poor diet and the milk is undoubtedly low in thiamin. As in the case of adults, several clinical syndromes may be observed, both acute and chronic. The acute cardiac form predominates and is initiated frequently by an infection. It begins with anorexia, vomiting, restlessness, insomnia, and pallor. Oliguria is noted frequently. Suddenly, the infant becomes cyanotic and dyspneic and the pulse rapid and weak. Death may occur within 24 to 48 hours. Partial or complete aphonia is characteristic in severe cases. The child appears to be crying, but no sound is heard or perhaps only a whine. Other common findings are vomiting, abdominal pain, convulsions, and coma. In the chronic condition, vomiting, inanition, neck contraction, and opisthotonus may develop. Constipation and meteorism are usually present.

The description by Albert of acute cardiac beriberi as quoted by Ramalingaswami is worthy of repetition.[13]

The baby around three months of age, apparently in good health, nursed entirely by its mother, is abruptly seized with an attack of screaming. As he utters his loud piercing cry his body stretches, the abdomen becomes hard, the pulse thready, respiration labored, his face either deadly white or cyanotic and an expression of profound terror or suffering grips the entire being. This state may last anywhere from one half to one hour and disappear spontaneously only to reappear with increasing severity and frequency until death supervenes or specific treatment is given promptly.

A pseudomeningitic type of beriberi has been described with CNS signs such as strabismus, nystagmus, spasmodic contraction of the facial muscles, convulsions, and fever. This is more common in infants aged 7 to 9 months. The spinal fluid is essentially normal except for being under increased pressure.

BIOCHEMICAL FINDINGS

The concentration of pyruvic acid in the blood is increased to several times normal. The ratio of lactic acid to pyruvic acid becomes abnormal and is of some value in diagnosis. The excretion of thiamin in the urine decreases and may be as low as 0 μg to 14 μg/24 hours. Early signs of deficiency may occur when excretion is less than 40 μg daily. The concentration of thiamin in whole blood falls in deficiency but not to a degree that is useful in making a definitive diagnosis in an individual subject. Thiamin concentration in beriberi has been reported to average 3.2 μg/100 ml. In thiamin deficiency, tests for methylglyoxal (pyruvic aldehyde) are positive in both blood and urine and also in the milk of mothers whose infants develop beriberi. One of the most useful tests in the diagnosis of thiamin deficiency is the measurement of transketolase activity in erythrocytes. This procedure is sensitive to mild degrees of depletion.[11]

TREATMENT

Treatment includes institution of a good diet and administration of thiamin. Few foods are rich in this vitamin. Lean pork, beans, nuts, and certain whole grain cereals are the best sources; kidney, liver, beef, eggs, and fish contain moderate amounts.

In infantile beriberi, 2 mg to 5 mg thiamin may lead to marked improvement within a few hours. In adult beriberi, it is customary to give larger doses of thiamin, particularly when cardiac findings predominate. In such instances, 10 mg to 20 mg thiamin should be given intramuscularly several times daily. Similar therapy should be used in Wernicke's encephalopathy and Korsakoff's syndrome.

In severe heart failure, or when convulsions or coma occur in infants, 25 mg to 50 mg thiamin can be given intravenously, very slowly, followed by daily intramuscular doses. In critically ill adults, 50 mg to 100 mg may be administered intravenously followed by the same amount intramuscularly for the next few days. After improvement has occurred, oral therapy may be instituted.

In the treatment of polyneuropathy, 5 mg to 10 mg thiamin three times daily is usually adequate. Thiamin should be continued in these amounts until maximum improvement has been achieved.

Patients with beriberi may have deficiency of vitamins of the B complex in addition to thiamin. Accordingly, it is advisable to administer some form of the whole vitamin B complex, such as a multivitamin tablet, brewer's yeast, liver extract, wheat germ, rice polishings, rice bran, or yeast extract.

Riboflavin Deficiency

PREVALENCE

Riboflavin deficiency is a relatively common disorder in practically all parts of the world, including the United States. It occurs primarily as the result of an inadequate dietary intake but may develop when some conditioning factor increases requirement or impairs absorption or utilization of the vitamin. Riboflavin deficiency is frequently observed in association with pellagra. In fact, lesions of riboflavin deficiency were considered to be part of the pellagra syndrome for many years. Deficiency is more frequent during periods of physiologic stress, such as rapid growth in childhood or during pregnancy and lactation. It may be the result of pathologic stress, including burns, surgical procedures, and other types of trauma. It occurs also in chronic debilitating illness (*e.g.,* tuberculosis, rheumatic fever) and in the course of congestive heart failure, hyperthyroidism, and malignancy. Malabsorption may be observed in chronic diarrheal diseases or following operations on the GI tract. Poor utilization may be the result of cirrhosis of the liver.

A relationship has been noted between the retention of riboflavin and that of protein. When protein is broken down, negative nitrogen balance occurs and urinary excretion of riboflavin increases. This has been reported in acute starvation, uncontrolled diabetes mellitus, and following trauma.

CLINICAL FINDINGS

Riboflavin deficiency is characterized by lesions of the lips (cheilosis), angular stomatitis, seborrheic dermatitis, and glossitis. In addition, ocular symptoms and signs that respond to administration of riboflavin have been reported.

Early symptoms of deficiency are soreness and burning of the lips, mouth, and tongue and—at times—photophobia, lacrimation, and burning and itching of the eyes. Cheilosis begins with redness and denudation of the lips along the line of closure. The lips become dry and chapped and shallow ulcers may appear. Maceration and pallor develop at the angles of the mouth followed by fissures that may extend out from the mucous membrane for a centimeter or more. The fissures may be covered with yellow crusts. Following healing, scars may remain at the angles of the mouth, and the lips may become atrophic.

The seborrheic dermatitis of riboflavin deficiency has a red, scaly, greasy appearance. The areas involved are the nasolabial and nasomalar folds, the alae nasi and vestibule of the nose, the ears, and the skin around the outer and inner canthi of the eyes. Fine, filiform comedones may be seen over the bridge of the nose, on the malar prominences, and on the chin. Dermatitis of the scrotum and vulva may develop with redness, scaling, and desquamation as characteristic findings. Similar changes occur in adjacent areas of the thigh.

The tongue is purplish red or magenta in color and often deeply fissured. The papillae may be swollen, flattened, or mushroom shaped, causing a pebbled appearance. Atrophy of the papillae may occur in long-standing deficiency. It is difficult to differentiate the glossitis of riboflavin deficiency from that due to lack of niacin, folic acid, or vitamin B_{12}.

Superficial vascularization of the cornea may be observed. Early lesions consist of injection and proliferation of the vessels of the limbic plexus and can be seen only with a slit lamp. Later, circumcorneal injection may be visible without magnification. The capillaries of the limbic plexus proliferate and extend into the superficial layers of the cornea, anastomosing to form tiers of loops. Superficial punctate opacities and ulcerations have been observed, the latter being demonstrable with fluorescein staining. Iritis has been reported. The conjunctiva may be grossly inflamed and the eyelids red, swollen, and matted together with exudate. Photophobia may be severe.

None of the lesions described are pathognomonic of riboflavin deficiency. Lesions of the lips have been observed in experimental niacin deficiency, following administration of desoxypyridoxine, and—rarely—in iron deficiency anemia. Fissures at the angles of the mouth may be the result of poorly fitting dentures or malocclusion. Cheilosis may be due to allergy or to wind and cold. Superficial vascularization of the cornea is found in association with infections, trauma, and deficiency of dietary substances other than riboflavin.

In experimental deficiency produced by the administration of analogues of riboflavin, Lane, Alfrey, and their colleagues report not only glossitis and seborrheic dermatitis, but also anemia and neuropathy late in the deficiency.[18] The anemia was macrocytic and normochromic and was associated with a reduction in the reticulocyte count and hypoplasia of the bone marrow. The anemia may be related to disturbances of folic acid metabolism. Decreased levels of folic acid in serum and liver have been reported, and conversion of folic acid to 5-N-methyltetrahydrofolic acid is impaired. These abnormalities are probably the result of diminished activity of flavoprotein enzymes that are required for utilization of folic acid.

BIOCHEMICAL FINDINGS

The urinary excretion of riboflavin falls to less than 50 μg daily in deficiency. An excretion of less than 27 μg riboflavin/g creatinine has been proposed as indicative of deficiency, although the excretion of 27 μg to 79 μg is considered low. Administration of a 1-mg test dose of riboflavin subcutaneously followed by measurement of excretion in the urine for 4 hours is useful in estimating tissue stores of riboflavin. In experimental deficiency, the excretion in 4 hours was 19 μg after 48 months of a diet that furnished 0.6 mg riboflavin daily. In subjects receiving 0.7 mg to 1.1 mg riboflavin daily, the 4-hour excretion was 56 μg to 81 μg. Subjects who received 1.6 mg riboflavin daily excreted an average of 235 μg.

Determination of flavoprotein enzymes in blood is not of much assistance in the diagnosis of deficiency. The concentration of riboflavin in erythrocytes decreases, and levels of less than 14 μg/100 ml have been suggested as indicative of potential deficiency. The activity of the enzyme erythrocyte glutathione reductase, and the magnitude of the increase in activity of this enzyme after ingestion of riboflavin, correlates with the dietary intake of the vitamin. The extent of stimulation of erythrocyte glutathione reductase activity *in vitro* by flavin adenine dinucleotide (FAD) is useful as an indicator of riboflavin nutriture.

Diagnosis of riboflavin deficiency is made by correlating dietary, clinical, and laboratory findings since there are no pathognomonic signs of this disorder.

TREATMENT

Treatment consists of institution of a good diet and administration of the vitamin. The best food sources of riboflavin are milk, liver, meat, eggs, and some of the green leafy and yellow vegetables. A quart of milk furnishes approximately 2 mg of the vitamin. Cereals and bread contain very little riboflavin, but enrichment of flour, bread, and cereals, as carried out in the United States, contributes significantly to the dietary supply.

Riboflavin should be administered orally in amounts of 5 mg, two or three times daily. In persons being fed parenterally, riboflavin should be included in the formula. The lesions of riboflavin deficiency heal rapidly, usually within a few days to a week or two.

Niacin Deficiency—Pellagra

PREVALENCE

Pellagra has occurred primarily in parts of the world in which corn is the staple cereal and has been noted chiefly among the poor. It has become relatively rare except in a few areas of the world where maize remains the principal constituent of the diet. It was common in the southern United States in the early 1900s, and the mortality was high. It is now seen in this country largely in association with chronic alcoholism (see Chap. 15). It occasionally develops in association with cirrhosis of the liver or in chronic diarrheal diseases, diabetes mellitus, neoplasia, prolonged febrile illnesses, and thyrotoxicosis. Pellagra may develop in patients who are fed parenterally without niacin supplementation.

Pellagra is due to an inadequate dietary intake of niacin and its precursor, the amino acid tryptophan. The association of corn diets with pellagra is due in large part to the low tryptophan content of this cereal. In addition, niacin is present in corn and certain other cereals in bound form and may not be available to the organism unless it is released by treatment with alkali. In certain areas, such as Central America, where it is common practice to treat corn with lime before incorporation in the diet, the incidence of pellagra is low, even when corn supplies a large percentage of the total food intake. Amino acid imbalance has been suggested as another factor in the pathogenesis of pellagra. Gopolan and his associates in India produced experimental deficiency in animals with diets high in leucine.[22] In some instances, isoleucine counteracted this effect. Oral administration of leucine appears to inhibit synthesis of niacin adenine dinucleotide. Pellagra is found in India in association with the ingestion of millet (jowar), which is high in leucine. Some years ago it was suggested that corn contained an inhibitory factor. If this is the case, it appears to have a minor role in the etiology of human pellagra.

Sunlight and heavy work appear to precipitate pellagra. The seasonal incidence in the spring months may be the result of a decrease in niacin intake during the winter, followed by exposure to the sun and increased physical activity. Pellagra is still endemic in some countries in the Near East, Africa, southeastern Europe, and southern Asia, namely, the Arab Republic of Egypt, Lesotho, South Africa, Yugoslavia, and India.

Niacin deficiency may occur in patients with malignant carcinoid tumors because of a decrease in availability of tryptophan for conversion to niacin since a large percentage is converted to 5-hydroxytryptophan (serotonin). Deficiency develops occasionally during therapy with isoniazid. In these instances, pyridoxine deficiency induced by isoniazid results in a decrease in the conversion of tryptophan to niacin.

CLINICAL FINDINGS

Pellagra is characterized by dermatitis, inflammation of mucous membranes, diarrhea, and psychic disturbances. In its endemic form, it occurs characteristically in the spring of the year with an occasional second outbreak in the fall. This appears to be explained largely on the basis of diet, but increased physical activity—which may elevate requirement—and exposure to sunlight probably both play a role.

Early symptoms of deficiency include lassitude, weakness, loss of appetite, mild digestive disturbances (especially heartburn), and psychic and emotional changes (*e.g.,* anxiety, irritability, and depression). Soreness of the tongue and mouth, aggravated by highly seasoned or acid food, is a frequent complaint.

Signs of advanced niacin deficiency vary with the severity and duration of depletion. The dermatitis of acute pellagra resembles ordinary sunburn in the early stages. The skin is red, and large blebs or blisters may develop. If these break, secondary infection may occur. The skin often peels away leaving large areas of denudation that resemble a severe sunburn. As deficiency progresses, the skin becomes darkly pigmented. Dermatitis is most often found on the face and neck, backs of the hands and forearms, and the anterior surfaces of the feet and legs. The lesions are usually bilateral and symmetric, and the damaged skin is clearly demarcated from the uninvolved portion. Dermatitis of the neck has been designated Casal's necklace due to its distribution and in recognition of the physician who first described it. Other areas of the skin may be involved, particularly those subjected to irritation and trauma, such as the axilla, groin, perineum, genitalia, elbows, knees, and areas under the breasts.

Skin changes of chronic pellagra are somewhat different. They are characterized by thickening, scaling, hyperkeratinization, and pigmentation. The face and neck are less often involved. Lesions are most common on the feet, hands, and points of pressure, such as the elbows and knees. Chronic pellagrous dermatitis has been confused with changes due to allergy, stasis, or irritation.

In acute pellagra, the mucous membranes of GI and GU tracts are severely inflamed and fiery red in appearance. The tongue is sore, swollen, and scarlet in color, and the lingual papillae become atrophic. Chewing and swallowing are so painful that even liquids may be refused. White areas appear on the mucous membrane of the mouth, probably due to death of superficial tissue. Secondary infection with fungi or Vincent's organisms is common. Inflammatory changes also occur in the esophagus, stomach, and small and large intestines. Symptoms include heartburn, indigestion, diarrhea, abdominal pain, and soreness of the rectum. The stools are watery and may contain blood. Achlorhydria is characteristic. The patient complains that he feels sore from the mouth to the rectum. Due to the severe inflammatory process and hypermotility of the GI tract, nutrients are poorly absorbed, and this results in profound weight loss.

Inflammation of the lower urinary tract causes urethritis with burning, pain, and frequency of urination. In the female, severe vaginitis is observed, and amenorrhea is common.

The psychic manifestations of pellagra are variable. Common early findings are anxiety, irritability, and depression. In more advanced deficiency, confusion, disorientation, delusions, and hallucinations may appear. Some patients are fearful, hyperactive, and manic; others are apathetic, lethargic, and stuporous. As the disease progresses, delirium ensues, and the patient may die in coma.

Other changes observed in pellagra include cheilosis, angular stomatitis, and seborrheic dermatitis, which may be due to niacin deficiency alone or to concomitant riboflavin deficiency. Anemia may occur and may be either macrocytic or microcytic and hypochromic. Neither of these types of anemia responds to niacin. The macrocytic anemia appears to be due to folic acid deficiency and the hypochromic anemia to an inadequate supply of iron.

Descriptions of pellagra in the older literature lists neurologic abnormalities (*e.g.*, incoordination, tremor, ataxia, reflex disturbances, and even sensory changes) as findings, but although these may have been manifestations of advanced niacin deficiency, they were more probably due to deficiency of other vitamins in the B complex. Neurologic changes have not been reported in experimental niacin deficiency.

Niacin Deficiency Other Than Pellagra

CLINICAL FINDINGS

Early, mild niacin deficiency, in contrast to pellagra, may have as its only manifestation redness of the tongue with a slight atrophy or hypertrophy of the papillae.

Two syndromes other than pellagra have been described that appear to be due to acute, severe niacin deficiency. One of these is characterized by confusion, hallucinations, and disorientation, and the clinical picture resembles an acute toxic psychosis. The other syndrome is an acute encephalopathy characterized by clouding of consciousness, cogwheel rigidity of the extremities, and uncontrollable grasping and sucking reflexes. These syndromes may occur singly or in combination. They have been observed in malnourished subjects following IV administration of glucose without concomitant administration of niacin. Occasionally, they develop during the course of serious infections. Both syndromes respond dramatically to administration of niacin. Death may occur if treatment is not initiated promptly.

BIOCHEMICAL FINDINGS

Urinary excretion of niacin metabolites falls to low levels in pellagra, usually to less than 3 mg/day. The excretion of niacinamide is little changed, but there is a marked decrease in the excretion of N^1-methylniacinamide (N^1-ME) and pyridone. The niacin-containing coenzymes in erythrocytes are not decreased significantly in pellagra, but coenzyme concentrations in liver and muscle decrease progressively as the disease advances. However, these estimates are not usually carried out in diagnosing niacin deficiency.

Measurement of excretion of N^1-ME in a random specimen of urine in relation to creatinine output gives useful information. An excretion of 0.5 mg N^1-ME/1 g creatinine is suggestive of deficiency, as is an excretion of less than 0.2 mg N^1-ME in 6 hours.

DIAGNOSIS

Mild niacin deficiency is characterized by glossitis, diarrhea, and nonspecific psychic disturbances. If there are no skin lesions, the diagnosis may be suspected on the basis of a dietary history indicating a poor intake of niacin and tryptophan. Diagnosis of acute pellagra is relatively easy, but the skin lesions of chronic pellagra may be confused with numerous other conditions, such as chronic irritation, stasis, or allergic dermatitis. Measurement of the urinary excretion of niacin metabolites is useful in establishing the diagnosis. Occasionally, a controlled therapeutic test is desirable.

TREATMENT

Niacin should be administered orally in most instances, the amount varying with the severity of the deficiency state. In acute pellagra, it is customary to give 300 mg to 500 mg niacin or niacinamide/day in divided doses of 50 mg to 100 mg each. If stomatitis and dysphagia are severe, 100 mg niacinamide should be given intramuscularly two or three times daily for the first 2 days. After subsidence of the acute symptoms, the dose may be decreased to 50 mg to 100 mg two or three times daily orally. Therapy should be continued until all lesions have healed.

In the treatment of mild niacin deficiency, administration of 50 mg niacinamide three times daily should be sufficient. Niacinamide is preferable to niacin since it does not induce vasodilating reactions. Niacin should not be given intravenously except in dilute solutions nor in amounts in excess of 25 mg. Niacinamide is safe for IV use.

In the treatment of severe pellagra, bed rest is essential. The diet must be liquid or soft at first because of stomatitis and pain associated with swallowing. Milk, eggs, strained cereals, and pureed vegetables are usually well tolerated. Skim milk powder may be added to whole milk to increase the protein and tryptophan content. As symptoms improve, the diet should be increased to include lean meat, glandular organs, vegetables, and fruits. Foods that are rich in niacin include lean meat (especially organ meats), legumes, nuts, and certain fish. Potatoes, some green vegetables, and whole wheat cereal and bread are fair sources of the vitamin. Refined white flour, cornmeal, and grits are low in niacin, but in the United States these cereals are enriched with niacin and accordingly add significant amounts to the diet. Not much niacin is present in milk or eggs, but these foods are high in tryptophan, as are most animal proteins with the exception of gelatin. Of the vegetable proteins, peanuts, beans, peas, and other legumes are good sources of both niacin and tryptophan.

If pellagra is complicated by deficiency of other vitamins of the B group, as is often the case, it is advisable to prescribe a tablet containing 5 mg thiamin, 5 mg riboflavin, 5 mg vitamin B_6, and 10 mg pantothenic acid, to be given once or twice daily. Brewer's yeast is an alternate and inexpensive supplement that may be given in amounts of 10 g to 30 g daily.

Folic Acid (Folacin) Deficiency

PREVALENCE

Folic acid deficiency is a widespread disorder that occurs throughout the world, particularly in the tropics, but not infrequently elsewhere. It is probably the most common hypovitaminosis of man. In underdeveloped countries where poor socioeconomic and dietary conditions prevail, the majority of the general population suffer from dietary folic acid deficiency often associated with cobalamin deficiency. In the United States it has been estimated that 45% of adult patients who are indigent or in the low income group are deficient in folic acid as reflected by low serum concentration of folate derivatives. In western countries, mild folic acid deficiency appears to be not uncommon among elderly patients.

Dietary deficiency of folic acid causes nutritional macrocytic anemia. This anemia is encountered in infants (megaloblastic anemia of infancy), during pregnancy, in sprue, and in a number of other malabsorption syndromes. Megaloblastic anemia of infancy, which develops in infants up to age two, is a major problem in developing countries. The role of folic acid deficiency in the development of this anemia is well established although other nutrients may be involved. In these same countries, macrocytic anemia of pregnancy occurs in as high as 20% of pregnant women, and significant megaloblastic changes in the bone marrow may be found in more than 50%. Folic acid deficiency often occurs in chronic alcoholism. Anorexia in a number of chronic diseases may result in deficiency.

Deficiency may be encountered in some of the hemoglobinopathies, in certain inborn errors of metabolism, and following the administration of drugs, particularly several used in the treatment of epilepsy (see Chap. 19). Hemoglobinopathies in which folic acid deficiency has been observed include sickle cell disease, thalassemia major, and combined sickle cell and thalassemia traits. Administration of folic acid antagonists in the treatment of leukemia may produce the picture of folic acid deficiency. Folic acid deficiency can arise from the use of oral contraceptive agents.

CLINICAL FINDINGS

Folic acid deficiency is characterized by macrocytic anemia, megaloblastosis of the bone marrow, diarrhea, and glossitis. Weight loss occurs frequently. All of the signs associated with anemia and tissue anoxemia may develop, including weakness, syncopal attacks, severe pallor of the skin, and cardiac enlargement with congestive heart failure.

Macrocytic anemia of pregnancy is usually due to folic acid deficiency and rarely to lack of vitamin B_{12}. This syndrome appears to be due to dietary deficiency upon which pregnancy superimposes an increased need (see Chap. 29). Rarely, it may result from malabsorption of folic acid. Clinical findings in nutritional macrocytic anemia of pregnancy often include glossitis and diarrhea. The tongue is sore and red, and the papillae may be atrophic. Fever has been reported. The bone marrow is megaloblastic. There is leukopenia, with hypersegmentation of the polymorphonuclear leukocytes, and thrombocytopenia.

Megaloblastic anemia of infancy usually occurs between the ages of 6 months and 1 year (see Chap.

32). As observed in the United States, this anemia was found in children who received diets inadequate in ascorbic acid. Patients responded to treatment with folic acid, but the anemia could be prevented with ascorbic acid. A role of ascorbic acid in the conversion of folic acid to coenzyme form would explain the pathogenesis of this anemia. Megaloblastic anemia responding to folic acid has been reported in infants with protein–calorie malnutrition.

Sprue and gluten-induced enteropathy are malabsorption syndromes in which macrocytic anemia and megaloblastosis of the bone marrow are observed. Tropical sprue is endemic in India, the Far East, the Caribbean area, and is seen—at times—in the United States. The pathogenesis of tropical sprue is not understood in spite of extensive investigation. Although folic acid deficiency is a constant finding, it cannot be the sole cause of the condition. Signs of deficiency appear early, namely, macrocytic anemia, megaloblastosis of the bone marrow, and glossitis. The steatorrhea of tropical sprue may persist after folic acid therapy.

Folic acid deficiency is inconstant in gluten-induced enteropathy and appears to be a secondary phenomenon. Megaloblastic anemia that responds to folic acid may be associated with the disorders of the small intestine, such as diverticulosis, Whipple's disease, stricture and anastomoses, and resections.

BIOCHEMICAL FINDINGS

An abnormal amount of formiminoglutamic acid (FIGLU) is excreted in the urine. An intermediate in the breakdown of the amino acid histidine to glutamic acid, FIGLU accumulates when folic acid coenzymes that are needed for this metabolic process are lacking. The normal excretion of FIGLU is 0 to 6 μg/ml of urine or 0 to 4 mg in 24 hours. Excretion is usually measured after administration of histidine, given in three 5 g doses in 24 hours. Normal FIGLU excretion with this test is less than 25 μg/ml of urine and less than 25 mg in 24 hours. In folic acid deficiency, excretion is greater than 30 μg/ml of urine and greater than 35 mg in 24 hours.

Measurement of folic acid concentration in serum by microbiologic assay using *Lactobacillus caseii* as the test organism is useful in the diagnosis of deficiency. It has been suggested that less than 3 ng/ml is indicative of deficiency. Folic acid can be measured also in whole blood, using several microorganisms, and in erythrocytes. Normal levels in erythrocytes are 160 ng/mg to 650 ng/ml. Levels of 100 ng/mg to 160 ng/ml are considered low, and concentrations less than 100 ng/ml are indicative of deficiency.

Plasma clearance and absorption tests for estimating folic acid nutrition have been suggested but have not been widely used. Determination of folate derivatives in serum is a reasonably satisfactory method of detecting folic acid deficiency unless cobalamin (vitamin B_{12}) deficiency coexists. Erythrocyte folate levels are useful in some instances.

TREATMENT

In the past, therapy of folic acid deficiency consisted of oral administration of 5 mg daily to infants and 5 mg two or three times daily to adults. Recent studies indicate that much smaller doses are often effective, as little as 25 μg to 100 μg in certain syndromes. The oral route is satisfactory in most instances. Clinical and hematologic response is rapid. Within a few days, the patient feels better, and his appetite improves. There is an increase in the reticulocyte count and a gradual return of the blood picture to normal. Recurrence of megaloblastic anemia in subsequent pregnancies should be prevented by administration of 5 mg folic acid daily.

Folic acid is particularly abundant in green leafy vegetables, yeast, and liver. Other good sources are green vegetables, kidney, beef, and wheat. Many of the folates in food are labile and are easily destroyed by cooking, the loss being related to the amount of reducing agent in the food. Folates in food are classified into two main groups: (1) *free* folates, which are available without pretreatment with conjugase, and (2) total folates, consisting of free folates and the polyglutamates that are available only after conjugase treatment. Free folates make up about 25% of dietary folate and are readily absorbed. Much more information is needed on the amount and forms of folate in foods and of conjugase and conjugase inhibitors in the diet.

Vitamin B_{12} (Cobalamin) Deficiency

PREVALENCE

Dietary deficiency of vitamin B_{12} is rare, occurring almost exclusively in vegetarians who do not include any foods of animal origin in the diet. Pernicious anemia is the most important condition resulting from vitamin B_{12} deficiency. In this disease, deficiency is caused by failure of absorption of vitamin B_{12} from the intestinal tract due to lack of intrinsic factor in the gastric juice. Pernicious anemia has a familial incidence that is high in persons of northern European ancestry. It is more common in older age groups and rare in childhood. Gastrectomy, total or at times partial, leads to vitamin B_{12} deficiency, because the stomach is the organ that forms the intrinsic factor. Vitamin B_{12} is absorbed in the ileum, hence resection of this area results in deficiency. Fish tapeworm infestation may cause vitamin B_{12} deficiency from competition of the parasite with the host for the vitamin. Vitamin B_{12} deficiency may also occur in a number of malabsorption syndromes, such as sprue, gluten-induced enteropathy, intestinal inflammation, strictures, and anastomoses. In these conditions, folic acid deficiency is usually present as well. Occasionally, megaloblastic anemia in chronic liver disease responds to vitamin B_{12} administration, but improvement is more likely after folic acid.

CLINICAL FINDINGS

The most important manifestations of vitamin B_{12} deficiency are macrocytic anemia, megaloblastosis of the bone marrow, glossitis, and neurologic abnormalities, including subacute combined degeneration of the spinal cord and peripheral neuritis.

The earliest neurologic complaints are paresthesias involving the hands and feet. Degeneration of the posterior and lateral columns of the spinal cord results in loss of vibratory and position sense in the lower extremities, incoordination of the legs, and loss of fine coordination of the fingers. Romberg's sign is positive, as is the Babinski reflex. Spasticity and either increased or decreased deep tendon reflexes (DTRs) may be noted. Sphincter disturbances may occur. Typical findings of peripheral neuritis may be observed, including loss of sensation beginning in the feet and extending upward, muscular weakness and atrophy, and loss of the DTRs. Mental changes such as irritability, memory disturbances, and depression may occur.

The tongue is often bright red in color and smooth, the papillae being atrophic. When the anemia is severe, prominent features are weakness, fatigue, symptoms of cerebral anoxemia, or cardiovascular complaints (*e.g.,* dyspnea, chest pain, slight edema, or even chronic congestive heart failure). Low-grade fever is present at times. In pernicious anemia, an additional finding is lemon yellow pallor of the skin. Gastrointestinal symptoms may occur, including anorexia, nausea and vomiting, vague indigestion, and midepigastric pain. Weight loss occurs occasionally. Diarrhea is common.

BIOCHEMICAL AND OTHER LABORATORY FINDINGS

Vitamin B_{12} deficiency is associated with a macrocytic anemia and megaloblastosis of the bone marrow. The mean corpuscular volume is greater than normal, that is, $100 \mu^3$ to $160 \mu^3$. The macrocytes are oval in shape, and nucleated red cells may be seen in the peripheral blood smear. The white cell count is low, and the polymorphonuclear neutro-

philic leukocytes are multilobular. Platelets are usually reduced in number. The bone marrow is hyperplastic and contains large numbers of megaloblasts.

In pernicious anemia, no free hydrochloric acid is found in the gastric juice after stimulation with histamine and intrinsic factor is absent from the gastric juice. Serum bilirubin is slightly increased as is excretion of urobilinogen in the urine and stool. These findings are due to a decrease in the survival time of erythrocytes. A number of abnormal phenolic compounds are found in the urine also.

In vitamin B_{12} deficiency, the serum concentration of vitamin B_{12} may range from 0 to less than 100 pg/ml. There is an increase in urinary excretion of methylmalonic acid. Normal excretion in 24 hours is about 3 mg, but excretions of greater than 4 mg have been noted in patients with low levels of serum vitamin B_{12}. Excretion of more than 5 mg is considered indicative of vitamin B_{12} deficiency.

The cause of vitamin B_{12} deficiency can be determined by dietary history, the presence of some disease that influences the absorption or utilization of the vitamin, the clinical findings, and measurement of absorption of radioactive vitamin B_{12}. The most common test of absorption is that devised by Schilling in which a small dose of radioactive vitamin B_{12} (0.5 μg of cobalt 60 or 57 labeled B_{12}) added to 1.5 μg of unlabeled vitamin is administered orally and radioactivity is measured in the urine for 24 hours thereafter. A flushing dose of 1000 μg of the nonlabeled vitamin is given an hour after the oral dose. Normal individuals excrete at least 10% to 40% of the vitamin in 24 hours, often more. In pernicious anemia, usually less than 2% is excreted. In such patients, the test is repeated, a concentrate of intrinsic factor being given in conjunction with the oral dose of radioactive vitamin B_{12}. This results in an increase in excretion to normal levels. In malabsorption syndromes of other causation, there is no increase in excretion when intrinsic factor is administered. Accordingly, two tests must be carried out to establish the diagnosis of pernicious anemia or of other malabsorption syndromes. When malabsorption is due to conditions other than intrinsic factor deficiency, GI x-rays may be useful in diagnosis. Biopsies of the intestinal mucosa may also be of assistance.

TREATMENT

Treatment in most instances consists of parenteral administration of the vitamin. With severe deficiency, in which macrocytic anemia or neurologic abnormalities, or both, are present, vitamin B_{12} is given in amounts of 50 μg to 100 μg three times a week until findings have returned to normal. Patients with pernicious anemia, gastrectomy, or post ileectomy syndromes need a maintenance dose of vitamin B_{12} for the remainder of their lives. The usual dose is 50 μg to 100 μg once a month. Patients can be maintained satisfactorily on 1000 μg parenterally every two or three months. Vitamin B_{12} can be given orally and is effective in pernicious anemia if sufficiently large doses are prescribed, but it is expensive therapy and is seldom used. Oral treatment is not recommended except in the management of dietary deficiency.

Administration of vitamin B_{12} is followed by a reticulocyte response that reaches a maximum in 5 to 8 days. There is a gradual return of the blood count to normal in several months. Megaloblastosis of the bone marrow disappears rapidly, often within 24 hours. Subjective improvement occurs in the first few days. There is an increase in appetite and a sense of well-being, mental symptoms—if present—disappear, and glossitis recedes rapidly. Neurologic lesions heal slowly, but if they have not been too long in duration, complete recovery may occur. Improvement may continue for as long as a year or more.

Vitamin B_6 Deficiency

PREVALENCE

Primary vitamin B_6 (pyridoxine) deficiency in man is extremely rare. It was reported some years ago in infants fed an autoclaved commercial milk formula low in vitamin B_6. Experimental deficiency has been produced in adult subjects who received diets low in the vitamin and were also given a pyridoxine antagonist. A vitamin B_6-dependent syndrome of genetic origin has been reported in infants. Cases of pyridoxine-responsive anemia have been described. Vitamin B_6 deficiency may occur in chronic alcoholism. A relationship between vitamin B_6, steroid hormones, oral contraceptives, and premenstrual symptoms has been observed, and abnormalities of vitamin B_6 metabolism have been noted during pregnancy.[26] Vitamin B_6 requirement may be increased in patients with hyperthyroidism. The administration of isonicotinic acid hydrazide (INH), a vitamin B_6 antagonist, may lead to deficiency.

CLINICAL FINDINGS

In infants, deficiency is characterized by irritability and convulsive seizures with abnormalities of the EEG. In experimental deficiency in two infants, convulsions developed in one instance and a macrocytic hypochromic anemia in the other. Some infants who develop convulsions shortly after birth respond to administration of pyridoxine. This appears to be a genetic pyridoxine deficiency or dependency syndrome.

In experimental deficiency in adults, the subjects became irritable, depressed, and somnolent. Seborrheic dermatitis appeared about the eyes, in the nasolabial folds, and around the mouth. In some instances, the lesions involved the face, forehead, eyebrows, and skin behind the ears. Occasionally, the scrotal and the perineal regions were involved. Intertrigo was noted under the breast and in other moist areas. In two subjects, pigmented scaly dermatitis resembling pellagra developed on the arms and legs. Glossitis, cheilosis, and angular stomatitis indistinguishable from the lesions of niacin and riboflavin deficiency occurred in some subjects. A few patients developed peripheral neuritis. Weight loss was noted in all subjects, and there was a tendency to develop infections, particularly of the GU tract. High intakes of protein appear to hasten the onset of vitamin B_6 deficiency. Several reports of pyridoxine-responsive anemia classified as sideroblastic anemia have been published.

BIOCHEMICAL FINDINGS

The urinary excretion of xanthurenic acid is determined after administration of a tryptophan load test (2 g L tryptophan). Normal subjects excrete less than 30 micromoles xanthurenic acid in 24 hours. Excretion is increased in vitamin B_6 deficiency. There is also an increase in the excretion of kynurenine, 3-hydroxykynurenine, kynurenic acid, acetylkynurenine, and quinolinic acid. The levels of vitamin B_6 in plasma and blood, as well as the urinary excretion of the vitamin and of its metabolite 4-pyridoxic acid, fall with decreased dietary intake. In deficiency, there is a decrease in glutamic oxaloacetic transaminase (GOT) and glutamic pyruvic transaminase (GPT) activities in blood. Women taking steroid hormones for contraceptive purposes excrete increased amounts of tryptophan metabolites following a tryptophan load test. During pregnancy, women may excrete abnormal amounts of kynurenine, xanthurenic acid, and 3-hydroxykynurenine. The concentration of the urea nitrogen in blood after administration of 30 g alanine should return to normal within 12 hours but may be delayed if pyridoxine is not available in adequate amounts.

TREATMENT

Vitamin B_6 deficiency can be prevented by the ingestion of a diet furnishing 2 mg vitamin B_6 daily for adults; 2.5 mg is recommended for pregnancy and lactation. Requirement is related to protein intake. In the treatment of deficiency, 10 mg to 150 mg/day have been used. The hypochromic anemia responds to 10 mg to 15 mg pyridoxine daily. Neuritis occurring in persons receiving INH can be prevented and treated with a daily dose of 50 mg to 100 mg. Therapy for various genetic and metabolic disturbances involving vitamin B_6 must be determined individually. Pyridoxine has been employed in the treatment of hyperoxaluria and recurrent oxalate kidney stones. The toxicity of pyridoxine is extremely low.

Pantothenic Acid Deficiency

PREVALENCE

Pantothenic acid is so widely distributed in food that dietary deficiency of the vitamin is exceedingly rare. Deficiency may develop in association with multiple B complex deficiency states, but clear-cut evidence for this has not been presented.

CLINICAL FINDINGS

Deficiency has been produced experimentally in man by Bean, Hodges, and their collaborators by marked restriction of pantothenic acid intake and by a combination of restricted diet and administration of an antagonist, ω-methyl pantothenic acid.[27,28] The clinical picture included personality changes, fatigue, malaise, sleep disturbances, and neurologic manifestations, such as numbness, paresthesias, and muscle cramps. Burning of the feet was observed occasionally. Motor coordination was impaired, resulting in a peculiar staggering gait. Personality changes included irritability, restlessness, and quarrelsomeness. At times, the subjects were sullen and petulant. Gastrointestinal complaints were common, including nausea, epigastric burning sensations, abdominal cramps, and occasional vomiting. The three most constant and annoying symptoms were fatigue, headache, and weakness. Some subjects had evidence of cardiovascular instability, for instance, tachycardia and lability of the blood pressure, with a tendency to orthostatic hypotension. Infections were common in some subjects but not in others.

Pantothenic acid has been reported to have a role in stress. A deficiency of pantothenic acid may be responsible for the burning foot syndrome encountered in certain parts of the world, including prisoners of the Japanese during World War II. The syndrome is characterized by bilateral paresthesias affecting the feet and lower legs and severe shooting pains that are aggravated by exertion or warmth and alleviated by cold. No muscle wasting, paralysis, or areflexia was observed. The condition is reported to improve with the administration of pantothenic acid.

BIOCHEMICAL FINDINGS

In experimental human deficiency, the eosinopenic response to ACTH was impaired and the sedimentation rate elevated. Adrenocortical function appeared to remain normal. There was increased sensitivity to insulin. Antibody protection against tetanus was impaired. The combination of pantothenic acid and pyridoxine deficiency aggravated the impaired antigenic response when bacterial antigens were used.

There are no satisfactory tests for detecting pantothenic acid deficiency. Urinary excretion of less than 1 mg/day is considered abnormally low in adults. In patients with chronic malnutrition, including alcoholics, levels of pantothenic acid in blood and urine tend to be low.

TREATMENT

No clearly defined therapeutic use of pantothenic acid has been presented. It would seem desirable to provide pantothenic acid in multivitamin preparations employed for IV use and probably for oral administration as well. Diets of adults in the United States usually supply 10 mg to 15 mg pantothenic acid daily. The Food and Nutrition Board suggests that 5 mg to 10 mg daily is probably adequate for both children and adults. The best food sources of pantothenic acid are yeast, liver, and eggs. Some meats, skim milk, and sweet potatoes, tomatoes, and molasses are fairly high in the vitamin.

Biotin Deficiency

PREVALENCE

It is unlikely that spontaneous biotin deficiency will be observed in man. Biotin is obtained not only from the diet but also from synthesis by intestinal bacteria, so that urinary and fecal excretion together often exceeds dietary intake. Biotin deficiency can occur if bizarre diets containing large amounts of raw egg are ingested. Low biotin levels have been found in some segments of the population such as the elderly, athletes, and epileptics.[30,31]

CLINICAL FINDINGS

Experimental biotin deficiency was produced in man by Sydenstricker and associates, who fed a diet rich in raw egg white to human volunteers.[33] Raw egg white contains avidin, a protein that has the ability to inactivate biotin. The subjects developed a grayish pallor of the skin, a nonpruritic dermatitis, depression, lassitude, somnolence, muscle pains, and hyperesthesias. Later manifestations were anorexia, nausea, anemia, hypercholesterolemia, and changes in the ECG. All signs and symptoms disappeared in a few days following parenteral therapy with 150 μg to 300 μg biotin concentrate daily.

Inborn errors of metabolism of biotin have now been well defined with symptoms of aciduria, acidemia, rash, alopecia, progressive neuromuscular disorders, and general debilitation that may eventuate in early death.[29] Treatment requires some 10 mg of biotin daily. Newer techniques of enzyme analysis and studies of fibroblasts now facilitate diagnosis *in utero* so that the earliest possible treatment can be instituted.[32]

TREATMENT

In the usual case of deficiency due to ingestion of large amounts of raw egg white, biotin administration is indicated. Biotin has been reported to be useful in the treatment of seborrheic dermatitis in infants including Leiner's disease (see Chap. 35).

Ascorbic Acid Deficiency—Scurvy

PREVALENCE

Scurvy occurs in infants in many parts of the world, but it is less frequent than in former years. It develops primarily in infants who have been fed cow's milk and—rarely—in breast-fed infants, unless the mother's diet has been very inadequate. The disease appears usually between the ages of 6 and 12 months. Scurvy is also seen in adults, particularly in persons living alone on very restricted diets. It may be found in chronic alcoholism and in diarrheal diseases. Thyrotoxicosis may increase the utilization of ascorbic acid.

CLINICAL FINDINGS

INFANTS

The disease occurs in non-breast-fed infants because of failure to include ascorbic acid in the feeding regimen. With the introduction of formulas containing ascorbic acid for infant feeding, scurvy has become a relatively rare disease. Early symptoms include poor appetite, increased irritability, and minimal growth failure. Then, tenderness of the legs and pseudoparalysis, usually involving the lower extremities, appears. Bleeding into the skin or gums is a fairly frequent manifestation.

In advanced scurvy, the clinical picture is characteristic. The marked tenderness of the legs results in failure of the infant to move them, causing pseudoparalysis. The infant lies quietly with the legs flexed at the knees and the hips flexed and externally rotated. The slightest jar or motion induces

crying because of severe pain due to subperiosteal hemorrhage, usually in the distal femur. Similar pseudoparalysis of the arms can occur. Small and large hemorrhages may appear almost anywhere in the body, most frequently under the periosteum of the long bones or in the gums, skin, and mucous membranes. Subperiosteal hemorrhages occur in about two thirds of the infants and are most frequent at the lower end of the femur and proximal end of the tibia. Hemorrhage of the gums is common if the teeth have erupted or are about to erupt. The gums are swollen, tense, livid, and bleed easily. Infection and ulceration may occur and the teeth may become loose and fall out. Petechiae and ecchymoses are seen in the skin near the bone lesions and on the eyelids and forehead. Hematuria, hematemesis, and bloody diarrhea may be found. Meningeal hemorrhage occurs occasionally. The scorbutic infant is often febrile.

Costochondral beading is the most frequent finding and may be confused with rickets. The deformity feels sharp on palpation, the so-called "bayonet" deformity, as compared with the rounded type of beading noted in rickets. This change occurs as a result of fractures and replacement of the growing ends of the ribs by fibrous tissue. The cartilaginous portion of the anterior chest wall is pulled toward the spine during breathing.

Radiographic examination shows characteristic changes at the cartilage–shaft junction, appearing earliest at the sites of most active growth, that is, the sternal ends of the ribs, distal end of the femur, proximal end of the humerus, both ends of the tibia and fibula, and the distal ends of the radius and ulna. Radiologic diagnosis is made by recognizing a group of characteristic changes, no one of which is diagnostic by itself. The cortex is thin and may be absent as it approaches the cartilage–shaft junction. The trabecular structure of the medulla atrophies and assumes a "ground glass" appearance. The zone of provisional calcification is widened and more dense than normal. Immediately shaftward, an area of decreased density appears, at first near the periphery, the "corner sign" of Park. This area is the site of multiple small fractures and disorganization. It may collapse and result in impaction of the calcified cartilage onto the shaft. The brittle zone of provisional calcification may break into two or more pieces, or it may be detached from the shaft and displaced several centimeters with the epiphysis. Subperiosteal hemorrhages may be visible; these calcify with healing. Eventually, the normal architecture of the bone is restored.

ADULTS

Adult scurvy is relatively rare, and the severe type observed in the previous century is seldom encountered. It is now seen primarily in the food faddist, the alcoholic, and the psychiatric patient. The time required for development of scurvy is 4 to 7 months after institution of a grossly insufficient diet. Nonspecific findings appear first: weakness, lassitude, irritability, and vague aching pains in joints and muscle. The muscle fatigue has been related to impaired carnitine biosynthesis that may influence the capacity of muscle to sustain contraction.[54] Weight loss may occur. The earliest physical sign in experimental scurvy was perifollicular hyperkeratotic papules, which appeared first on the buttocks, thighs, and legs and later on the arms and back. Subsequently, the hairs became buried in the lesions and petechiae appeared around the follicles. The petechiae then became generalized over the lower legs. The only early change in the gums was an interruption of the lamina dura shown on x-rays of the teeth.

In more advanced deficiency, the tendency to hemorrhage becomes marked. Symptoms are dependent on the number, amount, and location of the hemorrhages. They are found most frequently in the skin, muscles, and gums and may be accompanied by edema. The involved areas of the legs tend to ulcerate. Ulcers and other wounds do not heal normally. Scars of previous trauma may become red and break down. Interstitial hemorrhages occur in the muscles, primarily in the thigh and leg, especially around the knee joint. Suppuration may develop in hematomas and lead to formation of large abscesses. Hemarthrosis may occur, in which case the joint becomes swollen, hot, and painful, and motion is limited. Bleeding from the mucous membranes of the GI, GU, or respiratory tracts may occur. Hemorrhagic fluid may be found in the pleural and pericardial cavities. At times, intracranial hemorrhage may develop.

Changes in the gums are a relatively late manifestation of scurvy. They become swollen, red, and spongy, bleeding easily. Such lesions occur only in the presence of teeth. Thromboses of vessels and infarcts of the gums may lead to ulceration and sloughing. The teeth may become loose and fall out due to the loss of gum tissue and softening of the bony structure of the alveolus.

Anemia is seen in both infantile and adult scurvy. It may be hypochromic in type caused by iron deficiency secondary to blood loss. In severe scurvy, particularly in infants, the anemia may be macrocytic with megaloblastosis of the bone marrow. In some instances this type of anemia responds to ascorbic acid. However, the administration of folic acid stimulates more-prompt blood regeneration and restoration to normal. The iron deficiency anemia may be related to the intake of cow's milk rather than to bleeding.

BIOCHEMICAL FINDINGS

The concentration of ascorbic acid in plasma falls to practically zero in scurvy. This occurs before clinical signs appear. The concentration of ascorbic acid in the white cell–platelet layer of blood decreases to 2 mg/100 g or less when scurvy develops, but this determination is difficult and is seldom available. A useful test is the administration of a large dose of ascorbic acid orally, followed by measurement of changes in blood concentration or urinary excretion in a given period of time. A load test that is simple to use in infants is administration of 200 mg ascorbic acid intramuscularly, determining serum concentration before and 4 hours after the dose. In scurvy, the 4-hour value is usually less than 0.2 mg/dl, indicating depleted tissue stores. In infants with poor recent intake but no tissue depletion the 4-hour value often rises to 1 mg/dl.

Clinical manifestations of scurvy have been seen in subjects with vitamin C plasma levels between 0.13 and 0.24 mg/100 ml; the threshold in leukocyte vitamin C concentration is about 10 μg/10^8 cells. In studies with healthy volunteers it has been shown that a daily intake of 100 mg of vitamin C for a nonsmoker and 140 mg for a smoker will maintain an adequate vitamin C level of 0.8 to 0.9 mg/100 ml. Low plasma and leukocyte vitamin C levels have been found in groups such as the elderly, the institutionalized, the hospitalized, and in patients with various diseases.[57]

TREATMENT

In treating infantile scurvy, 25 mg ascorbic acid may be administered four times daily added to the milk. Some pediatricians prescribe 50 mg to 100 mg four times daily. After a week, the amount of ascorbic acid may be reduced to about 30 mg/day. This can be given in the form of orange juice or as ascorbic acid *per se.* In the therapy of adult scurvy, 250 mg should be administered four times daily. This amount is sufficient to replenish body stores, which amount to 2 g to 3 g, within less than a week. The dose may then be decreased to 50 mg to 100 mg several times daily until healing is complete.

The diet should be adequate in all respects. Excellent sources of ascorbic acid are citrus fruits, oranges, grapefruit, lemons, limes, and pineapple. Other good sources are strawberries, cabbage, tomatoes, and green vegetables. Other fruits and vegetables contain some ascorbic acid; even turnips and potatoes are useful in large amounts. Much of the vitamin C in foods may be lost in cooking and storage because of destruction by heat and oxidation. Ascorbic acid is relatively stable in canned and frozen foods.

Wound healing is impaired in vitamin C deficiency, because ascorbic acid is necessary for the formation of collagen. The amount of ascorbic acid in the diet is related to the strength of healing wounds and also to the concentration in scar tissue. A decrease in plasma ascorbic acid occurs following trauma or surgical procedures, apparently due to a shift of ascorbic acid from the serum to the site of wounding. Low ascorbic acid concentrations are found almost routinely in patients with wound disruption. Patients admitted to surgery with concentrations of less than 8 mg/100 g in the white cell–platelet layer of blood should receive extra ascorbic acid as there is an eight-fold increase in incidence of wound dehiscence in these patients.

Administration of ascorbic acid in amounts of several hundred milligrams has been found to increase the assimilation of food iron.[52] It may also function in the release of ferric iron from linkage to the plasma protein transferrin for subsequent incorporation into tissue ferritin.

Abruptio placenta was found to occur in 7 out of 355 women (2%) who had plasma acorbate levels above 0.4 mg/100 ml, but in 6 out of 31 women (19.4%) with concentrations below 0.4 mg/100 ml. A marginal vitamin C deficiency and an accompanying high histamine level were thought to play a role in its etiology.[46] This data suggest that supplementation with vitamin C during pregnancy, particularly for those at risk, may be useful in preventing this disorder.

In patients with hemorrhagic ocular disease, plasma vitamin C levels were found to be in the range of 0.43 mg/dl to 0.56 mg/dl. Supplementation of the diet with vitamin C over 40 days improved the plasma levels of C toward normal levels and caused significant improvement in the hemorrhagic ocular phenomena.[50]

Pauling suggests administration of large doses of ascorbic acid, 1 g to 5 g daily, in the prevention of the common cold and even larger doses for its treatment.[56] Recent controlled studies indicate that these doses do not prevent the common cold but may slightly decrease its duration and the severity of symptoms.

In man, particularly in the elderly with low plasma vitamin C levels and hypercholesteremia, long-term administration of C in gram doses gradually replenished body stores and reduced the elevated cholesterol levels to normal.[48]

The controversy over the alleged effectiveness of gram amounts of vitamin C in cancer has continued, but accumulating data suggest that its value may be very limited. However, the daily administration of 3 g vitamin C for 13 months has been shown to have a beneficial effect in the disappearance of rectal polyps in patients with familial polyposis.[47]

TOXICITY

There is little evidence that ascorbic acid is toxic, for excess amounts are excreted by the kidney. However, large doses may cause GI irritation. Prolonged administration of ascorbic acid in amounts of several grams daily is without risk to human health.[53]

Vitamin D Deficiency

PREVALENCE

Vitamin D deficiency has become a rare disease in the United States, whereas at one time it was a common affliction of infancy and childhood. Eradication of this deficiency has been due largely to the widespread practice of feeding infants cow's milk or preparations based on cow's milk that are enriched with irradiated ergosterol so as to contain 400 units of vitamin D in the amount of food equivalent in calories to a quart of milk. Since the vitamin D requirement of infants approximates 100 to 150 units daily, the intake of a quart of milk by infants over 2 to 3 months of age provides a considerable margin of safety. Breast-fed infants require supplementary vitamin D unless they are exposed to adequate amounts of ultraviolet irradiation. It is common practice to prescribe 400 IU daily in the form of vitamin concentrates.[59]

Vitamin D deficiency in older children and adults is unusual if they are exposed to sunlight and to minimal dietary sources of the vitamin. Vitamin D deficiency during pregnancy is seen primarily in countries where cultural patterns prevent women from receiving exposure to sunlight.

RICKETS

Clinical Findings. Manifestations of vitamin D deficiency in infants are due to reduction of serum ionized calcium with resultant tetany and convulsions or to deficient mineralization of growing bones leading to skeletal deformities and retardation of growth. Evidence of deficiency rarely appears before 3 to 4 months of age. An early finding is hypocalcemia, which is rarely symptomatic. If vitamin D deficiency continues, the clinical picture of infantile rickets develops.[60]

The major manifestations of rickets are progressive bony deformities, resulting from the mechanical weakness of bone and the response of growing bone to deforming stresses. The earliest sign of rickets in the infant under 6 months of age is craniotabes. This consists of areas of softening of the skull, usually located in the occipital and parietal bones along the lambdoidal sutures. Pressure of the fingers on the skull causes indentation and the bone seems to snap back when pressure is released. In chronic rickets, the skull becomes thickened, with enlargement of the frontal and parietal areas causing "bossing" of the skull. Enlargement of the costochondral junctions of the ribs produces the "rachitic rosary." Retraction of the rib cage at the attachment of the diaphragm results in what is known as Harrison's groove. The growing ends of the long bones are widened at the wrists and ankles. As the child stands and walks, a deformity of the pelvis develops, which may result in serious problems in the female in childbearing later in life. The bones of the lower extremities may become bent and twisted causing bowing of the legs and abnormalities of gait with a characteristic waddling appearance. Scoliosis of the spine may develop with sitting. In advanced rickets, the costal cartilages may be pulled in causing the sternum to protrude, producing the pigeon breast deformity. The teeth are delayed in eruption, and enamel development is defective. The final result of rickets is a deformed child with reduced stature.

Roentgenograms are useful in the diagnosis of rickets in advanced stages. Abnormal findings may be seen at the cartilage–shaft junction and in the shafts of the bones. The former are characterized by cupping, spreading, fringing, and stippling, which may be seen first at both ends of the fibula and the lower end of the ulna. Similar findings due to weakness of the cartilage–shaft junction have been noted in the lower end of the radius, both ends of the tibia, and ·the lower end of the femur. In the shaft the trabecular meshwork becomes coarse, and in severe rickets there is a loss of bone density. The cortex may appear abnormally thin in advanced cases, but at times it is thickened or duplicated. Curvature of the long bones may be seen on x-ray. Following treatment with vitamin D, a characteristic transverse line of radio-opacity (Mueller's line) makes its appearance, crossing the cartilage in advance of the end of the shaft and parallel to it. This represents newly calcified cartilage.

Biochemical Findings. Hypocalcemia is the earliest manifestation. This is associated with normal or slightly reduced concentrations of serum phosphorus, which differentiates it from hypoparathyroidism. Serum alkaline phosphatase is elevated to 20 to 30 Bodansky units or more. As vitamin D deficiency progresses, the serum phosphate concentration decreases to values as low as 2 mg to 3 mg/100 ml. When hypophosphatemia develops, the serum calcium concentration rises to approach normal values, although it usually remains slightly low.

OSTEOMALACIA

Clinical Findings. In the United States, osteomalacia due to primary deficiency of vitamin D is extremely rare. It is usually secondary to defective intestinal absorption or to abnormalities of renal function. It is found most often in association with chronic steatorrhea in which faulty digestion and absorption of fat lead to formation of insoluble calcium salts that are lost in the stool along with vitamin D. Pregnancy and lactation intensify the symptoms.

The most frequent complaint is pain in the bones, particularly in the lower part of the back and in the legs, which is often worse while standing and walking. These symptoms are due to microfractures and compression of the weight-bearing bones, the vertebrae, and lower extremities. The bones become soft from failure of mineralization as they undergo remodeling. Wide zones of demineralized osteoid tissue are found at the junction of mineralized bone and the layer of osteoblasts. Defects of bone structure, pseudofractures, occur at the sites of muscle attachment. Cyst-like zones of demineralization may be seen in the metaphyseal region. Muscular weakness is a common finding. The bones are sensitive to light pressure, for instance, over the ribs, hips, and thighs. The tendency of the bones to bend leads to a waddling gait. Tetany may develop. Roentgenograms show extensive decalcification. Deformities of the pelvis and sacrum are common. In the long bones, the cortex is thin and separated into many layers. The bones may become curved and show fractures or pseudofractures. Biochemical findings are similar to those found in rickets.

TETANY ASSOCIATED WITH OSTEOMALACIA AND RICKETS

Tetany is characterized by hyperirritability of the nervous system and is evidenced by carpopedal spasm, convulsions, and—occasionally—laryngospasm. Chvostek's sign is positive, and Trousseau's phenomenon can be demonstrated. Galvanic stimulation shows anodal reversal and an anodal opening reaction with a stimulus of less than 5 ma. In tetany, protein-bound calcium is normal. Total serum calcium measures 7 mg to 7.7 mg/100 ml and ionized calcium is less than 4.3 mg/100 ml.

TREATMENT

In the treatment of infantile rickets, administration of vitamin D in amounts of 1200 IU daily is usually sufficient. Evidence of healing will be noted in the x-ray after about 3 weeks of therapy. Mueller's line, which indicates calcium salt deposition in the cartilage, will appear, and the concentration of phosphorus in plasma will rise. If rickets is severe, it may be advisable to give larger amounts of the vitamin, such as 5000 IU daily. It is safe to continue to administer these higher doses for 5 to 6 weeks. Treatment should be continued until the bone ends have filled in, at which time dosage should be decreased to the preventive level, that is, 400 IU daily.

In the treatment of osteomalacia, vitamin D has been given in amounts of 5,000 IU to 20,000 IU or more daily. Calcium may be prescribed in the form of milk, or as calcium gluconate or lactate, 5 g three times daily dissolved in water.

The immediate treatment of acute tetany is the injection of a calcium salt intravenously. Calcium gluconate may be given, 10 ml to 20 ml, in 10% solution, 1 g gluconate providing 90 mg calcium. After relief of the acute episode, calcium may be given orally in association with vitamin D as outlined above.

SECONDARY VITAMIN D DEFICIENCY OWING TO INCREASED REQUIREMENT

Rickets and osteomalacia may occur in subjects who have been receiving what are ordinarily adequate amounts of vitamin D as a result of poor absorption from the intestinal tract due to the malabsorption of fats (*e.g.*, as a consequence of lack of bile salts) or to small intestinal disease (*e.g.*, gluten-induced enteropathy or pancreatic disease).

Increased vitamin D requirement may result from hepatic disease because the initial step in the conversion of cholecalciferol or ergocalciferol to the physiologically active compound is 25-hydroxylation by a liver enzyme. In severe renal disease, osteodystrophy is due in large part to increased requirement of vitamin D, presumably because of a block in the formation of 1,25-dihydroxycalciferol. Increased requirement of vitamin D may also result from a genetically determined abnormality in metabolism at the final site of action of vitamin D, so-called vitamin D-dependent rickets. Antivitamin D factors may operate through unknown mechanisms. Some patients with epilepsy who receive multiple anticonvulsant drugs have an increased need for vitamin D to prevent hypocalcemia, hypophosphatemia, rickets, and osteomalacia (see Chap. 3).

TOXICITY

Vitamin D is toxic in doses of 2000 IU to 5000 IU (50 µg to 125 µg) per kg per day if taken over a period of several weeks. Important manifestations of toxicity include hyperabsorption of calcium, hypercalcemia, and hypercalciuria. The latter two findings result in renal calcinosis and injury, which may result in progressive renal insufficiency. Symptoms are polyuria and polydipsia, anorexia, nausea, vomiting, constipation, and hypertension. Drowsiness and coma may be observed owing to extreme hypercalcemia or to hypertensive encephalopathy. Calcium is deposited in the blood vessels and around the joints, findings that may be visible on x-ray. There is increased density at the growing ends of bones with diminished density in the shaft. Dense metaphyseal lines may be seen. Hypercalcemic levels in serum are 12 mg/100 ml or more.

Treatment consists of correction of dehydration and electrolyte loss and administration of cortisone. The latter should be continued until calcium levels in the serum are less than 12 mg/100 ml.

Vitamin E (Tocopherol) Deficiency

PREVALENCE

Although evidence indicates that vitamin E is essential in human nutrition, deficiency is not observed in healthy subjects who consume and absorb the constituents of an average American diet. In newborn and premature infants, the tocopherol concentration in blood and tissues is low. Breast feeding results in a prompt rise to normal levels, but cow's milk, which has a lower tocopherol concentration, is less effective. Tocopherol deficiency may occur in children with cystic fibrosis of the pancreas or with congenital atresia of the bile ducts. Adult subjects with either malabsorption syndromes and steatorrhea or xanthomatous biliary cirrhosis may develop tocopherol deficiency (see Chap. 3) and a betalipoproteinemia.

CLINICAL AND BIOCHEMICAL FINDINGS

In premature infants, anemia and a syndrome consisting of edema, skin abnormalities, an elevated platelet count, and morphologic changes in the red cells has been attributed to deficiency of vitamin E.

Infants and children with cystic fibrosis of the pancreas have low levels of serum tocopherol and an increased susceptibility of erythrocytes to hemolysis. In some instances, creatinuria is observed, accompanied by a decrease in plasma creatine and an increase in muscle creatine. Ceroid pigment has been found in increased amounts in children with cystic fibrosis of the pancreas and in patients with celiac disease and sprue. Similar pigment has been found in vitamin E-deficient animals.

Infants with congenital atresia of the bile ducts have low concentrations of plasma tocopherol, abnormal erythrocyte hemolysis tests, and creatinuria. Focal lesions resembling those seen in several animal species with vitamin E deficiency have been found in muscle.

Recent studies in children with chronic cholestasis, who gradually developed a symptom complex of neuromuscular disease including ataxia, dysmetria, areflexia, loss of vibratory sensation, and ophthalmoplegia, were found to have low serum vitamin E concentrations. They characteristically had abnormal pharmacokinetics in their response to various forms of high doses of vitamin E but over months showed progressive improvement in maintaining blood levels of vitamin E and in the regression of their symptoms.[61]

In adults with malabsorption syndromes, beta-lipoproteinemia and steatorrhea, low serum tocopherol concentrations, and increased susceptibility of erythrocytes to hemolysis may be observed. Comparable findings plus creatinuria have been reported in xanthomatous biliary cirrhosis.

Experimental vitamin E deficiency in man was produced by Horwitt and associates in subjects who received a diet high in polyunsaturated fats for several years.[63] In addition to changes in the level of serum tocopherol and in erythrocyte susceptibility to hemolysis, a slight decrease in erythrocyte survival time was observed. When tocopherol was administered, a small increase in reticulocytes in the peripheral blood was noted.

PREVENTION AND TREATMENT

Vitamin E requirement appears to be related to the polyunsaturated fat content of a diet. A recommended intake of 10 mg to 30 mg/day for adults, depending on the type of fat in the diet, has been suggested. It is desirable to keep the level of tocopherol in serum above 0.5 mg/100 ml. In the treatment of tocopherol deficiency, 30 mg to 100 mg or more may be prescribed daily. Toxicity of this vitamin has not been reported even in persons receiving more than a gram a day for many months. Benefits claimed for therapy with large doses of vitamin E have not been substantiated. Vegetables and seed oils are the largest contributors of tocopherol to the diet.

The pharmacologic action of vitamin E is currently under study with noteworthy results in two important areas. One is in the administration of 100 mg daily to preterm infants who are receiving oxygen therapy in order to reduce the severity of the retrolental fibroplasia that may develop.[62] The other is in women with fibrocystic disease of the breast in whom 600 mg daily has been reported to cause regression of the pathology.[64]

Vitamin K Deficiency

PREVALENCE

Vitamin K deficiency due solely to an inadequate diet has not been reported. In conjunction with synthesis of vitamin K by intestinal bacteria, the average diet provides adequate amounts.

The newborn infant has low serum levels of prothrombin and several other coagulation factors related to vitamin K. Deficiency of this vitamin develops in the absence of bile from the intestinal tract and is found in chronic biliary fistula and obstructive jaundice. Inadequate absorption of vitamin K also occurs in the steatorrheas, for example, sprue, gluten-induced enteropathy, various lesions of the small intestine, short circuiting operations, and chronic pancreatic diseases. Deficiency may result from prolonged administration of antibiotics or sulfonamides. In patients receiving salicylates, hypoprothrombinemia has been reported.

CLINICAL AND BIOCHEMICAL FINDINGS

In newborn infants, a low level of prothrombin and other coagulation factors in serum has been observed. In normal infants, prothrombin concentration may decrease to as low as 20% in the second and third day of life and then gradually increase to normal adult values over a period of weeks. If values fall below 10%, hemorrhagic disease of the newborn may occur. The situation in the infant may be due to delay in establishing bacterial flora for vitamin K synthesis, insufficient bile in the first few days of life for vitamin K absorption, or delay in manufacture of prothrombin by the liver.

The clinical manifestation of vitamin K deficiency in all age groups is hemorrhage. In patients with obstructive jaundice, hemorrhage is most apt to occur after surgical intervention and is usually noted between the first and fourth postoperative days. Slow oozing from the operative incision is common, as is bleeding from the gums, nose, or GI tract. The prothrombin clotting time is prolonged. Hemorrhage also occurs in various intestinal disorders in which vitamin K absorption is impaired or in patients who have received prolonged antibiotic therapy.

In the presence of severe liver damage, a marked prolongation of prothrombin time that is not responsive to administration of vitamin K may be observed. This failure of response has been used as a test of liver function.

Diagnosis of vitamin K deficiency is dependent on detection of diminished prothrombin activity in the blood. In most instances, prothrombin activity has fallen to less than one third of normal before bleeding occurs. The technique developed by Quick, or some modification thereof, is frequently used to determine prothrombin clotting time.

PREVENTION AND TREATMENT

It is commonly recommended that the infant be given a dose of 1 mg to 2 mg vitamin K shortly after birth to prevent hemorrhagic disease of the newborn. As an alternative, it has been suggested that 2 mg to 5 mg vitamin K be given to the mother prior to delivery, but the value of this therapy is controversial.

The treatment of hypothrombinemia due to vitamin K deficiency consists of administration of the vitamin in doses of 2 mg to 5 mg daily.

Synthetic water-soluble preparations of vitamin K or menadione are equally effective. Water-soluble preparations are preferable when deficiency is due to absence of bile from the intestinal tract or in the steatorrheas. If menadione is given, it must be used in conjunction with 1 g to 3 g bile salts to facilitate absorption.

In the preparation of patients with obstructive jaundice for surgery, vitamin K should be given even if prothrombin activity is normal. A postoperative decrease in prothrombin can be prevented by 1 mg to 2 mg vitamin K daily. If prothrombin time is prolonged, larger doses (up to 5 mg daily) should be given. The vitamin may be administered intravenously in similar amounts if bleeding is present. Transfusions are needed when hemorrhage is severe to combat shock and provide a temporary supply of prothrombin. The amount of prothrombin furnished by transfused blood is effective for about 6 to 12 hours. In the therapy of hypoprothrombinemia due to administration of anticoagulants, vitamin K_1 has been found to be the most effective preparation.

TOXICITY

The administration of large amounts of vitamin K to newborn infants, particularly in water-soluble form, may be responsible for hemolytic anemia, hyperbilirubinemia, and kernicterus. Prematurity and vitamin E deficiency increase the susceptibility to the toxic effects of vitamin K. In adults, 20 mg to 40 mg vitamin K daily have been given for several weeks without evidence of toxicity. Quantities larger than this may cause vomiting. Very large doses have been associated with porphyrinuria and albuminuria. Occasionally, such doses of vitamin K have been reported to depress prothrombin activity in patients with severe disease of the liver.

References

VITAMIN A

1. Bauernfeind JC: The Safe Use of Vitamin A—A Report of the International Vitamin A Consultative Group. Washington, D.C., The Nutrition Foundation, 1980
2. Brubacher G, Vuilluemier JP, Ritzel G, et al: Early signs of hypovitaminosis A. Ernährung 6: (in press)
3. Dicken CH, Connolly SM: Systemic retinoids in dermatology. Mayo Clin Proc 57:51–57, 1982
4. Hodges RE: Hematopoietic studies in vitamin A deficiency. Am J Clin Nutr 31:876–885, 1978
5. Hume EM, Krebs HA: Vitamin A requirements of human adults. Medical Research Council Special Report Services (Lond) 664, 1949
6. McClaren DS: Malnutrition and the Eye. New York, Academic Press, 1963
7. McClaren DS, Oomen HAPC, Escaponi H: Ocular manifestations of Vitamin A deficiency in man. Bull WHO 34:357–361, 1966
8. Oomen HAPC: An outline of xerophthalmia. Int Rev Trop Med 1:131–213, 1960
9. Peto R, Doll R, Buckley JD, Sporn MB: Can dietery beta–carotene materially reduce human cancer rates? Nature 290:201–208, 1981

THIAMIN

10. Blankenhorn MA: The diagnosis of beriberi heart disease. Ann Int Med 23:398–404, 1945
11. Brin M: Thiamin deficiency and erythrocyte metabolism. Am J Clin Nutr 12:107–116, 1963
12. Goldsmith GA: The B vitamins, thiamin, riboflavin, niacin. In Beaton GH, McHenry EW (eds): Nutrition: A Comprehensive Treatise, Vol 2, pp 109–206. New York, Academic Press, 1964
13. Ramalingaswami V: Beriberi. Fed Proc 17(2):43–46, 1958
14. Williams RR: Toward the Conquest of Beriberi. Cambridge, Harvard University Press, 1961

RIBOFLAVIN

15. Bro–Rasmussen F: The riboflavin requirements of animals and man and associated metabolic relations. Nutr Abstr Rev 28:369–386, 1958
16. Goldsmith GA: Clinical aspects of riboflavin deficiency. In Rivlin RS (ed): Monograph on Riboflavin. New York, Plenum Publishers, 1975
17. Horwitt MK, Liebert E, Kreisler O, et al: Investigations of human requirements for B-complex vitamins. National Research Council Bulletin 116, 1948

18. Lane M, Alfrey CP, Mengel CE, et al: The rapid induction of human riboflavin deficiency with galactoflavin. J Clin Invest 43:357–373, 1964

NIACIN

19. Goldsmith GA: Experimental niacin deficiency in man. J Am Diet Assoc 32:312–316, 1956
20. Goldsmith GA: Niacin–tryptophan relationships and niacin requirements. Am J Clin Nutr 6:479–486, 1958
21. Goldsmith GA: Niacin: Antipellagra factor, hypocholesterolemia agent. JAMA 194:116–176, 1965
22. Gopolan C: Some recent studies in the nutrition research laboratories, Hyderabad. Am J Clin Nutr 23:35–51, 1970
23. Manual For Nutrition Survey, Interdepartmental Committee on Nutrition for National Defense. Washington, D.C., US Government Printing Office, 1957

VITAMIN B$_6$ DEFICIENCY

24. Coursin DB: Present status of vitamin B$_6$ metabolism. Am J Clin Nutr 9:304, 1961
25. Mueller JF, Vilter RW: Pyridoxine deficiency in human beings induced with desoxypyridoxine. J Clin Invest 29:193–201, 1950
26. Taylor RW, James CE: The clinician's view of patients with premenstrual syndrome. Curr Med Res Opin 6 Suppl 5:46–51, 1979

PANTOTHENIC ACID

27. Bean WB, Hodges RE, Daum K: Pantothenic acid deficiency induced in human subjects. J Clin Invest 34:1073–1084, 1955
28. Hodges RE, Bean WB, Ohlson MA, et al: Human pantothenic acid deficiency produced by omega-methyl pantothenic acid. J Clin Invest 38:1421–1425, 1959

BIOTIN

29. Bonjour JP: Biotin-dependent enzymes in inborn errors of metabolism in humans. World Rev Nutr Diet 38:1–88, 1981
30. Krause KH, Berlit P, Bonjour JP: Reduction of biotin level as a possible factor in the mode of action of anticonvulsants. Arch Psychiatr Nervenkr 231:141–148, 1982
31. Roth KS: Biotin in clinical medicine—a review. Am J Clin Nutr 34:1967–1974, 1981
32. Roth KS, Yang W, Allan L, et al: Prenatal administration of biotin in biotin-responsive multiple carboxylase deficiency. Pediatr Res 16:126–129, 1982
33. Synderstricker VP, Singai SA, Briggs AP, et al: Observations on the "egg white injury" in man. JAMA 118:1199–1200, 1942

FOLIC ACID

34. Blakely RL: The Biochemistry of Folic Acid and Related Compounds, New York, American Elsevier, 1969
35. FAO–WHO Expert Group: Requirements of ascorbic acid, vitamin D, vitamin B$_{12}$, folate, and iron. WHO Tech Sym Ser 452:43, 1970
36. Goldsmith GA, Hunter FM, Prevatt AL, et al: Vitamin B$_{12}$ and the malabsorption syndromes. Am J Gastroenterol 32:453–466, 1959
37. Herbert V: Experimental nutritional folate deficiency in man. Trans Assoc Am Physicians 75:307–320, 1962
38. Herbert V: Nutritional requirements for vitamin B$_{12}$ and folic acid. Am J Clin Nutr 21:743–752, 1968
39. Herbert V: Folic acid deficiency: Introduction. Am J Clin Nutr 23:841–842, 1970
40. Luhby AL, Cooperman JM: Folic acid deficiency in man and its interrelationship with vitamin B$_{12}$ metabolism. In Advances in Metabolic Procedures, pp 263–334. New York, Academic Press, 1964

VITAMIN B$_{12}$

41. Baker SJ: Nutrition and diseases of the blood: The megaloblastic anemias. In Goldsmith GA (ed): International Encyclopedia of Food and Nutrition. London, Pergamon Press, 1977
42. Beck WS: The metabolic functions of vitamin B. N Engl J Med 266:708–714, 1962
43. Herbert V: The Megaloblastic Anemias. New York, Grune & Stratton, 1959
44. Schilling RF: Intrinsic factor studies. J Lab Clin Med 42:860–866, 1953

ASCORBIC ACID

45. Barnes AE, Bartley W, Frankaw IM, et al: Vitamin C requirements of human adults. (Compiled by Bartley W, Krebs HA, O'Brien JP) Medical Research Council Special Report Services (Lond) 280, 1953
46. Clemetson CAB, Cafaro V: Abruptio Placentae. Int J Gynaecol Obstet 19:453–460, 1981
47. Decosse JJ, Adams MB, Kuzma JF, et al: Effect of ascorbic acid on rectal polyps of patients with familial polyposis. Surgery 78:608–612, 1975
48. Ginter E, Bobek P: The influence of vitamin C on lipid metabolism. In Counsell JN, Hornig DH (eds): Vitamin C–Ascorbic Acid, pp 269–347. Englewood, NJ, Applied Science Publishers, 1981
49. Goldsmith GA: Human requirements for vitamin C and its use in clinical medicine. Ann NY Acad Sci 92:1, 230–245, 1961
50. Greco AM, Fioretti F, Rimo A: Relationship between hemorrhagic ocular diseases and vitamin C deficiency: Clinical and experimental data. Acta Vitaminol Enzymol 2 ns (1–2):21–25, 1980
51. Hodges RE, Baker EM, Hood J, et al: Experimental scurvy in man. Am J Clin Nutr 22:535–548, 1969
52. Hallberg L: Effect of vitamin C on the bioavailability of iron from food. In Counsell JN, Hornig DH (eds): Vitamin C–Ascorbic Acid, pp 49–61, Englewood, NJ, Applied Science Publishers, 1981
53. Hornig DH, Moser U: The safety of vitamin C intakes in man. In Counsell JN, Hornig DH (eds): Vitamin C–Ascorbic Acid, pp 225–248. Englewood, NJ, Applied Science Publishers, 1981
54. Hughes RE: Recommended daily amounts and biochemical roles—the vitamin C, carnitine, fatigue relationship. In Counsell JN, Hornig DH (eds): Vitamin C–Ascorbic Acid, pp 75–86. Englewood, NJ, Applied Science Publishers, 1981
55. Lind J: A treatise of the scurvy. In Stewart CP, Gutherie

D (eds): Lind's Treatise on Scurvy, Edinburgh, University Press, 1953

56. Pauling L: Vitamin C and the Common Cold, San Francisco, WH Freeman & Co, 1970
57. Shorah CJ, Tormey WP, Brooks GH, et al: The effect of vitamin C supplements on an elderly population. Am J Clin Nutr 34:871–876, 1981
58. Woodruff CW: Ascorbic acid—scurvy. In Goldsmith GA (ed): International Encyclopedia of Food and Nutrition, London, Pergamon Press, 1976

VITAMIN D

59. DeLuca HF, Suttie JW (eds): The Fat Soluble Vitamins, Madison, University of Wisconsin Press, 1969
60. Park EA: Vitamin D and rickets. In Jolliffe N (ed): Clinical Nutrition, pp 506–564, New York, Harper & Row, 1962

VITAMIN E

61. Guggenheim MA, Ringel SP, Silverman A, et al: Progressive neuromuscular disease in children with chronic cholestasis and vitamin E deficiency: Diagnosis and treatment with alpha tocopherol. J Pediatr 100:51–58, 1982
62. Hittner HM, Godio LB, Rudolph AJ, et al: Retrolental fibroplasia: Efficacy of vitamin E in a double-blind clinical study of preterm infants. N Engl J Med 305:1365–1371, 1981
63. Horwitt MK, Harvey CC, Duncan GD, et al: Effects of limited tocopherol intake in man with relationships to erythrocyte hemolysis and lipid oxidations. Am J Clin Nutr 4:408–419, 1958
64. London RS, Sundaram GS, Schultz M, et al: Endocrine parameters and alpha tocopherol therapy of patients with mammary dysplasia. Cancer Res 41:3811–3813, 1981
65. Vitamin E. Minneapolis, General Mills, 1973

VITAMIN K

66. Dam H: Vitamin malnutrition, vitamins E and K. In Goldsmith GA (ed): International Encyclopedia of Food and Nutrition. London, Pergamon Press, 1977
67. Martius C: The metabolic relationships between the different K vitamins and the synthesis of the ubiquinones. Am J Clin Nutr 9:97–102, 1961

13
Parenteral Nutrition— Principles, Nutrient Requirements, Techniques, and Clinical Applications

H. C. Meng

An adequate intake of nutrients is necessary to maintain an optimal state of nutrition and health. This is no less true in patients with trauma, severe burns, or major surgical procedure. Such patients are hypercatabolic, with a marked increase in energy expenditure and nitrogen loss, and are usually anorexic or unable to eat. In some instances, such as injury, surgery, or disease of the gastrointestinal tract, oral feeding can aggravate the disease or be detrimental to wound healing. For these reasons, parenteral nutrition is an important, or sometimes the only, form of therapy to meet the nutritional needs.

Parenteral nutrition, or intravenous feeding, by definition concerns the administration of nutrients by routes other than the gastrointestinal tract. This excludes feedings by the gastric or intestinal tube or by the rectal route. Since the amounts of nutrients and the volume of nutrient solutions are necessarily large, it is not convenient to use subcutaneous, intramuscular, or intraperitoneal routes. In addition, the absorption of the major foodstuffs (carbohydrate, protein, and fat) is slow, time-consuming, and not without discomfort. Thus, the only practical route for the introduction of all nutrients in adequate amounts is intravenous administration.

In terms of cellular nutrition, it makes little difference whether the nutrients are supplied orally or intravenously. However, it should be recognized that with the administration of nutrients directly into the blood circulation, the gastrointestinal tract is being bypassed. The physico-chemical form of nutrients given intravenously must be suitably modified (*e.g.,* protein in the form of free amino acids or hydrolysates, carbohydrates as monosaccharides, and fat or oil as an oil-in-water emulsion), and the total amount and rate of administration must be regulated within the body's capacity to metabolize. Solutions or preparations for intravenous or parenteral administration, of course, must be sterile and nonpyrogenic. In addition, small bowel hypoplasia, changes in gastrointestinal hormone secretion, and decrease in intestinal enzyme activity have been observed in dogs, rabbits, and rats maintained on total parenteral nutrition. The question has been raised, therefore, about the importance or necessity of direct contact of food to maintain normal morphologic and functional integrity of the gastrointestinal tract. A consideration of such consequences following long-term total parenteral nutrition is necessary in the planning of subsequent oral alimentation.

Historical Background

Although a variety of substances administered intravenously has been recorded since the middle part of the 17th century, it was not until 1911 that Kausch reported the use of intravenously infused glucose to a patient following surgery. The use of fat emulsion in dogs was accomplished by Marlin and Riche in 1915 and by Yamakawa and associates in patients in 1920. Henriques and Anderson demonstrated nutritional utilization of hydrolyzed protein after intravenous injection in animals in 1913. In 1939, Elman and Weiner were the first to give protein hydrolysate to a patient. Schohl and Blackfan infused a mixture of synthetic crystalline amino acids into infants in 1940.

Clark and Brunschwig were the first to administer solutions containing the three major nutrients—carbohydrate, protein, and fat intravenously to adult patients in 1942. Another documented success of parenteral nutrition in an infant was reported by Helfrick and Abelson in 1944. However, subsequent attempts to provide complete parenteral nutrition met with failure. In 1949, Meng and associates were the first to provide dogs with complete parenteral nutrition, including all six essential nutrient groups: (1) protein, (2) fat, (3) carbohydrate, (4) vitamins, (5) electrolytes and some inorganic trace minerals, and (6) water.[101] They demonstrated that a patient fed by long-term "complete" parenteral nutrition, exclusively by continuous infusion into the superior vena cava through an indwelling catheter, is capable of achieving weight gain, positive nitrogen balance, general health, and a sense of well-being. Research in the field of parenteral nutrition progressed at a slow pace, although much enthusiasm existed in the development of fat emulsions as a concentrated energy source in the 1950s and early 1960s. Because of the adverse effects encountered after long-term administration of Lipomul, a 15% cottonseed oil emulsion, physicians were compelled to return to the conventional intravenous therapy, which consists of 5%-10% glucose and occasional protein hydrolysate.

Parenteral nutrition entered into a new era in the late 1960s. In 1968, Dudrick and colleagues demonstrated in puppies, in an infant, and in postoperative patients, that normal growth, development and positive nitrogen balance can be achieved by continuous administration, by means of an indwelling catheter into the superior vena cava, of a solution containing protein hydrolysate and concentrated glucose along with vitamins and minerals.[43] Further work reported by Dudrick and associates confirmed these favorable results, and during the period from 1969 to 1975 many other reports also appeared in the literature documenting the effectiveness of this procedure in achieving body weight gain, positive nitrogen balance, wound healing, and spontaneous closure of enterocutaneous fistulas in patients after surgery or with various diseases.[7,41,42,43,48,104,157,158] Today, parenteral nutrition has wide use in the practice of medicine as a means of therapy for nutritional support in patients who cannot or should not eat by mouth. In addition, many medical centers have established parenteral nutrition units or nutritional support services as one of the services to improve patient management.

In the United States prior to 1975, total parenteral nutrition was administered without fat. For this reason, a large amount of carbohydrate, in the form of glucose in high concentrations, had to be given to meet the energy need. The availability of fat emulsions suitable for intravenous use has made "complete," total parenteral nutrition possible. In addition, parenteral nutrition can be administered in some instances into a peripheral vein as well as through a central venous catheter.

Parenteral Nutrition Indication

Parenteral nutrition is indicated when patients are unable to eat by mouth and tube feeding is contraindicated or has failed. Indications are as follows:

1. Abnormality of gastrointestinal tract
   a. Ingestion of food impossible or unwise, for instance, obstruction, peritonitis
   b. Inability to retain ingested food, for example, vomiting, diarrhea, or fistula
   c. Impaired digestion and absorption, for example, malabsorption syndromes, regional enteritis, or ulcerative colitis
   d. Trauma or elective surgery, for instance, short bowel syndrome, edema due to severe malnutrition
2. Preparation for surgery in nutritionally depleted and emaciated patients
3. After surgery or trauma, especially in burns or multiple fractures with complications such as sepsis
4. Renal failure, especially those in acute phase
5. Coma, anorexia nervosa, or refusal to eat
6. Supplementation of inadequate oral feeding in patients with cancer, especially those receiving chemotherapy or radiation therapy, and those with renal or hepatic failure, or other diseases

Careful consideration should be given to the nutritional status, clinical condition, and gastrointestinal function of the patient, in order to assess whether total parenteral nutrition through a central vein is necessary. Peripheral parenteral nutrition, plus intravenous fat emulsion, may be adequate, or tube feeding with appropriate defined formula diet may be indicated. Once the choice of total parenteral nutrition is made, it is important to institute the therapy as early as possible to check starvation and prevent further deterioration. Consideration must be given to administer all nutrients, protein, carbohydrate, fat, vitamins, electrolytes, and water in adequate amounts and in proper proportion, because efficient utilization of one nutrient requires the presence of others. However, one should consider the specific disease condition of the patient and prescribe for him according to his needs rather than follow a standard formulation for all patients and remember that rehabilitation of nutritionally depleted patients is slow. Once parenteral nutrition is initiated, it should be pursued with vigor to improve the patient's nutritional status, assist his recovery, and permit prolonged treatment of underlying disease states. In some cases, the objective of nutritional therapy may be just for maintenance, because of the patient's clinical condition and nutritional needs. Substitution of intravenous feeding for oral feeding requires meticulous care and is inconvenient, time consuming, and expensive. Therefore, total parenteral nutrition (TPN) should be replaced by oral feeding as soon as the patient is able to eat a reasonable amount of food in an appropriate form.

In this chapter, the principles, nutrient requirements, techniques, and clinical use of parenteral nutrition in adults are briefly presented. For further information, readers are referred to reviews, proceedings of symposia, and books on this subject.[46,47,59,84,88,103,125,134,162,165]

Nutrient Requirements

The nutritional requirements in adults are generally similar when age, sex, height, and weight are considered. (For pediatric patients, see Chap. 14.) However, the principle of furnishing adequate nutrients to meet the needs of the specific patient should be the goal of nutritional support.

PROTEIN

Based on the nitrogen loss from all sources and other factors, the protein allowance for maintenance suggested by the (FAO/WHO) report is 0.6 g/kg/day of high quality protein. The allowance for the "mixed" proteins (proteins of high biological value and those of low biological value) of the United States diet is 0.8 g/kg/day. Thus, the allowance for a 70 kg man is 56 g of protein/day, and for a 55 kg woman, 44 g.[123] Expressed in terms of nitrogen, this is approximately 9.0 g/day.

Extreme environmental stress, infection, fever, trauma, and surgical procedure can result in substantial urinary loss of nitrogen. In illness or trauma that has led to severe protein depletion, requirement of proteins for repletion of wasted tissues is increased; this is comparable to infants and children who are in the state of rapid growth. The available information on any special increase in protein requirement in elderly people is not con-

clusive.[30,112,159,174] Cheng and colleagues and Zanni and associates show that the same amount of dietary protein per kilogram of body weight will bring both young and old into nitrogen equilibrium.[30,174] In the case of total parenteral nutrition, the nitrogen requirement has been reported to be 200 mg/kg/day to 416 mg/kg/day, as crystalline amino acids, to achieve nitrogen equilibrium. It has also been stated that the total nitrogen need in adult patients is 8 g to 16 g/day regardless of their age. Loirat and co-workers, studying stressed patients, have shown that nitrogen 9 g/M^2/day to 18 g/M^2/day are necessary to maintain nitrogen equilibrium. Burn patients required as much nitrogen as 20.7 g/M^2/day to 25.5 g/M^2/day during the acute catabolic phase. In my experience, 12 g/day to 13 g/day have been found adequate to maintain positive nitrogen balance in most of the patients except those with severe trauma, such as major burns and sepsis.[104,157] Recently, Shizgal and Forse have demonstrated that with the calorie intake of 50 Cal/kg/day, 1.28 g protein equivalent, or 200 mg nitrogen kg per day as crystalline amino acids, produced significant improvement in cell mass as shown by body composition studies after 14 days of total parenteral nutrition in malnourished patients.[142] The degree of stress, possible hypercatabolic state, and the special clinical condition, for instance, renal failure and hepatic insufficiency of the patient, affect the protein need and tolerance. In addition, adequate energy administered concurrently with nitrogen is of paramount importance to promote the nitrogen of amino acids utilization for protein synthesis.

SOLUTIONS FOR SUPPLYING NITROGEN IN PARENTERAL NUTRITION

Currently available preparations used as a nitrogen source in parenteral nutrition are protein hydrolysates, crystalline amino acids, plasma, and serum albumin.

Protein Hydrolysates. Four preparations of protein hydrolysates are currently available in the United States. They are prepared by either enzymatic hydrolysis of casein (Hyprotigen, CPH, and Travamin) or by acid hydrolysis of plasma fibrin (Aminosol). They are fortified by adding certain amino acids that have been destroyed during hydrolysis. In these preparations of partially hydrolyzed proteins, as much as 40% of the total amino acids may be in the form of short peptides of 2 to 4 amino acids. Utilization of the intravenously administered peptides is not as efficient as that of free amino acids, and their loss in the urine may be considerable.

In general, protein hydrolysates are fairly well tolerated, although mild adverse reactions such as nausea and vomiting are occasionally encountered. Decreasing the rate of infusion usually reduces the incidence of reactions. One gram of protein hydrolysate is equivalent to about 0.75 g protein. Such preparations are usually available as a 5% to 10% solution. Thus, protein hydrolysate of 75 g/day to 100 g/day, or 1.0 g to 1.5 g, or 20 ml/kg body weight/day to 30 ml/kg body weight/day should be sufficient for most of the patients except those with major burns or sepsis. However, the formulated amino acid solutions that are commonly used in the United States are considered as a better nitrogen source than the protein hydrolysate.

Crystalline Amino Acid Mixture. Recently, the use of crystalline amino acid mixtures in parenteral nutrition has been revived. The advantages of using amino acids are the following: (1) pure starting material, (2) composition of amino acids can be formulated according to needs, and (3) lack of peptides, which increases the usable nitrogen and re-

duces the urinary loss. Currently, four crystalline amino acid solutions are commercially available in the United States: (1) Aminosyn, (2) FreAmine III, (3) Travasol, and (4) VeinAmine. The amino acid composition of these solutions is shown in Table 13-1. There are several amino acid solutions available for parenteral nutrition in European countries (*e.g.*, Vamin and Aminofusin) and in Japan. In addition to the amino acid solutions for general use, preparations are available for patients with renal failure (see Table 13-2). A solution containing a high concentration of branch chain and a low concentration of aromatic amino acids has been used experimentally in animals and in patients with hepatic insufficiency (see Table 13-3).

PLASMA AND SERUM ALBUMIN

For the purpose of intravenous protein nutrition, neither plasma, nor serum albumin is a preparation of choice.

TABLE 13-1
Amino Acid Content of Solutions for Parenteral Nutrition in the US (mg/100 ml)*

Amino Acid†	Aminosyn‡ (7%)	Freamin III (8.5%)	Travasol‡ (8.5%)	Veinamine (8%)
Essential				
Isoleucine	510	590	406	493
Leusine	660	770	526	347
Lysine	510§	624§	492 (as HCl)	667 (as HCl)
Methionine	280	450	492	427
Phenoalanine	310	480	526	400
Threonine	370	340	356	160
Tryptophane	120	130	152	80
Valine	560	580	390	230
Nonessential				
Alanine	900	600	1760	—
Arginine	690	810	880	749
Histidine	210	240	372	237
Proline	610	950	356	107
Serine	300	500	—	—
Glycine	900	1190	1760	3387
Cysteine	—	20	—	—
Aspartic	—	—	—	400
Glutamic	—	—	—	426
Tryrosine	44	—	34	—
Total Nitrogen (g)	1.10	1.25	1.42	1.33

*Aminosyn (Abbott Laboratories), FreAmine III (American McGaw), Travasol (Travenol Laboratories), VeinAmine (Cutter Laboratories).

†Amino acids are in L-form.

‡Amino acid solution of other concentrations and with or without added electrolytes are also available.

§Does not include acetate salt.

(Chen WJ, Ohasi E, Kasai M: Amino acid metabolism in parenteral nutrition with special reference to the calorie: nitrogen ratio and the blood urea nitrogen level. Metabolism 23:1117, 1974. By permission of Grune & Stratton, NY)

TABLE 13-2
Composition of Amino Acid Solutions for Renal Failure

Amino Acid	Nephramine* (mg/100 ml)	Aminosyn–RF† (mg/100 ml)
L-isoleucine	560	462
L-leucine	880	726
L-lysine	900	535
	(acetate salt)	(Does not include acetate salt)
L-methionine	880	726
L-phenylalanine	880	726
L-threonine	400	330
L-tryptophan	200	165
L-valine	650	528
L-arginine	—	600
L-histidine	—	429

*American McGaw, 5.1 g amino acids and 0.58 g nitrogen/100 ml.
†Abbott Laboratories, 5.25 g amino acids and 0.78 g nitrogen/100 ml.

Selection of Solutions. When selecting an amino acid solution for parenteral nutrition, it is important to consider the following factors:

1. Total nitrogen given should be adequate.
2. All eight essential amino acids should be present in adequate amounts to meet the requirement (see Table 13-4) and in proper balance (see Table 13-5).
3. The E/T ratio (essential amino acids in grams divided by the total amount of nitrogen in grams) should be considered. This ratio in whole egg protein or a high quality protein is 3:2.
4. The percent of essential amino acids of total amino acids is also important. This ratio for adults and for infants is about 0.20 (20%) and 0.40 (40%), respectively, but suggestions have been made that it should be about 40% in adult patients given total parenteral nutrition, except for those with renal failure or hepatic insufficiency.
5. The presence of several nonessential amino acids is more effective in maintaining nitrogen balance than is the use of only one.[55,112] However, the amount of glycine should not be excessive in order to avoid an increase in blood ammonia.
6. L-amino acids are better employed than those in DL-form. Histidine has been found essential for growth in infants and perhaps also in uremic adults. Adequate amounts of arginine are needed to prevent hyperammonemia, and proline, after hydroxylation, is required for the synthesis of collagen, which is necessary for wound healing. In addition, alanine is the main form of transport for amino nitrogen between tissues, and it seems preferable to include this as a major part of the nonessential amino acids for parenteral nutrition.

TABLE 13-3
Amino Acid Solution for Hepatic Failure* (8% Amino Acids)

Component	Amount/100 ml
Amino Acids	
Essential:	
L-isoleucine	900 mg
L-leucine	1100 mg
L-lysine	610 mg
(as lysine acetate)	
L-methionine	100 mg
L-phenylalanine	100 mg
L-threonine	450 mg
L-tryptophan	66 mg
L-valine	840 mg
Nonessential:	
L-alanine	770 mg
L-arginine	600 mg
L-histidine	240 mg
L-proline	800 mg
L-serine	500 mg
Glycine	900 mg
L-cysteine·HC1·H$_2$O	< 20 mg
Phosphoric Acid, NF	115 mg
Sodium Bisulfite, USP	< 100 mg
Glacial Acetic Acid	Adjust pH to 6.5
Water for Injection, USP	qs

*Hepatamine™, Product of American McGaw. Has been approved by FDA for clinical use. All amino acids are U.S.P. This solution also contains the following electrolytes in mEq/liter: Na$^+$, 10; Cl$^-$ < 4; HPO$_4^{-2}$, 20; and acetate, 63. Nitrogen content, 1.21 g/100 ml. Protein equivalent, 7.6 g/100 ml.

A quantitative comparison of the amino acid content of the commercially available amino acid solutions with that of the whole egg protein is shown in Table 13-6, and comparison of the branch chain amino acid content with that of the whole egg protein is shown in Table 13-7. At the present, data from objectively controlled clinical studies are lacking to suggest any one of the available amino acid solutions as superior to others. When one is dealing with a specific clinical condition such as renal failure, hepatic insufficiency, or sepsis, it may be appropriate to select a preparation which could be more efficient and safe even if the documented evidence is less than conclusive. It may be pointed out also that the cost of crystalline amino acid solution is higher than that of protein hydrolysates, and cost factors may become important in selecting a particular crystalline amino acid solution.

ENERGY (CALORIES) REQUIREMENT

The Recommended Dietary Allowances (see Appendix Table A-1) suggest 2700 Cal and 2000 Cal/day for a young man or woman, respectively, be-

TABLE 13-4
The Requirement of Essential Acids in Human Adults*

| Requirement | Adult Women (Hegsted)† mg/kg | Adult Men | | Estimated for Repletion (Steffee et al)‡ mg/kg |
		(Rose)† mg/kg	(Inque et al.)† mg/kg	
Histidine	—	—	—	7.4
Isoleucine	10	10	11	10
Leucine	13	11	14	39
Lysine	10	9	12	54
Methionine & Cysteine	13	14	11	16
Phenylalanine & Tyrosine	13	14	14	57
Threonine	7	6	6	11
Tryptophan	3.1	3.2	2.6	4.3
Valine	11	14	14	20
Total Essential Amino Acids	80	81	85	219

*Results were obtained in studies with oral feeding.

†Summarized by Munro HN: Protein hydrolysate and amino acids. In White PL, Nagy ME (eds): Total Parenteral Nutrition, Acton, Publishing Sciences Group, 1974.

‡Calculated by Shenkin A, Wretlind A: Parenteral nutrition. World Rev Nutr Diet 28:1, 1978; from data of Steffee CH, Wissler RW, Hamphreys EM, et al: Studies in amino acid utilization. V. The determination of minimum daily essential amino acid requirements in protein-depleted adult male rats. J Nutr 40:483, 1950.

tween 23 and 50 years of age, who is engaged in moderate physical activities. The estimation of total caloric requirement is shown in Table 13-8. The energy expenditure is progressively decreased with age. Calories given should be adequate to maintain the body weight in patients who are in a reasonably good nutritive state; this is about 35 Cal/kg/day. In patients who have lost considerable weight, more calories are necessary to achieve weight gain; in some cases, 55 Cal/kg a day or more need to be given (see Table 13-9). As illustrated in Figures 13-1, 13-2 and 13-3, energy expenditure, as well as nitrogen loss, is further increased in patients with severe trauma or sepsis.[85,121] Utilization of amino acids or nitrogen for protein synthesis cannot be accomplished to the fullest extent without concomitant administration of adequate calories. On the other hand, further prevention of nitrogen loss cannot be achieved with a daily energy intake beyond 900 Cal if no protein is administered (see Fig. 13-4).

Although some amino acids are used for energy, it is suggested that only nonprotein calories should be considered. Since the monohydrate of glucose is used in the United States, 3.4 Cal/g should be used for calculation. Each gram of fat and ethanol furnishes 9 and 7 Cal respectively, if completely oxidized.

SOURCE

Glucose (Dextrose). In the common American diet, carbohydrates are consumed primarily as starch. Some sucrose and a small amount of lactose are also ingested. After digestion in the intestine, monosaccharides, which consist typically of about 80% glucose, 15% fructose, and 5% lactose, are formed. Generally, carbohydrates of American diets supply about 35% to 60% of the total daily calories. In a healthy individual the brain may require about 120 g to 140 g glucose per day. Nervous tissue also fills about 20% to 30% of its energy requirement with glucose. Without glucose, gluconeogenesis from amino acids will be increased, and ketosis will occur. Thus, glucose is used as the nonprotein energy source of choice in parenteral nutrition. Concentrations of commercially available glucose solutions are 5% to 70% for parenteral nutrition. However, the glucose concentration of solutions given to patients maintained on central venous parenteral nutrition is usually 20% to 45%. This is necessary in order to supply the daily need of about 3000 Cal when fat is not given. Excessive amounts of glucose may result in increased fat synthesis and storage, and in excessive carbon dioxide production, leading to severe respiratory distress in some patients.[10,27]

TABLE 13-5
Ideal Dietary Essential Amino Acid Pattern, Whole Egg, FAO Recommendation and the Minimum Requirement of Rose*

Amino Acid	Ideal Protein†	Whole Egg	FAO‡	Rose§
Isoleucine	4.5	5.6	4.5	4.2 (0.70)
Leucine	6.8	6.4	5.1	6.6 (1.10)
Lysine	5.2	5.0	4.5	4.8 (0.80)
Methionine	3.7	2.9	2.4	
Methionine + Cysteine	5.5	4.5	4.5	6.6 (1.10)
Phenylalanine + Tyrosine	8.0	7.5	6.0	6.6 (1.10)
Tryptophan	1.0	0.9	1.5	1.5 (0.25)
Valine	4.3	5.1	4.5	4.8 (0.80)
Threonine	3.0	3.0	3.0	3.0 (0.50)

*Relative figures achieved by setting threonine at 3 to make comparison.

†Longenecker JB: In Albanese AA (ed): New Methods of Nutritional Biochemistry. New York, Academic Press, 1963.

‡Protein Requirement. Report of a Joint FAO/WHO Experts Group, WHO Technical Report series, No. 301, 1965.

§Rose WC: The amino acid requirements in adult man. Nutr Abst Rev 27:631, 1957. Figures in parentheses are minimum requirements of Rose. The values of methionine and phenylalanine were attained when no cysteine or tyrosine was added to the diet; cysteine was found to spare methionine requirement by 80% to 89%, and tyrosine was found to spare phenylalanine requirement by 70% to 75%.

TABLE 13-6
Amino Acid Content of Solutions for Parenteral Nutrition in the US (g per 16 g nitrogen)

Essential Amino Acid	Whole Egg	Aminosyn*	FreAmine III†	Travasol‡	VeinAmine‖
Isoleucine	6.6	7.4 (112)§	7.3 (111)§	4.5 (69)	4.2 (63)
Leucine	8.8	9.6 (109)	9.5 (111)	5.9 (67)	5.9 (67)
Lysine	6.4	7.4 (116)	7.6 (119)	5.9 (91)	6.4 (100)
Methionine	3.1	4.1 (131)	5.5 (178)	5.9 (189)	5.1 (165)
Cysteine	2.4	—	0.24 (10)	—	—
Phenylalanine	5.8	4.5 (78.0)	5.9 (102)	5.9 (102)	4.8 (82)
Tyrosine	4.2	0.96 (23)	—	0.40 (9)	—
Threonine	5.1	5.4 (105)	4.2 (82)	4.0 (78)	1.9 (37)
Tryptophan	1.6	1.7 (109)	1.6 (100)	1.8 (113)	0.96 (60)
Valine	7.3	8.1 (112)	6.9 (94)	4.4 (60)	3.0 (41)
Total Essential a.a./16 g nitrogen	51.3	49.2	48.7	38.6	32.5

Nonessential Amino Acid					
Alanine	7.4	13.0 (176)	7.4 (100)	20.9 (282)	—
Arginine	6.1	10 (164)	10 (164)	10.5 (172)	9.0 (147)
Histidine	2.4	3.1 (129)	3.0 (123)	4.4 (183)	2.8 (117)
Proline	8.1	8.9 (110)	11.7 (144)	4.2 (52)	2.8 (16)
Serine	8.5	4.4 (52)	6.2 (72)	—	—
Glutamic Acid	16.0	—	—	—	5.1
Aspartic Acid	9.0	—	—	—	4.8
Glycine	—	13.1	14.7	19.7	40.6
% Nitrogen from Glycine	—	15.2	16.8	23.0	47.5
Total Nonessential a.a./16 g Nitrogen	57.5	52.3	53.0	59.8	63.6
Total a.a. per 16 g Nitrogen	109	102	101.7	98.3	96
E/T Ratio	3.2	3.1	3.2	2.4	2.4
% Essential of Total a.a.	47	48	48	39	33.7

*Abbott Laboratories
†American McGaw
‡Travenol Laboratories
‖Cutter Laboratories
§Figure in parentheses represents % of the whole egg.
Modified from Rusho WJ, Standish R, and Bair JN: A comparison of crystalline amino acid solutions in parenteral nutrition. Hospital Formulary, Jan 1981, p 29.

TABLE 13-7
Branched-Chain Amino Acids in Amino Acid Solutions for Parenteral Nutrition in the US (g per 16 g nitrogen)

Branched-Chain Amino Acid	Egg	Aminosyn*	FreAmine III†	Travasol§	VeinAmine‡
Isoleucine	6.6	7.4	7.3	4.5	4.2
Leucine	8.8	9.6	9.5	5.9	5.9
Valine	7.3	8.1	6.9	4.4	3.0

*Abbott Laboratories
†American McGaw
§Travenol Laboratories
‡Cutter Laboratories
From Rusho WJ, Standish R, and Bair JN: A comparison of crystalline amino acid solutions in parenteral nutrition. Hospital Formulary, Jan 1981, p 29.

TABLE 13-8
Estimated Total Caloric Need

Requirement	Patient		
	1	*2*	*3*
Calculated basal*	1449	1701	1853
Fever (8% of basal/1°F)	81	272	444
Specific dynamic action (8% of basal)	135	136	148
Bed activity (30% of basal)	506	510	556
Total estimated	2171	2619	3001
Total measured†	2422	2653	2925

*From the DuBois chart on the basis of the height, age, and sex of the patient

†Determined by Jones Metabolism apparatus. From Rice CD, Orr B, and Enquist L: Parenteral nutrition in surgical patients as provided from glucose, amino acids and alcohol—the role played by alcohol. Ann Surg 131:289, 1950

TABLE 13-9
Daily Caloric Intake of Average (70 kg) Man Under Normal and Surgical Conditions*

Condition	Normal BMR	Measured Resting Expenditure		Caloric Intake (RME + 50%)
		ΔBMR (%)	*Cal*	
Normal	1,800			
Postoperative	1,800		1,800	2,700
Multiple fractures	1,800	+20	2,160	3,240
Major sepsis	1,800	+40	2,520	3,780
Major burn	1,800	+80	3,240	4,860

*From Kinney JM: Energy requirement for parenteral nutrition. In Fischer JE (ed): Total Parenteral Nutrition p 135, Boston, Little, Brown, 1976

BMR, basal metabolic rate

RME, resting metabolic expenditure

Fructose (Levulose). Since glucose intolerance exists in many conditions such as severe trauma, major surgery, diabetes mellitus, hepatic disease, uremia, sepsis, and excessive stress, studies on the use of glucose substitutes have been conducted, including fructose and invert sugar. Fructose is also a physiologic sugar; its quantity in the body is smaller than glucose. Fructose is less insulin dependent, does not produce hyperglycemia, and its loss in the urine is small. It is rapidly transformed into glycogen in hepatocytes, and inhibits gluconeogenesis in the liver, and thus spares amino acids. It has been reported that intravenous administration of fructose produced lactic acidosis, hyperuricemia, and depletion of adenosine triphosphate. These changes are observed in studies involving administration of relatively larger amounts of fruc-

tose injected in short periods of time. It is not likely, however, that fructose will replace glucose as the sole source of calories in long-term parenteral nutrition. Fructose intolerance has been reported in some individuals. Dietary history must rule out this possibility before fructose is administered.

INVERT SUGAR OR COMBINATION OF GLUCOSE AND FRUCTOSE

Invert sugar is a hydrolytic product of sucrose composed of equal amounts of fructose and glucose. Recent observations at Vanderbilt University Medical Center suggest that the use of a mixture consisting of 10% fructose and 10% glucose is better tolerated than is a 20% glucose solution in premature and postoperative infants. Meng and co-

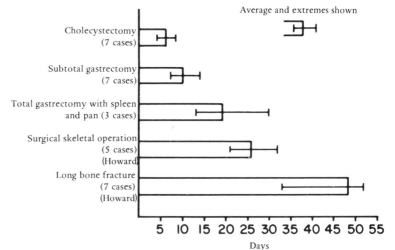

FIG. 13-1 Duration of negative nitrogen balance following surgically uncomplicated operation or trauma. (Randall HT: Indications for parenteral nutrition in postoperative catabolic states. In Meng HC, Law DH (eds): Parenteral Nutrition, p 13. Springfield, Ill., Charles C Thomas, 1970)

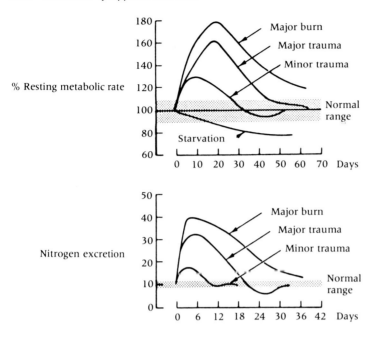

FIG. 13-2   Hypermetabolism and increased nitrogen excretion are closely related following minor or major trauma or major burn injury. Patients received 12 g nitrogen intake per day. (Adapted by Wilmore DW: The Metabolic Management of Critical Ill, New York, Plenum Book Company, 1977.) Data from Kinney JM: Energy deficits in acute illness and injury. In Morgan AP (ed): Proceedings of a Conference on Energy Metabolism and Body Fuel Utilization, p 150, Cambridge, Harvard University Press, 1966. Courtesy Plenum Medical Book Company, New York.

workers have also observed better tolerance in adult postoperative patients for esophageal cancer given a combination of 15% fructose and 10% glucose than in those given 25% glucose.[106] Further study on the use of a mixture of fructose and glucose of various ratios and of invert sugar is warranted. Currently, 5% and 10% fructose, and invert sugar, are commercially available. Invert sugar must not be given to patients with fructose intolerance.

Sorbitol and Xylitol.   Sorbitol is a 6-carbon sugar alcohol. It is oxidized to fructose and then converted to glucose; it is metabolized as such thereafter. Sorbitol, as 5% to 30% solution, has also

been used in parenteral nutrition in Europe. Urinary loss has been found as high as 25% of the total amount administered intravenously. It is not commercially available in the United States.

Xylitol is a 5-carbon sugar alcohol. Conversion of xylitol to glycogen occurs by means of the pentose phosphate pathway. As high as 86% of xylitol may be transformed into glucose, and it has a strong antiketogenic effect. Xylitol is also less insulin dependent. Clinical use of xylitol in parenteral nutrition has been reported in Germany and Japan. Owing to toxicities (*e.g.*, hyperuricemia, hyperbilirubinemia and renal insufficiency) observed following the intravenous administration of xylitol,

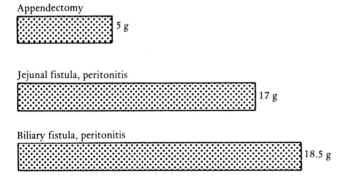

Appendectomy
5 g

Jejunal fistula, peritonitis
17 g

Biliary fistula, peritonitis
18.5 g

Ruptured aortic aneurysm, renal failure, sepsis
21 g

FIG. 13-3   Comparative daily nitrogen losses after surgery of a 70-kg man. (Lawson LJ: Bri J Surg 52:795, 1965. Courtesy John Wright and Sons, Bristol, England)

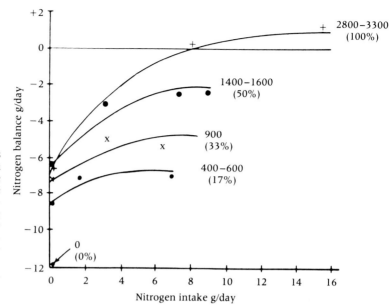

FIG. 13-4 Nitrogen balance increases with the addition of energy or nitrogen to the diet. The range of caloric intake is listed to the right of each isobar. The number in parentheses below each calorie-intake value expresses total calorie intake as a percentage of total daily metabolic expenditure. (Data from Calloway DH, Spector H: Am J Clin Nutr 2:405, 1954. Adapted by Wilmore DW: The Metabolic Management of Critical Ill, New York, Plenum Book Company, p 197, 1977)

its clinical use for parenteral nutrition in the United States has been cautious and hesitant. However, long-term studies in dogs show that xylitol is fairly well tolerated when the total daily dosage is not excessive (10 g/kg/day), the infusion rate is not more than 0.4 g/kg/day, and the concentration of the solution is not above 15%.[99] It has also been reported that when giving xylitol in combination with other sugars (glucose, fructose, and sorbitol), adverse effects have not been encountered.

Maltose. It has been reported that intravenous (IV) maltose is metabolized. An advantage of IV maltose is that it is less osmolar as compared to glucose of the same concentration. Signer and associates report that maltose is tolerated by dogs and can be used for parenteral nutrition.[141] Recently, Andersen and associates have given 12% of total daily energy as glucose or maltose in growing miniature pigs.[9] Based on the chemical analyses of the urine, both glucose and maltose are used, although maltose was used less well (87%) than glucose (99%). Growth and body composition data also indicate maltose utilization. Maltose use may minimize the adverse effects frequently encountered in patients given hyperosmolar glucose. The use of maltose for parenteral nutrition in man has not been studied.

Glycerol. The caloric value of glycerol is approximately the same as that of glucose. Given as a diluted solution in moderate dosages, glycerol is

tolerated by man and animals. Large doses of glycerol can cause hemolysis, hypotension, central nervous disturbances, and convulsions. Its substitution for glucose in parenteral nutrition does not appear warranted except for special reasons. Currently, glycerol at a concentration of 2.25% or 2.5% is used in the preparation of fat emulsions to make them isotonic. The utilization of the intravenously infused glycerol or of glycerol in Intralipid has been reported.[170]

Alcohol (Ethanol). Ethyl alcohol supplies 7 Cal/g if completely oxidized. The liver is the main site of its metabolism, and the rate of metabolism has been estimated to be 100 mg/kg/hr to 200 mg/kg/hr, but the range of individual differences is large. Evidence for utilization of the intravenous alcohol as an energy source has been reported. It is usually given as a 2.5% to 5% solution. Rice and associates have used alcohol in parenteral nutrition and have demonstrated its nitrogen-sparing effect.[124] However, the rate of alcohol infusion must be carefully controlled so that blood levels are not higher than 0.08% or even 0.05% in order to avoid intoxication and urinary loss. It should be remembered that hepatotoxic effects have been noted despite the consumption of an adequate diet (see Chap. 15). It has also been reported that older debilitated patients often do not tolerate even diluted solutions of alcohol well. Thus the use of alcohol in parenteral nutrition is not recommended, although there may be times when it seems appropriate because of its tranquilizing effect.

TABLE 13-10
Composition of Fat Emulsions

Component	Fat Emulsion			
	Intralipid*		Liposyn†	
	10%	20%	10%	20%
Soy bean oil (g)	10	20	—	—
Safflower oil (g)	—	—	10	20
Egg yolk phosphatides (g)	1.2	1.2	1.2	1.2
Glycerol (g)	2.25	2.25	2.5	2.5
Water to (ml)	100	100	100	100

*Cutter (Vitrum) Laboratories
†Abbott Laboratories

FATS

Fat, as an important or essential nutrient, should be given in parenteral nutrition to make the intravenous feeding regimen "complete." It is not only a concentrated source of energy (9 Cal/g), providing a large amount of calories in a small volume of water, which may be advantageous in some patients, but it also supplies essential fatty acids. Essential fatty acid deficiency has been observed in adult patients as well as infants and children on long-term parenteral nutrition devoid of fat and in those who are fasting in a variety of diseases. [11,31,64,114,126] Fat emulsions, as prepared, are isotonic and may be infused into a peripheral vein.

Currently, two fat emulsions (Intralipid and Liposyn) for parenteral nutrition are available in the United States. The composition of these fat emulsions and the major fatty acid composition of soybean, safflower, and corn oils, are shown in Tables 13-10 and 13-11. Much work has been done on the safety and efficacy of Intralipid[61,95,96,106,171] and of Liposyn.[15,34,149] They are well tolerated and are

TABLE 13-11
Fatty Acid Composition of Corn, Safflower and Soybean Oils

Major Fatty Acids*	Percent of Total Fatty Acids		
	Corn	Safflower	Soybean
Palmitic, 16:0	13	7	11
Oleic, 18:1ω9	28	13	23
Stearic, 18:0	2.5	2.5	4
Linoleic, 18:2ω6	55	75–78	52–54
α-Linolenic, 18:3ω3	0.8	0–0.5	8
Arachidonic, 20:4ω6	Trace	Trace	Trace

*Short hand notations of fatty acids: the number preceding the colon represents the number of carbons in the fatty acid molecule; the number immediately following the colon denotes the number of double bonds; the number after the Greek letter *omega*, ω, indicates the carbon position of the double bond from the methyl terminal of the molecule.

effective as a source of essential fatty acids and calories. Severe toxic effects, such as *overloading syndrome,* which were observed in some patients given Lipomul, a 15% cottonseed oil emulsions were not encountered.[90,102] (Lipomul was withdrawn from the market by the manufacturer in 1964.) Other fat emulsions are available in other countries, for instance, Lipofundin S. (Germany), Lipophysan (France), and Intrafat and Intralipos (Japan). In addition, two fat emulsions are available in Europe that also contain added amino acids: Nutrifundin (Germany) and Trivemil (France). These preparations are not available in the United States.

ESSENTIAL FATTY ACIDS

Certain polyunsaturated fatty acids have been found essential for growth, proper health maintenance, and biological processes (see Chap. 2). Their functions in the maintenance of skin, hair, and integrity of cell membrane, regulation of cholesterol metabolism, among others, are well known. Essential fatty acid deficiency delays wound healing and may increase the susceptibility to infection.[70] It has been recognized that many polyunsaturated fatty acids have essential fatty acid activities, but the three most important are linoleic (18:2ω6), α-linolenic (18:3ω3), and arachidonic (20:4ω6). The numbers in parentheses are shorthand notations for the acids. The number preceding the colon represents the number of carbons, and the number immediately following the colon denotes the number of double bonds; the number after the Greek letter omega (ω) indicates the carbon position of the double bond from the methyl terminal of the molecule. Although arachidonic acid is listed as an essential fatty acid and may be the most important polyunsaturated fatty acid for the mammal, it does not need to be supplied in the diet; under normal conditions mammalian tissue has the ability to convert linoleic to arachidonic acid (except in the cat). However, linoleic acid cannot be synthesized by the mammal and must be supplied in the diet.

It is well known that dihomo-gamma-linolenic acid (20:3ω6), which is converted from linoleic (18:2ω6) and the immediate precursor of arachidonic acid, is the precursor of the series 1-prostaglandins (*e.g.,* PGE$_1$). Arachidonic acid (20:4ω6) is the precursor of the series 2-prostaglandins (*e.g.,* PGE$_2$, PGF$_2\alpha$). Alpha-linolenic acid (18:3ω3) is considered essential, but its requirement is probably small. It supports growth of rats but does not effectively cure dermal changes in animals deprived of linoleic or arachidonic acid. Alpha-linolenic acid is converted mainly to the docosahexaenoic acid (22:6ω3) of glycerophosphatides, which are thought to be necessary to maintain membrane integrity of the cell and its organelles. The immediate precursor of docosahexaenoic is Δ-eicosapentaenoic acid (20:5ω3), which serves as a precursor of the series 3-prostaglandins (*e.g.*, PGE_3). It has been found difficult to deplete tissue docosahexaenoic acid in animals fed diets deprived of α-linolenic acid.

In patients or animals fed a fat-free diet or deprived of essential fatty acids, saturated fatty acids are biosynthesized in the body. Plasma palmitoleic (16:1ω7) and oleic (18:1ω9) are usually elevated. Oleic acid is converted to $\Delta^{5,8,11}$-eicosatrienoic (20:3ω9). Eicosatrienoic acid (20:3ω9) in plasma or tissue is very low or not detectable in persons consuming adequate essential fatty acids. However, it is elevated, and linoleic and arachidonic acids are decreased, in patients maintained on a fat-free diet, or on total parenteral nutrition devoid of fat. Therefore, the triene (eicosatrienoic acid, 29:3ω9) to tetraene (arachidonic acid, 20:4ω6) ratio (T/T) is increased. T/T of 0.4 or greater has been considered as a biochemically essential fatty acid deficiency; this ratio has been lowered to 0.2 or greater, since the plasma eicosatrienoic acid (20:3ω9) in individuals consuming normal American diets is rarely detectable.

The exact requirement of essential fatty acids in man is not clearly defined. Collins and associates suggest that at least 7.5 g linoleic acid/day, furnishing 2.2% of the total caloric intake, are necessary to correct essential fatty acid deficiency.[31] However, at this intake, the plasma T/T (eicosatrienoic acid, 20:3ω9 to arachidonic acid, 20:4ω6) remained greater than 0.3. When 22.5 g of linoleic acid per day furnishing 6.4% of the total caloric intake were given, the percentage of eicosatrienoic acid decreased from 9.9% to 1.2% of the total plasma fatty acids after the first day of treatment. Jeejeebhoy and co-workers suggest that 25 g linoleic acid per day may be required.[75] Perhaps the essential fatty acid requirement in man is within the ranges of 7.5 g/day to 25 g/day. However, this range may represent the requirement for therapy and not that for maintenance. The severity of deficiency and the period of time necessary for correction may affect the dosage required. It is interesting that Press and associates have daily applied and rubbed 230 mg sunflower oil (containing 120 mg linoleic acid) on the surface of one forearm of 3 adult patients with essential fatty acid deficiency.[119] They found that this treatment was capable of increasing the levels of linoleic and arachidonic acids, and decreasing eicosatrienoic acid (20:3ω9) in the serum toward normal. These results suggest that the daily requirement of essential fatty acids may be as low as 2 mg/kg/day to 3 mg/kg/day. It seems generally agreed that the optimal requirement for linoleic

acid in infants and children is 4% of the total caloric intake, as originally suggested by Holman and associates.[67] It should be recognized that the increase in metabolic demand associated with growth, hypermetabolism following injury, sepsis, or stress in adults aggravates or accentuates essential fatty acid deficiency. According to the experience of the author and other investigators, 500 ml of a 10% fat emulsion twice or three times a week should be adequate in *nonstress* patients to maintain the normal essential fatty acid status. However, daily infusion of 500 ml of a 10% fat emulsion may be needed for the correction of essential fatty acid deficiency. In patients maintained on home parenteral nutrition who can take some food by mouth, 10 ml corn or safflower oil three times a day should be adequate to prevent biochemical essential fatty acid deficiency.

OPTIMAL REQUIREMENT

The optimal requirement of fat in terms of calories is not known. Based on the daily fat intake in the United States, it is about 1.5 g/kg to 2.5 g/kg in individuals consuming 2500 to 3500 Cal. The importance of fat or triglyceride in nutrition other than as a source of essential fatty acids was suggested by Deuel and colleagues. In later communications the same group of workers reported that greater growth was found in rats fed 30% cottonseed oil diets than in those on a low-fat diet supplemented with an optimum quantity of methyl linoleate or a combination of methyl linoleate and methyl arachidonate. Meng and Youmans showed that more calories are required per gram of weight gain/day in rats fed a fat-free diet than in those given diet containing 5% or 25% fat. These authors also administered isonitrogenous nutrients through a central vein to dogs; only those receiving fat emulsion gained weight.[98,108] Administration of adequate amounts of methylesters of linoleic and arachidonic acids to the dogs receiving total parenteral nutrition without fat prevented the essential fatty acid deficiency but did not correct the weight loss. Recently, Heird and associates analyzed the data on the relationship between caloric intake and weight gain, and nitrogen balance in infants receiving parenteral nutrition, as reported by Borresen and associates.[63] They state that despite administration of fewer total calories (86 Cal/kg/day–100 Cal/kg/day) and less nitrogen, the weight gains and nitrogen balances were equivalent to those demonstrated by Dudrick and associates, giving 115 Cal/kg/day to 120 Cal/kg/day, and 4 g of protein/kg/day. The difference in the two regimens was that fat as a soybean oil emulsion (Intralipid), in a dosage of 3 g/kg/day to 4 g/kg/day was given along with amino acids and other nutrients by Borresen and co-workers, while fat was not administered by Dudrick and associates. Jeejeebhoy and associates reported that only 35 Cal/kg/day supplied by soybean oil emulsion (also Intralipid) and carbohydrate seemed adequate to maintain weight and nitrogen equilibrium; in this study fat furnished 40% to 50% of the total caloric intake.[75] Fat as a calorie source for protein sparing has also been demonstrated by others. However, the importance of fat as a calorie source in comparison with glucose in parenteral nutrition may depend on the nutritional state and clinical condition of the patient. Long and colleagues have presented results obtained from studies in critically ill patients maintained on total parenteral nutrition showing that inclusion of fat emulsion did not affect the nitrogen excretion at any level of carbohydrate intake when a nitrogen intake was maintained constant at 11.7 g/M^2/day.[92] They suggested that when a primary clinical goal is nitrogen conservation, carbohydrate calories should be given in amounts approximating the resting metabolic rate. Additional calories can be given as intravenous fat emulsion. On the other hand, Jeejeebhoy and associates compared the two different calorie sources in patients who were markedly depleted because of severe gastrointestinal diseases, evaluating each regimen during a one-week study and then switching to the other regime.[73] With an isonitrogenous intake, no difference was observed when comparing fat-rich intravenous nutrition with the isocaloric carbohydrate administration. Wolfe and associates conducted studies evaluating fat and carbohydrate calories in normal fasting subjects.[170] Nitrogen equilibrium or positive nitrogen balance was associated with the quantity of nitrogen and energy administered regardless of the energy source. It seems that fat is not as effective as carbohydrate in promoting nitrogen equilibrium in hypercatabolic patients, but these two energy sources are equally effective in starved, depleted patients. It is clear that fat alone is not as effective as glucose in protein-sparing. In fact, it may cause further increase in nitrogen loss in some patients. Thus, fat emulsion should not be administered without amino acids and glucose in parenteral nutrition, but must be given in combination with carbohydrate with adequate nitrogen for protein synthesis.

The daily dosage of fat given to most adult patients receiving parenteral nutrition is 1.0 g/kg to 2.5 g/kg body weight. However, some investigators have given as much as 6.6 g/kg/day to adult patients; this is not recommended. It should be remembered that the daily dosage of fat given should be below the metabolic capacity of the patient receiving long-term parenteral nutrition so that a margin of safety is preserved to avoid "overloading" or other adverse effects.

Various fat emulsions administered intravenously are known to result in deposition of pigments, the so-called *intravenous fat pigments,* in the reticuloendothelial cells of the bone marrow, lymph nodes, spleen, and the liver of man and animals. To date, no adverse effects can be attributed to these histologic changes.

Fat emulsions are contraindicated in patients with hyperlipidemia or with disorders leading to failure in clearing triglycerides from the blood circulation. Occasionally, fat emulsion may produce leucopenia, thrombocytopenia, and anemia. Patients with marked decrease in platelets or leucocytes should be monitored closely. Close monitoring is also necessary in patients with hyperbilirubinemia. Severe liver damage has been considered as a contraindication for fat emulsion. However, Intralipid up to 100 g of fat/day has been given to patients with moderate to severe liver disease without deleterious effect on liver function.

CARBOHYDRATE–FAT CALORIE RATIO

The optimal ratio of carbohydrate to fat calorie ratio is not known. In newborn infants on breast milk, 50%, 38% and 12% of the total caloric intake is supplied by fat, carbohydrate, and protein, respectively. Based on the average daily consumption of fat per person in the United States, the calories contributed by fat range from 30% to 55% of the total intake in most individuals. Since the percent of calories supplied by protein is usually 10% to 15%, the carbohydrate fraction probably ranges between 60% and 30%. It has been suggested that with adequate nitrogen and energy, the carbohydrate:fat calorie ratio should be close to 1:1. In some countries, the dietary fat intake is low, contributing about 10% to 15% of the total caloric intake. It is clear that the carbohydrate to fat calorie ratio of food consumed orally varies widely, and it is difficult to suggest what may be the optimal carbohydrate to fat calorie ratio for parenteral nutrition. It seems, however, that a minimum of 10% to 15% and a maximum of 60% of the total caloric intake may be given as fat with 20% to 50% of the total caloric intake supplied as fat a reasonable suggestion. In protein-depleted rats given total parenteral nutrition, Stein and associates observed that a nonprotein energy intake supplied by glucose, 75%, and by fat, 25%, was superior to 100% as glucose or 100% as fat.[152] Our findings concur. Although as much as 80% of total calories as fat have been given in some recent studies, the needs and disease states of the individual patients must be taken into consideration.

CALORIE–NITROGEN RATIO

The importance of the energy–nitrogen relationship is exemplified in Table 13-12. It is noted that giving only 5% or 10% glucose without nitrogenous nutrients does not provide adequate calories, and would result in a marked negative balance. Increasing both nitrogen and caloric intake can significantly reduce the nitrogen loss. Calloway and Spector review the relationship between nitrogen and energy intake and nitrogen equilibrium.[25] Their findings show that for normal, young, active men on a protein-free diet, the negative nitrogen balance can be maximally reduced by supplying about 700 to 900 nonprotein calories; further protein-sparing effect is not observed, even if the intake is increased to as high as 2800 Cal in the absence of protein. When the energy intake is 2800 Cal, nitrogen equilibrium is achieved with a daily nitrogen intake of about 8.5 g; the energy-nitrogen ratio in this case is about 410:1. The energy–nitrogen relationship observed by Calloway and Spector as modified by Wilmore is shown in Figure 13-4.[165] Using the estimations on body weight loss as results of fasting, elective surgery, trauma, and sepsis, Kinney suggests a calorie–nitrogen ratio of about 120:1 to 180:1.[79] At Vanderbilt University Medical Center, patients (excluding those with major burns) given parenteral nutrition, receive a daily intake of nonprotein (glucose) calories and nitrogen (crystalline amino acids), which is approximately 2532 (42 Cal/kg per day) and 12.5 g (210 mg/kg per day) respectively; the calorie–nitrogen ratio is 202:1. The protein contribution to the total caloric intake (glu-

cose + protein) is about 11%. In one later study, it was found that nitrogen equilibrium was achieved with a daily nitrogen intake of about 270 mg/kg and 35 Cal/kg/day (see Fig. 13-5).[24] Wilmore reports that the nitrogen requirement is 21 g/M^2 body surface/day to 25 g/M^2 body surface/day during the period of 30 to 40 days postburn. With the combination of tube feeding and intravenous nutrition, 4000 Cal to 8000 Cal were given daily. This amount was able to correct the negative nitrogen balance. The nitrogen–calorie ratio of these regimens is certainly greater than 200:1.

Recently, Chen and associates studied the energy–nitrogen relationship in dogs given total parenteral nutrition.[29] They found that with an amino acid intake of 250 mg/kg/day to 300 mg/kg/day remaining constant, blood urea nitrogen was decreased when the caloric intake was increased until a nitrogen to energy ratio of 450:1 is reached. Figure 13-6 shows this relationship. Johnston has reviewed the calorie–nitrogen relationship and nitrogen balance.[77] Findings of Peters and Fischer show that a calorie to nitrogen ratio of 163 appeared to be most efficacious in stable patients receiving total parenteral nutrition.[118] Recently, Smith and associates reported that caloric and nitrogen of 53.4 Cal and 360 mg/kg/day, respectively, are required to prevent net body loss of protein; the calorie to nitrogen ratio is 135:1.[146] As Table 13-13 shows, the primary factor of importance to achieve positive nitrogen balance depends on the adequacy of nitrogen and energy intake. Nitrogen to energy ratio may be of secondary consideration. When either calorie or nitrogen is relatively low, a calorie to

TABLE 13-12
Nitrogen Balance of Patients on Parenteral Nutrition: Nitrogen–Energy Relationship

Author	Surgical Procedure	Nitrogen Intake (g/kg)	Cal/kg	Operation	1	2	3	4	Cumulative Nitrogen Balance
				Daily Nitrogen Balance (g)					
Krieger *et al*§	Subtotal	0 (10)*	13	− 13.7	− 11.6	− 12.4	− 10.7	− 12.8	− 57.9 (− 11.6)†
	Gastric	0.17 (6)	23	− 2.6	− 9.4	− 9.4	− 8.2	− 8.6	− 38.2 (− 7.6)
	Resection	0.28 (10)	38	− 3.3	− 1.2	− 1.2	− 3.2	− 2.9	− 7.3 (− 1.5)
Wadstrom,	Cholecystectomy	0 (10)	10						− 11.9 (− 6.0)†
Wirklund‖		0.10	10						− 4.8 (− 2.4)
		0.10	35						− 1.2 (− 0.6)
Heller#	Hysterectomy	0 (10)	0	− 7.4	− 9.3	− 6.8			− 23.5 (− 7.8)†
		50‡ (9)	0	− 4.5	− 4.3	− 3.7			− 12.5 (− 4.2)
		50‡ (19)	1000**	− 3.4	− 2.3	− 2.3			− 8.0 (− 2.7)

*Figures in parentheses are the number of patients

†Figures in parentheses represent average nitrogen balance per day

‡50 g amino acids as Aminofusin L-600, which represents about 7.6 g nitrogen/day et al:

§Krieger H, Abbott WE, Leavy S, et al: The use of a fat emulsion as a source of calorie in patient requiring intravenous alimentation. Gastroenterol 33:807, 1957

‖Wadstrom LB, Wirklund PE: Effect of fat emulsion on nitrogen balance in the postoperative period. Acta Chir Scand. 325:50, 1964

#Heller L: Clinical and experimental studies on complete parenteral nutrition. Scand J Gastroenterol (4 suppl) 3:7, 1969

**1000 Cal/day/patient

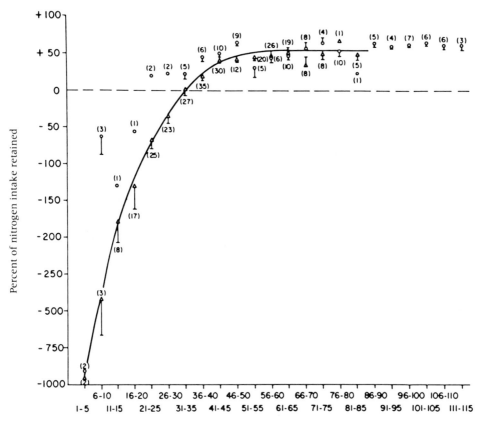

FIG. 13-5   Effect of increasing the daily nonprotein caloric intake on the percent of infused amino acid nitrogen retained. Mean ± SEM (number of patients). O, children. Δ, adults. (Caldwell MD, O'Neill JA Jr, Meng HC: Ann Surg 185:153, 1977)

nitrogen ratio of 200:1 seems more efficacious. In addition, one must consider the amino acid pattern and the condition of patient. It may be pointed out that the objectives of total parenteral nutrition should be considered: body weight gain, positive nitrogen balance, or improvement of body composition, such as increase in lean body mass, intracellular nitrogen, and potassium retention.

VITAMINS

The knowledge of vitamin requirements in total parenteral nutrition is meager. In addition, patients who require total parenteral nutrition are under stress, nutritionally depleted, critically ill, septic, or any combination of these. Such conditions may further alter vitamin requirements. Vitamin deficiency will result if vitamin-free parenteral nutrition is administered, especially in nutritionally depleted patients. Generally, vitamins given to patients

receiving parenteral nutrition are based on assumptions made from oral requirements previously established. In addition, the dosages of vitamins are also subject to the availability of preparations that can be obtained commercially. Parenteral vitamin preparation administered rapidly as a separate injection or infusion may result in high concentration in the blood that exceeds the renal threshold, and much will be lost in the urine. Thus, it may be advantageous to administer the vitamins simultaneously with all nutrients. Some vitamins added to the parenteral nutrition solution may lose their activity during storage.[69] Adsorption of some vitamins to the infusate containers (glass bottle or plastic bag) also occurs. In the author's practice, 0.7 ml Multivitamin Injection (MVI) Concentrate is added to 1 liter of amino acid–glucose solution, and 3 liters of this solution, or 2.1 ml of the 5 ml-vial MVI, are given daily to an adult patient. Folate, 200 μg, B_{12}, 5 μg, and vitamin K, 0.2 mg are added to 1 liter of infusate (see Table 13-

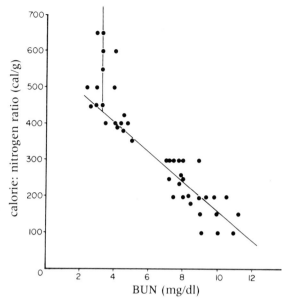

FIG. 13-6 Data were obtained from three dogs demonstrating an inverse linear correlation between the blood urea nitrogen levels and the calorie:nitrogen ratios of the infusates up to a ratio of 450. (Chen WJ, Ohashi E, Tasai M: Metabolism 23:1117, 1974. With permission of Grune and Stratton, Inc., New York)

folic acid, 2 or 3 weeks were required to achieve normal levels. With 15 μg/day, serum B_{12} was higher than normal.

Nichoalds et al. gave MVI-12 (multivitamin infusion), which provides 10 IU vitamin E to patients with cancer requiring parenteral nutrition. At this daily dosage, serum vitamin E was maintained at low-normal levels that appear to be satisfactory (personal communication).

Bone disease has been reported in some adult patients receiving long-term parenteral nutrition at home.[80,135] The vitamin D intake was 250 IU/day in one study, and it was as high as 1000 IU in the other. The laboratory findings varied in these patients. Serum calcium was elevated or normal; hypercalciuria and negative calcium balance were common; serum phosphorus and plasma 25-hydroxy–vitamin D levels were normal or elevated; plasma parathyroid hormone was normal or low. The mechanism of this bone disease is complex and may be related to vitamin D or its metabolites, and perhaps to calcium and phosphorus supplementation.

Biotin deficiency has been reported in a child receiving total parenteral nutrition.[109] However, biotin has not been added to parenteral nutrition solution in most studies until recently; it is now included in both commercial multivitamin formulations that are commonly used for parenteral nutrition. Although mixed American diets are thought to provide a biotin intake of 100 μg to 300 μg per day, a daily dosage of 60 μg should be adequate for maintenance in patients with normal vitamin status.

Although choline is considered an essential nutrient for many laboratory animals, currently it is not added to the parenteral nutrition infusate. It

14). Figure 13-7 shows the serum levels of six of the vitamins measured at weekly intervals in patients maintained on total parenteral nutrition supplied with this vitamin formulation.[113] It seems that vitamins A, E, C, and B_{12} were within the normal ranges. However, vitamin A showed a tendency to increase after the fourth and fifth weeks of total parenteral nutrition, and vitamin E remained at low-normal levels. At a daily dosage of 600 μg of

TABLE 13-13
Nitrogen and Calorie Relationship to Achieve Positive Nitrogen Balance
After Elective Surgery

Investigators*	Nitrogen/kg/day (g)	Calories/kg/day (Cal)	Calorie: Nitrogen Ratio	Nitrogen Balance
Abbott et al (1959)	0.20	35	175:1	—
Johnston et al (1966)	0.16	33	219:1	—
Van Larsen, Brockner (1969)	0.24	32	133:1	—
Tweedle, Johnston (1971)	0.23	45	196:1	+
Johnston (1972)	0.223	38	170:1	0
Meng et al (1972)	0.210	42	200:1	+
Meng et al (1976)	0.228	48	221:1	0 or +
Caldwell et al (1977)	0.27	35	167:1	+
Moghissi et al (1980)	0.2–0.25	40–45	200:1	+
Shizal, Force (1980)	0.20	50	250:1	+
Peters, Fischer (1980)	0.265	52	163:1†	+
Smith, Burkinshaw, Hill (1982)	0.36	53	135:1	+

*See references.

†As reported

TABLE 13-14
Composition of Vitamin Formulations

Vitamin	Daily Dosage of Vanderbilt Formulation*	RDA†	AMA Advisory Group Recommendation‡
A, IU	4,200	4000-5000	3,300
D, IU	420	200-300	200
C (ascorbic acid) (mg)	210	45	100
E, IU	2.1	12-15	10
K	0.6	—	—
Thiamin (mg)	21	1.0-1.5	3
Riboflavin (mg)	4.2	1.1-1.8	3.6
Pyridoxine (mg)	6.3	1.6-2.0	4.0
Niacin (mg)	42	20	40
Pantothenic Acid (mg)	10.5	5-10	15
Folate (μg)	600	400	400
Cyanocobalamin (μg)	15	3	5
Biotin (μg)	—	150-300	60

*M.V.I. Concentrate, 0.7 ml was added to one liter of TPN solution. Amount shown is the content in three liters. Vitamin K (as Synkavite), folate, and B$_{12}$ are added to (TPN) separately.
†Recommended Dietary Allowances, Food and Nutrition Board, National Research Council, National Academy of Science
‡Suggested by the Advisory Group, Foods and Nutrition Department, American Medical Association

has been reported that serum choline levels are decreased in patients maintained on total parenteral nutrition.[23] However, specific adverse effects attributable to choline deficiency in patients have not been identified. Although egg phosphatide in IV fat emulsions contains choline, it is not known whether it is readily available for utilization because of its slow turnover rate. Perhaps it should be given at a daily dosage of 300 mg to 500 mg added to the parenteral nutrition solution. The composition of two commercial multivitamin formulations, Multivitamin Additive (Abbott Laboratories), and MVI-12 (USV Laboratories), is based on the requirements suggested by the Nutrition Advisory Group of the American Medical Association as shown in Table 13-14.

ELECTROLYTES AND INORGANIC TRACE MINERALS

The requirements for electrolytes vary widely in individual patients depending on volume and type of fluid loss, preexisting deficits, cardiovascular, renal, gastrointestinal, and endocrine status, and type and amount of nutrients given. It is essential to monitor plasma electrolyte levels at frequent intervals to afford a rational basis for adjusting dosages until the preexisting deficits and abnormal acid-base balance are corrected. It should be pointed out also that the dosages of electrolytes given by various investigators vary. The article on minerals by Shils may be consulted.[139]

SODIUM AND POTASSIUM

In patients without excessive loss, supplies of 60 mEq sodium/day to 100 mEq sodium/day are adequate, although a wider range up to 150 mEq/day has been suggested. Less sodium should be given to patients with renal insufficiency or cardiovascular disease, and more should be given to those known to have large sodium losses or who are markedly sodium depleted. Sodium may be given as chloride or acetate. Sodium bicarbonate should not be added because of reactions of biocarbonate with other ions.

Potassium is needed during glucose infusion. Davidson and associates report that hyperaminoaciduria occurred in the presence of potassium deficiency but disappeared when potassium was replaced.[39] Cannon and co-workers have shown that administration of protein hydrolysate to potassium-depleted rats will not promote growth; the addition of potassium results in growth and nitrogen balance.[26] The ratio between urinary potassium and nitrogen during fasting is 10 mEq:1 g; a ratio similar to this is also found in normal muscle (6:1-7:1, or a minimum of 3.5:1). In the author's practice, 120 mEq/day or 1.5 mEq/kg/day to 2.0 mEq/kg/day are given to an adult patient.

MAGNESIUM AND CALCIUM

The precise requirement for magnesium in parenteral nutrition is not known. A daily dosage of 15

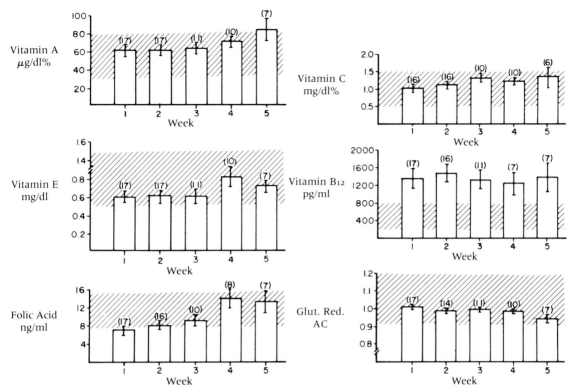

FIG. 13-7 Circulation blood levels of vitamins in patients receiving total parenteral nutrition with the daily dosages shown in Table 13-14 (Glut. Red. AC = glutathione reductase activity coefficient, an index of riboflavin nutriture). Crosshatched areas delimit normal ranges. Figures in parentheses indicate number of patients, and thin vertical lines represent SEM. (Adapted from Nichoalds GE, Meng HC, Caldwell MD: Arch Surg 112:1061, 1977. Courtesy of American Medical Association)

mEq to 30 mEq or 0.3 mEq/kg to 0.5 mEq/kg/day should be adequate unless extensive losses are present. The magnesium (as magnesium sulfate) concentration of the parenteral nutrition infusate currently used at Vanderbilt University Medical Center is 10 mEq/liter, or 30 mEq/day in an adult patient. The quantity of calcium required in parenteral nutrition to maintain balance, bone mineralization, and normal function of the parathyroid gland has not been established. Wittine and Freeman reported that 0.25 mEq/kg/day calcium maintained either an equilibrium or a positive balance during parenteral nutrition.[169] Similar findings have also been observed by Grant.[59] The parenteral nutrition solution currently used at Vanderbilt University Medical Center contains 4.5 mEq (90 mg) calcium/liter as calcium gluconate or glucoceptate; in a patient receiving 3 liters of infusate, the total calcium intake is 13.5 mEq or 270 mg/day, a value that appears to be satisfactory. According to Sloan and Brennan this dosage may be slightly low.[144] Shils suggests 200 mg calcium/day to 400 mg calcium/day for an adult patient.[138] It should be pointed out that immobilization increases urinary excretion and that the presence of intestinal drainage also contributes to its loss. In this case, 400 mg/day to 500 mg/day may be needed.

PHOSPHORUS, CHLORIDE, AND ACETATE

The infusate used at Vanderbilt University Medical Center contains 465 mg (15 mEq) elemental phosphorus as a mixture of potassium acid and dibasic phosphate; the total daily dosage in an adult patient is 1395 mg (45 mEq). Although inorganic phosphate given by investigators varies widely, it is likely that this daily dosage is large for most patients. Half of this amount may meet the daily requirement in most of the patients if there is no excessive loss.

The parenteral nutrition infusate that we used contains 48 mEq chloride and 70 mEq acetate/liter. Excessive chloride should be avoided, in order to prevent hyperchloremia. A considerable amount of anions should be given as acetate. It is a good bicarbonate precursor and maintains acid–base equilibrium.

INORGANIC TRACE MINERALS

Preexisting iron deficiency anemia should be corrected with intramuscular or intravenous injection of iron. Maintenance iron may be added to parenteral nutrition infusate, 1 mg/liter as Imferon (iron–dextran complex). Iodine has not been given to patients receiving parenteral nutrition. However, it should be given to patients on long-term parenteral nutrition. It has been suggested that the requirement of iodine may be in the order of 100 μg to 150 μg/day for goiter control. Other inorganic trace elements, such as zinc, copper, manganese, chromium, nickel, cadmium, molybdenum, selenium, and vanadium, have been reported as essential nutrients, but the requirements for these metals in man are not known. The RDA is 15 mg zinc daily for an adult.[123] Based on current knowledge regarding the absorption of zinc after oral ingestion, 4 mg to 10 mg elemental zinc/day should be given intravenously to an adult. Usually 5 mg zinc sulfate is added to each liter of parenteral nutrition infusate; 3 liters of this infusate supply 15 mg zinc sulfate or about 5 mg zinc. This intake is low for therapy in deficient patients; but *bona fide* zinc deficiency has not been documented by the author. Zinc deficiency has been reported by others in patients receiving parenteral nutrition without supplementation of this element.[52,93,95]

Copper deficiency has been observed in patients on long-term TPN.[52,93,95,136,160] It is recommended that copper be added to the infusate for parenteral nutrition. However, the precise copper requirement in humans is not known. According to the suggestion of the WHO Expert Committee, the estimated requirements are 80 μg/kg/day for infants, 40 μg/kg/day for older children, and 30 μg/kg/day for adult men.[156] Vilter and colleagues administered 1 mg copper as copper sulfate to a 56-year-old woman who had copper deficiency as the result of long-term parenteral nutrition.[160] She responded to the treatment immediately with an increase in white blood cell count and in neurophilic leucocytes in bone marrow. Shike and associates

studied copper requirement in patients with gastrointestinal diseases receiving total parenteral nutrition and found it to be 0.3 mg/day in patients with normal amounts of gastrointestinal excretion.[136] In the presence of diarrhea, or increased fluid loss through gastrointestinal stoma or fistula, the copper requirements for total parenteral nutrition are 0.4 mg/day to 0.5 mg/day.

Chromium deficiency has also been reported in a patient receiving long-term parenteral nutrition.[72] It seems reasonable to assume that chromium should be given to these patients. The urinary loss, which constitutes the major portion of the daily loss of chromium, is 5 μg to 10 μg/day; this amount could be considered the minimum requirement and must be replaced in order to maintain balance in an adult.[156] According to the available information from toxicity studies in various laboratory animals, a daily dosage of 10 μg to 20 μg chromium is not likely to produce any toxic effect in man. Selenium deficiency in patients receiving total parenteral nutrition has been reported in a country where the serum selenium of the general population is low. Estimated needs of some trace minerals are shown in Table 13-15 as a general guide.

WATER

Since all nutrients given for parenteral nutrition are administered in aqueous solutions or oil-in-water emulsion, it is clear that problems of hydration and excretion must be met to achieve successful therapy and to avoid overhydration or dehydration. Consideration should be given first to correct any preexisting abnormality, especially in the presence of water deficits, extensive water loss from fistulas of the gastrointestinal tract, denuded body surfaces, or severe diarrhea. The quantity of water that fulfills the need of excretions (urine and stools), insensible water loss, and proper tissue hydration of a normal adult is approximately 100 ml/100 Cal/day or about 2600 ml. The fluid volume usually given to an adult patient is about 3 liter/day or 30 ml/kg/day to 45 ml/kg/day. However, in patients with renal or pulmonary disease or cardiac decompensation, a large volume of fluid cannot be tolerated. In general, if one avoids osmotic diuresis, water requirements usually present no problems. Careful attention to urinary output and observation of fluid retention should provide information on appropriate daily fluid loads.

Techniques and Procedures

Law has compiled the composition of several solutions used by various investigators who have documented their effectiveness in correcting nega-

Table 13-15
Suggested Requirement of Inorganic Trace Minerals in Adults

Mineral	Amount (per day)
Iron	0.5–2.0 mg/day
Iodide	0.05–0.12 mg/day
Copper	0.4–1.0 mg/day
Manganese	0.2–0.5 mg/day
Chromium	10–20 μg/day
Zinc	4–10 mg/day
Selenium	120 μg/day

tive nitrogen balance, achieving weight gain, and promoting wound healing.[84] Parenteral nutrition solutions of similar composition have also been used by other workers.[134] However, because of a lack of objective methods for the evaluation of the efficacy of these preparations, it is difficult to select any one of them as superior to the others. Objective assessment of nutritional therapy may be improved by the development and use of refined procedures for the measurement of body composition changes.[65, 142,143] Typically, the total amino acid concentration is 30 g to 50 g and glucose concentration is 200 g/liter to 250 g/liter, with various amounts of electrolytes, trace minerals, and vitamins as described previously. The composition of the parenteral nutrition solution currently given to adult patients at Vanderbilt University Medical Center is shown in Table 13-16. Each liter of this solution contains 250 g glucose (dextrose monohydrate, United States Pharmacopeia [USP]), furnishing about 850 Cal (1 g dextrose monohydrate yields 3.40 Cal). The nitrogen, at a concentration of 5.5 g/liter, is supplied as a formulated mixture of essential and nonessential amino acids with a protein equivalent of 34.4 g. Three liters of this solution provide 16.5 g nitrogen, 105 g amino acids, or 103.2 g protein equivalent, and 2550 Cal. The nitrogen and caloric intake is about 275 mg and 42 Cal/kg body weight/ day, respectively. The nonprotein calorie to nitrogen ratio is 154:1, supplied by glucose. With additional calories from 500 ml of a 10% fat emulsion, the calorie to nitrogen ratio will be about 190:1.

The need of adequate calories for amino acid utilization for protein synthesis is well known. To achieve the effectiveness of both calories and nitrogen, they must be administered concurrently. The importance of the temporal relationship of nitrogen and calorie administration has been demonstrated. This temporal relationship may be also applicable to vitamins and electrolytes in the utilization of amino acids, carbohydrates, and fats.

PREPARATION OF SOLUTIONS

As suggested by Burke, the preparation of solutions for parenteral nutrition should be the responsibility of the pharmacy staff.[22] However, the justification for setting up a parenteral nutrition program depends on the individual hospital. In hospitals that wish to establish such programs, the guidelines suggested by Shils may be helpful.[138] In addition, there are a number of publications that may be useful.[18,59,84,134] It may be emphasized that it is of utmost importance to prepare all solutions for parenteral nutrition using strict aseptic procedures and a laminar air flowhood. All solutions are sterile. Vanderbilt University Medical Center uses

TABLE 13-16
Solution for Parenteral Nutrition

Component	Amount/Liter	Amount/Day
Glucose (monohydrate)	250 g	750 g
Glucose calories*	850 Cal	2550 Cal
Amino acids†	35 g	105 g
Nitrogen	5.5 g	15.5 g
Protein equivalent	34.4 g	103.2 g
Na^+	35 mEq	105 mEq
K^+	40 mEq	120 mEq
Ca^{2+}	4.5 mEq	13.5 mEq
Mg^{2+}	10 mEq	30 mEq
Cl^-	48 mEq	144 mEq
Acetate$^-$	70 mEq	210 mEq
P (inorganic phosphorus)	465 mg	1395 mg
$ZnSO_4$	5 mg	15.0 mg
Iron	1.0 mg	3.0 mg
Vitamins‡	1.4 ml	4.2 ml

*Glucose Monohydrate (U.S.P.) was used, and 3.4 Cal/1 g glucose was used for the calculation of calories/liter.

†Aminosyn® 7% with electrolytes was used.

‡Vitamins were given as aqueous multivitamin infusion solution (MVI) 5 ml-ampule (see Table 13-14). Folate and B_{12} were added to the infusate separately. Iron was added as Imferon.

the following procedures to prepare parenteral nutrition solutions:

1. Aminosyn 7% of crystalline amino acids with electrolytes is used. Appropriate amounts of calcium gluconate, potassium acetate, magnesium sulfate, and zinc sulfate in sterile solutions are mixed to obtain the desired concentration in the final infusate; this solution is filtered through a cellulose ester membrane filter (Millipore filter, pore size 0.22 μ).
2. Folic acid, vitamin B_{12}, vitamin K (as Synkavite), and Iron-Dextran in appropriate volumes are added to the electrolyte solution (step 1 above).
3. MVI Concentrate is added to 500 ml Aminosyn.
4. The electrolyte–vitamin mixture (step 2 above) is also added to the amino acid solution, Aminosyn.
5. The amino acid solution containing electrolytes–vitamins (step 4) is transferred to a partially filled 1-liter bottle containing 500 ml 50% glucose. Thirty 60-liter bottles are prepared in one lot. The solution is then capped, labeled, dated, and sampled at random for sterility and pyrogenicity before being released for infusion. This is considered *standard TPN solution* (see Table 13-16). The solution is stored at 4°C for no more than one month. In addition to the standard TPN solution, there are also individually tailored solutions with modified electrolytes, halfstrength with reduced concentration of glucose for peripheral TPN, and Aminosyn RF—40% glucose solution for renal failure.

Another procedure is the use of commercially available hyperalimentation kits, which consist of either protein hydrolysate or crystalline amino acid solution and 50% glucose. One solution is transferred into the other; electrolytes and vitamins are then added under a laminar air flowhood. This procedure may be convenient in hospitals where only a small number of patients are given total parenteral nutrition.

ADMINISTRATION

CENTRAL VENOUS CATHETER

In order to meet the daily nitrogen and energy requirements with a tolerable volume of fluid, the solutions currently used for TPN are hyperosmolar. To prevent or minimize damage to the vein, a central vein must be used for infusion. The selection of a central vein and procedures for the placement of a central venous catheter are described in detail by Parsa and associates, Ryan, and Grant.[59,116,130] In general, the technique introduced by Wilmore and Dudrick is the most widely used.[167] At Vanderbilt the procedure is to place a 1.6-mm Silastic catheter into the subclavian or an external jugular vein percutaneously or through a cutdown; the catheter is then directed into the superior vena cava. The position of the catheter must be verified radiographically and then is sutured to the skin. The use of a brachial, axillary, or femoral vein is not recommended. The small lumen of a peripheral vein permits little blood flow between the vessel wall and the catheter, and would thus contribute to the occurrence of phlebitis. Furthermore, a long catheter is an inconvenience to the patient and may increase the possibility of contamination. Placement of the central venous catheter must be done in accordance with strict aseptic techniques. Povidone–iodine solution is applied to the skin surrounding the catheter entry site, and a completely occlusive sterile dressing is applied. Dressings are changed daily, or at least every 48 hours. All procedures must be done with meticulous care to avoid infection. It is suggested that the dressing changes be done by a limited number of staff physicians or nurses who know the procedure well.

PERIPHERAL VENOUS INFUSION

Recently, peripheral veins have been used for parenteral nutrition; this is termed *peripheral parenteral nutrition* (PPN). PPN may be given when occasionally it is impossible or unwise to use a central venous catheter. It may also be given as a temporary measure for severely depleted patients or in patients who are fairly well-nourished but require parenteral nutrition for a relatively short period of time—less than 7 to 10 days. PPN may be also useful to supplement inadequate oral intake or tube feeding. Three liters of a solution containing 10% glucose and 3.5% amino acids along with vitamins and electrolytes supplying about 1020 Cal and 16.5 g nitrogen (114 g protein equivalent) may not be beneficial owing to an inadequate caloric intake. Van Way, Meng, and Sandstead have shown that the intake of nitrogen as crystalline amino acids and calories of less than 8 g and 1800 Cal/day, respectively, did not significantly improve the negative nitrogen balance over that observed in patients receiving no nitrogen and only 550 Cal/day (see Fig. 13-8).[158] Therefore, an addition of 1000 Cal supplied by 1 liter 10% fat emulsion should be given. The fat emulsion and glucose–amino acid solution should be administered concurrently through a Y tube connected to the central venous catheter. Since fat emulsion dilutes the glucose–amino acid solution, the concentration of amino acid can be slightly decreased. Issacs and associates give a solution that has been used with apparently good results.[71] In addition to amino acids, glucose, and electrolytes, cortisol and heparin are also added to the infusate to prevent phlebitis and formation of thrombus. The use of fat emulsion–amino acid–glucose in peripheral parenteral nutrition can achieve positive nitrogen balance and weight gain as shown in Figure 13-9, provided both calories and nitrogen are adequate.[155] Total parenteral nutrition by peripheral vein has been used successfully in infants, children, and in adults, by Borressen, Coran, Knutrud, by our group, and by others.[14,17,54,115] However, it may be cautioned that the use of the peripheral vein for parenteral nutrition may not be as trouble-free as it appears. Care and skill in maintaining a peripheral line are needed. In addition, the use of large doses of fat requires careful monitoring.

USE OF ARTERIOVENOUS SHUNT

The external arteriovenous shunt that is used for hemodialysis has been modified for TPN by Shils and associates and by Scribner and associates with apparent success.[132,140] The use of an internal arteriovenous shunt for parenteral nutrition has also been reported.[64] However, it is not recommended when placement of a central venous catheter is possible or when peripheral parenteral nutrition is capable of providing adequate support. In rare occasions this may be the only possible route available.

USE OF IN-LINE FILTER AND PUMPS

Generally, the nutrient solution is delivered from a bottle or plastic bag to a patient by gravity. An

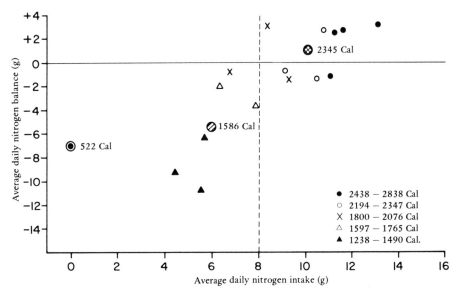

FIG. 13-8 Relationship between nitrogen intake and nitrogen balance in patients receiving varying caloric intake. (Van Way CW III, Meng HC, Sandstead HH: Arch Surg 110:272, 1975. Courtesy American Medical Association)

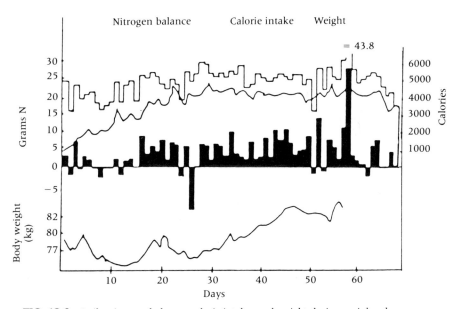

FIG. 13-9 Daily nitrogen balance, caloric intake, and weight during peripheral venous parenteral nutrition, including Intralipid. (Thompson WR: In Meng HC, Wilmore DW (eds): Fat Emulsion in Parenteral Nutrition, p 61. American Medical Association, Department of Foods and Nutrition, 1976)

in-line Millipore filter about 2.5 cm in diameter interposed between the infusion tubing and the catheter is a helpful addition. A filter with a porosity of 0.22 μ provides absolute sterility, but a peristaltic pump must be used to overcome the resistance exerted by the filter and to assure constant and adequate flow. Since the use of a pump creates the risk of air embolization, close supervision is strongly recommended. The use of filters of this porosity is not recommended for the infusion of fat emulsion. Millipore filters with a porosity of 0.45 μ will prevent the passage of some microorganisms and particulate matters; they do not accomplish absolute sterility. The use of in-line filter is discouraged by some workers, as reviewed by Grant.[59]

Changes of Infusion Tubing and Administration of Drugs. The infusion bottle that contains 1 liter parenteral nutrition solution should be changed every 12 hr, even if it is not completely empty. The infusion tubing from the bottle down to the catheter hub must be changed at least once every 24 hr. To prevent contamination and to avoid physical or chemical incompatibility between parenteral nutrition solution and drugs, especially antibiotics, nothing should be added to the bottle or injected into the infusion line. Transfusion or withdrawal of blood through the catheter must be avoided. Such practices usually are responsible for infection, or for plugging of the catheter.

Rate of Infusion. The optimal infusion rate for glucose is 0.5 g/kg/hr to 0.75 g/kg/hr, although 0.35 g has been proposed to avoid hyperglycemia and urinary spillage. The rate depends on the clinical condition of the individual patient. Insulin must be administered to some patients. The dosage of insulin is based on urinary glucose loss or blood sugar levels given at appropriate intervals. Some investigators prefer to add insulin into the infusate—1 unit insulin to 7 g to 10 g glucose. The addition of insulin to parenteral nutrition solution is also discussed by Grant.[59]

Information concerning urinary loss of amino acids during infusion of protein hydrolysate or amino acid solutions at different rates is not available. It has been proposed that nitrogen, 0.02 g/kg/hr to 0.03 g/kg/hr may be given continuously during a 24-hr period with no adverse effects. In most patients, except those with renal and cardiac disease, 3 liters of the solution shown in Table 13-16 are given during the 24-hr period. On the first day about 1 liter is administered, 2 liters on the second day, and 3 liters on the third and succeeding days. Additional fluid is given when needed during the first 2 days. A continuous infusion rate of 125 ml/hr provides 3 liters in 24 hr. In a study by Grant, measurements were made of electrolytes, glucose, urea, protein, and osmolality in blood drawn through a catheter with its tip positioned 2 cm to 3 cm below the tip of the subclavian catheter for TPN at an infusion rate of 125 ml/hr, and similarly in blood drawn from a peripheral vein.[59] The concentration of these substances in the blood drawn simultaneously from these two sites were quite similar. The results indicate adequate dilution of the hyperosmolar infusate in the blood below the tip of the catheter. If the infusion should falter, the resulting deficit may be corrected by increasing the rate of administration slowly. If the infusion stops completely, measures must be taken to avoid reactive hypoglycemia, especially when insulin has been added to the infusate; usually 5% or 10% glucose should be given. The rate of infusion of fat emulsion may be maintained at 0.1 g/kg/hr to 0.5 g/kg/hr. Regardless of the daily dosage, the infusion rate should be maintained at about 0.5 ml to 1 ml/minute during the first 15 to 30 min to avoid possible adverse effects. The initial dosage of fat should be given at 0.5 gm/kg/day; it is increased stepwise to 1, 1.5, 2, and 2.5 g/kg/day in 4 or 5 days. Plasma triglyceride or optical density should be measured before each increment is made. The increase in dosage should be delayed when hyperlipidemia or hypertriglyceridemia is observed. In fact, the dosage may be reduced or administration of fat emulsion temporarily discontinued when hyperlipidemia persists. For further information the readers are referred to reviews and proceedings of a symposium on this subject.[96,97,107]

Clinical Application in Various Disease States

In the past 15 years, parenteral nutrition has become increasingly used. It has been given not only to post-operative or post-traumatized patients, but also to those with a variety of disease states. Both Fischer, and Shenkin and Wretlind review these subjects further in detail.[46,47,134]

SURGERY AND TRAUMA

Well-nourished patients with uncomplicated major surgery or moderately severe trauma may not need an extensive TPN program. In these cases, a well-planned IV therapy is sufficient to maintain adequate circulatory volume and provide fluid, electrolytes, and glucose for preventing dehydration, electrolyte imbalance, and continued body protein loss.[120] Moore suggests that vigorous attempts at TPN may be deleterious by delaying the return of appetite and intestinal functions.[110] Blackburn and colleagues introduced the protein-sparing concept (see Chap. 11) and have proposed peripheral venous nutrition with 3.5% amino acid solution containing adequate vitamins and electrolytes but devoid of glucose.[16] The primary source of energy is the mobilized triglyceride from the adipose tissue in the form of free fatty acids. However, in patients who are severely debilitated because of chronic disease or prolonged malnutrition, or in those who are unable to eat for an extended period of time as the result of severe trauma, sepsis, or complications of surgery, vigorous TPN must be carefully planned and initiated. These patients present substantial weight loss, with marked reduction of both skeletal muscle mass and total body protein. In addition, energy depots in the adipose tissue are depleted. Lawson has observed that an acute loss of 30% of body weight was uniformly fatal in a series of severely ill surgical patients.[85] Randall has estimated that the nitrogen loss that a patient can sustain acutely and still have sufficient muscle strength to survive is about one third of his total protein nitrogen or somewhat less than 50% of skeletal muscle protein.[122] This would be a negative nitrogen balance of about 350 g, representing 2200 g protein or 13 kg muscle. It is apparent that a patient with a negative nitrogen balance of this magnitude is usually unable to survive for more than 2 weeks if adequate nutritional support is not given.

Parenteral nutrition that can significantly decrease nitrogen loss at the peak of catabolic response was demonstrated by many investigators prior to 1968. Many reports have been published showing the effectiveness of TPN since Dudrick and co-workers first introduced the technique of intravenous hyperalimentation.[43] The following cases

are presented to exemplify the importance and effectiveness of maintaining adequate TPN in surgical and traumatized patients.

Patient H.O. received TPN for 30 days (see Fig. 13-10). Six years before admission, the patient, a 70-year-old man, had undergone total gastrectomy with *en bloc* resection of omentum, spleen, left hemidiaphragm, left lower lobe of the left lung, body and tail of the pancreas, left lobe of the liver, left adrenal gland, and splenic flexure of the colon. The pathologic diagnosis was reticulum cell carcinoma of the stomach. His preoperative weight was about 70 kg, but was subsequently stabilized at around 55 kg. He had persistent anemia and hypoalbuminemia. During the previous 2 to 3 years, he had begun to lose weight gradually so that he weighed only 45 kg on admission. There was no evidence of a recurrent tumor. A course of TPN was elected and continued for 30 days. During the period of parenteral nutrition his average daily caloric intake was 2865 Cal with an average daily nitrogen intake of 13.4 g as crystalline amino acids. Thus, the caloric and nitrogen intake were about

FIG. 13-10 Daily caloric intake, nitrogen intake, body weight, and nitrogen balance of patient H.O. (Van Way CW III, Meng HC, Sandstead HH: Ann Surg 177:103, 1973)

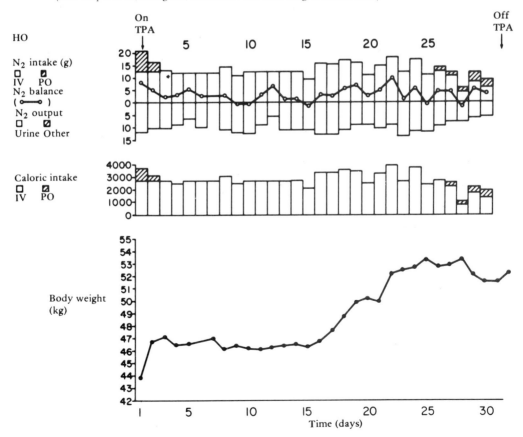

61 Cal and 285 mg/kg/day, with a calorie to nitrogen ratio of 214:1 during the early part, and 50 Cal and 244 mg/kg/day with a calorie to nitrogen ratio of 205:1 during the later part of the total parenteral nutrition period, respectively. The average daily nitrogen retention was 3.32 g, and he gained 9.6 kg body weight in a month; most of the weight gain occurred during the second half of the parenteral nutrition period. He required diuretic therapy for control of pedal edema during this period, but showed no other signs of fluid overload. As his general condition improved, he was able to maintain his weight by oral alimentation. One month after discharge from the hospital he weighed 53 kg.

During the period of TPN in a 32-year-old woman with achalasia, the average daily nitrogen intake was 17.9 g given as a protein hydrolysate and the average daily caloric intake was 2656 Cal. Both continued weight gain and persistent positive nitrogen balance were observed (see Fig. 13-11).

A 28-year-old chemical plant worker with phosphorus burns on 70% of the body surface involving the trunk and all four extremities received nutritional therapy (see Fig. 13-12). About 30% of the body had full-thickness skin loss. Following stabilization of the initial fluid and electrolyte imbalances, 6 days after the burn, he was placed on parenteral nutrition as a part of the program of nutritional supplementation, which included oral feedings of hospital diets and oral feeding of an

elemental diet (Vivonex–100). Except for days 3 and 7, the caloric intake furnished by oral and parenteral routes was about 3000 Cal/day during the first 10 days of nutritional therapy; the average daily caloric intake during the 35-day period was 4137 Cal. The average daily nitrogen intake was 15.3 g with a net nitrogen loss of 15.8 g/day during the first 10 days. The weight loss during this period was very rapid with an average of 1.7 kg/day. From days 11 to 35 the body weight was maintained between 73 and 77 kg. The average daily nitrogen and caloric intake was 16.5 g and 4684 Cal, respectively, with an average net nitrogen loss of 3.4 g/day. Further weight loss was observed when parenteral nutrition was discontinued and oral intake was resumed, but was inadequate. This patient represents a fairly typical major burn case. Such patients have an astounding catabolic drain. Despite attempts made to institute a program for vigorous nutritional supplementation by all routes available, he still lost a total of 16 kg during the 35-day period on TPN. This was due, in part, to difficulties encountered in administering enough nitrogen and calories to meet extensive loss. The nitrogen loss during the first 6 days on nutritional therapy was 30 g to 35 g/day. Beginning from the eighth day of nutritional therapy, the nitrogen balance was almost maintained, and body weight was stabilized. Nutritional supplementation in the range of 4000 Cal/day to 6000 Cal/day with a nitrogen intake of 20 g to 30 g as amino acids is necessary

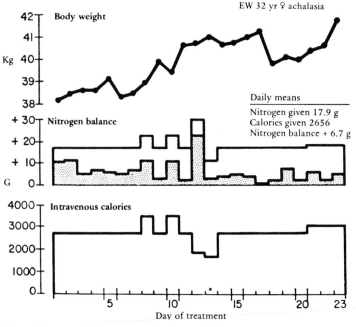

EW 32 yr ♀ achalasia

Daily means
Nitrogen given 17.9 g
Calories given 2656
Nitrogen balance + 6.7 g

*Operation

FIG. 13-11 Continued weight gain and persistent positive nitrogen balance accompanied by successful esophagomyotomy on day 13 in patient with achalasia, tuberculosis, and recurrent staphylococcal infections. (Dudrick SJ, Wilmore DW, Vars HM, Rhoads JE: Ann Surg 169:974, 1969)

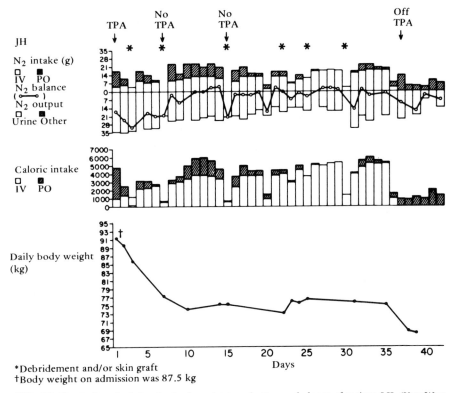

FIG. 13-12 Daily caloric intake, body weight, and nitrogen balance of patient J.H. (Van Way CW III, Meng HC, Sandstead HH: Ann Surg 177:103, 1973)

to maintain a patient with severe burns in nutritional balance after the initial 10 to 14 days. Wilmore and associates have shown that with daily intakes of 4000 Cal to 8000 Cal, by combined IV-enteral nutritional support, weight gain was achieved in some patients in the latter phase of severe burns.[165] It may be pointed out that marked changes in hormone secretion and response occur in burned and traumatized patients.[59,165] These hormonal changes in relation to the time of initiation of, and the kind of nutrients given in, parenteral nutrition to severely stressed hypercatabolic patients should also be considered.

GASTROINTESTINAL DISEASES

Maldigestion and malabsorption are invariably associated with diseases of the gastrointestinal tract, especially chronic inflammatory disease of the bowel such as regional enteritis. Short bowel syndrome and fistula formation may result following surgical intervention. The occurrence of intestinal cutaneous fistulas is associated with significant morbidity; mortality rates have been reported as high as 65%. In addition, complications of fluid and electrolyte imbalances, infection, starvation, and skin

erosion often lead to progressive deterioration of the patient's condition. Excessive weight loss, marked reduction of serum albumin, and delayed wound healing are encountered. Failure to ameliorate or correct the abnormal conditions, even when the bowel was put at rest, has been attributed by some to the lack of proper nutrition. The importance of nutrition during fistula therapy was first emphasized by Chapman and associates in 1964.[28] They reported that at caloric intakes of 1500 Cal/day to 2000 Cal/day, the mortality rate of their patients was considerably improved. Sheldon and co-workers further emphasized the importance of adequate nutrition in the treatment of intestinal fistulas.[133] MacFayden reported a study of 62 patients with 78 GI fistulas who were treated with TPN and bowel rest as an adjuvant to conventional surgical measures.[94] Spontaneous fistula closure occurred in 70.5%, and of the patients requiring operation, successful closure occurred in 94%. The overall mortality rate in this series was 6.45%.

The balance studies obtained from a patient D.B. are shown in Figures 13-13 and 13-14. This patient was a 28-year-old man with a five year history of regional enteritis involving duodenum, jejunum, ileum, and colon. He also had a draining fistula from the perirectal area to the back of the right thigh. A gastrojejunostomy and vagotomy were performed for the posterior duodenal ulcer about 3 years prior to the present admission. Oral intake of food was intolerable because of frequent diarrhea. The patient was anorexic and mentally depressed. He had lost more than 40 kg body weight since the beginning of his illness. Total parenteral nutrition was given for 38 days during which time he received nothing by mouth except water. The total intake of amino acids and glucose by the IV route was 3.06 kg and 29.04 kg, respectively. The average daily nitrogen intake was 11.85 g and the average daily caloric intake 3056 Cal. Figure 13-13 shows the caloric intake, body weight gain, nitrogen balance, and the progressive decrease in nitrogen loss from the fistula drainage. It can be noted that he gained about 1.5 kg body weight after 14 days of parenteral nutrition, furnishing 2700 Cal/day from nonnitrogen sources (47 Cal/kg/day). Increasing nonnitrogen calories to 3600 (60 Cal/kg/day) seemed to improve the curve of body weight gain. The total weight gained was 7 kg with an average daily gain of 0.19 kg. The nitrogen balance was maintained positive throughout the period of TPN except for the last 3 days when caloric and nitrogen intakes were reduced. The daily average of nitrogen retention was 4.14 g. The volume of (and the nitrogen loss from) fistula drainage were progressively decreased throughout the period of TPN.

The fluid balance was calculated as the difference between the sum of water intake by mouth, plus the volume of parenteral nutrition given by vein and the sum of urinary output plus fistula drainage. The insensible water loss was not considered. It is seen from Figure 13-14 that, in general, there was considerable water retention. The average daily amount of water retained was 1652 ml. Sodium, potassium, and magnesium balances were maintained positive except for the last 3 days when intakes of these electrolytes were reduced, resulting in negative balance. The daily average of sodium, potassium, and magnesium retention was 17.8 mEq, 36.2 mEq and 8.1 mEq, respectively; the ratios of nitrogen to potassium and nitrogen to magnesium were 4.14:36.2 (or approximately 1:9) and 4.14:8.1 (or approximately 1:2), respectively. Table 13-17 shows the increase in total body potassium during the period of total parenteral nutrition. Increase in intracellular potassium has been observed in recent studies in patients receiving total parenteral nutrition.[65,142] Figure 13-15 shows the appearance of the enterocutaneous fistula before and after the period of TPN. The size of skin erosion was reduced and the erosion appeared dry at the end of the parenteral nutrition period. The fistula was closing. Dressner and associates and Aguirre and associates also have presented radiologic evidence documenting spontaneous closure of intestinal fistulas in patients given TPN.[7,40] Grant has summarized the results of total parenteral nu-

FIG. 13-13 Daily caloric intake, body weight, nitrogen balance, and nitrogen loss from fistula drainage of patient D.B. during the total parenteral nutrition period. (Meng HC, Sandstead HH: Long-term total parenteral nutrition in patients with chronic inflammatory diseases of the intestines. In Wilkinson AW (ed): Parenteral Nutrition, p 213. Edinburgh, Churchill Livingstone, 1972)

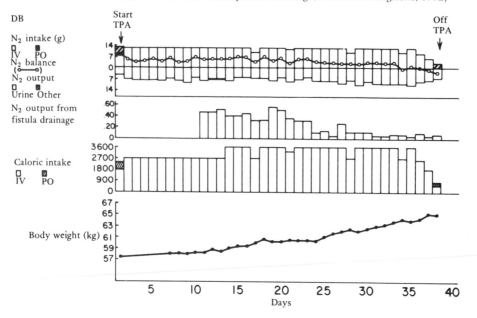

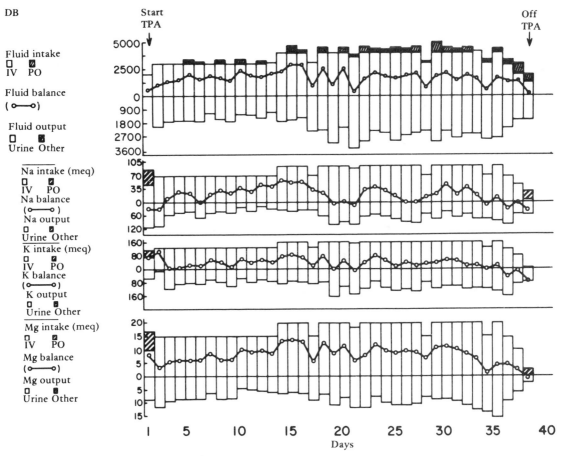

FIG. 13-14 Fluid, sodium, and potassium and magnesium balances of patient D.B. during the total parenteral nutrition period. (Meng HC, Sandstead HH: Long-term parenteral nutrition in patients with chronic inflammatory diseases of the intestines. In Wilkinson AW (ed): Parenteral Nutrition, p 213. Edinburgh, Churchill Livingstone, 1972)

TABLE 13-17
Total Body and Serum Potassium (D.B.)*
During Total Parenteral Nutrition (TPN)

Days on TPN	Potassium	
	Total Body (mEq)†	Serum (mEq/l)
Day 3	2367	4.6
Day 14	2758	3.8
Day 31	2859	4.1
Day 38	3191	3.8

*From Meng HC, Sandstead HH: Long-term total parenteral nutrition in patients with chronic inflammatory diseases of the intestine. Wilkinson AW, 1972. Reproduced with permission of Churchill Livingstone, Edinburgh and London.

†Total body potassium was measured by the method of Brill AB, Sandstead HH, Price RR, et al: Changes in body composition after jejunoileal bypass in morbidly obese patients. Am J Surg 123:49, 1972

trition in patients with enterocutaneous fistulas; total parenteral nutrition is effective in spontaneous closure of the fistulas and is capable of maintaining a good nutritional state.[59]

However, Aguirre and associates stated that under certain conditions, such as the presence of distal intestinal obstruction, bowel discontinuity as demonstrated by contrast-radiographic studies, undrained intraabdominal abscesses, and lack of fistula closure after 30 to 90 days of total parenteral nutrition, early surgical intervention is necessary.[7] Fischer and co-workers have considered hyperalimentation as a primary therapy for inflammatory bowel disease, and Layden and associates have observed the reversal of growth arrest in adolescents with Crohn's disease after parenteral nutrition.[48,87] It has also been reported that when total parenteral nutrition was given to patients with Crohn's disease limited to the small intestine, 60% to 80% remission in symptoms was demonstrated and sur-

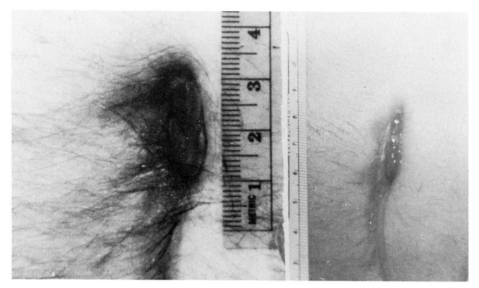

FIG. 13-15 The enterocutaneous fistula of patient D.B. before and at the end of the total parenteral nutrition period. (Meng HC, Sandstead HH: Long-term parenteral nutrition in patients with chronic inflammatory diseases of the intestines. In Wilkinson AW (ed): Parenteral Nutrition, p 213. Edinburgh, Churchill Livingstone, 1972)

gery was avoided. In patients with granulomatous colitis with or without involvement of the small intestine, 30% to 60% of the cases responded with clinical remission. On the other hand, patients with ulcerative colitis responded poorly with very few remissions, although the nutritional status was improved. Other abdominal diseases in which total parenteral nutrition may be beneficial are acute pancreatitis, peritonitis, and prolonged paralytic ileus.

CANCER

Loss of weight is common in patients with cancer and cachexia owing, in part, to anorexia. In addition, impaired intestinal absorption often accompanies malignant tumors. The nutritional state of the host is further affected by gastrointestinal and other side-effects of chemotherapy, radiation therapy, or surgical procedure, such as loss of appetite, nausea, vomiting, and diarrhea. Thus, a vicious cycle results: (1) chemotherapy or radiation therapy produces malnutrition because of its toxic effects, and (2) malnutrition further delays wound healing and decreases immune responses, leading to infection and other complications. Provision of adequate nutrients by TPN can interrupt this vicious cycle (see Chap. 36).

Nutritional rehabilitation of cancer patients was attempted by Terepta in 1956.[154] Adults presenting a variety of neoplasms were forced fed, with weight gain demonstrated in 7 out of 9 patients, and positive nitrogen balance shown in all patients. In 1971, Schwartz and colleagues gave combined parenteral nutrition and systemic chemotherapy to a group of ten patients with widespread malignant disease.[131] They showed that almost all patients had decreased analgesic requirements, improved performance, increased appetite and oral intakes, and reversal of the downward weight trend. In addition, there was a striking absence of GI toxicity despite the administration of extremely large doses of chemotherapeutic agents over prolonged periods of time. Recently, Copeland and co-workers observed a possible correlation between nutritional status and response to chemotherapy in patients with adenocarcinoma or squamous cell carcinoma of the lung.[37] The GI toxic side-effects of chemotherapy are better tolerated, even at high dosages, in patients receiving parenteral nutrition with weight gain, as compared to those receiving no nutritional therapy. Similar results were obtained in patients with head and neck cancer in response to radiation therapy as well as chemotherapy.[38] Copeland and co-workers also report that adequate parenteral nutrition improved the immune response. They further demonstrated that the use of central venous parenteral nutrition did not increase the incidence of catheter-related sepsis, even in patients on chemotherapy.[36] This is an important finding since it has been reported that chemotherapy invariably causes leucopenia and immunodepression.[56] We have also demonstrated that adequate parenteral nutrition is capable of improving the nutritional status, achieving weight gain and a positive nitrogen balance in cancer patients with little or no oral intake.[100] Therapy with a second chemotherapeutic agent can be given following nonresponsiveness to the first during long-term parenteral nutrition. Lanzotti and co-workers suggest that the response to chemotherapy in patients with cancer is related to concurrent IV hyperalimentation.[83]

The following questions have been raised: (1) Does good nutrition promote the growth of tumors? Steiger and associates have shown that hyperalimentation stimulated tumor growth in rats.[151] However, no apparent increase in cancer cell replication has been documented in human subjects receiving adequate parenteral nutritional support.[35] (2) Should patients with terminal disease, unresponsive to all therapeutic measures, be given total parenteral nutrition even if they will at times show an improved but temporary well-being upon initiation of this treatment? This question cannot be easily answered, and will depend on certain circumstances as discussed by both Fischer and Grant.[46,59] The issue of selection of patients with cancer for total parenteral nutrition is also discussed by Brennan.[18,19]

RENAL FAILURE

In spite of improvements in the management of patients with renal failure, malnutrition continues to be a problem (see Chap. 34). The intake of protein, sodium, and water is necessarily restricted because of the difficulty in the disposal of these substances and nitrogenous metabolites. In addition, these patients are usually anorexic and also may have disturbances of intestinal absorption. Readers are referred further to the review by Abel.[3] The generally agreed upon concept of dietary management of renal failure is to give a small amount of nitrogen, as protein of high biological value, or essential amino acids and relatively high caloric intake. Endogenous urea as well as exogenous nitrogenous compounds can be used for protein synthesis when essential amino acids and adequate calories are given. The discussion of parenteral nutrition in renal failure patients is here divided into two parts: acute and chronic renal failure.

ACUTE RENAL FAILURE

Lawson and co-workers have given diets supplying 1200 Cal to 1400 Cal and up to 40 g protein of high biologic value to patients with acute renal failure; they observed no significant increase in blood urea.[86] Other similar dietary regimens have

been designed to maintain the nutritional status of acute renal failure patients.[13] However, frequently one must treat patients with hypercatabolic acute renal failure in whom only the IV route is possible. Thus, TPN with or without fat emulsion has been used and found successful.[89] With low dietary nitrogen furnished as essential amino acids, and with a relatively high caloric intake, Wilmore and Dudrick demonstrated in 1969 that weight gain, wound healing, and positive nitrogen balance may be achieved by TPN in a patient with acute renal failure and severe abdominal injuries.[168] Furthermore, blood urea remained stable and other symptoms of uremia were resolved.

From 1970 through 1974, Abel and associates gave TPN to a large number of patients with acute renal failure at the Massachusetts General Hospital.[1,3-6] From this experience the following conclusions were drawn: (1) in certain instances of nonoliguric acute renal failure, with TPN, dialysis may become unnecessary, or the frequency with which it is generally employed may be decreased; (2) the BUN-lowering effects of the Giordano–Giovannetti diet (see Chap. 11) are confirmed in a variety of clinical situations; (3) TPN therapy may be particularly helpful following aortoiliac surgery with the onset of acute renal failure, under conditions of and prolonged adynamic ileus; (4) serum potassium, phosphate, and magnesium decreased in association with therapy; these effects avert demise from ionic intolerance or toxicity; (5) in certain instances of reversible acute renal failure, treatment with essential L-amino acids and hypertonic glucose IV may result in improved survival; (6) recovery of renal function appeared to be more rapid in patients with acute tubular necrosis than in a matched group of control patients receiving hypertonic glucose alone; (7) there is an apparent rapid clearance from the blood of the administered amino acids, suggesting full use of the exogenous amino acids.

The following observations were made in a representative patient (see Fig. 13-16). Six days after abdominal aortic aneurysmectomy, parenteral nutrition was instituted with a solution consisting of the eight essential L-amino acids in 47% glucose by constant infusion into the superior vena cava. Despite a continuing rise in the serum creatinine level, the BUN value began to decline. Because of the unavailability of the essential amino acid solution, glucose alone was given for a brief period. This was accompanied by a recurrent increase in BUN, which was again brought under control by the 17th day, coincident with the reinstitution of essential amino acid administration. Stabilization of BUN value continued to the 25th day postoperatively, and a gradual improvement in renal

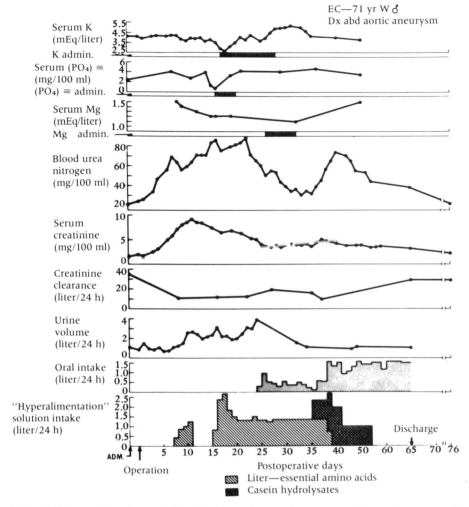

EC—71 yr W ♂
Dx abd aortic aneurysm

Serum K (mEq/liter)
K admin.
Serum (PO₄) ≡ (mg/100 ml)
(PO₄) ≡ admin.
Serum Mg (mEq/liter)
Mg admin.
Blood urea nitrogen (mg/100 ml)
Serum creatinine (mg/100 ml)
Creatinine clearance (liter/24 h)
Urine volume (liter/24 h)
Oral intake (liter/24 h)
"Hyperalimentation" solution intake (liter/24 h)
Discharge
ADM.
Operation
Postoperative days
Liter—essential amino acids
Casein hydrolysates

FIG. 13-16 Renal function and electrolyte determinations in a 71-year-old man in acute renal failure following resection of an abdominal aortic aneurysm. (Abel RM, Abbott, WM, Fischer JE: Arch Surg 103:513, 1971. Courtesy of American Medical Association)

function was observed at that time. By the 28th day the patient's prolonged adynamic ileus had resolved, and he was able to tolerate some oral feedings. Supplementary parenteral nutrition, with casein hydrolysate and 23% glucose, was given on the 35th day, and an increase in BUN to 75 mg/100 ml was observed. However, after reducing the total nitrogen intake, the BUN level slowly returned to normal. During the parenteral nutrition period, serum potassium was decreased, requiring replacement therapy to maintain the normal levels. Marked hypophosphatemia and hypomagnesemia also occurred, requiring replacement therapy.

The composition of the parenteral nutrition solution given to patients with acute renal failure at Vanderbilt University Medical Center has been a solution containing the eight essential amino acids and 40% to 44% glucose. This solution is prepared by mixing one unit of 250 ml Nephramine (see Table 13-2 for amino acid composition) with 600 ml 70% glucose solution. After the addition of vitamin and electrolyte solutions, an appropriate volume of sterile distilled water is added to make a total volume of 1 liter. One liter of the infusate contains 420 g glucose and 13.1 g essential L-amino acids (1.46 g nitrogen) furnishing about 1500 Cal. The amounts of the eight essential amino acids per liter solution furnish twice the minimal requirement of Rose.[128] Vitamins given were the same as shown in Table 13-14. Electrolytes are usually added according to the patient's need. The volume of the solution given depends on the tolerance of the patient; it may be as much as 3 liter/day to 4 liter/day.

The amino acid solution more recently used at Vanderbilt is Aminosyn–RF, the composition of which is shown in Table 13-2. In this solution, histidine and arginine are included in addition to the eight essential amino acids.

CHRONIC RENAL FAILURE

Severe nutritional depletion is frequently experienced in patients with chronic renal failure. Most of the chronic uremic patients can tolerate some oral intake, but usually it is far from adequate. In some cases oral consumption of food or even tube-feeding is impossible because of complications; TPN must be instituted. Lee and associates have shown the beneficial effect of TPN in chronic uremic patients.[89] By administering approximately 1 liter solution per day, as described above, for patients with acute renal failure, similar results have been observed in our studies.

It is appropriate to point out the possible essential role of histidine in chronic uremic patients. This amino acid is essential for infants (see Chap. 2). Giordano and associates indicated that small amounts of histidine added to a low-nitrogen diet increased the rate of amino acid incorporation into hemoglobin in chronic uremic patients.[57] They also reported an initially decreased concentration of serum histidine in these patients and concluded that the anemia associated with chronic uremia may be related to a relative histidine deficiency. Josephson and associates made similar observations in a group of chronic uremic patients who improved following the addition of histidine to a solution of the eight essential L-amino acids.[78] Bergstrom and associates also found improvement of nitrogen balances when histidine was administered in addition to the eight essential amino acids.[22] However, evidence has been reported showing no significant differences in fasting blood concentration of histidine between normal and uremic subjects, although elevation of 3-methylhistidine was observed in severely uremic patients.[33] The plasma amino acid pattern observed in acute renal failure patients by Abel and co-workers also demonstrated no deficiency in histidine and arginine.[6] Thus, the requirement of histidine in renal failure patients requires further definitive study. In the meantime, it is suggested that histidine at a dosage of 1 g/day be given to patients with severe uremia.

The nitrogen-free alpha-keto analogs of leucine, isoleucine, valine, methionine and phenylalanine, included along with the remaining essential amino acids, have been given to renal failure patients.[161] Beneficial results were observed comparable to those studies in which all the essential amino acids were given. These alpha-keto compounds probably are converted to their respective amino acids by transamination using endogenous nitrogen by uremic patients. Additional work remains to be done to sustain their clinical effectiveness.

The requirement of vitamin B_6 may be increased in uremic patients, necessitating supplementation; 25 mg B_6 seems to be adequate.[153]

HEPATIC FAILURE

Malnutrition is usually presented in patients suffering from hepatic failure. The oral intake of protein may induce hepatic encephalopathy in some susceptible patients with chronic liver disease. The generation of ammonia, various mercaptans, and probably other nitrogenous substances from protein by bacteria, occurs within the gut. In addition, ingested protein is converted to urea by the liver, and the urea, which undergoes an enterohepatic circulation in the gut, is hydrolyzed by bacterial urease to ammonia.[171] Thus, the relationship between protein intake, bowel flora, and ammonia-induced hepatic coma seems fairly well defined. Theoretically, therefore, administration of nitrogen directly into the blood circulation should bypass the intestinal bacterial flora and allow better nutrition without the risks of encephalopathy.

Freeman and MacLean reported their experience with four patients (two of whom were comatose) suffering from advanced liver disease.[55] Of the 24-hour fluid requirement, 90% was given as hypertonic glucose and the remainder as protein hydrolysate. If no changes occurred in the BUN, blood ammonia, or neurologic status, more protein hydrolysate was substituted for glucose until the conventional 750–350 mixture was attained. "Surprising success" with this treatment was achieved. The frequency of glycosuria did not appear to be increased when patients with liver disease were given hypertonic glucose. In 1972, Host, Serlin, and Rush first reported their attempts in treating 11 cirrhotic patients with parenteral nutrition.[68] The solution they used contained either protein hydrolysate or crystalline amino acids, glucose (20%), vitamins, and electrolytes and was administered through a central venous catheter. Some beneficial effect was achieved. However, positive nitrogen balance was not accomplished, owing in part, to the inadequate intake. Blood ammonia levels were increased, but no adverse mental symptoms occurred. Sodium intolerance and acidosis were also observed. Intravenous feeding has also been found beneficial in liver failure patients by Silvis and Badertscher.[144] Fischer and co-workers, using a mixture or essential amino acids (formerly FreAmine E, currently Nephramine) used for renal failure of a mixture of essential and nonessential amino acids (FreAmine), found that although the tolerance of cirrhotic patients to amino acid infusion was greater than tolerance to similar amounts of protein given orally, the daily total intake of patients receiving infusions was not very much greater than that of patients on oral protein-restricted diets.[52] Encephalopathy was observed in all cirrhotic patients regardless of the route of protein administration, orally or IV as crystalline amino acids. The important finding in this study is the significant imbalance in plasma amino acids in patients given either FreAmine or FreAmine E (Nephramine). This finding of plasma amino acid imbalance is consistent with other clinical and experimental observations showing elevations of phenylalanine, methionine, and tyrosine, and decreases in the branched-chain amino acids, leucine, isoleucine, and valine. In dogs with chronic end-to-side portacaval shunts, survival may be related to the feeding of different diets, survival being the shortest with a meat diet and the longest with a milk diet.[32] The length of survival is related inversely to the content of aromatic amino acids such as phenylalanine, tyrosine, and tryptophan in various diets; meat diets have the highest content of these amino acids, and the milk diet the lowest.[32] Blood was less well tolerated than casein when given in isonitrogenous amounts to patients with hepatic insufficiency, or similar amount of protein given as meat.[45] This difference in tolerance could be related to the amino acid compositions in these proteins.

Fischer suggests the following requirements in treating patients suffering from liver disease with parenteral nutrition: (1) provide adequate nitrogen and calories; (2) avoid plasma amino acid imbalance; (3) maintain electrolyte and acid-base balance; (4) prevent neurologic or encephalopathic symptoms; and (5) administer the volume of fluid tolerable to patients.[8,49] Based on these criteria, Fischer and associates have developed a solution of crystalline L-amino acids for parenteral nutrition in dogs and in patients with liver disease.[49,50] The amino acid composition of this solution, Hepatamine (formerly, FO80), is shown in Table 13-3. One liter of the infusate used contained 38 g protein equivalent (6 g nitrogen) either as FreAmine II or Hepatamine (FO80), hypertonic glucose (23%), 40 mEq HCl, 30 mEq sodium acetate, 6 mEq magnesium sulfate, 25 mEq phosphate, and 4 mEq calcium. The results showed that normalization of the plasma amino acids, which could be achieved by the administration of Hepatamine (FO80), may be of value in controlling the hepatic encephalopathy in dogs with portacaval shunts and in humans as well.

OTHER ILLNESSES

There are other illnesses that affect the dietary intake, leading to malnutrition or nutritional deficiency. Among these, cardiac disease is noteworthy. As Abel points out, an increasing percentage of older hospitalized patients have moderate to severe impairment of cardiac function.[2] About 50% of these patients in the age group of over 60 years may require parenteral nutrition therapy regardless of their primary manifestation, surgical or medical. However, the management of parenteral nutrition in this group of patients is complex. It requires a thorough understanding of the physiopathologic status of their cardiac, renal, pulmonary, and liver functions, hormonal and metabolic changes, and fluid and electrolyte tolerance in order to achieve a successful objective.

Severe pancreatitis with impaired intestinal function leads to malnutrition or semistarvation. Experimental studies have shown reduction of gastrointestinal, exocrine pancreatic, and biliary secretion during parenteral nutrition.[62] Thus, total parenteral nutrition may be able to set the pancreas at rest and maintain patients at a reasonably good nutritional state. Positive nitrogen balance can be achieved in patients with acute pancreatitis given jejunal tube feeding or parenteral nutrition.[58,82] Although parenteral or enteral nutrition may not play a direct role in the improvement of the pancreatitis or inflammatory process, it seems reasonable to suggest that good nutritional support is capable of preventing or correcting malnutrition in patients with severe pancreatitis. Parenteral nutrition should be initiated when jejunal feeding is not possible or tolerable.[163]

Parenteral nutrition may be very beneficial prior to major surgery in patients who are nutritionally depleted and have lost a significant amount of weight. (See Chap. 36.) Patients included in this category may have a variety of diseases, particularly malignant neoplasms. Meng and co-workers observed that presurgery total parenteral nutrition resulted in a greater positive nitrogen balance and weight gain over those observed during the postoperative period even if the nitrogen and caloric intake were the same for both pre- and postsurgical period.[106]

In some patients with psychiatric problems, such as anorexia nervosa, hysterical vomiting, pathologic food faddism, and the obstetric syndrome of hyperemesis gravidarum, parenteral nutrition support may be useful in preventing severe morbidity and even death. In addition, use of parenteral nutrition has been reported in patients with tetanus, post-vagotomy gastric stasis, and protein enteropathy due to idiopathic intestinal lymphangiectasis.

Long-Term Parenteral Nutrition at Home—The Concept of an Artificial Gut

Because of the potential risks of infection and metabolic disturbances and the complex procedures in the preparation of nutrient infusate and catheter care, most of the patients receiving parenteral nutrition are hospitalized. In some instances, for example, short gut syndrome as the result of radiation, resection, or certain diseases, impairment of GI function is presented that may result in death. The combination of long-term access to the circulation by means of arteriovenous shunts and extensive experience with use of self-administered hemodialysis at home resulted in the proposal for long-term TPN at home, which Scribner and colleagues describe as "the concept of artificial gut."[132] Following the work of Scribner and associates, Shils also reported a patient to whom long-term parenteral nutrition was given through an external arteriovenous shunt.[140] However, the use of arteriovenous shunts for long-term parenteral nutrition at home has generally proved less than satisfactory. Nonetheless, Heizer and Orringer have successfully maintained a patient with short bowel syndrome on home TPN for 5 years.[64] Broviac and associates designed a right arterial catheter suitable for long-term use.[20] The catheter developed by Hickman, the so-called Hickman catheter, which has been used routinely in marrow transplant recipients, has also been used for home TPN. Jeejeebhoy and co-workers have also given long-term parenteral nutrition to patients at home and observed excellent results.[73,75] Solassol and associates have developed and used still another type of catheter and technique for long-term parenteral nutrition with success.[148] The home TPN program has grown significantly since 1970.[53,60,81,127] Currently, there are about 500 patients registered in this program of therapy in the United States. However, it has been said that a realistic estimate may be 1000 or more.

To assure the success of long-term parenteral nutrition at home, the following basic principles must be considered:

1. Selection of a method of circulatory access or a catheter system for continuous IV infusion of concentrated nutrient solution.

2. Selection of available sterile nutrient solutions that can be mixed easily and safely by the patient or some member of the family immediately prior to infusion; the composition of the infusate is predetermined and has been adapted to the patient during hospitalization.

3. Selection of a suitable delivery system, preferably with pump and alarm device to provide a constant infusion rate and to warn the patient that the infusion bottle is nearly empty. This is necessary especially if the infusions are given during the night.

4. The suitability of the patient for long-term parenteral nutrition at home must be carefully considered for insuring proper execution of the procedure.

Shils suggests the following additional criteria:[137]

1. A relatively stable clinical state with expectancy of a reasonably comfortable home life for many months.

2. A suitable home environment with supportive family members or other individuals who are conversant with all aspects of the techniques.

3. Availability of a trained nurse to visit the home periodically, to follow the clinical status, and to supervise the change of filters (if applicable) and dressings, the care of the catheter, and the mixing of the infusate, for an initial period.

4. When the patient lives some distance from the hospital, cooperation of a physician in the town of residence, who will assume responsibility for medical care, is important.

In addition, the patient and the individual(s) who will assist him or her at home must be trained to perform the mixing of the infusate and to care for the delivery system. The patient must be given an infusate with the same or quite similar composition as the one used in the hospital to ensure metabolic adaptation and to avoid complications at home. Some biochemical tests, for instance, blood glucose and serum electrolytes, should be done before discharge of the patient to his home, and dietary programs must be carefully planned to assure the tolerance of any oral intake both from the quantitative and qualitative points of view. Clinical and biochemical monitoring at reasonable intervals should be provided to ascertain that the patient is doing well.

The home parenteral nutrition program originally suggested by Broviac and Scribner was to mix two 500-ml bottles of amino acid solution (FreAmine II) with 1000 ml 60% glucose.[21] The glucose solution is in a half-filled, 2-liter bottle in vacuum. Vitamins and electrolytes are added using aseptic procedures. Two liters of this solution containing 600 g glucose and 85 g crystalline L-amino acids (12.5 g nitrogen), along with appropriate amounts of vitamins and electrolytes, are given during the night on a 5-nights-a-week schedule. The infusion usually is started at about 7:00 or 8:00 pm and is completed in about 12 hr. The program currently used by Scribner and his colleagues in Seattle is more flexible, in that it is designed according to the nutritional needs of the individual patient in terms of the amino acid and glucose content of the infusate.* The patient is free to visit or even to work during the day. The organization and the training program are discussed by Shils, Solassol and Joyeux, and others.[137,147] It is essential to consider all aspects of the problems before the parenteral nutrition at home is initiated. In addition to the preparation of infusate by the patient or a family member that Scribner and associates prefer, there are two other alternatives: (1) infusate may be prepared by a pharmacist in the hospital of the patient's physician. The infusate in bottles or bags can be picked up at intervals and stored in the refrigerator at the home of the patient, and (2) infusate may be prepared by one of the qualified home health-care companies with the approval of the attending physician.

Laboratory Findings

BIOCHEMICAL, PHYSIOLOGICAL, AND CLINICAL MONITORING

All aspects of the patient's condition must be monitored: vital signs, mental state, daily body weight, daily fluid intake, and daily fluid output—including fistula or wound drainage, urine, stools, GI aspirates, and other losses. The patient's state of hydration must be considered. Serum sodium, potassium, chloride, bicarbonate, and urea should be monitored daily at first and then once weekly when stabilized. Serum magnesium, calcium, phosphorus, and plasma protein should be measured, and a hemogram should be done at weekly intervals. In critically ill patients, it is often necessary to measure blood gasses, pH, and osmolarity. Liver function tests including serum glutamic-oxaloacetic transaminase (SGOT), serum glutamic-pyruvic transaminase (SGPT), lactic dehydrogenase (LDH), serum bilirubin, serum alkalkine phosphatase, and prothrombin time should be obtained at weekly or biweekly intervals. Nitrogenous compounds (besides urea) that should be monitored are serum creatinine, uric acid, and ammonia.

Frequent monitoring of blood and urinary glucose should be done during the early days of the parenteral nutrition period, especially in debilitated, elderly, stressed, or diabetic patients. Adjustments must be made in the infusion if the urinary glucose exceeds 2 plus. In patients with renal dysfunction, the urinary glucose value may be misleading and a blood Dextrostix reading is more valuable than fractional urine determinations. In order to prevent the urinary loss of glucose, the rate of administration should be reduced or insulin should be given, with insulin dosage based on the blood glucose level or urinary loss. Subcutaneous administration of eight units regular insulin every 4 to 6 hr with stepwise increment of 5 to 10 units/dose as needed, has been found to give better control than a sliding scale of insulin dosage based on the urinary glucose level. Because of the great variation of the renal threshold for glucose, even in patients with normal renal function, treatment must be individualized to maintain the blood glucose level below 180 mg/100 ml. As stated previously, some physicians prefer to add insulin to the infusate at ratios of one unit insulin to 7 to 10 g glucose. When fructose or invert sugar is given, serum lactate should also be determined at frequent intervals.

When fat emulsion is used, a plasma lipid profile including triglycerides, phospholipids, cholesterol, and free fatty acids should be determined at weekly intervals. If laboratory facilities are limited, it is acceptable to use the plasma optical density as a qualitative index of plasma triglyceride before each dosage increase, and then at weekly intervals. However, the measurement of optical density or light scattering is not reliable in the presence of endogenous hyperlipoproteinemia. In this case, plasma triglyceride should be determined by a chemical method. When parenteral nutrition is given without fat, serum total fatty acid patterns should be monitored for the possible development of essential fatty acid deficiency. In addition to lipid profiles, liver enzymes, and platelet count, coagulation time, partial thromboplastin time, and prothrombin time must be measured at weekly intervals in patients receiving fat emulsion over a long period of time.

As a means to avoid morbidity in the patient who is receiving TPN, walking should be encouraged if possible. A patient may walk while guiding a mobile IV infusation pole; this type of activity will assist in the maintenance or restoration of muscle tone, and skeletal and vascular competence. Ambulation while receiving parenteral nutrition is possible even if the use of a light-weight, portable, battery-operated pump is necessary. Activity is important, but the patient must have adequate control of his physical and mental facilities.

*Personal communication, 1975.

Complications

The impressive beneficial effects of parenteral nutrition have not occurred without hazard to patients. However, the incidence of complications has decreased in recent years as the techniques and knowledge in nutrient requirements and metabolism have advanced. For historic interest and prevention of complications, readers are referred to several reviews and books on the subject.[46,59,84,116, 130,134,162] Complications have occurred in the following areas.

CENTRAL VENOUS CATHETER

CATHETER PLACEMENT (SUBCLAVIAN APPROACH)

The central venous catheter (subclavian approach) has been found responsible for various complications, including perforation of the heart and laceration of major vessels, with extravasation of blood or solutions, obstruction of the major vessels, pneumothorax, as well as air embolism, hemothorax, and nerve injury. In addition, thrombosis or thrombophlebitis may develop around the catheter, especially if it is introduced into an arm vein. The formation of a fibrin sleeve around the catheter may cause pulmonary embolus.

CATHETER SEPSIS

Catheter-related sepsis, bacterial or fungal, is one of the most common dangerous complications, ranging from skin infection to fatal septicemia. The most prevalent serious infection appears to be yeast or fungal involvement. At the onset of an unexplained fever or signs of sepsis, the catheter should be withdrawn, and the tip as well as the blood, cultured. Serial blood cultures 2 to 3 days after withdrawal of the catheter may help decide the subsequent course of therapy.

Patients with septic foci may seed infection to their IV catheter. Infection also may occur from contamination of the delivery system, especially if additives or medications are given through the infusion line. However, long-term parenteral nutrition with a very low incidence of 1% to 4% sepsis is possible.

METABOLIC DISTURBANCES

Hyperglycemia is a common problem, particularly in patients with glucose intolerance. Hyperglycemia may lead to osmotic diuresis, dehydration, and nonketotic hyperosmolar syndrome progress-

ing to coma. On the other hand, hypoglycemia has been observed with excessive insulin administration when technical failure of the infusion system occurs. Hypoglycemia may also occur after abrupt cessation of infusion of parenteral nutrition infusate containing hypertonic glucose.

Elevation of the blood urea nitrogen level has been observed in some patients secondary to excessive administration of nitrogeneous nutrients, or to dehydration. Hyperammonemia also has been observed. This may be due to the presence of a large amount of free ammonia or ammonia ion in protein hydrolysate or to an inadequate amount of arginine in amino acid solutions. This can be corrected by the administation of additional arginine. Abnormal liver function indicated by the elevation of liver enzymes also may be a factor.

ELECTROLYTE IMBALANCE

Electrolyte imbalance usually results from administration of a standard solution without consideration of the patient's special needs. Hyponatremia may occur in the presence of increased loss or inadequate intake of sodium. Hypernatremia may be secondary to prerenal azotemia associated with excessive diuresis or to the hyperosmolar syndrome. Hypophosphatemia has been a common finding in patients receiving TPN containing concentrated glucose solutions that have little or no phosphate.

Hyperchloremic acidosis has been observed, especially in infants. This is primarily due to high chloride content in the infusate. Chloride ion is present in protein hydrolysates. It is also present in crystalline amino acid solutions; some amino acids are in HCL form. In addition, the use of sodium and potassium as chloride salts further increases the supply of this anion. It is recommended that some sodium and potassium be given as acetate. Recent attempts have also been made to use amino acids, such as lysine, in a base form.

DEFICIENCY OF ESSENTIAL FATTY ACIDS AND MICRONUTRIENTS

The incidence of clinical essential fatty acid deficiency, as demonstrated by the occurrence of severe skin lesion, has decreased since fat emulsions have become available. However, biochemical essential fatty acid deficiency, as judged by the increase in T/T ($20:3\omega9/20:4\omega6$), remains high. This results in part from the poor nutritional or hypercatabolic condition of the patients requiring TPN support or from inadequate dosage of linoleic acid administered. Although the physiologic or metabolic significance is under investigation and still unclear, the biochemical abnormality in plasma fatty acid composition should be corrected.

As stated previously, biotin deficiency has been observed in a child given TPN.[109] It is suggested that this vitamin should be given. This is also true for choline, which may be added to the infusate to prevent its decrease in the serum.[23] Bone disease in patients maintained on home TPN has been reported. Although the cause of this complication is unknown, excessive vitamin D intake may be one of the etiologic factors. Serum level and urinary excretion of calcium and phosphorus should be measured, and vitamin D dosage may need to be adjusted. Deficiency of inorganic trace minerals such as zinc or copper has been described earlier in this chapter.

OTHER COMPLICATIONS

Allergic reactions following the administration of protein hydrolysate have been observed rarely in some patients. When this occurs, the particular hydrolysate should be discontinued, and another protein hydrolysate or crystalline amino acid solution should be substituted. Anemia is a common finding in patients with protein–calorie malnutrition. It may be due to a deficiency of iron, folate, vitamins B_{12} and E, or copper. In order to correct anemia, all these nutrients should be provided along with adequate protein and calorie nutrition. In severe cases, it may be advisable to give blood transfusion.

Psychological effects of TPN, particularly in patients maintained on long-term home parenteral nutrition support, have also been reported.[117]

Conclusion

Conventional IV nutrition with 5% to 10% glucose, saline, and occasionally protein hydrolysate, is grossly inadequate to meet the needs of a stressed and hypercatabolic patient. Today, long-term TPN with adequate calories and nitrogenous nutrients is possible. The calories and nitrogen are given as a solution containing concentrated glucose (20% to 40%) and protein hydrolysate or crystalline amino acid mixture with vitamins, electrolytes, and trace minerals. Because of the hyperosmolarity of these solutions, they are infused continuously into a central vein, usually the superior vena cava, through an indwelling catheter during a 24-hr period. The method is effective in maintaining nitrogen balance and promoting weight gain and wound healing in patients with a variety of disease states. The use of fat emulsion (Intralipid, 10% or 20% soybean oil emulsions; and Liposyn, 10% or 20% safflower oil emulsions) has been found beneficial to correct or prevent essential fatty acid deficiency; it also furnishes additional calories. To ensure safe and effective parenteral nutrition, the following aspects should be considered.

In the planning of parenteral nutrition, it is of paramount importance to consider the condition of the patient and his nutritional needs. Nitrogen as protein hydrolysate or crystalline amino acids should be adequate. In addition, ample calories along with vitamins, electrolytes, and inorganic trace minerals should be given concurrently with the nitrogenous nutrients to achieve maximum amino acid utilization for protein synthesis. The total fluid volume and the amount of each nutrient given should be considered and the rate of administration regulated. In general, nitrogen, 12 g to 13 g (200 mg/kg/day–240 mg/kg/day) as crystalline amino acids and 2500 Cal/day–3000 Cal/day (32 Cal/kg/day–50 Cal/kg/day) with a calorie (nonprotein) to nitrogen ratio of about 200:1 are adequate for relatively stable patients. Fat emulsion should also be given at a daily dosage of 1 g/kg to 2 g/kg in adults and 2 g/kg to 4 g/kg in infants and young children.

Constant, meticulous care must be given to the central venous catheter and its site of insertion in order to avoid infection. In addition, the clinical condition and mental state of the patient must be assessed frequently. Serum electrolytes must be monitored frequently. In older, debilitated, diabetic, and stressed patients who may have glucose intolerance or inadequate insulin secretion, the administration of exogenous insulin may be required to maintain blood sugar levels between 100 mg/dl to 180 mg/dl to avoid hyperglycemia, osmotic diuresis, and hyperosmolar syndrome.

References

1. Abbott WE, Abel RM, Fischer JE: Intravenous essential L-amino acids and hypertonic dextrose in patients with acute renal failure. Effects on serum potassium, phosphate and magnesium. Am J Surg 123:632, 1972
2. Abel RM: Parenteral nutrition for patients with severe cardiac illness. In Fischer JE (ed): Total Parenteral Nutrition, p 171. Boston, Little, Brown, & Co., 1976
3. Abel RM: Parenteral nutrition in the treatment of renal failure. In Fischer JE (ed): Total Parenteral Nutrition, p 143. Boston, Little, Brown & Co 1976
4. Abel RM, Abbott WM, Fischer JE: Acute renal failure: Treatment without dialysis by total parenteral nutrition. Arch Surg 103:513, 1971
5. Abel RM, Beck CH Jr, Abbott WM, et al: Improved survival from acute renal failure after treatment with intravenous essential L-amino acids and glucose. N Engl J Med 288:695, 1973
6. Abel RM, Shik VE, Abbott WM, et al: Amino acid metabolism in acute renal failure: Influence of intravenous essential L-amino acid hyperalimentation therapy. Ann Surg, 180:350, 1974

7. Aguirre A, Fischer JE, Welch CE: The role of surgery and hyperalimentation in therapy of gastrointestinal cutaneous fistulae. Ann Surg 180:393, 1974
8. Aguirre A, Funovics J, Wesdrop RIC, Fischer JE: Parenteral nutrition in hepatic failure. In Fischer JE (ed): Total Parenteral Nutrition, p 219. Boston, Little, Brown & Co, 1976
9. Andersen DW, Wu–Rideout MYC, Filler LJ, Jr, et al: Utilization of intravenously administered maltose by growing miniature pigs. J Nutr 111:1185, 1981
10. Askanazi J, Rosenbaum SH, Hyman AI, et al: Respiratory changes induced by the large glucose loads of total parenteral nutrition. JAMA 243:1444, 1980
11. Barr LH, Dunn GD, Brennan MF: Essential fatty acid deficiency during total parenteral nutrition. Ann Surg 193:304, 1981
12. Bergstrom J, Bucht J, Furst P, et al: Intravenous nutrition of amino acid solutions in patients with chronic uremia. Acta Med Scand 191:359, 1972
13. Berlyne GM, Bazzard FJ, Booth EM, et al: Dietary treatment of acute renal failure. Q J Med 35:59, 1967
14. Berman ML, Homrell CE, Lagasse LD, et al: Parenteral nutrition by peripheral vein in the management of gynecologic oncology patients. Gynecol Oncology 7:318, 1979
15. Bivins BA, Rapp RP, Record K, et al: Parenteral safflower oil emulsion (Liposyn 10%): Safety and effectiveness in treating or preventing essential fatty acid deficiency in surgical patients. Ann Surg 191:307, 1980
16. Blackburn GL, Flatt JP, Clowes GHA, et al: Peripheral intravenous feeding with isotonic amino acid solutions. Am J Surg 125:447, 1973
17. Borresen HC, Coran AG, Knutrud O: Metabolic results of parenteral feeding in neonatal surgery: A balanced parenteral feeding program based on a synthetic L-amino acid solution and a commercial fat emulsion. Ann Surg 172:291, 1970
18. Brennan MF: Total parenteral nutrition in the cancer patient. N Eng J Med 305:375, 1981
19. Brennan MF: Total parenteral nutrition in the management of the cancer patient. Annu Rev Med 32:233, 1981
20. Broviac JW, Cole JJ, Scribner BH: A silicone rubber arterial catheter for prolonged parenteral nutrition. Surg Gynecol Obstet 136:602, 1973
21. Broviac JW, Scribner BH: Prolonged parenteral nutrition in the home. Surg Gynecol Obstet 139:24, 1974
22. Burke WA: Preparation and guidelines to utilization of solutions. In White PL, Nagy ME (eds): Total Parenteral Nutrition, p 329, Acton, Publishing Sciences Group, 1974
23. Burt ME, Hanin I, Brennan MF: Choline deficiency associated with total parenteral nutrition. Lancet 2:638, 1980
24. Caldwell MD, O'Neill JA Jr, Meng HC, et al: Evaluation of a new amino acid source for use in parenteral nutrition. Ann Surg 185:153, 1977
25. Calloway DH, Spector H: Nitrogen balance as related to caloric and protein intake in active young men. Am J Clin Nutr 2:405, 1954
26. Cannon PR, Frazier LE, Hughes RH: Influence of potassium on tissue protein synthesis. Metabolism 1:49, 1952
27. Carpentier YA, Askanazi J, Elwyn DH, et al: Effects of hypercaloric glucose infusion on lipid metabolism in injury and sepsis. J Trauma 16:649, 1979
28. Chapman R, Foran R, Dunphy JE: Management of intestinal fistulas. Am J Surg 108:157, 1964
29. Chen WJ, Ohashi E, Kasai M: Amino acid metabolism in parenteral nutrition with special reference to the calorie–nitrogen ratio and the blood urea nitrogen level. Metabolism 23:1117, 1974
30. Cheng AH, Gomez RA, Bergen JG, et al: Comparative nitrogen balance study between young and aged adults using three levels of protein intake from a combination of a whey–soy–milk mixture. Am J Clin Nutr 31:12, 1978
31. Collins FD, Sinclair AJ, Royle JP, et al: Plasma lipids in human linoleic acid deficiency. Nutr Metab 13:150, 1971
32. Condon RE: The effect of dietary protein on symptoms and survival in dogs with an Eck fistula. Am J Surg 121:107, 1971
33. Condor JR, Asatoor AM: Amino acid metabolism in uremic failure. Clin Chim Acta 32:333, 1971
34. Connors RH, Coran AE, Wesley JR: Pediatric TPN: Efficacy and toxicity of a new fat emulsion. JPEN, 4:384, 1981
35. Copeland EM, MacFayden BV Jr, Dudrick SJ: Intravenous hyperalimentation in cancer patients. J Surg Res 16:241, 1974
36. Copeland EM, MacFayden BV Jr, Dudrick SJ: The use of hyperalimentation in patients with potential sepsis. Surg Gynecol Obstet 138:377, 1974
37. Copeland EM, MacFayden BV Jr, Lanzotti VJ, et al: Intravenous hyperalimentation as an adjunct to cancer chemotherapy. Am J Surg 129:167, 1975
38. Copeland EM, MacFayden BV Jr, MacComb WS, et al: Intravenous hyperalimentation in patients with head and neck cancer. Cancer 35:606, 1975
39. Davidson LAG, Flear CTG, Donald KW: Transient amino aciduria in severe potassium depletion. Br Med J 1:911, 1968
40. Dressner TA, O'Grady WP, Throbjarnarson B: Parenteral hyperalimentation and multiple gastrointestinal fistulas. NY State J Med 71:665, 1971
41. Dudrick SJ, Rhoads JE: New horizon for intravenous feedings. JAMA 215:939, 1971
42. Dudrick SJ, Wilmore DW, Vars HM, et al: Can intravenous feeding as the sole means of nutrition support growth in the child and restore weight loss in an adult? An affirmative answer. Ann Surg 169:974, 1969
43. Dudrick SJ, Wilmore DW, Vars HM, et al: Long-term total parenteral nutrition with growth, development, and positive nitrogen balance. Surgery 64:134, 1968
44. Fekl W: Some principles of modern parenteral nutrition. Scand J Gastroenterol (4 Suppl.) 3:3, 1969
45. Fenton JCB, Knoght EJ, Humpherson PL: Milk and cheese diet in portal-systemic encephalopathy. Lancet 1:164, 1966
46. Fischer JE: Hyperalimentation. Adv Surg 11:1, 1977
47. Fischer JE (ed): Total Parenteral Nutrition. Boston, Little, Brown & Co, 1976
48. Fischer JE, Foster GS, Abel RM, et al: Hyperalimentation as primary therapy for inflammatory bowel disease. Am J Surg 125:164, 1973
49. Fischer JE, Funovics JM, Aguirre A, et al: The role of plasma amino acids in hepatic encephalopathy. Surgery 78:276, 1975
50. Fischer JE, Rosen HM, Ebeid AM, et al: The effect of normalization of plasma amino acids on hepatic encephalopathy in man. Surgery 80:77, 1976

51. Fischer JE, Yoshimura N, Aguirre A, et al: Plasma amino acids in patients with hepatic encephalopathy: Effects of two amino acid solutions. Am J Surg 127:40, 1974
52. Fleming CR, Hodges RE, Hurley LS: A prospective study of serum copper and zinc levels in patients receiving total parenteral nutrition. Am J Clin Nutr 29:70, 1976
53. Fleming CR, McGill DB, Berkner S: Home parenteral nutrition as primary therapy in patients with extensive Crohn's disease of the small bowel and malnutrition. Gasteroenterology 73:1077, 1977
54. Freeman JB: Peripheral parenteral nutrition. Can J Surg 21:489, 1978
55. Freeman JB, MacLean LD: Intravenous hyperalimentation: A review. Can J Surg 14:180, 1971
56. Freii E: Combination cancer therapy: Presidential address. Cancer Res 32:2593, 1972
57. Giordano C, DePasquale C, DeSanto NG, et al: Disorder in the metabolism of some amino acids in uremia. Proceedings of the Fourth International Congress of Nephrology 2:196, 1969
58. Goodgame JT, Fischer JE: Parenteral nutrition in the treatment of acute pancreatitis: Effect of complications and mortality. Ann Surg 186:651, 1977
59. Grant JP: Handbook of Total Parenteral Nutrition, Philadelphia, WB Saunders, 1980
60. Grundfest S, Steiger E: Experience with the Broviac catheter for prolonged parenteral alimentation. JPEN 3:45, 1979
61. Hallberg D, Schuberth O, Wretlind A: Experimental and clinical studies of fat emulsions for intravenous nutrition. In Meng HC, Law DH, (eds) Parenteral Nutrition, p 376. Springfield, IL, Charles Thomas, 1970
62. Hamilton RF, Davis WC, Stephenson DV, et al: Effect of parenteral hyperalimentation on upper gastrointestinal tract secretion. Arch Surg 102:348, 1971
63. Heird WC, Driscoll JM Jr, Schullinger JN, et al: Intravenous alimentation in pediatric patients. J Pediatr 80:351, 1972
64. Heizer WD, Orringer EP: Parenteral nutrition at home for 5 years via arteriovenous fistulae: Supplemental intravenous feedings for a patient with severe short bowel syndrome. Gastroenterology 72:527, 1977
65. Hill GL, King RFGJ, Smith RC, et al: Multi-element analysis of the living body by neutron activation analysis—application to critically ill patients receiving intravenous nutrition. Brit J Surg 66:868, 1979
66. Holman RT: Essential fatty acid deficiency in humans. In Calli C, Jacini G, Pecile A (eds): Dietary Lipids and Postnatal Development, p 127. New York, Raven Press, 1973
67. Holman RT, Carter WD, Wiese HF: The essential fatty acid requirement of infants and the assessment of their intake on linoleate by serum fatty acid analysis. Am J Clin Nutr 10:70, 1964
68. Host WR, Serline O, Rush BF: Hyperalimentation in cirrhotic patients. Am J Surg 123:57, 1972
69. Howard L, Chu R, Feman S, et al: Vitamin A deficiency from long-term parenteral nutrition. Ann Intern Med 9:576, 1980
70. Hulsey TU, O'Neill JA Jr, Neblett WR, et al: Experimental wound healing in essential fatty acid deficiency. J Pediatr Surg 15:505, 1980
71. Issac JW, Millikan WJ, Stackhouse J, et al: Parenteral nutrition of adults with a 900 miliosmolar solution via peripheral veins. Am J Clin Nutr 30:552, 1977.
72. Jeejeebhoy KN, Chu RC, Marliss EB, et al: Chromium deficiency, glucose intolerance and neuropathy reversed by chromium supplementation in a patient receiving long-term total parenteral nutrition. Am J Clin Nutr 30:531, 1977
73. Jeejeebhoy KN, Langer B, Tsallas, G, et al: Total parenteral nutrition at home: Studies in patients surviving for 4 months to 5 years. Gastroenterology, 71:945, 1976
74. Jeejeebhoy KN, Marliss EB, Anderson GH, et al: Lipid in parenteral nutrition: Studies of clinical and metabolic features. In Meng HC, Wilmore DW (eds): Fat Emulsions in Parenteral Nutrition p 45. Department Foods and Nutrition, AMA, 1976
75. Jeejeebhoy KN, Zohrab WJ, Launger B, et al: Total parenteral nutrition at home for 23 months, without complication and with good rehabilitation. Gastroenterology 65:811, 1973
76. Johnston IDA (ed): Advances in Parenteral Nutrition, Lancaster, England, Medical and Technical Publishing Co, 1978
77. Johnston IDA: Metabolic foundations of intravenous nutrition. In Johnston IDA (ed): Advances in Parenteral Nutrition, p 3. Lancaster, England, MTP Press Ltd, 1978
78. Josephson B, Bergstrom J, Buckt H, et al: Intravenous amino acid treatment in uremia. Proc of the Fourth International Congress of Nephrology 2:203, 1969
79. Kinney JM: Energy requirement for parenteral nutrition. In Fischer JE (ed): Total Parenteral Nutrition, Boston, Little, Brown & Co, 1976
80. Klein GL, Ament ME, Bluestone R et al: Bone disease associated with total parenteral nutrition. Lancet 2:1041, 1980
81. Ladefoged K, Jarnum S: Long-term parenteral nutrition. Br Med J 2:262, 1978
82. Lanson, DW, Daggett, WM, Civetta, JM et al: Surgical treatment of acute necrotizing pancreatitis. Ann Surg 172:665, 1970
83. Lanzotti VJ, Copeland EM III, George SL, et al: Cancer chemotherapeutic response and intravenous hyperalimentation. Cancer Chem Rep 59:437, 1975
84. Law DH: Total parenteral nutrition. Adv Int Med 18:389, 1972
85. Lawson LJ: Parenteral nutrition in surgery. Br J Surg 52:795, 1965
86. Lawson LJ, Blainey JD, Dawson–Edwards et al: Dietary management of acute oliguric renal failure. Br Med J 1:293, 1962
87. Layden T, Rosenberg J, Nemchausky B, et al: Reversal of growth arrest in adolescents with Crohn's disease after parenteral nutrition. Gastroenterology 70:1017, 1976
88. Lee HA (ed): Parenteral Nutrition in Acute Metabolic Illness, New York, Academic Press, 1974
89. Lee HA, Sharpstone P, Ames AC: Parenteral nutrition in renal failure. Postgrad Med J 43:81, 1967
90. Levenson SM, Upjohn JL, Sheehy TW: Two severe reactions following the long-term infusion of large amounts of intravenous fat emulsion. Metabolism 6:807, 1967
91. Loirat PH, Rohan JE, Chapman A, et al: Positive nitrogen balance in hypercatabolic states: Results obtained with parenteral feeding after major surgical procedures. European Journal Intensive Care Medicine 1:11, 1975
92. Long JM, Wilmore DW, Mason AD Jr, et al: Intravenous feeding. Ann Surg 185:417, 1977
93. Lowry SF, Smith JC Jr, Brennan MF: Zinc and copper replacement during total parenteral nutrition. Am J Clin Nutr 34:1853, 1981

94. MacFayden BV Jr, Dudrick SJ, Ruberg RL: Management of gastrointestinal fistulas with parenteral hyperalimentation. Surgery 74:100, 1973

95. McGarthy DM, May RJ, Mather M, et al: Trace metal and essential fatty acid deficiency during total parenteral nutrition. Am J Dig Dis 23:1009, 1978

96. Meng HC: Fat emulsions. In White PL, Nagy ME (eds): Total Parenteral Nutrition, p 155. Acton, Publishing Sciences Group, 1974

97. Meng HC: Fat emulsions in parenteral nutrition. In Fischer JE (ed): Total Parenteral Nutrition, p 305. Boston, Little, Brown & Co, 1976

98. Meng HC: Preparation, utilization and importance of fat emulsion in intravenous alimentation. In Majjar V (ed): Fat Metabolism: A Symposium on the Clinical Aspects of Fat Utilization in Health and Disease, p 69. Baltimore, Johns Hopkins Press, 1954

99. Meng HC: Sugars in parenteral nutrition. In Sipple HL, McNutt KW (eds): Sugars in Nutrition, p 528. New York, Academic Press, 1974

100. Meng HC, Caldwell MD, Sandstead HH: Total parenteral nutrition in patients with cancer. Am J Clin Nutr 29:481, 1976

101. Meng HC, Early F: Studies of complete parenteral alimentation in dogs. J Lab Clin Med 34:1121, 1949

102. Meng HC, Kaley JS: Effects of multiple infusions of a fat emulsion on blood coagulation, liver function and urinary excretion of steroids in schizophrenic patients. Am J Clin Nutr 16:156, 1965

103. Meng HC, Law DH (eds): Proceedings of an International Symposium on Parenteral Nutrition. Springfield, IL, Charles C Thomas, 1970

104. Meng HC, Law DH, Sandstead HH: Some clinical experiences in parenteral nutrition. In Berg G (ed): Advances in Parenteral Nutrition, p 64. Prague, Georg Theime Verlag, Stuttgart, 1970

105. Meng HC, Sandstead HH: Long-term total parenteral nutrition in patients with chronic inflammatory diseases of the intestines. In Wilkinson AW (ed): Parenteral Nutrition, Part 1, p 213. Edinburgh, London, Churchill Livingstone, 1972

106. Meng HC, Wang PY, Lu KS: The use of fructose and glucose as an energy source in total parenteral nutrition. Int J Vitam Nutr Res 15:252, 1976

107. Meng HC, Wilmore DW, eds: Fat Emulsions in Parenteral Nutrition, Department of Foods and Nutrition, AMA, 1976

108. Meng HC, Youmans JB: Indispensibility of fat in parenteral alimentation in dogs. J Clin Nutr 1:372, 1953

109. Mock DM, Delorimer AA, Liebman WM, et al: Biotin deficiency: An unusual complication of parenteral nutrition. N Engl J Med 304:820, 1981

110. Moore FD: Surgical nutrition—parenteral and oral. In Committee on Preoperative and Postoperative Care of the American College of Surgeons: Manual of Preoperative and Postoperative Care, p 66. Philadelphia, WB Saunders, 1967

111. Munro HN: Amino acid requirements and metabolism and their relevance to parenteral nutrition. In Wilkinson AW (ed): Parenteral Nutrition, London, Churchill Livingstone, 1972

112. Munro HN: Protein hydrolysate and amino acids. In White PL, Nagy ME (eds): Total Parenteral Nutrition, p 59. Acton, Publishing Sciences Group, 1974

113. Nichoalds GE, Meng HC, Caldwell MD: Circulating levels of vitamins in adult patients receiving total parenteral nutrition. Arch Surg 112:1061, 1977

114. O'Neill JA, Caldwell MD, Meng HC: Essential fatty acid deficiency in surgical patients. Ann Surg 185:535, 1977

115. O'Neill JA Jr, Meng HC, Caldwell MD, et al: Variations in intravenous nutrition in the management of catabolic states in infants and children. J Pediatr Surg 9:889, 1974

116. Parsa MH, Ferner JM, Hatif DV: Safe central venous nutrition guidelines for prevention and management of complications. Charles C Thomas, Springfield IL, 1974

117. Perl M, Hall RCW, Dudrick SJ, et al: Psychological aspects of long-term home hyperalimentation. JPEN 4:554, 1980

118. Peter C, Fischer JE: Studies on calorie to nitrogen ratio for total parenteral nutrition. Surg Gynecol Obstet 151:1, 1980

119. Press H, Hartop PJ, Prottey C: Correction of essential fatty acid deficiency in man by the cutaneous application of sunflower seed oil. Lancet 1:597, 1974

120. Randall HT: Fluid and electrolyte therapy. In Committee on Preoperative and Postoperative Care of the American College of Surgeons: Manual of Preoperative and Postoperative Care, p 15. Philadelphia, WB Saunders, 1967

121. Randall HT: Indications for parenteral nutrition in postoperative catabolic states. In Meng HC, Law DH (eds): Parenteral Nutrition, p 13. Springfield IL, Charles C Thomas, 1970

122. Randall HT: Nutrition in surgical patients. Am J Surg 119:530, 1970

123. Recommended Dietary Allowances. A Report of the Food and Nutrition Board 9th ed. National Research Council, National Academy of Science, 1980

124. Rice CO, Orr, B, Enquist I: Parenteral nutrition in surgical patients as provided from glucose, amino acids and alcohol—the role played by alcohol. Ann Surg 131:289, 1950

125. Richards JR, Kinney JM (eds): Nutritional Aspects of Care in Critically Ill, Edinburgh, Churchill Livingstone, 1977

126. Richardson TJ, Sqoutas D: Essential deficiency in four adult patients during total parenteral nutrition. Am J Clin Nutr 28:258, 1975

127. Riella MC, Scribner BH: Five years' experience with a right atrial catheter for prolonged parenteral nutrition at home. Surg Gynecol Obstet 134:205, 1976

128. Rose WC: The amino acid requirements in adult man. Nutr Abst Rev 27:631, 1957

129. Rusho WI, Standish R, Bair JN: A comparison of crystalline amino acid solutions for parenteral nutrition. Hospital Formulary, Jan: 29, 1981

130. Ryan JA Jr: Complications of total parenteral nutrition. In Fischer JE (ed): Total Parenteral Nutrition. Little, Brown & Co, p 55. Boston, 1977

131. Schwartz FG, Green HL, Bendon ML, et al: Combined parenteral hyperalimentation and chemotherapy in the treatment of disseminated tumors. Am J Surg 121:169, 1971

132. Scribner BH, Cole JJ, Christopher G, et al: Long-term total parenteral nutrition. JAMA 212:457, 1970

133. Sheldon GF, Gardiner BN, Way LW, et al: Management of gastrointestinal fistulas. Surg Gynecol Obstet 133:385, 1971

134. Shenkin A, Wretlind A: Parenteral nutrition. World Rev Nutr Diet 28:1, 1978

135. Shike M, Harrison JE, Sturtridge WD, et al: Metabolic bone disease in patients receiving long-term total parenteral nutrition. Ann Int Med 92:343, 1980

136. Shike M, Roulet M, Kurian R, et al: Copper metabolism and requirements in total parenteral nutrition. Gastroenterology 81:290, 1981
137. Shils ME: A program for total parenteral nutrition at home. Am J Clin Nutr 28:1429, 1975
138. Shils ME: Guidelines for total parenteral nutrition. JAMA 220:1721, 1972
139. Shils ME: Minerals. In White PL, Nagy ME (eds): Total Parenteral Nutrition, p 257. Acton, Publishing Sciences Group, 1974
140. Shils ME, Wright WL, Turnbull A, et al: Long-term parenteral nutrition through an external arteriovenous shunt. N Engl J Med 282:341, 1970
141. Signer R, Stanford W, Levenson SM, et al: Maltose in parenteral alimentation. Am J Clin Nutr 26:28, 1973
142. Shizgal HM, Force RA: Protein and calorie requirements with total parenteral nutrition. Ann Surg 192:562, 1980
143. Shizgal HM, Milne CA, Spanier AH: The effect of nitrogen-sparing intrvenous fluids on postoperative body composition. Surgery 85:496, 1979
144. Silvis SE, Badertscher V: Treatment of severe liver failure with hyperalimentation. Am J Gastroenterol 59:416, 1973
145. Sloan GM, Brennan MF: Positive calcium balance in patients receiving total parenteral nutrition. Clin Res 28:621A, 1980
146. Smith RC, Burkinshaw L, Hill GL: Optimal energy and nitrogen intake for gastroenterological patients requiring intravenous nutrition. Gastroenterology 82:445, 1982
147. Solassol CI, Joyeux H: Ambulatory parenteral nutrition. In Fischer JE (ed): Total Parenteral Nutrition, p 285. Boston, Little, Brown, & Co, 1976
148. Solassol CI, Joyeux H, Etco L, et al: New techniques for long-term intravenous feeding: An artificial gut in 75 patients. Ann Surg 179:519, 1974
149. Somani P, Leathem WD, Barlow AL: Safflower oil emulsion: Single and multiple infusions with or without added heparin in normal human volunteers. JPEN 4:307, 1980
150. Steffee CH, Wissler RW, Hamphreys EM, et al: Studies in amino acid utilization. V: The determination of minimum daily essential amino acid requirements in protein-depleted adult male rats. J Nutr 40:483, 1950
151. Steiger E, Oram–Smith J, Miller E, et al: Effects of nutrition on tumor growth and tolerance to chemotherapy. J Surg Res 18:455, 1975
152. Stein TP, Buzby GP, Leskin MJ, et al: Protein and fat metabolism in rats during repletion and total parenteral nutrition. J Nutr 111:154, 1981
153. Stone WJ, Warnock LG, Wagner C: Vitamin B_6 deficiency in uremia. Am J Clin Nutr 28:950, 1975
154. Terepka AR, Waterhouse C: Metabolic observation during the forced feeding of patients with cancer. Am J Med 20:225, 1956
155. Thompson WR: Peripheral venous TPN in the treatment of critically ill surgical patients. In Meng HC, Wilmore DW (eds): Fat Emulsions in Parenteral Nutrition, Department of Foods and Nutrition, AMA, 1976
156. Trace Elements in Human Nutrition. Report of WHO Expert Committee, World Health Organization Technical Report Series No. 532, Geneva, 1973
157. Van Way CW III, Meng HC, Sandstead HH: An assessment of the role of parenteral nutrition in the management of surgical patients. Ann Surg 177:103, 1973
158. Van Way CW III, Meng HC, Sandstead HH: Nitrogen balance in postoperative patients receiving parenteral nutrition. Arch Surg 110:272, 1975
159. Vauy R, Scrimshaw NS, Young VR: Human protein requirements: Nitrogen balance response to graded levels of egg protein in elderly men and women. Am J Clin Nutr 31:779, 1978
160. Vilter RW, Bozian RC, Hess EV et al: Manifestations of copper deficiency in patient with systemic sclerosis on intrvenous hyperalimentation. N Engl J Med 291:188, 1974
161. Walser M: Keto acids in the treatment of uremia. Clin Nephrol 3:180, 1975
162. White PL, Nagy ME (eds): Total Parenteral Nutrition. Acton, Publishing Sciences Group, 1974
163. White TT, Heimbach DM: Sequestrectomy and hyperalimentation in the treatment of hemorrhagic pancreatitis. Am J Surg 132:270, 1976
164. Wilkinson AW (ed): Parenteral Nutrition. Edinburgh, London, Churchill Livingstone, 1972
165. Wilmore DW: The Metabolic Management of Critical Ill, New York, Plenum Medical Book Company, 1977
166. Wilmore DW, Curreri PW, Spitzer KW, et al: Supranormal dietary intake in thermally injured hypermetabolic patients. Surg Gynecol Obstet 132:881, 1971
167. Wilmore DW, Dudrick SJ: Safe long-term venous catheterization. Arch Surg 98:256, 1969
168. Wilmore DW, Dudrick SJ: Treatment of acute renal failure with intravenous essential L-amino acid. Arch Surg 99:669, 1969
169. Wittine MF, Freeman JB: Calcium requirements during total parenteral nutrition in well nourished individual. JPEN 1:152, 1977
170. Wolfe BM, Culebras JM, Sim AJW, et al: Substrate interation in intravenous feeding: Comparative effects of carbohydrate and fat on amino acid utilization in fasting man. Ann Surg 186:518, 1977
171. Wolpert E, Phillips SF, Summerskill WHJ: Ammonia production in the human colon. Effects of cleansing, neomycin and acetohydroxamic acid. N Engl J Med 283:159, 1970
172. Wretlind A: Fat emulsions. In White PL, Nagy ME (eds): Tota; Parenteral Nutrition, p 201. Acton, Publishing Sciences Group, 1974
173. Young EA, Weser E: The metabolism of infused maltose and other sugars. In Jeanes A, Hodges J (eds): Physiological Effects of Food Carbohydrates, p 73. Washington, DC, American Chemical Society Symposium Series 15, 1975
174. Zanni E, Calloway DH, Zezulka A: Protein requirement of elder men. J Nutr 109:513, 1979

14
Parenteral Nutrition—
Pediatrics

William C. Heird
Robert W. Winters

One of the earliest documented uses of total parenteral nutrition (TPN) in infants was published by Helfrick and Abelson in 1944.[31] Their patient was a 5-month-old male with severe marasmus—so severe, in fact, "all observers agreed that he would not survive more than a day or two at most." Using alternate infusions of a mixture of 50% glucose, 10% casein hydrolysate, electrolytes, and an olive oil-lecithin homogenate, these investigators were able to deliver 130 Cal in 150 ml/kg/day by peripheral vein infusions. Despite repeated thrombophlebitis, TPN was maintained for 5 days. Toward the end of this period, "the fat pads of the cheeks had returned, the ribs were less prominent, and the general nutritional status was much improved." In addition, "[his] former expression of dire misery was gone." The patient ultimately survived.

During the next 20 or so years, many investigators tried to duplicate this impressive performance, usually without success. The hypertonicity of the nutrient infusate necessitated such frequent changing of peripheral vein infusion sites that all available sites were soon used, often without prevention of thrombophlebitis. Alternatively, the volumes of less-concentrated infusates required for anabolism exceeded the infant's tolerance for fluid.

In 1966, Dudrick and associates reported a relatively simple technique that made TPN a practical reality—that is, a method allowing a catheter to be inserted and maintained for long periods of time in the superior vena cava.[16] Since the blood flow in this central vein is high, these investigators reasoned that giving the hyperosmolar nutritive fluid by a slow, continuous infusion would result in immediate dilution, thereby preventing damage to the vein. By using this type of delivery system to administer a hypertonic mixture of glucose, protein hydrolysate, electrolytes, minerals, and vitamins, Dudrick and associates demonstrated good growth and development, first in beagle puppies and subsequently in an infant.[16,54] This dramatic demonstration provided the stimulus for the now widespread use of TPN in pediatric patients.

Central Vein Total Parenteral Nutrition

CLINICAL EXPERIENCE

There is little doubt that central vein TPN as described by Dudrick and colleagues successfully produces growth in infants and children and regrowth of depleted adults.[16,54] In infants, a regimen delivering 2.5 g/kg/day of amino acids or protein hydrolysate and 110 Cal/kg/day to 120 Cal/kg/day reliably produces weight gains of 12 g/kg/day to 15 g/kg/day, nitrogen retention of approximately 200 mg/kg/day, and normal increments in both length and head circumference.[30] In adolescents, weight gains in excess of 1 kg/week can be achieved by provision, intravenously, of protein and energy intakes approximately 20% above resting requirements. Weight gains of younger children are intermediate between those of infants and adolescents.

TPN has been used widely in infants and children who require multiple operative procedures for correction of congenital or acquired anomalies of the intestinal tract and in patients with intractable diarrhea.[30] The technique has also been used in low-birth-weight infants, either as the sole source of nutritional support or as a supplement to tolerated enteral nutrients.[7,14] More recently, it has been used in older patients with chronic gastrointestinal disease, for instance, inflammatory bowel disease, and in patients with various malignancies, particularly those requiring abdominal radiation or chemotherapeutic regimens that result in nausea or intestinal dysfunction.[10,53] Special modifications of the technique have been used in adult patients with either renal or hepatic failure.[1,19]

It is difficult to ascribe improvements in either mortality or morbidity directly to TPN. On the other hand, the mortality of infants with surgically correctable anomalies of the gastrointestinal tract (*e.g.,* gastroschisis), as well as infants with intractable diarrhea, is less than 10% today, whereas mortality from both conditions was as high as 70% to 90% prior to routine use of TPN. Because this improved survival coincides with the advent of TPN, and since there have been no major changes in the primary therapy for these conditions, it is likely that TPN has played a major role in reduction of mortality in these groups of infants.

The improved survival of infants with surgically correctable gastrointestinal anomalies and intractable diarrhea seems to result primarily from improved nutritional management. There is no convincing evidence that parenterally administered nutrients result in improved intestinal function. Although intestinal morphology may improve during periods of exclusive parenteral intake, return of completely normal gastrointestinal morphology or function does not occur until enteral feeding is resumed.[25,35,46] Normal animals, when changed from enteral to parenteral feeding, undergo marked atrophy of the intestinal mucosa.[17,35,36] Further mucosal atrophy does not occur in animals that receive parenteral nutrients following a period of starvation; however, the increase in mucosal mass that occurs when previously starved animals are refed does not occur in animals that are refed parenterally.[17] Whether or not atrophy of intestinal mucosa occurs in otherwise normal infants (low-birth-weight infants) when only parenteral nutrients are given is not known. If atrophy does occur, it appears to be readily reversible, because few unexpected feeding difficulties are encountered when such infants are fed (or refed) enterally.

It is clear that TPN effectively produces normal weight gain in low-birth-weight infants.[14] However, it is not clear that this technique improves either survival or morbidity of this group of infants. The additional problems with parenteral nutrition in this group of infants, in fact, have led many to feel that the risks of the technique outweigh the benefits.

One important clinical benefit of parenteral nutrition in patients with either surgical complications or inflammatory bowel disease is that the closure of fistulas is hastened.[5] This beneficial clinical result is thought to occur because the intestinal tract is bypassed, thereby reducing secretions and consequently the flow of intestinal contents through the fistulas. In many patients, a period of parenteral nutrition results in closure of fistulas without surgical intervention.

Parenteral nutrition improves the overall nutritional status of patients with malignancies and may allow administration of greater doses of both chemotherapeutic agents and radiation (see Chap. 36).[10] Although such therapy may prolong survival, there is no evidence that it improves overall mortality rate.

In patients with renal failure, provision of essential amino acids along with sufficient calories and other nutrients results in recycling of nitrogenous wastes for endogenous production of nonessential amino acids. These endogenously produced nonessential amino acids, together with administered essential amino acids and other required nutrients, result in growth or regrowth in pediatric and adult patients, respectively.

Abel and co-workers demonstrated that survival of adult patients with acute renal failure given a parenteral glucose-essential amino acid regimen was better than that of patients given glucose alone.[1] Further, the glucose-essential amino acid regimen seemed to result in more rapid return of normal renal function. Other investigators have shown that a regimen of glucose plus organic acid analogues of essential amino acids is equally efficacious.[52] The organic acid analogues, in fact, may elicit a more marked anabolic response than essential amino acids.[51]

Use of an amino acid mixture containing a high percentage of branched-chain amino acids results in marked improvement of the state of consciousness of adult patients with coma secondary to severe liver disease.[19] This improvement is thought to be due to changes in brain amino acid patterns and subsequent changes in the concentrations of various neurotransmitters.[18] No effect on overall mortality of patients with severe hepatic dysfunction has been demonstrated.

Successful therapy in patients with either renal or hepatic failure seems to rely upon the mixture of amino acids used, not on the route of delivery. However, the limitation of fluid intake imposed by renal failure often makes enteral delivery of sufficient calories to promote anabolism impossible. Thus, parenteral delivery of glucose concentrations of up to 50% is often necessary for success. Similarly, parenteral delivery is often required in patients with severe coma secondary to liver disease.

NATURE OF WEIGHT GAIN

Despite apparently normal weight gain during periods of total parenteral nutrition, a number of factors suggest that the composition of this added tissue may be more hydrated than that achieved with conventional enteral nutrition. Although frank edema is uncommon, most patients receiving only parenteral nutrients develop a characteristic Cushingoid appearance. Further, the weight loss observed following cessation of TPN is greater than would be expected solely on the basis of decreased nutrient intake.

Changes in body composition during TPN have been estimated using actual intake, weight gain, and nitrogen retention data plus assumptions concerning either resting energy expenditure and the energy cost of growth or the relationship between protein and water content of lean body mass (LBM).[30,37] These data all suggest that the increase in body mass achieved with TPN is hyperhydrated. An example of the probable magnitude of this hyperhydration, based on assumptions of resting energy expenditure and the energy cost of growth, is shown in Figure 14-1. Animals nourished exclusively by the parenteral route certainly retain excessive fluid.[43] Failure to detect these changes clinically is probably related to the available methodology.

COMPLICATIONS OF CENTRAL VEIN TPN

There are two general types of complications associated with parenteral nutrition: those related to presence of the indwelling catheter (catheter-related complications) and those related to the infusate (metabolic complications).

Catheter-related complications include thrombosis (including superior vena cava thrombosis), dislodgment, perforation, and infection. While all can be controlled, it has been difficult to totally prevent any of these complications. The most common such complication has been infection, with infection rates as high as 40% to 50% having been reported.[12]

Some of the metabolic complications result from the patient's limited metabolic capacity for the various components of the nutrient intake. These are easily controlled with appropriate monitoring, as indicated below. Others are related to lack of

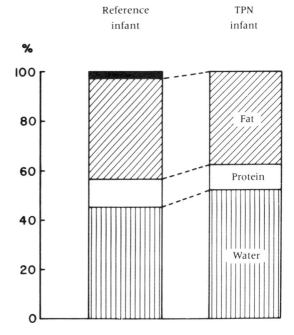

FIG. 14-1 Composition of weight gain during the total parenteral nutrition period (*TPN*) in comparison to that of Fomon's male reference infant over the first 4 months of life. (Fomon SJ: Body composition of the male reference infant during the first year of life. Pediatrics 40:863, 1967.) (Reproduced, with permission, from Levy JS et al: Total parenteral nutrition. In Kretchmer N, Brasel JA (eds): Biomedical and Social Bases of Pediatrics, p 185. New York, Masson Publishing, 1981)

knowledge about the differences between enteral and parenteral requirements and the fact that appropriate infusate components are not available. Both types of metabolic complications are summarized in Table 14-1.

The abnormal plasma aminogram that results from use of all currently available amino acid mixtures is one of the most troubling metabolic complications.[55] This problem involves both safety and efficacy. The long-recognized coexistence of mental retardation and elevated plasma amino acid concentrations in patients with various inborn errors of metabolism (*e.g.,* phenylketonuria and maple syrup urine disease, see Chap. 25) is the major reason for concern about safety. Since elevated plasma amino acid concentrations (*e.g.,* methionine, glycine) occur routinely in patients receiving TPN, this concern is valid. However, the low plasma concentrations of other amino acids (*e.g.,* tyrosine, cysteine, branched-chain amino acids, lysine) may be of equal or greater importance—particularly in terms of efficacy. Tyrosine and cysteine, both thought to be essential amino acids for the newborn, are only sparingly soluble; thus, no available

TABLE 14-1
Metabolic Complications of Total Parenteral Nutrition and Their Usual Causes

Metabolic Disorder	Usual Cause
Disorders related to patient's metabolic capacity	
Hyperglycemia	Excessive intake (either concentration or infusion rate)
	Change in metabolic state (*e.g.,* sepsis, surgical stress)
Hypoglycemia	Sudden cessation of infusion
Azotemia	Excessive nitrogen intake
Electrolyte disorders	Excessive or inadequate intake
Mineral (major and trace) disorders	Excessive or inadequate intake
Vitamin disorders	Excessive or inadequate intake
Disorders related to infusate components	
Acid–base disorders (hyperchloremic metabolic acidosis)	Use of hydrochloride salts of cationic amino acids
Hyperammonemia	Inadequate arginine intake
Abnormal plasma aminograms	Amino acid pattern of nitrogen source
Hepatic disorders	Unknown

amino acid mixture contains an appreciable amount of either.[47,48] Failure to provide either these or provision of other amino acids in amounts sufficient to result in elevated plasma concentrations might limit the ongoing protein synthesis.[49] The degree of cerebral protein deficit of parenterally nourished animals seems to be related to the degree of abnormality of both the plasma and cerebral free amino acid patterns.[39]

CENTRAL VEIN CATHETER TECHNIQUE

CATHETER INSERTION AND CARE

Specific techniques for inserting central vein catheters, either through one of the jugular veins or percutaneously through the subclavian vein, are readily available.[15,29] In either instance, absolutely sterile surgical technique is mandatory. A silicon rubber (Silastic) catheter is preferable, and the position of its tip should be verified radiographically before it is used for administration of hypertonic nutrient infusates.

Regular meticulous care of the central vein catheter is imperative for prolonged, safe, and complication-free use. Most believe that this aspect of the

technique is the most important in preventing infection. In general, the catheter should never be used for purposes other than infusion of the nutrient solution. It is particularly important that it not be used for administering blood or obtaining blood samples. The catheter exit site should be dressed at least three times weekly. On each occasion the skin site should be cleaned with acetone then scrubbed with both an antiseptic agent (*e.g.,* Betadine) and alcohol. An antiseptic ointment should then be applied to the catheter exit site, and an occlusive dressing should be applied.

With strict adherence to the above measures of catheter maintenance, a single catheter can function for up to 90 days, often longer. In our hands the average life of a catheter is approximately 30 days.

THE NUTRIENT INFUSATE

The nutritional infusate obviously should include a nitrogen source as well as calories, electrolytes, minerals, and vitamins. A suitable solution for pediatric patients is shown in Table 14-2.

Hydrolysates of both fibrin and casein as well as several crystalline amino acid mixtures have been used successfully as the nitrogen source for parenteral nutrition. A crystalline amino acid mixture is used more commonly. Although there is no evidence that they are more efficacious, their composition is controlled more rigidly than is that of the hydrolysates. Amino acid intakes ranging from 2 g/kg/day to 4 g/kg/day have been used. Although the magnitude of nitrogen retention during TPN appears to be related directly to the magnitude of nitrogen intake, an amino acid intake of 2.5 g/kg/day results in nitrogen retention comparable to that observed in enterally fed normal infants.[30] Moreover, greater nitrogen intakes often result in azotemia.

Glucose, alone or with fat emulsions, is the most commonly used calorie source. A total daily caloric intake of at least 110 Cal/kg/day to 120 Cal/kg/day is necessary for "normal" growth. Although glucose intakes greater than 15 g/kg/day usually are not tolerated on the first day of therapy, intake often can be increased by roughly 5 g/kg/day until the desired intake is achieved. Until the metabolism of intravenously administered lipid emulsions is better understood, it seems desirable to limit intake of these preparations to 3 g/kg/day.

Convenient additive preparations of electrolytes, minerals, and vitamins have been available for many years. More recently, commercially available trace mineral preparations have also become available. The requirements for all these nutrients obviously vary from patient to patient. Thus, the amounts shown in Table 14-2 cannot be interpreted as absolute requirements. Almost certainly the suggested amount of calcium is inadequate for optimal skeletal mineralization. On the other hand, addition of more calcium will result in precipitation of calcium phosphate.

The suggestions for vitamin and trace mineral intakes are the most tenuous of the suggested intakes. We have provided the suggested vitamin intake for the past 10 years without recognizing obvious clinical vitamin deficiencies or excesses; however, sophisticated monitoring has not been conducted. Currently, it is clear that both zinc and copper deficiency occur relatively frequently if these nutrients are not included in the TPN regimen.[26,32] Thus, intakes of both are recommended, particularly if TPN is likely to be the sole source of nutrients for 2 weeks or more. It is likely that other trace minerals are also required, but data on which to base recommendations are not available.

Total Parenteral Nutrition by Peripheral Vein Infusion

CLINICAL RESULTS

Perhaps because of the time and effort required to contain both metabolic and catheter-related complications of total parenteral nutrition at an acceptable level, infusion of nutritional mixtures by peripheral vein has increased in popularity.[8,11] Since concentrations of glucose exceeding 10% cannot easily be infused by peripheral vein, this technique obviously mandates use of less concentrated nutrient infusates. Therefore, greater fluid intakes are required to deliver the quantity of nutrients, particularly calories, than can be delivered by central vein. To compensate, most peripheral vein regimens include an intravenous lipid emulsion which has a caloric density of 1.1 Cal/ml. Nonetheless, if fluid intake is limited to a total volume of 150 ml/kg/day (assuming that a glucose concentration of 10% is not exceeded) and intravenous fat intake is limited to 3 g/kg/day, the maximum caloric intake that can be delivered is approximately 80 Cal/kg/day. Obviously, the growth achieved with this regimen is less than that achieved with conventional central vein TPN. In general, weight gains of 8 g/kg/day to 10 g/kg/day without obvious fluid overload are observed.[11] Benner and associates recently reported successful use of a 12% glucose, amino acid, and lipid (4 g/kg/day) regimen that delivered approximately 110 Cal/kg/day with fluid intakes of less than 200 ml/kg/day.[4] The growth achieved with this regimen approached that achieved with central vein regimens.

TABLE 14-2
Composition of Infusates for Central Vein Delivery

Component	Daily Amount (per kg)
Nitrogen source	2.5–3 g
Protein hydrolysate or mixture of crystalline amino acids	
Calories	120–125
Glucose*	20–30 g
Lipid	0.5–3 g
Electrolytes and minerals	
Sodium (as chloride)	3–4 mEq
Potassium (as phosphate and chloride)†	2–4 mEq
Calcium (as gluconate)	1–4 mEq
Magnesium (as sulfate)	0.25 mEq
Phosphorus (as potassium phosphate)†	1.36 mmole
Zinc (as sulfate)	150–300 µg
Copper (as sulfate)	20–40 µg
Vitamins	
Multivitamin preparation‡	1–2 ml/day
Volume	120–130 ml

*For peripheral vein infusion, glucose concentration must be limited to 10%.

†Potassium, as phosphate, should be limited to 2 mEq/kg/day; additional potassium should be provided as the chloride salt.

‡MVI (USV Pharmaceutical Corp, Tuckahoe, NY) plus folic acid, 1–2 mg IM/2 wk; vitamin B_{12}, 50 µg IM monthly; vitamin K_1, 1 mg IM/2 wk.

The only study of peripheral vein nutrition regimens that includes nitrogen retention data is that of Anderson and colleagues.[2] The average nitrogen retention of low-birth-weight infants who received only 60 Cal/kg/day plus amino acids (2.5 g/kg/day) during the first week of life was approximately 150 g/kg/day. No statistically significant differences in weight gain were noted between these infants and control infants who received 60 Cal/kg/day as glucose. The obvious anabolism achieved with addition of amino acids to what is otherwise conventional fluid therapy for these infants, although somewhat surprising, is preferable to the obvious catabolism of infants who receive only glucose. Further, it seems reasonable to conclude that such peripheral vein nutrition regimens, at the very least, will adequately maintain existing body composition of older infants.

TECHNIQUE

Any of the usual peripheral vein infusion techniques can be used for infusing parenteral nutrients. On the other hand, when hypertonic (often caustic) nutrient infusates are used, more careful observation of the infusion site is necessary. Failure to terminate the infusion at the first suggestion of infiltration is likely to result in skin or subcutaneous tissue sloughs. This appears to be particularly true for the low-birth-weight infant. The composition of a suitable nutrient infusate for peripheral vein infusion is shown in Table 14-3.

COMPLICATIONS

There are considerably fewer infectious complications with peripheral infusion than with central vein infusion. However, maintenance of peripheral infusions with hypertonic infusate for longer than 2 weeks is difficult. After this period, subcutaneous and skin sloughs secondary to infiltration of the nutrient mixture become a major problem.

The metabolic complications are the same as those encountered with central vein delivery of the virtually identical infusate. One obvious exception is glucose intolerance; the lower glucose concentration of peripheral vein infusates makes hyperglycemia a less common problem.

In our experience, successful administration of parenteral nutrition by peripheral vein is neither easier nor less time consuming than successful parenteral nutrition by central vein. The nursing supervision required is identical for the two techniques. The time and effort necessary to maintain functioning peripheral vein infusions are greater

TABLE 14-3
Composition of Nutritional Infusate for Peripheral Vein Infusion

Component	Daily Amount (per kg)
Nitrogen Source	2.5–3 g
Protein hydrolysate crystalline amino acid mixture	
Calories	Approximately 75
Glucose	10–15 g
Lipid	0.5–3 g
Electrolytes and Minerals	
Sodium (as chloride)	3–4 mEq
Potassium (as phosphate and chloride)*	2–4 mEq
Calcium (as gluconate)	1–4 mEq
Magnesium (as sulfate)	0.25 mEq
Phosphorus (as potassium phosphate)*	1.36 mMol
Zinc (as sulfate)†	150–300 μg
Copper (as sulfate)†	20–40 μg
Vitamins	
Multivitamin Preparation‡	1–3 ml/d
Volume	150 ml

*Potassium, as phosphate, should be limited to 2 mEq/kg/day; additional potassium should be provided as the chloride salt.

†Optional.

‡MVI (U.S.V. Pharmaceutical Corp., Tuckahoe, NY) plus Folic Acid, 1–2 mg IM/2 wk; vitamin B_{12}, 50 μgm IM monthly; vitamin K_1, 1 mg IM/2 wk.

than with the central vein technique. The only study comparing the complication rates of the two routes of delivery supports this opinion.[33] The overall complication rate per day of therapy, including metabolic complications as well as complications related to the infusion technique, was similar with the two techniques. Thus, as suggested by these investigators, the choice of delivery route should be based not on which technique is thought to be easier but on the patient's clinical condition and nutritional needs.

Choice of Peripheral versus Central Vein Total Parenteral Nutrition

Currently, most physicians agree that parenteral nutrients, either as the sole or partial source of nutritional support, are indicated for any patient who is unable to tolerate sufficient enteral feedings for a significant period of time.

There is less agreement, however, concerning the definition of *significant period of time.* A reasonable guideline is to provide parenteral nutrients prior to erosion of the patient's endogenous nutrient stores. For example, it is unlikely that the well-nourished term newborn or older infant who must forego enteral feedings for only two or three days will require any form of parenteral nutrition. However, even this short period without nutrient intake is likely to result in significant depletion of the limited endogenous stores of very small infants or infants with preexisting nutritional depletion.

Since parenteral nutrition regimens that can be delivered by peripheral vein almost certainly maintain existing body composition, this route of delivery is a reasonable choice for the normally nourished infant who can be fed within a short period of time, that is, less than 2 weeks. Infants or older children who are expected to be intolerant of enteral feedings for longer than 2 weeks, regardless of initial nutritional status, are better candidates for central vein TPN. It is usually difficult to maintain peripheral vein infusates for more than 2 weeks. Further, a central vein regimen will support normal growth rather than merely maintain existing body composition.

Many pediatric patients seem to require parenteral nutrition for 10 to 18 days (*e.g.,* postoperative complications, necrotizing enterocolitis, many surgically correctable lesions, intractable diarrhea). In these patients it is difficult or impossible to choose between peripheral and central vein TPN strictly on the basis of how long they are expected to be intolerant of enteral feedings. Nutritional status, duration of illness, and clinical course prior to beginning parenteral nutrition are additional factors that must be considered. The larger infant who becomes intolerant of enteral feedings within the first few days of life (*e.g.*, the term infant with a surgically correctable lesion), provided there is a reasonable possibility of maintaining peripheral vein infusions for up to 2 weeks, might be assigned to a peripheral vein regimen. On the other hand, central vein TPN seems a more logical choice for the smaller neonate (*e.g.*, a low-birth-weight infant with the same surgically correctable lesion) or one who requires parenteral nutrition later in life after a clinical course necessitating prolonged intravenous infusions (*e.g.*, the infant with intractable diarrhea). Such infants are less likely to tolerate peripheral infusions for an additional 2 weeks and are also likely to be nutritionally depleted.

Use of Intravenous Fat Emulsions

It is now well established that infants who receive fat-free TPN develop essential fatty acid deficiency.[41] Preterm infants and nutritionally depleted infants develop essential fatty acid deficiency within days, particularly if growth is rapid. Thus, use of intravenous (IV) fat emulsions to prevent essential fatty acid deficiency seems indicated.* However, the amount required for this purpose (*i.e.*, 0.5 g–1 g/kg/day) is considerably less than the amount used as a nonglucose caloric source (*i.e.*, 3–4 g/kg/day).

Use of large amounts of fat emulsions (*i.e.*, 3 g–5 g/kg/day) apparently has not caused severe adverse effects. Nonetheless, several theoretical possibilities should be considered. These include the consequences of failure to metabolize the infused emulsion as well as the consequences of increased plasma fatty-acid concentrations secondary to metabolism. In addition, the relative nitrogen-sparing effects of carbohydrate and fat calories must be considered.

The rate of metabolism of IV fat emulsions appears to be variable, particularly in infants.[27,28] Neither the mechanisms for clearing intravenously infused lipid from the bloodstream (by the enzyme lipoprotein lipase with phagocytosis by the reticuloendothelial cells playing a secondary role) nor the mechanisms for subsequent metabolism to glycerol and free fatty acids are well developed in newborn infants.[3,21] The ability to use IV fat emul-

*A recent report casts doubt on the ability of at least one currently available lipid emulsion to prevent essential fatty acid deficiency completely.[22] Despite elevated tissue content of linoleic acid, the tissue arachidonic acid content of infants who died after long-term infusion was low. Further, these infants had a lower urinary concentration of a prostaglandin metabolite than normally fed infants. Obviously, much further research is needed concerning the ability of the human infant (even the human adult) to convert linoleic acid to arachidonic acid.

sions is related directly to maturity.[45] Lipoprotein lipase, for example, is very low prior to 27 weeks of gestation.[13] However, the stressed patient, regardless of maturity (even adults), also behaves as if this enzyme were low.[42] The infant who is small for gestational age, regardless of gestational age, is less able to use these preparations than is the infant whose size is appropriate for gestational age.[3,45] Based on this latter observation, the nutritionally depleted older child would not be expected to use IV fat as well as a nondepleted patient; however, this possibility has not been studied directly.

In both animals and adult volunteers, administration of large doses of fat emulsion has been associated with decreased pulmonary diffusion capacity.[24] This results, presumably, from accumulation of small lipid droplets within the pulmonary capillaries. The same phenomenon, of course, could result from smaller doses, if the rate of administration exceeded the rate at which the fat could be metabolized. Lipid droplets have also been demonstrated at autopsy in both pulmonary and hepatic macrophages—a situation that may interfere with reticuloendothelial function and thereby decrease resistance to infection.[23,40] Thus, use of large doses of IV lipid, depending upon its rate of metabolism, may be hazardous for infants with pulmonary disease or infection.

Metabolism of IV fat emulsions results in increased plasma concentrations of free fatty acids. Because free fatty acids compete with bilirubin and other substances for binding to albumin, use of large doses of IV lipid may also be hazardous for infants with hyperbilirubinemia.[50]

The relative nitrogen-sparing effects of carbohydrate and lipid calories have not been studied directly in infants. However, a large body of information from studies in adults and animals suggests that fat calories are less efficacious than are carbohydrate calories in promoting nitrogen retention.[6] In one recent study, addition of IV lipid to a parenteral nutrition regimen was found to have no effect on nitrogen retention of stressed patients unless at least 85% of the measured energy expenditure was met by carbohydrate calories.[38] In another study, however, little difference in nitrogen retention of nutritionally depleted adults was observed between isocaloric regimens of 100% glucose or 83% lipid and 17% glucose.[34] The patient populations of these two studies differed with respect to underlying clinical conditions, degree of on-going stress, and nutritional status; thus, any one or a combination of these variables might explain the discrepancy in results.

The possibility that fat calories are not as efficacious as carbohydrate calories in promoting nitrogen retention must be considered in the design of nutritional regimens to be delivered by peripheral vein. If, in fact, a minimal carbohydrate calorie intake is required for optimal nitrogen retention, this carbohydrate intake must be determined and included in such regimens.

Requirements for Successful Parenteral Nutrition

Successful parenteral nutrition, whether infused by central vein or peripheral vein, is not simple to achieve. Success cannot be achieved if either technique is approached merely as a modification of routine fluid therapy. Realization that the techniques are deceptive in their simplicity and require dedicated personnel as well as specialized facilities enhances the likelihood of success. Most have found that success is more likely to be achieved if the responsibility for administering this form of nutritional support is specifically delegated to a parenteral nutrition or clinical nutrition support team (see Chap. 9).

The key member of such a team is the physician, who is responsible for all of the team's activities. This physician must have an interest in the general problems of parenteral nutrition and nutritional support as well as a thorough knowledge of nutritional metabolism. He or she should have sufficient time to supervise the day-to-day details of the nutrition support program and to educate other hospital staff on the intricacies of parenteral nutrition and the potential advantages, disadvantages, indications, and contraindications of all nutritional support techniques. Many institutions now have established nutrition support teams with full-time directors. This practice appears to have markedly improved the overall practice of parenteral nutrition as well as the overall nutritional management of hospitalized patients.

The team must also include one or more nurses who work exclusively with patients requiring nutritional support. These individuals can serve primarily an educational role, especially in larger institutions that have several patients requiring nutritional support at any one time. Alternatively, they can assume responsibility for all nursing aspects of the care of patients requiring parenteral nutrition. Such duties include the frequent dressing changes required with central vein TPN as well as assisting the responsible physician in all aspects of the program.

Successful parenteral nutrition also requires availability of a flexible system for mixing the nutrient infusates. While standard solutions, which can be mixed routinely and stored until needed, are useful for some situations (*e.g.*, many peripheral vein regimens), ability to change the infusate in response to biochemical monitoring or to provide special requirements for individual patients is also necessary. Such a requirement implies that a pharmacist or similar person trained in aseptic mixing techniques is available and able to devote considerable time to preparation of the infusates. It also implies that special facilities needed for aseptic fluid preparation are available (*e.g.*, a laminar flow hood).

A number of responsive and convenient laboratories are also necessary for successful TPN. The chemical monitoring required for safe parenteral nutrition in pediatric patients mandates availability of microchemistry laboratory facilities. A responsive microbiological laboratory is also a necessity; however, neither routine microbiological cultures of the nutrient infusate nor routine blood cultures appear to be necessary.

Such a system has been used for the past 10 years at Babies Hospital, New York. With compulsive adherence to the system, preventable metabolic and catheter-related complications have been virtually nonexistent, and a catheter-related infection rate of less than 10% has been maintained. Unless the technique is approached in this way, the resulting complications are likely to be so great as to render the technique clinically useless, if not actually hazardous.

MONITORING REQUIREMENTS

Adequate monitoring to detect both metabolic and catheter-related complications is obviously necessary. However, parenteral intake and clinical results of this intake must also be monitored carefully if the full potential of the technique is to be realized. Adequate clinical monitoring usually requires that the patient be housed in an intensive care or semi-intensive care setting. Nursing observation necessary to prevent infiltration of the nutritional infusate delivered by peripheral vein and to assure proper, long-term function of the central vein catheter usually cannot be provided in the ordinary clinical setting. Adequate monitoring also requires personnel familiar with the intricacies of the IV infusion apparatus, including the many varieties of constant infusion pumps that are an absolute necessity for both central vein and peripheral vein delivery.

The suggested schedule for chemical monitoring shown in Table 14-4 will allow detection of metabolic complications in sufficient time to permit correction by altering the infusate.

Plasma osmolality can be predicted easily from the concentration of plasma electrolytes. In the absence of hyperglycemia, plasma osmolality can be estimated sufficiently accurately as twice the plasma sodium concentration; thus, this determination is not necessary.

All available amino acid mixtures result in some derangement of the plasma aminogram; specific derangements are largely a function of the particular mixture of amino acids used.[55] Thus, this expensive and difficult to obtain determination is not mandatory.

Although the consequences of the hepatic dysfunction that develops during the course of TPN are not known, the fact that evidence of dysfunction occurs in approximately 75% of all patients who receive parenteral nutrition makes careful assessment and monitoring necessary.[9]

The monitoring required to ensure safe and efficacious use of IV fat emulsions is unknown. The usual clinical practice is to inspect the plasma periodically for presence of lipemia. Alternatively, nephelometry is substituted for visual inspection. However, it is unlikely that either method effectively detects elevated plasma triglyceride or free fatty acid concentrations.[44] Thus, complete and adequate monitoring requires actual chemical determinations of both serum triglyceride and free fatty acid concentrations. Since microtechniques for these assays are not routinely available, and since they are performed by most laboratories only two or three times per week, such monitoring is not likely to be practical. A reasonable compromise is daily inspection or nepholometry for detecting lipemia, with less frequent determination of actual triglyceride and free fatty acid concentrations.

Home Parenteral Nutrition

Considering the many difficulties of TPN in hospitalized patients, the potential problems of home TPN, at first glance, appear formidable. Nonetheless, both patients who can tolerate some enteral intake and patients who can tolerate only parenteral nutrients have been treated successfully with home administration of parenteral nutrients for several months to years.[55] In many cases sufficient nutrients can be administered at night, allowing the patient to pursue reasonably normal daytime activities. Novel devices, including small portable infusion pumps that can be enclosed in vests, handbags, or the like have been developed, allowing even the patient who requires constant infusion of parenteral nutrients to pursue a reasonably normal life. Obviously, home parenteral nutrition is more applicable for the older child, adolescent, or adult. The youngest pediatric patient for whom the technique has been used successfully was 27 months old.

In general, the catheter used for home TPN is

TABLE 14-4
Suggested Monitoring Schedule During Total Parenteral Nutrition

Variables to be Monitored	Frequency (per wk)*	
	Initial Period	Later Period
Growth variables		
Weight	7	7
Length	1	1
Head circumference	1	1
Metabolic variables		
Blood or plasma		
Sodium, potassium, chloride	3–4	1
Calcium, magnesium, phosphorus	2	1
Acid–base status	3–4	1
Urea nitrogen	2	1
Albumin	1	1
Lipids	2	2
Urine glucose	2–6/d	2/d
Hepatic function	1	1
Prevention and detection of infection		
Clinical observations (activity, temperature)	Daily	Daily
WBC count and differential	As indicated	As indicated
Cultures	As indicated	As indicated

*Initial period is the time during which a full caloric intake is being achieved. Later period implies that the patient has achieved a metabolic steady state. In the presence of metabolic instability, the more intensive monitoring outlined under initial period should be followed.

the Broviac catheter, which can be implanted under the skin. These catheters can be used for much longer periods than the usual Silastic catheter. Usually, standard nutrient infusates are obtained from the hospital pharmacy on a regular basis (weekly or biweekly) and stored in a small, home refrigerator. However, some patients (or a family member) have been taught to prepare their infusates at home. More recently, a number of commercial concerns, often without hospital affiliation, have taken over the routine care of patients who require home TPN. As yet, no data are available for evaluation of this practice.

Most patients who are candidates for home parenteral nutrition have reached the point at which requirements are reasonably stable. Thus, less frequent monitoring is required. Interestingly, rebound hypoglycemia does not seem to be a problem, even in patients who receive parenteral nutrition at home only during the evening. All the usual metabolic and catheter-related complications occur with home TPN but appear to be much less frequent than in the hospitalized patient.

References

1. Abel RM, Beck CH Jr, Abbott WM, et al: Acute renal failure: Treatment with intravenous acids and glucose. N Engl J Med 288:695, 1973
2. Anderson TL, Muttart CR, Bieber MA, et al: A controlled trial of glucose versus glucose and amino acids in premature infants. J Pediatr 94:947, 1979
3. Andrew G, Chan G, Schiff D: Lipid metabolism in the neonate: I. The effects of intralipid infusion on plasma triglyceride and free-fatty acid concentration in the neonate. J Pediatr 88:273, 1976
4. Benner JW, Coran AG, Weintraub WH, et al: The importance of different calorie sources in intravenous nutrition of infants and children. Surgery 86:429, 1979
5. Byrne WJ, Ament ME: Home parenteral nutrition: Results of its use in the management of enterocutaneous and rectovaginal fistulas. JPEN 3:25, 1979
6. Calloway DH, Spector H: Nitrogen balance as related to caloric and protein intake in active young men. Am J Clin Nutr 2:405, 1954
7. Cashore WJ, Sedaghatian MR, Usher RH: Nutritional supplements with intravenously administered lipid, protein hydrolysates and glucose in small premature infants. Pediatrics 56:8, 1975
8. Cohen IT, Dahms B, Hayes DM: Peripheral total parenteral nutrition employing a lipid emulsion (Intralipid): Complications encountered in pediatric patients. J Pediatr Surg 12:837, 1977
9. Collins JC, Pulito AR, Heird WC: Hepatic dysfunction during total parenteral nutrition (TPN). Pediatr Res 11:442, 1977
10. Copeland EM, Daly JM, Dudrick SJ: Nutrition as an adjunct to cancer treatment in the adult. Cancer Res 37:2451, 1977
11. Coran AG: The long term total intravenous feeding of infants using peripheral veins. J Pediatr Surg 8:801, 1973
12. Curry CR, Quie PF: Fungal septicemia in patients receiving parenteral hyperalimentation. N Engl J Med 285:1221, 1971
13. Dhanireddy R, Hamosh M, Sivarubramanian KN, et al: Postheparin lipolytic activity and Intralipid clearance in very low birth weight infants. J Pediatr 98:617, 1981
14. Driscoll JM Jr. Heird WC, Schullinger JN, et al: Total intravenous alimentation in low-birth-weight infants: A preliminary report. J Pediatr 81:145, 1972
15. Dudrick SJ, Copeland E: Parenteral hyperalimentation. In Nyhus LM (ed): Surgery Annual, p 69, New York, Appleton–Century–Crofts, 1973
16. Dudrick SJ, Wilmore DW, Vars HM, Rhoades JE: Long-term total parenteral nutrition with growth, development, and positive nitrogen balance. Surgery 64:134, 1968
17. Feldman EJ, Dowling RH, McNaughton J, et al: Effects of oral versus intravenous nutrition on intestinal adaptation after small bowel resection in the dog. Gastroenterology 70:712, 1976
18. Fischer JE, Baldessarini RJ: False neurotransmitters and hepatic failure. Lancet 2:75, 1971
19. Fischer JE, Yoshimura N, Aguirre A, et al: Plasma amino acids in patients with hepatic encephalopathy: Effects of amino acid infusions. Am J Surg 127:40, 1974
20. Fomon SJ: Body composition of the male reference infant during the first year of life. Pediatrics 40:863, 1967
21. Forget PP, Fernandes J, Begemann PH: Utilization of fat emulsion during total parenteral nutrition in children. Acta Paediatr Scand 64:377, 1975
22. Friedman A, Frolich JC: Essential fatty acids and major urinary metabolites of the E prostaglandins in thriving neonates and infants receiving parenteral fat emulsions. Pediatr Res 13:932, 1979
23. Friedman Z, Danon A, Stahlman MT, et al: Rapid onset of essential acid deficiency in the newborn. Pediatriacs 58:640, 1976
24. Greene HL, Hazlett D, Demarec R: Relationship between intralipid-induced hyperlipemia and pulmonary function. Am J Clin Nutr 29:127, 1976
25. Greene HL, McCabe DR, Merenstein GB: Protracted diarrhea and malnutrition in infancy: Changes in intestinal morphology and disaccharidase activities during treatment with total intravenous nutrition or oral elemental diets. J Pediatr 87:695, 1975
26. Greene HL, Van Der Vorm D, Helinek GL, et al: Trace elements in parenteral feeding of infants. In Visser HKA (ed): Nutrition and Metabolism of the Fetus and Infant, p 377. Boston, Martinus Nijhoff Publishers BV, 1979
27. Gustafson A, Kjellmer I, Olegard R, et al: Nutrition in low birth weight infants: I. Intravenous injection of fat emulsion. Acta Pediatr Scand 61:149, 1972
28. Gustafson A, Kjellmer I, Olegard R, et al: Nutrition in low birth weight infants: II. Repeated intravenous injections of fat emulsion. Acta Paediatr Scand 61:177, 1974
29. Heird WC, MacMillan RW, Winters RW: Total parenteral nutrition in the pediatric patient. In Fischer JE (ed): Total Parenteral Nutrition, p 253, Boston, Little, Brown & Co, 1976
30. Heird WC, Winters RW: Total intravenous alimentation: State of the art. J Pediatr 86:2, 1975
31. Helfrick FW, Abelson NM: Intravenous feeding of a complete diet in a child: Report of a case. J Pediatr 25:400, 1944
32. Heller RM, Kirchner SG, O'Neill JA Jr, et al: Skeletal changes of copper deficiency in infants receiving prolonged total parenteral nutrition. J Pediatr 92:947, 1978
33. Jakabowski D, Ziegler MD, Periera G: Complications of pediatric parenteral nutrition: Central versus peripheral administration. JPEN 3:29, 1979
34. Jeejeebhoy KN, Anderson GK, Nakhooda AF, et al: Metabolic studies in total parenteral nutrition with lipid in man: Comparison with glucose. J Clin Invest 57:125, 1976
35. Johnson LR, Copeland EM, Dudrick SJ, et al: Structural and hormonal alterations in the gastrointestinal tract of parenterally fed rats. Gastroenterology 68:1177, 1975
36. Levine GM, Deren JJ, Steiger E, et al: Role of oral intake in maintenance of gut mass and disaccharidase activity. Gastroenterology 67:975, 1974
37. Levy JS, Heird WC, Winters RW: Total parenteral nutrition. In Kretchmer N, Brasel JA (eds): Biomedical and Social Bases of Pediatrics, p 185. New York, Masson Publishing USA, 1981
38. Long JM III, Wilmore DW, Mason AD Jr, et al: Effect of carbohydrate and fat intake on nitrogen excretion during total intravenous feeding. Ann Surg 185:417, 1977
39. Malloy MH, Rassin DK, Gaull GE, et al: Cerebral growth and development during total parenteral nutrition. Pediatr Res 13:360, 1979
40. Nordenstrom J, Jarstrand C, Wiernik A: Decreased chemotactic and random migration of leukocytes during intralipid infusion. Am J Clin Nutr 32:2416, 1979
41. Paulsrud JR, Pensler L, Whitten CF, et al: Essential fatty acid deficiency in infants inducted by fat-free intravenous feedings. Am J Clin Nutr 25:897, 1972

42. Person B: Lipoprotein lipase activity of human adipose tissue in health and in some diseases with hyperlipidemia as a common feature. Acta Med Scand 193:457, 1973

43. Pulito AR, Nicholson JF, Heird WC: Nature of weight gain during total parenteral nutrition. Pediatr Res 10:359, 1976

44. Schreiner RL, Glick MR, Nordschow CD, et al: An evaluation of methods to monitor infants receiving intravenous lipids. J Pediatr 94:197, 1979

45. Shennan AT, Bryan MH, Angel A: The effect of gestational age on intralipid tolerance in newborn infants. J Pediatr 91:134, 1977

46. Shwachman H, Lloyd–Still JD, Khaw KT, et al: Protracted diarrhea of infancy treated with intravenous alimentation. II. Studies of small intestinal biopsy results. Am J Dis Child 125:365, 1973

47. Sturman JA, Gaul G, Raiha NCR: Absence of cystathionase in human fetal liver: Is cystine essential? Science 169:74, 1970

48. Synderman SE: The protein and amino acid requirements of the premature infant. In Jonxis JHP, Visser HKA, Troelstra JA (eds): Nutricia Symposium, Metabolic Processes in the Fetus and Newborn Infant, p 128. Leiden, Stenfert Kroese, 1971

49. Taub F, Johnson TC: The mechanism of polyribosome disaggregation in brain tissue by phenylalanine. Biochem J 151:173, 1975

50. Thiessen H, Jacobsen J, Brodersen R: Displacement of albumin-bound bilirubin by fatty acids. Acta Paediatr Scand 61:285, 1972

51. Walser M, Bodenlos LJ: Urea metabolism in man. J Clin Invest 38:1617, 1959

52. Walser M, Dighe S, Coulter AW, et al: The effect of keto-analogues of essential amino acids in severe chronic uremia. J Clin Invest 52:678, 1973

53. Werlin SL, Grand RJ: Severe colitis in children and adolescents: Diagnosis, course and treatment. Gastroenterology 73:828, 1977

54. Wilmore DM, Dudrick SJ: Growth and development of an infant receiving all nutrients by vein. JAMA 230:860, 1968

55. Winters RW, Heird WC, Dell RB, et al: Plasma amino acids in infants receiving parenteral nutrition. In Clinical Nutrition Update—Amino Acids, p 147. Chicago, American Medical Association, 1977

Application
of
Nutrition
to
Clinical
Specialties

15
Alcoholism

Spencer Shaw
Charles S. Lieber

The relationship between nutrition and alcohol is complex, stemming from many levels of interaction. Alcoholic beverages are themselves nutrients, predominantly providing caloric food value, but in an intricate way. Ethanol affects the level of food intake by its displacement of required nutrients in the diet, by its effect on appetite, and by its multiple actions on almost every level of the gastrointestinal (GI) tract. The obligatory metabolism of ethanol by the liver alters this organ and profoundly affects the metabolism of many nutrients. Ethanol alters the storage, mobilization activation, and metabolism of nutrients and has a significant effect on almost every organ. Thus, ethanol alters nutrition extensively at the level of supply and demand.

Alcohol is directly toxic to many bodily tissues.[67] The synergism of malnutrition and alcohol in this regard, especially in alcoholic liver injury, has not yet been fully clarified. With the increase in alcoholism, the extent of related physical damage to members of our society has dramatically increased. The resulting pathologic alterations represent an enormous medical burden requiring complex nutritional therapy. Alcoholism remains one of the major causes of nutritional deficiency syndromes in the United States. Nutritional therapy in the alcoholic is often a balance between maximizing recovery and avoiding iatrogenic complications. For example, patients with alcoholic liver disease may develop encephalopathy with levels of dietary protein below the daily requirements; since tolerance in a given patient may change from day to day, daily evaluation is often necessary. The multitude of physiologic systems affected by alcohol makes a simple prescription difficult. Although much information is available about pathophysiology and the problems of iatrogenic complications, few well-controlled clinical studies are available. This chapter is devoted to providing a current basis for the diagnosis and management of nutritional problems in the patient with alcoholism.

Nutritive Aspects of Alcohol

NUTRITIONAL VALUE OF ALCOHOL

Calorimetrically, the combustion of ethanol liberates 7.1 Cal/g, but ethanol does not provide food value that is calorie-for-calorie equivalent to carbohydrates. Isocaloric substitution of ethanol for carbohydrate as 50% of total calories in a balanced diet results in a decline in body weight (see Fig. 15-1). When given as additional calories, ethanol causes less weight gain than calorically equivalent carbohydrate (see Figs. 15-2 and 15-3). Support for the view that ethanol increases the metabolic rate is provided by the observation that ingestion of ethanol increases oxygen consumption in normal subjects, and this effect is much greater in alcoholics.[149] Oxidation without phosphorylation, through stimulation of the microsomal ethanol oxidizing system or other catabolic pathways, remains a possible explanation for the observed differences. Evidence for interference with digestion or absorption as the explanation for caloric value differences is lacking. The estimated contribution

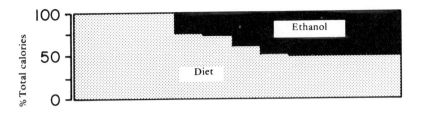

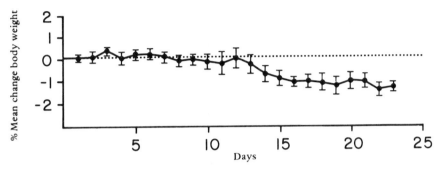

FIG. 15-1 Body weight changes after isocaloric substitution of carbohydrate by ethanol in 11 subjects (means ± standard errors). *Dotted line,* mean change in weight in control period. (Pirola RC, Lieber CS: Pharmacology 7:185, 1972. Permission from S Karger AG, Basel)

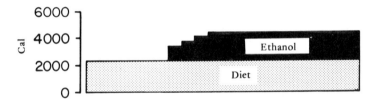

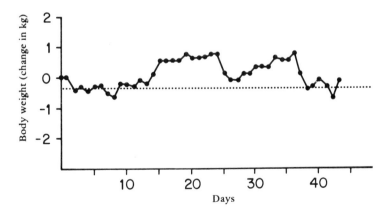

FIG. 15-2 Effect on body weight of adding 2000 Cal/day as ethanol to diet of one subject. *Dotted line,* mean change during control period. (Pirola RC, Lieber CS: Pharmacology 7:185, 1972. Permission from S Karger AG, Basel)

of alcohol to the average American diet is 4.5% of total calories, based on national consumption figures.[134] The share of dietary calories is much greater in heavy drinkers, generally estimated to be more than 50% of their daily caloric intake.

Alcoholic beverages differ little in nutritive value except for carbohydrate content, which varies considerably, trace amounts of B vitamins (especially niacin and thiamin), and iron content.[58] The significance of congeners in beverages remains largely

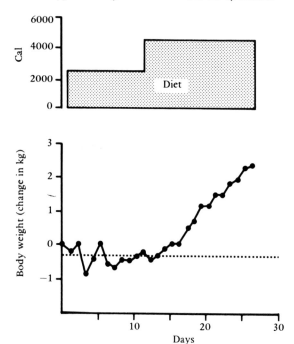

FIG. 15-3 Effect on body weight of adding 2000 Cal/day as chocolate to diet of same subject as in Figure 15-2. *Dotted line,* mean change during control period. (Pirola RC, Lieber CS: Pharmacology 7:185, 1972. Permission from S Karger AG, Basel)

unexplored, except for occasional instances in which harmful amounts of iron, lead, or cobalt may be present.

In summary, alcoholic beverages provide little nutritive value aside from calories; as such, alcohol is not as physiologically adequate as equivalent calories of carbohydrate.

NUTRITIONAL STATUS OF ALCOHOLICS

The nutritional status of alcoholics is generally considered to be very poor. Iber estimated that 20,000 alcoholics suffer major illnesses due to malnutrition requiring hospitalization each year, accounting for 7.5 million hospital days.[53] The spread of alcoholism to various socioeconomic classes, and, possibly, the greater availability and enrichment of foods, have modified the traditional nutritional view of the alcoholic. Neville found no evidence of marked change between nutritional status of the alcoholic and the nonalcoholic matched for socioeconomic and health history.[98] The impact of drinking patterns on dietary intake was studied by Bebb, who found little significant impact on nutrition as a result of moderate ethanol consumption.[9] However, heavier consumption of alcohol may lead to a decrease in food intake, and the

caloric load of alcohol has been postulated as a cause of appetite suppression.[163] Other factors that may limit intake in the alcoholic include gastritis and depressed consciousness. Sample selection may have accounted for previous stereotypes; also, there is often a lack of correlation of biochemical, dietary, and clinical data. In a recent epidemiological study, hospitalized alcoholics with liver disease were found to have poor dietary protein intakes.[108] Such studies, however, fail to take into account cause and effect, since liver disease and its complications (*e.g.*, encephalopathy and ascites) may lead to poor dietary protein intake. Although the stereotype of the malnourished alcoholic may be unfounded as it applies to the millions of alcoholics in the United States, alcohol remains one of the few causes of florid nutritional deficiency in our society. The impact of more subtle nutritional alterations produced by alcohol, as they relate to ethanol-induced and other disease states, remains to be elucidated. Alcohol-related diseases requiring hospital and outpatient dietary therapy have become one of the largest health care problems in the United States. The theory of nutritional deficiency as a cause of alcoholism has not been proven valid, and nutritional therapy as a cure for alcoholism has not been successful.[49]

Liver Injury

PATHOGENESIS

RESPECTIVE ROLES
OF ALCOHOL AND MALNUTRITION

The role of nutrition in the pathogenesis of alcoholic liver injury (fatty liver, hepatitis, and cirrhosis) is a very significant question in terms of prevention and therapy. Patek and co-workers and Morrison have demonstrated the efficacy of a normal protein, normal fat, vitamin-enriched diet in the treatment of cirrhosis as measured by clinical response and longevity.[96,106] Erenoglu and associates, extending previous work, treated cirrhotic patients with 198 ml ethanol daily and an adequate diet.[98] They found no adverse effects and a possible benefit from higher dietary protein. Hartroft and Porta conducted parallel studies in experimental animals demonstrating the importance of nutritional factors in pathogenesis and prevention.[44] The role of nutrition in the genesis of alcoholic liver injury has also been implicated by analogy: the fatty liver of kwashiorkor, the frequency of cirrhosis in underdeveloped countries where malnutrition is common, and fatty liver and possible progression to cirrhosis after intestinal bypass.[86]

The studies that demonstrated no adverse effects of ethanol in the presence of adequate nutrition generally can be criticized because of the use of dosages of alcohol much below those of heavy drinkers. Experimental models of nutritional injury may not be relevant to humans, especially with regard to lipotropes. Epidemiologic studies have not borne out a relationship between cirrhosis and malnutrition in underdeveloped countries, and liver biopsies of severely malnourished prison camp victims of World War II revealed only minimal abnormalities.[22] By contrast, a direct relationship between alcohol consumption and frequency of cirrhosis has been demonstrated in studies dealing with prohibition in the United States and during the rationing of alcoholic beverages during World War II.[150]

Furthermore, the studies of Lelbach clearly showed a linear relationship between the incidence of cirrhosis in an alcoholic population and amount of alcohol intake, whereas no role for dietary deficiency was revealed.[64] A similar statistical relationship of the incidence of cirrhosis to the amount of alcohol consumed (but not to protein malnutrition) was shown by Pequignot in France.[109] In fact, the individuals surveyed had developed cirrhosis despite an average daily dietary protein intake of 100 g or more. In another epidemiological study, hospitalized alcoholics reported a history of a poorer protein intake.[108] However, one cannot conclude from such an observation to what extent, if any, low protein intake contributed to the liver complications. In addition to showing that even diets relatively rich in protein do not preclude the development of alcoholic cirrhosis, the studies of Pequignot also revealed that the incidence of cirrhosis increased markedly when the daily intake of alcohol reached 160 g. This was interpreted by some to indicate a threshold of toxicity of alcohol at that level.

More recent studies of Pequignot and associates have also shown that daily intake of alcohol as low as 40 g in men and 20 g in women resulted in a statistically significant increase of the incidence of cirrhosis in a well-nourished population.[110] Because of individual variations, the exact toxic level for a given subject is usually unknown. However, the public should be made aware of the fact that even with adequate diets, amounts of alcohol previously considered innocuous may indeed harm the liver. This is particularly pertinent in the case of women, whose increased susceptibility was also indicated by a higher incidence of cirrhosis for a given intake. Wilkinson and co-workers found women to be more susceptible than men to the development of alcoholic cirrhosis.[164] Nutrition again did not play an appreciable role in causing liver disease, and cirrhosis was not found to be more common among the lowest socioeconomic groups.[164] A more recent study found the incidence of chronic advanced liver disease to be higher among women than among men for a similar history of alcohol abuse.[94] Menghini shows that in sufficient quantity ethanol decreases the clearance of hepatic fat.[87] More significantly, alcohol has been shown to be directly hepatotoxic histologically (light and electron microscope) and biochemically in both the alcoholic and nonalcoholic regardless of dietary variation in fat, protein, vitamins, and lipotropes.[126] Recently, fatty liver and cirrhosis have been produced in a primate model given alcohol in the presence of an adequate diet.[69]

Ethanol and nutrition may interact with respect to their effects on the liver. The role of nutrition in the recovery from alcoholic liver injury has been alluded to before and will be discussed subsequently. Erenoglu pointed out that alcoholics are unable to drink in moderation; therefore, in spite of his data indicating that limited consumption was not harmful, he recommended abstinence.[28] The evidence for the direct toxicity of ethanol makes such advice especially warranted. Alcohol is metabolized predominantly by the liver and profoundly alters the metabolic function of this organ. As such, it affects the metabolism of almost every nutrient. The significance of congeners, moderate dosages of alcohol, genetic factors, and marginal nutritional deficiencies in alcoholic liver injury remains to be clarified. The long pathogenesis, the unreliability of alcoholic populations, the difficulty of nutritional evaluation, and the variability of disease expression make the resolution of these questions difficult.

Experimental, clinical, and epidemiological evidence indicates that even when adequate diets are consumed, ethanol exerts liver toxicity, whereas the role of malnutrition in the development of human cirrhosis remains elusive. Nutritional deficiencies should of course be prevented and, if present, should be corrected. It is not clear, however, that one can slow down or prevent the process of cirrhosis if alcohol abuse is continued. Therefore, one must also focus on the control of the alcohol intake. Recent studies have shown that even in well-nourished population, amounts of alcohol much lower than hitherto suspected must be considered as potentially cirrhogenic, particularly in women.

LIPOTROPES

The question of the significance of and requirements for lipotropes in alcoholism is beset by confusion because of inappropriate extrapolations from animal models. Although in growing rats deficien-

TABLE 15-1
Fatty Liver—Clinical Aspects*

Findings	Occurrence
Hepatomegaly	75%
Tenderness	18%
Jaundice	15%
Spider nevi	8%
Splenomegaly	4%
Biochemical tests (*e.g.*, alkaline phosphatase, SGOT, SGPT, prothrombin time) are usually minimally elevated.	

*From Leevy CM: Fatty liver: A study of 270 patients with biopsy proven fatty liver and a review of the literature. Medicine (Baltimore) 41:249, 1962.

cies in dietary protein and lipotropic factors (choline and methionine) can produce fatty liver, primates are far less susceptible than rodents to protein and lipotrope deficiency.[50] Clinically, treatment with choline of patients suffering from alcoholic liver injury has been found to be ineffective in the presence of continued alcohol intake, and experimentally, massive supplementation of choline failed to prevent fatty liver produced by alcohol in volunteers.[126] This is not surprising because there is no evidence that a diet deficient in choline is deleterious to adult man. Unlike rat liver, human liver contains very little choline oxidase activity, which may explain the species difference in choline deficiency. The phospholipid content of the liver represents another key difference between the ethanol and the choline-deficient fatty liver. After the administration of ethanol, hepatic phospholipids increase.[95] In the fatty liver produced by choline deficiency, they decrease. Thus, hepatic injury in-

TABLE 15-2
Alcoholic Hepatitis—Clinical Aspects*

Findings	Occurrence
Hepatomegaly	81%
Anorexia	77%
Nausea and vomiting	59%
Abdominal pain	46%
Jaundice	46%
Ascites	35%
Fever	28%
Encephalopathy	11%
Malnutrition (*e.g.*, weight loss, muscle wasting, overt vitamin deficiency)	55%
Leukocytosis	34%
Frequently elevated alkaline phosphatase, moderate elevations of SGPT, SGOT	

*Lischner MW, Alexander JF, Galambos JT: Natural history of alcoholic hepatitis. Am J Dig Dis 16:481, 1971

duced by choline deficiency appears to be primarily an experimental disease of rats, with little if any relevance to human alcoholic liver injury. Even in the rat, massive choline supplementation failed to prevent fully the ethanol-induced lesion, whether alcohol was administered acutely or chronically.[68] Although excess lipotropes are of no proven value in recovery from liver injury, they may prove harmful as an excess nitrogen load.[112]

CLINICAL SPECTRUM

Alcohol-related liver injury includes fatty liver, hepatitis, and cirrhosis. These morphologic categories may overlap, as do the clinical findings characteristic of each group. The most severe complications, such as encephalopathy and ascites, occur most frequently in cirrhosis but are well documented in the presence of fatty liver alone. Liver injury, especially cirrhosis, is the most common clinical problem resulting from alcohol that requires nutritional therapy. Each patient must also be evaluated for associated problems.

FATTY LIVER

Fatty liver is a benign reversible condition characterized by deposition of lipid within hepatocytes. It is an early stage of liver injury indicating a severe metabolic derangement that is felt to be a forerunner of more severe parenchymal injury.[72] Most persons do not seek or require medical attention. Clinical findings are variable, depending on population selection. Typical findings in a series of 270 hospital patients are shown in Table 15-1.

ALCOHOLIC HEPATITIS

This stage of liver disease is characterized morphologically by extensive necrosis and inflammation. The onset usually follows a bout of heavy drinking. Patients tend to require medical attention more often than with fatty liver. Typical clinical findings in a series of hospitalized patients are presented in Table 15-2.

CIRRHOSIS

Cirrhosis is characterized morphologically by scarring and regeneration. It represents the most advanced and least reversible stage of liver injury. Patients may have the highest incidence of associated complications, or they may be completely asymptomatic. Stigmata of chronic liver disease, such as spider nevi, liver palms, muscle wasting, testicular atrophy, gynecomastia, parotid enlargement, ascites, and collateral venous abnormalities, are common in this group. Biochemical abnormalities (including hypoalbuminemia, bromsulphalein (BSP) retention, and prolongation of the prothrombin time) are also common. Clinical problems of encephalopathy, sodium and water retention, renal failure, and specific nutritional deficiencies must be evaluated carefully in this group.

TREATMENT

Since the work of Patek, little has been added to the dietary armamentarium for specific therapy of alcoholic liver disease. Advances have been made in the understanding and avoidance of iatrogenic problems and the therapy of associated conditions, such as sodium and water retention and encephalopathy. The basic diet of normal protein and fat content with vitamin supplements remains the mainstay of therapy.

PREVENTION

Ethanol consumed in large amounts has been shown to be directly hepatotoxic despite adequate nutrition with high-protein, low-fat, vitamin-enriched, and lipotrope-supplemented diets. Problem drinkers are generally felt to be unable to drink in moderation. There is no established prophylactic regimen except abstinence. Liver injury is time- and dose-related. Although a moderate level of consumption may be safe in a number of individuals, a no-effect dose level has not been established clinically.

FATTY LIVER AND ALCOHOLIC HEPATITIS

Therapy for fatty liver includes abstinence and a regular diet. Specific nutritional deficiencies or clinical problems are treated, if present. Patients who are acutely ill with fever, nausea, vomiting, and encephalopathy may require fluid and electrolyte replacement and parenteral alimentation. Specific nutritional therapy is as listed below.

CALORIES

Calories must be provided in sufficient quantity to allow regeneration and to maximize nitrogen sparing. Estimates for a reasonable minimum are 25 Cal/kg or approximately 1600 Cal/day.[34] A level of approximately 2600 Cal, depending on activity and associated problems, is desired. Intravenous glucose may be necessary to supplement dietary calories if nausea, vomiting, and anorexia persist for a long period of time. The nitrogen-sparing effect of calories prevents endogenous protein catabolism.

PROTEIN

Finding the optimal dietary protein level is one of the most difficult aspects of nutritional therapy in patients with alcoholic liver injury, because protein intake must be adequate to prevent nitrogen wasting but not so great as to precipitate hepatic coma. Nitrogen-balance studies have revealed essentially normal protein requirements in cirrhosis, and some studies have even suggested increased nitrogen retention.[36,127] Dietary requirements for specific amino acids may be altered as evidenced by plasma levels and clearance rates. In general, patients with alcoholic liver disease have been found to have depressed plasma branched-chain amino acids and increased clearance of these amino acids, along with increased levels of aromatic amino acids and decreased clearance of these amino acids.[33] Amino acids may differ in their ability to produce ammonia and are tolerated to a different extent in hepatic encephalopathy.[128]

In patients with hepatic encephalopathy, the tolerance to dietary protein may be related to the amino acid content of the protein administered. Blood is less well tolerated than isonitrogenous protein in the form of casein. Meat protein is less well tolerated than isonitrogenous milk or casein.[41] These differences have been attributed to the increased content of aromatic amino acids present in meat and blood proteins.

Greenberger and associates in 1977 demonstrated clinical improvement in patients with hepatic encephalopathy given vegetable protein diets as compared to animal protein diets.[41] The benefits of such diets on nitrogen balance and long-term survival remain to be demonstrated.

Fischer and colleagues studied hepatic encephalopathy in the dog with an experimentally produced end-to-side portacaval anastomosis.[33] He found improved survival after infusion of amino acid mixtures rich in branched-chain amino acids and low in aromatic amino acids, compared to isonitrogenous infusions of Freamine or plasma. In a recent communication this same group has reported clinical improvement in humans with hepatic encephalopathy given a mixture of amino acids rich in branched-chain amino acids and low in aromatic amino acids.

Maddrey and co-workers demonstrated clinical improvement in patients with encephalopathy given keto analogones of essential amino acids.[85] Such modalities are being evaluated clinically and are discussed more completely in the section on metabolism of amino acids.

Initially 0.5 g/kg/day high-quality protein may be tried (approximately 30 g/day–35 g/day) unless encephalopathy is present. This may be increased with increments of 10 g/day to 15 g/day every 5 to 7 days until a level of approximately 70 g/day is reached. Benefit from dietary protein above this level is not established, and the risk of encephalopathy is increased. A zero-protein regimen, which may be indicated initially when hepatic encephalopathy is present, should not be continued for more than a few days in order to minimize resultant endogenous protein catabolism. If a minimum of 20 g/day to 35 g/day is not tolerated, neomycin or lactulose or both should be employed (see section on Hepatic Encephalopathy).

FAT

Low-fat diets, although of theroretical interests, are not advocated because of the lack of palatability of such regimens, especially in an already anorectic patient.[20] Resulting inadequate caloric intake promotes protein catabolism. Fat is generally not restricted unless gastrointestinal (GI) intolerance develops because of jaundice, pancreatic insufficiency, or other causes of steatorrhea.

VITAMINS

Specific deficiencies should be corrected immediately (often with parenteral administration). Usually, patients are treated with B vitamins. Suggested amounts are approximately five times the daily requirements listed in Appendix Table A-1, although several times these amounts are commonly given without apparent harm or proven efficacy. Generally, fat-soluble vitamins are not deficient. Vitamin K may be administered intramuscularly (10 mg/day for 3 days) if the prothrombin time is prolonged. Failure to correct a prolonged prothrombin time indicates severe hepatocellular injury.

Small, infrequent feedings may be useful in maintaining an adequate diet. Value of lipotrope therapy is not established and may be harmful in excess. Trace elements remain of theoretic interest except in extreme deficiency states.

Alcohol and the Gastrointestinal Tract

STOMACH

Ethanol affects the stomach by increasing acid secretion, impairing motility, and altering the mucosa. Secretory changes may be due to direct stimulation, vagal effects, and gastrin release.[17] Chronic ethanol administration first increases mean daily acid secretion and then gradually decreases it.[18] Increased acid secretion may result in enhanced iron absorption.[15] Alcohol delays gastric emptying.[7] Ethanol disrupts the mucosal barrier and may act synergistically with other drugs in producing injury in this way.[21] It is an accepted cause of acute gastritis, but its role in the pathogenesis of duodenal ulcer, gastric ulcer, and chronic gastritis remains controversial.[81] Acute gastritis may decrease appetite and produce iron deficiency through hemorrhage.

SMALL INTESTINE

Alcohol has been shown to be directly injurious to the small intestine.[125] Acute administration of ethanol (1 g/kg) by mouth (PO) results in endoscopic and morphologic lesions in the duodenum.[38] Previous failure to observe such lesions may have been due to their transient and patchy nature.[116] Experimentally, such lesions appear to be related to the concentration of ethanol used, with the greatest damage resulting from those solutions with the highest concentration of ethanol.[8] Acute administration of ethanol may impair the absorption of many nutrients and experimentally results in alterations in mucosal enzymes.[49] Studies with orally and intravenously administered alcohol have revealed an inhibition of type I (impeding) waves in the jejunum and an increase in type III (propulsive) waves in the ileum.[123] These changes have been proposed as one possible mechanism of the diarrhea observed in binge drinkers. Ingestion of ethanol has been demonstrated to result in release of secretin from the duodenum.[142]

The effect of chronic ethanol consumption on intestinal function is complicated by the concomitant effects of nutrition. Indeed, malnutrition itself may lead to intestinal malabsorption and folate depletion, which is common in alcoholics.[43] Impaired absorption of folate, thiamin, B_{12}, xylose, and fat has been described in chronic alcoholics, with recovery after withdrawal from alcohol and institution of a nutritious diet. Depressed levels of intestinal lactase and consequent lactose intolerance have been observed in apparently well-nourished chronic alcoholics with recovery following withdrawal from alcohol (see Figs. 15-4 and 15-5).[111] In this latter study an apparent racial difference in susceptibility to this injurious effect of ethanol was observed. In patients with alcoholic gastritis or in alcoholics with peptic ulcer disease, milk products must be prescribed for the diet with caution.

Chronic ethanol administration, along with an adequate diet, results in impairment of B_{12} absorption in well-nourished volunteers despite supplementary pancreatin and intrinsic factor.[77]

The acute and chronic effects of alcohol upon small intestinal function may be potentiated by concomitant alterations in pancreatic function, bile salts, and small intestinal flora. However, in patients with cirrhosis, steatorrhea (fecal fat greater than 30 g/24 hr on a 100-g fat/day diet) is relatively uncommon and in one series was present in only 9% of cases.[79] Furthermore, creatorrhea or excess excretion of fecal nitrogen is only rarely reported in the alcoholic.[2] Portal hypertension has also been postulated as a cause of malabsorption.[83] Finally, specific therapeutic interventions, such as neomycin, may by themselves cause malabsorption.[30]

PANCREAS

Pancreatic function may be altered by acute and chronic ethanol administration. Oral administration of ethanol causes chiefly an increase in pancreatic secretion of water and bicarbonate. This may result from ethanol-stimulated gastric acid secretions reaching the duodenum and causing release of secretin. If gastric juice is prevented from reaching the duodenum, IV or intragastric ethanol administration results in a decrease in stimulated water, bicarbonate, lipase, and chymotrypsin secretion. Although acute ethanol administration causes an increase in tone at the sphincter of Oddi, the ethanol-induced decrease in pancreatic secretion persists when the pancreatic duct is directly cannulated in dogs.[8]

Many theories have been offered to explain the occurrence of pancreatic insufficiency in the alcoholic. The older hypotheses proposed that stimulation of pancreatic flow against increased resistance resulted in hypertension, ductular rupture, and glandular autodigestion. According to this theory, pancreatic stimulation depends on acid-mediated release of the hormone secretin, and increased ductal resistance is due to alcohol-induced

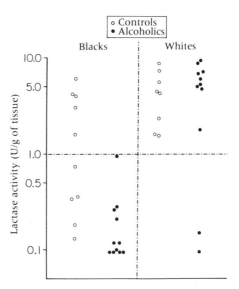

FIG. 15-4 Effects of chronic alcohol consumption on intestinal lactase activity. Black alcoholics were found to be especially sensitive to the effects of ethanol in lowering intestinal lactase activity (Perlow W, Baraona E, Lieber CS: Symptomatic intestinal disaccharidase deficiencies in alcoholism. Gastroenterology 72:680, 1977)

duodenitis or increased tone in Oddi's sphincter. More recently, it has been suggested that chronic alcohol consumption may alter the composition of pancreatic juice by increasing cholinergic tone.[147] Hypersecretion of protein in the juice would result from these factors. Subsequent precipitation of proteinaceous plugs and their calcification might, in turn, lead to ductular blockage, metaplasia, and rupture. Whether chronic pancreatitis in the alcoholic is due to alcohol *per se* or to concomitant malnutrition remains an important but ill-defined aspect of this disorder. Although protein plugs are

FIG. 15-5 Effect of withdrawal from alcohol upon intestinal lactase. A significant increase in intestinal lactase was observed following 1 to 3 weeks of withdrawal from alcohol. A similar effect was noted for intestinal sucrase activity. (From Perlow W, Baraona E, Lieber CS: Symptomatic intestinal disaccharidase deficiencies in alcoholism. Gastroenterology 72:680, 1977)

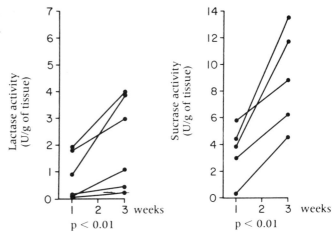

common in the chronic pancreatitis of kwashior-kor (implying that poor nutrition might also be an etiologic factor in alcoholic pancreatitis), epidemiologic surveys of premorbid dietary patterns in alcoholic chronic pancreatitis have revealed that these patients had diets that were enriched, rather than deficient, in protein and fat.[130]

Chronic pancreatitis has important effects on nutrition. When pancreatic damage is sufficiently extensive, hyposecretion of bicarbonate and enzymes may result in maldigestion of fat and protein. Despite steatorrhea, deficiencies of fat-soluble vitamins are unusual in patients with pancreatic insufficiency.[29] Defects in the absorption of vitamin B_{12} have also been described in chronic pancreatitis.[148] Vitamin B_{12} malabsorption has been attributed to a failure of pancreatic juice to inactivate nonintrinsic factor binders of the vitamin.[157] As expected, pancreatic extract is effective in restoring vitamin B_{12} absorption. Since vitamin B_{12} deficiency is unusual in patients with chronic pancreatitis, the clinical relevance of these findings is uncertain.

CLINICAL CONSIDERATIONS

Alcoholics may have acute or chronic pancreatitis. The dietary management of acute pancreatitis includes intravenous fluid and electrolyte administration associated with nasogastric suction. Diet is initiated slowly to minimize pancreatic stimulation. Clear liquids are generally given first. The major therapeutic considerations for chronic pancreatitis are discussed below. Glucose intolerance with both acute and chronic pancreatitis should be looked for.

BILE SALTS

Intraluminal bile salts are decreased by the acute administration of ethanol into the jejunum or intravenously. Experimentally, ethanol feeding prolongs the half time of excretion of cholic acid and chenodeoxycholic acid, increases slightly the pool size, and decreases daily excretion.[63] In the same model, hepatic esterified cholesterol and serum free and esterified cholesterol, are increased. In cirrhotics, bile salt-related steatorrhea may be due to decreased cholic acid synthesis, decreased total bile acid pools, diminished concentrations of bile salts in bowel juice, and deconjugation of bile salts in the upper GI tract by altered flora.[156] In patients with alcoholic cirrhosis deoxycholate may be markedly diminished in the bile; one explanation for this is the impaired conversion of cholate to deoxycholate by the intestinal bacteria in these patients.[57] Alcohol-induced ileal dysfunction has been suggested as a cause of decreased cholic acid pools.[23]

Increased gallstone formation in alcoholic liver disease and increased tone in the sphincter of Oddi with acute ehthanol administration have been observed.

MALABSORPTION

Malabsorption, especially steatorrhea, may occur with acute or chronic alcoholism. Malabsorption may be caused by the acute effects of alcohol on intestinal mucosa, bile salts, pancreatic function, intestinal motility, and specific intestinal absorptive processes. These acute alterations generally revert to normal with abstinence. Steatorrhea in cirrhosis is infrequent and in one series was present in only 9%.[79] Folate deficiency of subjects with megaloblastic intestinal changes may cause malabsorption that responds to folic acid administration. Pancreatic insufficiency due to chronic alcoholic pancreatitis may result in steatorrhea. Replacement therapy with pancreatic extract may result in improvement. Altered bile salts and abnormal GI flora may contribute to fat malabsorption. A low-fat diet and treatment with medium-chain triglycerides may be helpful. Medium-chain triglycerides are triglycerides that contain fatty acids with carbon skeletons of 6 to 12 atoms. They have several advantages over long-chain triglycerides normally found in the diet with respect to digestion and absorption: increased enzyme hydrolysis within the GI tract, greater water solubility and thus decreased bile salt requirement, some direct absorption without hydrolysis, and portal transport as medium-chain fatty acids as opposed to lymphatic transport for long-chain fatty acids.[42] However, in the alcoholic, central nervous system (CNS) sensitivity and difficulty in handling the appreciable sodium load present in some preparations must be considered.[79]

The main dietary consideration with respect to jaundice is the effect impaired bile salt secretion has on fat absorption. Dietary fat may have to be restricted in symptomatic patients. Portal hypertension has been postulated as a possible cause of malabsorption.[83] Specific therapeutic interventions, such as neomycin, may themselves cause malabsorption.[30] The effect of congeners on the GI tract is unknown. Alcoholics may have other coincidental causes of malabsorption (see Chap. 21).

Metabolic Effects of Alcohol

PROTEIN

The metabolism of protein in alcoholism is especially relevant to the role of protein in recovery from injury and to its potential for producing encephalopathy. Nitrogen-balance studies have revealed essentially normal protein requirements in cirrhosis, and some studies suggest increased nitrogen retention.[36,127] Experimentally, ethanol has a complex effect on nitrogen balance, depending on dietary conditions. Given as supplementary calories it may be nitrogen sparing, but given as an isocaloric substitute for carbohydrate it increases urea excretion in the urine.

Acute ethanol administration may inhibit lipoprotein and albumin synthesis in experimental models, with reversal of some of these effects following amino acid administration.[133] Chronic ethanol feeding, however, is associated with increased synthesis of lipoproteins. In addition, chronic ethanol administration results in hepatic accumulation of hepatic transport proteins such as albumin and transferrin (see Fig. 15-6). This effect may be mediated by the action of ethanol or its metabolites on hepatic microtubules.[6]

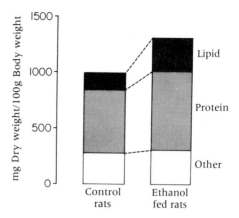

FIG. 15-6 Effect of ethanol feeding on hepatic dry weight; lipid and protein content. The increase in hepatic weight due to protein was comparable to that due to fat. (From Baraona E, Leo MA, Barowsky SA, et al: Alcohol hepatomegaly: Accumulation of protein in the liver. Science 190:794, 1975)

AMINO ACIDS

Numerous alterations in amino acid metabolism in relation to both acute and chronic alcohol administration as well as alcohol liver disease have been extensively described and reviewed.[36,102] The clinical relevance of the majority of observations, however, has not been established.

Impairment of intestinal absorption, as well as hepatic uptake of amino acids, has been observed in the presence of ethanol.[56,115] Impairment of hepatic uptake may be related to the metabolism of ethanol.[115] However, increased nitrogen excretion in the stool is only rarely observed with chronic alcohol consumption, and both protein and urea synthesis are increased with chronic alcohol feeding. Therefore, the significance of the observed effects of ethanol on amino acid transport to the liver and hepatic amino acid metabolism must be questioned.

The hepatic metabolism of amino acids may be altered by chronic alcohol consumption or the presence of liver disease. While alterations have been demonstrated for almost every amino acid studied, several amino acids are of particular interest.[102]

Chronic alcohol administration for 3 to 10 days to protein-deficient rats results in an increase in enzymes related to the degradation of methionine.[32] This is of interest because of the role of methionine as a lipotrope in rodents and because of the recent observation of increased α-amino-η-butyric acid (a product of methionine catabolism) in the plasma following chronic alcohol consumption.[138]

Increased catabolism of methionine after alcohol may be explained, at least in part, by ethanol-induced hepatic lipid peroxidation and glutathione depletion.[137] Methionine is a precursor of glutathione, and the latter is consumed during lipid peroxidation.

Tryptophan metabolism has aroused considerable interest because of its catabolism to the neurotransmitter serotonin as well as nicotinic acid. Urinary excretion products have been measured, but conflicting results have been observed regarding the effect of alcoholism on these competing pathways of catabolism.[102] This is not surprising in light of the many nutritional variables that may play a role, such as pyridoxine availability.

In cirrhosis there is decreased conversion of phenylalanine to tyrosine, and abnormal tyrosine tolerance tests; elevated plasma tyrosine may be markedly elevated in the plasma along with tyramine (a decarboxylation product of tyrosine).[31] Severe liver disease has also been associated with elevated levels of tyrosine, methionine, phenylalanine, and tryptophan.[31,33] In fulminant liver disease a generalized nonspecific increase in amino acids has been observed. The aromatic amino acids may be especially important for the pathogenesis of hepatic encephalopathy.[33]

Branched-chain amino acids (BCAA) have been observed to be decreased in the plasma of patients with alcoholism or liver injury as well as in the muscle of patients with cirrhosis. Furthermore, BCAA clearance from the plasma is increased in cirrhosis. Recently, it has been observed that depressed BCAA levels in patients are due to dietary protein deficiency (see Fig. 15-7) rather than to alcoholism or liver disease *per se.*[138] By contrast, chronic alcohol consumption along with an adequate diet results in a striking increase in BCAA as well as α-amino-η-butyric acid relative to BCAA, regardless of the presence of liver disease or of the

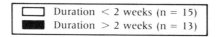

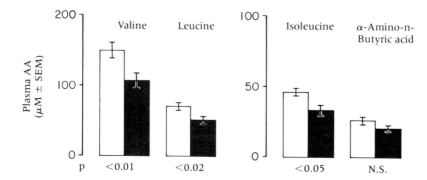

FIG. 15-7 Effects of dietary protein deficiency upon plasma amino acids *(AA)* in the alcoholic. Branched-chain amino acids valine, leucine, and isoleucine as well as α-amino-η-butyric acid were depressed to a similar degree by dietary protein deficiency. (From Shaw S, Lieber CS: Plasma amino acid abnormalities in the alcoholic: Respective role of alcohol, nutrition, and liver injury. Gastroenterology 74:677, 1978)

nutritional status in both human patients and experimental animal models (see Fig. 15-8).[139]

Selective mixtures of essential amino acids (high in branched-chain amino acids, low in aromatic amino acids) or keto analogs of amino acids have been proposed for the treatment of hepatic insufficiency.[33,85] The long-term efficacy of these therapies on survival and nitrogen balance has not been determined. Special vigilance is required in order to avoid precipitation of hepatic coma. Dietary protein low in aromatic amino acids (generally vegetable as opposed to animal protein) has been advocated for patients with hepatic encephalopathy.[41]

CARBOHYDRATES

Glucose homeostasis is impaired in alcoholic liver disease. With severe decompensation and with prolonged fasting following heavy drinking, symptomatic hypoglycemia may occur. Possible mechanisms include autonomic dysfunction, impaired gluconeogenesis, glycogen depletion, and endocrine effects.[1] On the other hand, alcoholics with fatty liver or cirrhosis have impaired glucose tolerance, elevated insulin levels, and abnormal responses to glucagon.[121] Alcohol has a priming effect on glucose-mediated insulin release and directly causes glucose intolerance itself.[88,113] These and other endocrine effects of ethanol are reviewed by Axelrod.[5] The absorption and digestion of carbohydrates in alcoholism are generally regarded as normal, although experimentally chronic alcohol administration impairs jejunal mucosal uptake and transport of carbohydrates.[34] The effect of alcohol on the intermediary metabolism of carbohydrates has been reviewed by Arky.[1]

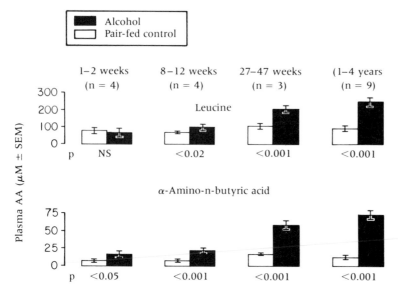

FIG. 15-8 Effect of chronic alcohol feeding on two plasma amino acids *(AA)* in the presence of an adequate diet. Branched-chain amino acids and α-amino-η-butyric acid were increased by chronic feeding. A representative branched-chain amino acid, leucine, is shown, but similar results were observed for valine and isoleucine. (From Shaw S, Lieber CS: Plasma amino acid abnormalities in the alcoholic: Respective role of alcohol, nutrition, and liver injury. Gastroenterology 74:677, 1978)

URIC ACID

The clinical observation of the relationship between alcohol and gout has stimulated investigations of uric acid metabolism in alcoholism. Acute administration of oral or IV alcohol has been shown to produce hyperuricemia in patients without known disorders of renal function or uric acid metabolism.[70] Since the elevations of serum uric acid were significantly above normal levels and persisted in some instances for several days, a physician unaware of this effect of ethanol might inadvertently treat hyperuricemia of this secondary type. The mechanism by which hyperuricemia occurs appears to be most clearly related to decreased urinary excretion of uric acid secondary to elevated serum lactate. This is illustrated in data from one patient in Figure 15-9. Lactate is reduced in the liver from pyruvate by the action of nicotinamide-adenine dinucleotide (NADH), which is generated from NAD in the metabolism of ethanol by alcohol dehydrogenase. Depending on the metabolic state of the liver, this inward NADH generation either enhances hepatic lactate production or prevents the liver from completing the Cori cycle and using lactate originating in peripheral tissues, especially lactate produced from muscle activity in alcoholic

withdrawal.[99] Other possible causes of hyperuricemia include alcohol-induced hyperlipemia and ketogenesis and starvation-induced ketosis. The mechanism by which increased serum lactate decreases urinary uric acid secretion is unclear. It is known that it is not due to a *p*H effect on the urine, and that it occurs despite probenecid administration.[70,84] Acute gouty attacks have been observed in patients with gout in relation to changes in serum uric acid associated with alcohol administration or starvation.[84]

LIPIDS

ALTERED HEPATIC LIPID METABOLISM

The metabolism of ethanol in the liver by alcohol dehydrogenase results in an increase in the ratio of NADH/NAD. In addition, metabolism of alcohol results in mitochondrial damage within the liver. These two alterations may in large part account for the observed increased hepatic ketogenesis, decreased fatty acid oxidation, and increased fatty acid synthesis that are observed effects of alcohol.[66] Triglycerides are thus produced in excess and may either accumulate in the liver (and thus create a fatty liver) or be released into the blood as lipo-

FIG. 15-9 Blood and urine studies with oral ethanol. (Lieber CS, Jones DP, Losousky MS et al: J Clin Invest 41:1863, 1962)

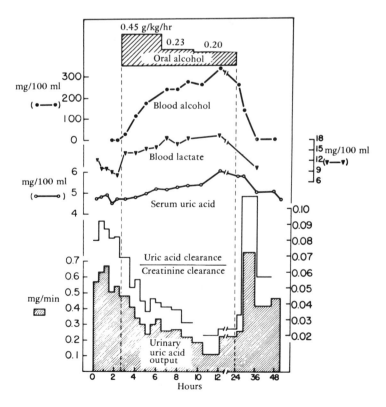

proteins. The effect of ethanol on intestinal production of very-low-density lipoproteins may also
be contributory, although this factor appears to play
only an insignificant role.[9] Ethanol increases hepatic cholesterogenesis and decreases bile salt secretion, and may thereby elevate the serum cholesterol.[63]

HYPERLIPIDEMIAS

The administration of ethanol to humans consistently results in hyperlipidemia; the response is
modified by associated dietary and pathologic conditions. The major elevation occurs in the serum
triglycerides, and this response may be greatly enhanced by a fat-containing meal.[166] When alcohol
is administered for several weeks at a dosage of
300 g/day, the initial several-fold increase in triglycerides gradually returns to normal (see Fig. 15-

10).[71] One explanation for this observation is that
continued ethanol administration results in hepatic
impairment. Hyperlipemia is usually absent with
severe liver injury (*e.g.*, cirrhosis), and hypolipe-
mia is usually present.

A characteristic feature of alcohol-induced hyperlipemia is that all of the lipoprotein fractions
are increased, although to a variable degree. Alcoholic hyperlipemia is usually classified as type IV
according to the International Classification of Hyperlipidemias and Hyperlipoproteinemias. The increased particulate fat behaves predominantly as
very-low-density lipoproteins. In 8% of patients,
chylomicrons or chylomicronlike particles can be
increased even in the fasting state. These patients
are classified as type V. Furthermore, 6% of alcoholics have hypercholesterolemia due to hyper-β-
lipoproteinemia classified as type II. Alcohol-induced hyperlipemia may change rapidly, with

FIG. 15-10 Effect of prolonged alcohol intake on serum lipids in seven chronic alcoholic
individuals. (Lieber CS, Jones DP, Mendelson J et al: Trans Assoc Am Physicians 76:289,
1963)

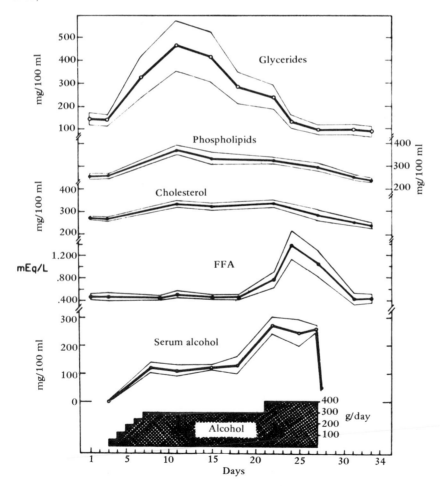

clearance of triglycerides being most rapid and cholesterol and phospholipids slower; thus, it is difficult to classify alcoholic hyperlipemia in a single group (see Fig. 15-11).

Some patients may demonstrate a marked sensitivity to the hyperlipidemic effects of alcohol. This may be observed in patients with type IV familial or carbohydrate-induced hyperlipidemia.[37]

Elevations of serum cholesterol and triglycerides have been directly attributed to alcohol in epidemiologic studies.[103] Moderate ethanol dosage may increase serum lipids in patients with type IV hyperlipidemias. The significance of such elevations as possible risk factors in coronary artery disease remains to be clarified. Ethanol may unmask a subclinical hyperlipidemia and should be excluded as a cause or contributing factor in an observed hyperlipidemia. Marked hyperlipidemias may be accompanied by hemolysis, which is transient and clears at the same time as the hyperlipidemia.[167] The constellation of hyperlipemia, alcoholic fatty liver, jaundice, and hemolysis constitutes what has been termed *Zieve syndrome.* Abdominal pain may occur with hyperlipidemia; differentiation of a primary effect from associated pancreatic, hepatic, or GI pathology may be exceedingly difficult. Dietary lipids may alter intrahepatic fat accumulation; however, a low-fat diet may not be practical in a clinical setting because its lack of palatability may result in inadequate caloric intake.[20]

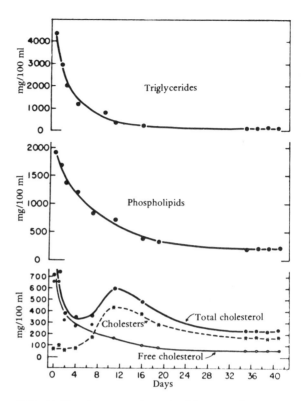

FIG. 15-11 Changes in plasma lipid fractions of a patient during recovery from alcoholic hyperlipemia. (Losowsky MS, Jones DP, Davidson CS et al: Am J Med 35:794, 1963)

WATER-SOLUBLE VITAMINS

Vitamin metabolism demonstrates the many levels at which alcohol may impair nutrition. Abnormalities of ingestion and absorption have been discussed. Decreased hepatic stores of folate, nicotinic acid, B_6, and B_12 have been described, and decreased hepatic affinity, as measured by displacement studies, has been demonstrated for folate.[16,62] Impaired utilization of folic acid, thiamin, and vitamin B_6 has been reported.[27,143] Pyridoxine is normally converted by the liver to pyridoxal phosphate, which is the active coenzyme form of the vitamin. Evidence has been presented that decreased activation of pyridoxine is due to displacement of pyridoxal phosphate from hepatic cytosol binding proteins by acetaldehyde produced by ethanol metabolism. This facilitates hydrolysis by pyridoxal phosphatase and results in a net decrease in activation. Mitchell and co-workers observed increased clearance of serum pyridoxal phosphate in cirrhosis.[92] Circulating levels of vitamins reveal abnormalities in 40% of chronic malnourished alcoholics, with folate and pyridoxine being most often depressed.[61] Clinical correlations are greatest with megaloblastic and sideroblastic anemias and

with neurologic syndromes related to thiamin deficiency. Although vitamins are clearly important in such cellular processes as DNA synthesis, the significance of mild deficiencies and massive vitamin therapy in altering recovery from liver injury remains unclear. Vitamin deficiencies have been proposed as causes of alcoholism, and vitamin therapy has been suggested as a cure.[165] The animal evidence used for these studies, however, is subject to many serious criticisms.[49] Since trace elements such as zinc and magnesium play a role in the function of some water-soluble vitamins, alcohol-related deficiencies of these elements may further exacerbate borderline insufficiencies. Increased requirements for vitamins have not been established in alcoholism, except perhaps for folate.

BERIBERI HEART DISEASE

Specific nutritional heart disease in the alcoholic occurs in the form of beriberi heart disease. Symptoms classically include those of congestive heart failure accompanied by a hyperkinetic circulation.[13] Low urinary thiamin and red blood cell transketolase confirm the clinical diagnosis. Other symptoms of thiamin deficiency may be present (see Chap. 12). Therapy with 5 mg to 10 mg thiamin three times daily is probably adequate, although larger doses may be given. The B vitamins are usually given as a group along with an adequate diet to the alcoholic whether or not a specific diagnosis is made.

NEUROLOGIC DISEASES

Alcoholics remain one of the few patient groups in the United States to present clinically with nutritional deficiency syndromes, the most dramatic of which involve the neurologic manifestations. The interaction of diet and alcohol in producing these deficiencies needs further investigation. Hypovitaminosis of the B vitamins remains the most well-delineated of the deficiency states. Administration of carbohydrates, such as IV glucose, to a marginally vitamin-depleted alcoholic may precipitate a florid syndrome if supplementary vitamins are not provided. Although dramatically responsive to replacement therapy and pathogenetically fascinating, the deficiency syndromes are relatively rare, constituting only 1% to 3% of alcohol-related neurologic admissions (see Chap. 27).[24]

POLYNEUROPATHY

This syndrome is characterized by generalized symmetric involvement of peripheral nerves which spreads proximally. First symptoms include discomfort and fatigue in the anterior tibial muscles and paresthesias in the feet. These symptoms are usually followed by weakness in the toes and ankles, diminished ankle jerks, and decreased fine movements and vibratory sense. Finally, glove and stocking hypoesthesia, hypalgesia, and severe weakness may result.[51] Thiamin deficiency has been most strongly implicated in etiology, but other B vitamins have also been implicated. Pyridoxine, B_{12}, nicotinic acid, and riboflavin deficiency can be associated with peripheral neuropathy, and pantothenic acid deficiency may produce symptoms of peripheral nerve disease.[51] Although the optimal therapeutic dosage has not been established, one recommendation is 10 times the normal daily requirement for the first week, and 5 times the daily requirement thereafter.[51] The daily requirements of the vitamins are presented in Appendix Table A-1.

WERNICKE–KORSAKOFF SYNDROME

The Wernicke–Korsakoff syndrome may be the most common CNS-related neurologic problem in the alcoholic. Wernicke's encephalopathy is characterized by weakness of eye movements, gait disturbance, and confusion. Horizontal nystagmus, paralysis of external recti, paralysis of conjugate gaze, and ataxia of gait and stance may be observed. Korsakoff's psychosis is characterized initially by anterograde amnesia, retrograde amnesia to a lesser extent, a disordered time sense, and often confabulation in the acute stages. Cognitive deficits have also been observed.[153] Ophthalmoplegia in Wernicke's encephalopathy responds rapidly to thiamin administration, while the ataxia and confusion respond more slowly. Although 2 mg to 3 mg may be sufficient, usually larger doses (50 mg) are given. Rapidity of response depends upon the conversion of thiamin to its active form in the liver, and patients with advanced liver disease such as cirrhosis may therefore have a delayed response.

The association of Korsakoff's psychosis with Wernicke's encephalopathy has led to their inclusion in one syndrome. However, while Wernicke's encephalopathy is a thiamin-responsive illness, the relationship of Korsakoff's psychosis to thiamin deficiency in terms of pathogenesis and treatment is not clearly delineated. Korsakoff's psychosis as well as Wernicke's encephalopathy are rarely seen in clinical thiamin deficiency without alcoholism.[118] It has been postulated that this difference may be related to the impact of alcohol on the balance and amount of dietary calories.[118] The Wernicke–Korsakoff syndrome is characterized by symmetrical CNS lesions in the periaquaductal and perivestibular areas of the diencephalon and midbrain and the cerebellum.[97] Symmetrical and bilateral lesions are also observed in experimental thiamin deficiency in animals.[25] It is not surprising, therefore, that the psychosis and some aspects of the encephalopathy are only minimally or slowly responsive to thiamin treatment, in view of the structural lesions which may be found.[114] In addition to the structural similarity of lesions, the theory that Korsakoff's psychosis is related to thiamin deficiency, or at least nutritional deficiency, is supported by the observation that the majority of alcoholics with memory and learning defects have a history of dietary deficiency.[154]

Clinical and pathological evidence supports the concept that Wernicke's encephalopathy and the pathological lesions associated with it are decreasing in association with improvement in nutrition in recent years.[97] Recent studies also have demonstrated an abnormal enzyme of transketolase in fibroblasts from patients with the Wernicke–Korsakoff syndrome, suggesting the importance of genetic factors in producing this illness.[11] Previous studies have supported the importance of alcohol in producing learning deficits in rodents, analogous to those seen in the Wernike–Korsakoff syndrome, but recent studies have supported the importance of thiamin deficiency alone in this respect.[139a, 158-160] The precise interrelation of alcohol, thiamin, and the Korsakoff's psychosis awaits further clarification.

NUTRITIONAL AMBLYOPIA

This disorder is characterized by central or centrocecal scotomata. Evidence is highly suggestive of a B vitamin deficiency, but a specific etiology has not been established.[153] Oral or parenteral B vitamins, abstinence from alcohol, and regular diet are indicated.

PELLAGRA

Neurologic symptoms in pellagra include psychosis, dementia, posterior and lateral column disease, and neuropathy. Skin changes and diarrhea accompany the neurologic findings. Pellagra is rare now, probably because of enrichment of bread. Nicotinic acid is specific, but B vitamins are generally administered as a group.

Nutritional factors are generally felt to be unrelated to states of acute alcohol intoxication and withdrawal. The role of nutritional factors in central pontine myelenosis, Marchiafava–Bignami syndrome, alcoholic cerebellar degeneration, and other rarer syndromes remains speculative. The response of cerebellar degeneration to massive thiamin administration has been reported.[40] Vitamin B administration in any alcohol-related neurologic state seems prudent.

HEMATOLOGIC CONSIDERATIONS

Hematologic abnormalities are among the most clearly delineated pathologic alterations resulting from an interaction of alcohol and diet. The frequency and nature of observed abnormalities are highly dependent on the population selected. Small amounts of pyridoxine and folic acid in the diet may prevent megaloblastic and sideroblastic anemias. In one series of 65 patients admitted for alcoholism and not selected for hematologic problems, 40% had megaloblastic erythropoesis secondary to folate deficiency, 30% had sideroblasts in the erythroid marrow, and a small percentage had iron deficiency anemia. A total of 75% had either anemia or bone marrow abnormalities. In middle- and upper-class alcoholics folate levels are generally normal.[26] Small amounts of folic acid (150 µg by mouth) prevent megaloblastic changes, and 1 mg pyridoxine/day prevents sideroblastic changes during ethanol administration. However, pharmacologic doses of folic acid do not prevent vacuolization of erythroid elements in patients fed alcohol with an adequate diet.[75] Thus, alcohol has

a direct toxic effect on the bone marrow. The timing of a bone marrow examination is important in establishing a diagnosis because improvement of bone marrow abnormalities may be rapid.

ANEMIAS

Anemia, low serum folate, and megaloblastic marrow with or without sideroblasts may be used to diagnose folate and pyridoxine-related hematologic abnormalities. Therapy includes abstinence and vitamin supplementation. Smaller doses may be adequate, but many times the daily requirement of folate and pyridoxine are generally administered. Although B_{12} absorption may be affected by acute alcohol administration, B_{12} deficiency anemia is not very common among alcoholics and will not be discussed here (see Chap. 23).

PLATELETS AND WHITE BLOOD CELLS

Thrombocytopenia and granulocytopenia have been described in alcoholics with varying frequency depending on patient selection. Causes of thrombocytopenia in the alcoholic include a direct effect of acute alcohol ingestion, folate deficiency, hypersplenism, infection, and disseminated intravascular coagulation. Ethanol causes a depression in circulating platelets despite the concomitant administration of a nutritious diet and vitamin supplements, including large doses of folic acid.[75] In addition, chronic alcohol administration, along with an adequate diet and folate supplements, impairs platelet function.[46] Granulocytopenia has been reported in alcoholics associated with alcohol intoxication without folate deficiency, hypersplenism, or infection and with rapid recovery after alcohol withdrawal.[74] However, in patients given chronic alcohol administration in the absence of nutritional deficiency, granulocytopenia does not develop.[75] Acute alcohol administration impairs leukocyte mobilization.[12]

FAT-SOLUBLE VITAMINS

Fat-soluble vitamins are usually not deficient in the alcoholic, but marginal nutrition, severe steatorrhea, altered GI flora, and hepatocellular injury may act synergistically to cause deficiencies. The major vitamins to be considered are vitamin K and vitamin D.

VITAMIN A

Vitamin A is absorbed and stored within the liver as retinol but must be oxidized to its active form, retinal, within target organs by alcohol dehydrogenase. It is necessary for dark adaptation and spermatogenesis, both of which may be impaired in the alcoholic.[105,152] Alcoholics may have impaired metabolism of vitamin A at several levels, including decreased absorption, steatorrhea, impaired storage, and diminished activation by alcohol dehydrogenase. The latter might occur through competition of retinol and ethanol for alcohol dehydrogenase in the liver, retina, and testes.[89,151]

VITAMIN D

Vitamin D metabolism in conjunction with calcium metabolism is of special interest in the alcoholic. Alcoholic populations have been observed to have decreased bone density, increased susceptibility to fractures, and increased frequency of osteonecrosis compared with other populations.[100,132,141] Vitamin D metabolism may be affected at many levels in the alcoholic. In addition to decreased dietary intake, decreased absorption may occur owing to pancreatic insufficiency and bile salt abnormalities. Similarly, calcium absorption may be impaired. Patients with alcoholic cirrhosis have been found to have decreased clearance of plasma cholecalciferol and decreased urinary glucuronide conjugates.[4] The liver is the first site of hydroxylation of vitamin D_3 (cholecalciferol), which is necessary for its activation; thus, hepatocellular injury may result in deficient activation of dietary vitamin D and resistance to parenteral vitamin D therapy.[3] Other postulated mechanisms of possible alterations in vitamin D metabolism include increased degradation of activated vitamin D by the cytochrome P 450 system (which may be stimulated by alcohol), and decreased storage depots of fat and muscle in debilitated patients with chronic liver disease.[3] The increased urinary losses of calcium induced by alcohol, ethanol-induced hypercorticism, and parathyroid stimulation secondary to calcium-binding proteins in cirrhosis are other mechanisms by which bone metabolism may be altered. The extent to which altered vitamin D metabolism specifically contributes to clinical musculoskeletal diseases in alcoholic populations and the site or sites of the abnormalities involved is unknown.

VITAMIN K

Vitamin K deficiency may result from dietary deficiency, malabsorption, or decreased synthesis by intestinal flora. Failure of clotting factor synthesis owing to alcoholic liver injury may result in prolongation of the prothrombin time. Although deficiency-related abnormalities are uncommon in the alcoholic, vitamin K may correct a prolonged pro-

thrombin time resulting from interaction of the above factors.[122] Generally, vitamin K is given intramuscularly (10 mg/day) for 3 consecutive days. Failure to correct the prothrombin time indicates severe parenchymal injury.

IRON

IRON FUNCTION IN THE LIVER

The question of the metabolism of iron in the alcoholic is particularly relevant because of the association of hepatic injury with excess iron. Acute alcohol administration may increase iron absorption, possibly through stimulation of gastric acid secretion, resulting in increased solubility of ferric ion in the small intestine.[15] Alcoholics may receive excessive dietary iron from the beverages they drink, such as certain wines or through inadvertent treatment with iron-containing vitamin preparations. In addition, anemias unrelated to iron deficiency may be incorrectly treated with iron. Pancreatic insufficiency, folate deficiency, portosystemic shunting, and cirrhosis may increase iron absorption.[39] The potential for excess iron to produce tissue injury and the finding of increased iron stores in a significant percentage of patients with alcoholic cirrhosis make this an important area for future investigation.

IRON DEFICIENCY ANEMIA

Iron deficiency anemia is uncommon in alcoholics unless factors such as GI bleeding from varices, ulcers and gastritis, repeated phlebotomies, dietary extremes, and chronic infections are present.[27] However, as discussed above, alcoholics have a propensity to develop increased iron stores that may potentiate tissue injury in the liver and other organs. Transfusions and iron therapy should be used with caution and only to the point of correcting deficiencies. Routine iron supplements are not indicated.

MINERALS AND ELECTROLYTES

PATHOGENESIS

Alcoholics with chronic liver disease may have disorders of water and electrolyte metabolism. Sodium and water retention may be the most common abnormalities that present clinically as ascites, edema, and portal hypertension, hypoalbuminemia, altered renal hemodynamics, endocrine abnormalities, and changes in lymph flow.[144] Low body potassium stores may result acutely from vomiting and diarrhea or as a result of hyperaldosteronism, muscle wasting, renal tubular acidosis, and diuretic therapy. Depletion of potassium may be especially significant because of consequent increased renal vein ammonia and worsening of hepatic coma.[140] Alcoholics may have decreased plasma levels of zinc, calcium, and magnesium resulting from ethanol-induced renal losses and decreased dietary intake.[119] The similarity of the neuromuscular excitability of hypomagnesemia and acute alcoholic withdrawal has aroused considerable interest; however, as with other trace elements, clinical correlations have not been significant, and florid deficiency states remain exceedingly rare.[47] Abnormalities of other trace elements, such as manganese and copper, in chronic liver disease have been discussed by Prasad.[119] They remain chiefly of investigative interest at present.

ASCITES AND EDEMA

The alterations leading to salt and water retention in liver disease have been discussed. Increasing abdominal girth, weight gain, a dragging sensation in the abdomen, shortness of breath, and swelling of the ankles may be typical presenting symptoms. The presence of shifting dullness, pitting edema, effusions on chest x-ray film, and the finding of fluid on paracentesis confirm the diagnosis. Dietary regimen is adjusted according to the severity of salt and water retention. Severe symptoms and refractory cases may require rigid sodium restriction (250 mg/day).

Restriction at this level is advocated even if mild hyponatremia is present, that is, if the serum sodium level is 125 mEq/liter to 130 mEq/liter.[35] Symptomatic hyponatremia with serum sodium below this level may require intervention with hypertonic saline and rigid water restriction. Fluid restriction of 1500 ml to 200 ml/day (including all liquids taken with medications) is recommended, especially if hyponatremia is present. With less severe retention, sodium restriction of 500 mg/day to 200 mg/day may be tried. Daily weights and serum electrolytes are necessary to guide therapy. Summerskill recommends not exceeding a weight loss of 5 kg/week by dietary or diuretic therapy.[194] In refractory cases, especially with symptoms such as severe dyspnea, paracentesis may be necessary. Two liters per 24 hr have been recommended as a safe rate of removal; more vigorous therapy may cause acute depletion of albumin, salt, and water and result in cardiovascular collapse. Replacement therapy with IV albumin and saline may be required during such therapy. Diuretics may be used with attention to the possible development of hypokalemia and hyponatremia. Following restriction, diuresis and improved handling of dietary so-

dium may result. A ceiling of 2500 mg of sodium in the diet has been suggested.[34]

Associated Conditions

RENAL FUNCTION

Patients with chronic liver disease may have difficulty in handling fluid loads. A daily total volume of 1500 ml to 2000 ml is recommended with observation for adequate urine output, weight gain, and hyponatremia. Oliguria, azotemia, and elevated creatinine may indicate deteriorating renal function. Patients with alcoholic liver disease are especially susceptible to acute tubular necrosis through such complications as variceal bleeding. Spontaneous renal failure or the so-called hepatorenal syndrome may also occur. Rising serum urea due to renal failure may present a special problem in the patient with alcoholic liver disease. Urea is secreted into the GI tract and hydrolyzed to ammonia; thus, it acts like any nitrogenous compound. With increasing levels of urea the resultant ammonia becomes a significant problem and may worsen or precipitate hepatic coma. In this case antibiotics may be given to prevent conversion of urea to ammonia, and enemas may decrease the total load of nitrogenous compounds absorbed. Administration of limited amounts of mixtures of essential amino acids to patients with diminished protein tolerance because of renal failure has been advocated.[144] The dietary management of acute renal failure is otherwise the same as in other etiologies and will be discussed elsewhere (see Chap. 34).

HEPATIC ENCEPHALOPATHY

Hepatic encephalopathy represents a neuropsychiatric syndrome secondary to liver disease, with a wide clinical spectrum ranging from personality changes to deep coma. Confusion, apathy, irritability, and other personality changes may represent the earliest findings. Constructive apraxia, hypothermia, asterixis, and electroencephalogram (EEG) changes may provide clinical evidence. The stages of hepatic coma and concomitant clinical findings are presented in Table 15-3. The etiology and pathogenesis of encephalopathy are complex. The major dietary considerations for the clinician include exogenous and endogenous nitrogen loads and potassium and acid–base balance.[135]

Acutely, protein restriction, correction of hypokalemia and alkalosis, and prevention of endogenous protein catabolism are the major interventions. Hypokalemia increases renal vein ammonia

TABLE 15-3
Stages in the Onset and Development of Hepatic Coma

Grade or Stage	Mental State	Tremor	EEG Changes
Stage 1: Prodrome (often diagnosed in retrospect)	Euphoria, occasionally depression: fluctuant, mild confusion; slowness of mentation and affect; untidy; slurred speech; disorder in sleep rhythm	Slight	Usually absent
Stage 2: Impending coma	Accentuation of Stage 1: drowsiness; inappropriate behavior; able to maintain sphincter control	Present (easily elicited)	Abnormal generalized slowing
Stage 3: Stupor	Sleeps most of the time, but is rousable; speech is incoherent; confusion is marked	Usually present (if patient can cooperate)	Always abnormal
Stage 4: Deep coma	May or may not respond to noxious stimuli	Usually absent	Always abnormal

through a direct effect of increased renal ammonia production and possibly through the increased back diffusion of ammonia from alkaline urine.[140] Parenteral or oral potassium may be given in a dosage of approximately 100 mEq to 200 mEq/day until deficits are corrected, provided that normal renal function is present. Nitrogen sparing should be maintained through IV glucose if caloric intake is not adequate. Since 5% dextrose contains only 200 Cal/liter, it may be necessary to administer hypertonic glucose through a large-bore catheter, especially if fluid restriction is a consideration. Dietary protein may be eliminated completely at first but must be resumed after a few days to prevent endogenous protein catabolism. Neomycin, lactulose, enemas, and divided small feedings may enhance protein tolerance. Neomycin inhibits the action of GI flora that convert protein and urea to ammonia and other potentially toxic nitrogenous products within the gut. Decreased renal function, as in the hepatorenal syndrome, may result in ototoxic and nephrotoxic blood levels of neomycin; dosage must be markedly lowered or the drug discontinued under such circumstances. Lactulose may act though acidification of bowel contents with resultant ammonia trapping (as ammonium) or through increased motility, but the precise mechanism has not been clarified.[52] Constipation and hypercatabolic states, such as with infections, may diminish tolerance and worsen encephalopathy by creating an endogenous nitrogen load.

Protein tolerance may vary, and so daily evaluation is required. Special considerations for protein of different types as well as special amino acid mixtures of ketoanalogues of amino acids are discussed above. A composite sheet with the patient's daily signature, the construction of figures such as a clock face and a record of performance of serial sevens, number connection tests, and the degree of asterixis may provide a useful way of following patient status. Medications that cause hypokalemia must be used with caution. Patients with portacaval shunts may be especially sensitive to dietary protein.

ALCOHOLIC CARDIOMYOPATHY

The chronic alcoholic may present with symptoms of congestive heart failure and clinical features of cardiomyopathy. Essentially, by process of exclusion, a diagnosis of alcoholic cardiomyopathy may be made. In contrast to beriberi heart disease, low cardiac output and peripheral vasoconstriction are usually present. Characteristic electron microscopic changes in the myocardium have been described that have been compared to those produced experimentally in hypomagnesemic rats.[48,145] This has heightened interest in a possible nutritional etiology. However, chronic alcoholics without evidence of heart disease or nutritional deficiency have been found to have abnormal left ventricular function when stressed.[120] Acute and chronic alcohol alters myocardial metabolism.[162] Acute alcohol in adequate doses (blood level of 150 mg/dl) causes a rise in end-diastolic pressure and decreases stroke output. Chronic alcohol administration in the face of a normal diet causes similar changes that persist for several weeks after withdrawal.[120] Cardiomyopathy in the alcoholic, even with an equivocal diagnosis of alcoholic cardiomyopathy, is prudently treated with complete abstinence from alcohol and vitamin supplements. Diet therapy chiefly entails sodium restriction and is similar to other cardiomyopathies in this regard (see Chap. 17).

It is possible that alcohol and nutritional factors may combine to produce alcoholic cardiomyopathy. Such a case is illustrated by the cobalt-mediated cardiomyopathy in beer drinkers. The combination of small quantities of cobalt combined with heavy ethanol abuse produces a fulminant cardiomyopathy in beer drinkers.[95] However, cobalt or ethanol alone, taken in amounts comparable to those ingested by patients who developed cobalt-beer-drinker's heart, does not produce this disorder.

INTERACTIONS WITH DRUGS, CARCINOGENS, AND DISEASE STATES

Alcoholism may interact with other clinical states and complicate therapy. Pregnancy and birth control pills may potentiate folate deficiency in the alcoholic.[49] The hyperuricemia induced by alcohol must be considered in the patient with gout. Alcohol-induced glucose intolerance, hypoglycemia, ketosis, and acidosis may make the management of the diabetic more difficult. Ethanol may interact with many drugs and so alter the management of many disease states. Ethanol can be oxidized in the liver by a microsomal system that shares many properties with the microsomal drug detoxifying systems.[54] Competition for this system may explain the inhibition of drug metabolism by ethanol.[124] Chronic alcoholism causes increased clearance of drugs, which may be explained by stimulation of this system.[90] Clinically, alcoholics may have delayed clearance of many drugs if they drink at the same time. This is especially significant for hypnotic-sedative drugs the depressant effects of which may be potentiated by alcohol. On the other hand, chronic alcoholism may result in increased metabolism of many drugs, which may thus require dosage adjustment. Drugs such as barbiturates, anesthetics, phenothiazines, Coumadin, oral hypoglycemics, and many others may be affected. Finally, through a similar mechanism of accelerated metabolism, the alcoholic may be susceptible to toxic agents, such as CCl_4, acetaminophen, and isoniazid.[46,131]

Epidemiologic studies support an association of alcoholism with cancers of the head and neck, esophagus, liver, and colon. The respective roles of alcohol and associated nutritional deficiency in carcinogenesis is an area of current investigation. Since it has been established that microsomal systems activate a variety of procarcinogens, the induction of microsomal enzyme activity by ethanol, with an associated increased conversion of procarcinogens to carcinogens and enhanced mutagenicity, may constitute a level at which alcohol and carcinogens interact.[93,136] It is also possible that carcinogenesis may be influenced by the nutritional consequences of alcoholism, since it is well known that diet modifies tumor formation in laboratory animals.[19,161] In human beings, chronic deficiency of iron may play a role in the etiology of gastric cancer, and zinc deficiency has been related to the high incidence of esophageal carcinoma in Iran.[56,155]

References

1. Arky RA: The effect of alcohol on carbohydrate metabolism: Carbohydrate metabolism in alcoholics. In Kissin B, Begleiter H (eds): Biology of Alcoholism, Vol 1, p 197. New York, Plenum Press, 1974
2. Atwater WO, Benedict FG: An experimental inquiry regarding the nutritive value of alcohol. Proc Natl Acad Sci USA 8:231, 1896
3. Avioli LV, Haddad JG: Vitamin D: Current concepts. Metabolism 22:507, 1973
4. Avioli LV, Lee SW, McDonald JE et al: Metabolism of $D_3 - ^3H$ in human subjects: Distribution in blood, bile, feces and urine. J Clin Invest 46:983, 1967
5. Axelrod DR: Metabolic and endocrine aberrations in alcoholism. In Kissin B, Begleiter H (eds): Biology of Alcoholism, Vol 3, p 291. New York, Plenum Press, 1974
6. Baraona E, Leo MA, Borowsky SA et al: Alcoholic hepatomegaly: Accumulation of protein in the liver. Science 190:794, 1975
7. Barboriak JJ, Meade RC: Effect of alcohol on gastric emptying in man. Am J Clin Nutr 23:1151, 1970
8. Bayer M, Rudick J, Lieber CS et al: Inhibitory effect of ethanol on canine exocrine pancreatic secretion. Gastroenterology 63:619, 1972
9. Bebb HT, Houser HB, Witschi JC et al: Calorie and nutrient contribution of alcoholic beverages to the usual diets of 155 adults. Am J Clin Nutr 24:1042, 1971
10. Best CH, Hartroft WS, Lucas CC et al: Liver damage produced by feeding alcohol or sugar and its prevention by choline. Br Med J 2:1001, 1949
11. Blass JP, Gibson GE: Abnormality of a thiamine-requiring enzyme in patients with Wernicke–Korsakoff syndrome. N Engl J Med 297:1367, 1977
12. Brayton RG, Stokes PE, Schwartz MS et al: Effect of alcohol and various diseases on leukocyte mobilization, phagocytosis and intracellular bacterial killing. N Engl J Med 282:123, 1970
13. Burch GE, Giles TD: Alcoholic cardiomyopathy. In Kissin B, Begleiter H (eds.): Biology of Alcoholism, Vol 3, p 435. New York, Plenum Press, 1974
14. Chait A, February W, Mancine M et al: Clinical and metabolic study of alcoholic hyperlipidaemia. Lancet 2:62, 1972
15. Charlton RW, Jacobs P, Seftel H et al: Effect of alcohol on iron absorption. Br Med J 5422:1327, 1964
16. Cherrick GR, Baker H, Frank O et al: Observations on hepatic avidity for folate in Laennec's cirrhosis. J Lab Clin Med 66:446, 1965
17. Chey WY: Alcohol and gastric mucosa. Digestion 7:239, 1972
18. Chey WY, Kosay S, Lorber SH: Effects of chronic administration of ethanol on gastric secretion of acid in dogs. Dig Dis Sci 17:153, 1972
19. Chu EW, Malmoren RA: Inhibitory effect of vitamin A on the induction of tremors of forestomach and in the Syrian hamster by carcinogenic polycyclic hydrocarbons. Cancer Res 25:884, 1965
20. Crews RH, Faloon WW: The fallacy of a low-fat diet in liver disease. JAMA 181:754, 1962

21. Davenport HW: Gastric mucosal hemorrhage in dogs—effects of acid, aspirin, and alcohol. Gastroenterology 56:439, 1969

22. Davidson CS: Nutrition, geography and liver diseases. Am J Clin Nutr 23:427, 1970

23. Desai HG, Merchant PC, Zaveri MP et al: Mechanism of steatorrhea in cirrhosis of liver: Correlation between cholate concentration and BSP retention and vitamin B_1 excretion. Indian J Med Res 60:1464, 1972

24. Dreyfus PM: Diseases of the nervous system in chronic alcoholics. In Kissin B, Begleiter H (eds): Biology of Alcoholism, Vol 3, p 265. New York, Plenum Press, 1974

25. Dreyfus PM, Victor M: Effects of thiamine deficiency on the central nervous system. Am J Clin Nutr 9:414, 1961

26. Eichner ER, Buchanan B, Smith JW et al: Variations in the hematologic and medical status of alcoholics. Am J Med Sci 263:35, 1972

27. Eichner ER, Hillman RS: The evolution of anemia in alcoholic patients. Am J Med 50:218, 1971

28. Erenoglu E, Edreira JG, Patek AJ Jr: Observations on patients with Laennec's cirrhosis receiving alcohol while on controlled diets. Ann Intern Med 60:814, 1964

29. Evans WB, Wollaeger EE: Incidence and severity of nutritional deficiency states in chronic exocrine pancreatic insufficiency: Comparison with non-tropical sprue. Am J Dig Dis 11:594, 1966

30. Faloon WW: Metabolic effects of nonabsorbable antibacterial agents. Am J Clin Nutr 23:645, 1970

31. Faraj BA, Bowen PA, Isaacs JW: Hypertyraminemia in cirrhotic patients. N Engl J Med 294:1360, 1976

32. Finkelstein JD, Cello JP, Kyle WE: Ethanol induced changes in methionine metabolism in rat liver. Biochem Biophys Res Commun 61:525, 1974

33. Fischer JE, Funovics JM, Aguirre A et al: The role of plasma amino acids in hepatic encephalopathy. Surgery 78:276, 1975

34. Gabuzda GJ: Nutrition and liver disease. Med Clin North Am 54:1455, 1970

35. Gabuzda GJ: Cirrhosis, ascites and edema: Clinical course related to management. Gastroenterology 58:546, 1970

36. Gabuzda GJ, Shear L: Metabolism of dietary protein in hepatic cirrhosis. Am J Clin Nutr 23:479, 1970

37. Ginsberg H, Olefsky J, Farquhar JW: Moderate ethanol ingestion and plasma triglyceride levels: A study in normal and hypertriglyceridemic persons. Ann Intern Med 80:143, 1974

38. Gottfried E, Korsten MA, Lieber CS: Gastritis and duodenitis induced by alcohol: An endoscopic and histologic assessment. Am J Gastroenterol 70:587, 1978

39. Grace ND, Powell LW: Iron storage disorders of the liver. Gastroenterology 67:1257, 1974

40. Graham JR, Woodhouse P, Read FH: Massive thiamine dosage in an alcoholic with cerebellar cortical degeneration. Lancet 2:107, 1971

41. Greenberger NJ, Carley J, Schenker S et al: Effect of vegetable and animal protein diets in chronic hepatic encephalopathy. Am J Dig Dis 22:845, 1977

42. Greenberger NJ, Skillman TG: Medium chain triglycerides, physiologic considerations and clinical implications. N Engl J Med 280:1045, 1969

43. Halsted CH, Robles EA, Mezey E: Intestinal malabsorption in folate-deficient alcoholics. Gastroenterology 64:526, 1973

44. Hartroft SW, Porta EA: Alcohol, diet and experimental hepatic injury. Can J Physiol Pharmacol 46:463, 1968

45. Hasumura Y, Teschke R, Lieber CS: Increased carbon tetrachloride hepatotoxicity and its mechanism, after chronic ethanol consumption. Gastroenterology 66:415, 1974

46. Haut MJ, Cowan DH: The effect of ethanol on hemostatic properties of human blood platelets. Am J Med 56:22, 1974

47. Heaton FW, Pyrah LN, Beresford CC et al: Hypomagnesaemia in chronic alcoholism. Lancet 2:802, 1962

48. Hibbs RG, Ferrans VJ, Black WC et al: Alcoholic cardiomyopathy: An electron microscopic study. Am Heart J 69:766, 1965

49. Hillman RW: Alcoholism and malnutrition. In Kissin B, Begleiter H (eds): Biology of Alcoholism, Vol 3, p 513. New York, Plenum Press, 1974

50. Hoffbaure FW, Zaki FG: Choline deficiency in baboon and rat compared. Arch Pathol 79:364, 1965

51. Hornabrook RW: Alcoholic neuropathy. Am J Clin Nutr 9:398, 1961

52. Hubel KA: Lactulose works, but why? Comment. Gastroenterology 65:349, 1973

53. Iber FL: In alcoholism, the liver sets the pace. Nutrition Today 6:2, 1971

54. Ishii H, Joly J-G, Lieber CS: Effect of ethanol on the amount and enzyme activities of hepatic rough and smooth microsomal membranes. Biochim Biophys Acta 291:411, 1973

55. Kessler JI, Kniffen JC, Janowitz HD: Lipoprotein lipase inhibition in the hyperlipemia of acute alcoholic pancreatitis. N Engl J Med 269:943, 1963

56. Kmet J, Mahboubi E: Esophageal cancer in the Caspian littoral of Iran: Initial studies. Science 175:846, 1972

57. Knodell RG, Kinsey D, Boedeker EC et al: Deoxycholate metabolism in alcoholic cirrhosis. Gastroenterology 71:196, 1976

58. Leake CD, Silverman M: The chemistry of alcoholic beverages. In Kissin B, Begleiter H (eds): Biology of Alcoholism, Vol 1, p 575. New York, Plenum Press, 1974

59. Lederman S: Alcohol, Alcoholisme, Alcoholisation. Paris: Institut national d'etudes demographiques, Travaux et Documents, Cahier No. 41, Presses Universitaires de France, 1964

60. Leevy CM: Fatty liver: A study of 270 patients with biopsy proven fatty liver and a review of the literature. Medicine (Baltimore) 41:249, 1962

61. Leevy CM, Baker H, tenHove W et al: B-complex vitamins in liver disease of the alcoholic. Am J Clin Nutr 16:339, 1965

62. Leevy CM, Thompson A, Baker H: Vitamins and liver injury. Am J Clin Nutr 23:493, 1970

63. Lefevre AF, DeCarli LM, Lieber CS: Effect of ethanol on cholesterol and bile acid metabolism. J Lipid Res 13:48, 1972

64. Lelbach WK: Cirrhosis in the alcoholic and its relation to the volume of alcohol abuse. Ann NY Acad Sci 252:85, 1975

65. Lieber CS: Interaction of ethanol with drug toxicity. Am J Gastroenterol 74:313, 1980

66. Lieber CS: Effects of ethanol upon lipid metabolism. Lipids 9:103, 1974

67. Lieber CS: Medical Disorders of Alcoholism: Pathogenesis and Treatment, Philadelphia, WB Saunders, 1982

68. Lieber CS, DeCarli LM: Study of agents for the prevention of the fatty liver produced by prolonged alcohol intake. Gastroenterology 50:316, 1966

69. Lieber CS, DeCarli LM: An experimental model of al-

cohol feeding and liver injury in the baboon. J Med Primatol 3:153, 1974

70. Lieber CS, Jones DP, Losowsky MS et al: Interrelation of uric acid and ethanol metabolism in man. J Clin Invest 41:1863, 1962

71. Lieber CS, Jones DP, Mendelson J et al: Fatty liver, hyperlipemia and hyperuricemia produced by prolonged alcohol consumption, despite adequate dietary intake. Trans Assoc Am Physicians 76:289, 1963

72. Lieber CS, Rubin E: Alcoholic fatty liver. N Engl J Med 280:705, 1969

73. Lieber CS, Seitz HK, Garro AJ et al: Alcohol related diseases and carcinogenesis. Cancer Res 39:2863, 1980

74. Lindenbaum J, Hargrove RL: Thrombocytopenia in alcoholics. Ann Intern Med 68:526, 1968

75. Lindenbaum J, Lieber CS: Hematologic effects of alcohol in man in absence of nutritional deficiency. N Engl J Med 281:333, 1969

76. Lindenbaum J, Lieber CS: Effects of ethanol on the blood, bone marrow, and small intestine of man. In Roach MK, McIsaac WM, Creaven PJ (eds): Biological Aspects of Alcohol, Vol 3, p 27. Austin, University of Texas Press, 1971

77. Lindenbaum J, Lieber CS: Effects of chronic ethanol administration on intestinal absorption in man in the absence of nutritional deficiency. Ann NY Acad Sci 252:228, 1975

78. Lindenbaum J, Shea N, Saha JR et al: Alcohol-induced impairment of carbohydrate (CHO) absorption. Clinical Research 20:459, 1972

79. Linscheer WG: Malabsorption in cirrhosis. Am J Clin Nutr 23:488, 1970

80. Lischner MW, Alexander JF, Galambos JT: Natural history of alcoholic hepatitis. I. The acute disease. Am J Dig Dis 16:481, 1971

81. Lorber SH, Dinoso VP, Chey WY: Diseases of the gastrointestinal tract. In Kissin B, Begleiter H (eds): Biology of Alcoholism, Vol 3, p 339. New York, Plenum Press, 1974

82. Losowsky MS, Jones DP, Davidson CS et al: Studies of alcoholic hyperlipemia and its mechanism. Am J Med 35:794, 1963

83. Losowsky MS, Walker BE: Liver disease and malabsorption. Gastroenterology 56:589, 1969

84. MacLachlan MJ, Rodnan GP: Effects of fast food and alcohol on serum uric acid and acute attacks of gout. Am J Med 42:38, 1967

85. Maddrey WC, Weber FL, Coulter AW et al: Effects of keto analogues of essential amino acids in portal-systemic encephalopathy. Gastroenterology 71:190, 1976

86. McGill DB, Humphreys SR, Baggenstoss AH et al: Cirrhosis and death after jejunoileal shunt. Gastroenterology 63:872, 1972

87. Menghine G: L'Aspect morpho-bioptique du foie de l'acoolique (non cirrhotique) et son évolution. Bull Schweiz Akad Med Wiss 16:36, 1960

88. Metz R, Berger S, Mako M: Potentiation of the plasma insulin response to glucose by prior administration of alcohol. Diabetes 8:517, 1969

89. Mezey E, Holt PR: The inhibitory effect of ethanol on retinol oxidation by human liver and cattle retina. Exp Mol Pathol 15:148, 1971

90. Misra PS, Lefevre A, Ishii H et al: Increase of ethanol, meprobamate and pentobarbital metabolism after chronic ethanol administration in man and in rats. Am J Med 51:346, 1971

91. Mistilis SP, Ockner RK: Effects of ethanol on endogenous lipid and lipoprotein metabolism in small intestine. J Lab Clin Med 80:34, 1972

92. Mitchell D, Wagner C, Stone WJ et al: Abnormal regulation of plasma pyridoxal 5-phosphate in patients with liver disease. Gastroenterology 71:1043, 1976

93. Mitchell JR, Jollow DJ: Role of metabolic activation in chemical carcinogenesis and in drug induced hepatic injury. Gerok W, Sickinger K (eds): Drugs and the Liver, 3rd International Symposium, p 395. Stuttgart–New York, Schattauer Verlag, 1975

94. Morgan MY, Sherlock S: Sex-related differences among 100 patients with alcoholic liver disease. Br Med J 1:939, 1977

95. Morin Y, Daniel P: Quebec beer-drinkers cardiomyopathy: Etiological considerations. Can Med Assoc J 97:926, 1967

96. Morrison LM: The response of cirrhosis of the liver to an intensive combined therapy. Ann Intern Med 24:465, 1946

97. Neubueger KT: The changing neuropathologic picture of chronic alcoholism. Arch Pathol 63:1, 1957

98. Neville JN, Eagles JA, Samson G et al: Nutritional status of alcoholics. Am J Clin Nutr 21:1329, 1968

99. Newcombe DS: Ethanol metabolism and uric acid. Metabolism 21:1193, 1972

100. Nilsson BE: Conditions contributing to fracture of the femoral neck. Acta Chir Scand 136:383, 1970

101. Olson RE: Nutrition and alcoholism. In Wohl MG, Goodhart RS (eds): Modern Nutrition in Health and Disease, pp 1037–1050. Philadelphia, Lea & Febiger, 1964

102. Orten JM, Sardesa VM: Protein nucleotide and porphyrin metabolism. In Kissin B, Begleiter H (eds): Biology of Alcoholism, Vol 1, p 229. New York, Plenum Press, 1974

103. Ostrander ID, Lamphiear MA, Block WD et al: Relationship of serum lipid concentrations to alcohol consumption. Arch Intern Med 134:451, 1974

104. Palasciano G, Tiscornia O, Hage G et al: Chronic alcoholism and endogenous CCK-PZ. Biomedicine 29:94, 1974

105. Patek AJ, Haig C: The occurrence of abnormal dark adaptation and its relation to vitamin A metabolism in patients with cirrhosis of the liver. J Clin Invest 18:609, 1939

106. Patek AJ, Post J: Treatment of cirrhosis of the liver by a nutritious diet and supplements rich in vitamin B complex. J Clin Invest 20:481, 1941

107. Patek AJ, Post J, Ratnoff OD et al: Dietary treatment of cirrhosis of the liver. JAMA 138:543, 1948

108. Patek AJ, Toth EG, Saunders MG et al: Alcohol and dietary factors in cirrhosis. Arch Intern Med 135:1053, 1975

109. Pequignot G: Die rolle des alkohols bei der atiologie von leberzirrhosin in Frankreich. Munchen Med Wochschr 103:1464, 1962

110. Pequignot GA, Tuyns AJ, Berta JL: Ascitic cirrhosis in relation to alcohol consumption. Int J Epidemiol 7:113, 1978

111. Perlow W, Baraona E, Lieber CS: Symptomatic intestinal disaccharidase deficiencies in alcoholism. Gastroenterology 72:680, 1977

112. Phear EA, Ruebner B, Sherlock SA et al: Methionine toxicity in liver disease and its prevention by chlortetracycline. Clin Sci 15:93, 1956

113. Phillips GB, Safrit HF: Alcoholic diabetes: Induction of glucose intolerance with alcohol. JAMA 217:1513, 1971

114. Phillips GB, Victor M, Adam RD et al: A study of the nutritional defect in Wernicke's syndrome: The effect of a purified diet, thiamine and other vitamins on the clinical manifestations. J Clin Invest 31:859, 1952

115. Piccirillo VJ, Chambers JW: Inhibition of hepatic uptake of alpha aminoisobutyric. Res Commun Chem Pathol Pharmacol 13:297, 1976

116. Pirola RC, Bolin TD, Davis AE: Does alcohol cause duodenitis? Am J Dig Dis 14239, 1969

117. Pirola RC, Lieber CS: The energy cost of the metabolism of drugs including alcohol. Pharmacology 7:185, 1972

118. Platt BS: Thiamine deficiency in human beriberi and in Wernicke's encephalopathy. In Wolstenholme GEW (ed): Thiamine Deficiency: Biochemical Lesions and Their Clinical Significance, pp 138–145. Boston, Little, Brown & Co, 1967

119. Prasad AS, Oberleas D, Rajasekaran G: Essential micronutrient elements: Biochemistry and changes in liver disorders. Am J Clin Nutr 23:581, 1970

120. Regan TJ, Levinson GE, Oldewurtel HA et al: Ventricular function in noncardiacs with alcoholic fatty liver: Role of ethanol in the production of cardiomyopathy. J Clin Invest 48:397, 1969

121. Rehfeld JF, Juhl E, Hilden M: Carbohydrate metabolism in alcohol-induced fatty liver (evidence for an abnormal insulin response to glucagon in alcoholic liver disease). Gastroenterology 64:445, 1973

122. Roberts HR, Cederbaum AI: The liver and blood coagulation: Physiology and pathology. Gastroenterology 63:297, 1972

123. Robles EA, Mezey E, Halsted CH et al: Effect of ethanol on motility of the small intestine. Johns Hopkins Med J 135:17, 1974

124. Rubin E, Gang H, Misra PS et al: Inhibition of drug metabolism by acute ethanol intoxication. A hepatic microsomal mechanism. Am J Med 49:801, 1970

125. Rubin E, Rybak BJ, Lindenbaum J et al: Ultrastructural changes in the small intestine induced by ethanol. Gastroenterology 63:801, 1972

126. Rubin E, Lieber CS: Alcohol-induced hepatic injury in non-alcoholic volunteers. N Engl J Med 278:869, 1968

127. Rudman D, Akgun S, Galambos JT et al: Observations of the nitrogen metabolism of patients with portal cirrhosis. Am J Clin Nutr 23:1203, 1970

128. Rudman D, Galambos JT, Smith RB et al: Comparison of the effect of various amino acids upon the blood ammonia concentration of patients with liver disease. Am J Clin Nutr 26:916, 1973

129. Sarles H: Chronic calcifying pancreatitis—chronic alcoholic pancreatitis. Gastroenterology 66:604, 1974

130. Sarles H, Sarles J–C, Camatte R et al: Observations of 205 confirmed cases of acute pancreatitis, recurring pancreatitis, and chronic pancreatitis. Gut 6:545, 1965

131. Sato C, Matsuda Y, Lieber CS: Increased hepatotoxicity of acetaminozolien after chronic alcohol consumption. Fed Proc 38:916, 1979

132. Saville PD: Changes in bone mass with age and alcoholism. J Bone Joint Surg (Am) 47:492, 1965

133. Schapiro RH, Drummey GD, Shimizu Y et al: Studies on the pathogenesis of the ethanol-induced fatty liver, II: Effect of ethanol on palmitate-1-C^{14} metabolism by the isolated perfused rat liver. J Clin Invest 43:1338, 1964

134. Scheig R: Effects of ethanol on the liver. Am J Clin Nutr 23:467, 1970

135. Schenker S, Breen KJ, Hoyumpa AM: Hepatic encephalopathy: Current status. Gastroenterology 66:121, 1974

136. Seitz HJ, Garro AJ, Lieber CS: Effect of chronic ethanol ingestion on intestinal metabolism and mutagenicity of benzo(α)pyrene. Biochem Biophys Res Commun 85:1061, 1978

137. Shaw S, Jayatilleke E, Ross WA et al: Hepatic lipid peroxidation and glutathione depression after ethanol. Gastroenterology 77:A41, 1979

138. Shaw S, Lieber CS: Plasma amino acid abnormalities in the alcoholic: Respective role of alcohol, nutrition, and liver injury. Gastroenterology 74:677, 1978

139. Shaw S, Stimmel B, Lieber CS: Plasma alpha-amino-η-butyric acid to leucine ratio: An empirical biochemical marker of alcoholism. Science 194:1057, 1978

139 a. Shaw S, Gorkin BD, Lieber CS: Effects of chronic alcohol feeding on thiamin status: Biochemical and neurological correlates. Am J Clin Nutr 34:856–860, 1981

140. Shear L, Gabuzda GJ: Potassium deficiency and endogenous ammonium overload from kidney. Am J Clin Nutr 23:614, 1970

141. Solomon L: Drug induced arthropathy and necrosis on the femoral head. J Bone Joint Surg (Br) 55:246, 1973

142. Straus E, Urbach H–J, Yalow RS: Alcohol-stimulated secretion of immunoreactive secretin. N Engl J Med 293:1031, 1975

143. Sullivan LW, Herbert V: Suppression of hematopoiesis by ethanol. J Clin Invest 43:2048, 1964

144. Summerskill WHJ, Barnardo DE, Baldus WP: Disorders of water and electrolyte metabolism in liver disease. Am J Clin Nutr 23:499, 1970

145. Susin M, Herdson PB: Fine structural changes in rat myocardium induced by thyroxine and by magnesium deficiency. Arch Pathol 83:86, 1967

146. Thomson AD, Baker H, Leevy CM: Patterns of ^{35}S-thiamine hydrochloride absorption in the malnourished alcoholic patients. J Lab Clin Med 76:34, 1970

147. Tiscornia OM, Singer M, Mendes de Oliveira JP et al: Exocrine pancreas response to a test meal in the dog. Am J Dig Dis 22:769, 1977

148. Toskes PP, Hansell J, Cerda J et al: Vitamin B$_{12}$ malabsorption in chronic pancreatic insufficiency: Studies suggesting the presence of a pancreatic intrinsic factor. N Engl J Med 284:627, 1971

149. Tremolierer J, Carre L: Etudes sur les modalities d'oxydation de l'alcool chez l'homme normal et alcoolique. Rev Alcoolisme 7:202, 1961

150. United States Bureau of the Census: Vital statistics rates in the United States, 1900–1940. Washington, DC, Government Printing Office, 1943

151. Van Thiel DH, Lester R: Alcoholism: Its effect on hypothalamic pituitary gonadal function. Gastroenterology 71:318, 1976

152. Van Thiel DH, Gavaler J, Lester R: Ethanol inhibition of vitamin A metabolism in the testes: Possible mechanism for sterility in alcoholics. Science 186:941, 1974

153. Victor M, Adams RD: Neurological and hepatic complications of alcoholism. Etiology of the alcoholic neurologic diseases with special reference to the role of nutrition. Am J Clin Nutr 9:379, 1960

154. Victor M, Adams RD: On the etiology of the alcoholic neurologic diseases with special reference to the role of nutrition. Am J Clin Nutr 9:379, 1961

155. Vitale JJ, Gottlieb LS: Alcohol and alcohol-related deficiencies as carcinogens. Cancer Res 35:3336, 1975

156. Vlahcevic SR, Juttijudata P, Bell CC et al: Bile salt metabolism in patients with cirrhosis. II. Cholic and chenodeoxycholic acid metabolism. Gastroenterology 62:1174, 1972

157. Von der Lippe G, Andersen K–J, Schjonsby H: Pancreatic extract and the intestinal uptake of vitamin B_{12}, III. Stimulatory effect in the presence of a non-intrinsic factor vitamin B_{12} binder. Scand J Gastroenterol 12:183, 1977

158. Vorhees CV, Barrett RJ, Schenker S: Increased muricide and decreased avoidance and discrimination learning in thiamine deficient rats. Life Sci 16:1187, 1975

159. Walker DW, Freund G: Impairment of shuttle box avoidance learning following prolonged alcohol consumption in rats. Physiol Behav 7:773, 1971

160. Walker DW, Freund G: Impairment of timing behavior after prolonged alcohol consumption in rats. Science 182:597, 1973

161. Weisburger JH: Chemical carcinogenesis. In Casavett LS, Doull J (eds): Toxicology, the Basic of Poisons, p 333. New York, Macmillan, 1979

162. Wendt VE, Wu C, Ajluni R et al: The acute and chronic effects of alcohol on the myocardium (abstr). Ann Intern Med 62:1068, 1965

163. Westerfeld WW, Schulman MP: Metabolism and caloric value of alcohol. JAMA 170:197, 1959

164. Wilkinson P, Santamaria JN, Rankin JG: Epidemiology of alcoholic cirrhosis. Aust Ann Med 18:222, 1969

165. Williams RJ: Alcoholism—The Nutritional Approach, p 1. Austin, University of Texas Press, 1959

166. Wilson DA, Schreibman PH, Brewster AC et al: The enhancement of alimentary lipemia by ethanol in man. J Lab Clin Med 75:264, 1970

167. Zieve L: Jaundice, hyperlipemia and hemolytic anemia: A heretofore unrecognized syndrome associated with alcoholic fatty liver and cirrhosis. Ann Intern Med 48:471, 1958

16
Burns: Metabolism and Nutritional Therapy in Thermal Injury

Joseph A. Molnar,
Robert R. Wolfe,
John F. Burke

At the turn of the century, clinicians noted that the majority of deaths following thermal burns occurred in the first 72 hours after injury. Subsequent advances in fluid resuscitation have come to minimize this early mortality from hypovolemic shock. Further knowledge in both topical and systemic antibiotic therapy, as well as improvements in methods of wound closure, has also prolonged survival. As a result, the clinical course of major thermal injury has changed from one of a brief illness with a uniformly tragic ending to one of a prolonged illness manifesting some of the greatest metabolic alterations of any disease treated by modern physicians. These metabolic alterations have been the subject of intense research that forms the foundation of our approach to the nutritional support of the thermally injured.

Nonetheless, the present available data do not indisputably prove that nutritional support can alter the mortality rate of thermal injury. However, three lines of evidence suggest that such therapy may be helpful.[55] First, without adequate dietary intake, burn patients suffer from rapid weight loss in the weeks before wound closure. While normal man may well tolerate brief periods of caloric restriction, individuals losing weight in excess of 10% of body weight demonstrate significant physiologic consequences. Increased mortality due to surgical stress is seen at greater than 20% weight loss, and 40% weight loss is thought to be lethal. Aggressive implementation of nutritional support has been able to minimize the weight loss of thermal injury. Second, a major cause of morbidity and mortality in

burn patients continues to be infection, which is a reflection of decreased immunocompetence.[40] Nutritional support would appear to maximize immunocompetence and improve survival from infections.[10] Third, severe protein malnutrition, as well as deficiencies of other specific nutrients, interferes with normal wound repair. It would seem valuable to avoid severe malnutrition to aid repair of the large wounds of thermal injury even though excessive therapy would not be advantageous. A discussion of the precise nutrient requirements of the burn patient on the basis of presently available evidence and the potential complications of nutrient excess is the topic of this chapter.

Metabolic Response to Thermal Injury

Cuthbertson has conveniently divided the metabolic response to injury into two major periods: the *ebb period* of traumatic shock and the *flow period* of hypermetabolism.[15] The ebb period is characterized by decreased metabolic rate and inadequacy of cardiac output. Mediation of this early response in burns likely involves the massive fluid loss from the wound, release of endogenous pyrogens, and cellular breakdown products as well as neurologic elements.[59] Hormonal changes generally described include elevated corticosteroids, catecholamines, and antidiuretic hormone, and a decreased responsiveness to insulin.[16,71] The resultant substrate alterations are characterized by a tendency toward hyperglycemia, elevated serum lactate, and free fatty acids.[16,45]

The duration of the ebb phase is generally brief, lasting minutes to days depending on the nature of the stimulus and the success of treatment. Medical management during this period is primarily one of critical care medicine and fluid resuscitation. Multiple reviews of this subject are available.[1,22,40] With successful support of the patient through the period of traumatic shock, he passes on to the flow phase of injury.

In contrast to the ebb phase, the flow phase is characterized by hypermetabolism, hyperthermia, increased pulse and respiratory rates, as well as accelerated losses of nitrogen, sulfur, phosphorus, and potassium, and continued hormonal and substrate alterations.[16,45] Furthermore, the flow phase in thermal injury may continue unabated for months, and it is this period of metabolic alteration that becomes relevant to nutritional support.

HYPERMETABOLISM IN BURNS

While all forms of trauma and infection exhibit an elevation in metabolic rate, burns are unique in the magnitude of this response. Metabolic rates of 100% to 150% above normal have been reported, although in our experience metabolic rates greater than 50% above basal are uncommon (see Fig. 16-1).[35,68] Some of the apparent discrepancy of reported values may be a result of differences in treatment modalities. The degree of hypermetabolism has been described to be modified by both burn size and ambient temperature (see Fig. 16-2).

Early inquiries into the etiology of this uniquely high metabolic rate dealt with the concept of increased energy loss from the burn wound. When normal man is exposed to a cold environment, he responds initially with a decrease in perspiration and peripheral vasoconstriction. When these first two lines of defense are overburdened, he finally responds with an increase of thermogenesis to maintain normal body temperature.[75] Since the burn patient suffers from a lack of the normal water impermeable barrier of the stratum corneum of the skin and is unable to respond through vasoconstriction or decreased perspiration in the burn wound, it was logical to assume that the observed hypermetabolism was merely a response to maintain thermal neutrality.[62] The physiologic importance of this can be appreciated if one realizes that the evaporation of 1 ml water consumes 0.576 Cal of heat. Assuming a loss of 2.5 liters to 4.0 liters of water from the patient's skin daily, he would need to generate 1440 Cal to 2300 Cal to maintain thermal equilibrium.[23] Since the evaporative losses

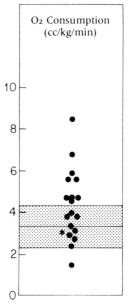

FIG. 16-1   Resting oxygen consumption in burn patients as compared to mean ± 2 SD for normal volunteers. (Wolfe RR, Durkot MJ, Allsop JR et al: Glucose metabolism in severely burned patients. Metabolism 28:1031, 1979. Reproduced by permission, Grune and Stratton)

would be dependent upon the size of the burn, this could explain the described relationship between the percent of the body surface area burned and the metabolic rate, as well as the decrease in metabolic rate observed with healing of the wounds.

To determine the contribution of water vaporization to metabolic rate, several studies have ex-

FIG. 16-2   Relationship between metabolic rate, burn size, and ambient temperature. (Wilmore DW, Long JC, Mason AD, et al: Catecholamines: Mediator of the hypermetabolic response to thermal injury. Ann Surg 180:653, 1974)

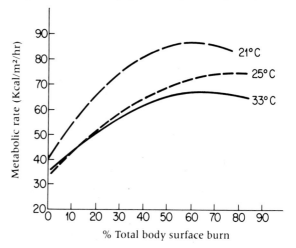

amined the effect of covering the burn wounds with a water-impermeable barrier. Neely demonstrated decreased metabolic rates that did not return to normal with such treatment.[41] Zawacki, however, found no consistent correlation between decreased evaporative water loss and metabolic rate.[75] While this study has been criticized, it would appear that the hypermetabolism of burns arises from more than a response to evaporative cooling.[24]

To further investigate the relationship of metabolic rate and environmental heat exchange, the effect of variation of ambient temperature has been examined. The evidence suggests that treating burn patients in higher environmental temperatures (32°C) decreases metabolic rate to some degree (see Fig. 16-2).[61,62] The relative magnitude of the influence of ambient temperature on metabolic rate has been debated. However, it has been demonstrated that burn patients allowed to control environmental temperature will choose a comfort zone higher than controls.[61] This suggests that at least some portion of the chronic hyperpyrexia ("traumatic fever") of thermal injury is secondary to a reset of the hypothalamus similar to that described in infectious disease. In order to meet the higher core temperature demanded by the hypothalamus, metabolic rate must be increased. However, determination of cause and effect becomes very difficult, because elevation of temperature will also increase metabolic rate. While the hypothalamus may play some role in the orchestration of the hypermetabolism of burns, the magnitude of its importance remains unknown.

Mediators of the hypermetabolism of thermal injury have been investigated. Neural afferents appear to be of secondary importance, and hormonal factors such as endogenous pyrogens, prostaglandins, and catecholamines have been implicated. Catecholamines have received special attention since they are generally elevated during the flow phase of burns and β-adrenergic blockade has demonstrated a lessening of metabolic rate.[61] This is an attractive idea, since it could help explain such phenomena as the observed mitochondrial uncoupling and the substrate cycling which may be major contributors to the hypermetabolism of thermal injury.

PROTEIN METABOLISM

One of the well-recognized metabolic responses to trauma is the tendency toward negative nitrogen balance in excess of local tissue damage.[15] This is not unique to trauma but is shared by infectious illness and even psychic stress.[6,11,16] The major route of this nitrogen loss is increased urinary urea nitrogen. This is true even in burns despite the sig-

nificant protein losses from the wound and elevated nonurea urinary nitrogen. Cuthbertson observed that the increased urea nitrogen loss was accompanied by increased losses of sulfur, potassium, phosphorus, and creatinine, and postulated increased muscle catabolism as the cause "to meet both the exigencies of repair and of maintenance."[14]

Subsequent investigations have borne out this basic premise and have led to the concept of a peripheral to visceral redistribution of protein and other nutrients in the stressed patient.[6,45] Under this paradigm, catabolism of the carcass provides nutrients to support the increased synthetic process of the viscera and wound, recognizing that catabolism and anabolism may be elevated simultaneously in the stressed individual (see Fig. 16-3). From this it is suggested that the flow phase of injury is characterized by a surfeit of nutrients for the immediate needs of trauma even without nutritional support.

Studies in starved man suggest that the major currency of nitrogen transfer from muscle to viscera is alanine, although glutamine may play a role. This transfer of alanine would allow synthesis of nonessential amino acids by transamination of α-keto-derivatives in the liver. It would appear that alanine is synthesized in the muscle with branch-chain amino acids being the primary nitrogen donor.[19] It has been suggested that there is an increased catabolism of branch-chain amino acids and that the release of alanine and glutamine is increased in stressed states that interfere with utilization of free fatty acids and ketone bodies as an energy source. This has prompted attempts to demonstrate decreased muscle catabolism with the exogenous administration of branch-chain amino acids. The success of these trials is consistent with the mechanism proposed above, although further investigation is required.

Since the carbon skeleton of alanine can provide a precursor for glucose synthesis, a second benefit of the transfer of this amino acid from the periphery to the viscera is to facilitate gluconeogenesis. The glucose may then be used as an energy source for erythrocytes, leukocytes, and repairative tissue which use glucose exclusively as a fuel, or it may be cycled back to muscle. Glycolytic degradation may then provide more three-carbon compounds for gluconeogenesis or transamination to alanine (see Fig. 16-4). While elevated blood alanine and increased release of alanine from burned extremities have been observed in burn patients, the contribution to gluconeogenesis appears to be minimal.

Description of hormonal mediation for this redistribution of substrates is not yet comprehensive.

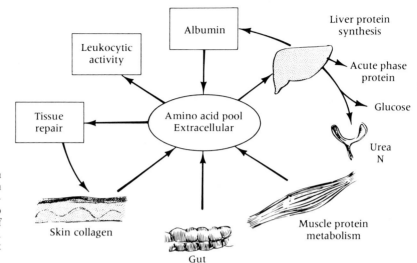

FIG. 16-3 Alterations in protein metabolism with injury create a functional redistribution of proteins from skin, gut, and muscle to aid increased synthetic activity of the viscera and healing wound. (Adapted from Benotti et al: Crit Care Med 7:520, 1979)

Catecholamines are elevated in thermal injury and have been implicated as producing the decreased insulin to glucagon ratios that have been described.[56,61] Unfortunately, the mechanism is not this simple since β stimulation increases pancreatic insulin release while α stimulation inhibits it.[43] Glucagon is known to be ureagenic, but apparently it is not catabolic to muscle.[56] However, recent evidence indicates a potentially important role of glucagon in stimulating glucose production after burn injury.[63] Corticosteroids are elevated and are thought to have a permissive effect on other hormones as well as being anabolic to the liver and catabolic to

muscle.[16] Overall, one must be cautious in the interpretation of data based on blood concentrations of hormones, since this may not always reflect end-organ response. While a combination of these factors is at play here, it is likely that substrate interactions are as important as hormonal factors in orchestrating these alterations of metabolism.

While there are similarities in protein metabolism with various forms of infection and trauma, they are not identical. By using isotopic tracer technology, it has been possible to look at relative rates of whole-body protein synthesis and degradation in various pathologic conditions. It would appear

FIG. 16-4 Glucose–lactate (Cori cycle) and glucose–alanine cycle.

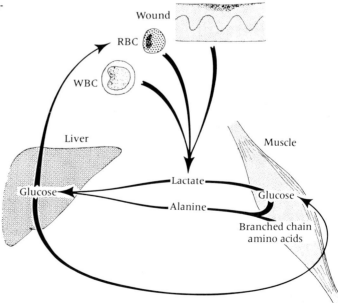

that immediately following elective surgery, net whole-body protein synthetic rates decrease while net catabolic rates remain constant.[33] However, similar studies performed in septic patients showed that both synthetic rates and catabolic rates increased, but the net result was one of catabolism. Examination of protein turnover in thermally injured children demonstrated that protein synthesis and catabolism are both elevated in burns much as described in sepsis (see Fig. 16-5). Furthermore, turnover rates were positively correlated with the percent body surface area burn, percent third degree burn, percent open wound, and the metabolic rate (see Fig. 16-6).[31,32] It should be emphasized, however, that the amount of elapsed time from injury until study period may influence the results of the study. It is likely that protein turnovers would be decreased immediately after thermal injury. Nonetheless, it is significant that in those pathologic conditions demonstrating the highest metabolic rates—sepsis and burns—both synthesis and catabolism are increased. Because protein synthesis requires energy expenditure for polypeptide bond formation, the high rates of protein synthesis may contribute to the elevation of metabolic rates.[32]

While the above studies examine whole-body protein turnover, they do not illuminate localization of the turnover. N[t]-methylhistidine, an amino acid found almost exclusively in muscle, is excreted in the urine unmetabolized and has proven to be a useful index of muscle catabolism. Uncomplicated trauma does not demonstrate increased N[t]-methylhistidine excretion, while major burns and infection do.[7] From the studies of Williamson, one

might suggest that the increased muscle catabolism in burns and infection might involve their inability to keto-adapt, although the evidence for this is not solid.[54] Such differences in the protein metabolism of burns compared to other forms of stress may prove to have important implications in nutritional management.

GLUCOSE METABOLISM

It has been demonstrated that increased gluconeogenesis is one of the fundamental alterations of metabolism in thermal injury as well as in other forms of trauma and sepsis.[45,66,68,69] While blood glucose concentrations may be elevated in burn patients, the magnitude of the gluconeogenesis is much greater than the observed hyperglycemia may account for.[68] Thus, it is logical to assume that not only must glucose production be elevated but there must also be a similar increase in cellular uptake. This has proven to be the case in both animal models and burned patients (see Fig. 16-7).[68,69] However, glucose clearance from the blood and uptake by the cells do not necessarily mean that there is increased glucose oxidation to CO_2 because the glucose skeleton may also be transaminated to amino acids, be used for glycogen and triglyceride synthesis, or cycled through lactate or alanine (see Fig. 16-4). Intravenous glucose tolerance tests have demonstrated this increased glucose turnover but give little insight into the ultimate fate of glucose carbons, and the results may be misleading.[65]

Labeled isotope studies of glucose metabolism have demonstrated in both animals and human

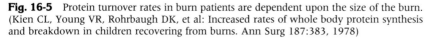

Fig. 16-5 Protein turnover rates in burn patients are dependent upon the size of the burn. (Kien CL, Young VR, Rohrbaugh DK, et al: Increased rates of whole body protein synthesis and breakdown in children recovering from burns. Ann Surg 187:383, 1978)

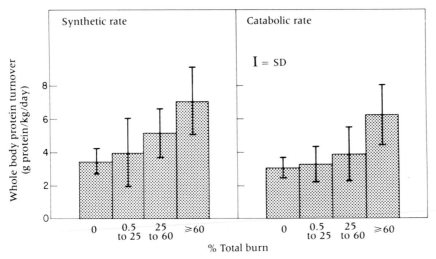

burn patients that despite the elevated glucose uptake, oxidation to CO_2 did not increase in a corresponding manner, and that there was a greater percentage of glucose carbons undergoing recycling (see Fig. 16-8).[66,68,69] Isotopically labeled lactate studies did not demonstrate increased lactate turnovers in minimally burned animals, although the turnover increased with exogenous glucose administration.[67] Indirect evidence of increased Cori-cycle activity has been produced from studies of lactate production in injured extremities. It has been observed that glucose uptake and lactate production are increased in extremities of animals with large surface wounds and in the burned extremities of humans.[58] These studies would suggest that at least one source of lactate production is in the burn wound itself. This is consistent with the proposed glycolytic activities of wound repairative cells in their anaerobic environment. However, the relative contribution of the burn wound to glucose cycling and gluconeogenesis is not known. Although glucose substrate cycling requires energy expenditure and generates heat, the possible contribution of this phenomenon to the hypermetabolism and thermogenesis of the burn patient probably is not great. As we will discuss later, these alterations of glucose metabolism have important implications regarding the limits of utilization of exogenously supplied carbohydrate.

It has been difficult to correlate any of the observed hormonal changes of thermal injury with the alterations in glucose metabolism.[68] In the past, corticosteroids were thought to play a key role in gluconeogenesis but are now thought to have pri-

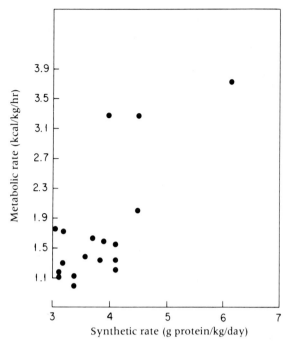

FIG. 16-6 Protein synthetic rates in burn patients correlate with metabolic rates. (Kien CL, Rohrbaugh DK, Burke JF, et al: Whole body protein synthesis in relation to basal energy expenditure in healthy children and in children recovering from burn injury. Pediatr Res 12:211, 1978)

FIG. 16-7 Basal production, disappearance, and clearance of glucose in 15 severely burned patients, as compared to mean ±2 SD from normal volunteers. (Wolfe RR, Durkot MJ, Allsop JR et al: Glucose metabolism in severely burned patients. Metabolism 28:1031, 1979. Reproduced by permission, Grune and Stratton)

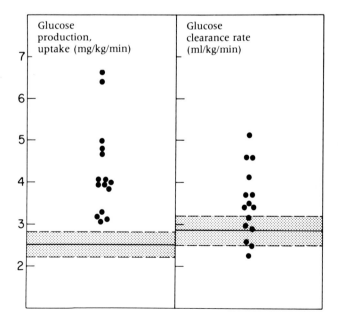

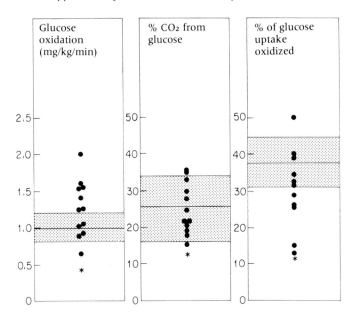

FIG. 16-8 Basal rate of glucose oxidation, the percent of CO_2 from glucose, and the percent of glucose uptake oxidized in human patients, as compared to mean ± 2 SD from normal volunteers. (Wolfe RR, Durkot MJ, Allsop JR et al: Glucose metabolism in severely burned patients. Metabolism 28:1031, 1979. Reproduced by permission, Grune and Stratton)

marily a permissive effect upon the actions of other hormones.[16] Catecholamines are observed to be elevated in burn patients, but the known glycolytic effects are not likely to play an important role in prolonged stress. Catecholamines are said to inhibit insulin release from the pancreas and stimulate glucagon release, but, as previously mentioned, this is an oversimplification. However, serum insulin levels have been demonstrated to be increased in burns as well as glucagon.[68] Unger has suggested that the insulin to glucagon ratio is the important factor in the control of glucose homeostasis.[52] The observed decreases in the insulin to glucagon ratio in thermal injury would favor gluconeogenesis. However, restoration of glucagon to insulin ratio in burned patients infused with somatostatin does not normalize glucose metabolism.[63]

The "insulin resistance" of stress has received much attention. Even in thermal injury there is a tendency toward elevation of blood glucose disproportionate to serum insulin.[68] Peripheral resistance to insulin in a burned animal model has been described.[50] In burn patients it would appear that there is a diminished responsiveness to the hypoglycemic effect of insulin because of decreased sensitivity both at the liver and peripherally.[68] It should not be concluded, however, that insulin is without effect in the burn patient. In fact, all expected responses to insulin seem to be elicited in the burn patient; insulin resistance refers to the fact that a greater concentration of insulin than normal is needed to elicit those responses.

LIPID METABOLISM

Unlike protein and carbohydrate metabolism, one is unable to discuss with any assurance the alterations in lipid metabolism in thermal injury. Dynamic studies are lacking, and many inferences must be made from other types of stress. It is generally agreed that serum free fatty acid and triglyceride levels tend to be elevated. These changes may be secondary to the elevated catecholamines and glucagon in the face of decreased peripheral insulin activity, resulting in increased mobilization of fat stores as described in other forms of trauma. Elevated triglyceride levels may also involve inhibition of lipoprotein lipase as demonstrated by the response to heparin. The increased availability of free fatty acids would have the adaptive advantage of providing fuel for synthetic processes in muscle and viscera and thus spare lean body mass. It has been suggested that fat is the major fuel source in burns as it is in some circumstances in normal man.[58]

Elevation of ketone bodies appears to be a normal response to trauma and may have a protein-sparing role by inhibiting muscle catabolism. However, it would appear that ketone bodies are not always elevated in burns. Furthermore, the onset of infection appears to inhibit ketogenesis such that the septic patient is likely to have more accelerated muscle wasting compared to other forms of stress if lacking in nutritional support.

Serum cholesterol levels are suggested to be decreased after burn injury coincident with a decrease in low-density β-lipoprotein.[8] Perhaps, this is indicative of an alteration in the release of lipoprotein from the liver.

In summary, the metabolic response to thermal injury may be conveniently divided into a hypometabolic *ebb* period and a hypermetabolic *flow* phase. Principles of critical-care medicine and fluid resuscitation are the keys to successful support during the relatively short ebb phase. The flow phase of thermal injury may last weeks and is the period relevant to nutritional support. The etiology of the hypermetabolism of this phase may include such factors as evaporative water loss, hypothalamic reset to a higher core temperature, and increased substrate turnover, as well as other mechanisms of thermogenesis. Protein metabolism is characterized by a peripheral to visceral redistribution as well as simultaneous increases in anabolism and catabolism. Alterations in glucose metabolism include increased gluconeogenesis and increased Cori-cycle activity. Relatively little is known about alterations in fat metabolism in burns, but serum levels of triglycerides and fats are elevated, and free fatty acids may be an important fuel source. Hormonal changes generally include elevated catecholamines as well as corticosteroids and decreased insulin to glucagon ratios. The term *insulin resistance* is often applied to the burn patient, but this should not be taken to mean an absolute resistance, nor should one assume that peripheral and visceral responses to insulin are necessarily of the same magnitude. Despite the abundant research on this topic, it is extremely difficult to correlate substrate alterations to changes of blood levels of specific hormones.

Nutritional Support of the Burn Patient

In the past, nutritional support in burn patients was limited by the post-traumatic fickleness of the GI tract. This often meant that the sickest patients could not be fed. With the advent of total parenteral nutrition, such hindrances were eliminated, and the clinician was then left to decide which of the burn patients are most likely to benefit from aggressive metabolic support. The NIH Consensus Development Conference in Supportive Therapy in Burn Care suggested that special emphasis be placed on those burn patients with (1) greater than 20% body surface area burn, (2) preinjury malnutrition, (3) complications such as sepsis or associated injury, and (4) those patients with a weight loss in excess of 10% of the premorbid weight.[40]

Timing is the next important factor in the nutritional support of the burn patient. Alimentation, if

Burn Patients Requiring Aggressive Nutritional Support
1. Greater than 20% body surface area
2. Individuals with preinjury malnutrition
3. Septic complications
4. Associated injury, including pulmonary
5. Threat of greater than 10% weight loss

needed, should begin immediately after cessation of the ebb phase of trauma, which is usually within 3 to 4 days of injury.[40] Earlier metabolic intervention is probably of no clinical advantage and would be complicated during the period of fluid resuscitation. However, it is imperative that nutritional support not be delayed unnecessarily so that the physician is not faced with the added difficulties of meeting the requirements of a burn patient with malnutrition. Having answered these questions, the clinician is ready to ask what nutrients to give the patient.

MEETING CALORIC REQUIREMENTS

The most direct and accurate approach to determination of energy requirements of the burn patient is to measure metabolic rate by means of indirect calorimetry. This maneuver has proven to be helpful in the management of both a variety of surgical patients as well as in thermal injury.[5] While ultimately this approach would hopefully gain greater acceptance, the required equipment is presently not widely available. As a result, multiple mathematical approaches to estimating caloric requirements have been devised. Recommendations of 32 Cal/kg/day (slightly above normal metabolic rate) to 100 Cal/kg/day (nearly four times basal metabolic rate) have been made.[73] Some of this apparent discrepancy is eliminated when one realizes that the weight of the patient is only one of the many variables determining the patient's metabolic rate. The ideal equation would include such additional factors as age, sex, percent body surface burn, percent open wound, presence of infection, ambulatory status, and presence of pain or psychic stress. Since such an approach would be extremely cumbersome, most formulas include only a few of the major variables.

Long (see Table 16-1) has suggested an approach based on an adaptation of the Harris–Benedict Equation and thus includes factors for age, sex, weight, and height. The activity factor allows one to adjust for the ambulatory status of the patient. However, based on our experience, the injury factor of 2 would seem to be somewhat larger

TABLE 16-1
Formulas for the Estimation of Caloric Requirements of Burn Patients

Source	Formula	Comments
Long*	Men: BMR = $(66.47 + 13.75W + 5\,H - 6.76A)$ $\times$ (activity factor) $\times$ (injury factor) Women: BMR = $(55 + 9.56W + 1.85H - 4.68A)$ Activity factor: Confined to bed 1.2 Out of bed 1.3 Injury factor Severe thermal burn 2.1 Skeletal trauma 1.35 Major sepsis 1.6 Minor operation 1.2	1. Based on Harris–Benedict equation and includes age, weight, height, and sex adjustments 2. Activity factor useful 3. Does not relate to size of burn 4. Injury factor large—likely overestimates requirements in smaller burns
Curreri†‡	Adults: Caloric intake = $(25 \times W) + (40 \times \%TBSB)$ Children: Caloric intake = $(B \times W) + (40 \times \%TBSB)$ B = 100 at 1 yr old, decreases to 25 at 15 yr old	1. Adjusts for age and weight 2. Does not adjust for sex 3. Includes factor for %TBSB
Wilmore§	Caloric intake = $2000 \times BSA$	1. Adjusts for height and weight 2. Does not adjust for %TBSB
Present Authors	Caloric intake = $2 \times BMR$	1. Adjusts for age, sex, height, and weight 2. Does not adjust for %TBSB 3. Likely to be excessive for smaller burns

Key: TBSB = total body surface burn; H = height in cm; W = weight in kg; A = age in years; BMR = basal metabolic rate; BSA = body surface area (m^2)

*Long CL: Energy expenditure of major burns. J Trauma 19:904, 1979

†Curreri PW: Nutritional replacement modalities. J Trauma 19:906, 1979

‡Curreri PW, Richmond D, Marvin J et al: Dietary requirements of patients with major burns. Research 65:415, 1974

§Wilmore DW: Nutrition and metabolism following thermal injury. Clin Plast Surg 1:603, 1974

TABLE 16-2
Basal Metabolic Rate—Children

Age, 1 wk–10 mo		Age, 11–38 mo			Age, 3–16 yr		
	Metabolic Rate (Cal/hr)		Metabolic Rate (Cal/hr)			Metabolic Rate (Cal/hr)	
Weight (kg)	♂ or ♀	Weight (kg)	♂	♀	Weight (kg)	♂	♀
3.5	8.4	9.0	22.0	21.2	15	35.8	33.3
4.0	9.5	9.5	22.8	22.0	20	39.7	37.4
4.5	10.5	10.0	23.6	22.8	25	43.6	41.5
5.0	11.6	10.5	24.4	23.6	30	47.5	45.5
5.5	12.7	11.0	25.2	24.4	35	51.3	49.6
6.0	13.8	11.5	26.0	25.2	40	55.2	53.7
6.5	14.9	12.0	26.8	26.0	45	59.1	57.8
7.0	16.0	12.5	27.6	26.9	50	63.0	61.9
7.5	17.1	13.0	28.4	27.7	55	66.9	66.0
8.0	18.2	13.5	29.2	28.5	60	70.8	70.0
8.5	19.3	14.0	30.0	29.3	65	74.7	74.0
9.0	20.4	14.5	30.8	30.1	70	78.6	78.1
9.5	21.4	15.0	31.6	30.9	75	82.5	82.2
10.0	22.5	15.5	32.4	31.7			
10.5	23.6	16.0	33.2	32.6			
11.0	24.7	16.5	34.0	33.4			

From Altman PL, Dittmer DS (eds): Metabolism. Bethesda, Federation of American Societies for Experimental Biology, 1968, p 344.

and would probably lead to caloric excess in smaller burns. This equation is also adaptable to other forms of trauma by adjusting the injury factor.

Curreri (see Table 16-1) recommends a formula based on a summation of proposed normal caloric requirements plus a factor for percent body surface burn.[40] This emphasis is based on the correlation of metabolic rate with the size of the burn (see Fig. 16-2). While correcting for the size of the burn wound may be helpful, this too has its limitations, since individual variability may obscure this association in any given patient. Adjustments are made for age and weight but not for sex. This formula has been demonstrated clinically to maintain body weight within 5% of admission weight.[49]

Wilmore has recommended an approach based simply on body surface area (BSA).[57] This method is shown in Table 16-1. Using the correct nomograms, one may readily adjust for height and weight. However, this formula does not adjust directly for the possible influence of the size of the burn wound.

Presently we are providing a caloric intake to our acutely ill patients at twice the basal energy expenditure as calculated by the Harris–Benedict Equation or as shown in Tables 16-2 and 16-3. This method has the advantage of adjusting for age, sex, height, and weight, although it does not adjust for the size of the burn. While grossly this method would seem to be excessive for smaller surface area burns, it should be recognized that these individuals will have a higher degree of physical activity than those with larger burns and thus will increase caloric requirements. This inverse correlation between physical activity and the percent BSA burn and percent open wound tends to equalize somewhat the caloric requirements. However, by the time the individual is convalescent from the acute trauma and once again ambulatory these rules no longer apply, and caloric requirements may more closely resemble premorbid values.

It should also be emphasized that providing calories at two times the calculated basal metabolic rate is not the same as providing calories at two times the measured metabolic rate. The measured oxygen consumption of these individuals is quite high but does not exceed twice the basal metabolic rate (see Fig. 16-1) and probably varies little throughout the day in most burn patients because they are always at bedrest and have little variation in their physical activity. Providing calories at twice the calculated basal metabolic rate ideally would be approximately equal to measured values of true metabolic rate. In our experience, twice the basal metabolic rate slightly exceeds metabolic needs of an acutely burned patient on bedrest.

The problem often arises in the burn patient in deciding upon the proper value to use for patient

TABLE 16-3
Basal Metabolic Rate—Adults

Age (yr)	Men	Women
	Metabolic Rate (Cal/m²/hr)	
17	41.9(36.1–47.7)	36.2(31.2–41.2)
18	40.5(34.9–46.1)	35.7(30.8–40.6)
19	40.1(34.6–45.6)	35.4(30.5–40.3)
20	39.8(34.3–45.3)	35.3(30.4–40.2)
21	39.4(34.0–44.8)	35.2(30.3–40.1)
22	39.2(33.8–44.6)	35.2(30.3–40.1)
23	39.0(33.6–44.4)	35.2(30.3–40.1)
24	38.7(33.4–44.0)	35.1(30.3–39.9)
25	38.4(33.1–43.7)	35.1(30.3–39.9)
26	38.2(32.9–43.5)	35.0(30.2–39.8)
27	38.0(32.8–43.2)	35.0(30.2–39.8)
28	37.8(32.6–43.0)	35.0(30.2–39.8)
29	37.7(32.5–42.9)	35.0(30.2–39.8)
30	37.6(32.4–42.8)	35.0(30.2–39.8)
31	37.4(32.2–42.6)	35.0(30.2–39.8)
32	37.2(32.1–42.3)	34.9(30.1–39.7)
33	37.1(32.0–42.2)	34.9(30.1–39.7)
34	37.0(31.9–42.1)	34.9(30.1–39.7)
35	36.9(31.8–42.0)	34.8(30.0–39.6)
36	36.8(31.7–41.9)	34.7(29.9–39.5)
37	36.7(31.6–41.8)	34.6(29.8–39.4)
38	36.7(31.6–41.8)	34.5(29.7–39.3)
39	36.6(31.5–41.7)	34.4(29.7–39.1)
40	36.5(31.5–41.5)	34.3(29.6–39.0)
45	36.3(31.3–41.3)	33.9(29.2–38.6)
50	36.0(31.0–40.0)	33.4(28.8–38.0)
55	35.4(30.5–40.3)	32.9(28.4–37.4)
60	34.8(30.0–39.6)	32.4(27.9–36.9)
65	34.0(29.3–38.7)	31.8(27.4–36.2)
70	33.1(28.5–37.7)	31.3(27.0–35.6)
75 +	31.8(27.4–36.2)	31.1(26.8–35.4)

From Altman PL, Dittmer DS (eds): Metabolism. Bethesda, Federation of American Societies for Experimental Biology, 1968, p 345.

weight when making these calculations. Measured weights may be deceiving owing to variable amounts of fluid retention as well as the presence of dressings and other supportive paraphernalia. Weight by history is also unreliable. To circumvent these problems we use the ideal body weight for these calculations as a closer representation of the lean body mass (LBM) than actual weight. In general, this will tend to minimize the number of calories provided. Furthermore, obese individuals will receive fewer calories than they would if calculations were based on measured weights. This should promote maximum utilization of adipose stores. Similarly, those individuals who were underweight prior to injury will receive more calories than they would based on measured weight. Thus, using ideal body weight in these calculations automatically adjusts to some degree for premorbid malnutrition. However, one must be able to individualize estimations,

TABLE 16-4
Autopsy Findings of Patients Treated with Very High Glucose Infusions

Patient	Sex	Age	Percent BSA Burned	Muscle Atrophy	Hypercal for 3 wk Before Death	Rate of IV Glucose (mg/kg/min)	Liver Weight at Autopsy (percent above normal)
1	M	11	80	0	yes	13.5	254
2	F	14	66	0	yes	14.8	246
3	F	10	86	0	yes	9.3	164
4	M	13	54	0	yes	10.8	309
5	F	16 mo	47	0	yes	17	291
6	M	10 mo	39	0	yes	17	324
7	M	3	85	0	yes	13.1	440
8	F	4	70	0	yes	14.3	331

From Burke JF, Wolfe RR, Mullany CF et al: Glucose requirements following burn injury. Ann Surg 190:274, 1979.

since the use of actual body weight would be more appropriate for muscular individuals with increased LBM.

Some evidence suggests that burn patients may actually do quite well receiving even fewer calories than recommended above. Examining the caloric intakes of four burned children, positive nitrogen balance could be obtained with caloric intakes similar to the RDA for normal children of the same age.[73] This emphasizes that some of the elevated caloric expenditure as a result of the trauma may be offset by the energy conserved by the inactivity of the critically ill patient.

CARBOHYDRATE REQUIREMENTS

Carbohydrate is an important part of any dietary regimen as a means to meet caloric requirements and spare nitrogen. However, it has recently been recognized that caloric excess may be associated with adverse consequences. Hepatic abnormalities manifested as changes in serum liver enzymes and serum bilirubin, cholestasis, and fatty metamorphosis have been associated with the use of parenteral nutrition for periods of one to three weeks.[9,36] While amino acid imbalances and essential fatty acid deficiencies may play a role in this pathology, infusion excess of both calories and carbohydrate have been implicated as etiologic agents. It is thought that constant glucose infusion leads to a chronic hyperinsulinemia that interferes with lipid mobilization both peripherally and in the liver. Postmortem examination of burn patients receiving caloric excess of carbohydrate has demonstrated significant fatty changes of the liver (see Table 16-4).[9] Cyclic hyperalimentation may be a method to avoid this problem; however, excess carbohydrate also presents a potential pulmonary stress in that high rates of glucose intake require a corresponding increase in elimination of CO_2. Patients with compromised pulmonary function may be further endangered.[9,46] Furthermore, overfeeding is known to increase metabolic rates in both normal and hypermetabolic humans, regardless of the route of administration. Figure 16-9 demonstrates that while glucose oxidation results in a respiratory quotient of 1, the use of excess carbohydrate to synthesize fat results in a dramatic increase

FIG. 16-9 (*A*) The complete oxidation of 1 mole of glucose produces an amount of CO_2 equivalent to oxygen consumed, yielding an RQ of 1. Energy is made available in this process in the form of ATP or reducing equivalents. (*B*) The synthesis of fatty acids from glucose yields more CO_2 than O_2 consumed, resulting in a potential RQ of 8.7. However, due to the combination of metabolic conversions of substrates, an RQ of 8.7 will not be attained *in vivo*. Unlike the oxidation of glucose that liberates energy for metabolic work, the synthesis of fatty acids requires energy input as ATP or reducing equivalents. (Further discussion of the biochemistry involved may be found in Wolfe RR, O'Donnell TF, Stone MD et al: Investigation of factors determining the optimal glucose infusion rate in total parenteral nutrition. Metabolism, in press.)

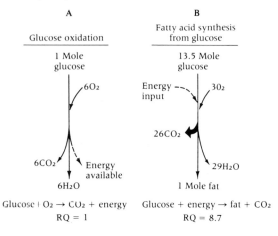

A

Glucose oxidation

1 Mole glucose

$6O_2$

$6CO_2$

Energy available

$6H_2O$

Glucose + O_2 → CO_2 + energy
RQ = 1

B

Fatty acid synthesis from glucose

13.5 Mole glucose

Energy input

$3O_2$

$26CO_2$

$29H_2O$

1 Mole fat

Glucose + energy → fat + CO_2
RQ = 8.7

in CO_2 production, elevating the respiratory quotient, as well as a concurrent loss of energy in the synthetic process. It is possible that the extremely high caloric intakes of 8,000 Cal/day to 10,000 Cal/day frequently administered to burn patients in the past may have contributed in part to the high measured metabolic rates.

While the minimal level of carbohydrate intake to spare protein was established by Gamble at approximately 100 g/day in fasting man, little information is available on the maximal beneficial intake for hypermetabolic man.[21] The mechanism of the favorable effects of administered carbohydrate to spare nitrogen are either through providing calories and thus minimizing amino acid breakdown as an energy source or through suppression of endogenous glucose production and thus decreasing the necessity of mobilization of amino acid as gluconeogenic precursors. Studies on the intravenous infusion of glucose in normal man and postoperative patients demonstrate maximal suppression of gluconeogenesis at rates of infusion of 4 mg/kg/min.[64,70] Further studies in postoperative patients demonstrated maximal glucose oxidation rates at infusion of glucose at 7 mg/kg/min. Infusion rates higher than this showed continued increase in glucose clearance but no significant increase in oxidation (see Fig. 16-10). This information, coupled with measured respiratory quotients greater than 1, suggests that the continued cellular glucose uptake was being used for fatty acid synthesis.

Similar studies in burn patients have demonstrated maximum glucose oxidation rates at infusions of approximately 5 mg/kg/min (see Fig. 16-11).[9] Infusion rates of 4.7 mg to 6.8 mg/kg/min supported maximal protein synthesis with no further benefit at higher infusion rates.

This data would suggest that there is an optimum rate of glucose infusion in the burn patient receiving adequate protein intake and that this rate appears to be approximately 5 mg/kg/min. Rates below this do not maximize protein sparing, and rates above this lead to excessive triglyceride synthesis that will be deposited in the liver, leading to hepatic dysfunction. In addition, the elevated respiratory quotient coincidentally produced (see Figs. 16-9 and 16-12) reflects the increased CO_2 production which will add an additional burden of pulmonary clearance. Whether these precise mechanisms are at play in enteral nutrition has not been documented by controlled studies. However, it would seem prudent to limit carbohydrate intake regardless of the route of administration.

Relevant to the issue of carbohydrate intake is the value of administration of exogenous insulin concurrent with large carbohydrate loads. Our studies in burn patients show no increase in oxi-

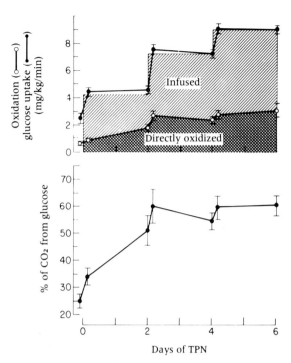

FIG. 16-10 Glucose infusion rates above 4 mg/kg/min demonstrate no increase in glucose oxidation in postoperative patients. (Wolfe RR, O'Donnell TF, Stone MD et al: Investigation of factors determining the optimal glucose infusion rate in total parenteral nutrition. Metabolism, in press. Reproduced by permission, Grune and Stratton)

dation of infused glucose with the addition of exogenous insulin.[9] It has also been suggested that in burns and other trauma insulin exerts a protein-sparing effect independent of its effects upon carbohydrate metabolism.[72] Indeed, insulin appears to have a direct anabolic effect on muscle *in vitro*. On the basis of this information, insulin may prove to be a helpful adjunct in some patients to minimize protein catabolism. However, if one administers insulin for the purpose of providing calories as carbohydrate in excess of needs, little will be accomplished except the synthesis of excess fat.

PROTEIN REQUIREMENTS

The exact protein requirement of the burn patient is still unknown. This is not surprising in light of the difficulty in determining this value in normal man.[74] Sutherland has reported that positive nitrogen balance can be attained in burned children at protein intakes similar to those of normal children of the same age.[49] However, there are multiple reasons to suspect that the nitrogen requirement of the burn patient is higher than normal.[73]

First, there are the obvious nitrogen losses through

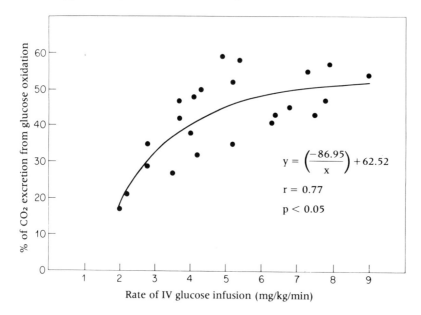

$$y = \left(\frac{-86.95}{x}\right) + 62.52$$

$$r = 0.77$$

$$p < 0.05$$

FIG. 16-11 Correlation between percent CO_2 production from glucose oxidation and rate of intravenous glucose infusion (mg/kg/min). (Burke JF, Wolfe RR, Mullany CJ et al: Glucose requirement following burn injury. Ann Surg 190:274, 1979)

wound transudate and exudate. Normal adults have estimated integument losses of less than 5 mg N/kg/day.[74] Maximally, this would account for less than 10% of total daily obligate nitrogen loss. Burn wound fluid may contain 4 g to 6 g of protein per 100 ml, and thus losses from the wound may account for as much as 25% to 50% of total daily nitrogen losses. However, wound contribution to nitrogen loss will be highly dependent upon size of the burn and the percent open wound (see Table 16-5), and thus protein requirements should diminish with convalescence.[32]

Secondly, both urea and nonurea urinary nitrogen losses are increased after burn trauma as part of the generalized alterations of protein metabolism. The extent of this contribution will depend upon the presence or absence of infection, the administration of exogenous calories to minimize use of protein as a caloric source and as a gluconeogenic substrate, the percent body surface burn, and the percent open wound.

The relationship of burn wound healing and protein requirement was investigated by Soroff.[48] Using linear regression analysis of nitrogen bal-

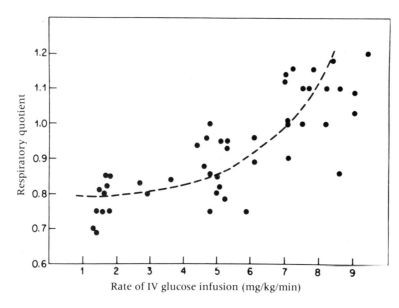

FIG. 16-12 Respiratory quotient as a function of glucose infusion rate. RQ increases rapidly in burn patients with infusion rates in excess of approximately 5 mg/kg/min. (Burke JF, Wolfe RR, Mullany CJ et al: Glucose requirements following burn injury. Ann Surg 190:274, 1979)

ance, nitrogen requirements were calculated according to four postburn time periods. While early requirements were nearly six times the recommended dietary allowances for healthy individuals, this diminished to normal levels upon healing of the wounds.

In a recent study we evaluated protein requirements of burned children using nitrogen balance methods.[73] Protein intakes of 3.2 g/kg/day–5.5 g/kg/day administered with adequate total caloric intake to provide a kilocalorie to nitrogen ratio of 110–180:1 allowed maintenance of a positive nitrogen balance.

Expressing the protein and energy requirements as a ratio (Cal:g nitrogen, or protein as percent of energy intake) is a useful concept to emphasize that the requirement for exogenous protein will increase if adequate caloric intake is not maintained, since protein itself will by necessity be used as an energy source. While caloric requirements will be met in this manner, the price that one pays is an increase in urea production. (This would be particularly troublesome in the patient with renal compromise.) Recommended Cal:N ratios for burn patients range from 75 to 200, indicating the lack of consensus.[40] Presently, we provide our patients with 2 g protein/kg/day to 3 g protein/kg/day with Cal:N ratio of approximately 100:1. However, one must not be led astray by providing macronutrients using only the Cal:N ratio as a guide. First, one must realize that all calories are not equal. One would not expect to get the same results in nitrogen balance by supplying the nonprotein calories as isocaloric amounts of only carbohydrate or only fat. As discussed in the next section, a minimum amount of carbohydrate should be supplied to all patients. Furthermore, multiple values of calories and nitrogen can yield the same Cal:N ratio. For example, a patient receiving 3400 Cal and 34 g of nitrogen would have the same Cal:N ratio as an individual receiving 340 Cal and 3.4 g of nitrogen. While the former regimen may be quite adequate for proper nutritional support, the latter regimen would be grossly inappropriate.

THE ROLE OF FAT

There are presently two major indications to supply fat as part of the dietary regimen of the burn patient. The most obvious is to supply calories and thus minimize the need for mobilization of endogenous proteins. Despite the evidence that free fatty acids may be used preferentially by muscle and liver as a fuel source in trauma including burns, there is controversy over whether isocaloric substitution of fat for carbohydrate yields the same nitrogen-sparing effect.[9] Some evidence suggests

TABLE 16-5
Estimates of Wound Nitrogen (N) Loss in Patients with Varying Burn Sizes

Patients Grouped by Burn size	Wound N Loss* (g N/kg/day)
PERCENT TOTAL BURN	
I (0–24%) (n=4)	0.01 ± 0.01
II (25–59%) (n=9)	0.04 ± 0.02
III (≥60%) (n=10)	0.09 ± 0.07
PERCENT OPEN WOUND	
I (≤10%) (n=8)	0.02 ± 0.02
II (11–30%) (n=6)	0.05 ± 0.02
III (≥31%) (n=6)	0.12 ± 0.06

*Results represent means ± SD (F-test $p<0.01$) from Kien CL, Young VR, Rohrbaugh DK et al: Ann Surg 187:383, 1978

that in normal humans carbohydrate has a unique action to maximize net protein synthesis not shared by fat (although this may be a time-dependent effect).[51] Similar results have been obtained in trauma patients including those with burns, although this has not been consistent.[29,36] Some of the apparent discrepancy stems from the fact that Intralipid, one of the readily available forms of intravenous fat emulsion, contains glycerol, which is a 3-carbon gluconeogenic precursor. While investigations have noted a nitrogen-sparing effect of Intralipid, that effect is not greater than that of equal amounts of glycerol alone when studied in normal man not receiving protein. Nonetheless, a limited number of studies in burn patients receiving constant protein intake and varied amounts of carbohydrate and fat demonstrate a superior nitrogen-sparing effect for carbohydrate.[36] While further research is required, at present it would appear that there is a minimum carbohydrate intake required to maximize nitrogen retention. Additional calories may be supplied as fat to meet the total caloric requirement. However, the relative benefit of isocaloric replacement of carbohydrate for fat beyond the minimum required for protein sparing is unknown.

The second indication for the administration of fat is to provide essential fatty acids. Due to the large adipose stores of adults, they are relatively immune to essential fatty acid (EFA) deficiency, and thus the first human cases were described in infants. However, in 1971, Collins presented an adult maintained on intravenous therapy without fat who developed both clinical and biochemical abnormalities of EFA deficiency.[12] Subsequently, biochemical changes of EFA deficiency have been demonstrated in trauma and burn patients.[25] It would appear that the requirement for producing adult EFA deficiency is a high-carbohydrate diet lacking in fat. The proposed mechanism is that high-carbohydrate diets lead to a chronic hyperinsulinemia inhibiting lipolysis and mobilization of EFA stores. Patients receiving enteral nutrition are less prone to develop a deficiency, because they are unlikely to be receiving a fat-restricted diet, even though they may be chronically hyperinsulinemic.

The precise EFA requirement in burn patients is unknown. Furthermore, clinically recognized (as opposed to biochemical) EFA deficiency has not been described in burns. However, in light of the diverse deleterious effects of EFA deficiency, such as alterations in wound repair and hepatic pathology including a fatty liver, it seems judicious to avoid this problem. Cyclic hyperalimentation may be one solution. By temporarily halting intravenous glucose infusions, insulin levels will drop, allowing mobilization of endogenous EFA from adipose stores. Alternately, it has been recommended to supply a minimum of 2% of the caloric intake as EFA in patients receiving total parenteral nutrition. Deficiency states in infants have also been corrected with cutaneous application of sunflower seed oil.

Presently, we include fats as part of nearly every patient's dietary regimen. Carbohydrates are administered at 5 mg/kg/min and proteins at 2 g/kg/day to 3 g/kg/day. The remaining calories are supplied as fat to meet the total calculated caloric requirement of the patient (see Table 16-1). This protocol appears to be useful in meeting macronutrient and caloric requirements of the patient while also avoiding excess carbohydrate or calories.

Enteral Alimentation

Enteral alimentation is always the preferred route of nutritional support in the burn patient over parenteral routes owing to the lower incidence of complications, lower cost and potentially superior utilization of nutrients, and visceral organ sparing.[26] Unfortunately, oral intake is often hampered by the anorexia of illness as well as facial burns that make mastication uncomfortable. Taste preferences are an additional problem, especially in children. Often these obstacles may be overcome by preparing foods meeting the gustatory needs of the patient, assisting the patient in eating, and providing nutrient-dense supplements. Nonetheless, it is frequently impossible to meet the high protein and calorie requirements of the burn patient through the oral route, and then tube feedings become a viable alternative.

Three types of tubes have commonly been employed in tube feedings. Polyvinyl chloride nasogastric tubes are mentioned only to discourage their use. The stiff plastic and large size are conducive to mechanical irritation of both pharyngeal and gastric mucosa. Gastric irritation is especially undesirable in patients prone to stress ulceration. The more recently available polyurethane and silastic feeding tubes are considerably more pliable and better tolerated by the patient. However, it must be emphasized that any tube used must readily allow aspiration to determine gastric residual volume during the course of feeding. This is an extremely important method for monitoring gastric emptying to minimize vomiting and pulmonary aspiration.

Tube feeding formulas are for four basic types. (1) *Chemically defined and elemental diets* probably have few indications in the nutritional support of burns. Burn patients typically have a normal gastrointestinal tract prior to injury and are capable of digesting complex macronutrients. In addition, elemental diets have a high osmolarity and are more expensive than equivalent products. Occasionally these products may be indicated to minimize bowel movements or in individuals with preburn gastrointestinal pathology. (2) *Meal replacement formulas* are the most commonly available. They are manufactured from a variety of complex carbohydrate, fat, and protein sources and usually have a caloric density of 1 Cal/ml and a relatively high carbohydrate content. More caloric dense products are available when fluid restriction is desirable. The advantage of meal replacement formulas is that they provide a balance of macronutrients, vitamins, and trace elements while still being palatable enough for use as an oral supplement. (3) *Modular formulas* are distinguished by using separate sources for carbohydrate, protein, and fat, which allows preparation of a diet specific for the patient's needs. The protein supplements may occasionally be useful to meet the high requirements of the burn patient. (4) *Blenderized and ''homemade'' diets* are a final alternative. Blenderized diets have the advantage of adding bulk to the diet as well as necessary micronutrients. Because of their high viscosity they may be cumbersome in tube feeding, but they are an excellent oral supplement. Various homemade diets may be constructed by the dietitian. One found particularly useful is described in Table 16-6. Polycose, a partially hydrolyzed starch, provides carbohydrates while not increasing osmolarity. As a result, it lacks the distressing gastrointestinal symptoms of hypertonic glucose. Egg supplies a protein source of low cost and high biologic value without evidence of deleterious effects in the burn patient.[30] Corn oil and safflower oil provide calories and are excellent sources of essential fatty acids. This mixture can be diluted with water to meet fluid requirements and with the possible addition of vitamins, potassium, and calcium can meet all

TABLE 16-6
Egg-rich Tube Feeding

Substrate	Rate of Administration	Source
Carbohydrate	5 mg/kg/min	Polycose powder
Protein	2 g–3 g/kg/day	Powdered egg
Fat	Remainder of calories	Corn oil or olive oil

the nutrient requirements of the burn patient at a lower cost than that of meal replacement formulas.

Three types of complications arise with tube feedings.[26] The most devastating of the mechanical problems is pulmonary aspiration. This complication may be minimized by employing constant infusion feedings with a mechanical pump. The head of the bed should be elevated 30°, and tubes should be checked for proper placement and gastric residuals at regular intervals. Gastrointestinal symptoms include regurgitation, diarrhea, and cramping pains. By using constant infusion feedings and less concentrated formulas these complications can be virtually eliminated. Diarrhea may also be controlled with a variety of constipating agents. Metabolic complications of tube feedings are similar to those of total parenteral nutrition (TPN) and include hyperglycemia, fluid overload, and electrolyte imbalances, as well as excessive CO_2 production secondary to the high carbohydrate content. Hyperglycemia and hyperosmolar coma are more apt to occur with more caloric dense formulas of 1.5 to 2 calories/ml. Fluid and electrolyte imbalances can be avoided with proper monitoring.

Using the guidelines provided above, enteral alimentation provides an effective means of meeting the nutrient requirements of many burn patients.

TOTAL PARENTERAL NUTRITION

While enteral alimentation is the preferred route to provide nutrients to the burn patient, there are definite indications for parenteral support, and nearly all of the more extensively burned patients will require this therapy at some time during their hospital stay. Adynamic ileus is one of the most frequent complications of thermal injury necessitating nutrition by parenteral routes. The ileus may result from a prolonged response to the original injury or may be secondary to a septic complication. Furthermore, patients requiring frequent escharectomy and skin grafting will suffer from multiple brief episodes of loss of intestinal motility that will have the additive effect of a prolonged ileus. A second indication for parenteral nutrition is as an adjunct to enteral support in the patient who is

unable to meet his total nutrient requirement through this route. Various types of gastrointestinal pathology, both preburn and postburn, are indications for total parenteral nutrition (TPN). Relevant to this is some evidence that suggests that stress ulcers may be minimized by adequate nutritional support.

Indications for TPN in Treatment of Burns
1. Adynamic ileus
   a. Post-trauma
   b. Postsurgery
   c. Sepsis
2. Unable to meet nutrient requirements by other routes
3. Postburn gastrointestinal pathology
   a. Curling's ulcer
   b. Other
4. Preburn gastrointestinal pathology

A variety of parenteral solutions is now available to supply the complete nutrient requirements of patients. The preparation and composition of these solutions have been extensively reviewed and need not be discussed here.[20] In order to meet the great protein and energy requirements of the burn patient without exceeding fluid balance, one must frequently employ the more concentrated amino acid and glucose solutions (see Chap. 13).

The complications associated with application of TPN generally fall into the categories of technical, metabolic, and septic.[20] Technical complications are those associated with catheter placement and include pneumothorax, hemothorax, thrombosis, and embolus. Metabolic complications include hyperglycemia, amino acid imbalances, hyperchloremic metabolic acidosis, and micronutrient excesses and deficiencies, as well as excess CO_2 production. Hyperglycemic complications and excess CO_2 production are likely to be minimized following the guidelines for glucose administration described above. By employing proper surveillance methods, metabolic complications may be minimized. In general, the incidence of metabolic and technical complications is similar to that of other patient populations. The etiology and methods of avoiding these complications have been reviewed.[20]

The infectious complications of TPN are of major importance in the burn patient. Catheter-related sepsis in general patient populations receiving TPN has an overall incidence of roughly 7%. However, in one study of 26 burned children receiving parenteral alimentation, 14 out of 19 episodes of recorded sepsis seemed to be related directly to central venous catheters.[42] The most frequent organism cultured from the blood was *S. aureus* followed by *P. aeruginosa* and *Candida* species. No infectious complications were associated with placement of catheters through unburned skin, while 50% of subclavian catheterizations through burn wounds had septic complications. Five patients in this series developed fatal septic thrombophlebitis and associated septic cardiac lesions. Wilmore noted that 23 of 26 burn patients on TPN had septic episodes, but the relationship to use of central venous catheters was not determined.[60] Dergane noted that sepsis was also a major problem in their patients and that the same organism was usually cultured simultaneously from blood, catheter tip, and burned tissue, making it difficult to demonstrate that the septic episode was due to the catheter alone.[17] However, resolution of clinical sepsis upon removal of the hyperalimentation catheter, with positive cultures of blood and catheter tip when no other septic locus can be identified, suggests catheter-related sepsis.

Multiple reasons for catheter sepsis have been suggested, including decreased host immunocompetence and the ability of infecting organisms to grow in the alimentation solutions. However, the most important cause is likely to be the growth of organisms along the cutaneous vascular prosthesis.[20] Hence, the burn patient is prone to cathether sepsis on two accounts—he is immunocompromised and the wound provides a ready source of infecting organisms. It is not surprising, therefore, that placement of catheters through burn wounds is associated with a higher infection rate. Unfortunately, in the extensively burned patient one may not have the luxury of a site for central venous catheterization that is not burned.

Candida sepsis is a particularly worrisome complication of the use of TPN. Mortality rates of disseminated candidiasis as high as 72% have been reported. MacMillan noted that over 50% of a series of 427 burn patients had culture-proven *Candida* infections at some time during their hospitalization.[39] Of 65 deaths, 14 had disseminated candidiasis on autopsy. Of 14 episodes of catheter-related septic episodes in burned children, 8 were associated with *Candida* organisms.[42] Limitation of the use of systemic antibiotics is useful in minimizing overgrowth of this opportunistic organism. Since the two major portals of entry are through intravenous catheters and the gastrointestinal tract, prophylactic therapy would be aimed at decreasing the number of organisms at these sites. Proper catheter care has been described.[20] Breaks in protocol are definitely associated with an increased incidence of infectious complications. The technique of *amphotericin flush* has been recommended specifically as a means to combat *Candida* catheter sepsis. At present, we administer oral nystatin to suppress the growth of gastrointestinal *Candida*. We also employ nystatin bladder irrigations for those patients on long-term broad-spectrum antibiotics. A multiple oral antibiotic regimen has demonstrated slowing of burn wound colonization.[28]

The onset of clinical signs of sepsis in a patient receiving parenteral alimentation requires thorough examination for a focus of infection. If no focus is found, the catheter must be removed, followed by culturing blood, catheter tip, and infusion solution. Peripheral hypotonic solutions may be administered for 24 hr, and then TPN may resume at another central venous catheter site. Usually septic symptoms resolve spontaneously, but if an anatomic site of catheter seeding is present, appropriate antibiotics may be instituted. Amphotericin B is currently the treatment of choice for systemic candidiasis.

PERIPHERAL ALIMENTATION

Peripheral intravenous alimentation may occasionally prove to be advantageous in the burn patient. While it is difficult to deliver all of the required nutrients by this route, it may be a useful method to supplement enteral alimentation to reach total nutrient requirements.

Two types of isotonic solution are available for peripheral administration. Three percent amino acid solutions have been demonstrated to be valuable for a variety of patients to maintain positive nitrogen balance.[20] Intravenous lipid emulsions provide calories and EFA.

Much as in the use of central venous catheters, care must be taken to avoid septic complications with the administration of solutions through peripheral veins.

MICRONUTRIENTS

Knowledge of the requirements of micronutrients in burns is still embryonic, and thus administration of these nutrients is often on an entirely empirical basis. While this is not the forum for a complete treatise on micronutrients, a few comments on the vitamin and mineral requirements of burn patients will be made.

VITAMINS

Among the water-soluble vitamins, the role of vitamin C in collagen synthesis makes it particularly interesting to surgeons. Lund noted abnormalities of ascorbic acid metabolism in severe burn patients that seemed to parallel alterations in nitrogen metabolism and suggested that burn patients receive 1 g to 2 g of ascorbic acid daily.[38] Others have demonstrated an eightfold increase in wound dehiscence in ascorbate-deficient patients and recommended daily administration of 100 mg to 300 mg of vitamin C to postoperative patients. Ascorbate levels in leukocytes and urine are decreased in postoperative patients in a manner suggesting a requirement that is related to the magnitude of the trauma, yet precise requirements in the burn patient are unknown. Furthermore, there is no evidence to prove that extremely large doses are advantageous. While most physicians administer ascorbate in excess of normal requirements, prudence would suggest moderation to prevent potential side-effects.

Owing to the relationship of folate to nucleic acid metabolism and protein synthesis, there is often an increased requirement in the individual undergoing growth and tissue repair. Measuring blood levels of folate and using a functional test of folate adequacy, Barlow has presented evidence to suggest increased folate requirements in burned children.[3] Similar recommendations have been made in a variety of surgical and postoperative patients. While B_{12} is intimately related to folate metabolism, deficiency is unlikely owing to the large body stores.

Nicotinic acid, biotin, pyridoxine, and thiamin metabolism have also been demonstrated to be altered in thermal injury.[2,4,38] Thiamin requirements may be increased by the high caloric and carbohydrate intake of burn patients.

Vitamin K is likely to be deficient only in the burn patient receiving antibiotics that suppress normal gastrointestinal flora. The need to administer vitamin K may be assessed by routinely monitoring coagulation studies.

Vitamin A has recently been implicated as having a protective effect against stress ulceration. An association has been made between hypovitaminosis A and stress ulceration in burn patients.[44]

Vitamin E is an important antioxidant and its requirement is at least in part dependent upon polyunsaturated fat intake. While the use of fat emulsions for a major portion of caloric intake may increase the requirement for this nutrient, there are no indications for vitamin E megadose therapy in burns.

TRACE ELEMENTS

The role of trace elements in nutrition is the subject of many recent investigations. Zinc has received much attention, particularly its proposed importance in wound repair. Certain lines of evidence would suggest that zinc requirements are increased after thermal injury. Since 20% of the body store of zinc is located in the skin, significant loss of skin would be associated with an important loss of total body zinc.[47] Furthermore, urinary losses of zinc increase after thermal injury, and there is a functional redistribution of zinc with inflammation.[6,47] In addition, zinc requirements are increased during periods of increased cell turnover and growth, and both blood and hair levels have been shown to decrease after thermal injury.[34,47] While administration of zinc in pharmacologic doses has been suggested to improve wound repair, the evidence is not conclusive. Adequate zinc replacement is necessary in burns, but large doses do not seem indicated on the basis of present evidence.

Magnesium deficiency has been reported in burn patients and is attributed to increased losses from wounds and urine.[18] One should be certain that the burn patient receives adequate magnesium supplementation, especially when receiving TPN.

Ultimately, the need for providing exogenous vitamins and trace elements is dependent upon the route of alimentation. On an enteral diet, the patient will receive a major portion, if not all, of the requirements for vitamins and trace minerals. An exception may be the patient receiving an elemental diet. Nonetheless, most physicians empirically order an additional multiple vitamin preparation and additional ascorbic acid for the burn patient, although there is little scientific basis for this. The patient receiving nutrition entirely through TPN must receive exogenous vitamins and minerals. Deficiencies of zinc, copper, chromium, and selenium have been documented in patients receiving parenteral nutrition.[18,47] However, time of onset may be weeks to months. General recommendations for micronutrient supplementation with TPN have been made (see Chap. 13).[37,53]

Nutritional Assessment

As discussed above, there are many inaccuracies in our estimations of nutrient requirements of the burn patient. As a result, one must have a method to monitor the efficacy of the therapeutic regimen employed. However, this is difficult with burn patients. For example, anthropomorphic measurements such as triceps skin fold and arm circumference are invalid in burn patients owing to the variable edema as well as the obvious inapplicability to burned extremities. Weight measurements are subject to many variables on a day-to-day basis, including fluid balance, dressing changes, and supportive paraphernalia. Major excisions of skin and subcutaneous fat will further invalidate weight measurements. However, general trends in the weight of the patient will be helpful to assess the

Nutritional Assessment Sheet

Name _____ Age _____ Sex _____

% Body surface area burn_____

| Actual admission weight (kg) _____ | Ideal body weight _____ | Weight by history _____ |

Height (cm) _____ Basal metabolic rate (from tables) _____

Surface area (M²) _____ Estimated caloric requirement _____

24-Hour intake—Week of_____

	Clinical Ideal	Mon	Tues	Wed	Thur	Fri	Sat	Sun
Body weight								
% Weight loss								
% Open wound								
Caloric intake								
Carbohydrate intake mg/kg/min/total								
Carbohydrate calories								
Protein intake gm/kg/day/total								
Protein calories								
Fat intake gm/kg/day/total								
Fat calories								
Nitrogen balance								
Nitrogen intake								
Nitrogen excretion								
Balance								

FIG. 16-13 Nutritional flow sheet is used as an aid in assessing the efficacy of nutritional support in burn patients.

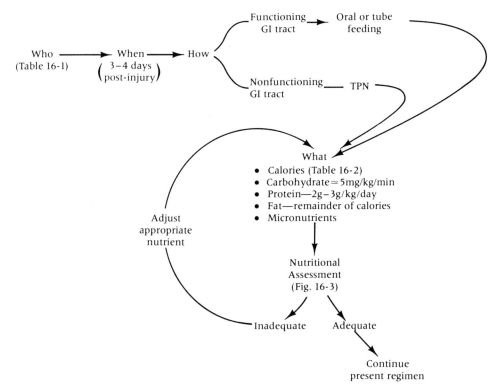

FIG. 16-14 Flow chart for nutritional support in burns.

efficacy of the nutritional support if efforts are made to account for misleading variables. Measurements of serum albumin and transferrin have been used as an estimate of visceral protein status. It would be extremely difficult to apply these parameters to the burn patient receiving blood and albumin infusions. However, nitrogen balance is a widely available and valid metabolic study for assessment of protein status. Appropriate adjustments must be made in the burn patient for wound nitrogen loss (Table 16-5). Erythrocyte intracellular sodium has been reported as an objective measurement of the effectiveness of nutritional support in burn patients. However, this has not gained wide acceptance. The preliminary report of Hiebert and co-workers on the value of delayed hypersensitivity testing to predict mortality in burn patients suggests that this may be a useful tool for nutritional assessment.[27] Further studies are required on the relationship of this parameter to metabolic support in the thermally injured.

Careful recording of the patient's daily dietary intake is important to determine if the patient is really receiving the planned nutritional support. Figure 16-13 displays the method we find useful for daily assessment of dietary intake. With the help of the dietitian, the physician can rapidly deter-

mine if the patient is receiving an appropriate amount of carbohydrate, fat, and protein, as well as adequate total caloric intake. While not necessarily reflective of metabolic status, such measures are a helpful adjunct to avoid iatrogenic malnutrition.

Summary

This chapter has reviewed the metabolic alterations of thermal injury and the nutritional support modalities that currently appear to benefit patient response. Enteral routes are preferred, but parenteral nutrition is often mandatory in these critically ill patients. Further research is needed to elaborate the exact requirements for all nutrients in the burn patient. Present evidence suggests that requirements are increased, but the physician should avoid nutritional excess because even the most innocuous of nutrients may have harmful side-effects when supplied in quantities beyond needs.

The general steps in the nutritional support of the burn patient are outlined in Figure 16-14. Identifying those patients requiring the greatest attention is the first step in nutritional therapy. Timing is also important, and the physician must know *when* to start alimentation. Nutritional support of the burn patient should begin immediately after the period of fluid resuscitation. It is of paramount importance to institute aggressive nutritional therapy as soon as possible in order to avoid significant malnutrition. Usually within 3 to 4 days postinjury the patient is beyond the shock period of fluid resuscitation, and nutritional support may begin. *How* to supply nutrients is a question of route of administration and is dependent on the clinical condition of the patient. Enteral alimentation is always the preferred route when possible.

What to give the patient is still a difficult question to answer, and one that must be tempered by information gained by nutritional assessment. Our present recommended approach is to supply calories at twice the calculated basal metabolic rate based on ideal body weight and the Harris–Benedict Equation. Protein is supplied at roughly 2 g/kg/day to 3 g/kg/day and carbohydrate at less than 5 mg/kg/min. Fats are provided to meet the deficit of calories. However, at least 1% to 2% of the calories should be supplied as EFA. In this manner, one should minimize both nutrient excess and deficiency. However, the discerning reader will recognize that such recommendations are subject to reappraisal based on further research on the metabolism and nutrient requirements of the burn patient.

References

1. Artz CP, Moncrief JA, Pruitt BA (eds): Burns, A Team Approach. Philadelphia, WB Saunders, 1979
2. Barlow GB, Dickerson JA, Wilkinson AW: Plasma biotin levels in children with burns and scalds. J Clin Pathol 29:58, 1976
3. Barlow GB, Wilkinson AW: 4-amino-imidazole-5-carboxamide excretion and folate status with burns and scalds. Clin Chim Acta 29:355, 1970
4. Barlow GB, Wilkinson AW: Plasma pyridoxal phosphate levels and tryptophan metabolism in children with burns and scalds. Clin Chim Acta 64:79, 1975
5. Bartlett RH, Allyn PA, Medley T et al: Nutritional therapy based on positive caloric balance in burn patients. Arch Surg 112:974, 1977
6. Beisel WR: Interrelated changes in host metabolism during generalized infectious illness. Am J Clin Nutr 25:1254, 1972
7. Bilmazes C, Kien CL, Rohrbaugh DK et al: Quantitative contribution by skeletal muscle to elevated rates of whole-body protein breakdown in burned children as measured by N+-methylhistidine output. Metabolism 27:671, 1978
8. Birke G, Carlson LA, von Euler VS et al: Lipid metabolism, catecholamine excretion, basal metabolic rate, and water loss during treatment of burns with warm dry air. Acta Chir Scand 138:321, 1972
9. Burke JF, Wolfe RR, Mullany CJ et al: Glucose requirements following burn injury. Ann Surg 190:274, 1979
10. Chandra RK, Newberne PM: Nutrition, Immunity and Infection. New York, Plenum Press, 1977
11. Clowes CHA, O'Donnell TF, Blackburn GL et al: Energy metabolism and proteolysis in traumatized and septic man. Surg Clin North Am 56:1169, 1976
12. Collins FD, Sinclair AJ, Royle JP et al: Plasma lipids in human linoleic acid deficiency. Nutrition and Metabolism 13:150, 1971
13. Curreri PW, Richmond D, Marvin J et al: Dietary requirements of patients with major burns. Research 65:415, 1974
14. Cuthbertson DP: The disturbance of metabolism produced by bony and non-bony injury, with notes on certain abnormal conditions of bone. Biochem J 24:1244, 1930
15. Cuthbertson DP: Observations on the disturbance of metabolism produced by injury to the limbs. Q J Med 1:233, 1932
16. Cuthbertson DP: Physical injury and its effects on protein metabolism. In Munro HN, Allison JB (eds): Mammalian protein metabolism, Vol 2, pp 373–414. New York, Academic Press, 1969
17. Dergane M: Parenteral nutrition in severely burned children. Scand J Plast Reconstr Surg 13:195, 1979
18. Domres R, Heller W, Koslowski L et al: Serum levels of magnesium and zinc after a controlled thermal trauma of the rat. Langenbecks Arch Chir 343:107, 1977
19. Felic P: The glucose–alanine cycle. Metabolism 22:179, 1973
20. Fischer JE (ed): Total Parenteral Nutrition. Boston, Little, Brown & Co, 1976
21. Gamble JL: Chemical Anatomy, Physiology and Pathology of Extracellular Fluid. Cambridge, Harvard University Press, 1954
22. Goodenough R, Burke JF: Burns. In Tinker J, Rapin M (eds): Care of the Critically Ill Patient. New York, Springer–Verlag, *in press*
23. Gump FE, Kinney JM: Caloric and fluid losses through the burn wound. Surg Clin North Am 50:1235, 1970
24. Gump FE, Kinney JM: Energy balance and weight loss in burned patients. Arch Surg 103:442, 1971
25. Helmkamp GM, Wilmore DW, Johnson AA et al: Essential fatty acid deficiency in red cells after thermal injury: Correction with intravenous fat therapy. Am J Clin Nutr 26:1331, 1973
26. Heymsfield SB, Bethel RA, Ansley JD et al: Enteral hyperalimentation: An alternative to central venous feeding. Ann Intern Med 90:63, 1979
27. Hiebert JM, McGough M, Rodeheaver G et al: The influence of catabolism on immunocompetence in burned patients. Surgery 86:242, 1979
28. Jarrett F, Balish E, Moylan JA et al: Clinical experience with prophylactic antibiotic bowel suppression in burn patients. Surgery 83:523, 1977
29. Jeejeebhoy KN, Marliss EB, Anderson GH et al: Lipid in parenteral nutrition: Studies of clinical and metabolic features. Symposium: Fat emulsions in parenteral nutrition. Chicago, American Medical Association, 1975
30. Kaufman T, Brook GJ, Hirshowitz B et al: Effect of an egg-rich diet on plasma lipids and proteins in severely burned patients. Isr J Med Sci 14:736, 1978
31. Kien CL, Rohrbaugh DK, Burke JF et al: Whole body protein synthesis in relation to basal energy expenditure in healthy children and in children recovering from burn injury. Pediatr Res 12:211, 1978
32. Kien CL, Young VR, Rohrbaugh DK et al: Increased rates of whole body protein synthesis and breakdown in children recovering from burns. Ann Surg 187:383, 1978
33. Kien CL, Young VR, Rohrbaugh DK et al: Whole body

protein synthesis and breakdown rates in children before and after reconstructive surgery of the skin. Metabolism 27:27, 1978

34. Larson DL, Maxwell R, Abston S et al: Zinc deficiency in burned children. Plast Reconstr Surg 46:13, 1970
35. Long CL: Energy balance and carbohydrate metabolism in infection and sepsis. Am J Clin Nutr 30:1301, 1977
36. Long JM, Wilmore DW, Mason AD et al: Effect of carbohydrate and fat intake on nitrogen excretion during total intravenous feeding. Ann Surg 185:417, 1977
37. Lowry SF, Goodgame JT, Smith CJ et al: Abnormalities of zinc and copper during total parenteral nutrition. Am Surg 189:120, 1979
38. Lund CC, Levenson SM, Green RW: Ascorbic acid, thiamine, riboflavin and nicotinic acid in relation to acute burns in man. Arch Surg 55:557, 1947
39. MacMillan BG, Law EJ, Holder IA: Experience with *Candida* infections in the burn patient. Arch Surg 104:509, 1972
40. N.I.H. Consensus Development Conference in Supportive Therapy in Burn Care. J Trauma 19:855, 1979
41. Neely WA, Petro AB, Holloman GH et al: Researches on the cause of burn hypermetabolism. Ann Surg 179:291, 1974
42. Popp MB, Law EJ, MacMillan BG: Parenteral nutrition in the burned child. A study of twenty-six patients. Ann Surg 179:219, 1974
43. Porte D: β-adrenergic stimulation of insulin release in man. Diabetes 16:150, 1967
44. Rai K, Courtemanche AD: Vitamin A assay in burned patients. J Trauma 15:419, 1975
45. Ryan NT: Metabolic adaptations for energy production during trauma and sepsis. Surg Clin North Am 56:1073, 1976
46. Sheldon GF, Petersen SR, Sanders R: Hepatic dysfunction during hyperalimentation. Arch Surg 113:504, 1978
47. Solomons NW: Zinc and copper in human nutrition. In Karcioglu Z, Sarper R (eds): Zinc and Cooper in Medicine. Springfield, Ill, Charles C Thomas, 1980
48. Soroff HS, Pearson E, Artz CP: An estimation of the nitrogen requirements for equilibrium in burned patients. Surg Gynecol Obstet 112:159, 1961
49. Sutherland AB, Batchelor ADR: Nitrogen balance in burned children. Ann NY Acad Sci 150:700, 1968
50. Thomas R, Aikawa N, Burke JF: Insulin resistance in peripheral tissues after a burn injury. Surgery 86:742, 1979
51. Thomson WST, Munro HN: The relationship of carbohydrate metabolism to protein metabolism. J Nutr 56:139, 1955
52. Unger RH: Glucagon and the insulin: glucagon ratio in diabetes and other catabolic illnesses. Diabetes 20:834, 1971
53. vanRij AM, Godfrey PJ, McKenzie JM: Amino acid infusions and urinary zinc excretion. J Surg Res 26:293, 1979
54. Williamson DH, Farrell R, Kerr A et al: Muscle–protein catabolism after injury in man, as measured by urinary excretion of 3-methylhistidine. Clin Sci Mol Med 52:527, 1977
55. Wilmore DW, Kinney, JM: Panel report on nutritional support of patients with trauma or infection. Am J Clin Nutr, 34:1213, 1981
56. Wilmore DW: Hormonal responses and their effect on metabolism. Surg Clin North Am 56:999, 1976
57. Wilmore DW: Nutrition and metabolism following thermal injury. Clin Plast Surg 1:603, 1974
58. Wilmore DW, Aulick LH, Mason AD et al: Influence of the burn wound on local and systemic responses to injury. Ann Surg 188:444, 1977
59. Wilmore DW, Aulick LH, Pruitt BA Jr: Metabolism during the hypermetabolic phase of thermal injury. Adv Surg 12:193, 1978
60. Wilmore DW, Curreri PW, Spitzer KW et al: Supranormal dietary intake in thermally injured hypermetabolic patients. Surg Gynecol Obstet 132:881, 1971
61. Wilmore DW, Long JC, Mason AD et al: Catecholamines: Mediator of the hypermetabolic response to thermal injury. Ann Surg 180:653, 1974
62. Wilmore DW, Mason AD, Johnson DW et al: Effect of ambient temperature on heat production and heat loss in burn patients. J Appl Physiol 38:593, 1975
63. Wolfe RR, Durkot MJ, Burke JF: Effect of somatostatin infusion in severely burned patients. Presented at American Burn Association, San Antonio, Texas, 1980
64. Wolfe RR, Allsop JR, Burke JF: Glucose metabolism in man: Responses to intravenous glucose infusion. Metabolism 28:210, 1979
65. Wolfe RR, Allsop JR, Burke JF: Fallibility of the intravenous glucose tolerance test as a measure of endogenous glucose turnover. Metabolism 27:217, 1978
66. Wolfe RR, Burke JF: Effect of burn trauma on glucose turnover, oxidation and recycling in guinea pigs. Am J Physiol 233:E80, 1977
67. Wolfe RR, Burke JF: Effect of glucose infusion on glucose and lactate metabolism in normal and burned guinea pigs. J Trauma 18:800, 1978
68. Wolfe RR, Durkot MJ, Allsop JR et al: Glucose metabolism in severely burned patients. Metabolism 28:1031, 1979
69. Wolfe RR, Miller HI, Elahi D et al: Effect of burn injury on glucose turnover in guinea pigs. Surg Gynecol Obstet 144:359, 1977
70. Wolfe RR, O'Donnell TF, Stone MD et al: Investigation of factors determining the optimal glucose infusion rate in total parenteral nutrition. Metabolism, *in press*
71. Wolfe RR, Spitzer JJ, Miller HI et al: Effects of insulin infusion on glucose kinetics in normal and burned guinea pigs. Life Sci 19:147, 1976
72. Woolfson AM, Heatley RV, Allison SP: Insulin to inhibit protein catabolism after injury. N Engl J Med 300:14, 1979
73. Young VR, Motin KJ, Burke JF: Energy and protein metabolism in relation to requirements in the burned pediatric patient. In Suskind RM (ed): Pediatric Nutrition. New York, Raven Press, *in press*
74. Young VR, Scrimshaw NS: Nutritional evaluation of proteins and protein requirements. In Milner M, Scrimshaw NS, Wang DIC (eds): Protein Resources and Technology, pp 23–43. Westport, Conn, AVI Publishing Corp, 1976
75. Zawacki BF, Spitzer KW, Mason AD et al: Does increased evaporative water loss cause hypermetabolism in burned patients? Ann Surg 171:236, 1970

The authors wish to thank Lois Burgess, Stacey Bell, R.D., and Nancy Kurz, R.N., for their respective contributions in the preparation of this manuscript.

17
Cardiovascular Disease
Scott M. Grundy

There are few issues of greater importance in the field of medicine than the "diet–heart question." Despite a significant drop in cardiovascular mortality in recent years in the United States, heart disease remains the foremost cause of death in the United States and in several other countries throughout the world. Indeed, outside the United States, deaths from heart disease seem to be on the rise. Since mortality from heart disease is greatest in affluent societies, many have suggested that disorders of the heart are related to life-style or environmental factors. The factor most often implicated is diet, but others—smoking, sedentary habits, and stress—also may be involved. A fundamental question is whether an alteration of eating habits will reduce the high incidence of heart disease in affluent societies. The major focus of this chapter, therefore, will be on the role of diet in prevention of heart disease. However, the diet in therapy of different categories of established cardiovascular disease also will be discussed.

Atherosclerotic Cardiovascular Disease

The most common forms of cardiovascular disease are those due to narrowing of the arterial supply to vital organs. This narrowing is usually the consequence of a particular form of arterial disease called *atherosclerosis*. Atherosclerotic involvement of the coronary arteries causes ischemic heart disease—either angina pectoris or myocardial infarction. Atherosclerosis of carotid or cerebral arteries

is responsible for transient cerebral ischemia or stroke. Finally, the blood supply to the lower limbs, kidneys, or bowel can be compromised by atherosclerotic narrowing.

Ischemic heart disease secondary to atherosclerosis is responsible for approximately one third of all deaths in the United States. Beyond age 65, deaths due to cardiac ischemia are twice as common as those caused by cancer.[3] To these statistics must be added a substantial mortality from atherosclerotic cerebrovascular disease. Thus, an understanding of the pathogenesis of atherosclerosis must be considered one of the foremost problems of medical research. The most abundant component of the atherosclerotic plaque is cholesterol, and the early finding that feeding of cholesterol to several species of experimental animals induced arterial accumulation of cholesterol gave rise to the hypothesis that dietary factors may contribute to atherosclerosis in humans. The importance of cholesterol in atherosclerosis is emphasized by the fact that the first stage in the development of an atherosclerotic plaque is the fatty streak; this lesion is characterized by accumulation of cholesterol-filled cells (foam cells) in the subintimal region of the artery.[32] Foam cells are thought to arise from both smooth muscle cells and macrophages, and their lipid-filled droplets contain mainly cholesterol oleate.[43]

The second-stage lesion, the fibrous plaque, shows that factors other than cholesterol also participate in atherogenesis. In this lesion, a fibrous cap containing smooth muscle cells and collagen cover a central region of foam cells and extracellular lipids. The accumulation of extracellular lipids contains mainly cholesterol linoleate. As the fibrous plaque grows, it is transformed into a more complex lesion characterized by calcification, necrosis, ulceration, and thrombosis.[32] Although a fibrous plaque may narrow a small artery, such as a coronary artery, sufficiently to produce distal ischemia, clinical disease frequently results from events occurring in a complex lesion—weakening of the wall with aneurysmal dilatation, rupture of a plaque with cholesterol embolization, or superimposition of a thrombosis causing obstruction of the arterial lumen.

The two most important pathologic processes in development of atherosclerosis are accumulation of cholesterol and proliferation of smooth muscle cells.[3] The available data suggest that most arterial cholesterol is derived from plasma cholesterol. The causes of proliferation of smooth muscle cells and deposition of a connective tissue matrix are unknown; they might be a response to lipid accumulation or to some other stimuli such as a recently discovered, mitogenic growth factor released from platelets. The factors responsible for proliferation of connective tissue in arterial lesions represent an important area of research in molecular biology.

Development of clinical atherosclerotic disease appears to be related to certain factors referred to as *risk factors*. The concept of risk factors is important because their modification may prevent or delay the onset of atherosclerotic disease. Factors associated with premature atherosclerotic disease include abnormalities in lipid transport, hypertension, smoking, hyperglycemia (diabetes mellitus), and obesity.[39] Appropriate modification of a risk factor obviously depends on the particular factor, but dietary change can alter several of these factors favorably. Therefore, in the discussion to follow, each of the risk factors will be examined, and the possible role of diet in its modification will be considered.

ABNORMALITIES OF LIPID TRANSPORT

LIPOPROTEINS

Several abnormalities in transport of lipids have been implicated in the pathogenesis of atherosclerosis. Current evidence indicates that most cholesterol found in atherosclerotic plaques is derived from plasma cholesterol. Although deposition of some plasma cholesterol in arteries appears to be a universal phenomenon, accumulation is increased greatly with certain abnormalities in transport of plasma cholesterol. To outline these abnormalities and how they are influenced by dietary factors, it is first necessary to review the mechanisms for plasma lipid transport. Since plasma lipids are insoluble in aqueous solutions, they do not circulate freely in plasma but are complexed with specialized proteins called *apoproteins* (see Table 17-1). The resulting lipid–apoprotein complexes are designated *lipoproteins*. The lipoproteins are composed of a central core of neutral lipids (cholesterol esters and triglycerides) and a membranous coating of unesterified cholesterol, phospholipids, and apoproteins. The lipoproteins, or their precursors, are produced in both the liver and the gut. In the following discussion the metabolism of each of the major lipoproteins will be considered along with available evidence of their role in atherogenesis.

Chylomicrons. The intestine produces lipoproteins called *chylomicrons*. Most of the lipids in chylomicrons are derived from the digestion of dietary fats (triglycerides). Dietary triglycerides are hydrolyzed in the intestinal lumen to fatty acids and monoglycerides; these in turn are taken up by the intestinal mucosa and resynthesized into triglycerides. Mucosal triglycerides, along with any absorbed cholesterol, are incorporated into large lipoproteins, or chylomicrons. The major *structural* apoprotein of chylomicrons is apoprotein B-48 (apo B-48), but most soluble apoproteins also have been

TABLE 17-1
Plasma Apolipoproteins

Apolipoprotein	Lipoprotein	Origin	Function
B-100	VLDL, LDL	Liver	Binds LDL receptor
B-48	Chylomicron	Intestine	Binds hepatic chylomicron remnant receptor(?)
C-II*	Chylomicrons VLDL	Liver	Activates lipoprotein lipase
C-III*	Chylomicrons VLDL	Liver	Inhibits lipoprotein lipase (?)
E	Chylomicrons VLDL	Liver	Binds hepatic apo E receptor
A-I	Chylomicrons HDL	Intestine and liver	Activates LCAT
A-II	Chylomicrons HDL	Intestine and liver	?

*Apoproteins C-II and C-III are transferred and "stored" in HDL during lipolysis of chylomicrons and VLDL; they are transferred back to newly secreted, triglyceride-rich lipoproteins.

identified on the surface coat of these lipoproteins (see Table 17-1).

The metabolism of chylomicrons is outlined in Figure 17-1. These particles are secreted into the intestinal lymph, enter the blood stream through the thoracic duct, and pass through peripheral capillary beds, where they come into contact with an enzyme located on the surface of capillary endothelial cells. This enzyme, lipoprotein lipase, hydrolyzes triglycerides to fatty acids and glycerol; in this process "soluble" apoproteins and surface components of chylomicrons are released into the circulation, where they are taken up by the other lipoproteins. When lipolysis is almost complete, a cholesterol-rich residual lipoprotein, called a *chylomicron remnant,* is released back into the circulation and is cleared rapidly by the liver. The recognition of the chylomicron remnant for hepatic uptake may be mediated by specific receptors on liver cells for apo B-48, or perhaps for apo E.

The atherogenic potential of chylomicrons is a matter of dispute, but mechanisms have been postulated.[6] For example, as chylomicrons undergo lipolysis on the surface of vascular endothelial cells, some cholesterol could be released into the arterial intima. Also, cholesterol-rich chylomicron remnants might be atherogenic in humans as they are in cholesterol-fed rabbits.[6] On the other hand, however, patients who have isolated hyperchylomicronemia appear not to be at unusually high risk for coronary heart disease (CHD). Furthermore, if chylomicrons or their remnants are atherogenic, CHD should be greater in populations with a high intake of fat. It is true that CHD is uncommon in countries where total fat ingestion is low, but in some parts of the world where consumption of fat is relatively high, as in Crete, the incidence of CHD also is quite low.[29] In these latter places, a lack of CHD seems related more to low total plasma cholesterol than to the level of fat intake.

Very Low Density Lipoproteins. Like the gut, the liver secretes triglyceride-rich lipoproteins called very low density lipoproteins (VLDL). The metabolism of VLDL is outlined in Figure 17-2. VLDL resemble chylomicrons except that they are smaller. Most plasma triglycerides in the fasting state are carried in VLDL. As VLDL enter plasma they contain another structural apoprotein (apo B-100). Because this is the major form of apoprotein B in fasting plasma, it will be designated simply *apo B.* Other apoproteins on circulating VLDL are of the C and E species, and they are soluble in aqueous solutions. As VLDL circulate in plasma, triglycerides are removed by lipolysis, and the soluble apoproteins are released into plasma; in contrast, apo B remains with the uncatabolized particle.

Partially catabolized VLDL are called *VLDL remnants.* These particles, which contain lesser amounts of triglyceride and soluble apoproteins, can have two fates. Under certain circumstances VLDL remnants are removed by the liver similar to chylomicron remnants, but in the usual course of events most remnants are transformed to another category of lipoproteins—low-density lipoproteins (LDL).

Normal VLDL may not be atherogenic for two reasons. First, they are not rich in cholesterol, and second, they may be too large to penetrate the arterial intima easily. However, VLDL from hypertriglyceridemic and diabetic patients behave abnormally in tissue culture in that they tend to deposit lipids in fibroblasts, endothelial cells, and macrophages. Thus, even if normal VLDL are not atherogenic, those from hyperlipidemic or diabetic patients may be.

VLDL remnants are smaller than native VLDL and contain more cholesterol, either of which may

FIG. 17-1 Chylomicron metabolism. Chylomicrons are secreted from the intestine following ingestion of dietary fat. They contain mainly triglycerides (*TG*) and small amounts of cholesterol ester (*CE*). In their surface coat are unesterified cholesterol (*Ch*), phospholipids (*PL*), and apoproteins A and B. The apoprotein B of chylomicrons, designated B-48, appers to be unique to this species of lipoprotein. In plasma, chylomicrons acquire apoproteins E and C. The apoproteins are shown enclosed in small circles. As chylomicrons circulate in plasma, they come in contact with an enzyme, lipoprotein lipase (*LPL*), located on the surface of capillary endothelial cells. The triglycerides are hydrolyzed, releasing fatty acids and glycerol; in this process, apoproteins C, E, and A are released and enter the surface coat of high-density lipoproteins (*HDL*). After lipolysis is almost complete, a chylomicron remnant returns to the circulation and is rapidly cleared by the liver. (Kane A, Hardman DA, Paulus HE: Heterogeneity of apolipoprotein B: Isolation of a new species from human chylomicrons. Proc Natl Acad Sci USA 77:2465, 1980)

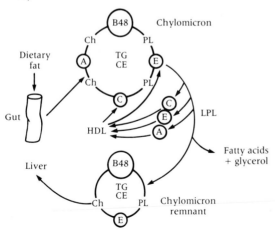

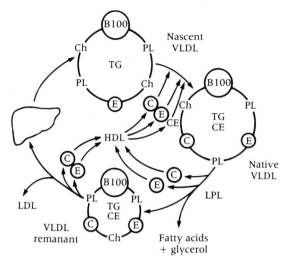

FIG. 17-2 Metabolism of very-low-density lipoproteins (*VLDL*). VLDL are secreted by the liver. They contain apoproteins B and E in their surface coat and triglycerides (*TG*) in their core. The apoprotein B of hepatic VLDL has been designated B-100 by Kane and associates (see legend, Fig. 17-1). As VLDL circulate in plasma, they acquire apoproteins C and E from high-density lipoproteins (*HDL*) along with cholesterol ester (*CE*). In this process, nascent VLDL are transformed into "native" VLDL, which in turn interact with lipoprotein lipase (*LPL*); this interaction leads to release of fatty acids and glycerol from TG and partial loss of apoproteins C and E to HDL. A smaller VLDL remnant is the product. Further catabolism of VLDL remnants results in transformation to low-density lipoprotein (*LDL*) or, in some circumstances, into direct uptake of remnants by the liver.

enhance their atherogenic potential. Evidence for the atherogenicity of VLDL remnants comes from three sources. First, many patients with CHD seem to have an increase in this class of lipoproteins. Second, in the genetic disorder, familial dysbetalipoproteinemia, VLDL remnants accumulate in plasma, and premature atherosclerosis is common; and third, cholesterol-fed animals, which rapidly develop atherosclerosis, have an increase in lipoproteins resembling VLDL remnants.[6]

Low-density Lipoproteins. Pathways of formation and removal of LDL are presented in Figure 17-3. As indicated above, LDL are derived largely from catabolism of VLDL. They are the major cholesterol-carrying lipoproteins in humans. Their core contains mainly cholesterol ester and very little triglyceride, and their surface coat has only one apoprotein, apo B (B-100). Recent evidence suggests that some LDL may be secreted directly by the liver, but this pathway may involve newly secreted, very small VLDL as precursors of LDL.

The means of removal of LDL from plasma has been a subject of great interest, and the basic mech-

anisms, as worked out in tissue culture, are outlined in Figure 17-3.[4] One pathway is a high-affinity, receptor-mediated uptake of LDL by cells. By this mechanism, the rate of uptake of LDL is a function of the number of binding sites; the lipoprotein first bound to the LDL receptor is internalized and digested by lysosomes; the cholesterol esters are hydrolyzed with release of cholesterol into the cytoplasm for use in cell membranes. When amounts of unesterified cholesterol exceed those needed for cell membranes, the excess will both inhibit the cell's own synthesis of cholesterol and be stored in the cell as inert cholesterol ester. Also, if a cell accumulates an excess of cholesterol because of large amounts of LDL in the media, synthesis of receptors is reduced, thereby reducing uptake of cholesterol.

Besides the uptake of LDL by means of the receptor mechanism, LDL can be degraded by other means as well. One example is bulk-phase phagocytosis of LDL. This pathway has been called the *scavenger pathway* because it may consist in part of phagocytic cells of the reticuloendothelial system.[4] This mechanism for LDL degradation is particularly important when the specific receptor pathway is saturated by high concentrations of LDL. Several types of nonreceptor pathways actually may be involved in LDL catabolism, and some of these probably are not part of the reticuloendothelial system.

FIG. 17-3 Formation and fate of low-density lipoproteins (*LDL*). Under normal circumstances most LDL are derived from catabolism of very-low-density lipoproteins (*VLDL*) (see Fig. 17-2). LDL, which contain apoprotein B-100 in their surface coat and mainly cholesterol ester in their core, can have at least four fates. They may be removed from the circulation by either the liver or extrahepatic tissues. Also, for each, tissue uptake can be either receptor mediated or receptor independent. The relative magnitudes of these different pathways have not been determined for humans.

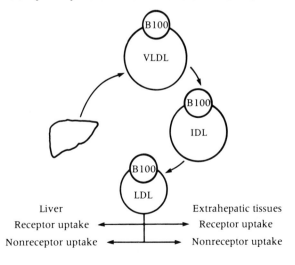

Recent studies indicate that circulating LDL can be removed from the circulation by both peripheral tissues and the liver. Peripheral catabolism of LDL is of interest because one site of uptake could be the arterial wall. There is increasing evidence that most lipid in atherosclerotic plaques, which consist mostly of cholesterol esters, is derived from LDL. Indeed, LDL appears to be the most atherogenic of all the plasma lipoproteins. The contribution of LDL to the arterial wall cholesterol might occur in at least four ways: (1) LDL–cholesterol could enter arterial smooth muscle cells through the receptor-mediated process; (2) LDL may be incorporated in arterial wall macrophages by the scavanger pathway; (3) LDL might become entrapped in extracellular spaces by interaction of LDL-apo B with mucopolysaccharide ground substance of the arterial intima; or (4) cholesterol may be released into extracellular spaces by death and rupture of foam cells.

High-Density Lipoproteins (HDL). Cholesterol entering peripheral cells during catabolism of LDL cannot be degraded, and thus, mechanisms must be provided for its transport back to the liver where it can be excreted. Although the pathways of this "reverse cholesterol transport" have not been defined fully, an attractive concept is that another lipoprotein, HDL, plays an important role. The basic pathways in the metabolism of HDL are presented in Figure 17-4. The formation of HDL is a multistep process that begins in the liver, and to a lesser extent in the intestine, and is completed in the plasma. Both the liver and gut seemingly secrete a particle called *nascent HDL*. This particle is composed mainly of apoproteins (A-I, A-II, and E) and phospholipids; it is shaped like a disk rather than a sphere.[21] Nascent HDL has an affinity for unesterified cholesterol that is obtained either from cell membranes or other lipoproteins. Following uptake of unesterified cholesterol into nascent HDL, this cholesterol undergoes esterification with a fatty acid. This reaction is catalyzed by an enzyme called *lecithin–cholesterol acyltransferase* (LCAT); it is so named because it transfers an acyl group (fatty acid) from lecithin to cholesterol. LCAT is activated by apo A-I. As cholesterol ester is formed, it enters the core of the lipoprotein, and the resulting particle takes on a spherical shape. The product of this sequence of steps appears to be a small lipoprotein designated HDL_3.

Finally, HDL_3 may undergo interaction with other lipoproteins of plasma. In the catabolism of triglyceride-rich lipoproteins (chylomicrons and VLDL), surface components (unesterified cholesterol, phospholipids, and C and E apoproteins) may be transferred to the surface coat of HDL. Also, HDL can exchange some of its cholesterol ester for triglycerides of VLDL.[46] The net result of these changes is the transformation of HDL_3 into a larger particle, HDL_2. The fate of HDL is poorly understood; whether it is removed intact from the circulation has not been determined.

The role of HDL in atherogenesis has become a subject of great interest in recent years. HDL are thought to be protective against development of atherosclerosis. Epidemiological studies have shown that low concentrations of HDL are associated with greater rates of CHD than are high concentrations.[15] Although the mechanisms by which HDL exert protective effects are not well understood, an attractive hypothesis is that these lipoproteins mobilize excess cholesterol from the arterial wall.

FIG. 17-4 Metabolism of high-density lipoproteins (*HDL*). Both the liver and the gut secrete nascent HDL. These particles are disc shaped and contain apoproteins A-I, A-II, and E combined with phospholipids (*PL*). As these particles enter the circulation, they first acquire unesterified cholesterol (*Ch*) from the surface of cells. Thereafter, they interact with an enzyme, lecithin cholesterol acyltransferase (*LCAT*), and the result is esterification of unesterified cholesterol. At the same time, the particles take on a spherical shape, and they obtain small amounts of apoproteins E and C from very-low-density lipoproteins (*VLDL*). The net result is a particle called HDL_3. As HDL_3 continues to circulate, they further enlarge by acquiring more cholesterol ester as well as triglycerides (from VLDL), and these larger HDL are called HDL_2. The fate of HDL_2 is not well understood.

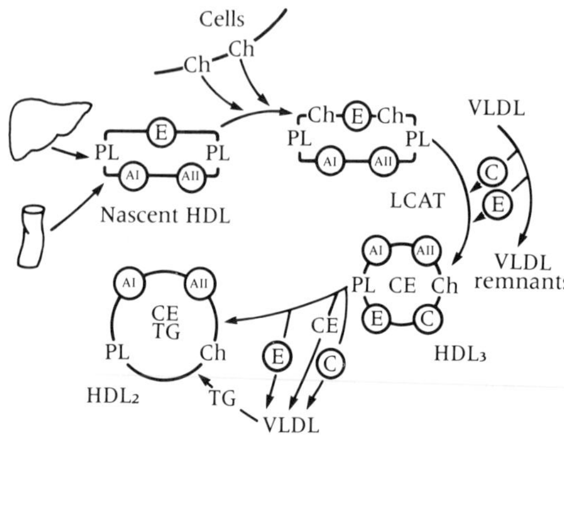

PLASMA CHOLESTEROL, LIPOPROTEINS, AND ATHEROSCLEROSIS

Total Plasma Cholesterol and CHD. Evidence of several kinds has implicated abnormalities of lipid transport in the development of atherosclerosis and CHD. A relation between hypercholesterolemia and atherosclerosis in experimental animals is well established. Also, epidemiological studies in humans have shown a significant correlation between plasma cholesterol levels and the incidence of CHD.[29] In cross-culture studies, populations with relatively low plasma cholesterol (*e.g.*, southern Europeans, North American Indians, and Japanese) have a correspondingly low prevalence of CHD. In contrast, populations with higher cholesterol concentrations, such as northern Europeans and North American whites and blacks, have higher CHD rates. Of interest, comparisons of Japanese living in Japan, Hawaii, and San Francisco have shown that serum cholesterol levels are about 12% greater in Hawaii and 21% higher in San Francisco than in Japan. As compared to Japan, death rates from CHD were 1.7 times higher in Hawaii and 2.8 times greater in San Francisco.[26] Thus, in a population with a high degree of genetic homogeneity, serum cholesterol correlated highly with CHD mortality.

One important epidemiological study in the United States population was the *Pooling Project*, in which results from several similar epidemiological studies were combined.[39] The CHD risk was compared to serum cholesterol through five steps of increasing cholesterol levels in men aged 40 to 64 years. The quintiles and relative CHD risk are shown in Table 17-2. No differences were noted between quintiles I and II, but CHD risk increased progressively with higher cholesterol levels.

The Desirable Range of Plasma Cholesterol.
Although a correlation between plasma cholesterol and coronary atherosclerosis undoubtedly exists, the result of the Pooling Project suggests that the relationship to CHD risk may not be linear over a broad range of cholesterol levels. Apparently, in the United States the risk for CHD increases significantly at cholesterol levels above 220 mg/dl and the desirable level clearly would be below 220 mg/dl.[39] Furthermore, if multicountry epidemiological studies are taken into consideration, a reduction of serum cholesterol below this value may further decrease risk, and therefore, it is reasonable to say that the desirable cholesterol is below 200 mg/dl.[26,29] Recently, a group of epidemiologists, clinical investigators, and experimental pathologists were requested to develop a consensus on the ideal cho-

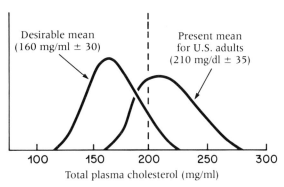

FIG. 17-5 Population distribution curves for total plasma cholesterol in present U.S. adults and for the desirable distribution.

lesterol level.[45] Taking all the available evidence into consideration, this group proposed that the ideal level for adults would be in the range of 130 mg/dl to 190 mg/dl (mean 160 mg/dl). This proposed ideal range is well below the distribution of plasma cholesterol in United States adults today (see Figure 17-5); at least 50% to 60% of adult American men have concentrations greater than 200 mg/dl, and these levels would seem to be in the zone of accelerating risk for CHD.[24]

LDL–Cholesterol and CHD. In epidemiological studies, total cholesterol concentrations are a good reflection of LDL–cholesterol, and the high correlation between plasma cholesterol and CHD suggests that high concentrations of LDL are atherogenic. The relation between LDL and atherosclerotic diseases has been confirmed recently in several epidemiological studies in which both clinical manifestations of CHD and angiographic proof of atherosclerosis were compared to LDL levels.

LDL-apo B and CHD. The exclusive apoprotein of LDL is apo B, and it is this apoprotein that directs the uptake of LDL by cells. Rates of interaction between LDL-apo B and LDL receptors thus may be one factor controlling clearance of LDL from plasma and thereby regulating LDL concentrations. Another factor influencing LDL levels is the rate of synthesis of apo B by the liver. Finally, apo B of LDL may be responsible for the interaction and deposition of LDL in extracellular spaces of the arterial intima through its interaction with mucopolysaccharides. Thus, the metabolism of apo B seemingly plays a key role in regulation of LDL concentrations, and preliminary studies suggest that LDL-apo B may be a better predictor of CHD risk than LDL–cholesterol.[44]

HDL and CHD. Epidemiological studies in the United States and northern Europe have shown an

TABLE 17-2
Results of the Pooling Project

Quintile	Plasma Cholesterol (mg/dl)	Relative CHD Risk
I	<194	1
II	194–218	1
III	219–240	1.50
IV	241–268	1.64
V	>268	1.99

Data from Pooling Project Research Group: Relationship of blood pressure, serum cholesterol, smoking habit, relative weight and ECG abnormalities to incidence of major coronary events: Final Report of the Pooling Project. J Chronic Dis 31:201–306, 1956.

inverse correlation between CHD rates and HDL.[15] The concept thus has developed that high concentrations of HDL may be protective against atherosclerosis, possibly by promoting removal of cholesterol from the arterial wall. While this hypothesis may be valid, low HDL may not increase risk for CHD in populations in which LDL concentrations also are low. Examples of a lack of increased CHD risk with low HDL are found in American Indians, Asians, and southern Europeans.

VLDL, Triglycerides and CHD. As indicated previously, elevations of triglyceride-rich lipoproteins may not be atherogenic. On the other hand, many patients with CHD have raised triglycerides, and hypertriglyceridemia probably signifies increased risk for CHD in some patients. Although the mechanisms linking triglycerides to CHD have not been defined, several possibilities can be considered. First, raised triglycerides are associated with reduced HDL, and the latter is a known risk factor. Second, high triglycerides may be accompanied by an increase in VLDL remnants (or beta-VLDL), which also may be atherogenic. Finally, most cases of hypertriglyceridemia are due to overproduction of VLDL, and this excess synthesis can lead to elevations of either LDL–cholesterol or LDL-apo B. Thus, in many patients, high plasma triglycerides may be a marker for increased risk for CHD even though triglycerides *per se* are not atherogenic.[25]

CLASSIFICATION OF ABNORMALITIES OF LIPID TRANSPORT ASSOCIATED WITH CHD

Several lipoproteins can participate in atherogenesis, particularly when they are associated with clinical abnormalities in lipid transport. These lipoprotein syndromes can have different origins. Some have a genetic basis and are due to either monogenic or polygenic defects. Others are caused mainly by dietary excess, or represent interaction between dietary and genetic factors. A brief description of lipoprotein disorders accompanied by increased risk for CHD is presented below. Most of these are associated with some degree of hypercholesterolemia, and the major causes of elevated plasma cholesterol are outlined here:

1. Mild hypercholesterolemia (total cholesterol = 225 to 275 mg/dl; LDL–cholesterol = 150 to 200 mg/dl)
   a. Dietary
   b. Hereditary
   c. Mixed (dietary + hereditary)
   d. Hyperapobetalipoproteinemia
2. Moderate hypercholesterolemia (total choles-

terol = 275 to 350 mg/dl; LDL–cholesterol = 200 to 275 mg/dl)
   a. Polygenic hypercholesterolemia
   b. Familial combined hyperlipidemia
   c. Monogenic hypercholesterolemia (predominant overproduction of LDL)
   d. Familial dysbetalipoproteinemia
   e. Secondary hypercholesterolemia (hypothyroidism, Cushing's syndrome, anorexia nervosa, acute intermittent porphyria, and nephrotic syndrome)
3. Severe hypercholesterolemia (total cholesterol >350 mg/dl; LDL–cholesterol >275 mg/dl)
   a. Familial hypercholesterolemia (predominant clearance defect for LDL)

Mild Hypercholesterolemia. Cholesterol levels over 200 mg/dl to 220 mg/dl are accompanied by accelerating risks for CHD, and for this reason levels above this range cannot be called "normal" even when they may fall in the normal distribution for the United States population.[24,39] Because of the association with increased risk, total cholesterol in the range of 225 mg/dl to 275 mg/dl might reasonably be called *mild hypercholesterolemia*. This assumes, of course, that LDL–cholesterol is increased proportionally (*e.g.*, 150 mg/dl–200 mg/dl). In some cases, especially in women, a high HDL may be associated with a plasma LDL–cholesterol concentration below 150 mg/dl even when total cholesterol is over 225 mg/dl. The same is true in patients with hypertriglycericemia, but in these patients, VLDL–cholesterol can be treated as equivalent to LDL–cholesterol.

The causes of mild hypercholesterolemia have not been determined completely. Many workers postulate that most cases are of dietary origin, and it is true that diets rich in saturated fats and cholesterol may elevate LDL–cholesterol into the range of mild hypercholesterolemia.[20] Still, many other people on such diets do not have LDL concentrations in the mildly elevated range, and thus genetic factors probably contribute as well. A question of some interest is whether mildly elevated LDL is due to increased production or decreased clearance of LDL. Recent studies from our laboratory indicate that most cases of mild hypercholesterolemia are associated with increased synthesis of LDL-apo B and not with decreased removal.[27] The relative contributions of diet and heredity to overproduction of apo B remain unknown.

Hyperapobetalipoproteinemia with Normal Cholesterol. A recent observation of importance is that many patients with CHD have increased concentrations of LDL-apo B despite a normal LDL–cholesterol.[44] This could reflect an elevation in the number of *atherogenic* LDL particles that are relatively poor in cholesterol. In other words, LDL-apo B levels may be a better estimate of the number of LDL, and hence the risk associated with this fraction, than LDL–cholesterol. The discovery of the existence of increased LDL-apo B (with normal LDL–cholesterol) may help to explain why many patients with premature CHD have normal cholesterol levels. Our preliminary studies suggest that hyperapobetalipoproteinemia is the result of overproduction of apo B.

Moderate Hypercholesterolemia. Moderate hypercholesterolemia can be defined as a total cholesterol in the range of 275 mg/dl to 350 mg/dl (LDL–cholesterol = 200 mg/dl to 275 mg/dl). Most patients with this disorder have a genetic defect although dietary excess may contribute to the rise in LDL–cholesterol. The genetic defect may be either monogenic or polygenic.[13,14] Several examples have been defined. The most common cause of moderate hypercholesterolemia probably is *polygenic hypercholesterolemia.* Family studies of patients with this disorder reveal that less than 10% of first-degree relatives have hypercholesterolemia; thus, it is unlikely to be a monogenic disorder.[13,14] Our studies indicate that overproduction of LDL-apo B is probably the underlying defect in most patients, but the role of decreased clearance of LDL needs further evaluation.[27]

Several monogenic disorders also can cause moderate hypercholesterolemia.[13,14] One of these is *familial combined hyperlipidemia.* Families with this metabolic disease have multiple lipoprotein patterns: some family members have high LDL only, others have increased VLDL only, and still others have increases in VLDL and LDL. Xanthomas do not occur, but affected individuals, regardless of their lipoprotein pattern, have enhanced risk for CHD. It has been estimated that about 10% of all patients with CHD have familial combined hyperlipidemia. The primary defect in familial combined hyperlipidemia seemingly is a monogenic overproduction of apo B, but the expression of the disorder (*i.e.,* increased VLDL, LDL, or both) may be modulated by other genetic or environmental factors affecting triglyceride metabolism.[7] We have shown recently that most hypertriglyceridemic patients with this disease have an increased synthesis of VLDL–triglyceride; this seemingly occurs in addition to overproduction of apo B.[1,7] Whether some families have only an overproduction of apo B (without abnormalities in triglyceride metabolism) has not been determined, but if so, they should have pure hypercholesterolemia.

A less common cause of moderate hypercholesterolemia is *familial dysbetalipoproteinemia.* This is a disorder characterized by increased plasma beta–VLDL, a subspecies of VLDL remnants. The primary defect appears to be a deficiency of an isoform of apo E called *apo E_3.*[5] This isoform may be involved in the normal transformation of VLDL remnants to LDL. Although the underlying abnormality in this disorder is accumulation of beta-VLDL due to defective remnant processing, the hyperlipidemia is accentuated greatly in patients who have a concomitant overproduction of VLDL–apo B. Patients with familial dysbetalipoproteinemia have orange discoloration of palmar and digital creases, tuberous or tuberoeruptive xanthomas, and premature atherosclerosis (particularly of peripheral vessels).

Finally, moderate hypercholesterolemia can occur with other diseases. The most common probably is hypothyroidism, in which clearance of LDL is reduced. Other causes of increased LDL are Cushing's syndrome, anorexia nervosa, acute intermittent porphyria, and nephrotic syndrome. Obesity and diabetes mellitus may be associated with increased secretion of VLDL–apo B, but alone they rarely raise LDL into the range of moderate hypercholesterolemia.

Severe Hypercholesterolemia. The usual cause of a plasma cholesterol over 350 mg/dl is *familial hypercholesterolemia.* It is an autosomal dominant disorder affecting about 1 person in 500. Almost all affected persons are heterozygotes for the disease. The primary abnormality is a lack of, or a defect in, the gene for the LDL receptor, and heterozygotes have only half the normal number of receptors.[4] The consequence is a defective clearance of plasma LDL. Hypercholesterolemia is present at birth, and LDL concentrations remain elevated throughout life. High LDL levels lead to premature atherosclerosis, and myocardial infarctions are common in the third and fourth decades, particularly in men. Another characteristic clinical feature is tendon xanthomas, which are almost pathognomonic of this disorder in a hypercholesterolemic patient.

Hypoalphalipoproteinemia. A low level of HDL (alpha-lipoproteins) predisposes a person to premature CHD, particularly when the LDL is in the high-normal or elevated range.[15] The normal concentration of HDL–cholesterol in United States men is 40 mg/dl to 50 mg/dl, and in women 55 mg/dl to 65 mg/dl. A low HDL apparently occurs in some families, suggesting a genetic defect (primary hypoalphalipoproteinemia); it is not known whether the low HDL is the result of a monogenic or polygenic disorder. The consequences can be premature and severe CHD. A reduction in HDL also can be secondary to other factors, for instance, obesity, hypertriglyceridemia, lack of exercise, smoking, androgens, and possibly polyunsaturated fats. Whether secondary hypoalphalipoproteinemia is associated with accelerated atherosclerosis is not known.

Hypertriglyceridemia. An elevation of plasma triglyceride can be associated with a variety of disorders. Increased triglyceride-rich lipoproteins can be the result of overproduction or decreased clearance, or both.[1] The risk for CHD associated with hypertriglyceridemia appears to be determined by the type of abnormality.

An overproduction of VLDL occurs in hypertriglyceridemic patients with *familial combined hyperlipidemia*; these patients have increased synthesis of both VLDL–triglycerides and VLDL-apo B, and they seem to be at greater than normal risk for CHD.[1,5] Their increased risk probably is related to a high production of apo B; whether this overproduction is driven by excess synthesis of VLDL–triglycerides has not been determined.[7] It is not yet certain whether enhanced synthesis of triglycerides can occur without increased apo B synthesis; however, dissociation of triglyceride and apo B synthesis has been claimed for some patients with *familial hypertriglyceridemia,* and these patients may not have increased CHD risk.[5]

Elevated plasma triglycerides also can be due to decreased clearance. Defective clearance of chylomicrons occurs when there are defects in the lipoprotein lipase system; these can be consequences of a familial deficiency of lipoprotein lipid itself or of apo C-II, which is required for the activation of this enzyme. The causes of reduced triglyceride clearance without overt deficiency of lipoprotein lipase or apo C-II have not been determined. Other lipolytic defects apparently exist, and when they are of genetic origin, patients can be said to have *familial hypertriglyceridemia.* The clearance capacity for VLDL–triglycerides in the general population varies widely. Some patients with high production rates of VLDL develop marked hypertriglyceridemia because of a relatively poor ability to clear triglycerides, whereas others with a high removal capacity to not develop elevated triglycerides despite overproduction of VLDL.[1] Hypertriglyceridemia caused entirely by decreased clearance of triglycerides does not appear to be associated with an increased risk for CHD, possibly because of a lack of atherogenicity of most triglyceride-rich lipoproteins.

Secondary hypertriglyceridemia due to overproduction of VLDL–triglycerides can result from obesity, diabetes mellitus, excess intakes of alcohol or carbohydrates, oral contraceptives, emotional stress, and, rarely, from glycogen-storage disease and acromegaly. Marked hypertriglyceridemia occurs in patients with one of these disorders combined with a primary defect in clearance of VLDL–triglycerides. Secondary decreased removal of plasma triglyceride occurs in many patients with renal failure. Whether secondary hypertriglyceridemia causes atherosclerosis is not known.

EFFECTS OF DIETARY FACTORS ON PLASMA LIPOPROTEINS

Saturated Fats. Of all dietary nutrients, saturated fats have the greatest potential for raising plasma cholesterol. The increase occurs mainly in the LDL, but cholesterol in VLDL, and probably HDL, rises to a lesser extent. According to equations developed by Keys and associates, plasma cholesterol is raised by 2.7 mg/dl for every 1% of total calories derived from saturated fats.[28] This increase is in relation to carbohydrates, which usually are considered to have no effect on plasma cholesterol. The actions of different types of saturated fatty acids may not be identical; for example, palmitic acid apparently raises plasma cholesterol more than does stearic acid.[23]

Saturated fatty acids are obtained from animal meats (beef and pork), dairy products (milk, butter, and cheese), eggs, bakery goods, and the hard fats of plants (coconut oil, cocoa butter, and hard margarines). All fatty acids from these products are not saturated, and a significant portion can be monounsaturated; however, these sources contribute most of the saturated fatty acids in the American diet.

Polyunsaturated Fats. The polyunsaturated fatty acids have the opposite effect on plasma cholesterol. In contrast to saturated fats, their major action is to lower LDL–cholesterol, but smaller reductions can occur in VLDL and HDL as well. For every 1% of calories from polyunsaturated fatty acids, total plasma cholesterol should fall about 1.35 mg/dl.[28] Again, this is relative to a baseline of carbohydrates. The mechanisms for LDL lowering by polyunsaturated fats have been a subject of intense investigation and controversy. Early workers suggested that these fats reduce plasma cholesterol by promoting excretion of cholesterol or its catabolic products, the bile acids. Although increased excretion of cholesterol or bile acids undoubtedly occurs in some patients, this effect is not universal and probably cannot adequately explain the reduction in LDL cholesterol.[17,18] Another postulated mechanism is that polyunsaturates decrease the cholesterol-carrying capacity of LDL because of *steric exclusion* of cholesterol by polyunsaturated fatty acids; however, our recent studies have shown that these fats do not alter the lipid or protein composition of LDL, and the reduction of LDL–cholesterol is associated with an equivalent decline in all the lipid and protein constitutents of this lipoprotein. Finally, polyunsaturates might lower LDL by changing the metabolism of apo B. A recent report claimed that polyunsaturated fatty acids increase the clearance of LDL-apo B in normal subjects, but reduced synthesis of apo B may contribute to LDL lowering in some patients with hyperlipidemia.

Although there was an early enthusiasm for increasing polyunsaturates in the American diet, a more cautious attitude has recently been assumed by most investigators. Since mechanisms for cholesterol lowering have not been defined fully, some workers are concerned that alterations in lipoprotein metabolism by these fats may not be beneficial. For example, decreased plasma cholesterol is not necessarily associated with reduced tissue cholesterol, especially arterial wall cholesterol. Furthermore, possible untoward effects of polyunsaturated fats have been suggested (*e.g.*, an increased incidence of cholesterol gallstones, cocarcinogenicity, and detrimental changes in lipid composition of cell membranes). Although none of these potentially dangerous effects has been proven in humans, neither has a large population consumed large amounts of polyunsaturated fats for long periods. Thus, the concept has evolved that polyunsaturated fatty acids probably should not exceed 10% of total calories.

Monounsaturated Fats. In contrast to polyunsaturates, little attention has been given to increasing monounsaturated fats in the American diet. The influence of these fats on plasma cholesterol seems to be the same as for carbohydrates. Thus for each 1% of calories substituted by monounsaturates for saturates, the plasma cholesterol should fall about 2.7 mg/dl. Although this is significant reduction, it may be only two thirds that produced by polyunsaturates.

Most monounsaturated fatty acids in the American diet come from fats that also contain saturated fatty acids. A rich source of monounsaturates is olive oil, which is consumed in large amounts in the Mediterranean region without apparent adverse effects.[29] Thus, there is no evidence that large amounts of monounsaturated fatty acids are harmful, and in fact, the human body synthesizes monounsaturates from saturated fatty acids. Still, the mechanisms by which monounsaturates lower LDL have not been determined, and more studies are needed.

Carbohydrates. Dietary carbohydrates, like monounsaturates, are assumed to have a neutral influence on plasma cholesterol causing neither an increase nor a decrease. In comparison with saturated fats, however, they reduce cholesterol levels. Alterations in lipoprotein metabolism responsible for the fall in LDL–cholesterol require further elucidation. As compared to fats, carbohydrates raise plasma triglycerides, an action due to stimulation of synthesis of VLDL–triglycerides but apparently not of VLDL-apo B.

Dietary carbohydrates can be either complex carbohydrates or simple sugars. Most authorities believe that complex carbohydrates are preferable to simple sugars because they are not associated with dental caries, they avoid surges of hyperglycemia that can occur with simple sugars, and provide bulk to the diet. Although different types of carbohydrates (*e.g.*, glucose, fructose, sucrose, and starch) have varying effects on plasma triglycerides in animals, corresponding differences have not been shown conclusively for humans.

Protein. In experimental animals the type of dietary protein can influence the plasma lipids. In some species, protein from vegetable sources (*e.g.*, soybean protein) can lower the plasma cholesterol compared to animal proteins. Also, exchange of soy protein for animal protein has been reported to lower plasma cholesterol in humans by about 5%. Our recent studies in man revealed that soy protein lowers VLDL when substituted for casein, but reductions in LDL–cholesterol usually were not seen.

Alcohol. For many Americans, alcohol constitutes a significant portion of total calories. Alcohol can alter the metabolism of two lipoproteins—VLDL and HDL. It stimulates synthesis of triglycerides in liver and thereby promotes secretion of VLDL–triglycerides. In patients with an inherent defect in VLDL clearance, alcohol can produce a marked hypertriglyceridemia. Alcohol also raises HDL–cholesterol in many people. The reasons for this increase have not been worked out, and its implications for CHD risk are not known. Alcohol apparently affects LDL concentrations little, if at all.

Total Caloric Intake. Effects of total caloric load on lipid metabolism depend on a person's metabolic state. In those with a high energy expenditure, large numbers of calories are needed to maintain the body weight, and apparently the metabolism of lipids is not altered adversely. With low energy expenditure, high caloric intake leads to weight gain and frequently to detrimental changes in lipoproteins. For instance, cholesterol synthesis is increased in obesity; this increase causes a greater flux of cholesterol into plasma and bile. The former can promote hyperlipidemia, and the latter increases risk for cholesterol gallstones.[2] Also, obese patients have overproduction of VLDL–triglycerides.

While metabolic adjustments can prevent hyper-triglyceridemia in many obese patients, those with defective clearance of VLDL will develop high triglyceride levels. Obesity raises LDL concentrations in some patients, probably because of increased synthesis of apo B. Finally, the obese state usually lowers HDL–cholesterol. Thus, excess calories in obese persons can adversely affect all lipoprotein fractions. These changes can be reversed by caloric restriction and weight loss.

Dietary Cholesterol.   The influence of dietary cholesterol on plasma cholesterol in humans has been a subject of great interest and dispute. In many animals species, including subhuman primates, ingestion of cholesterol can raise plasma cholesterol and produce atherosclerosis. Cholesterol feeding in humans, however, generally does not markedly enhance plasma cholesterol. Indeed, some have questioned whether dietary cholesterol contributes in any way to human atherogenesis. This question is based on claims that cholesterol in the diet has little or no effect on plasma cholesterol, but carefully controlled metabolic studies show otherwise. For example, Keys and co-workers reported that the cholesterol concentration is raised by 1.5 mg/dl times the square root of the number of milligrams of cholesterol per 1000 calories.[28] A similar response was noted by Hegsted and co-workers, who reported an increase of 0.068 mg/dl per milligram of cholesterol in the diet.[23] Accordingly, 250 mg of dietary cholesterol (roughly equivalent to 100 mg/1000 Cal) should increase cholesterol levels by 17 mg/dl. Mattson and associates found a similar response.[31] In cholesterol-fed primates, some animals are responsive to dietary cholesterol and show a marked rise in plasma cholesterol, while others are nonresponders, that is, they are resistant and fail to increase cholesterol levels. A similar variability has been proposed for humans, but the studies of Mattson and associates suggest that for normal subjects, at least, the response to dietary cholesterol is fairly uniform for all.[31] The same, however, may not be true for hyperlipidemic subjects.

The rise in plasma cholesterol from dietary cholesterol occurs mainly in LDL, but lesser increases have been reported for VLDL– and HDL–cholesterol. In several types of primates, dietary cholesterol induces an abnormally large LDL, which is highly atherogenic; the same has not been observed in humans. Still, it must be asked whether dietary cholesterol might be atherogenic in ways not revealed by its effect on fasting levels of cholesterol. For example, large intakes of cholesterol could enhance cholesterol content of chylomicron remnants, which could be atherogenic; also dietary cholesterol may induce abnormal lipoproteins (*e.g.,* beta-VLDL) that could promote atherosclerosis in the postprandial state, but not during fasting.

Fiber.   A great interest has been expressed in the possible role of dietary fiber in protection against a variety of diseases including CHD. The term *fiber* encompasses several types of different nondigestible polysaccharides which may have differing actions. For instance, bran fiber does not alter plasma cholesterol and excretion of cholesterol products. On the other hand, pectin polysaccharides may interfere with reabsorption of bile acids and thereby mildly reduce LDL levels. Even though most types of dietary fiber change lipid metabolism only slightly, this does not exclude the possibility that they could be useful in prevention of other diseases such as colon cancer or diverticulitis.

RELATION OF DIET TO CORONARY HEART DISEASE

Evidence for a relationship between diet and CHD comes from several sources. No single source provides unequivocal proof for this link, but when all data are considered, the case for an association is strong. This evidence can be reviewed briefly.

Experimental Atherosclerosis.   Dietary cholesterol can induce atherosclerosis in several species of experimental animals. The degree of atherosclerosis generally depends on the rise in plasma cholesterol. With marked hypercholesterolemia, atherosclerosis can be severe; but in animals without significant rises in cholesterol, atherosclerosis usually is minimal. The role of dietary cholesterol in experimental atherogenesis, however, cannot necessarily be extrapolated to humans. In susceptible animals, the height of cholesterol levels far exceeds that induced by dietary cholesterol in humans. Also, in animals the increase occurs in highly atherogenic, cholesterol-rich lipoproteins (beta-VLDL or large LDL) that are not found in appreciable amounts in humans. Nevertheless, the finding that relatively small quantities of dietary cholesterol can significantly increase plasma cholesterol and induce atherosclerosis in nonhuman primates provides suggestive evidence that humans also may be susceptible to cholesterol in the diet.

Population Surveys.   Comparisons of different populations can be considered clinical trials of nature, and they can have distinct advantages over man-made trials. Especially, they can include large numbers of people who have consumed the same diet over many years. Both number and duration usually are insufficient in intervention trials. Still, epidemiological studies usually contain confounding variables that can lead to misinterpretation of results. Although many population surveys have been carried out, some stand out as showing a likely relation between diet and CHD. One extensive study examined severity of atherosclerosis at autopsy in 21,000 people in 15 countries.[33] The results suggested a high correlation between estimated level of dietary fat intake in these countries and extent of atherosclerosis.

In the Seven-Countries Study, a high correlation likewise was noted between percent calories as saturated fats and CHD deaths in several different populations.[29] The Ni-Hon-San Study compared CHD rates in Japanese living in Japan, Hawaii, and San Francisco.[26] In this study, serum cholesterol concentrations were higher in proportion to greater intakes of saturated fats and cholesterol in Hawaii and San Francisco, and there were corresponding increases in rates of CHD; thus, in this population with genetic homogenity, the composition of the diet correlated significantly with both serum cholesterol and CHD mortality. Another study compared CHD mortality in Seven Day Adventists, who are mainly lacto-ovo-vegetarians, with an age-matched group of Californians.[47] The vegetarians had both lower cholesterol levels and lesser rates of CHD.

Finally, the Western Electric Study compared diet, serum cholesterol, and CHD rates in 1900 middle-aged men over a period of 20 years; in this prospective study, a positive correlation between dietary factors (cholesterol and saturated fatty acids) and CHD rates was reported.[40] Although other factors may have contributed to differences in CHD rates among the different comparisons in the above studies, the results taken as a whole strongly suggest that high intakes of saturated fats and cholesterol contribute significantly to atherosclerosis and CHD.

Dietary Intervention Trials. Although epidemiological studies support the concept that diet contributes to CHD risk, they do not reveal whether a change in diet can retard atherogenesis. Therefore, several intervention trials have been carried out to test the "lipid hypothesis." These trials generally have tested effects of diets rich in polyunsaturated fats. One trial was carried out in Helsinki, Finland, in which institutionalized men were compared on a diet low in saturated fats with one high in polyunsaturates.[35] Over a six-year period, the cholesterol-lowering diet was associated with reduced CHD mortality rates. A similar trial was carried out in a Minnesota mental hospital; a preliminary report indicated that rates of coronary events were reduced in men under 40 years by the cholesterol-reducing diet, but rates were not different in control and diet-treatment groups for older men and women.[11] Positive results with cholesterol-lowering diets also were reported from a study done at the Veterans Administration domiciliary facility in Los Angeles and from another in a free-living population in Oslo, Norway.[8,30] Although the experimental design and execution of all these studies can be criticized, particularly because of an inadequate number of patients studied for too short a period, they nevertheless have been uniform in showing a favorable trend toward decreasing rates of CHD on cholesterol-lowering diets. Unfortunately, for many reasons it is unlikely that a major dietary trial of sufficient duration and patient number can be carried out to prove beyond doubt that dietary alteration at some point in life can reduce the chances of developing CHD.

Diet-Induced Hypercholesterolemia in Humans. Despite the failure of epidemiological surveys and dietary intervention trials to prove conclusively that dietary change can retard development of CHD in high risk populations, the fact remains that dietary saturated fats and cholesterol can raise the total cholesterol and LDL–cholesterol. Thus, the unequivocal relationship between these dietary factors and plasma LDL levels and between LDL levels and atherosclerosis provides an extremely strong case that diet *can* contribute to atherogenesis in humans. Unfortunately, precise knowledge as to how much cholesterol lowering is needed and for how long in order to significantly decrease rates of CHD in the United States population may never be known. For this reason, we are left with the general principle that diet contributes to the relatively high concentrations of plasma cholesterol in the United States population and that the increased risk associated with higher levels should be reduced by diet-induced lowering of plasma cholesterol. It is upon this principle that dietary therapy of hypercholesterolemia can be justified.

DIETARY TREATMENT
OF LIPID TRANSPORT DISORDERS

Mild Hypercholesterolemia. The aim of dietary therapy for mild hypercholesterolemia is to reduce plasma cholesterol (and LDL–cholesterol) into the desirable range, that is, to below 200 mg/dl. In the majority of patients it should be possible to accomplish this goal by strict adherence to diet. The primary dietary change should be to decrease intake of saturated fats and cholesterol. If a patient is obese, total caloric intake also should be decreased, preferably by curtailing intakes of saturated fats. If obesity is not present, removal of saturated fats requires replacement with other nutrients. Three substitutes can be considered, namely, carbohydrates, polyunsaturated fats, and monounsaturates. Combinations also can be used. The major kinds of diet for treatment of mild hypercholesterolemia can be summarized briefly.

A low-fat, high-carbohydrate diet is recommended by the American Heart Association (AHA); basically, saturated fats are replaced mainly by carbohydrates. The current American diet contains about 40% of total calories as fat, of which approximately 17% is saturated, 17% monounsaturated, and 5% polyunsaturated. The average cholesterol intake is about 500 mg/day, or slightly lower. The AHA recommends the following: (1) a reduction of total fat to 30%, (2) an increase of carbohydrate to 55%, (3) a decrease of saturates and monosaturates to 10% each, (4) an increase of polyunsaturates to 10%, (5) a decrease in cholesterol intake to not more than 300 mg/day, and (6) reduction of body weight to the desirable range. The postulated effects of such changes on plasma cholesterol can be estimated from the equations of Keys and associates.[28] A decrease of saturated fats from 17% to 10%, along with an increase in polyunsaturates from 5% to 10%, should decrease total plasma cholesterol by approximately 26 mg/dl. Also, a reduction in cholesterol intake from 500 mg/day to 300 mg/day should lower cholesterol by about 14 mg/dl. Finally, weight loss to the desirable range probably should reduce plasma cholesterol by about 10 mg/dl, and at the same time raise HDL. Thus, a change to the AHA-recommended diet should decrease cholesterol by 40 mg/dl to 50 mg/dl, and for most patients with mild hypercholesterolemia, this reduction would put the plasma cholesterol near or into the ideal range. Furthermore, this could be accomplished without a radical change in diet or creating danger of long-term side-effects from diet.

Since polyunsaturated fats have a greater potential for cholesterol lowering than do carbohydrates, some investigators believe that it would be better to keep the fat intake at 40% of calories but to replace saturated fats as much as possible with polyunsaturated fats. A somewhat greater decrease in total cholesterol should in fact occur on such a diet. For instance, if saturated fats were decreased to 10% and polyunsaturates were increased to 20% of total calories, the fall in plasma cholesterol from this change alone should be about 39 mg/dl instead of the 26 mg/dl achieved by changing diet composition to the AHA diet. At the same time, the increased fat intake might make the diet more palatable to many people. On the other hand, the long-term consequences of a very high intake of polyunsaturates are unknown, and many investigators question the prudence of such a recommendation for the United States population.

In the Mediterranean region the diet is rich in monounsaturated fatty acids owing to the high intake of olive oil. Monounsaturates commonly compose 20%, and in Crete up to 25%, of total calories. Plasma cholesterol concentrations in this region are relatively low as are CHD mortality rates. Since monounsaturates have about the same potential for cholesterol lowering as carbohydrates, the effects of a diet high in these fats should be about the same as for a high-carbohydrate diet. Although no rich source of monounsaturated fats is readily available in the United States, one potential source is the partial hydrogenation of plant oils. Unfortunately, hydrogenation produces significant amounts of unnatural trans-monounsaturated fatty acids, and the metabolic effects of these acids have not been determined.

Dietary therapy of mild hypercholesterolemia can be justified on the grounds that affected patients are at increased risk for CHD. The question, however, can be asked whether dietary change should be recommended for the whole United States population. For example, many people apparently have cholesterol levels in the desirable range, and dietary change should be of little benefit. Furthermore, young people seem to be relatively protected against clinical atherosclerotic disease before puberty and thereafter into early adulthood, as do women before menopause. Thus, is it necessary to recommend dietary change for all these people? Those who support a generalized dietary change for the United States population list the following reasons. First, a massive effort would be required to screen patients for cholesterol concentrations, and facilities are not currently available to carry out such screening. Second, a single estimation of plasma lipids is not sufficient to separate individuals from high-risk and low-risk groups; multiple determinations over a considerable period of time are needed to clearly define a person's lipoprotein status. Third, in order to change the dietary habits of people at higher risk, it would be necessary to carry out a major change in the eating patterns of the nation. Fourth, there is evidence to suggest that the lower the cholesterol level, the lower the CHD risk; and therefore, many people with relatively low concentrations might still benefit from a further reduction in plasma cholesterol. And fifth, even for children and women, there is an increasing risk with aging. Development of favorable eating habits early in life may establish prudent eating patterns for later in life when risk increases. Thus, if specific patients can be identified who have mild hypercholesterolemia, the need for a change in diet can be emphasized, but even for those who appear to be at relatively low risk, a modified eating pattern can be considered prudent.

Moderate Hypercholesterolemia. In patients with higher levels of plasma cholesterol, dietary changes alone may not be adequate to bring concentrations into the desirable range. This is because genetic factors also can raise cholesterol levels. Nevertheless, even in this category strict adherence to diet may lower concentrations to acceptable levels. One approach is to recommend marked dietary changes, such as decreasing total fat intake to 20% or less of total calories and cholesterol intakes to about 100 mg/day. The American Heart Association supports this approach to dietary therapy of moderate hypercholesterolemia. Although clinical trials testing the potency of very low fat diets are lacking, epidemiological surveys in other populations suggest that they usually are associated with low cholesterol concentrations.

Failure of dietary therapy to normalize cholesterol levels in patients with genetic hypercholesterolemia does not mean that strict dietary change is without value. Many patients obtain a substantial lowering through diet, and the use of drugs in combination with diet may bring plasma cholesterol to the desirable range. In patients with *polygenic hypercholesterolemia,* the use of bile acid sequestrants (cholestyramine or colestipol), in addition to dietary change, can be recommended for LDL lowering. In those with *familial combined hyperlipidemia,* who have increases in both LDL and VLDL, bile acid sequestrants can be combined with either nicotinic acid or fibric acid derivatives (clofibrate or gemfibrozil). Commitment of a patient with moderate hypercholesterolemia to long-term drug therapy should not be taken lightly or as substitute for strict dietary treatment. Patients on hypocholesterolemic drugs must be followed frequently for therapeutic response and side-effects.

Severe Hypercholesterolemia. Most patients in this category have *heterozygous familial hypercholesterolemia,* and while dietary therapy may be helpful, most patients required drug treatment as well. Most respond best to combined drug therapy; this should include a bile acid sequestrant plus another drug such as nicotinic acid, neomycin, or, less desirable, a fibric acid. Some younger patients may be considered for an ileal exclusion operation for satisfactory lowering of cholesterol levels. Because of the great risk for CHD in patients with *familial hypercholesterolemia,* they should not be treated with dietary change alone.

HYPERTENSION

A second major risk factor for CHD is hypertension. A hypertensive study group in 1971 indicated that the prevalence of hypertension in United States adults is 15% to 20%, and at least 50% of this population has hypertensive heart disease. Fortu-

nately, more and more patients with hypertension are being treated, and control of hypertension may have contributed to the decline in cardiovascular mortality in the past decade.

DEFINITION OF HYPERTENSION

A precise definition of hypertension has been difficult to obtain because, as with plasma cholesterol, the relation between blood pressure and cardiovascular disease seems to extend over a broad range of blood pressures, including those which were previously thought to be in the normal range. The World Health Organization has defined definite hypertension in adults as a systolic pressure over 160 mm Hg or a diastolic pressure greater than 95 mm Hg and borderline hypertension as a pressure between 140/90 mm Hg and 160/95 mm Hg. The ideal range for blood pressure has not been defined adequately, but if the effects of blood pressure on atherogenesis are considered, it probably should be near 120/80 mm Hg or below.

PATHOLOGIC CONSEQUENCES OF HYPERTENSION

A prolonged increase in blood pressure can cause damage to many organ systems. Perhaps the most serious complication of hypertension is acceleration of atherosclerosis. The mechanisms whereby hypertension enhances atherogenesis have not been elucidated, but several have been postulated. For example, increased blood pressure may cause damage to the endothelial lining of arteries, which in turn may promote proliferation of smooth muscle cells or infiltration of lipoproteins into subendothelial spaces. Also, increased pressure may directly force more LDL into the arterial intima. The requirement of a threshold level of blood pressure for atherogenesis is revealed by the fact that atherosclerosis does not develop in veins or in pulmonary arteries (except with pulmonary hypertension).

Hypertension has other adverse effects on the cardiovascular system besides accelerating atherosclerosis. It can induce hypertrophy of the left ventricle of the heart, and this complication, with or without concomitant coronary atherosclerosis, can cause heart failure. Elevated blood pressure is often present in patients with cystic medial necrosis of the aorta resulting in dissecting aneurysm. Hypertension also can damage the kidneys through its effect on the small vessels (arteriolar nephrosclerosis). The cerebral consequences of hypertension are several: cerebral atherosclerosis and stroke, vasospasm causing ischemia, and cerebral hemorrhage.

ETIOLOGY OF HYPERTENSION

Over 90% of cases of hypertension are of unknown cause, hence the term *essential hypertension.* Less commonly, high blood pressure can be due to secondary disorders—renovascular disease, preeclampsia and eclampsia, primary aldosteronism, Cushing's syndrome, acromegaly, hypercalcemia, and coarctation of the aorta. A common cause of elevated blood pressure is use of estrogen-containing oral contraceptives; these agents may activate the renin-angiotensin-aldosterone system, possibly through estrogen stimulation of hepatic synthesis of renin substrate, which promotes production of antiotensin II and secondary aldosteronism.

The etiology of essential hypertension is an important but unresolved question in medicine. Both hereditary and environmental factors have been implicated. Hereditary factors almost certainly play a role in essential hypertension because many normal people, who are exposed to the same environmental influences as hypertensive patients, do not develop elevated blood pressure. Specific genetic defects contributing to essential hypertension have not been demonstrated but have been postulated to involve enhanced neurogenic outflow of sympathetic impulses, inability to excrete a salt load, or overactivity in the renin-angiotensin-aldosterone system. The importance of hereditary influences is reflected by the more common occurrence of hyptertension in blacks than in whites. Several environmental factors also have been implicated in the etiology of hypertension, including emotional stress, family size, and crowding. Two dietary factors, which are of interest in this chapter, are high intakes of salt and obesity. Each may be discussed separately.

Salt and Hypertension. The intake of sodium chloride in the United States population averages much more than is needed for normal body function. Intakes of sodium as low as 0.4 g/day (1 g/day salt) are compatable with health in most adults. Exceptions are individuals engaged in strenuous exercise who can loose large amounts of sodium through perspiration. Sodium consumption in United States adults averages between 4 g/day and 6 g/day (10 g/day–15 g/day salt). About one third of this total is inherent in natural foods of our diet; another third comes from industrial processing of food, and the remainder is added by cooking at home or with the salt shaker.

The potential role of salt in causing hypertension comes from studies in experimental animals, epidemiological studies, and a number of clinical investigations in humans. Chronic hypertension has been induced by high intakes of sodium in a variety of species of animals. In some strains of rats, salt-induced hypertension can persist indefinitely even after removal of excess sodium from the diet.

In several populations around the world, salt intakes are habitually very low (0.2 g/day–0.7 g/day sodium); hypertension rarely develops in these groups. In contrast, other populations exemplified by people in certain areas of Japan have very high intakes of sodium (*e.g.,* 10 g/day); such high intakes may be responsible for an increased prevalence of hypertension and stroke.[34] In the United States and Western Europe, salt consumption is intermediate as is the prevalence of high blood pressure. Finally, certain homogenous populations can have striking differences in sodium intakes because of geographical separation; in those eating low-sodium diets, hypertension rarely occurs, whereas those with high intakes of sodium have an increase of elevated blood pressure.[10]

Clinical investigations demonstrating that salt can directly raise the blood pressure in humans are limited, and more studies are needed to determine the incidence of salt-induced hypertension in the United States. Evidence that salt *can* cause hypertension is found in a few studies in which very large amounts of salt were administered to a few individuals.[36] Also, the blood pressure in patients with renal failure and on hemodialysis can be controlled by the quantity of salt in the dialysate. A reduction in blood pressure of hypertensive patients by sodium restriction provides further evidence that salt contributes directly to high blood pressure.

From studies of the types outlined above, several prominent investigators have concluded that the United States population should reduce its average intake of salt. They have postulated that a decrease of sodium intake to about one third its present level, that is, to less than 2 g/day sodium, or 5 g/day salt, would dramatically decrease the prevalence of hypertension in the United States, perhaps to as low as 3%. Obviously, if such a reduction in the incidence of high blood pressure could be achieved, the potential for decrease in CHD mortality in the United States would be considerable.

However, other investigators maintain that any recommendations to the general public about changing salt intake are premature. Several reasons are cited. First, evidence that decreasing salt intake to about 5 g/day would result in a remarkable decrease in the prevalence of hypertension in the United States is inadequate; although the available data are suggestive, much more research is needed for proof. Second, a marked change in the eating habits of Americans would be required to achieve a sodium intake of less than 2 g/day, and many are skeptical that such a change is possible. Not only would removal of most salt from processed foods be needed, but almost complete elimination of salt at home would be required. Third, since the incidence of salt-sensitive hypertension is not extremely high, almost certainly less than 15% of the population, the remaining 85% would have altered their diet for nothing. Those who voice the latter reservation usually suggest that a better approach to hypertension is to detect individuals with high blood pressure and treat them appropriately.

In spite of these arguments against the recommendation of universal reduction in sodium intake, the potential for decreasing CHD risk by sodium restriction could be considerable. For instance, if the mean blood pressure in the United States population could be reduced by an average of 10 mm Hg to 15 mm Hg, this should decrease overall risk for CHD significantly. The reason is that there appears to be a linear relationship between CHD risk and blood pressure even down into the normal ranges. Therefore, more research is needed to define the extent to which the average level of blood pressure can be reduced by restriction of salt.

Another indication for salt restriction is in treatment of established hypertension. The success of the Kempner rice diet for lowering blood pressure was due primarily to low sodium intakes. Although the major emphasis on treatment of essential hypertension during the past two decades has been on use of drugs, there is a renewed interest in dietary therapy and reduction in sodium intake. In milder cases of essential hypertension, normalization of blood pressure can sometimes be achieved by decreasing sodium intake to less than 2 g/day. In more severe cases, the action of diuretics can be enhanced by simultaneously decreasing intakes of sodium. However, in patients treated for hypertension with diuretics, care must be taken not to deplete the body of sodium reserves by salt restrictions; if this is done, a decreased availability of sodium may impair renal function.

Obesity and Hypertension. Although more attention has been given to the role of salt than to that of obesity in the causation of hypertension, the latter actually may be more important.[9,42] Several lines of evidence implicate obesity in elevation of blood pressure: (1) epidemiological studies show a positive correlation between body weight and blood pressure within relatively homogenous population groups, (2) the rise of blood pressure with age roughly parallels gain in body weight, and (3) weight reduction usually causes a decrease in blood pressure in patients with hypertension. The fall in blood pressure with weight loss is not necessarily related to reduced sodium intake, as shown by the fact that caloric restriction can decrease blood pressure in the presence of a high salt intake.

The mechanisms by which obesity raises blood pressure have not been determined.[42] It may enhance cardiac output by increasing blood volume in the presence of a "normal-sized" arterial tree. This could be due in part to increased sodium intake associated with a higher food intake. Also, there could be alterations in neuroendocrine regulation of blood pressure in obesity. For instance, it is known that the obese state is associated with changes in the metabolism of insulin, catecholamines, and thyroid hormones, and some of these changes may affect blood pressure regulation.

If obesity indeed is an important factor in many cases of hypertension, then the potential for control of elevated blood pressure through weight loss is great. Several studies have now confirmed that caloric restriction can be used as an effective therapy for mild essential hypertension. Thus, weight reduction plus sodium restriction someday may prove to be effective dietary measures for control of hypertension; this in turn should decrease the risk for CHD.

SMOKING

Smoking is closely linked to diet because it represents a form of oral gratification. It also can be used as a substitute for food because body weight often increases dramatically when a person gives up smoking. Smoking is a major risk factor for CHD.[39] It clearly increases the severity of atherosclerosis although the mechanisms are not well understood. The primary atherogenic action of smoking probably is not mediated through the plasma lipoproteins, although it does cause a small lowering of HDL levels. Other postulated mechanisms are adverse effects on platelet adhesiveness, damage to the arterial endothelium, reduction of arterial oxygen transport and utilization, and increase in the blood pressure. In patients with established heart disease smoking also may enhance susceptibility to ventricular dysrhythmias.

Avoidance of smoking almost certainly will reduce the risk for CHD. It has been reported that those who quit smoking have less than half the risk for CHD death as those who persist in the habit.[16] Fortunately, adult men in the United States, who are the population at greatest risk, appear to be reducing the smoking habit. On the other hand, the prevalence of smoking in women and teenage girls has been increasing, a rise that eventually may increase atherosclerotic disease in women. When the powerful effect of smoking on CHD risk is taken into consideration, it is obvious that the impact of any dietary change will be lessened in any patient who persists in smoking. Therefore, one of the major goals of dietary therapy must be to eliminate smoking simultaneously with any alteration of the diet.

DIABETES MELLITUS

Fasting hyperglycemia has been claimed to be a risk factor for CHD and stroke. Although atherosclerosis appears to be accelerated in diabetics, this disease also has other adverse effects on the cardiovascular system; two of these are microvascular injury and cardiomyopathy. These pathologic processes must be differentiated, and all should not be attributed to atherosclerosis. The mechanisms by which diabetes promotes atherogenesis are not known. Diabetes can affect the plasma lipoproteins in several ways; it stimulates synthesis of VLDL and can cause hypertriglyceridemia; it can raise LDL slightly or lower HDL. All of these changes could accelerate atherosclerosis. Diabetes also can damage the arterial microvasculature, which may allow increased filtration of lipoproteins into the arterial wall.[16] Other changes—endothelial damage, glycosylation of arterial wall proteins, increased proliferation of collagen—may participate in atherogenesis as well.

An important question is whether dietary control of hyperglycemia or other alterations in diet in diabetics can reduce the risk for CHD. Without conclusive evidence, two dietary changes seem prudent. First, weight reduction in obese diabetics will decrease hyperglycemia, lower plasma triglycerides, and raise HDL levels. Second, removal of saturated fats and cholesterol from the diet will lower LDL concentrations. In most diabetic patients the diet proposed for treatment of mild hypercholesterolemia and recommended by the American Heart Association for the general public should be satisfactory. A detailed description of dietary therapy in diabetes is provided in Chapter 18. Besides dietary control of increased plasma glucose and lipids, the modification of other risk factors (*e.g.*, hypertension and smoking) should be given special attention in diabetics.

OBESITY

Whether obesity is an independent risk factor for cardiovascular disease is a matter of dispute. A common clinical impression is that obesity is frequently associated with heart disease, but this apparent relationship has not always been confirmed by epidemiological studies. Without doubt, many obese people never develop heart disease, but many

others do. The problem in establishing a link seems to be that obesity directly contributes to other risk factors, as discussed above, and when these contributions are factored out, little independent action of obesity on CHD risk remains.

Indeed, it is difficult to visualize a mechanism whereby an excess of adipose tissue might directly affect events occurring in the arterial wall; any action probably would be indirect and through other factors. Furthermore, the influence of obesity cannot be separated from the general nutritional status. To maintain the obese state, an excess of calories must be ingested. While the level of caloric intake does not necessarily exceed, and may even be less than, that of nonobese people with greater energy expenditures, it nevertheless is greater than the number of calories needed to maintain the obese person's desirable weight. Thus, the nutrient composition of this excess caloric intake could have a direct effect on the major risk factors.

If the diet of obese persons contains an excess of saturated fats and cholesterol, this will cause a rise in the plasma level of LDL–cholesterol, which may accelerate atherosclerosis. Recent studies from our laboratory indicate that the relatively high concentrations of LDL seen frequently in obese patients are related more to the nutrient composition than to total caloric intake.[48] A more direct action of obesity is a reduction of HDL–cholesterol, another known risk factor; our studies suggest that HDL levels are related more to the degree of obesity than to the composition of the diet.[48]

The total caloric intake also affects plasma levels of VLDL. Excess calories raise triglycerides by increasing VLDL synthesis.[19] This action raises the question of whether increased plasma flux of lipoproteins might affect atherogenesis independently of their concentrations. A recent study from our laboratory showed that patients with coronary heart disease frequently have increased plasma flux of LDL-apo B even when their concentrations of LDL–cholesterol were in the normal range. In other words, overproduction of lipoproteins could overload their degradation systems, which might promote accumulation of arterial cholesterol even with only minimal increases in plasma lipids.

As discussed above, obesity also can accentuate hyperglycemia and hypertension. In either case, weight reduction modifies these risk factors in a favorable direction. Thus, caloric restriction in obesity and maintaining weight in the desirable range must be an important aim in the controlling of established risk factors. The treatment of obesity is discussed elsewhere in this volume (see Chap. 28). However, two points might be made as they pertain to obesity and CHD risk. First, even relatively mild degrees of obesity can aggravate risk factors in those who are genetically susceptible to dietary excesses. Particularly for people with mild to moderate obesity it is by no means futile to attempt to achieve weight loss to the desirable range. Second, when treating obese patients, the composition of the diet should be altered in addition to reducing intake of total calories. In particular, ingestion of saturated fats, cholesterol, and salt should be restricted. A change in diet composition will help to alter risk factors independently of caloric restriction and thus provide benefit even when weight loss is slow.

Dietary Therapy of Active Heart Disease

ANGINA PECTORIS

Patients with angina pectoris can be considered to be at increased risk for myocardial infarction because of danger of progression of atherosclerotic lesions. Therefore, modification of existing risk factors—lipoprotein disorders, hypertension, smoking, and diabetes mellitus—can be recommended. The alteration of these risk factors may require therapy with both diets and drugs. Also, weight loss in obese patients may lessen the frequency and duration of chest pain associated with myocardial ischemia. Sometimes chest pain is brought on by eating, which increases the cardiac output; if eating is associated with anginal pain, large meals should be avoided.

It is not necessary to proscribe use of alcohol in moderation, especially if the patient clearly derives a benefit from it; on the other hand, alcohol can induce arrythmias in susceptible people and in large amounts may depress cardiac function. Smoking is another matter; patients with angina pectoris definitely should not smoke because smoking accelerates the development of atherosclerosis and also may cause arrhythmias.

ACUTE MYOCARDIAL INFARCTION

For the first 24 to 48 hours after an acute myocardial infarction the patient should be given a liquid or soft diet. If complications develop it may be necessary to extend this period. Small meals should be given to prevent increases in cardiac output. The patient usually can feed himself. As soon as possible after the first two days bulk should be added to the diet to prevent constipation. Also, a stool softener such as dioctyl sodium sulfosuccinate, 200 mg daily, should be used, and if necessary, a bulk laxative or milk of magnesia can be given. However, since one may safely delay a bowel movement for several days after infarction, laxatives are not needed immediately and may not be needed at all. If congestive heart failure is present, a low-sodium diet should be ordered, and if diuretics are needed, dietary potassium should be increased.

The convalescence period after a myocardial infarction is perhaps the best time to induce a patient to change his dietary habits. If the patient is obese, he should be encouraged to restrict the total caloric intake. Any elevation in plasma lipids should be treated with appropriate dietary changes. However, in the postinfarction period, plasma lipids may be deceptively low, and only after the patient has returned to his usual nutritional state may the lipids be elevated. Thus, plasma lipids should be determined 3 to 4 months after the myocardial infarction to obtain a more reliable indication of the patient's usual lipoprotein profile. During the convalescence period, every effort should be made to correct any existing risk factor; in particular, if the patient is a smoker, he should be encouraged strongly to discontinue the habit.

HEART FAILURE

One of the hallmarks of chronic heart failure is retention of excessive sodium and water. Although the accumulation of fluid may precipitate clinical complications, for instance, congestive heart failure, it also contributes to maintaining adequate cardiac output. Fluid retention thus appears to be a compensatory response to a low cardiac output. On the other hand, excessive retention of fluid in patients with heart failure can be life threatening.

The two fundamental principles of treatment of chronic heart failure are to enhance the myocardial contractility with digitalis and to promote excretion of excess body fluid. The latter usually is achieved through use of diuretics bolstered by reduction of sodium intake. The thiazide diuretics are the first-line therapy of cardiac edema. When the effects of these are less than optimal, more potent diuretics, such as ethacrynic acid or furosemide, can be tried. In those who respond poorly to these drugs alone, their action can be potentiated through the addition of other diuretics—spironolactones, triampterene, or amiloride.

The diuretics also can be made more effective by reducing the sodium intake. Therefore, patients who fail to respond adequately to diuretics should be urged to decrease dietary sodium. This is particularly so for patients in severe heart failure, who may have to reduce sodium to as low as 500 mg/day or less. In these patients, no salt can be added in cooking or at the table; canned or processed foods must be eliminated; and even certain natural foods, like milk, cheese, cereals, and salt-containing vegetables, must be avoided. It is usually not necessary to restrict water intake except in patients with severe heart failure, who may have dilutional hyponatremia. Finally, weight loss should be encouraged in any obese patient with chronic heart failure.

References

1. Beil U, Grundy SM, Crouse JR et al: Triglyceride and cholesterol metabolism in primary hypertriglycerides. Arteriosclerosis 2:44–57, 1982
2. Bennion LJ, Grundy SM: Effects of obesity and caloric intake on biliary lipid metabolism in man. J Clin Invest 56:996–1011, 1975
3. Bierman EL: Atherosclerosis and other forms of arteriosclerosis. In Isselbacher KJ, Adams RD, Braunwald E, et al (eds): Harrison's Principles of Internal Medicine, Vol 9, pp 1156–1166. New York, McGraw–Hill, 1980
4. Brown MS, Goldstein JL: Familial hypercholesterolemia: A genetic defect in the low density lipoprotein receptor. N Engl J Med 294:1386–1390, 1976
5. Brunzell JD, Schrott HG, Motulsky AG et al: Myocardial infarction of familial forms of hypertriglyceridemia. Metabolism 25:313–320, 1976
6. Castelli MP, Doyle JT, Gordon T et al: HDL cholesterol and other lipids in coronary heart disease. The cooperative lipoprotein phenotyping study. Circulation 55:767–772, 1977
7. Chait A, Albers JJ, Brunzell JD: Very low density lipoprotein overproduction in genetic forms of hypertriglyceridemia. Eur J Clin Invest 10:17–22, 1980
8. Dayton S, Pearce ML, Hashimoto S et al: A controlled clinical trial of a diet high in unsaturated fat in preventing complications of atherosclerosis. Circulation (Suppl 2) 40:1–63, 1969
9. Dustan HP: Obesity and hypertension in childhood. In Lauer RM, Skekelle RB (eds): Prevention of Atherosclerosis and Hypertension, pp 305–312. New York, Raven Press, 1980
10. Fodor JG, Abbott EC, Rusted IE: An epidemiological study of hypertension in Newfoundland. Can Med Assoc J 108:1365–1368, 1973
11. Franz ID Jr, Dawson EA, Kuba K et al: The Minnesota coronary survey: Effect of diet on cardiovascular events and death (abstr). Circulation (Suppl 2) 52:4, 1975
12. Friedman GD, Petitta DB, Bawol RD et al: Mortality in cigarette smokers and quitters. Effect of base-line differences. N Engl J Med 304:1407–1410, 1981
13. Goldstein JL, Schrott HG, Hazzard WR et al: Hyperlipidemia in coronary heart disease II. Genetic analysis of lipid levels in 176 families and delineation of a new inherited disorder, combined hyperlipidemia. J Clin Invest 52:1544–1568, 1973
14. Goldstein JL, Albers JJ, Schrott HG et al: Plasma lipid levels and coronary heart-disease in adult relatives of newborns with normal and elevated cord blood lipids. Am J Hum Genet 26, No. 6:727–735, 1974
15. Gordon T, Castelli WP, Hjortland MC et al: High density lipoprotein as a protective factor against coronary heart disease. Am J Med 62:707–714, 1977
16. Groszek E, Grundy SM: The possible role of the arterial microcirculation in the pathogenesis of atherosclerosis. J Chronic Dis 33:679–684, 1980
17. Grundy SM, Ahrens EH Jr: The effects of unsaturated dietary fats on absorption, excretion, synthesis, and distribution of cholesterol in man. J Clin Invest 49:1135–1152, 1970
18. Grundy SM: Effects of polyunsturated fats on lipid metabolism in patients with hypertriglyceridemia. J Clin Invest 55:269–282, 1975
19. Grundy SM, Mok HYI, Zech LA et al: Transport of very low density lipoprotein–triglycerides in varying degrees of obesity and hypertriglyceridemia. J Clin Invest 63:1274–1283, 1979
20. Grundy SM: Saturated fats and coronary heart disease. In Winick M (ed): Nutrition and the Killer Diseases, pp 57–78. John Wiley & Sons, 1981
21. Hamilton RL, Williams MC, Fielding CJ et al: Discoidal bilayer structure of nascent high density lipoproteins from perfused rat liver. J Clin Invest 58:667–680, 1976
22. Havel RJ: Familial dysbetalipoproteinemia: New aspects of pathogenesis and diagnosis. In Havel RJ (ed): Medical Clinics of North America on Lipid disorders. Philadelphia, WB Saunders, in press
23. Hegsted DM, McGandy RB, Myers ML et al: Quantitative effects of dietary fat on serum cholesterol in man. Am J Clin Nutr 17:281–295, 1965
24. Heiss G, Tamir I, Davis CE et al: Lipoprotein cholesterol distributions in selected North American populations: The Lipid Research Clinics Program Prevalence Study. Circulation 61:302–315, 1980
25. Hulley SB, Rosenman RH, Bowol RD et al: Epidemiology as a guide to clinical decisions: The association between triglyceride and coronary heart disease. N Engl J Med 302:1383–1389, 1980
26. Kagan A, Harris BR, Winkelstein W Jr et al: Epidemiologic studies of coronary heart disease and stroke in Japanese men living in Japan, Hawaii, and California: Demographic, physical, dietary, and biochemical characteristics. J Chronic Dis 27:345–364, 1974
27. Kesaniemi YA, Grundy SM: The significance of low density lipoprotein production in the regulation of plasma cholesterol levels in man. J Clin Invest 70:13–22, 1982
28. Keys A, Anderson JT, Grande F: Prediction of serum cholesterol responses of man to change in fats in the diet. Lancet 2:959–966, 1957
29. Keys A: Coronary heart disease in seven countries. Circulation (Suppl I) 41:1970
30. Leren P: Effect of plasma cholesterol lowering diet in male survivors of myocardial infarction. A controlled clinical trial. Acta Med Scand (Suppl) 466:1–92, 1966
31. Mattson FH, Erickson BA, Kligman AM: Effect of dietary cholesterol on serum cholesterol in man. Am J Clin Nutr 25:589–594, 1972
32. McGill HC, Geer JC, Strong JP: In Sandler M, Bourne GH (eds): Atherosclerosis and Its Origins. New York, Academic Press, 1963
33. McGill HC Jr: In McGill HC (ed): Geographic Pathology of Atherosclerosis, p 41. Baltimore, Williams & Wilkins, 1968
34. Miall WE, Oldham PD: Factors influencing arterial blood pressure in the general population. Clin Sci 17:409–444, 1958
35. Miettinen M, Turpeninen O, Karvonen MJ et al: Effect of cholesterol-lowering diet on mortality from coronary heart disease and other causes—a twelve-year clinical trial in men and women. Lancet 2:835–838, 1972
36. Murray RH, Luft FC, Block R et al: Blood pressure responses to extremes of sodium intake in normal man. Proc Soc Exp Biol Med 159:432–436, 1978
37. Oliver WJ, Cohen EL, Neel JV: Blood pressure, sodium

intake and sodium related hormones in the Yanomamo Indians, a "no-salt" culture. Circulation 52:146–151, 1975

38. Page LB, Danion A, Moellering RC Jr: Antecedents of cardiovascular disease in six Solomon Island societies. Circulation 49:1132–1146, 1974

39. Pooling Project Research Group: Relationship of blood pressure, serum cholesterol, smoking habit, relative weight and ECG abnormalities to incidence of major coronary events: Final report of the Pooling Project. J Chronic Dis 31:201–306, 1956

40. Shekelle RB, Shyrock AM, Olglesby P et al: Diet, serum cholesterol, and death from coronary heart disease: The Western Electric Study. N Engl J Med 304:65–70, 1981

41. Shepherd J, Packard CJ, Grundy WM et al: Effects of saturated and polyunsaturated fat diets on the chemical composition and metabolism of low density lipoproteins in man. J Lipid Res 21:91–99, 1980

42. Sims EAH, Berchtold P: Obesity and hypertension. JAMA 247:49–52, 1982

43. Small DM: Cellular mechanisms for lipid deposition in atherosclerosis. N Engl J Med 297:873–877, 924–929, 1977

44. Sniderman A, Shapiro S, Marpole D et al: Association of coronary atherosclerosis with hyperapobetalipoproteinemia. Proc Natl Acad Sci USA 77:604–608, 1980

45. Stamler J: Public health aspects of optimal serum lipid–lipoprotein levels. Prev Med 8:733–759, 1979

46. Tall AR, Small DM: Plasma high-density lipoproteins. N Engl J Med 299:1232–1236, 1978

47. West RO, Hayes OB: Diet and serum cholesterol levels—a comparison between vegetarians and nonvegetarians in a Seventh-Day Adventist group. Am J Clin Nutr 21:853–862, 1964

48. Wolf RN, Grundy SM: Effects of caloric restriction on plasma lipids and lipoproteins (abstr). Clin Res 28:55A, 1980

18
Diabetes Mellitus
*Kelly M. West**

Characteristics and Prevalence

The cardinal manifestation of diabetes is hypergly-cemia. Most, if not all, of the pathologic expressions of diabetes are probably attributable to insulin deficiency, either absolute or relative. There are many causes of diabetes, the most important of which are obesity and certain genetic diatheses. Separately or together these genetic and environmental factors lead to decompensation of the pancreatic β cells. Several different genetic attributes may increase susceptibility to diabetes. The genetic factors that increase susceptibility to typical child-hood-onset, insulin-dependent (ID) diabetes seem for the most part different from those that enhance susceptibility to the more common and less severe type of adult-onset, noninsulin-dependent (NID) diabetes. For example, certain histocompatibility antigens are associated with severe ID diabetes but not with the more common type that does not re-quire treatment with insulin. Obesity causes insensitivity to insulin in muscle, fat, and liver. This produces compensatory hyperinsulinism. One to four decades of hyperinsulinism often results in decompensation of β-cell function. Maturity-onset diabetes in obese subjects is typically characterized by mild to moderate hyperglycemia and little pro-

*While on a trip to China, Kelly West was stricken and removed to Hong Kong. He died there on July 29, 1980. Before he left for the Orient, he had sent to the editors his revision of the chapter on diabetes mellitus that he had contributed to the first edition. We are greatly indebted to Edwin L. Bierman, M.D., for his advice in readying for publication what must be among the last written words of our friend, Kelly M. West, M.D.

pensity to ketonemia. Particularly in the early stages of the disease, serum insulin levels of obese diabetics are often in the normal range, but they are seldom as high as in obese nondiabetics. As decompensation progresses, insulin levels frequently become subnormal. Complete β-cell failure is not common in this type of diabetes, but such cases frequently require treatment with insulin after one to two decades of diabetes.

In most affluent Western societies about 70% to 80% of diabetics are of the fat, NID type, while about 5% to 10% are lean ID cases, with little or no endogenous insulin and severe diabetes. About 10% to 20% have other types of diabetes.[18,37] Patients with severe diabetes require insulin therapy for survival because no dietary treatment can adequately control the severe metabolic abnormalities that attend total failure of β-cell function. The most characteristic and immediate expressions of this complete deficit of insulin are severe hypergly-cemia and ketonemia, but many other metabolic abnormalities attend total insulin deficiency, which if unchecked lead to diabetic ketoacidosis, coma, and death. Patients with mild hyperglycemia often have no symptoms. Characteristic symptoms in persons with moderate hyperglycemia include excessive urine (polyuria) and excessive thirst (polydipsia). With severe diabetes, weakness, weight loss, and excessive hunger (polyphagia) occur.

Serum lipid abnormalities are common in both of the main types of diabetes, and rates of atherosclerosis are excessive in all types of diabetes. In North America and Europe a substantial majority of NID cases are obese, but NID diabetes also occurs in lean adults and may be either mild, moderate, or severe. In ID cases, β-cell decompensation is occasionally incomplete in the early stages, resulting in mild diabetes for months or a few years, but severe diabetes usually follows.

Diabetes is among the most common afflictions of modern society. In the United States, rates of known diabetes are about 4% in middle-aged subjects and about 8% in the elderly. The rate in school-age children is roughly 0.1%. In preschool children the disease is even more rare. Roughly 1% of adults under 40 years of age are known to have diabetes. In North American adults the rate of undiscovered diabetes is at least as great as the rate of known diabetes. Diabetes has been diagnosed in about 2% of Americans (all ages).

About one fourth of known diabetics in the United States are being treated with insulin, about half are receiving oral agents, and about one fourth are not receiving any antidiabetic medication. With optimum long-term diet therapy only about 25% would require any kind of medication. The high frequency with which medications are used is largely a reflection of the infrequency with which long-term diet therapy is successfully implemented in obese diabetics.

The major cause of death in American diabetics is coronary disease, which is roughly two to three times more common in diabetics than in nondiabetics. Renal failure secondary to diabetic glomerulosclerosis is the most common cause of death in youth-onset cases. Fatal coronary disease is also common in youth-onset diabetics and now closely rivals glomerulosclerosis as the leading cause of death in this group. In certain age groups diabetes is the leading cause of new cases of blindness. This is mainly the result of diabetic retinopathy, but cataract is also especially common in diabetics. A major cause of morbidity in diabetics is gangrene secondary to occlusive vascular disease. Impaired sensation attributable to diabetic neuropathy is also a frequent contributing factor in the genesis of gangrene. Other frequent manifestations of neuropathy include pain in the extremities, muscle weakness, bladder weakness, or paresis, and, in males, sexual impotence. Diabetic coma is no longer a leading cause of death in diabetics, but death from ketoacidosis is by no means rare.

Many diabetics now live as long with diabetes as they would be expected to live without it. Yet, on the average, life expectancy at onset is still only about half of normal in ID cases and approximately 70% of normal in NID diabetics. There is still considerable uncertainty and controversy about the extent to which various types of therapy affect risk and degree of each of the several major manifestations of diabetes, but most agree that risk of death and morbidity are considerably reduced with well-conceived therapy. It is clear, however, that in preventing long-term complications, clinical modalities currently at hand are not completely effective.

Dietary Factors as Causes of Diabetes

The genetic mechanisms that cause diabetes are still poorly understood, but it has long been evident that hereditary factors are often etiologically important. Until recently the categorization of diabetes as a genetic disorder tended to lower the priority assigned to the study of the importance and character of environmental factors as etiologic agents. Although it seemed that rates of diabetes were different among certain societies, it was commonly thought that these differences were mainly attributable to racial factors. Moreover, it seemed quite possible that some of these differences were more apparent than real because of marked differences among societies in the frequency with which screening and diagnostic tests were performed. It is now clear, however, that environmental factors sometimes exert a profound influence on rates of diabetes. Prior to World War II, for example, it was widely believed that diabetes was common in Jews and rare in American Indians, but more recent studies have shown that in each of these races rates of diabetes vary as much as tenfold depending on environmental circumstances. These marked intraracial variations in rates of diabetes have also been confirmed in whites and blacks.[37] In general, recent epidemiologic evidence suggests that economic, cultural, and other environmental circumstances are more important than race in determining risk of adult-onset diabetes.[37]

Several considerations suggest that diet may play a very important role in determining susceptibility to diabetes. In adults, rates of diabetes are closely related to adiposity, both among and within populations.[37] Among populations there is an imperfect but general association between rates of diabetes and levels of consumption of fat.[37] It is not yet certain, however, to what degree this latter association is causal. Our studies in 12 populations show a decidedly negative correlation between starch consumption and prevalence of diabetes in adults.[37] This evidence does not necessarily mean that eating starch prevents diabetes but does suggest strongly that eating starch does not in itself incite diabetes, and it is possible that insofar as risk of diabetes is concerned, starch may be one of the most innocuous of the major foodstuffs. Generally speaking, societies with high protein intakes have high rates of diabetes, but certain exceptions suggest that this correlation may be coincidental. For example, in rural Uruguay, where protein consumption is high, diabetes is infrequent, and diabetes is also quite rare among primitive Eskimos, whose diets are very high in protein.[36]

In several populations, rising levels of sugar consumption have been attended by rising rates of diabetes. This has led some scientists to suspect sugar consumption as a cause of diabetes.[13] However, most epidemiologic evidence is negative in this respect.[9,23,37] In several populations no relationship has been found between sugar consumption and risk of diabetes.[37] The Pima Indians have extremely high rates of diabetes despite levels of dietary sugar that were considerably lower than those of the general United States population.

Diabetes rates have been low in many populations where fiber intake is high, but exceptions to this negative relationship have been observed. Diabetes and obesity are rife in Pima Indians despite a high-fiber diet, and diabetes is rare in primitive Eskimo tribes on diets with very little fiber.

Adiposity is the most important of the many factors that contribute to the genesis of diabetes in adults. In several populations the greater rates of diabetes in females were explained entirely by their greater adiposity.[37] After adjusting for fatness, interracial differences were slight. In two of these populations the association of parity and diabetes was probably also attributable to the greater fatness of the multiparous women. Although dietary factors undoubtedly have considerable importance in determining risk of obesity, it also seems likely that physical indolence plays a major role in the genesis of both obesity and diabetes.[37] Epidemiologic studies in diabetes are often rather difficult to interpret in some respects because certain variables tend to change simultaneously. In most societies where rates of diabetes have increased dramatically, sugar consumption has risen sharply, but usually there also has been a rise in fat consumption together with a decline in exercise and a rise in adiposity. This is true, for example, among certain East Indians, American Indians, Eskimos, and Polynesians, in each of which groups rates of diabetes have risen sharply.

Although fatness and family history of diabetes are in most societies the principal risk factors in NID diabetes, there are several other important etiologic agents. Keen and associates studied a group of fat African females in whom diabetes was uncommon.[23] Several possible explanations for this include genetic factors, relatively high levels of exercise (unusual but possible in obesity), and a relatively short duration of obesity (duration of obesity was not known in this latter group). In every lean society in which data are available, diabetes

has been uncommon. In several societies excessive consumption of iron leading to hemochromatosis is a major cause of diabetes (*e.g.,* in parts of Ghana and in certain Bantu communities). In most of the affluent societies in which diabetes rates are high, pancreatitis is a significant, but not a major, factor in producing the high rates. However, in a few lean societies where alcohol consumption is very high (*e.g.,* certain communities in Africa), pancreatitis is a leading cause of diabetes. In some disadvantaged communities of India and Africa a substantial portion of diabetes is the result of pancreatic disease associated with pancreatic fibrosis and calcification in persons who are not alcoholic. The etiology of this pancreatic disease is uncertain, but it may have its roots in nutritional deprivations of childhood and toxicity from high levels of consumption of cassava (tapioca) or other foods containing cyanide. In this type of diabetes, symptoms of diabetes typically began in adolescence or early adult life, but clinical diabetes is often antedated by other signs of exocrine pancreatic disease. Under some circumstances deprivation of certain trace metals (*e.g.,* chromiun and zinc) may have unfavorable effects on glucose tolerance. It is not yet certain, however, whether such deficiencies play a significant role in determining risk of clinical diabetes.

The extent to which nutritional factors influence risk of typical ID diabetes is not clear. Because this disorder is relatively uncommon, it has been difficult to gather and interpret epidemiologic data. It does seem that ID diabetes is substantially more common in North American than in Japan (the difference may be as much as fivefold). ID diabetes is also rare in rural Africa and India. Nutritional factors may or may not contribute to these geographic differences. Racial factors are an important determinant of susceptibility to this type of diabetes.

Nutritional Factors and the Manifestations of Diabetes

There is now considerable evidence that nutritional factors also play an important role in determining risk of certain complications of diabetes. In most affluent societies the major cause of death of diabetics is coronary disease. In both primitive and affluent societies, diabetics have more coronary disease than nondiabetics. Even so, clinical coronary disease is uncommon among diabetics in many underprivileged societies. The relative importance of various factors in enhancing rates of coronary disease among diabetics is not yet established. Among the possibilities is the unfavorable effect of diabetes on serum lipids.[37] Although both cholesterol and triglyceride levels in the serum are often within the normal range in individual diabetics, cholesterol levels tend to be somewhat higher in diabetics, and serum triglycerides are decidedly higer. There is a very impressive association in groups of diabetics between coronary disease and consumption of saturated fat.[37] In the multinational study of the World Health Organization it was found that coronary disease was several times more common in the diabetics of North American and European populations than in the diabetics of certain Asian populations.[22]

Under certain conditions the feeding of carbohydrate leads to elevations of fasting serum triglyceride levels. Also, in some studies the risk of coronary disease seems to be affected by serum triglyceride values. On the other hand, elevations in triglyceride levels produced by increasing dietary carbohydrates tend to decline with time unless calories are excessive. Moreover, prevalence of coronary disease in diabetics is generally lowest in societies where starch consumption is high.[37] For example, in Nigeria and Japan, both diabetics and nondiabetics derive a substantial majority of calories from starch, and coronary disease in diabetics is much less common than in diabetics of North America or Western Europe. Triglyceride levels are low in Japan and in certain Micronesian societies despite high starch diets.[30,35] Simpson and associates fed high-starch diets to diabetics with no unfavorable effects on serum triglyceride levels.

This and other evidence suggest that (1) serum triglyceride levels are in the long run much more responsive to calories than to starch itself; and (2) the very high rates of coronary disease in the diabetics of affluent Western societies are not the inevitable result of genetic diabetes, or even of hyperglycemia.[29] Rather, risk of coronary disease in diabetes is markedly affected by dietary factors. This does not exclude the possibility that risk of coronary disease may relate to intensity of hyperglycemia under certain conditions. However, in some circumstances coronary artery disease is uncommon even when hyperglycemia is considerable. In the World Health Organization study, rates of coronary disease were low in Asian diabetics, even among those with fasting plasma glucose values that were considerably elevated. Oklahoma Indians with mild hyperglycemia had much higher rates of coronary disease than Tokyo diabetics with moderate or severe hyperglycemia.[40] Saturated fat consumption was almost three times as great in Oklahoma as in Tokyo.

Diabetics also have more cerebral atherosclerosis than nondiabetics. Rates of cerebral thrombosis are about twice as common in diabetics as in nondiabetics. Vascular disease of the lower extremity is very greatly enhanced in diabetics. It is quite likely that some of the same factors discussed above account for increased amounts of atherosclerosis in large- and medium-sized arteries of the head and legs in diabetics. For example, gangrene is relatively uncommon in diabetics of Japan.[37,40] Studies of rates of clinical atherosclerosis in diabetics of various American Indian communities also suggest strongly the possibility that nutritional factors contribute significantly to the genesis of these lesions. Risk of cerebrovascular disease in diabetes in some circumstances may relate more to dietary sodium than to cholesterol or animal fat consumption. Stroke is less common in diabetics of North America than in diabetics of certain Japanese communities where sodium intake is very high.

Evidence is less impressive that risk and extent of diabetic microvascular disease are influenced by qualitative features of diet (*e.g.*, proportion of calories as carbohydrate). To the extent that diet is capable of mitigating hyperglycemia, it may reduce rates at which these lesions develop. In certain animals, for example, it has been shown that control of hyperglycemia produces favorable effects on the degree of nephropathy and retinopathy.[31] However, when groups of diabetics from populations observing diets that differ qualitatively are compared, differences in rates of microvascular disease are generally less than differences in atherosclerosis. In diabetics of Japan, for example, the rates and extent of microvascular disease seem to be similar to those observed in Western societies. As will be indicated below, dietary strategies other than carbohydrate restriction are important in controlling hyperglycemia. Under certain conditions, restriction of dietary fat may significantly improve retinal exudates, but immediate improvement of other manifestations of retinopathy is uncommon with diet therapy.

Ketosis seems to be peculiarly uncommon in the lean diabetics of certain societies. The reasons for this are incompletely understood. Probably dietary factors play a role, (*e.g.*, low levels of dietary saturated fat, paucity of body fat, and peculiarities of fat-cell function secondary to extreme nutritional deprivations of infancy). Little is known about the effect of diet on diabetic neuropathy, although some recent evidence suggests that the degree of hyperglycemia enhances at least some aspects of these pathologic changes in nerve tissue. Neuropathy seems to be quite common, however, in groups of diabetics observing diets that differ qualitatively widely (*e.g.*, Nigeria, Asia, and North America). Clements has observed improvement of neuropathy after increasing dietary myoinositol.[16]

It is of great importance that several groups of genetically susceptible individuals have largely escaped both diabetes and its vascular lesions. The microvascular lesions of diabetes are rife in certain communities of Jews, other whites, blacks, Indians, and American Indians.[37] However, when these races are protected by environmental and social conditions from developing hyperglycemia, they also escape the microvascular lesions. This epidemiologic evidence lends no support to the hypothesis that these microvascular lesions are independent of hyperglycemia, but rather suggests that prevention and control of hyperglycemia have potential for prevention and mitigation of these microvascular lesions. Thus, diet modification has great potential for preventing and ameliorating not only diabetes but also certain of its complications.

Diet Therapy

PRINCIPLES, OBJECTIVES, AND STRATEGIES

The history of concepts and practice of diet therapy has been reviewed in an interesting essay by Wood and Bierman.[42] Principles of modern therapy have been promulgated recently by the Nutrition Committee of the American Diabetes Association.[3] Good reviews of this subject include those of Reaven and co-workers and Ensinck and Bierman.[17,27]

Four therapeutic goals may be listed. The applicability and priority of each of these four objectives

in individual patients vary considerably, as will be explained below. Dietary objectives may include (1) reversal of the diabetic state toward or to normal with improvement in glucose tolerance and β-cell reserve, and amelioration of resistance to insulin; (2) mitigation and regulation of hyperglycemia, including the control of symptoms of diabetes, and prevention and therapy of hypoglycemia; (3) prevention or reduction in progression of certain complications of diabetes (*e.g.,* vascular disease, neuropathy, cataract, and ketosis), control of which both hyperglycemia and hyperlipidemia play a role; and (4) management of certain complications of diabetes (*e.g.,* pregnancy, renal failure, and hypertension). In typical obese patients the strategy with greatest potential for achieving the first three objectives is reduction of the excessive fat tissue. Table 18-1 contrasts objectives and strategies in the two most common types of diabetes.

EFFECTIVENESS AND FEASIBILITY OF DIET THERAPY

For centuries there has been controversy about dietary strategies and the extent to which any diet therapy is effective. There have been disagreements among authorities for at least several decades concerning what priority should be assigned to the limitation of starch and sugar. It has long been evident that the diabetic liver can readily make sugar

TABLE 18-1
Dietary Strategies for the Two Main Types of Diabetes*

Dietary Strategy	Obese Patients Who do not Require Insulin	Insulin-dependent Nonobese Patients
Decrease calories	Yes	No
Protect or improve β-cell function	Very urgent priority	Seldom important (β-cells usually extinct)
Increase frequency and number of feedings	Usually not†	Yes
Day-to-day consistency in intake of calories, carbohydrate, protein, and fat	Not crucial if average caloric intake remains in low range	Very important
Day-to-day consistency in ratios of carbohydrate, protein, and fat for each feeding‡	Not crucial	Desirable
Consistency in timing meals	Not crucial	Very important
Extra food for unusual exercise	Not usually appropriate	Usually appropriate
Use of food to treat, abort, or prevent hypoglycemia	Not necessary	Important
During complicating illness provide small, frequent feedings or IV CHO to prevent starvation ketosis	Often not necessary because of resistance to ketosis	Important

*Adapted from West KM: Ann Intern Med 79:425–434, 1973

†There are some theoretic advantages in dividing the diet into four or five feedings even in mild diabetes if this can be done without increasing caloric consumption. However, because limitation of calories has highest priority in obese diabetics, there are potential disadvantages in providing extra feedings. Giving fat people an opportunity to eat at bedtime is particularly risky if weight reduction is the primary goal.

‡The total daily insulin requirement is apparently not much affected when dietary constituents are changed under isocaloric conditions, but insulin requirement immediately after a high-carbohydrate meal is higher than immediately after a low-carbohydrate meal, even if the meal is isocaloric.

out of noncarbohydrate foodstuffs and that over-production of glucose plays a major role in maintaining hyperglycemia. This and other evidence led many to doubt the usefulness of limiting carbohydrates when they are entirely replaced with other calories.

Soon after the discovery of insulin a freely chosen diet was advocated by a few in lean patients with ID diabetes. In the 1940s, several groups advocated *free diet, unrestricted diet,* and *liberal diet,* basing their recommendations on several considerations and opinions. Some doubted that traditional diet therapy was effective in preventing the long-term complicatons of diabetes. Most who advocated free diet also argued that the vascular lesions of diabetes were probably unrelated to the degree of glycemia. They also pointed out that most patients didn't follow their prescribed diets. Some thought that conventional diets were often onerous and that under certain conditions ID diabetics observing traditional restrictive diets might be more susceptible to insulin reactions than those on less formal regimens. Studies by Knowles also cast doubt on whether certain traditional diets for ID diabetes were any more effective than less complex regimens similar to the normal diet.

Some well-qualified scholars still believe it appropriate to assume that moderate hyperglycemia is innocent until proven guilty. Most, however, believe that the possibility of guilt is sufficiently great to warrant attempts to mitigate hyperglycemia even in asymptomatic patients.[41] All agree that modest hyperglycemia is preferable to severe hypoglycemia, and most do not believe that the theoretic risks of minimal asymptomatic hyperglycemia warrant making life a perpetual and rigid metabolic clinic. There also is disagreement about the degree of danger attending hypoglycemic episodes that may be produced by aggressive therapy in lean insulin-treated patients.

Yet an increasing body of evidence suggests that hyperglycemia and its attendant metabolic aberrations may be noxious to small vessels, nerves, and perhaps to large arteries. Rates at which cataracts develop seem to be affected by degree of glycemia, but it is not clear at what level this untoward effect begins. Under certain conditions mitigation of hyperglycemia may improve glucose tolerance and protect overstrained β-cells from exhaustion. Diabetes may sometimes, in fact, be entirely reversed, with return of glucose tolerance to normal. Thus, to the extent that diet modification can ameliorate hyperglycemia, this is a useful objective, although by no means the only purpose of diet therapy. Among the arguments for dietary mitigation of hyperglycemia are the favorable effects on serum lipids induced by control of the blood glucose. The degree and character of these effects depend on many factors, but control of hyperglycemia often lowers cholesterol levels (to varying degrees) while regularly and substantially lowering serum triglycerides.[19]

Not surprisingly, physicians who know little about dietary strategies and techniques are more likely to doubt the feasibility and effectiveness of dietary measures in controlling hyperglycemia or reducing morbidity. It is well established that diet therapy of diabetes is ineffective when carried out clumsily and without enthusiasm, and there is considerable evidence that most diabetics do not follow their diet prescriptions very well. This raises the question as to whether effective diet therapy is really feasible. Under certain conditions, however, patients do follow their prescriptions, and measurable clinical benefits have been observed.[3,25,30]

Although certain areas of controversy remain, better understanding of the nature of diabetes and its complications has tended to mitigate the previous disagreements. Most of the previous controversy was based on poor definition and understanding of the issues. There is now, for example, better understanding of the very substantial differences between the dietary principles in the two main types of diabetes (see Table 18-1). No disagreement remains about the potentially great effectiveness of limiting calories in obese NID diabetics. Although some authorities still believe that carbohydrate restriction may have a favorable effect unrelated to its effect on caloric intake, most now give little priority to starch restriction in obese diabetics except as it may relate incidentally to caloric restriction. Thus, there is now a wide consensus that in this type of diabetes the prime objective is caloric restriction, irrespective of sources of calories. The importance of distinguishing between the diet prescription and the actual diet is now more widely appreciated. The failure of diet therapy to affect outcome is mainly attributable to the infrequency with which patients follow their prescriptions.[34]

Some of the previous arguments are due in part to semantic problems and misunderstandings concerning definitions. Most patients on so-called free diets, for example, were actually observing dietary modifications of varying degree. These often included proscribing or limiting intake of refined sugars and, in the case of ID patients, dividing feedings into more than three meals, or eating regularly at scheduled times. High rates of atherosclerosis in patients on conventional *strict* diets are probably attributable in part to the fact that these strict diets have not usually been strict in their allowance of cholesterol and animal fat. Rather, by limiting carbohydrate they have tended to increase consumption of fat and cholesterol. ID diabetics who have been told to follow unimaginative and impractical strict regimens often have a greater fluctuation from day to day in their actual eating patterns than certain patients who "follow no diet." ID diabetics who like their assigned diets are more likely to follow them regularly; and those on rigid diets often follow them carefully—part of the time. Sugar consumption is usually reduced in these strict or rigid prescriptions, but a major objective (achieving consistency of intake) is often frustrated. It is not evident that, in controlling blood–glucose levels of ID patients, regulation and predictability of diet are more important than proscription of any specific food items. Another problem is that there has been no unanimity about definitions of popular terms and expressions, such as "careful diet," "watch your diet," "strict diet," or "diabetic diet," but for the most part these expressions have been strongly associated with proscription and deprivation of carbohydrates. In ID patients, the need to trade food items imaginatively and to adjust continuously to the vagaries of exercise, illness, or work schedules suggests that the term *dietary regulation* fits the appropriate regimen better than terms such as *rigid diet* or *strict diet*. In formulating the diet prescription, the physician should keep in mind that the coronary arteries of Asian and African diabetics who were never seen by a physician or a dietitian usually look much better than those of patients in the United States who have had the "advantage" of traditional "diabetic diets" of the past.

In obese NID diabetics, diet has potential not only for controlling diabetes, but also for actually reversing the disease. Reduction in adiposity improves sensitivity to insulin and usually improves glucose tolerance and β-cell function. Diet only rarely returns glucose tolerance to normal, but the infrequency of this accomplishment is mainly the result of the rarity with which substantial and sustained weight reduction is achieved in these obese patients. It seems likely that complete reversal of diabetes would be commonplace if a substantial percentage of obese patients were able to lose all or most of their excess adiposity. Early in the course of obesity-related diabetes, abnormalities of insulin secretion and glucose tolerance are regularly corrected entirely by reversal of obesity.[25,28] Although successful treatment of obesity is uncommon, it is clear that under certain circumstances very significant rates of success have been achieved.[15,19] Amelioration of obesity also tends to normalize serum lipids of diabetics. In view of the profoundly beneficial effects of weight reduction in obese diabetics, a rather substantial effort is often justified. The management of obesity is reviewed in Chapter 28.

FORMULATING THE PRESCRIPTION

Tables 18-1 and 18-2 and the following list suggest many of the considerations that apply in developing, implementing, and adjusting the dietary prescription. Among the determinations to be made are the total number of calories; the characteristics and amounts of the specific foods to be allowed, encouraged, limited, or avoided; the number, characteristics, and relative sizes of the various feedings; and the timing of these feedings. The following check list may aid dietitians and physicians in formulating and implementing a diet prescription for a specific patient:[34]

1. In order of priority, what are the main general purposes (not strategies or methods) of this patient's prescription?
2. How much should the patient weigh? How much do the doctor, the dietitian, and the patient think he should weigh? How much would the patient like to weigh?
3. What is the appropriate level of caloric consumption for this patient?
4. Does the patient require insulin? If so, is the blood glucose relatively stable, moderately labile, or severely labile? What kind of insulin is to be given, at what time, in what amounts?
5. What and when and how much would the patient like to eat if he did not have diabetes? Are there any special considerations relating to economic factors or to family or cultural dietary propensities?
6. Is the level of carbohydrate to be fixed? To what level or range? To what extent and under what conditions, if any, are concentrated carbohydrates to be used?
7. Are there special requirements concerning levels of protein?
8. Are there any specific or general requirements with respect to levels of dietary fat, either saturated or unsaturated? Dietary fiber?
9. How much alcohol is to be permitted? Under what conditions? Should alcohol be exchanged for another food? If so, what kind and in what amounts?
10. If time distribution of food is of any importance, are there specific requirements concerning (1) the relative size and timing of each of the three main meals and (2) the timing, size and characteristics of any extra feedings?
11. To what degree is day-to-day consistency required in (1) total calories and (2) size and characteristics of specific feedings, such as lunch?
12. Are dietary adjustments to be made for exercise or marked glycosuria? Of what nature?

TABLE 18-2
Distribution of Major Nutrients in Normal and Diabetic Diets (as percentages of total calories)

	*Starch and Other Polysaccharides** *(%)*	*Sugars† and Dextrins* *(%)*	*Fat* *(%)*	*Protein* *(%)*	*Alcohol* *(%)*
Typical American diet	25–35	20–30	35–45 p:s ratio 1:3#	12–19	0–10
Traditional diabetic diets	25–30	10–15‡	40–45	16–21	0
Newer diabetic diets	35–45§	5–15‡	25–35§ p:s ratio 1:1#	12–23	0–6

*Almost all of these calories are starch, but complex carbohydrates also include cellulose, hemicellulose, pentosans, and pectin

†Monosaccharides and disaccharides, mainly sucrose, but also includes fructose, glucose, lactose, and maltose

‡Almost exclusively natural sugars, mainly in fruit and milk (lactose)

§The ideal diet is probably even higher in starch and lower in saturated fat, but in typical affluent Western Societies it is usually not feasible to achieve higher ratios of starch to fat than that shown on the bottom line of this table.

#Polyunsaturated:saturated (fatty acids)

13. Are there any special conditions unrelated to diabetes requiring diet modification (*e.g.*, gout, hyperlipidemia, and renal or cardiac failure)?
14. Can all elements of the prescription be reconciled, and how should this be done? (*E.g.*, it is usually not feasible to construct a palatable diet for a lean diabetic if the prescription calls for a diet that restricts both carbohydrate and fat.)
15. What kinds and what degree of changes are to be made subsequently by the dietitian without consulting the physician?
16. What should this patient do if he finds it necessary to postpone or modify a meal (*e.g.*, at a dinner meeting or social affair)? How should he adjust diet if his appetite fails (*e.g.*, during illness)?
17. The following tactical questions should be considered: (1) How much precision is required in the various elements of this prescription? (2) What foods can be freely allowed? (3) What foods, if any, are to be weighed or measured? (4) Are any modifications of the standard exchange system appropriate, such as simplification? (5) In general, is food to be unmeasured, estimated, measured, or weighed? (6) Is it necessary or desirable to teach this patient the carbohydrate, protein, and fat content of the common foods? (7) Under what circumstances are artificial or nutritive sweeteners and diet drinks to be used?
18. Has this patient's understanding of dietary principles and methods been systematically evaluated?

CALORIES

Caloric requirements of the prescription vary considerably depending on factors such as the weight, desirable weight, and activity of the patient. It is not urgent that a precise determination be made initially of level of calories to be prescribed. An estimate can be made, with subsequent appropriate adjustments on the basis of experience. Elsewhere in this book more detailed information may be found, relative to the assessment of caloric requirement. A few simple generalizations may be helpful. A typical young man weighing 70 kg (154 lb) who is moderately active requires about 2800 Cal/day (40 Cal/kg). While relatively inactive (*e.g.*, ambulatory, but hospitalized), he may require as few as 2100 Cal/day (30 Cal/kg). Men of this size who habitually engage in heavy exercise may require as much as 3500 Cal/day (50 Cal/kg). A typical young woman weighing 58 kg (128 lb) who is moderately active requires about 2000 Cal/day. Older patients usually require somewhat less in relation to body size. Children under 12 years of age require an average of 1000 Cal/day plus 100 Cal/day/year of age. Thus, a 7-year-old child would require roughly 1700 Cal/day. Because sizes and activity levels vary considerably in children of the same age, the formula above should be used only as a crude guideline.

A strategy commonly employed is to prescribe a number of calories somewhat less than the number intended for consumption under the assumption that there is a natural tendency to eat a bit more than the amount prescribed. In ID patients this is undesirable because it often leads to irregularity of intake. Underprescription of calories is also common when estimates are based mainly on the new diabetic's description of his normal diet. There is a general tendency toward underestimation, even by nonobese patients. The main reason for this is that many tend to underestimate the calories taken outside their typical meals (*e.g.*, alcohol, soft drinks, sugar and cream in coffee, candy, large meals on special occasions). New, lean diabetics often feel at first that the prescribed diet is generous or even excessive because foods high in calories (sugar and fat) are replaced by many foods that are less concentrated in calories, and because consumption of calories is now confined to prescribed feedings. In lean patients an initial prescription that is generous helps to make the point that the main objective is regulation rather than deprivation. In lean patients, satiety, appetite, and hunger are usually reliable guides to the caloric requirements; body weight is, of course, the definitive long-term guide.

Obese patients may, according to circumstances, be given prescriptions ranging from total starvation to as much as 2000 Cal/day, but long-term reduction diets typically provide 1000 Cal/day to 1400 Cal/day. These allotments should be raised when and if weight approaches an optimum level. Caloric requirements of obese patients are well related to weight, but these patients are usually less active than lean persons. In most, weight maintenance requires roughly 30 Cal/kg to 35 Cal/kg. If they are understood and followed, prescriptions of about 15 Cal/kg to 20 Cal/kg provide the desired weight reduction. Increasing exercise will, of course, be helpful.

SIZE, DISTRIBUTION, AND TIMING OF FEEDINGS

Typical diet prescriptions provide about 25% to 35% of total calories as lunch, 25% to 35% as supper, 10% to 30% as breakfast, and 0% to 25% as between-meal snacks. In most patients, allowances of some degree can be made for the preferences and life-style of the patient before fixing the distribution scheme. In ID patients consistency of timing and distribution have considerable priority, but there is usually some flexibility of alternatives in determining the distribution pattern to be regularly followed. For example, a farmer who prefers or requires an early breakfast of generous size may be given a greater portion of his daily allotment as breakfast (*e.g.,* as much as 30%). Such adjustments are often made possible by the substantial number of available alternatives in tactics of insulin therapy. The ID diabetic who prefers a small breakfast may receive a smaller dose of plain quick-acting insulin before breakfast or no rapidly-acting insulin at that time. Some persons who prefer or need a larger breakfast may be given a larger dose of the quick-acting insulin before breakfast, or the insulin may be given 30 min to 40 min before breakfast instead of 10 min to 30 min before eating. Patients who eat breakfast late and take no quick-acting insulin may do well with a small breakfast.

Most ID patients are more effectively treated when they have two to three snacks and smaller main meals. In ID patients, regular ingestion of a mid-afternoon snack often facilitates a better fit with the time–action characteristics of the intermediate-acting insulins, such as NPH or Lente. Occasionally, however, the midafternoon feeding may not be necessary (*e.g.,* when lunch is large or when the time interval between lunch and supper is relatively short). It is crucial that the character of these snacks fit the circumstances under which the patient is supposed to consume them. One may ask the patient, for example, if a coffee break is traditional in the afternoon at his place of employment, and what kinds of foods or drinks are most appealing and readily available on these occasions. When other options are cumbersome, it may be appropriate occasionally in an ID patient to prescribe modest amounts of concentrated carbohydrate on these occasions (*e.g.,* a doughnut, soft drink, or even sugar in coffee or tea). Of prime importance in ID patients is that these feedings be predictable in their size, timing, and general characteristics. If the patient consumed 8 ounces of a soft drink containing 27 g sugar at 3 p.m. on a regular and predictable basis, it would be much better than if he consumed irregularly a more conventional but less convenient snack. When the snacks are well suited to the patient's tastes and schedules, they are likely to become a pleasant habit and, therefore, a dependable element of the therapeutic program. This again introduces the point, often unappreciated, that the dietary objectives in lean, ID diabetics are regulation and consistency of distribution, not proscription and deprivation. Many of these patients and some physicians have erroneously concluded that the main point of the diet is to eat as little carbohydrate as possible. Table 18-1 outlines considerations concerning the temporal distribution of feedings in typical obese, NID diabetics. Usually snacks are unnecessary.

CARBOHYDRATES, FATS, AND PROTEINS

Table 18-2 shows the distribution of the major nutrients in traditional diets for diabetes, and compares this to the typical American diet and the "modernized" diet for diabetes. Until recently, carbohydrate restriction usually received priority in the dietary management of diabetes. As a matter of fact, the most widely used standard diets in America and Europe still recognize this priority. In 1950 the American Diabetes Association was joined by the American Dietetic Association and the United States Public Health Service in promulgating standard diets, all of which were low in carbohydrates and high in fats. Although a change in these standards has been endorsed recently by these agencies, the old diets are still in wide use. The Nutrition Committee of the American Diabetes Association, however, issued informational statements in 1971 and 1979 calling attention to the disadvantages of standard diabetic diets that are high in fat.[3] The 1979 publication also points out that when calories are controlled at appropriate levels, diets high in carbohydrate are well tolerated by diabetics. Several recent reports provide evidence indicating that insulin requirement is more closely related to caloric intake than to carbohydrate intake.[3,11,30,33] One of the reasons for this is the excellent capability of the diabetic liver for manufacturing glucose from a variety of noncarbohydrate sources. In some circumstances blood glucose levels have been lower on high-carbohydrate diets than on isocaloric traditional diets.

Indeed, under certain conditions, even high-sugar diets are well tolerated by diabetics.[10,11] However, several considerations have led most authorities to recommend that simple sugars (mono- or disaccharides) be proscribed or sharply limited in diabetic diets. When ingested in large amounts (*e.g.*, greater than 20 g), sugars tend to produce sharp elevations of the blood glucose, although these elevations tend to be evanescent when calories are appropriately limited.

On the other hand, high-starch diets are very well tolerated when calorie intake is appropriately controlled.[30] In obese patients who refuse to limit calories, fasting serum triglycerides tend to be higher when starch or sugar is substituted for much of the fat in equicaloric amounts. These elevations may abate with time, but they may persist to varying degrees, particularly if caloric intake remains excessive. However, postprandial triglyceride levels are usually higher when fat is substituted for carbohydrate.[29] Epidemiologic evidence has been cited earlier suggesting the favorable effects of high-starch, low-fat diabetic diets on both serum triglyceride levels and vascular disease. When calories are appropriately controlled, serum triglyceride levels of diabetics are no higher on high-starch diets than on traditional diets low in starch and carbohydrate.[30]

These considerations have led to the development of a ''modernized'' dietary regimen for diabetics of Western societies (see Table 18-2). About half of the calories of such diets are derived from carbohydrates, mainly starch. A small amount of sugar remains, principally as fruit, fruit juice, or milk lactose. These diets provide as much or more starch (*e.g.*, bread, cereals, vegetables) than the traditional American diets of nondiabetics. About 30% of calories are derived from fat. It is usually feasible to limit saturated fat (*e.g.*, meat, milk, eggs) to about one third of total fat (10% of total calories). The remaining two thirds of this fat can be derived from polyunsaturates (*e.g.*, vegetable oils, special margarines) and from monosaturates (*e.g.*, nuts, poultry fat, olive oil) in approximately equal amounts. This contrasts with the typical American diet (about 40% fat, of which about half is saturated). Limitation of saturated fat also tends to limit, incidentally, cholesterol consumption. Eggs are a particularly rich source of cholesterol. In some persons, limiting or eliminating the habitual consumption of eggs in itself substantially reduces total cholesterol consumption. Special egglike products free of cholesterol are now widely available. Most patients find it possible to reduce animal fat intake by 50% or more without making sacrifices they consider particularly onerous, provided they are allowed to participate in the consideration of alternatives. Appendix Table A-24 shows amounts of cholesterol and amounts and types of fatty acids in specific foods. In many patients, saturated fat intake can be reduced considerably by simply proscribing or limiting fried foods, or just by trimming most of the visible fat from meat. Another alternative attractive to some is frying in polyunsaturated oil. Several studies have demonstrated the feasibility and effectiveness of dietary measures in reducing serum lipid levels of diabetics, including in juveniles.[7,30]

Proteins usually provide about 17% to 20% of calories in these newer diabetic diets, but lower and higher amounts may be appropriate. In most adults a much smaller intake of protein, as low as 0.9 g/kg/day, would suffice, but the necessity to control fat intake and limit sugar tends to raise the level of protein in the diet. Patients who trim all gross fat from meat and those who eat leaner meat (*e.g.*, fowl and fish) often find it feasible and desirable to consume more protein to replace the calories in the fat contained in ordinary cuts of meat from which fat has not been trimmed. The old standard meat exchange of 1 ounce (see below) contains an average of 7 g protein and 5 g fat, while an ounce of very lean meat may contain as much as 9 g protein and as little as 2 g fat. In some patients, who find meat protein and certain polyunsaturates too expensive, starch can usually be substituted to replace much of the energy previously derived from sugar and fat. The mistaken notion that diabetic diets are necessarily expensive is based largely on the outmoded concept that starch is bad for diabetics and must be replaced with more expensive foods, such as meat and dairy products. Moreover, the protein requirement of adult diabetics is usually far below the amounts in the old standard diets. Protein consumption should, however, exceed 1.5 g/kg daily in children and in pregnant and lactating women (see Chaps. 29 and 32).

FIBER

High-fiber diets have recently been advocated for several reasons: (1) because of potentially favorable effects in preventing or treating conditions other than diabetes (*e.g.*, diverticulosis, hyperlipoproteinemia, colon cancer), (2) because of the possibility that such diets might reduce caloric intake, (3) because certain fibers may mitigate postprandial surges of hyperglycemia, and (4) because some believe that high-fiber diets may reduce insulin requirements.[6]

The purported benefits of high-fiber diet in diabetes have, in some circumstances, been attributable to changes in other dietary characteristics that have attended such diets (*e.g.*, higher levels of carbohydrate and lower levels of fat). Marked differences exist in the effects of different kinds of fiber. It is quite true, however, that certain fibers can reduce the rate of absorption of dietary carbohydrates. Pima Indians are very obese despite a high-fiber diet. The feasibility, acceptability, and utility of using fiber to improve control of diabetes and obesity remain to be established, but diets high in fiber are now commonly recommended.

Since the metabolism of alcohol does not require insulin, it would appear to offer some theoretic advantages in the diet therapy of diabetes. There are, however, several disadvantages. Alcohol is high in calories (7.1 Cal/g) and devoid of nutritional value, except as a source of calories. It frequently tends to promote hypertriglyceridemia. In some patients who take a sulfonylurea (particularly chlorpropamide), alcohol produces distressing symptoms, which include palpitation and flushing. The mechanism of these reactions is incompletely understood, but the symptoms are similar in some respects to those produced by the combination of alcohol and disulfiram (Antabuse). In fasting ID patients, alcohol in large amounts may precipitate hypoglycemia by abetting insulin in reducing liver glucose output, and this hypoglycemia may be unrecognized because symptoms are attributed to intoxication. Many alcoholic drinks (*e.g.*, beer and wine) also contain appreciable amounts of carbohydrate in amounts that may or may not be known and taken into account by the patient. The direct and indirect effects of alcohol on glucose tolerance under various circumstances are still incompletely understood, as are its indirect effects on insulin requirement. In some patients, alcohol is more difficult to ration and to regulate predictably than other

foods. Not infrequently, alcohol consumption is attended by irregularities in the timing of the regular feedings and of their amounts and characteristics.

Even so, in most patients an occasional drink can be permitted. A convenient method is to trade fat calories for alcohol calories. One advantage of this is to demonstrate how high in calories alcoholic drinks are (one drink equals 15 g–20 g fat or three to four fat exchanges). The use of alcohol in therapeutic diets has been the subject of a recent review.[38]

VITAMINS AND MINERALS

Special vitamin and mineral supplements are not ordinarily required. Diets of the type described above usually supply all nutritional requirements. There are a few exceptions. Very fat persons who consume diets containing less than 1000 Cal over a long period may need supplemental nutrients on a temporary basis. Poor patients on high-starch, low-fat, low-protein diets may at times require supplements, such as iron or additional calcium. Profound hyperglycemia over long periods can lead to nutritional deficits, including negative nitrogen balance and muscle wasting. Vitamin supplements, including thiamin and vitamin B_{12}, have frequently been given in the hope they might ameliorate diabetic neuropathy, but there is no evidence suggesting that they are effective. However, diabetics with diarrhea secondary to pancreatitis or diabetic neuropathy may require vitamin and mineral (*e.g.*, calcium) supplements. Feeding myoinositol may help neuropathy.[16] It has been suggested that metabolic aberrations of diabetes might lead to an increased need for ascorbic acid, a relative deficiency of which might contribute to the development of the microvascular lesions. However, this has been offered only as a hypothesis and not as a recommendation for therapy. There is no direct evidence at present that supplemental vitamin C is helpful in this respect. Profound deficiencies of potassium, chromium, and zinc have been associated with impairment of glucose tolerance, but replacement of these elements is seldom necessary as a regular part of the diabetic diet.

ADJUSTMENTS FOR UNUSUAL EXERCISE, POSTPONED MEALS, OR ILLNESS

All ID patients should have specific instructions on the need for extra food to balance episodes of unusual exercise. Usually no extra feedings are required for exercise of short duration or of modest intensity (*e.g.*, walking one half mile at a moderate pace), but more extensive exercise that is not habitually performed usually requires 10 g to 50 g of extra carbohydrate. A typical prescription might include 10 g/hr to 15 g/hr for moderate exercise (*e.g.,* hunting or playing golf) and 20 g/hr to 30 g/hr for vigorous exercise (*e.g.,* playing basketball or digging). Although the matter is in some dispute, it appears that the hypoglycemic effect of exercise in some circumstances may be somewhat greater when the exercise involves the anatomic part into which the subcutaneous insulin has been administered. Also, ID patients should have specific instructions on dietary measures to ensure that hypoglycemia does not occur while driving. Some who are relatively insensitive to the potential dangers to themselves or others are more responsive to the possibility of losing their driver's license. Patients with labile diabetes should be given specific instructions on what to do when meals are unavoidably delayed. Usually the ingestion of 15 g to 30 g carbohydrate (*e.g.,* a few crackers, a large glass of fruit juice, one soft drink) protects from hypoglycemia for 1 to 2 hr on these occasions.

When illness curbs appetite in ID patients, special measures are required. These should be prescribed to fit the circumstances, but some generalizations may be made. Consumption of carbohydrate in any form at the rate of about 50 g to 75 g/6 to 8 hr usually suffices to prevent the ketosis of starvation. Often the lessening of insulin requirement that attends diminished caloric intake is at least balanced by an increase in requirement induced by the illness. Nevertheless, small, frequent carbohydrate feedings are desirable as a means for protecting against hypoglycemia and ketosis.

In hospitalized ID patients whose food intake is unpredictable (*e.g.,* postsurgical state, gastrointestinal problems), it is desirable that there be some kind of standard operating procedure with respect to the replacement of prescribed food that is not consumed or retained at meal time. This standard operating procedure can, of course, be modified according to the prevailing circumstances, but there should be an understanding among physicians, dietetic staff, and nursing staff concerning what is to be done routinely if specific orders are not promulgated. A typical plan is to try to provide, in the 3-h period following the meal, enough food to bring intake of carbohydrate and calories to at least half that prescribed in the feeding. If this cannot be accomplished, the physician is informed, and he or she then determines whether additional measures, such as IV glucose or changes in insulin dosage or diet, are warranted. It is frequently desirable during such occasions to revise diet prescriptions temporarily to lighter and more digestible regimens that may contain a higher portion of simple sugars and lesser amounts of complex carbohydrates, proteins, and fats (*e.g.,* fewer vegetables, less meat, more

fruit juices). During some illnesses it may also be desirable to reduce calories in the prescription on a temporary basis. When sickness impairs appetite and digestion it is sometimes appropriate to permit or encourage simple sugars that are not ordinarily in the diet prescriptions, such as ginger ale or other soft drinks. In these situations priority should be given to avoidance of starvation and vomiting and to predictability of intake and retention; carbohydrate restriction itself has little or no priority. In hospitalized patients who are acutely ill or in a postsurgical state, one way to make this point with the dietetic and nursing staffs is to order that the diabetic diet be temporarily discontinued and replaced with a regimen along the lines described above. This temporary revision of priorities and strategies should also be explained to the patient.

SPECIAL TYPES OF DIABETES AND THE HYPERLIPIDEMIAS

Not all diabetics have features conforming to those of the two main classic types (fat, maturity-onset, NID and lean, youth-onset ID). A very small percentage of ID patients are also fat, and severe ID diabetes occasionally begins in later life. NID diabetes of mild to moderate degree is not infrequently observed in lean adults. Not much direct evidence is available to suggest the optimal diet for the latter group of patients. Most diabetologists advise these patients to give up refined carbohydrates, but there is less unanimity concerning the types of foods that should replace these sugar calories (in nondiabetics typically 10%–25% of the total). Based on considerations described above, a diet moderate in calories and low in sugars and animal fats with moderate to high levels of protein and vegetable fats and liberal amounts of starches can be recommended.

Patients with hyperlipoproteinemias may present special problems. Although special measures are sometimes warranted, in a substantial majority of cases good control of diabetes and the diets recommended above will substantially ameliorate or completely control these hyperlipidemias. In diabetics the most common type is an excess of very low-density lipoproteins with high serum triglyceride levels and with serum cholesterol levels that are in or somewhat above the normal range (type IV or mixed types) (see Chap. 17). Diabetics with type IV hyperlipidemia are usually obese. Only rarely does mitigation of obesity and hyperglycemia fail to ameliorate substantially the serum lipid abnormalities in such patients. This type of hyperlipoproteinemia has been referred to as a *carbohydrate-sensitive* condition based on the assumption that restriction of carbohydrate is helpful. It now appears, however, that most of this benefit is incidental to the decrease in caloric consumption that so often attends carbohydrate restriction. Thus, the most critical factor in the control of hypertriglyceridemia of obese diabetics is control of hyperglycemia and calories. Control of obesity and hyperglycemia also regularly mitigates the high cholesterol levels seen in patients with type II, type IIa, or type V lipid patterns. On the other hand, diabetics with high cholesterol levels not infrequently require additional measures, such as further reduction of dietary cholesterol and saturated fat, further increasing the ratio between unsaturated and saturated fat, and sometimes antilipemic medication.

PREGNANCY

Additional dietary requirements are few in diabetics who become pregnant (see Chap. 29). To ensure a daily protein level of at least 1.5 g/kg it may be necessary to raise levels of protein in the prescription. Patients who have been under poor control may require, temporarily, even higher levels of protein intake to repair deficits resulting from the negative nitrogen balance that attends marked hyperglycemia. In the last half of pregnancy, a modest increase in calories (300 Cal/day–800 Cal/day) is indicated in lean patients, but total weight gain should not exceed 30 lb. Because of the higher frequency of toxemia and polyhydramnios in diabetics, dietary salt conventially is limited routinely in the last trimester to levels below 4 g daily. This can usually be accomplished simply by discontinuing use of table salt and avoiding or limiting a few foods that are grossly salty, such as bacon (see Chap. 29).

DIETARY IMPLICATIONS OF COMPLICATING CONDITIONS

Provided one has a thorough understanding of the principles and priorities of diet therapy in diabetes, it is seldom difficult to adjust the diet prescription to meet the needs of other conditions requiring diet manipulation. Among the common coincidental conditions are renal failure, congestive heart failure, peptic ulcer, and other gastrointestinal disorders. The dietary requirements in these conditions are described in other sections of this book (see Chaps. 34, 17, and 21). Many of the previous difficulties and concerns about reconciling dietary objectives have been mitigated by the knowledge that dietary carbohydrate is well tolerated by diabetics so long as calories are controlled. It is now evident, for example, that in patients with severe renal failure the control of diabetes is not adversely affected by diets high in starch and low in protein, if calories are not excessive.

SUMMARY OF STRATEGIES FOR DEVELOPING AND MODIFYING THE DIET PRESCRIPTION

First, a determination of dietary objectives and priorities is made based on such factors as the degree of deficit of endogenous insulin secretion, obesity, age, type of drug therapy required, and the presence of any special requirements (*e.g.*, complicating illness, pregnancy, hyperlipoproteinemia). Then an analysis is made of the patient's attitudes, propensities, dietary preferences, preferred feeding patterns, and capacity for self-discipline. Having gained insights into both dietary requirements and dietary preferences, it is usually possible to construct a prescription that is suitable, attractive, and feasible. The best way of constructing the prescription is to begin with the diet that the patient would follow if he did not have diabetes, modifying this only to the degree necessary to meet the truly essential requirements imposed by the metabolic disorder. Unfortunately, few physicians know enough about dietetics to construct these *personalized* prescriptions, and few dietitians have a sufficient clinical acumen to evaluate all of the considerations that may determine dietary priorities and degree of precision required in a given patient. For example, the prescription for supper might appropriately provide exactly 4 ounces lean meat, 3 to 5 ounces, or an unlimited amount, depending on several factors, such as the severity of diabetes, age, and adiposity of the patient. For these reasons, it is usually best that the prescription be developed as a joint enterprise involving the physician, the dietitian, and the patient (see Chaps. 5 and 8). Tables 18-1 and 18-2 suggest the considerations that apply. The physician may, for example, tell the dietitian that the initial prescription should contain about 2400 Cal/day, of which roughly 10% should be derived from animal fat. He may add, however, that if problems of feasibility arise, these figures can be adjusted within certain limits, permitting 2200 Cal to 2600 Cal and 10% to 15% animal fat.

In a substantial majority of diabetics who are not insulin dependent, diet prescriptions and technical instructions can be quite simple. A typical prescription might provide only for limiting calories initially to a level in the range of 900 Cal/day to 1400 Cal/day, proscribing or sharply limiting simple sugars, and reducing saturated fat and cholesterol intake to roughly half of previous amounts. Because implementation of such a prescription does not require great precision, this patient might not be required to learn the details of the standard exchange system (see below). Time saved in simplifying the technical aspects of teaching these obese diabetics should be reinvested in the counseling required to change their entrenched attitudes and behavior, and in creating and strengthening incentives to develop new habits of diet and exercise. A highly simplified diet low in sugars and fat has been described, including specific instructions for patient and family.

Of great importance are continuing review and adjustment of the initial prescription. One reason for this need is that the feasibility, appropriateness, and effectiveness of the initial prescription can only be estimated. Subsequent experience is very helpful in determining how best to compromise the therapeutic objectives with the patient's preferences and changing patterns of living. The substantial discrepancies between the diet consumed and the diet prescribed are in no small measure attributable to the failure to make appropriate adjustments to fit changing conditions.

Mechanics of Implementing the Prescription

With few exceptions, it is best to give the patients written instructions summarizing the purposes and advantages of the diet as well as its characteristics and mechanics. In children, for example, it should be stressed that regularity and predictability of intake are more important than proscription. Written instructions usually include a list of foods that may be taken in any amount and a list of those that should be avoided entirely. Standard lists of this kind are widely available from the American Diabetes Association, and these can be modified if necessary to fit the specific needs of the patient at hand.[1] The size and characteristics of each meal are usually described, including the limits of variation permissible. These limits may be narrow or wide depending on the clinical circumstances. An elderly thin patient may be told, for example, that he may eat as he wishes, except that he should omit or limit a short list of foods that contain sugars. A middle-aged, obese patient with mild diabetes might be told only to omit a list of specified sweets and to reduce animal fat to about half of the previous amount.

A variety of methods have been employed to achieve precision and reliability while avoiding monotony. In ID patients who may require a high degree of constancy and predictability of dietary intake, the best method is to teach them the concentrations of carbohydrate, protein, and fat in common foods (*diet calculation*). This provides a wider range of attractive options than the simpler but less flexible standard exchange system described below. Patients or parents of juvenile diabetics, of average intelligence can usually learn how to formulate or select meals containing the appropriate amounts of fat, carbohydrate, protein, and calories. Often it is desirable in these patients to

begin at first with the standard exchange method before proceeding later to the more complex system of diet calculation. Weighing food portions is seldom necessary on a long-term basis, but patients, or mothers of juvenile diabetics, who have weighed and measured portions for a few weeks gain considerable precision in estimating portion weights and amounts.

STANDARD EXCHANGE SYSTEMS AND STANDARD DIETS

The standard exchange systems are designed to allow the patient a considerable degree of day-to-day flexibility of diet while achieving a moderate degree of constancy with respect to amounts and distributions of the major food elements (carbohydrate, protein, fat, and calories). The most widely used exchange system is that developed and promulgated by the American Diabetes Association, the American Dietetic Association, and the United States Public Health Service. This general method, with or without minor modifications, is used in most hospitals in the United States. Similar approaches have been employed in other countries, although details differ slightly. The details of these well-known "A.D.A." exchange lists are not presented here because they are already widely available in hospitals, diet manuals, and books on nutrition and diabetes. This system was revised in 1976 by the American Diabetes Association.[1] The newer revision is recommended. Guidelines also have been promulgated for uses of the exchange system by the American Diabetes Association.[2]

This standard American system involves the categorization of the foods allowed into six groups based on general characteristics. Foods consisting mainly of protein appear, for example, on a *meat exchange list*, and foods containing mainly fat appear on a *fat exchange list*. The lists indicate how much of each of these foods is equivalent to the standard exchange unit and how much carbohydrate, protein, and fat is in the unit. For example, the bread exchange list shows that one serving of potato, and of certain specified portions of the many other foods on this list, are each equivalent to one standard slice of bread, and that each contains about 15 g carbohydrate, 2 g protein, and negligible amounts of fat. For each feeding prescribed, the patient is told how many exchange units he may have from each of these lists. For example, breakfast might consist of two meat exchanges, three bread exchanges, two fat exchanges, two fruit exchanges, and one half milk exchange.

This system may be easily modified to fit the needs of specific patients. For instance, a certain patient may be told that he can have unlimited amounts of vegetables, except for those on the bread exchange list that are higher in calories. It may be appropriate to permit certain patients to make exchanges between the fruit list and the bread list under the assumption that one bread exchange is roughly equivalent to one and a half fruit exchanges. Amounts of fat in various meats differ greatly. Trimming gross fat from meat servings and selecting especially lean meats, such as chicken and certain fish, reduce fat from an average of 5 g per ounce to about 3 g per ounce, thereby reducing cholesterol consumption and calories as well. Some foods on the old meat exchange lists (*e.g.*, eggs and certain cheeses) contain as much as 6 g to 7 g fat per exchange. A new lean meat exchange list includes meats containing about 3 g of fat per ounce (30 g).[1] Saturated fat calories trimmed from the diet can be replaced, if necessary, with starch, vegetable fat, or protein.

A 1976 publication entitled *Meal Planning and Exchange Lists* is widely available and may be obtained from the American Diabetes Association or the American Dietetic Association. In addition to the exchange lists, this booklet contains standard lists of foods to be omitted and those that may be freely consumed. Several recipes and some general instructions are also included. Recipes are available in several cookbooks for diabetics from the American Diabetes Association.[8] These recipes yield food portions with defined amounts of carbohydrate, protein, and fat. Typically these constituents correspond to units or combinations of units of the standard exchange system.

The American Diabetes Association and the American Dietetic Association also promulgated nine standard diets ranging from 1200 Cal/day to 3500 Cal/day. These diets were conceived in the 1940s and reflect the priority given at that time to restriction of carbohydrate. Most authorities now believe that these standard diets contain too much fat. Endorsement of these traditional diets by these organizations was discontinued in 1976. These standard diets are, however, still very widely used. There are many hospital diet manuals from which they have not been removed. Another reason for the continuing popularity of standard diets is that most physicians have very limited capacity for developing individualized prescriptions, and their use often saves time initially. Moreover, they may serve as a framework for a more individualized prescription produced by modifying the standard regimen. But the two disadvantages of these old standard diets should be kept in mind, since their indiscriminate use may increase intake of saturated fat and militate against the development of a prescription based on the patient's individual preferences and metabolic needs. If used judiciously and modified appropriately, standard diets will continue to have utility, particularly after they are modernized along lines suggested in Tables 18-1 and 18-2.

SPECIAL FOODS AND FOOD SUBSTITUTES

No special low-carbohydrate foods are required in the diabetic diet. The use of special foods marketed as "dietetic" often leads to difficulties. Although most of these contain less carbohydrate and fewer calories than the food they are designed to imitate, many contain appreciable carbohydrate and calories, the amounts of which may not be specified or understood by the patient. However, when the constituents of these special foods are clearly stated and understood, they may have value in making the diet more attractive. Canned fruit without sugar may, for example, be useful and economical. The uses of low-cholesterol foods and of polyunsaturated fat products have been mentioned above.

With respect to the use of artificial sweeteners, two different approaches are possible. The patient may be encouraged to become accustomed to doing without sweets. One can point out, for example, that in cultures where sugar has been unknown people find their diets palatable and attractive because they are accustomed to these foods. Not infrequently, diabetic children, after a period of time, lose their craving for sweets. On the other hand, in many circumstances the use of artificial sweeteners is warranted. Many obese diabetics, for example, like artificially sweetened drinks about as well as the standard products. Some of these "dietetic" drinks can be allowed freely, but some contain appreciable amounts of sugar. Even so, if their composition is known, they may sometimes be included in the diet by exchanging other foods in the prescription for them. Older patients are often firmly attached to the sweetening of tea or coffee. Frequently they find saccharin or other substitutes quite acceptable as replacements for sugar. Some scientists are concerned that saccharin may be carcinogenic, even when ingested in ordinary amounts, but evidence to this effect is weak. The status of saccharin has been reviewed by Kalkhoff and Levin.[21]

Fructose has been suggested as a substitute for sucrose for two reasons: (1) under some, but not all, conditions, fructose is considerably sweeter than sucrose, by as much as 70%, so that a relatively small amount is required for sweetening; and (2) fructose does not require insulin for certain steps in its metabolism. Much of this advantage is, however, lost because of the capacity of the diabetic liver to convert substantial proportions of fructose and its metabolic products to glucose. Fructose has been used effectively under some conditions as part of the diabetic diet. Its role deserves further exploration, but the potential practical advantages that attend use of fructose products do not seem substantial.

Sorbitol has been widely used as a sugar substitute in dietetic foods because it is slowly absorbed and does not require insulin in the initial steps of its metabolism. Sorbitol contains approximately as many calories as the sugar it replaces, and it is only 60% as sweet as sucrose. It may produce diarrhea if consumed in large amounts. Sorbitol is metabolized to fructose, which in turn is partly converted to glucose. It is seldom recommended by diabetologists. The use of nutritive sweeteners including xylitol has been well reviewed by Talbot and Fisher and by Olefsky and Crapo.[26,32]

EDUCATING THE PATIENT

Emphasis has been placed on the importance of conveying to the patient an understanding of both the objectives and the mechanics of diet therapy. There is also need for a systematic program to identify any deficiencies of knowledge or misunderstandings. The checklist described previously was designed to help the physician and the dietitian in this respect. Group instruction may be helpful and economical, but the principles of diet therapy are quite different in the two main types of diabetes, and any group teaching must take this into account. A good argument can be made for separating entirely the dietary instruction of these two main subgroups. Instruction of hospital patients who are not acutely ill should be initiated on entry rather than at time of discharge. At the time of admission, the physician should, whenever possible, construct in consultation with the dietitian a prescription for both the hospital diet and the approximate diet anticipated on discharge. The education program should include the patient's spouse.

Under proper supervision and after adequate training, other professionals (see Chaps. 5–8), as well as nurses, physician's assistants, social workers, lay groups (*e.g., Weight Watchers, TOPS*), and diabetics themselves, can play effective roles in the dietary instruction of diabetics. The general dietary strategies pursued by the Weight Watchers organizations usually fit well the dietary requirements of obese diabetics.

The American Diabetes Association (1 West 48th Street, New York, NY 10020) publishes informative materials on diet therapy. Special teaching centers for diabetics have been developed by Davidson and Delcher.[14]

One of the few inconveniences in the diabetic diet is the need to abstain from certain mixed dishes served outside the home, the constituents of which are highly uncertain. I advise the obese diabetic

simply to decline these whenever feasible. When no alternatives are easily available, I advise the lean ID diabetic to accept the dish after crudely estimating its constituents and taking them into account, erring on the side of anticipated overconsumption. Subsequent urine testing readily identifies any need for compensatory adjustments in therapy. Gross and persistent aberrations of glycemia are never the result of miscalculation of the constituents of a single dish. Even dietary indiscretions of gross degree, if they are temporary (*e.g.*, a single feast), seldom lead to any serious immediate problems, such as ketosis. ID patients on completely free diets who eat regularly usually feel quite well if they get enough insulin to avoid gross polyuria and acidosis. Patients are often given exaggerated notions about the immediately deleterious effects of dietary indiscretions. *Patients should understand, therefore, the important distinction between the relatively innocuous short-term effects of overconsumption and the more deleterious effects that follow persistent dietary indiscretion.*

Obese patients seldom understand the degree to which their diabetes can be reversed with mitigation of adiposity. A major educational goal in such patients is to show them clearly the dangers of continued obesity and the profoundly beneficial effects of its reversal.

Ultimately, the patient treats himself. The role of the physician, the dietitian, and those who help them, is to teach the patient what he should do. This teaching, however, must extend well beyond technical details, such as the number of bread exchanges in lunch. The patient must understand the advantages to be gained by modifying the diet and the reasons for, and relative importance of, the various strategies employed.

A frequently overlooked point is that the more the patient knows about principles and details, the greater are his tactical options and the easier and more pleasant his regimen.

Unfortunately, only a minority of physicians have the time, inclination, and expertise to conceive and implement optimal diet therapy, and the dietitian who knows all about diet exchanges may have little understanding of certain important metabolic or clinical considerations. Even physicians who have considerable clinical sophistication are often quite ignorant about certain aspects of dietetics. When physicians and dietitians work closely together in designing and implementing the prescription and in teaching the patient, many of these difficulties are overcome. Insulin-dependent patients in particular require special expertise that is not possessed by most dietitians and most physicians. It is not difficult for the physician to learn these rudiments—they are not complex—but the physician who does not know the major nutritional constituents of common foods and how to calculate, modify, and individualize diets probably shouldn't attempt to treat patients with labile diabetes. And dietitians who are responsible for teaching ID diabetics also require special training in order to understand the principles and strategies, as well as the tactics, of diet therapy. The major role of the physician is to see that the patient learns these principles and how to implement them. Much of this responsibility can be delegated to dietitians or others with special knowledge in the field, but the physician must assume responsibility for developing these mechanisms and applying them to the specific needs of individual patients.

OTHER SOURCES OF INFORMATION

Many sources of information have been mentioned above and in the references. The H. J. Heinz Company and the Campbell Soup Company publish lists showing the composition of their soups. The publication of Church and Church gives details on the composition of foods, as does Handbook Number 8 of the Department of Agriculture.[12] The American Diabetes Association and the American Dietetic Association have published a cook book and a guide for eating in fast-food restaurants.[4,5] Anderson and Sieling have published a description of their high-fiber, high-carbohydrate diet and a publication on the composition of foods commonly used in diets of diabetics.[7,8] *Forecast* magazine, a publication of the American Diabetes Association, frequently contains useful information for diabetics and their families concerning nutrition and dietetics.

References

1. American Diabetes Association: Exchange Lists for Meal Planning. New York American Diabetes Association, Inc., and American Dietetic Association, 1976
2. American Diabetes Association: A Guide for Professionals: The Effective Application of "Exchange Lists for Meal Planning." New York American Diabetes Association, Inc, and American Dietetic Association, 1977
3. American Diabetes Association, Nutrition Committee: Special report: Principles of nutrition and dietary recommendations for individuals with diabetes mellitus: 1979. Diabetes 28:1027, November, 1979
4. American Diabetes Association, ADA Committee on Food and Nutrition and the Scientific Advisory Panel of the Executive Committee: Fast food restaurants: Policy statement. Diabetes Care 3, No. 3:389, March–April, 1980
5. American Diabetes Association: The American Diabetes Association and the American Dietetic Association's Whole-Family Diabetes Cookbook and General Nutritional Guide. New Jersey, Prentice-Hall, 1980
6. Anderson JW, Ward K: Long-term effects of high-carbohydrate, high-fiber diets on glucose and lipid metabo-

7. Anderson JW, Lin WJ, Ward K: Composition of foods commonly used in diets for persons with diabetes. Diabetes Care 1, No. 5:293, September–October, 1978
8. Anderson JW, Sieling B: HCF Diets: A Professional Guide to High Carbohydrate, High Fiber Diets, p 54. Lexington, University of Kentucky Diabetes Fund, 1979
9. Bierman EL: Carbohydrates, sucrose, and human disease. Am J Clin Nutr 32:2712, December 1979
10. Brunzell JD, Lerner RL, Hazzard WR et al: Improved glucose tolerance with high carbohydrate feeding in mild diabetes. N Engl J Med 284:521, 1971
11. Brunzell JD, Lerner RL, Porte D Jr et al: Effect of a fat free, high carbohydrate diet on diabetic subjects with fasting hyperglycemia. Diabetes 23:138, 1974
12. Church CF, Church HN: Food values of portions commonly used, 12th ed. Philadelphia, JB Lippincott, 1975
13. Cohen AM: Environmental aspects of diabetes. Isr J Med Sci 8:358, 1972
14. Davidson JK, Delcher HK: Policy and procedure manual, 3rd ed. Atlanta, Grady Hospital Diabetes Unit, 1979
15. Davidson JK: Plasma glucose lowering effect of caloric restriction in obesity-induced insulin treated diabetes mellitus. Diabetes (Suppl 1), 26:355, 1977
16. Clements RS Jr: Dietary myo-inositol and diabetic neuropathy. In Camerini–Davalos R, Hanover B (eds): Treatment of Early Diabetes. Adv Exp Med Biol 119:287, 1978
17. Ensinck JW, Bierman EL: Dietary management of diabetes mellitus. Annu Rev Med 30:155, 1979
18. Harris M, Cahill G, Expert Panel of the National Institutes of Health Diabetes Data Group: Classification and diagnosis of diabetes mellitus and other categories of glucose intolerance. Diabetes 28; No. 12:1039, 1980
19. Howard BV, Savage PJ, Nagulesparan M et al: Changes in plasma lipoproteins accompanying diet therapy in obese diabetics. Atherosclerosis 33:445, 1979
20. Jackson WPU, Goldberg MD, Marine N et al: Effectiveness, reproducibility and weight–relation of screening tests for diabetes. Lancet 2:1101, 1968
21. Kalkhoff RK, Levin ME: The saccharin controversy. Diabetes Care 1, No. 4:211, July–August, 1978
22. Keen, H, Jarrett RJ: The WHO Multinational Study of Vascular Disease in Diabetes: 2. Macrovascular disease prevalence. Diabetes Care 2, No. 2:187, March–April, 1979
23. Keen H, Thomas BJ, Jarrett RJ et al: Nutrient intake, adiposity, and diabetes. Br Med J 1:655, 1979
24. Mann JI: Diet and diabetes. Diabetologia 18:89, 1980
25. Olefsky J, Reaven GM, Farquhar JW: Effects of weight reduction on obesity: Studies of lipid and carbohydrate metabolism in normal and hyperlipoproteinemic subjects. J Clin Invest 53:64, 1974
26. Olefsky, J, Crapo P: Fructose, xylitol, and sorbitol. Diabetes Care 3, No. 2:390, March–April, 1980
27. Reaven GM, Coulston AM, Marcus RA: Nutritional management of diabetes. Med Clin N Am 63, No. 5, 927, September, 1979
28. Savage PJ, Bennion LJ, Flock EV et al: Diet-induced improvement of abnormalities in insulin and glucagon secretion and in insulin receptor binding in diabetes mellitus. J Clin Endocrinol Metab 48:999, 1979
29. Schellenberg B, Oster P, Vogel G et al: 24-hour patterns of blood sugar, plasma insulin and free fatty acids in patients with primary endogenous hyperlipoprotein-

emia on isocaloric diets containing 30, 43, and 79 cal% carbohydrates. Nutr Metab 23, No. 4:316, 1979

30. Simpson RW, Mann JI, Eaton J et al: Improved glucose control in maturity-onset diabetes treated with high-carbohydrate-modified fat diet. Br Med J 1:1753, 1979
31. Steffes MW, Brown DM, Mauer SM: The development, enhancement, and reversal of the secondary complications of diabetes mellitus. Hum Pathol 10, No. 3:293, 1979
32. Talbot JM, Fisher KD: The need for special foods and sugar substitutes by individuals with diabetes mellitus. Diabetes Care 1, No. 4:231, July–August, 1978
33. Viswanathan M, Snehalatha C, Ramachandran A et al: Effect of a calorie restricted high carbohydrate, high protein low fat diet on serum lipids in diabetes—A follow up study. J Assoc Physicians India 26:162, March, 1978
34. West KM: Diet therapy of diabetes: An analysis of failure. Ann Intern Med 79:425, 1973
35. West KM: Epidemiology of adiposity. In Vague J, Boyer J (eds): The Regulation of the Adopose Tissue Mass. Proceedings of the IV International Meeting of Endocrinology. International Congress Series No 315 of Excerpta Medica, Amsterdam, 1974
36. West KM: Diabetes in American Indians and other native populations of the new world. Diabetes 23:841, 1974
37. West KM: Epidemiology of Diabetes and Its Vascular Lesions. New York, Elsevier, 1978
38. West KM: Incorporating alcoholic beverages into therapeutic diets: Some potentialities and problems. In Gastineau CF, Darby WJ, Turner TB et al (eds): Fermented Food Beverages in Nutrition, pp 257–262. New York, Academic Press, 1979
39. West KM: Recent trends in dietary management. In Podolsky S (ed): Clinical Diabetes: Modern Management. New York, Appleton-Century-Crofts, 1980
40. West KM, Keen H, Jarrett RJ et al: Relationship of vascular disease to fasting plasma glucose (FPG) and other variables in 3583 with diabetes. Diabetes 29:(Suppl 1a), 1980
41. West KM, Erdreich LJ, Stober JA: A detailed study of risk factors for retinopathy and nephropathy in diabetes. Diabetes 29:501, 1980
42. Wood FC Jr, Bierman EL: New concepts in diabetic diabetics. Nutrition Today 7:4, 1972

19
Drug and Nutrient Interactions

Daphne A. Roe

In recent years, it has been shown that the therapeutic efficacy and safety of drugs are influenced by both diet and nutritional status. Drug–food and drug–alcohol incompatibilities are well recognized and can be prevented. Directly and indirectly, drugs can affect nutritional status by stimulating appetite, thereby increasing food intake, or by producing anorexia, malabsorption, hyperexcretion of nutrients, or impaired nutrient utilization.

Effects of Food on Drug Absorption and Metabolism

ABSORPTION

Absorption of drugs from the gastrointestinal tract may be increased or decreased by concomitant food intake.[47] Food or elements of food can delay or reduce drug absorption. Food may delay drug absorption because of changes in the motility of the gastrointestinal tract, because the drug takes longer to diffuse to the absorption site when food is present, and also because food fiber components may adsorb drugs. Previous studies have shown that the delaying effect of food on the absorption of acetaminophen may be due to the pectin content.[15] Delayed absorption of digoxin by food may be due to food bran. Tetracycline and related broad-spectrum antibiotics are less efficiently absorbed when taken with calcium or iron-containing foods.[27] Antibiotic complexes are formed with these mineral elements of the diet, and these chelates are poorly absorbed. If milk or other dairy foods are taken at the same time as tetracycline, the desired therapeutic effect of the drug is not achieved. This is an important consideration in adolescents and young adults receiving tetracycline for the treatment of acne. Drugs which are more slowly or less efficiently absorbed when taken with food are shown in Table 19-1.[34]

On the other hand, food may promote the absorption of drugs. Reasons for such enhancement of drug absorption are the following:

1. Prolonged contact of solid (pill) formulations of a drug with the gastric contents promote dissolution.[4]
2. Food delays gastric emptying time, which may allow metering out of a dissolved drug from the stomach to the optimal saturable absorption site in the small intestine.[14]
3. Specific nutrients can promote drug absorption, particularly absorption of lipid-soluble drugs. The antifungal agent, griseofulvin, is better absorbed when taken with a meal containing fat, probably because it is one of these lipid-soluble drugs, and because bile flow may enhance absorption.[9] Therapeutic diets may reduce or alter the efficiency of griseofulvin absorption. For example, low-fat diets prescribed for patients with hyperlipidemia, atherosclerotic heart disease, or diabetes mellitus may significantly reduce the absorption of griseofulvin. When low-fat diets have been prescribed, and it is necessary to administer griseofulvin for the control of extensive fungus infections of the skin, then either a micronized or ultramicronized form of the drug

TABLE 19-1
Drugs for Which Absorption is Delayed or Reduced by Food

Delayed	Reduced
Amoxicillin	Penicillin G
Cephalexin	Penicillin V (K)
Cephradine	Phenethicillin
Sulfanilamide	Ampicillin
Sulfadiazine	Amoxicillin
Sulfamethoxine	Tetracycline
Sulfamethoxypyridazine	Demethylchlortetracycline
Sulfisoxazole	Methacycline
Sulfasymazine	Oxytetracycline
Aspirin	Aspirin
Acetaminophen*	Propantheline
Digoxin	Levodopa
Furosemide	Rifampicin
Potassium ion	Doxycycline
	Isoniazid
	Phenobarbital

*Probable pectin effect
From Roe DA: Interactions between drugs and nutrients. Med Clin North Am 63:985–1007, 1979

should be used, or it should be given in a suspension in a small volume of corn oil.

4. Food increases splanchnic blood flow, and hence promotes drug absorption.[23]
5. Food enhances the bioavailability of certain drugs, including propranolol (Inderal). Since the absorption of propranolol is complete under fasting conditions, food or food components cannot actually promote absorption of this drug but may reduce first-pass extraction and in turn hepatic metabolism.[24] Drugs that are better or more efficiently absorbed in the fed state include the following:
   a. Griseofulvin
   b. Nitrofurantoin
   c. Riboflavin
   d. Propranolol
   e. Metoprolol
   f. Hydralazine
   g. Spironolactone
   h. Carbamazepine
   i. Propoxyphene

METABOLISM

The rates of metabolism of phenacetin, antipyrine, and theophylline are increased by the eating of charcoal-broiled beef.[7,17] Indolic compounds present in cabbage and Brussels sprouts can also speed up the rate of drug metabolism.[30,31]

Both hepatic and intestinal drug metabolism are affected by diet composition. Rates of *in vivo* metabolism of antipyrine and theophylline are in-

creased by high protein intake. Protein, when substituted either for dietary carbohydrate or fat, has a marked inducing influence on oxidative drug metabolism in human subjects.[1,18]

The degree to which diet composition or cooking method affects oxidative drug metabolism shows interpersonal variability. Intake of methylxanthine-containing foods and beverages significantly affects both the metabolism and elimination kinetics of theophylline.[26] The importance of the metabolism of therapeutic drugs by the gastrointestinal microflora is receiving recognition.

Microbial metabolism of drugs in the gut may produce an active compound with greater therapeutic effect than the parent drug, or may lead to the production of a toxic metabolite. Intestinal drug biotransformations by the gut bacterial flora involve degradative processes and reduction in molecular size, including deconjugation of glucuronides and glycosides, reduction of nitro- or azo-compounds and decarboxylation of phenolic acids. Changes brought about by bacteria in the gut modify the extent and nature of the enterohepatic circulation of drug metabolites. Whereas metabolism of drugs within the gut may be due to enzymes within the intestinal mucosa, the more extensive drug metabolism is microbial. It has been suggested that the increased toxicity of chloramphenicol to some individuals may be explained by the presence of a large gut population of enterobacteria, which leads to the production of a toxic metabolite of this drug.[38]

In the rat and in human subjects, salicylazosulfapyridine (SASP) is metabolized in the gut by reductive scission of the azo-bond brought about by the intestinal microflora. Colonic bacterial enzymes split this drug with the formation of 5-aminosalicylic acid (5-ASA) and sulfapyridine. Further metabolism of these daughter products leads to the formation of acetyl aminosalicylic acid and both acetylated and glucuronidated metabolites of sulfapyridine. The acetylation and glucuronidation of the metabolites of SASP are produced in the liver. While SASP is the drug most commonly used in the management of inflammatory bowel disease, including regional enteritis and ulcerative colitis and proctitis, its effectiveness is dependent upon the efficient microbial metabolism of the parent drug. Present information indicates that 5-ASA is the therapeutically active metabolite of SASP. In patients who have very active inflammatory bowel disease and an accelerated intestinal transit time with diarrhea, SASP is less effective in controlling the disease process. The relationship between intestinal transit time and effectiveness of SASP is explained in that if the intestinal transit time is very short, then insufficient time elapses for the microbial metabolism of SASP and production and absorption of 5-ASA. From the practical standpoint, it should be remembered that high intake of dietary fiber will reduce the intestinal transit time and could therefore diminish the effectiveness of SASP in control of cases of inflammatory bowel disease. Also, dietary changes that influence the microbial flora of the intestine may change drug efficacy by reducing the bacterial population which is responsible for azo-bond scission.[10,44]

Effects of Drugs on Food Intake and Nutritional Status

EFFECTS OF DRUGS ON APPETITE

HYPERPHAGIC AGENTS

Drugs can be used intentionally to stimulate appetite in debilitated children and adults. The most effective drug in this regard is cyproheptadine (Periactin), which has been shown to improve appetite and cause significant weight gain in children and adults recovering from catabolic disease. The advantage is that cyproheptadine is largely nontoxic, having only drowsiness as a significant side-effect.[5,28,42]

Psychotropic drugs improve appetite in disturbed psychiatric patients. Whereas chlorpromazine (Thorazine) has been used deliberately to improve appetite in agitated patients, more frequently the appetite-promoting effects of phenothiazines and benzodiazepines are recognized as an undesirable side effect of these psychotropic agents. While these tranquilizers when given in high dosage to disturbed psychotic patients often effect a marked increase in food intake, such that the patients become obese, these same drugs when given to geriatric patients may have an opposite effect, because they may reduce alertness and interest in food.

Tricyclic antidepressants and also monamine oxidase inhibitor antidepressants can also promote appetite and lead to undesirable weight gain. Depressed patients receiving amitriptyline (Elavil) or other related tricyclic drugs often describe a craving for sweets which they will consume in addition to their normal meals. Lithium carbonate intake also increases appetite and weight gain in many patients. Prevalence of obesity in patients in psychiatric institutions can, in part, be attributed to the uniform use of psychotropic drugs for behavioral control and management of mental disease.[2,12,16,29]

Appetite promotion by drugs may be a direct or indirect effect. Direct appetite stimulation occurs with administration of anabolic steroids and glucocorticoids. The appetite-stimulating effect of glucocorticoids is most notable when these drugs are given to patients with chronic adrenal insufficiency or used in the management of anterior pituitary insufficiency. When corticosteroids are used in the treatment of leukemia, appetite stimulation and weight gain only occur if the appetite depressant effects of chemotherapeutic agents do not outweigh the effects of glucocorticoids. In patients with acute or chronic infections, the disease process has an anorectic effect. Anti-infective drugs used to combat disease can lead indirectly to an improvement in appetite.[28]

HYPOPHAGIC AGENTS

Amphetamines of the unsubstituted or substituted types are used in the control of obesity because of their appetite suppressant effects. Since food intake in fat people is not necessarily related to appetite, the long-term effectiveness of these drugs as a means of weight control is unsatisfactory. Further, the central effect of amphetamines and the risk of addiction detract from their usefulness for the purposes of weight reduction.[25,46]

Hyperactive children receiving amphetamines such as dextroamphetamine or the related stimulant drug, methylphenydate, may show growth retardation. Slow weight gain and height gain are associated with lowered food intake. Effects are dose dependent. When these drugs are discontinued in these children, a growth spurt occurs and is proportional to the previous growth depression. There is evidence that the growth rebound is associated with an increase in food intake.[35–37]

Cancer chemotherapeutic agents commonly induce anorexia, which may be associated with nausea and vomiting. The incidence of these acute side-effects is dependent on the drug or drug combination employed, on the mode and rate of administration of the drug, and on patient characteristics. With single-bolus drug protocols, nausea and vomiting only occur in the hours following injection of the drug, or these symptoms may be prolonged or delayed. Occurrence of nausea and vomiting with cancer chemotherapy can result in a marked reduction in food intake as well as decreased retention of food. Awareness by the patient that chemotherapy will induce nausea and vomiting may discourage him from eating at times of drug administration. Further, aversion to certain foods may develop because, in the patient's mind, they are associated with postdrug periods of nausea. Anorexia, independent of nausea and vomiting, may be related to drug-induced loss of taste acuity. Loss of taste acuity frequently occurs in patients receiving Cis-platin (Cis-diamminedichloroplatinum). Reduction in food intake for any reason, in a patient receiving cancer chemotherapy, will contribute to malnutrition and lowered drug tolerance. Whether or not food aversion, anorexia, nausea, and vomiting seriously impair the patient's nutritional status during cancer chemotherapy is dependent on the severity and duration of symptoms, and on whether nutritional support therapy is instituted early and appropriately (see Chap. 36).[40]

D-penicillamine, which is used in the treatment of Wilson's disease, cystinuria, heavy metal poisoning, and rheumatoid arthritis, may produce anorexia associated with loss of taste. Loss of taste is most likely to occur in patients who are receiving this drug over a long period of time, as, for example, when penicillamine is used in the management of rheumatoid arthritis. Loss of taste with this drug has been attributed to zinc deficiency. Recent studies also indicate that copper deficiency may be a contributory factor. Loss of taste in patients with rheumatoid arthritis receiving penicillamine is frequently associated with diminished food intake and weight loss.[22]

Digitalis glycosides, given at high dosage levels, induce anorexia, nausea, and vomiting. Cachexia can ensue.[3]

Drugs affecting appetite and food intake are summarized in Table 19-2.

DRUG-INDUCED MALABSORPTION

Primary drug-induced malabsorption is defined as the direct effects of a drug on luminal events or on the intestinal mucosa. Secondary malabsorption occurs when a drug interferes with the absorption, disposition, or metabolism of one nutrient which in turn leads to malabsorption and deficiency of other nutrients. Causes and consequences of primary and secondary drug-induced malabsorption are summarized in Tables 19-3 and 19-4. Drugs which cause secondary malabsorption are those which (1) suppress vitamin D absorption or metabolism leading to malabsorption of calcium, and (2) cause malabsorption or impair utilization of folacin and, secondarily, malabsorption of other nutrients.[33]

Cytotoxic drugs used singly or in combination for the treatment of neoplastic disease have been shown to produce toxic effects on the mucosa of the small intestine. Among cancer chemotherapeutic drugs in common use, malabsorption has been most frequently reported with methotrexate. Biopsies from the jejunum of patients who have received single doses of methotrexate demonstrate ultrastructural changes. Malabsorption of d-xylose has been found in children with acute leukemia within seven days of receiving methotrexate. Current evidence suggests that malabsorption is cumulative with a dose of methotrexate received. However, this is difficult to evaluate when multi-

TABLE 19-2
Drugs Affecting Appetite and Food Intake

	Example
A. APPETITE AND FOOD INTAKE ARE INCREASED BY:	
1. Antihistamines	Cyproheptadine
2. Psychotropic agents	Tranquilizers [Phenothiazines and benzodiazepines] Antidepressants [MAO inhibitors, Tricyclic antidepressants] Other: Lithium carbonate
3. Steroids	Anabolic steroids Glucocorticoids
B. APPETITE AND FOOD INTAKE ARE DECREASED BY:	
1. Amphetamines and related stimulant drugs	Dextroamphetamine, Fenfluramine, Methyl phenidate
2. Cancer chemotherapeutic drugs	Cis-platin Methotrexate
3. Chelating agents	Penicillamine
4. Cardiac glycosides	Digitalis and derivatives

drug regimens are employed, as in the treatment of leukemia.[8]

Combination cancer chemotherapy may produce both structural and functional changes in the gastrointestinal tract. In cancer patients, combination chemotherapy with nitrogen mustard, vinblastine, procarbazine, and prednisone can impair d-xylose absorption and cause malabsorption of vitamin B_{12}. Under well-controlled studies, in which nutrient intake of patients was known, patients receiving cyclophosphamide, methotrexate, and 5-fluorouracil showed histological evidence of villous damage in intestinal biopsies taken after therapy. In this series, there were several biochemical indicators of malabsorption following chemotherapy and in patients in whom malabsorption was present prior to therapy, this condition became worse with drug administration.

Combination of radiation therapy and chemotherapy may have additive effects in causing intestinal maldigestion and malabsorption. The incidence of lactose intolerance caused by lactase deficiency has been shown to be much higher in patients receiving both chemotherapy and radiation therapy than in those receiving radiation therapy alone.[41]

DRUGS CAUSING MINERAL DEPLETION

Drug-induced mineral depletion is a common and often serious clinical problem. Hyperexcretion of minerals may be through the gastrointestinal (GI) tract or the kidney.

TABLE 19-3
Primary Intestinal Absorptive Defects Caused by Drugs

Drug	Usage	Malabsorption or Fecal Nutrient Loss	Mechanism
Mineral oil	Laxative	Carotene, vitamins A, D, K	Physical barrier, nutrients dissolve in mineral oil and are lost; micelle formation decreased
Phenolphthalein	Laxative	Vitamin D, Ca	Intestinal hurry; K depletion; loss of structural integrity
Neomycin	Antibiotic to "sterilize" gut	Fat, N, Na, K, Ca, Fe, lactose, sucrose, vitamin B_{12}	Structural defect; pancreatic lipase lowered; binding of bile acids (salts)
Cholestyramine	Hypocholesterolemic agent; bile acid sequestrant	Fat, vitamins A, K, B_{12}, D, Fe	Binding of bile acids (salts) and nutrients, *e.g.*, Fe
Potassium chloride	Potassium repletion	Vitamin B_{12}	Ileal *p*H lowered
Colchicine	Anti-inflammatory agent in gout	Fat, carotene, Na, K, vitamin B_{12}, lactose	Mitotic arrest; structural defect; enzyme damage
Para-amino salicylic acid	Antituberculosis agent	Fat, folacin, vitamin B_{12}	Mucosal block in B_{12} uptake
Salicylazosulfapyridine (Azulfidine)	Anti-inflammatory agent in ulcerative colitis and regional enteritis	Folacin	Mucosal block in folate uptake
Methyldopa	Antihypertensive agent	Folacin, vitamin B_{12}, iron	Autoimmune mechanism?

Adapted from Roe DA: Interactions between drugs and nutrients. Med Clin North Am, 63:985–1007, 1979

Phosphate depletion occurs in patients on high doses of antacids. Antacids producing phosphate depletion are those containing aluminum or magnesium hydroxide. Dietary phosphate combines with these antacids to form insoluble aluminum and magnesium phosphates, which are then excreted through the gastrointestinal tract. The risk of acute phosphate depletion is greatest in those whose intake of phosphate in the diet is low. Symptoms of phosphate depletion are profound muscle weakness, which may be limited to proximal limb muscles, malaise, paresthesia, anorexia, and convulsions. In some patients phosphate depletion leads to osteomalacia.[32,39]

Potassium depletion occurs with prolonged or high intake of oral diuretics including thiazides, furosemide, and ethacrynic acid. In the initial phase of potassium depletion, there is association between potassium loss and the development of hypokalemia. However, further potassium deficit is not accurately reflected in changes in serum potassium levels. Triamterene and spironolactone are potassium-sparing diuretics. Potassium depletion can occur with laxative abuse because large amounts of potassium are lost into the lumen of the large intestine. Drug-induced hypokalemia can also be due to glucocorticoids and certain antibiotics, including carbenicillin and penicillin. Potassium de-

TABLE 19-4
Drugs Causing Secondary Malabsorption

Drug	Usage	Malabsorption	Mechanism
Prednisone	Used in allergy	Calcium	Calcium transport ↓
Phenobarbital	Anticonvulsant	Calcium	Accelerated metabolism of vitamin D
Diphenylhydantoin	Anticonvulsant	Calcium	
Primidone	Anticonvulsant	Calcium	
Glutethimide	Sedative	Calcium	Impaired calcium transport
Methotrexate	Leukemia	Calcium	Acute folacin deficiency

Adapted from Roe DA: Interactions between drugs and nutrients. Med Clin North Am, 63:985–1007, 1979

TABLE 19-5
Mineral Depletion Induced by Drugs

Drug	Mineral Depleted
Diuretics	Calcium (not thiazides) Potassium Magnesium Zinc
Laxatives (laxative abuse)	Potassium Calcium
Glucocorticoids	Calcium Potassium
Chelating agents (penicillamine)	Zinc Copper
Cis-platinum	Magnesium Zinc
Antacids	Phosphates
Non-narcotic analgesics (aspirin, indomethacin)	Iron (by G.I. blood loss)

Adapted from Roe DA: Interactions between drugs and nutrients. Med Clin North Am 63:985–1007, 1979

ficiency is clinically manifested by weakness, anorexia, nausea, vomiting, listlessness, apprehension, and sometimes diffuse abdominal pain; other symptoms include drowsiness, stupor, and irrational behavior. In some patients, severe hypokalemia can occur without abnormal clinical findings, and this is particularly true in elderly patients. In the elderly, potassium depletion and hypokalemia are commonly the result of low potassium intake and renal wasting of potassium by use of diuretics. Misuse of laxatives in these patients is an additional cause of potassium depletion. Potassium depletion sensitizes patients to digitalis intoxication.

Magnesium and zinc are hyperexcreted by patients on oral diuretics and also by those receiving cardiac glycosides. Cis-platinum has also been shown to induce both magnesium and zinc deficiency, apparently through drug-induced impairment of renal tubular reabsorption. The nephrotoxic effect of Cis-platin, which induces excessive magnesium losses, can be minimized by concurrent use of mannitol and hydration of patients.[13,20,45]

Hypercalciuria occurs with intake of such oral diuretics as furosemide and ethacrynic acid, but not with thiazide diuretics. Hypercalciuria leading to severe loss of bone calcium may also occur with prolonged or high-dose intake of glucocorticoids.[11,34,43]

Iron deficiency may be induced by chronic intake of aspirin or other salicylates, or other non-narcotic analgesics such as indomethacin. These drugs cause erosions in the stomach and intestine that are associated with blood loss. Chronic blood loss into the GI tract causes iron-deficiency anemia.[6,21]

Mineral depletion, induced by drugs, is summarized in Table 19-5.

EFFECTS OF DRUGS ON NUTRIENT CATABOLISM

An increase in folacin catabolism has been suggested as a cause of folacin deficiency induced by drugs. Increased folacin catabolism has been induced by administration of diphenylhydantoin to mice. An earlier suggestion that vitamins might be catabolized more rapidly by different drugs that share the property of being microsomal enzyme inducers has not been borne out by the recent studies of mice that showed that phenobarbital does not affect the rate of metabolism of folacin.[19]

Drug–Food and Drug–Alcohol Incompatibilities

Acute toxic reactions occur when particular drugs are taken in combination with foods containing non-nutrients that potentiate or alter the pharmacologic effect of the drug, and similarly, toxic reactions can arise when certain drugs are taken with alcoholic beverages. Predisposition to these reactions may be due to pharmacogenetic factors, to allergy to chemicals contained in both drugs and food, or to hepatic or renal causes for slow drug elimination.

Recognition that these reactions may occur is a crucial element in the education of physicians, dietitians, and pharmacists. The clinician needs to be able to tell the patient whether a food or alcohol restriction is necessary with the drug to be prescribed. The dietitian should know what drugs a patient is taking, so as to avoid giving the patient foods having ingredients that interact with these drugs. The pharmacist who fills the prescription needs to be able to caution the patient about avoidance of certain foods and alcohol during the period when a specific drug with the potential of inducing such reactions is to be administered. With the increasing availability of interactive computer terminals, the pharmacist or physician could be cued about risk of drug–food or drug–alcohol incompatibilities (as well as risk of other adverse drug reactions) when patient information and drug prescription is "entered." Occurrence of these reactions would thereby be limited to those that are difficult or currently impossible to predict.

A summary of drug–food and drug–alcohol incompatibilities is presented in Table 19-6.

TABLE 19-6
Drug–Food and Drug–Alcohol Incompatibilities

Classification	Reactants		Effect
	1	*2*	
1. Tyramine reactions	*MAO Inhibitors*	High tyramine/ dopamine foods	
	Antidepressants, *e.g.,* Phenelzine, Procarbazine, Isoniazid (INH, Isonicotinic acid hydrazide)	Cheese	Flushing
		Red wines	Hypertension
		Chicken's liver	Cerebrovascular accidents
2. Disulfiram reactions	*Aldehyde dehydrogenase inhibitors*	*Ethanol*	
	Disulfiram	Beer	Flushing, headache
	(Antabuse)	Wine	Nausea, vomiting
	Calcium carbimide	Liquor	Chest and abdominal pain
	Metronidazole	Foods containing	
	Nitrofurantoin	alcohol	
	Sulfonylureas		
3. Hypoglycemic reactions	*Insulin releasors*		
	Oral hypoglycemic agents		Weakness
	Sugar (as in sweet mixes)		Mental confusion
			Irrational behavior
			Loss of consciousness
4. Flush reactions	*Miscellaneous*	*Ethanol*	
	Chlorpropamide		Flush
	(+ diabetes)		Dyspnea
	Griseofulvin		Headache
	Tetrachlorethylene		
5. CNS depression	*Drugs with sedative effects*	*Ethanol*	
	Antihistamines		Somnolence
	Narcotic analgesics		Inability to drive car or
	Tranquilizers		operate machinery
	Barbiturates		
	Tricyclic antidepressants		
	Tetrachloroethylene		
6. Loss of intended drug effect	*Anticonvulsants*	*Ethanol*	
	Diphenylhydantoin	Folic acid	Seizures
7. Potentiation of intended drug effect	*Anticoagulants*	*Ethanol*	
	Coumarin drugs	Acute drinking	Hemorrhage

Adapted from Roe DA: Interactions between drugs and nutrients. Med Clin North Am 63:985–1007, 1979

RISK AND PREVENTION

Risks of the adverse effects of drug–nutrient interactions in clinical practice are highest in patients who are taking the most drugs (*e.g.,* the elderly), in patients who are malnourished (*e.g.,* cancer patients), and in those whose ability to metabolize drugs and use nutrients is compromised (*e.g.,* alcoholics). Intervention to prevent undesired effects of drug–nutrient interactions is feasible provided that health professionals are aware of circumstances that lead to their occurrence, and as long as careful nutritional monitoring of patients on acute or chronic drug therapies is maintained. Concurrent monitoring of nutritional status and serum levels of drugs, as well as day-by-day recording of diet and food intake, is desirable if drug–nutrient interactions that result in untoward effects on therapeutic management are to be minimized.

References

1. Anderson KE, Conney AH, Kappas A: Nutrition and oxidative drug metabolism in man: Relative influence of dietary lipids, carbohydrate, and protein. Clin Pharmacol Ther 26:493, 1979

2. Arenillas L: Amitriptyline and body weight. Lancet 1:432, 1964
3. Banks T, Nayab A: Letter: Digitalis cachexia. N Engl J Med 290:746, 1974
4. Bates TR, Sequera JA, Tembo AV: Effect of food on nitrofurantoin absorption. Clin Pharmacol Ther 16:63, 1974
5. Bergen SS: Appetite stimulating properties of cyproheptadine. Am J Dis Child 108:270, 1974
6. Boardman PL, Hart ED: Side effects of indomethacin. Ann Rheum Dis 26:127, 1967
7. Conney AH, Pantuck EJ, Hsiao K-C et al: Enhanced phenacetin metabolism in human subjects fed charcoal-broiled beef. Clin Pharmacol Ther 20:633, 1976
8. Craft AW, Kay HEM, Lawson DN et al: Methotrexate-induced malabsorption in children with acute lymphoblastic leukaemia. Br Med J 2:1511, 1977
9. Crounse RG: Human pharmacology of griseofulvin: The effect of fat intake on gastrointestinal absorption. J Invest Dermatol 37:529, 1961
10. Das KM, Eastwood MA, McManus JPA et al: The metabolism of salicylazosulfapyridine in ulcerative colitis. I. The relationship between metabolites and response to treatment in in-patients; II. The relationship between metabolites and the progress of the disease studied in out-patients. Gut 14:631, 1973
11. Duarte GC, Winnacker JL, Becker KL et al: Thiazide-induced hypercalcemia. N Engl J Med 284:828, 1971
12. Gander DR, Lond MB: Treatment of depressive illnesses with combined antidepressants. Lancet 2:107, 1965
13. Gonzales–Vitale JC, Hayes DM, Cvitkovic E et al: The renal pathology of clinical trials of Cis-platinum. II. Diamminedichloride. Cancer 39:1362, 1977
14. Hunt JN: Gastric emptying in relation to drug absorption. Am J Dig Dis 8:885, 1963
15. Jaffe JJ, Colaizzi JL, Barry H: Effects of dietary components on GI absorption of acetaminophen tablets in man. J Pharm Sci 60:1646, 1971
16. Johns MP: Drug Therapy and Nursing Care, p 489. New York, Macmillan, 1979
17. Kappas A, Alvares AP, Anderson KE et al: Effect of charcoal-broiled meat on antipyrine and theophylline metabolism. Clin Pharmacol Ther 23:445, 1978
18. Kappas A, Anderson KE, Conney AH et al: Influence of dietary protein and carbohydrate on antipyrine and theophylline metabolism. Clin Pharmacol Ther 20:643, 1976
19. Kelly D, Weir D, Reed B et al: Effect of anticonvulsant drugs on the rate of folate catabolism in mice. J Clin Invest 64:1089, 1979
20. Krakoff IH: Nephrotoxicity of Cis-dichlorodiammine-platinum (II). Cancer Treat Rep 63:1523, 1979
21. Leonards JR, Leevy G: Gastrointestinal blood loss during prolonged aspirin administration. N Engl J Med 289:1020, 1973
22. MacFarlane MD: Penicillamine and zinc. Lancet 2:962, 1974
23. Mao CC, Jacobson ED: Intestinal absorption and blood flow. Am J Clin Nutr 23:820, 1970
24. Melander A: Influence of food on the bioavailability of drugs. Clin Pharmacokinet 3:337, 1978
25. Modell W: Status and prospect of drugs for overeating. JAMA 173:1131, 1960
26. Monks TJ, Caldwell J, Smith RL: Influence of methylxanthine-containing foods on theophylline metabolism and kinetics. Clin Pharmacol Ther 513, 1979
27. Neuvonen P, Mattila M, Gothini G et al: Interference of iron and milk with absorption of tetracycline (abstr). Scand J Clin Lab Invest (Suppl) 27:76, 1971
28. Pawan GLS: Drugs and appetite. Proc Nutr Soc 33:239, 1973
29. Paykel PS, Mueller PS, De La Vergne PM: Amitriptyline, weight gain and carbohydrate cravings: A side effect. Br J Psychiatry 123:501, 1973
30. Pentuck EJ, Hsiao KC, Loub WD et al: Stimulatory effect of vegetables on intestinal drug metabolism in the rat. J Pharmacol Exp Ther 198:278, 1976
31. Pentuck EJ, Pentuck CB, Barland WA et al: Effect of dietary brussel sprouts and cabbage on human drug metabolism. Clin Pharmacol Ther 25:88, 1978
32. Ravid M, Robson M: Proximal myopathy caused by iatrogenic phosphate depletion. JAMA 236:1380, 1976
33. Roe DA: Drug-Induced Nutritional Deficiencies. Westport, Conn, AVI Publishing, 1976
34. Roe DA: Interactions between drugs and nutrients. Symposium on Applied Nutrition in Clinical Medicine. Med Clin North Am 63:985, 1979
35. Safer DJ, Allan RP: Factors influencing the suppressant effects of two stimulant drugs on the growth of hyperactive children. Pediatrics 5:660, 1973
36. Safer D, Allan R, Barr E: Depression of growth in hyperactive children on stimulant drugs. N Engl J Med 287:7, 1972
37. Safer DJ, Allan RP, Barr E: Growth rebound after termination of stimulant drugs. J Pediatr Pharm Therap 86:113, 1975
38. Scheline RR: Metabolism of foreign compounds by gastrointestinal microorganisms. Pharmacol Rev 25:451, 1973
39. Shields HM: Rapid fall of serum phosphorus secondary to antacid therapy. Gastroenterology 75:1137, 1978
40. Shils ME: Nutrition and neoplasia. In Goodhart R, Shils M (eds): Modern Nutrition in Health and Disease, 6th ed. Philadelphia, Lea & Febiger, 1979
41. Shore MT, Spector MH, Ladman AJ: Effects of cancer, radiotherapy and cytotoxic drugs on intestinal structure and function. Cancer Treat Rev 6:141, 1979
42. Stiel JN, Liddle GW, Lacey WW: Studies on mechanism of cyproheptadine-induced weight gain in human subjects. Metabolism 19:192, 1970
43. Suki W, Yiem JJ, Von Minden M et al: Acute treatment of hypercalcemia with furosemide. N Engl J Med 283:836, 1970
44. Van Hees PAM, Tuente JHM, Van Rossum JM et al: Influence of intestinal transit time on azo-reduction of salicylazosulfapyridine (salazopyrine). Gut 20:300, 1979
45. Von Hoff DD, Schilsky R, Reichert CM et al: Toxic effects of Cis-dichlorodiammineplatinum (II) in man. Cancer Treat Rep 63:1527, 1979
46. Van Praag HM: Abuse of dependence on and psychoses from anorexigenic drugs. In Meyer L (ed): Drug Induced Diseases, pp 281–294. New York, North Holland Publishing, 1968
47. Welling PC: Influence of food and diet on gastrointestinal drug absorption: A review. J Pharmacokinet Biopharm 5:291, 1977

20
Endocrinology

Mark E. Molitch
William T. Dahms

Hormones have a direct effect on every aspect of the body's handling of nutrients, including appetite, absorption from the gastrointestinal (GI) tract, transport across cell membranes, and metabolism of substrates (storage, catabolism, and excretion). Conversely, changes in an individual's nutritional status have profound effects on the functioning of the endocrine system. Many of the concepts to be discussed below have been familiar for decades, particularly some of the physiologic effects of thyroxine, cortisol, and insulin. However, in the past decade, after the introduction of techniques for radioimmunoassay into endocrinology, these basic concepts have been greatly expanded, and it is now apparent that the metabolism of carbohydrate, fat, and protein is each influenced in some way by every major hormone. This chapter will focus first on those aspects of calcium and iodine metabolism in which endocrinology and nutrition directly affect each other, on the way in which the body deals with both an excess and a deficiency of calories, and finally on the more subtle aspects of nutrition and endocrinology.

Endocrine and Nutritional Control of Calcium and Magnesium Metabolism

Calcium (Ca) is one of the major ionic constituents in the body. The recommended levels of Ca intake (See Appendix Table A-1) may be somewhat below the optimal levels needed to prevent osteoporosis. Moreover, the high intake of phosphate associated with ingesting large amounts of meat and soft drinks may play a role in the development of osteoporosis in susceptible individuals. The control of serum Ca is closely regulated by the interaction between vitamin D and the parathyroid gland. The way in which vitamin D enhances intestinal Ca absorption has been clarified by the finding that an active form of vitamin D is produced by chemical reactions occurring in the liver and kidneys. This metabolically active form of vitamin D is important in treating bone disease associated with renal failure. The differential diagnosis of hypocalcemia and hypercalcemia involves a myriad of endocrine and nutritional diseases.

Magnesium (Mg) is mainly located within cells. Deficiency of Mg which may occur in alcoholism and many other diseases, may impair the release of parathyroid hormone (PTH) and thus produce hypocalcemia.

Phosphate deficiency is a clinically defined entity that may lead to poor formation of bones by its effect on calcium metabolism.

Mineral homeostasis is thus achieved by an intricate process in which dietary intake and excretory losses of Ca, phosphorus (P), and Mg are regulated by vitamin D and PTH. Before the nutritional aspects of Ca metabolism can be discussed, a brief review of recent advances in this field is appropriate.

ENDOCRINE CONTROL OF CALCIUM AND MAGNESIUM

CALCIUM HOMEOSTASIS

Over 90% of the 1000 g to 1200 g Ca in the body is located in the hydroxyapatite crystals of the skeleton, with the rest present in the extracellular fluid and within cells.

Vitamin D is the most important regulator of intestinal Ca absorption, but the dietary form of this vitamin must first be converted to an active form (see Fig. 20-1). Dietary vitamin D_3 is first hydroxylated in the liver to 25-hydroxycholecalciferol (25-OHD_3), which is then further hydroxylated in the kidney to 1,25-dihydroxycholecalciferol (1,25-$(OH)_2D_3$, which is the active form of vitamin D in the human being. Conversion to 1,25-$(OH)_2D_3$ is stimulated by a high serum PTH level and a low serum level of P. The 25-OHD_3 can also be hydroxylated in the 24 position to give 24,25-$(OH)_2D_3$, which is probably a metabolically inactive product. 1,25-$(OH)_2D_3$ itself stimulates the 24-hydroxylase enzyme and inhibits the 1 alpha hydroxylase enzyme. Finally, 24,25-$(OH)_2D_3$ can then be hydroxylated in the 1 position to give 1,24,25-$(OH)_2D_3$. This last compound may play a minor role in regulating the intestinal absorption of Ca, but more likely it is a degradation product.[6,25]

PTH is an 84 amino acid (9,500-dalton) peptide, initially synthesized in a larger precursor form. Hy-pocalcemia stimulates the intracellular conversion of precursor to PTH and the secretion of PTH into the blood. In turn, PTH increases the conversion of 25-OHD_3 to 1,25-$(OH)_2D_3$. Thus, hypocalcemia increases the peripheral blood concentrations of both PTH and the active form of vitamin D. Hypophosphatemia does not stimulate the release of PTH but does enhance the conversion of 25-OHD_3 to 1,25-$(OH)_2D_3$.[6]

In the intestine, bone, and kidney PTH and 1,25-$(OH)_2D_3$ interact to increase blood Ca (see Fig. 20-2). Dietary Ca and P are absorbed in the duodenum and upper jejunum. Absorption is promoted by 1,25-$(OH)_2D_3$, probably through the stimulation of the synthesis of an intracellular Ca-binding protein in the brush border of the intestine, and PTH probably influences absorption indirectly by stimulating synthesis of 1,25-$(OH)_2D_3$. In bone, PTH acts to increase bone resorption by increasing the activity and number of the osteoclasts while at the same time decreasing the activity of the osteoblasts. The activity of osteoclasts is enhanced by 1,25-$(OH)_2D_3$, thereby mobilizing Ca and P from mineralized bone. Each hormone needs the other's presence for max-

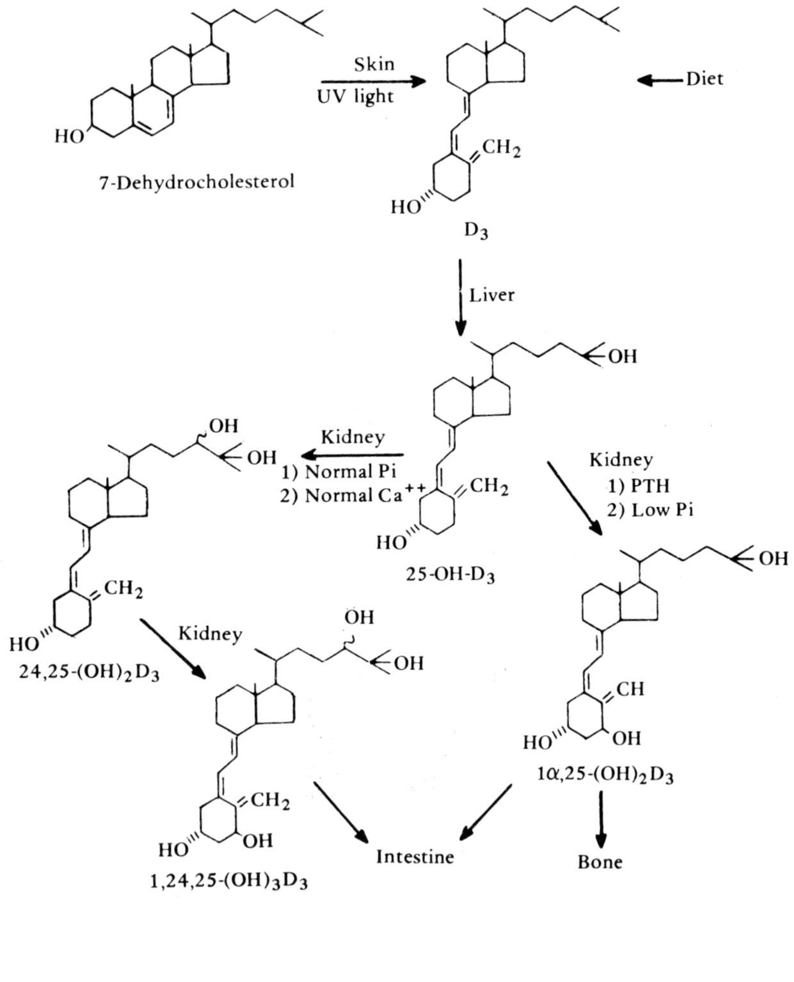

FIG. 20-1 Vitamin D metabolism in preparation for function. (DeLuca HP: Am J Med 58:42, 1975)

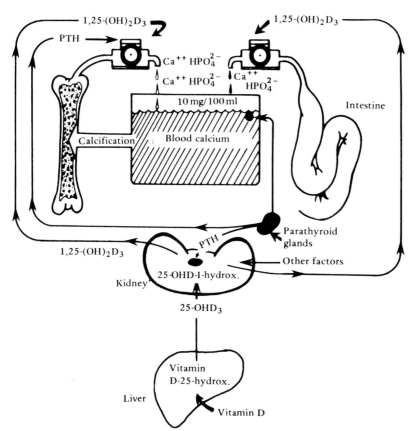

FIG. 20-2 Calcium homeostasis system, which includes regulation of kidney hydroxylase systems. Note that $1,25\text{-}(OH)_2D_3$ functions in intestine without presence of PTH, whereas its function in bone requires presence of that hormone. (Holick MF, Kleines–Bossaler A, Schnoes HK et al: J Biol Chem 248:6691, 1973)

imal action on bone. In the kidney, PTH acts in the proximal tubule to reduce the reabsorption of Ca and bicarbonate and, to a lesser extent, the reabsorption of amino acids, Mg, and potassium (K). In the distal tubule, PTH increases Ca absorption. The net effect on the kidney is to increase Ca reabsorption.[6]

Calcitonin is a 32-amino acid polypeptide secreted by the parafollicular "C" cells of the thyroid. It may be important in growing bone, but its physiologic role in adult humans is unclear. It may play a minor role in inhibiting bone resorption.[6]

MAGNESIUM HOMEOSTASIS

The total body content of Mg is about 21 g to 28 g, or about 2000 mEq. Half of it is found in the skeleton, 1% in the extracellular fluid, and the remainder within the cells. The average daily intake is about 25 mEq, and an intake of 0.30 to 0.35 mEq/kg body weight/day is necessary to maintain a positive Mg balance. The most common dietary source of Mg is green vegetables. Magnesium is absorbed primarily in the small intestine, but it can also be absorbed in the colon. The proportion of

intestinal Mg absorbed varies inversely with the intake. Renal losses of magnesium may be increased with the use of diuretics, persistent glycosuria, and alcohol ingestion.[49] In Mg deprivation, the renal loss is restricted to less than 1 mEq/day.[49] The mechanisms controlling serum concentrations of Mg are not well understood. Parathyroid hormone and vitamin D seem to be involved, but the experimental data are conflicting. Small changes in serum Mg affect PTH secretion as do similar changes in serum Ca. Prolonged Mg depletion, however, blocks both the release of PTH by the parathyroid glands and the action of PTH on the kidney.[6]

EFFECT OF NUTRITION ON CALCIUM METABOLISM

CALCIUM

In normal humans Ca balance is determined largely by whether the dietary intake is adequate because urinary excretion in the adult is relatively fixed. The main routes of losses are 100 mg/day to 200 mg/day in the urine, 140 mg/day to 175 mg/day in the biliary and pancreatic excretion, and 20 mg/

day in desquamated skin and sweat. The total daily loss in a normal individual is, therefore, 260 mg/day to 400 mg/day. During pregnancy, an additional 25 g to 30 g Ca is transferred to the fetus. In the postpartum period, lactation may account for the loss of another 750 mg/day. To balance these losses and maintain Ca balance, a high dietary intake must be maintained. The efficiency of absorption of Ca is inversely proportional to the dietary intake (see Table 20-1), with effects on absorption probably being mediated through PTH and vitamin D.[6] Calcium absorption also decreases linearly with age.[18] An intake well in excess of 1000 mg/day is required to maintain a positive Ca balance, and this level substantially exceeds the recommended daily allowance of 800 mg proposed by the National Research Council (see Appendix Table A-1). Dietary surveys of young adults in the United States have shown that the average intake is closer to 400 mg/day. Using the calculations of Lutwak and associates (see Table 20-1), the actual amount absorbed is thus between 150 mg/day and 200 mg/day, leaving a net daily loss of 50 mg to 100 mg.[31] Over 30 to 40 years this might produce a loss from the skeleton of up to 1000 g, or two thirds of the original amount of Ca present in the skeleton at the end of adolescence. Lutwak and his colleagues have proposed that this continued loss of Ca may be the major cause of osteoporosis in middle- and older-aged individuals, especially in women, who have a less dense bone matrix than men.[31] In addition, the presence of intestinal lactase deficiency in 47% of the Caucasian population with osteoporosis would further decrease the dietary intake of Ca.

The current American diet has an average Ca:P ratio of 1:4. This results from the low intake of milk, the high meat intake, and a high intake of carbonated soft drinks, which have a high P content. Beagle dogs placed on a diet in which the Ca:P ratio was 1:10 developed marked osteoporosis and secondary hyperparathyroidism.[31] When the Ca:P ratio was reduced to 1:1, the osteoporosis resolved. Because of these findings, Lutwak has recommended a diet containing at least 1000 mg Ca/day and a Ca:P ratio of 1:2 or less.

Intestinal malabsorption of fats can produce a negative Ca balance by causing a loss of the fat-soluble vitamin D. Calcium absorption may also be decreased after damage to the absorbing surface of the intestine.[25] A decrease in Mg absorption because of damage to the absorbing surface of the intestine may lead to decreased secretion of PTH as noted above. The diagnosis of hypocalcemia must be made with care in states of malabsorption, since 45% to 50% of Ca exists in serum bound to protein, and total serum proteins are often low in patients with malabsorption. A correction factor of 1

TABLE 20-1
Dietary Calcium and Calcium Absorption*

Subject	Dietary Intake (mg/d)	Efficiency of Absorption (% ± SD)	Absorbed Calcium (mg/d)
12	<150	59.3 ± 49.6	89
40	150–300	38.1 ± 22.5	114
34	300–400	35.2 ± 21.8	141
13	400–600	27.1 ± 24.7	163
16	600–800	26.5 ± 21.8	212
23	800–1000	23.9 ± 22.5	239
77	1000–1200	27.5 ± 16.6	330
30	1200–1400	20.9 ± 46.6	293
34	1400–1600	24.9 ± 23.0	398
32	>1600	25.2 ± 23.8	504

*Lutwak L, Singer FR, Urist MR: Ann Intern Med 80:639, 1974

mg Ca/1 g albumin below the average of 4 g may be used to correct for altered protein levels. In all states of hypocalcemia not caused by hypoparathyroidism, a secondary hyperparathyroidism develops, with effects on bone and kidney similar to those of primary hyperparathyroidism.

In addition to inadequate dietary Ca, a dietary deficiency of vitamin D may produce rickets in children and osteomalacia in adults. The recommended daily intake of 400 IU vitamin D is usually adequate for children and adults; clinical osteomalacia may be produced when the intake is less than 70 IU/day. The best natural sources for vitamin D are eggs, butter, cream, liver, and fish. Since in the United States it is standard practice to add 400 IU vitamin D to each quart of milk, simple vitamin D deficiency is rare in this country. However, infants who had only been breast fed and had not received vitamin D supplements developed rickets in the United States.[36]

There are several disease states in which the nutritional requirements for vitamin D are greatly increased. Intestinal malabsorption with steatorrhea and gastric surgery can often lead to malabsorption of vitamin D. In biliary cirrhosis, absorption of vitamin D may be reduced, and hydroxylation of vitamin D_3 to $25\text{-}OHD_3$ may also be impaired. The anticonvulsants phenobarbital and diphenylhydantoin interfere with the action of $1,25\text{-}(OH)_2D_3$, giving rise to osteomalacia in some instances; $1,25\text{-}(OH)_2D_3$ levels are normal in these patients.[25] The recommended daily allowance of vitamin D for patients on anticonvulsant drugs is now 8,000 IU/week to 10,000 IU/week.[25] When osteomalacia occurs, it is characterized by bone pain, proximal muscle weakness, and occasionally symptoms of hypocalcemia. Blood calcium levels are low to normal. The phosphate is low, alkaline phosphatase

TABLE 20-2
Vitamin D Preparations*

Name	Usual Dose (in Hypoparathyroidism)	Time to Restore Normocalcemia	Persistence after Stopping Drug
Cholecalciferol (D_3)	50–100,000 IU	4–8 wk	6–18 wk
Ergocalciferol (D_2)	50–100,000 IU	4–8 wk	6–18 wk
Dihydrotachysterol (DHT)	0.25–1.25 mg	1–2 wk	1–3 wk
25OHD$_3$	50–200 µg	2–4 wk	4–12 wk
1,25-(OH)$_2$D$_3$	0.5–2.5 µg	3–7 d	3–7 d
1αOHD$_3$	0.5–3 µg	1–8 wk	6–14 d

*Modified from Molitch ME: Endocrinology. In Molitch ME (ed): *Management of Medical Problems in Surgical Patients.* Philadelphia, F. A. Davis, 1982

is usually elevated, and parathyroid hormone levels are elevated. Bone biopsy reveals increased unmineralized osteoid.[46] Several preparations of vitamin D are now available for use; the most often used are cholecalciferol and 1,25-(OH)$_2$D$_3$ (see Table 20-2).

The gradual loss of bone mass that occurs with aging (osteoporosis) must be differentiated from true osteomalacia. Although the bone loss affects the entire skeleton, some areas are affected at different rates; for instance, bone loss from the vertebrae and long bones occurs earlier and at a greater rate than does loss from coritcal bone. In general, the rate of bone loss does not increase with age, but there is a steady fall of about 8% every decade in women and 3% every decade in men, with the loss starting earlier in women. The rate accelerates in women following menopause.[1,46] On bone biopsy, osteoporotic bone is characterized by normal osteoid mineralization (as opposed to osteomalacia) but a total decrease in bone volume. Features of osteomalacia are seen in over 30% of women with osteoporosis, however. On spine x-ray films, 29% of women and 18% of men between the ages of 45 and 79 years demonstrate osteoporosis.[1,46] These figures are low because at least 30% loss of bone mineral is needed before x-ray changes become evident. Clinically, patients present most often with back pain owing to vertebral collapse and usually have loss of height from vertebral compression and possibly some dorsal kyphosis. Other common sites of fracture include the neck of the femur and the radius.

The etiology of osteoporosis is far from clear and probably involves a multitude of factors, including estrogen loss at menopause and low Ca intake, high P intake, and occasionally low vitamin D intake.[1,46] An adequate intake of Ca (probably 1 g/day) and vitamin D may help to prevent the development of osteoporosis, and estrogen therapy started at the time of menopause may be helpful as well. Once osteoporosis is established and symptomatic, the mainstays of therapy are a high Ca intake of 1 g/day to 2 g/day and vitamin D intake of at least 1000 IU/day (possibly up to 10,000 IU/day).[1]

The easiest and most economical form of Ca supplement is calcium carbonate (see Table 20-3). Patients receiving Ca and vitamin D supplements should have periodic measurements of serum and 24-hr urinary Ca to avoid the complications of hypercalcemia or hypercalciuria. Estrogen or androgen therapy may be beneficial for up to 6 months initially because of demonstrated effects or decreasing bone resorption, but longer-term therapy causes a secondary decrease in bone formation. At present, fluoride and calcitonin therapies are experimental and cannot yet be recommended.

In renal failure, defective conversion of 25-OHD$_3$ to 1,25-(OH)$_2$D$_3$ occurs for two reasons: (1) the

TABLE 20-3
Calcium Supplement Preparations

Generic Name	Trade Name	Calcium Content	Route
Calcium carbonate	Oscal	250 mg/tablet	Oral
	Titralac	168 mg/tablet	Oral
Calcium glucobionate	Neocalglucon	115 mg/5 ml	Oral
Calcium lactate		80 mg/650 mg/tablet	Oral
Calcium gluconate 10%		9 mg/ml	Intravenous
Calcium glucoheptonate	Calcium Gluceptate	18 mg/ml	Intravenous

high level of P shuts off the conversion of 25-OHD$_3$ to 1,25-(OH)$_2$D$_3$ and (2) there is a relative lack of normal renal tissue to effect this conversion. Very large doses of vitamin D have been used to overcome these defects. However, administration of small amounts of the active 1,25-(OH)$_2$D$_3$ to uremic subjects also repairs the malabsorption of Ca. Several analogs of vitamin D in which the 1 position is hydroxylated are also effective in treating the bone disease found in patients with renal failure (see Chap. 34).

Vitamin D-dependent rickets is now thought to represent a defect in the conversion of 25-OHD$_3$ to 1,25-(OH)$_2$D$_3$. This syndrome is characterized by hypocalcemia, hypophosphatemia, and clinical rickets. It can be treated with 10,000 IU/day to 50,000 IU/day vitamin D$_3$ or with very small quantities of 1,25-(OH)$_2$D$_3$. Vitamin-D-resistant rickets, on the other hand, appears to be a defect in the renal tubular transport of P and is not really a deficiency state of vitamin D.[25]

PHOSPHATE

Dietary phosphate deficiency is less common than deficiency states for either Ca or vitamin D. Prolonged ingestion of phosphate-binding antacids and parenteral hyperalimentation are the most common causes of phosphate depletion, but other causes include diuretic use, alcoholism, diabetic ketoacidosis, vomiting, sepsis, and glucocorticoid use.[28] Hypophosphatemia stimulates the synthesis of 1,25-(OH)$_2$D$_3$, which increases the intestinal absorption of Ca and phosphate. Prolonged hypophosphatemia also increases urinary Ca excretion, decreases urinary losses of phosphate, and thus produces a net negative Ca balance. A low phosphate intake also decreases red blood cell 2,3-diphosphoglycerate (2,3-DPG) and adenosine triphosphate (ATP), with an associated decrease in the ability of the red cell to release oxygen to the tissue.[28] Clinically, the hypophosphatemic syndrome presents with vague complaints of weakness, anorexia, malaise, bone pain, and joint stiffness. When severe and prolonged, it can lead to severe osteomalacia and weakness.[28]

Phosphate depletion is best treated with oral supplements (see Table 20-4). Milk, which contains 60 g each of Ca and P per quart, can also be used. The various phosphate preparations should be given in three to four doses, the maximum dose being that which is tolerated by the patient. Diarrhea is usually the dose limiting factor. Severe hypophosphatemia (< 1 mg/dl) causing cardiac or respiratory muscle weakness, confusion, hemolysis, or severe bone pain may require parenteral phosphate in a dose of 2.5 mg/kg to 5 mg/kg (0.08

TABLE 20-4
Oral Phosphate Preparations*

Name	Dose to Provide 1 g Elemental Phosphorus	Cation (mEq) Na	Cation (mEq) K
Phospho–soda	6.2 ml	57	
Neutra–Phos	300 ml or 4 capsules	28.5	28.5
Neutra–Phos K	300 ml or 4 capsules		57
K–Phos	8 tablets		29.4
K–Phos Neutral	4 tablets	48	8.3
Hyper Phos K	6 tablets		57
Phos–tabs	6 tablets		52
Uro-KP-Neutral	6 tablets	36.9	21.8

*After Molitch ME: Endocrinology. In Molitch ME (ed): *Management of Medical Problems in Surgical Patients.* Philadelphia, F.A. Davis, 1982

mM/kg–0.16 mM/kg) body weight over 6 hours of any one of the parenteral preparations available.[29] Intravenous phosphate therapy has been associated with hypotension, hypocalcemia (with tetany), hyperkalemia, and metastatic calcification. To avoid such complications, intravenous phosphate should be given slowly, as indicated above, and the serum phosphorus should be measured and the clinical status assessed after each dose to ascertain whether further doses are needed. Intravenous phosphate should be avoided in patients with hypercalcemia or renal insufficiency (unless the hypercalcemic patient has not responded to other means of lowering the calcium and this is part of planned therapy).

MAGNESIUM

Magnesium deficiency in humans occurs in alcoholics who eat little food or in patients with intestinal malabsorption. Other less common causes of Mg depletion include protein–calorie malnutrition, hyperparathyroidism, hyperaldosteronism, thyrotoxicosis, diabetic ketoacidosis, early renal insufficiency, and diuretic therapy. As discussed above, Mg deficiency can lead to defective secretion or action of parathyroid hormone, or both, resulting in a hypocalcemic state that is responsive to Mg repletion alone. Clinically, Mg deficiency leads to neuromuscular hyperexcitability, with tetany, tonic-colonic seizures, ataxia, vertigo, tremors, weakness, depression, psychosis, and cardiac arrhythmias as the major manifestations.[27]

If severe central nervous system (CNS) symptoms or cardiac irritability can be accurately attributed to Mg depletion, then parenteral Mg therapy is indicated; 10 ml to 15 ml of 10% magnesium sulfate can be given intravenously over 15 min, followed by 500 ml of 2% magnesium sulfate intravenously over 6 hr. Alternatively 1 g of magnesium sulfate may be given intramuscularly every 4 to 6 hr. Magnesium levels should be checked twice daily during therapy, and deep tendon reflexes should be tested before each dose as Mg toxicity causes loss of these reflexes.[27]

EFFECTS OF ENDOCRINE DISEASE ON CALCIUM METABOLISM

HYPOCALCEMIA

Damage to the remaining parathyroid glands during surgery on the thyroid or parathyroid glands is the most common etiology for hypoparathyroidism. Neonatal immaturity, congenital absence of the parathyroid glands (along with the thymus in the DiGeorge's syndrome), idiopathic glandular failure, Mg deficiency, vitamin D deficiency, a defect in the receptor mechanism for parathyroid hormone (pseudohypoparathyroidism), and a defect in the hormone molecule itself are other etiologies for hypocalcemia. After surgical removal of a parathyroid adenoma, there is a transient (1–14 days) hypoparathyroidism, because secretion from the other glands was suppressed by the adenoma. In addition, postoperatively the bones affected with osteitis fibrosa in patients with hyperparathyroidism often avidly incorporate Ca. For both of these reasons, hypocalcemia may develop requiring treatment with extra Ca and sometimes with vitamin D for several weeks. In states of permanent hypoparathyroidism, requirements are very large for both Ca (1 g/day–2 g/day) and vitamin D (25,000 IU/day–200,0000 IU/day) in order to maintain the serum Ca at a normal level. The reason for this extraordinary vitamin D resistance appears to be that parathyroid hormone is necessary for the hydroxylation of vitamin D_3 in the 1 position. 1,25-$(OH)_2D_3$ has been used successfully in the treatment of hypoparathyroidism in doses of 0.5 μg/day to 2.5 μg/day.[6]

HYPERCALCEMIA

Elevated levels of parathyroid hormone are one cause for hypercalcemia and hypophosphatemia. In rare situations, a dietary deficiency of vitamin D can partially ameliorate this hypercalcemic response to excessive parathyroid hormone, but the histologic picture is confusing, showing combined osteomalacia and osteitis fibrosa. Secondary hyperparathyroidism is a usual accompaniment of vitamin D deficiency or renal failure, but hypercalcemia is not seen. In other causes of hypercalcemia, secretion of parathyroid hormone is suppressed.

Of special nutritional importance is vitamin D intoxication, which may result from 50,000 IU or more per day. Treatment consists of hydration and the administration of 100 mg hydrocortisone per day. In sarcoidosis there seems to be an increased sensitivity to the effects of vitamin D, yielding increased intestinal calcium absorption. The frequency of hypercalcemia, however, is probably quite low (2.2%) and is associated with widespread sarcoidosis. Sarcoid-induced hypercalcemia is readily reversible with glucocorticoids. The milk–alkali syndrome of Burnett consists of hypercalcemia due to the prolonged and excessive intake of milk and alkali, but the exact mechanism of the hypercalcemia is obscure. Ingestion of vitamin A in excess doses (>100,000 IU/day) over a period of years has been associated with hypercalcemia in rare instances. The hypercalcemia associated with malignancies usually is due to osseous metastases or the neoplastic production of PTH-like and other calcium mobilizing substances (*e.g.* prostaglandin E_2) and is not modified by dietary alterations.[6]

OTHER HORMONAL EFFECTS ON CALCIUM METABOLISM

In hyperthyroidism, there is an increase in bone remodeling with hypercalciuria and progressive loss of bone Ca. Hypercalcemia may occur in up to 17% of cases. In addition, there is decreased GI absorption of Ca, probably because of decreased transit time. For these reasons, osteoporosis is often present in long-standing hyperthyroidism. As mentioned above, glucocorticoids antagonize the action of vitamin D on the intestine and also stimulate bone resorption. In Cushing's syndrome, or when excessive doses of glucocorticoid are used in therapy, hypercalciuria and a negative Ca balance ensue, resulting in osteoporosis.[23] Growth hormone causes an increase in intestinal absorption of Ca and P, as well as hypercalciuria, and an increase in periosteal bone growth. However, growth hormone excess produces a decrease in cancellous bone formation. Estrogens administered exogenously in pharmacologic doses to osteoporotic postmenopausal women initially cause a decrease in bone resorption, but after 6 to 12 months, resorption of bone returns to pretreatment levels. The actions of estrogens in physiologic amounts on bone are unknown.

Iodine and Thyroid Metabolism

The importance of iodine in human thyroid metabolism has long been recognized. Major emphasis during most of the 20th century has been on providing adequate levels of iodine intake in those regions of the world where iodine deficiency is an endemic problem. With the introduction of iodized salt, the problem of iodine deficiency has largely disappeared, but in its place, people in many areas of the world now have higher intakes of iodine resulting from the addition of iodide to table salt and the use of iodate as a preservative in bread. The high intake of iodine in many regions of the United States has altered the interpretation of tests measuring the radioactive iodine uptake by the thyroid gland so that normal values are now lower than they were 10 years ago. The range of normal values for radioactive iodine uptake has been lowered to 5% to 30% in 24 hr, compared to the old normal range of 15% to 45%.[26] Excess iodine may be responsible for the decreased effectiveness of oral antithyroid drugs as a form of treatment for hyperthyroidism. The increased requirement for vitamins and minerals in hyperthyroidism is well recognized as is the reduced turnover that occurs when thyroid hormone is deficient.

IODINE AND THE THYROID

The only known function of iodine in animals is as part of the thyroid hormone molecule (see Fig. 20-3). Inorganic iodide derived from nutritional sources is actively transported into the thyroid, a process stimulated primarily by thyrotropin as well as by a complex intrathyroidal autoregulatory system. Additional iodide (about two thirds of the total free iodide in the gland) is liberated by the deiodination of the iodotyrosines that are formed when thyroglobulin is hydrolyzed. The free iodide in the thyroid is either discharged into the blood or reoxidized to iodine by peroxidase(s). The iodine is then "organified" into the tyrosine residues of thyroglobulin to form monoiodotyrosine (MIT) and diiodotyrosine (DIT). Finally, these two precursors are coupled within the thyroglobulin molecule to form triiodothyronine (T_3) and thyroxine (T_4). Proteolysis of thyroglobulin releases T_3 and T_4 into the blood, but the iodotyrosines are dehalogenated by iodotyrosine deiodinase. Several enzyme deficiencies can occur in this pathway, and most lead to goiter and hypothyroidism.

In the United States, dietary iodine intake averages 500 μg/day, and iodine deficiency is very rare. Iodine undergoes compartmentalization in the body (see Fig. 20-3). There is an exchangeable extrathyroidal pool of 250 μg iodide and an intrathyroidal pool of 8000 μg iodide. The circulating pool of T_4 and T_3 contains 600 μg iodine. Iodide is filtered and partially reabsorbed by the kidney. Renal iodide clearance is 30 ml/min to 40 ml/min, making this the major pathway for loss of iodine from the body. Minimal amounts of iodide are lost through the GI tract, except in states of malabsorption. In addition, large amounts of iodide and iodine can be lost through lactation.

Dietary iodine deficiency occurs where the soil has a low iodine content. The minimum daily requirement is 40 μg to 70 μg (see Table 20-5). Iodine deficiency usually results in a goiter and can be diagnosed when the urinary excretion is less

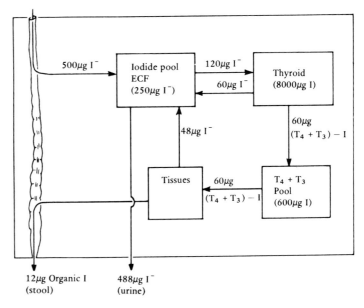

Fig. 20-3 Iodine metabolism in a state of iodine balance. Note that most (approximately 90%) of body iodine stores are present in thyroid (chiefly in organic form); approximately 10% are present as iodide. Arrows indicate daily flux of iodine. In this example, one fifth (120 μg/608 μg) of the iodide entering iodide space is accumulated by thyroid. Peak thyroid uptake of ^{131}I should be 20%, and the rate of turnover of thyronine–iodine peripherally 10% per day. (Ingbar SH, Woeber KA: The thyroid gland. In Williams RH (ed): Textbook of Endocrinology, 6th ed, p 121. Philadelphia, WB Saunders, 1974)

than 50 μg iodide/24 hr. Why some patients with iodine deficiency do not develop goiters and others do is unclear, but those with goiters have lower serum T_4 and higher serum thyroid-stimulating hormone (TSH). Most people in iodine-deficient regions are not clinically hypothyroid, even though their serum T_4 may be low because the synthesis of T_3 is increased. This appears to be an adaptive response of the thyroid to iodine deficiency. Some patients, of course, do become hypothyroid, and there is an increased incidence of cretinism in regions of iodine deficiency. Because these areas are usually in poorly developed countries with limited access to medical care, the standard treatment consists of injections of an iodized oil that releases iodide slowly over a period of 1 to 3 years.[26]

Hyperthyroidism occurs in areas of iodine deficiency, and the incidence of T_3 *toxicosis* (a state of hyperthyroidism due to excessive serum levels of T_3 and normal levels of T_4) is three times greater than in areas of normal iodine intake. When iodine is administered to a population with iodine deficiency, some patients become hyperthyroid due to the unmasking of a preexisting tendency toward hyperthyroidism that had been prevented by the deficiency.

Iodide therapy can also produce goiters in certain susceptible subjects. Excess iodide can inhibit thyroid hormone formation (Wolff–Chaikoff effect), but its effect is usually transient, and subjects treated with iodine usually "escape" from this inhibition after several days. The patients who develop goiters while on treatment with iodide apparently do not escape and become hypothyroid with goiter formation secondary to a rise in TSH. Patients with preexisting Hashimoto's thyroiditis,

in which there is a basic defect in organification of iodine, seem to be particularly susceptible to this form of goiter and can develop such goiters on the doses of iodide used in treatment of chronic lung disease. Since iodide can cross the placenta, iodide-induced goiters may also occur in newborn infants of mothers who have taken pharmacologic doses of iodides for pulmonary disease. Other side-effects of iodide therapy include skin rashes, coryza, fever, headache, dysgeusia, conjunctivitis, lymphadenopathy, and parotid swelling. Cardiac irritability has been seen in a case of massive iodide overdose.[26]

In recent years, lithium carbonate has been used extensively to treat patients with manic-depressive illness. Lithium is able to block the thyroidal release of T_3 and T_4, but the thyroid usually escapes from this effect, over a several month period. Here, again, some patients do not escape from this inhibition and develop lithium-induced hypothyroidism and goiters, which, at least in some cases, are reversible with the cessation of lithium therapy. There is some evidence that many of these patients may also have a defect in iodine organification (*e.g.*, an underlying Hashimoto's thyroiditis). It is important to note that this effect of lithium is not a dose-related effect and seems rather to reflect a defect within the thyroid itself.[26] This inhibitory effect of lithium has been used in recent years as part of the therapeutic armamentarium employed in the treatment of hyperthyroidism.[26] Although several foodstuffs are goitrogenic in animals, none have been proven to be clinically important in this regard in normally consumed amounts in the United States.

THYROID HORMONES

Secretion of thyroid hormone is regulated by thyrotropin (TSH), which is secreted by the anterior pituitary. The release of TSH, in turn, stimulated by the release of thyrotropin-releasing hormone (TRH) from the hypothalamus into the hypothalamic–pituitary portal blood system. A second hypothalamic inhibitory hormone called *somatostatin* inhibits TSH secretion. The active hormones secreted by the thyroid gland are T_4 and T_3. Although T_3 is secreted by the thyroid, approximately 70% to 80% of the circulating T_3 is derived from peripheral conversion from T_4, with only 20% to 30% being secreted directly by the thyroid. On a molar basis, T_3 is approximately four times more potent than T_4. Since the affinity of T_3 for thyroxine-binding globulin (TBG) is about one tenth that of T_4, and since the concentration of free T_3 in the serum is only one fifth of the concentration of free T_4, it has been estimated that these hormones con-

TABLE 20-5
Iodine Content of Some Foods*

Food	Iodine Content (μg/kg Fresh Weight)
Milk	26–370
Cheese	26–450
Eggs	6–20
Meat	21–420
Chicken	200–230
Saltwater fish	163–9860
Shellfish	150–2000
Freshwater fish	17–40
Cereals	14–80
Vegetables	9–201
Fruits	10–94
Beer	43–46
Wine	8–32

*Werner SC, Ingbar SH (eds): The Thyroid, p 410. New York, Harper & Row, 1971

tribute equally to biologic activity. Because many tissues have the ability to monodeiodinate T_4 to T_3, it is now thought that most of the biologic activity of the thyroid hormones is due to T_3. Whether T_4 has any intrinsic biologic activity is uncertain.[26] Reverse triiodothyronine (3,3',5' triiodothyronine) is a second major triiodothyronine that exists in plasma, and it is over 97% derived from peripheral conversion from T_4. Reverse T_3 (rT_3) is metabolically inactive. Several conditions, including reduced caloric intake, severe illness, and steroid administration, have now been shown to cause a decrease in serum T_3 levels while concomitantly causing an increase in rT_3 levels. It has been thought that this decrease in T_3 levels is due to decreased peripheral conversion of T_4 to T_3 and that the increase in rT_3 levels is due to a defect in metabolic clearance of rT_3. This change from metabolically active T_3 to metabolically inactive rT_3 is thought to be a compensatory phenomenon to decrease metabolic rate and energy substrate oxidation in the face of severe catabolic stress or inadequate nutrient intake.[8] Recently it has been shown that a large portion of these changes in thyroid hormone metabolism that occur in patients with severe illness is due to the reduced caloric intake associated with the illness.[41]

The thyroid hormones affect metabolic processes in all areas, although the precise mechanisms are unknown. These hormones stimulate an increase in oxygen consumption (*i.e,* basal metabolic rate). Thyroid hormones in physiologic amounts are necessary for protein synthesis and also promote nitrogen retention.

By affecting insulin-mediated synthesis of glycogen and epinephrine-mediated glycogenolysis, thyroid hormones in small amounts promote glycogen synthesis, whereas in excess amounts they promote glycogenolysis. In addition, thyroid hormones promote intestinal absorption of glucose and galactose and the uptake of glucose by adipocytes. The general metabolic rate controlled by thyroid hormones influences insulin degradation and can be important in states of thyroid overactivity and underactivity.

Thyroid hormones directly increase lipolysis and also sensitize adipose tissue to the actions of other lipolytic hormones. The mobilized free fatty acids and glycerol increase triglyceride synthesis, but the level of lipoprotein lipase is also higher so that the levels of triglycerides are not increased. Thyroid hormones, on the other hand, lower the serum cholesterol by increasing the removal of low-density lipoproteins, which are the main carriers of cholesterol. This occurs by increasing the conversion of cholesterol to bile acids and by increasing the excretion of cholesterol and bile salts in the feces. Thyroid hormones also promote cholesterol synthesis but to a lesser extent than its elimination so that the net effect is a lowering of serum cholesterol. The oxidation of the free fatty acids mobilized from fat tissues is also increased by thyroid hormones.

Thyroid Disease

HYPERTHYROIDISM

Hyperthyroidism results in an increased basal metabolic rate (BMR) and weight loss in spite of increased appetite and food intake. Increased perspiration, heat intolerance, and a slightly elevated basal body temperature may also be present.[30] The rise in cellular metabolism is reflected in the increased number and size of mitochondria. Protein synthesis is accelerated even more. In the child, acceleration of linear growth and bone maturation are an early manifestation of hyperthyroidism, but if the hypermetabolic state continues to the point of decreased nutrition and weight loss, growth may be retarded. When protein catabolism is severe, patients are often found to have myopathy with muscle wasting and weakness.

Glucose intolerance occurs frequently in hyperthyroidism. This appears to be due to (1) increased insulin degradation, (2) increased glycogenolysis, (3) increased intestinal absorption of glucose, and (4) increased gluconeogenesis from the protein catabolism. Preexisting diabetes can be made worse by hyperthyroidism.[30] Triglyceride levels are lowered in hyperthyroidism because of the increase in degradation.

Vitamin requirements are usually elevated in hyperthyroidism for the following two reasons: (1) the requirements for thiamine, riboflavin, B_{12}, ascorbic acid, pyridoxine, and vitamins A, D, and E are all increased because of enhanced cellular metabolism, and (2) degradation of many vitamins is accelerated in hyperthyroidism. Hyperthyroidism also stimulates Ca resorption from bone, with resultant hypercalciuria and osteopenia if the process is prolonged. Varying degrees of hypercalcemia develop at least transiently in up to 17% of patients with hyperthyroidism, probably on the basis of an increase in bone resorption greater than the renal excretion of Ca.

Increased dietary intake of iodine may influence the therapy of hyperthroidism. A review of the studies in which hyperthyroid patients were treated with antithyroid drugs has shown that the remission rate induced by these drugs has progressively declined from 50% to 60% in the 1950s to 13% in 1973. This change corresponds with a rise in iodine intake, suggesting that this phenomenon results from the increase in iodine intake. Rarely, an acute iodide load (usually the administration of iodide-containing radiographic contrast media) can precipitate hyperthyroidism in a predisposed individual.[26]

Because of the characteristic weight loss in patients with hyperthyroidism, both T_4 and T_3 have been used experimentally to induce weight loss in obese patients. Patients so treated predictably lose weight, but much of the weight loss is from catabolism of protein-containing lean body tissue. Surprisingly, patients treated with very large doses of T_3 (225 μg/day) and T_4 (900 μg/day) exhibited very few subjective manifestations of hyperthyroidism other than a minimal increase (6 beat/min) in heart rate and perspiration.[4]

HYPOTHYROIDISM

In hypothyroidism, there is a decrease in BMR. Clinically, patients gain weight in spite of a decreased appetite. Cold intolerance and a decreased basal body temperature also occur. Nitrogen balance is positive, indicating that the slowing of protein degradation is of a greater magnitude than the slowing of protein synthesis. Hypothyroidism in children results in delayed growth and bone maturation.

Oral glucose tolerance tests show a flattened response, possibly owing to slowed absorption of glucose from the intestine. Insulin secretion is also delayed as is its degradation; this latter effect accounts for the decreased insulin requirements in diabetics who become hypothyroid. Lipid metabolism is also decreased more than its synthesis so that triglycerides and cholesterol are increased in the blood. The concentration of the low-density lipoproteins, which are the main carriers of cholesterol, increases more than does the concentration of triglyceride-rich, very-low-density lipoproteins. In hypothyroidism, there is a decrease in the conversion of carotene to vitamin A, and serum carotene levels are often increased, giving the skin a yellowish hue. Hypothyroid patients are often hyponatremic with an impairment in the clearance of free water. This is probably due to the decreased glomerular filtration rate (GFR) and resulting low rate of delivery of filtrate to the distal diluting segment and possibly also to an increased secretion of antidiuretic hormone.[26]

Effects of Nutrition on the Endocrine System

An affluent society is associated with an increased frequency of obesity (see Chap. 28). The importance of obesity resides in part in its effects on high blood pressure, gallbladder disease, and diabetes mellitus. The diagnosis of many endocrine diseases in the presence of obesity can be a complex problem because corpulence itself modifies the response to many of the usual endocrine tests.[4]

At the other extreme from obesity is the problem of malnutrition, which occurs in many forms. One important variety of malnutrition and growth retardation results from maternal or environmental deprivation. Anorexia nervosa, a psychiatric complex appearing at puberty, may also cause malnutrition and requires careful evaluation to exclude organic forms of malnutrition (see Chap. 33).

The interaction of endocrine diseases with trace elements is complex and frequently difficult to assess.

OBESITY

INSULIN SECRETION

The islets of the pancreas are enlarged in obese patients. A similar hyperplasia of islet tissue has been demonstrated in experimental obesity produced by hypothalamic injury, as well as in genetically obese animals. Obese patients also have increased levels of insulin both while fasting and after meals. The degree of elevation in insulin is correlated with the degree of obesity. In addition to the increase in basal secretion of insulin, obese subjects almost uniformly show an increase in the secretion of insulin after the administration of glucose, the injection of glucagon, or the infusion of L-leucine. Patients with long-standing obesity show more impairment of glucose tolerance than those with recent onset of obesity. The rise in insulin of obese, normal, and diabetic subjects in response to glucose has been carefully analyzed, with the conclusion that the increment in insulin following an oral glucose load is comparable in these three groups if it is expressed as a percentage increment above the fasting or basal level. Other studies have indicated that in obese subjects the maximal rise in insulin is greater than in normal subjects, but that the concentration of glucose required to produce half of this maximal rise remains the same.[21]

The available data on the turnover and metabolism of insulin in obesity suggest that the increased concentration of insulin in obesity results from increased secretion and not from a reduced removal of this hormone. Since the increased basal levels of insulin reflect enhanced secretion, the question then becomes: by what mechanism is the secretion of insulin augmented? Both nutrients and neural factors can modify insulin secretion.

Increased concentrations of amino acids might increase basal insulin in obesity. Plasma arginine, leucine, tyrosine, phenyalanine, and valine are increased in the obese, but the remaining amino acids are normal. This increase in amino acids might be in part responsible for the enhanced insulin output. Both arginine and leucine are potent stimulators of insulin secretion. In addition, the small increase in leucine might act synergistically with glucose to stimulate insulin secretion.

The autonomic nervous system is one regulator of basal insulin levels in obesity. The infusion of epinephrine into normal subjects increases the concentration of glucose but blocks the rise in insulin. In obese patients, an infusion of epinephrine also increases the concentration of glucose and actually reduces the concentration of insulin below control levels. Blockade of the alpha receptors in the Islets of Langerhans by infusing phentolamine reverses the block to insulin release, and there is a rise in insulin in normal subjects. This implies that there is normally some sympathetic inhibition of insulin secretion. In obese patients, on the other hand, phentolamine does not significantly change the concentration of insulin, raising the possibility that tonic sympathetic activity is not suppressing insulin release in the obese patients. This would mean that a significant portion of the rise in basal insulin in obesity might represent withdrawal of tonic inhibition by the sympathetic nervous system.

The second problem to be examined is the paradox of an elevated glucose along with high levels of insulin. This phenomenon has been called *insulin resistance* and has been demonstrated in adipose tissue, liver, and muscle. Insulin exerts its effects only after binding to receptors on the surface of cells. Multiple studies have shown decreased insulin receptors in obesity, although some controversy exists.[37] This decrease in receptors probably accounts for most of the insulin resistance found in obesity. It has also been demonstrated that the decrease in insulin receptors correlates well with the degree of insulin resistance. Recent evidence suggests that insulin itself may be responsible for the decrease in receptors (down regulation) because acute insulin suppression in obese subjects causes an increase in lymphocyte insulin receptors.[21] It is therefore unclear whether the primary deficit is a decrease in insulin receptors causing a compensatory increase in insulin, or whether the increased insulin comes first and produces a decrease in insulin receptors. In this latter situation the cause of the insulin resistance is unclear but may be due to a postreceptor, intracellular mechanism.[21]

Composition of the diet is one factor that influences the sensitivity to insulin. Fat cells were obtained by needle aspiration of subcutaneous tissue from volunteers who were fed diets of known carbohydrate content before and after weight gain and in obese patients who were also fed controlled diets before and after weight loss. Large fat cells from either group were less responsive to insulin than small fat cells. When the size of the fat cells remained constant, however, increasing carbohydrate in the diet increased both the basal and insulin-stimulated metabolism of glucose.[45] Since adipose tissue accounts for less than 5% of *in vivo* glucose disposal, it is likely that this phenomenon plays only a minor role in total body insulin resistance.

Additional insights have been obtained as to the role of diet and weight gain on the development of insulin resistance in man. One group of investigators asked the following question: can the endocrine profile of spontaneous obesity be reproduced when lean subjects gain weight by a period of self-induced overeating?[45] The results of these studies are summarized in Table 20-6. Approximately 70% of the weight gained by these subjects was fat, and the remainder was water and protein. The fat was stored by increasing the size of preexisting fat cells. Plasma glucose was significantly increased. Of particular note is the fact that glucose was raised even when fat provided the entire caloric supplement used to produce weight gain. The basal levels of insulin were also increased after weight gain, regardless of the type of diet used to increase body weight. Cortisol secretion was elevated and the release of growth hormone in response to several stimuli was blunted. The concept that hyperinsulinemia and glucose intolerance are consequences of excess caloric intake is consistent with the improvement in glucose tolerance and the fall of insulin levels during weight loss.

GLUCAGON SECRETION

Studies on glucagon levels in obesity are conflicting. Basal levels of glucagon are unchanged by obesity, but the rise in glucagon after amino acid infusions has been found to be both larger and smaller in obese subjects than in lean controls. One possible explanation for these differences is diet. Since glucagon is a hormone of "glucose need," the level of carbohydrate in the diet might change the basal level as well as the stimulated level of glucagon in obese patients.

ADRENAL FUNCTION

The concentration of total and free cortisol is usually normal in the circulation of obese patients. In addition, the diurnal rhythm is preserved. Obese patients frequently show higher afternoon values

TABLE 20-6
Endocrine and Metabolic Changes in Spontaneous and Experimental Obesity*

Parameters	Spontaneous Obesity	Experimental Obesity	Parameters	Spontaneous Obesity	Experimental Obesity
Adipose tissue			Evidence of insulin resistance		
Cell size	↑	↑	Insulin: glucose ratio	↑	↑
Cell number	↑	U	Adipose tissue metabolism		
Caloric Balance			Sensitivity to insulin *in vitro*	↓	↓
Calories required to maintain obese state (Cal/m²)	1300	2700	Sensitivity to insulin *in vivo*	↓	↓
Return to starting weight	Rapid	Rapid	Forearm muscle metabolism		
Spontaneous physical activity	↓	↓			
Appetite late in the day	↑	↑	Insulin-stimulated glucose uptake	↓	↓
Fasting concentrations in blood			Insulin inhibition of release of amino acid		↓
Cholesterol	↑	↑	Hormones possibly affecting insulin resistance		
Triglycerides	↑	↑			
Free fatty acids	↑	U or ↓			
Amino acids	↑	↑	Glucocorticoids		
Glucose	N or ↑	↑	Plasma cortisol	N or ↓	U
Insulin	↑	↑	Cortisol production rate	↑	↑
Glucagon	N		Urinary 17-hydroxycorticoids	↑†	↑†
Growth hormone	N or ↓	U or ↓	Growth hormone		
Glucose tolerance			Response to glucose	↓	↓
Oral	↓	↓	Response to arginine	↓	↓
Intravenous	↓	↓	Nocturnal rises		↓
Insulin release					
After oral glucose	↑	↑			
After IV glucose	↑	↑			
After IV arginine	↑	↑			

*Horton ES, Danforth E Jr, Sims EAH et al: In Bray GA (ed): Obesity in Perspective, p 324. DHEW Publ No (NIK) 75–708, 1976
†Normal/kg body weight
U = unchanged
N = normal

of plasma cortisol than normal, but these are suppressed normally with dexamethasone. Obese patients in whom suppression does not occur are a small group for whom more complex procedures are needed to exclude the possibility of Cushing's syndrome. The response to most stimuli that release cortisol is normal in the obese patient.

Although plasma cortisol is usually normal, the cortisol production rate is frequently increased. Since the secretory rate is correlated with the body weight, expressing the data as mg/g creatinine/24 hr or mg/m² body surface area/24 hr will usually distinguish between obese patients and patients with Cushing's syndrome. The increased output of adrenal steroids is metabolized by the liver, and the increased quantity of metabolites is excreted in the urine. To promote this increased production of adrenal steroids the ACTH level is slightly higher in

obesity. Urinary free cortisol is, however, normal in obesity and is the best screening test to diagnose Cushing's Syndrome.[21]

GROWTH HORMONE SECRETION

The effects of obesity on growth hormone have been studied extensively. The basal concentrations of growth hormone are normal or reduced in obese subjects.[21] The induction of hypoglycemia with insulin usually does not stimulate a significant rise in growth hormone in obese patients, and a reduced growth hormone response to IV arginine has also been demonstrated.[28] The nocturnal rise in growth hormone associated with sleep is reduced significantly in obese children and nearly absent in obese adults.[28] Exercise, which also stimulates a rise of growth hormone in normal individuals, fails to do so in the obese.[21] In normal subjects, an acute reduction in plasma free-fatty acids is followed by a secondary rise in growth hormone 2 hr later. In obese subjects, a reduction in fatty acids has no significant effect on the level of growth hormone. The response to L-dopa, like the responses mentioned above, is also blunted in the obese. Thus, as a general rule, obesity blunts the responsiveness to all factors that normally stimulate the release of growth hormone.[21]

It has been conclusively shown that growth hormone dynamics are altered by weight gain in normal volunteers.[45] Three provocative tests were used for this demonstration: (1) the late rise in growth hormone after a glucose tolerance test, (2) the response to an infusion of arginine, and (3) the rise during sleep. With all three stimuli, the rise of growth hormone was blunted in lean volunteers who had gained 15% to 25% above their initial body weight. Conversely, responsiveness of growth hormone was restored after weight loss in these normal volunteers and in obese patients. In addition, growth hormone concentrations in very muscular but overweight men rose during an infusion of arginine, whereas obese patients showed very little response. Thus, the data strongly support the conclusion that the reduced response of growth hormone in the obese is secondary to the adipose tissue increase.

Growth hormone produces its growth-promoting effects by causing somatomedin production in the liver, which then exerts a direct effect on cartilage.[38] Despite the decreased growth hormone levels in obesity, somatomedin levels are normal and growth rate in obese children is normal or advanced. This suggests that in obesity somatomedin production is directly increased by either increased levels of insulin or increased protein intake.[38] Negative feedback on the pituitary by the increased somatomedin could explain the decreased growth hormone levels.

REPRODUCTIVE FUNCTION

In obesity, the onset of menstruation (menarche) and the regulation of menses may be deranged. The onset of menarche in obese girls frequently occurs at a younger age than in girls of normal weight. Frisch has proposed that puberty and menstruation are initiated in females when body weight or percent body fat reaches a critical level.[16] As the rate of growth accelerates in late childhood, the entrance into this critical weight range initiates the pubertal process. The teleologic explanation has been suggested that this allows the female to have adequate calorie stores to carry a pregnancy to term

successfully. In lean, very active ballet dancers there is a high frequency of primary and secondary amenorrhea and irregular menstrual cycles.[17] These abnormalities were most frequent in the dancers with the lowest lean body mass. Hypotheses have been suggested as to ways in which the percent body fat might affect the reproductive system by altering steroid metabolism, but they have not been tested.[15] Further studies on the role of percent body fat in the onset of puberty in humans are important because studies in rats show that percent body fat is not the only factor in determining the onset of puberty in the rat.

The obese patient often shows irregularity of menstrual cycles and an increase in the frequency of menstrual abnormalities. These abnormalities often correct themselves with weight loss. It would thus appear that alterations in body weight can influence both the onset of menstruation and the subsequent initiation of menstruation in women who have developed secondary amenorrhea.

An analysis of the menstrual cycle in six obese women reveals two abnormalities: (1) the rise in follicle-stimulating hormone (FSH) in the first half of the cycle was lower than normal, and (2) progesterone failed to rise normally in the second half of the menstrual cycle.[44] The mechanism of these distortions in obese women is unknown, but they are reversible after weight loss. Pulsatile gonadotropin release and pituitary luteinizing hormone (LH) and FSH reserve, as assessed by the response to luteinizing hormone releasing hormone (LH-RH), are normal in obese women.

Increased production rates of the adrenal androgens dehydroepiandrosterone and dehydroepiandrosterone sulfate are present in obese women. These androgens decrease after weight loss. They may exert a suppressive effect on the hypothalmus and lead to menstrual irregularities. Obese women also have increased conversion of androgens to estrogen, yielding increased circulating estrogens. This increase in estrogen levels may be responsible for the increased incidence of endometrial carcinoma in obese women.[33]

Obese men have decreased total serum testosterone, but when the biologically active free testosterone is measured, the values are normal. This is caused by a decrease in serum sex hormone binding globulin, which is the binding protein for testosterone. The reason for this decrease is not known. LH and FSH dynamics and testicular size are normal. Serum estrogen levels may be increased and this may be due to increased conversion from androgens by adipose tissue. Signs of estrogen excess, such as gynecomastia, are rarely present.[20]

ALDOSTERONE AND SALT WATER BALANCE

The inability of many obese patients, particularly those with extreme weight problems, to excrete both salt and water normally is now generally recognized. The problem of water retention in obesity is aggravated by carbohydrate intake and becomes more severe with refeeding at the end of a period of starvation. With the onset of fasting, there is an enhanced excretion of sodium, chloride, and potassium, which peaks at 2 to 4 days and then gradually subsides. With refeeding carbohydrate or protein, sodium excretion falls to very low levels and fluid retention occurs.

Several hypotheses have been advanced to explain the mechanism for salt loss during starvation and the retention of salt and water during refeeding with carbohydrate.[47] Since sodium excretion is partly under the control of aldosterone, changes in the circulating level of this hormone or in its action on the kidney could explain the alterations in sodium excretion. With short-term starvation, the secretion of aldosterone rises slowly and then gradually returns to normal. Upon refeeding, aldosterone may rise. In some studies the sodium retention with refeeding is blocked by spironolactone, which inhibits the action of aldosterone. The injection of aldosterone after 7 days of fasting reduced sodium excretion, indicating that the renal tubule can still respond to this hormone. Measurement of plasma renin shows no consistent changes during fasting, but a small rise is observed after refeeding.[47]

The acidosis that develops during starvation may play a role in the loss of sodium. If a metabolic acidosis is induced by giving ammonium chloride, the loss of sodium during subsequent starvation will be markedly reduced.

Finally, it has been proposed that glucagon may be important in the loss of sodium in starvation. During starvation, both glucagon and sodium excretion rise in parallel, but more importantly, infusing glucagon enhances sodium excretion to achieve the levels reached during fasting. Glucagon is thought to act by blocking the action of aldosterone at the distal tubule.[47] Plasma vasopressin levels are normal in obesity, but after water loading they do not suppress as much as in lean subjects. The clinical significance of these findings is unknown.

The following sequence may thus be constructed. The early loss of sodium occurs to provide cations for excretion of anions during the development of acidosis. If acidosis is produced before starvation begins, most of the initial salt loss is prevented. The retention of sodium with refeeding can be inhibited by spironolactone, implying that al-

dosterone plays an important role in the retention of sodium after carbohydrate or protein (but not fat) is given. The special effect of carbohydrate in shutting off sodium loss suggests that it may provide a necessary source of energy to the aldosterone-mediated transport of sodium in the renal tubule and that the glucagon rise may block aldosterone action.

MALNUTRITION

Malnutrition has profound effects on the endocrine system.[43] This section will consider the endocrine changes in four types of malnutrition: (1) acute starvation, (2) chronic malnutrition, (3) emotional deprivation, and (4) anorexia nervosa.

ACUTE STARVATION

As fasting begins, the levels of glucose and insulin decrease. In contrast, glucagon levels rise, promoting the breakdown of hepatic glycogen to provide glucose. However, in humans, glycogen stores are exhausted in less than 24 hr, and since glucose remains the primary energy source for brain and blood cells during a short fast, the body must make more glucose. The two carbon acetate fragments produced during the metabolism of fatty acids cannot be converted back into glucose. Thus, the liver is required to use amino acids for protein as the source of carbon for new glucose. If the body continued to use protein during prolonged starvation, the protein stores would be exhausted rapidly and death would occur. However, as starvation continues, the brain adapts to use ketones as a major energy source. Thus, nitrogen loss decreases after 30 days of fasting to one fifth of the value found during early fasting. This process is mediated by the complex interplay between hormones. The increase in circulating glucagon enhances the hepatic production of glucose-derived ketones, and the fall in insulin reduces glucose entry into most tissues.[9]

CHRONIC MALNUTRITION

Endocrine changes in chronic malnutrition have been studied in the childhood syndromes of marasmus and kwashiorkor.[19] The requirement of growing children for calories and protein makes them especially susceptible to deficits in nutrients (see Chap. 32).

Marasmus is characterized by inadequate calorie intake beginning in the first few months of life and is usually found in underdeveloped countries where breast feeding is discontinued early. Clinically, the patients are short for their age with an even greater decrease in weight. Fat stores are depleted and muscle wasting occurs. Serum albumin is normal or slightly decreased, and edema is not present.

This picture contrasts with that seen in patients with kwashiorkor in which the caloric intake is normal but the protein intake is severely deficient. This usually occurs after 1 year of age. The patients have edema and hepatomegaly, and serum albumin is low. The skin and mucous membranes are abnormal. However, the form of malnutrition frequently cannot be categorized this clearly, since elements of both marasmus and kwashiorkor are often present. Protein–calorie malnutrition (PCM) is thus a preferable term.

Because the pattern of malnutrition varies from country to country, endocrine studies are occasionally in conflict. When body weight is 30% or more below normal, a number of endocrine changes take place. The BMR is decreased. Plasma thyroxine (T_4) and the uptake of radioactive iodine (RAI) by the thyroid may be normal or slightly low. Thyroid-binding globulin is normal in marasmus but low in kwashiorkor. Free T_4, however, is normal or elevated in both. Plasma thyrotropin (TSH) is usually in the normal range and responds normally to the administration of hypothalamic-releasing factor (thyrotropin-releasing hormone). Exogenously administered TSH causes a normal increase in thyroid uptake of RAI by the thyroid gland.[22] In adults with malnutrition, plasma TSH and plasma T_4 are normal before and after refeeding. However, the free T_4 is high, and plasma T_3 is low before treatment, suggesting that in malnutrition, there is a peripheral defect in conversion of T_4 to the metabolically more active T_3.[8,41] The deficit is not permanent and is corrected by refeeding.

The levels of growth hormone in marasmus may be high, normal, or low. Regardless of the level, there is no increase after infusing arginine or injecting hypoglycemic doses of insulin, both of which normally increase growth hormone. In marasmus, growth hormone returns to normal with refeeding, and responsiveness to arginine and insulin-induced hypoglycemia returns. In kwashiorkor, growth hormone is very high but, as in marasmus, there is no response to provocative stimulation. After recovery in kwashiorkior, the fasting levels of growth hormone decrease to normal, and responsiveness to stimulation returns. Despite elevated levels of growth hormone, patients with kwashiorkor have low levels of somatomedin. During dietary treatment, somatomedin rises even though growth hormone is falling. Since it is believed to be made in the liver, somatomedin levels could be a reflection of hepatic dysfunction in kwashiorkor.

In both kwashiorkor and marasmus, plasma cortisol levels are increased, but a normal diurnal variation remains. Urinary excretion of free cortisol also remains normal. In malnourished adults, plasma cortisol is high with high urinary free cortisol. Plasma ACTH, however, is not suppressed by the elevated concentrations of cortisol and oral dexamethasone also fails to suppress cortisol normally. The responses to oral metyrapone and to IV ACTH are normal, and the metabolic clearance rate of cortisol is reduced. These findings suggest that the pituitary–adrenal axis is intact but is reset at a higher level with elevated plasma ACTH and cortisol levels. Children with kwashiorkor have elevated plasma aldosterone with normal aldosterone secretory rates.

In malnourished individuals glucose levels are normal or slightly low, and serum insulin levels are low. In PCM, patients generally show decreased tolerance to oral or IV glucose, with a blunted rise in serum insulin.

In men with PCM, the total and unbound plasma testosterone is low, with elevated levels of plasma LH and FSH. The rise in serum testosterone after IM human chorionic gonadotropin is subnormal. After refeeding, the testosterone and FSH levels return to normal, but the LH level may remain elevated. This suggests the Leydig cell function is diminished and that refeeding does not completely reverse the deficit.

EMOTIONAL DEPRIVATION

A group of pediatric patients with short stature, delayed bone age, decreased weight for height, and developmental retardation has been described.[19] All patients have an emotionally deprived home environment. Upon changing the environment to provide more emotional rewards, these patients become more responsive and resume normal growth. The syndrome has been divided into subgroups: patients who are less than 3 years old have been termed to have *maternal deprivation;* the older children have been termed to have *psychosocial deprivation.* It is not clear how much of a role primary malnutrition plays in the development of this clinical picture. In several patients with psychosocial deprivation, access to food was considered normal; indeed, in some, food intake was thought to be adequate for growth.[39] In the younger patients with maternal deprivation, it appeared that mothers were offering an inadequate diet. The hormonal changes in emotional deprivation are similar to those in malnourished children. Thyroid function is normal or low. In children with psychosocial deprivation, the growth hormone levels are low or normal, with an inadequate response to hypoglycemia. In younger patients with maternal deprivation, the rise in growth hormone in response to hypoglycemia is normal. The 11-deoxycortisol response to metyrapone is blunted when low doses are used but administration of 300 mg/m^2 for 2 days produces a normal response.

ANOREXIA NERVOSA

Anorexia nervosa is a clinical diagnosis characterized by an aversion to food usually occurring in females between 10 and 30 years of age (see Chap. 33).[43,50] These women reject food in all forms, even engaging in hiding of food and self-induced vomiting to avoid calorie consumption. In spite of the developing malnutrition, these patients remain physically active and may even increase activity with programs of vigorous exercise. They have a distorted body image, often believing themselves to be overweight, and view their developing emaciation as a positive accomplishment. The etiology of the disease is probably a combination of organic vulnerability and environmental stress.

It is common for females with anorexia nervosa to develop amenorrhea, often before they have lost much weight. Even during recovery, as weight is regained, there is frequently a delay before the resumption of menses, although some authors attribute the delay to dietary factors. This has focused interest on the reproductive system. Plasma LH and FSH are low in most patients. The 24-hr pattern of LH secretion is prepubertal; after weight gain, the pattern returns to normal. The low levels of the gonadotropins are reflected in the low urinary and serum estrogens in females and the low plasma testosterone in males. There is no increase in serum LH after the administration of clomiphene when the patient's weight is less than 80% of normal, but when the patient's weight rises to greater than 80% of normal, the response to clomiphene returns. The LH response after IV gonadotropin-releasing hormone (GnRH) has usually been found to be impaired when the patients are at their lowest weight, but after therapy, when the patients weigh 90% to 94% of ideal body weight, their responses are normal. The rise in FSH after IV GnRH is low to normal before, and returns to normal after, weight gain. The pattern of response to GnRH administered for several days shows that patients with anorexia nervosa revert to a prepubertal pattern of response that returns to normal after weight gain. These data suggest that the defect at the pituitary and hypothalamic level is secondary to the weight loss.

Fasting growth hormone levels are increased and the response to arginine infusion and induced hypoglycemia is subnormal. Despite increased growth hormone concentrations, somatomedin levels are normal. In some cases, a paradoxical rise in growth hormone occurs when glucose is given by mouth.

Plasma norepinephrine levels are low, which may be a reflection of diminished sympathetic neuronal activity. There is also a decrease in urine catecholamine metabolites, and these abnormalities can be reversed by weight gain.[43]

The BMR, serum T_4, and RAI uptake by the thyroid are all normal or slightly low, but plasma T_3 is very low, suggesting a defect in peripheral conversion of T_4 to T_3. Basal thyrotropin is normal, as is the rise in TSH when the thyrotropin-releasing hormone (TRH) is given.

Plasma cortisol is slightly elevated, but the secretory rate for cortisol, the response to ACTH, and metyrapone are all normal. The increased concentration of cortisol is not suppressed normally with administration of dexamethasone. These data suggest that the increase in cortisol is due to increased protein-bound hormone and not to increased physiologically active hormone. Other data suggest that the affinity of corticosteroid-binding globulin for cortisol is decreased.

Patients with anorexia nervosa have low fasting insulin levels and increased sensitivity to injected insulin. However, abnormal glucose tolerance tests with delayed clearance of glucose are also found. Insulin receptors on red blood cells are increased in number but have a normal affinity for insulin. Refeeding normalizes these changes.

The similarities between the thyroid, adrenal, growth hormone, and insulin systems in anorexia nervosa and malnutrition strongly suggest that the hormonal changes in anorexia nervosa are secondary to malnutrition.

In summary, endocrine responses to various types of malnutrition are complex. It is clear that these changes are not simply the result of pituitary insufficiency as was once believed. It is thought that these are adaptive changes that serve to slow metabolic rate and preserve lean body mass in the face of nutritional deprivation. Correction of these abnormalities should involve correction of the malnutrition and not direct efforts to alter hormone levels by medication.[43,50]

TRACE ELEMENTS

Knowledge is rapidly expanding in the field of trace elements and their importance in biological functions. Iodine, which is the most important trace element in endocrine function, has already been discussed in the section on the thyroid gland. Evidence is accumulating that zinc and chromium are also important for normal endocrine function.

ZINC

Zinc deficiency has been implicated as a cause of short stature and delayed sexual development.[7,24] The syndrome has been described in two groups: (1) in Iranian males who consumed large amounts of clay that chelated zinc in the intestine, and (2) in Egyptian males who had parasitic infestation producing chronic blood loss. Treatment of these patients with supplements of zinc increased the rate of growth and accelerated development of secondary sexual characteristics.

During a screening program for zinc deficiency in humans, 10 of 132 children living in Denver were found to have low levels of serum zinc.[24] Most of these patients had a poor appetite and showed decreased growth and taste acuity. Treatment with zinc produced normal taste acuity and increased the zinc level to normal. The effect on their short stature has not yet been reported. Zinc deficiency has also been found in short children with Crohn's disease.

Endocrine studies on zinc-deficient Egyptians showed decreased serum testosterone levels with a normal increase following administration of human chorionic gonadotropin.[11] This suggests that patients with zinc deficiency may have a defect in the release of pituitary gonadotropins. Growth hormone secretion was decreased in the zinc-deficient subjects after hypoglycemia, but it was decreased as well in control subjects without zinc deficiency. In adult rats zinc deficiency produces minimal effects on the hypothalamic–pituitary axis, however, in immature male rats gonadal growth is impaired and LH and FSH levels are increased. Further studies are needed to define the role of zinc in short stature and delayed sexual development.

CHROMIUM

Chromium is necessary for the normal metabolism of glucose in animals.[24] This has been shown not only *in vivo*, but also by using isolated adipose tissues *in vitro*. Chromium appears to act as a cofactor in the peripheral action of insulin. Brewer's yeast contains high concentrations of a specific chromium complex that has been purified and found to be more active than chromium alone in improving glucose metabolism. Studies in human beings with normal chromium nutrition have shown a rise in serum chromium during an oral glucose tolerance test. During an oral glucose tolerance test, urinary excretion of chromium is less in diabetics than in normal controls. Adults with high fasting blood glucose levels have low red blood cell chromium levels and a decreased postprandial increment in plasma chromium.[40] Chromium or brew-

er's yeast has been given to adults having insulin-dependent diabetes, with variable results. It has been found that some patients had improved glucose tolerance, but in other studies, chromium produced no change in glucose metabolism. Some differences may be accounted for by the labile characteristics of the active chromium factor. Chromium administered to malnourished children has improved IV glucose tolerance. These data suggest that in some human beings with decreased glucose tolerance, chromium deficiency may be a factor in the impaired metabolism of glucose, but there is as yet no clinical indication for use of chromium in treatment of diabetes.

Effects of the Endocrine System on Nutrition

PITUITARY–HYPOTHALAMUS

The hypothalamus and pituitary function as an integrated unit. This section will discuss the effect of the hypothalamic hormones and growth hormone on nutrition. The other pituitary hormones are discussed in the sections that deal with their target glands.

HYPOTHALAMUS

The hypothalamus controls the secretion of pituitary hormones by the elaboration of releasing factors and inhibiting factors. Some of these factors have been isolated and their chemical structures determined. Hypothalamic-releasing factors are abnormal in some, but not all, patients with the syndrome of generalized lipodystrophy.[32] This is a rare congenital disease characterized by a lack of all body fat, an early increase in growth, hyperpigmentation, elevated level of glucose, and hyperinsulinism. Although there is some evidence of increased circulating levels of the hypothalamic-releasing factors that release ACTH, gonadotropins, and melanocyte-stimulating hormone, this is of uncertain significance.[32] Following treatment with pimozide, a selective inhibitor of cerebral dopaminergic receptors, one patient had decreases in the circulating levels of hypothalamic-releasing factors, in triglycerides, and in insulin and glucose. Since hypophysectomy does not effect the long-term course of this disease, these data suggest that a hypothalamic hormone may have an important effect on the peripheral metabolism of fat.

Hypothalamic injury has produced syndromes of overnutrition and undernutrition. Hypothalamic obesity, which is characterized by the lack of satiation and chronic weight gain, occasionally follows hypothalamic tumors or surgery in this region of the brain and is very similar to the syndrome produced in animals by the destruction of the ventromedial region of the hypothalamus.[5] Most endocrine changes in hypothalamic obesity are the same as those present in obesity from other causes and are discussed in a previous section. One exception is that the concentration of insulin in serum is higher in hypothalamic obesity.

The diencephalic syndrome is characterized by a lack of cutaneous fat, normal or increased appetite, increased growth, hyperactivity, and euphoria and is associated with tumors of the hypothalamus or third ventricle. Increased fasting growth hormone levels are not suppressed after oral or IV administration of glucose, but this minor abnormality does not appear to account for the profound metabolic changes in these children. Increased levels of urinary norepinephrine and epinephrine have been described. The extreme loss of fat in the presence of a normal appetite and food intake suggests the possibility that there is a substance that blocks storage of calories in adipose tissue in this syndrome.

GROWTH HORMONE

Human growth hormone (hGH) is a polypeptide secreted by the pituitary under the control of the hypothalamus, which affects carbohydrate, fat, and protein metabolism throughout the body.[34] It increases cellular uptake of amino acids and facilitates incorporation of amino acids into protein. Replication of DNA and RNA is increased in cartilage. Conversion of proline to hydroxyproline for use in collagen synthesis is enhanced. All of these actions of hGH are mediated by somatomedins, growth hormone-dependent peptides produced in the liver that increase cellular utilization of glucose and decrease adipose cell lipolysis.[38] The insulin-like effects of somatomedins are in marked contrast to the anti-insulin effects of hGH itself. In pharmacologic doses, growth hormone decreases the uptake of glucose by adipose cells, increases the release of pancreatic insulin, increases lipolysis in adipose tissue, and elevates plasma free-fatty acids. It also increases Ca absorption from the GI tract and thus enhances retention of Ca in bone.

A group of children with familial dwarfism has been described; the children have very high concentrations of hGH and low serum levels of somatomedins. Their serum somatomedin levels do not rise after administration of hGH, suggesting a defect in somatomedin production. One tribe of African pygmies has been found to have normal levels of hGH and a selective deficiency of only one of the somatomedins (insulin-like growth factor I).[35] Low somatomedin levels in the presence of normal or high hGH levels may be responsible for poor growth in children taking glucocorticoids and in children with chronic renal failure.[38]

Patients with hGH deficiency have short stature, delayed bone age, hypoglycemia with increased glucose tolerance, and mild obesity. With the administration of hGH, they show positive nitrogen balance, increased growth rate, normal glucose tolerance, and decreased body fat. Since many patients with hGH deficiency have deficiencies of other pituitary hormones, these must be tested for and replaced as required. Thyroid hormone replacement is especially important because hGH is not effective in hypothyroidism.

Excessive secretion of hGH before epiphyseal closure results in gigantism. Excess hGH after epiphyseal closure produces acromegaly. Here the increase of bone growth is restricted to facial bones, particularly the mandible, and cortical portions of the membranous bones. In both syndromes, there is increased growth of connective tissue, body hair, cartilage, and enlargement of visceral organs (*i.e.,* liver, kidneys, spleen, and thyroid). In these patients, plasma hGH does not decrease after oral glucose. Glucose tolerance is occasionally impaired, but compensatory hyperinsulinism usually prevents overt diabetes.[14]

ADRENAL CORTEX

The adrenal cortex produces three groups of steroids: (1) the androgens, (2) the glucocorticoids, and (3) the mineralocorticoids. The androgenic steroids and their modes of action are discussed in a separate section. Cortisol, the principal glucocorticoid in humans, exerts far-reaching effects on protein, carbohydrate, and fat metabolism.[3] In muscle, glucocorticoids impair amino acid uptake, impair protein synthesis, enhance protein catabolism, and enhance the conversion of ketogenic and branched amino acids to the glycogenic amino acids alanine and glutamine. The net result is a glucocorticoid-induced rise in plasma amino acids, especially alanine and glutamine, which serve as substrates for hepatic gluconeogenesis. In addition, all of the enzymes required for hepatic gluconeogenesis are increased in both amount and activity (*i.e.,* glucose 6-phosphatase, fructose 1, 6-diphosphatase, pyruvate carboxylase, phosphoenolpyruvate carboxykinase, tyrosine aminotransferase, glutamine pyruvic transaminase, and tryptophan pyrrolase), some through direct glucocorticoid induction. Glucocorticoids stimulate glucagon release, which also enhances hepatic gluconeogenesis. In addition to these effects on the stimulation of glucose production, glucocorticoids cause a peripheral resistance to the action of insulin in some tissues, possibly through a decrease in binding of insulin to its receptor. Glucocorticoids inhibit fatty acid synthesis (*i.e.*, lipogenesis) and permit the enhanced lipolytic effects of catecholamines in some tissues (*e.g.*, the subcutaneous fat cells of the arms and legs), but in other tissues, glucocorticoids stimulate lipogenesis (*e.g.*, the dorsal and supraclavicular fat pads). In addition to their effects on intermediary metabolism, glucocorticoids are necessary for the excretion of dilute urine by the kidneys.[3]

Glucocorticoids also antagonize the effect of vitamin D on intestinal Ca transport, possibly in part by interfering with the conversion of vitamin D to its active metabolites.[23]

Aldosterone is the primary mineralocorticoid in humans. It regulates Na balance by the kidneys independently of the hypothalamic–pituitary axis. Secretion of aldosterone is regulated primarily by the renin–angiotensin system. Hyperkalemia also stimulates aldosterone secretion. Aldosterone acts primarily on the distal convoluted tubule and collecting tubules to increase the reabsorption of Na from the urine; the Na reabsorption, in turn, is coupled to the excretion of K and hydrogen ion.

EFFECTS OF EXCESSIVE ADRENAL CORTICOSTEROIDS

The administration of glucocorticoids (*e.g.*, cortisone, prednisone, dexamethasone) or the endogenous secretion of excess cortisol results in a state of *hypercortisolism* and can, therefore, be considered as a single entity for the purposes of this discussion. Increased concentrations of glucocorticoids exert an effect on carbohydrate, protein, and lipid metabolism. In about 15% of patients receiving exogenous steroids, a mild, nonketotic form of diabetes occurs, but 95% of patients with endogenous Cushing's syndrome have abnormal glucose tolerance. Catabolic effects on protein are often the most striking changes. Muscle wasting, thinning of the skin, dissolution of vertebral bone matrix, poor wound healing, and growth retardation in children are frequently found. The varying influences on lipid metabolism discussed above result in the peculiar truncal obesity seen in Cushing's syndrome, with loss of subcutaneous fat tissue from the arms and legs and excessive deposition in the dorsal and ventral fat pads, the supraclavicular and mediastinal areas, and the abdominal walls. Excessive cortisol stimulates the appetite and can thus contribute to the obesity. The antagonistic effects of glucocorticoids on the action of vitamin D produce a markedly negative Ca balance.

Patients receiving corticosteroids for a prolonged period should be treated with vitamin D (50,000 IU three times a week) plus Ca mg/day (500–1000 mg/day) in an attempt to prevent steroid-induced

osteopenia.[23] Along with the enhanced catabolism of protein, this may lead to the appearance of osteoporosis with vertebral fractures. Aseptic necrosis of the femoral head may also occur. High cortisol levels often exert a mineralocorticoidlike effect, even though the levels of aldosterone are not elevated. The result is hypertension, which may be associated with hypokalemic alkalosis. This mineralocorticoidlike effect is commonly seen in patients with neoplasms producing ACTH and is not usually seen in patients treated with the newer synthetic glucocorticoids. In a few reports, glucocorticoid therapy has also resulted in zinc depletion with resultant delayed wound healing. This is correctable using oral supplements of zinc. The effects of glucocorticoids on the metabolism of other trace metals and vitamins have not been adequately investigated.

Hyperaldosteronism, or Conn's syndrome, is a disease with excessive secretion of aldosterone. Metabolically, this results in hypertension and hypokalemic alkalosis. Thus, the possibility of high levels of aldosterone should be considered whenever low serum K is detected. Hypokalemia interferes with the release of insulin and may lead to abnormal glucose tolerance.

DEFICIENCY OF ADRENAL CORTICOSTEROIDS

Addison's disease can occur because of primary adrenal failure or because the pituitary fails to secrete ACTH.[3] Most cases of Addison's disease are *idiopathic* and probably result from an *autoimmune* adrenalitis in which the adrenal medulla is spared. Less than one third of cases are now caused by tuberculosis, histoplasmosis, or other infectious diseases. Patients with adrenal insufficiency frequently manifest anorexia, weight loss, weakness, loss of body hair in the female (loss of adrenal androgens), reactive hypoglycemia following a carbohydrate meal, and rarely hypercalcemia. Statistically, there is an increased incidence of both diabetes mellitus and Hashimoto's thyroiditis in patients with idiopathic Addison's disease.

Deficiency of aldosterone itself can occur congenitally, or it may appear in older diabetics with mild renal insufficiency. This latter form frequently is due to primary deficiency of renin with a secondary hypoaldosteronism. In all of these forms, the major manifestation is hyperkalemia with occasional modest hyponatremia and acidosis. Other metabolic effects are rarely seen.

ADRENAL MEDULLA

Epinephrine is the major catecholamine secreted by the adrenal medulla, but norepinephrine is also

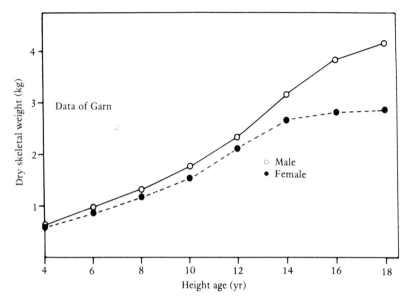

FIG. 20-4 Growth of skeleton versus height–age. Clearly, the greater gain in body and muscle of the male is associated with greater gain in skeletal mass. (Cheek DB: Body composition, hormones, nutrition and adolescent growth. In Grumbach MM, Grave GD, Mayer FE (eds): Control of the Onset of Puberty, p 430. New York, John Wiley & Sons, 1974)

released in smaller amounts.[13] Epinephrine stimulates both alpha and beta receptors, whereas norepinephrine predominantly activates the alpha receptors. The principal metabolic effect mediated through alpha receptors is the inhibition of insulin secretion. Stimulation of beta receptors, on the other hand, causes an increase in glycogenolysis in both muscle and liver, along with an inhibition of glycogen synthetase in muscle and a mild increase in insulin secretion. This process also activates hormone-sensitive lipase in fat cells and results in the breakdown of triglycerides with liberation of free fatty acids. Blockade of beta receptors by propranolol can result in impaired secretion of insulin and hyperglycemia in patients with a preexisting tendency to diabetes.

In patients with pheochromocytomas, epinephrine secretion is often greatly increased whereas norepinephrine is only modestly increased. In this disease, glucose tolerance is impaired because in-

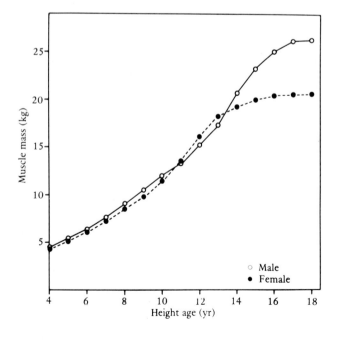

FIG. 20-5 Muscle mass (from creatinine excretion) is plotted against height–age for males and females. Note that muscle mass doubles in males from 10 to 17 years. (Cheek DB: Body composition, hormones, nutrition and adolescent growth. In Grumbach MM, Grave GD, Mayer FE (eds): Control of the Onset of Puberty, p 426. New York, John Wiley & Sons, 1974)

sulin release is blocked. Alpha receptor blockade with phenoxybenzamine restores insulin secretion to normal in these patients.

ESTROGENIC AND ANDROGENIC STEROIDS

In the male, the principal circulating androgen is testosterone. In most tissues, dihydrotestosterone (DHT) is the active form of testosterone. About 90% of DHT is produced from testosterone in peripheral tissues by the enzyme 5 α-reductase; the remaining 10% is produced by the testes.[2] This enzyme system has not been demonstrated in muscle, and testosterone itself is the active agent there. In women, the most important androgens are testosterone and androstenedione, which are secreted by the ovary and the adrenal gland and dehydroepiandrosterone, which is secreted by the adrenals. Most of the circulating testosterone, however, derives from the metabolism of androstenedione.[42]

In women, the main estrogen secreted by the ovary is estradiol. Estrone circulates in plasma at levels similar to those of estradiol and is largely a conversion product of androstenedione. The physiologic significance of estrone is uncertain, since it has much less estrogenic activity than estradiol. Progesterone is secreted by the ovary during the luteal phase and is only present in minimal amounts before puberty. Although there has been some controversy regarding naturally occurring estrogenlike substances in plant foodstuffs and cattle exposed to diethylstilbesterol, the actual amounts of estrogens from these sources appear to be physiologically insignificant.[48]

At the cellular level of responsive tissues, testosterone, dihydrotestosterone, and estradiol stimulate protein synthesis. In addition, these hormones also cause a decrease in protein catabolism, thus producing a positive nitrogen balance. In the secondary sex organs, muscle, and bone, androgen stimulation results in tissue growth and is reflected by a rise in lean body mass (LBM) and a decrease in fat mass at the time of adolescence. The LBM and skeletal mass at adolescence increase faster with age in males than in females. In boys and girls, the heights at each age are similar until about the age of 9 (*i.e.*, height, 137 cm), when the male height for age accelerates faster than that of the female.[10] Similarly, the skeletal mass (see Fig. 20-4) and muscle mass diverge at this point, with an eventual rate of growth in muscle that is three times faster in boys (see Fig. 20-5). Multiplication of muscle cells parallels these changes in muscle mass. As these increments in LBM occur, total caloric and protein intake increases concomitantly.

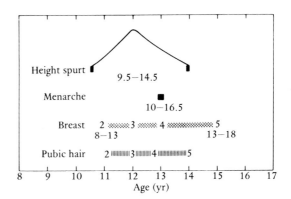

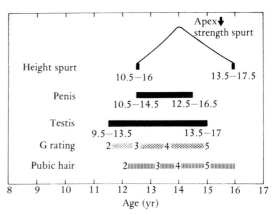

FIG. 20-6 Events at puberty. Average female (*upper*) and male (*lower*) are represented. Range of ages within which each event charted may begin and end is given by the figures placed directly below its start and finish. (Tanner JM: Sequences and tempo in the somatic changes in puberty. In Grumbach MM, Grave GD, Mayer FE (eds): Control of the Onset of Puberty, p 460. New York, John Wiley & Sons, 1974)

Figure 20-6 shows the spurt in height in relation to other pubertal changes in both sexes. It is felt that this increase in height and LBM in females is attributable to adrenal androgens, the smaller increment in total androgens in the female possibly accounting for the smaller increases in height and LBM. The role of increasing estrogen levels on linear growth at puberty is unclear but may be also important.

At the same time that androgens are stimulating bone growth, along with estrogens they also cause a maturation and eventual closure of the bony epiphyses. In precocious puberty and in the virilizing forms of congenital adrenal hyperplasia, there is a marked early increase in muscle mass and linear skeletal growth along with virilization. Because the androgens also accelerate closure of the epiphyseal centers, however, these children usually become

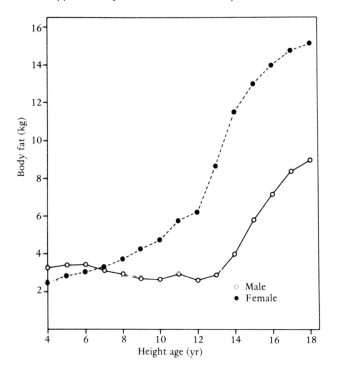

FIG. 20-7 Increasing fatness of males and females during adolescence. (Cheek DB: Body composition, hormones, nutrition and adolescent growth. In Grumbach MM, Grave GD, Mayer FE (eds): Control of the Onset of Puberty, p 426. New York, John Wiley & Sons, 1974)

short adults. Conversely, eunuchoid individuals with androgen deficiency often have a slow but continued growth without an adolescent growth spurt, so that they end up taller than predicted from early growth records.

In addition to the changes in LBM that occur at puberty, there are also changes in distribution of the body fat. The increase in fat is much greater in females than in males (see Fig. 20-7), and this occurs at about the same time as the divergence in lean body mass.[10] Estrogens are probably responsible for the development of the female body contour. However, Crawford and Osler have found similar changes of an increase in body fat with a decrease in body water in patients with gonadal dysgenesis (Turner's syndrome) who develop an increase in gonadotropins at the usual time of puberty.[12] Because of their streak ovaries, however, they do not have a significant rise in estrogens. This interesting data suggest that not all of the changes in fat at puberty may be due to estrogens, but that gonadotropins may also play a direct role or a nonovarian-mediated indirect role. Interestingly, Simeons first proposed using human chorionic gonadotropin for treating obesity because he thought that this substance might help to bring back the lost female body contour; neither he nor the subsequent users of this drug have ever substantiated the efficacy of human chorionic gonadotropin for the treatment of obesity.

References

1. Avioli LV: Senile and postmenopausal osteoporosis. Adv Intern Med 21:391–415, 1976
2. Bardin CW, Paulsen CA: The testes. In Williams RL (ed): Textbook of Endocrinology, 6th ed, pp 293–354. Philadelphia, WB Saunders, 1981
3. Baxter JD, Tyrrell JB: The adrenal cortex. In Felig P, Baxter JD, Broadus AE et al (eds): Endocrinology and Metabolism, pp 385–510. New York, McGraw-Hill, 1981
4. Bray GA: The Obese Patient. WB Saunders, Philadelphia, 1976
5. Bray GA, Gallagher TF Jr: Manifestations of hypothalamic obesity in man: A comprehensive investigation of eight patients and a review of the literature. Medicine 54:301–330, 1975
6. Broadus A: Mineral metabolism. In Felig P, Baxter JD, Broadus AD et al (eds): Endocrinology and Metabolism, pp 963–1079. New York, McGraw-Hill, 1981
7. Burch RE, Hahn HKJ, Sullivan JF: Newer aspects of the roles of zinc, manganese and copper in human nutrition. Clin Chem 21:501–520, 1975
8. Burman KD: Recent developments in thyroid hormone metabolism: Interpretation and significance of measurement of reverse T_3, 3,3' T_2, and thyroglobulin. Metabolism 27:615–630, 1978
9. Cahil GF Jr: Starvation in man. N Engl J Med 282:668–674, 1970
10. Cheek DB: Body composition, hormones, nutrition and adolescent growth. In Grumbach MM, Grave GD, Mayer FE (eds): Control of the Onset of Puberty, pp 424–442. New York, John Wiley & Sons, 1974
11. Coble YD Jr, Bardin CW, Ross GT et al: Studies of endocrine function in boys with retarded growth, delayed

sexual maturation, and zinc deficiency. J Clin Endocrinol Metab 32:361, 1971

12. Crawford JD, Osler DC: Body composition at menarche: The Frisch–Revelle hypothesis revisited. Pediatrics 56:449–458, 1975

13. Cryer PE: Diseases of the adrenal medullae and sympathetic nervous system. In Felig P, Baxter JD, Broadus AE, et al (eds): Endocrinology and Metabolism, pp 511–550. New York, McGraw–Hill, 1981

14. Daughaday WH: The adenohypophysis. In Williams RH (ed): Textbook of Endocrinology, 6th ed, pp 73–116. Philadelphia, WB Saunders, 1981

15. Fishman J: Fatness, puberty and ovulation. N Engl J Med 303:42–43, 1980

16. Frisch RE, McArthur JW: Menstrual cycle: Fatness as a determinant of minimum weight necessary for their maintenance on onset. Science 185:949–952, 1974

17. Frisch RE, Wyshak G, Vincent L: Delayed menarche and amenorrhea in ballet dancers. N Engl J Med 303:17–19, 1980

18. Gallagher JC, Riggs BL: Nutrition and bone disease. N Engl J Med 298:193–195, 1978

19. Gardner LI: Deprivational dwarfism. Sci Am 227:76–82, 1972

20. Glass AR, Swerdloff RS, Bray GA et al: Low serum testosterone and sex-hormone-binding-globulin in massively obese men. J Clin Endocrinol Metab 45:1211–1219, 1977

21. Glass AR, Burman KD, Dahms WT et al: Endocrine function in human obesity. Metabolism 30:89–104, 1981

22. Graham GG, Baertl JM, Claeyssen G et al: Studies in normal and severely malnourished infants and small children. J Pediatr 83:321–331, 1973

23. Hahn TJ: Corticosteroid induced osteopenia. Arch Intern Med 138:882–885, 1978

24. Hambridge KM: Zinc and chromium in human nutrition. J Human Nutr 32:99–110, 1978

25. Haussler MR, McCain TA: Basic and clinical concepts related to vitamin D metabolism and action. N Engl J Med 297:974–983, 1041–1050, 1977

26. Ingbar SH, Woeber KA: The thyroid gland. In Williams RH (ed): Textbook of Endocrinology, 6th ed, pp 117–247. Philadelphia, WB Saunders, 1981

27. Iseri LT, Freed J, Bures AR: Magnesium deficiency and cardiac disorders. Am J Med 58:837–846, 1975

28. Knochel JP: The pathophysiology and clinical characteristics of severe hypophosphatemia. Arch Intern Med 137:203–220, 1977

29. Lentz RD, Brown DM, Kjellstrand C: Treatment of severe hypophosphatemia. Ann Intern Med 89:941–944, 1978

30. Loeb JN: Hyperthyroidism: Metabolic changes. In Werner SC, Ingbar SH (eds): The Thyroid, 4th ed, pp 785–711. Hagerstown, Harper & Row, 1978

31. Lutwak K, Singer FR, Urist MR: Current concepts of bone metabolism. Ann Intern Med 80:630–644, 1974

32. Mabry CC, Hollingsworth DR, Upton GV et al: Pituitary–hypothalamic dysfunction in generalized lipodystrophy. J Pediatr 82:625–633, 1973

33. MacDonald PC, Edman CD, Hemsell DL et al: Effect of obesity on conversion of androstenedrone to estrone in postmenopausal women with and without endometrial cancer. Am J Obstet Gynecol 130:448–455, 1978

34. Merimee TJ, Rabin D: A survey of growth hormone secretion and action. Metabolism 22:1235–1251, 1973

35. Merimee JJ, Zapf J, Froesch ER: Dwarfism in the pygmy. An isolated defect of insulin-like growth factors I. N Engl J Med 305:965–968, 1981

36. O'Connor P: Vitamin D-deficiency rickets in two breast-fed infants who were not receiving vitamin D supplementation. Clin Pediatr 16:361–363, 1977

37. Olefsky JM: The insulin receptor: Its role in insulin resistance of obesity and diabetes. Diabetes 25:1154–1165, 1976

38. Phillips LS, Vassilopoulou–Sellin R: Somatomedins. N Engl J Med 302:371–380, 438–446, 1980

39. Powell GF, Brasel JA, Raiti S et al: Emotional deprivation and growth retardation simulating idiopathic hypopituitarism. II, Endocrinologic evaluation of the syndrome. N Engl J Med 276:1279–1293, 1967

40. Rabinowitz MB, Levin SR, Gonick HL: Comparisons of chromium status in diabetic and normal men. Metabolism 29:355–364, 1980

41. Richmand DA, Molitch ME, O'Donnell TF: Altered thyroid hormone levels in bacterial sepsis: The role of nutritional adequacy. Metabolism 29:936–942, 1980

42. Ross GT, VandeWiele RL: The ovaries. In Williams RL (ed): Textbook of Endocrinology, 6th ed, pp 355–411. Philadelphia, WB Saunders, 1981

43. Schwabe AD, Lippe BM, Chang RJ et al: Anorexia nervosa. Ann Intern Med 94:371–381, 1981

44. Sherman B, Korenman SG: Measurement of serum LH, FSH, estradiol and progesterone in disorders of the human menstrual cycle: The inadequate luteal phase. J Clin Endocrinol Metab 39:145–149, 1974

45. Sim EAH, Danforth E Jr, Horton ES et al: Endocrine and metabolic effects of experimental obesity in man. Recent Prog Horm Res 29:457–487, 1973

46. Singer FR: Metabolic bone disease. In Felig P, Baxter JD, Broadus AE et al (eds): Endocrinology and Metabolism, pp 1081–1118. New York, McGraw–Hill, 1981

47. Spark RF, Arky RA, Boulter PR et al: Renin, aldosterone, and glucagon in the natriuresis of fasting. N Engl J Med 292:1335–1340, 1975

48. Verdeal K, Ryan DS: Naturally-occurring estrogens in plant foodstuffs—A review. Journal of Food Protection 42:577–583, 1979

49. Wacker WEC, Parisi AF: Magnesium metabolism. N Engl J Med 278:658–663, 1969

50. Vigersky RA (ed): Anorexia Nervosa. New York, Raven Press, 1977

21
Gastroenterology
Keith B. Taylor

Until quite recently, scientific nutritional principles have not been applied suitably to the treatment of gastrointestinal (GI) disease. Inadequately tested diets in the management of peptic ulcer, colitis, and diverticulosis were widely used. In retrospect, many such diets suggest more the physician's treating himself than the patient. The results, furthermore, were not always harmless to the patient. At best, needless dietary hardship or monotony was imposed on patients and often on those who ate with them. At worst, severe and specific deficiencies or intoxications resulted. An extreme example is that reported by Hawkins of a woman 60 years of age who developed scurvy as a consequence of having been advised by a doctor 40 years earlier to eat no fruit or vegetables, as treatment for dyspepsia.[23] The doctor had subsequently died without rescinding his advice, so that she had been subjected to a dull and dangerous diet for her whole adult life. Another extreme example is the milk–alkali syndrome, now fortunately rare, which was a consequence of overenthusiastic application of treatment for effective relief of the pain of peptic ulcer.

In general, people have familial and cultural preconceptions about food, both in health and in disease. They expect to have such beliefs confirmed by their medical advisors or, if contrary advice is given, they require explanations couched in terms that they can grasp and that they consider to be intellectually sound. If the doctor fails to consider dietary matters, the patient will seek advice elsewhere. Surveys have shown that in the United States the public puts physicians at the top of the list of those from whom they would seek dietary advice. Health-food stores were not far behind.

In establishing a therapeutic regimen each component should be carefully scrutinized for adequacy, acceptability, potential value, and undesirable side-effects; this applies as well to nutritional and dietary factors, which are sometimes disregarded.

Gastrointestinal Diseases

The GI tract and liver play central roles in the digestion, absorption, and metabolism of aliments and their products. It is clear that alimentary or hepatic disease may profoundly disturb normal nutrition, and the affected patient may require nutritional support as an essential component of therapy.

Additionally, if the need for such support is not recognized early, nutritional abnormalities may occur which aggravate the original disease. Deficiency of vitamin B_{12} causes intestinal malabsorption, deficiency of zinc can cause failure of response of celiac sprue to gliadin exclusion or possibly of Crohn's disease to current therapies. Chronic iron deficiency induces epithelial changes in the foregut, including the buccal cavity, that can be premalignant.

Some dietary constituents may cause disease of the gastrointestinal tract or liver in subjects in whom there may be predisposing factors. Evidence that ethanol produces acute and chronic liver disease is strong; the extent to which nutritional deficiencies play a synergistic role is still uncertain. Cirrhosis may occur despite apparently adequate diet.[33] The fact that no more than approximately 20% of subjects who consume 150 ml/day ethanol or more develop cirrhosis clearly points to involvement of other factors, some of which may be nutritional deficiencies. This possibility is reinforced by increasing evidence that ingestion of ethanol impairs small bowel absorption. Wheat gliadin induces an enteropathy in susceptible subjects, and other food proteins such as β-lactoglobulin and soy may be responsible for small bowel disease in some subjects.

Important causes of abnormal nutritional states associated with diseases of the gastrointestinal tract and liver include the following: (1) recurrent infective enteritis in infants and young children; (2) esophagitis, stricture, esophageal carcinoma, and achalasia; (3) chronic peptic ulcer disease (less common in the past 2–3 decades); (4) gastrointestinal surgery, in the immediate postoperative period and in the long term; (5) small bowel malabsorption owing to pancreatic and biliary disease, abnormal bacterial flora, radiation enteritis, vascular insufficiency, inflammatory bowel disease, and surgical resection; (6) anorexia and other disturbances of function in the aged; and finally (7) acute and chronic liver diseases.

GASTROENTERITIS

Fortunately, acute enteritis no longer presents a major problem in modern communities with high standards of hygiene. Should diarrhea and vomiting lead to dehydration and loss of electrolytes, these can be restored intravenously while the acute infection is treated. The situation in societies in which undernutrition and poor hygiene go hand in hand is quite different. There is a significant correlation between attacks of enteric infection, reduced food consumption, and rates of growth in children of preschool age in such communities.[34]

ESOPHAGEAL DISEASES

Esophagitis occurs as a consequence of esophageal reflux of gastric contents caused by an impaired lower esophageal sphincter or, less commonly, as a result of opportunistic monilial infection occurring in immunologically comprised subjects or in those receiving large doses of corticosteroids. Dysphagia is usually present. If passage of a soft diet is too painful, frequent high-calorie–protein liquid feeds at body temperature should be given. Certain foods, such as citrus juices, may cause pain for unknown reasons, and others, such as chocolate and coffee, may encourage gastroesophageal reflux, possibly because of the action of the xanthines that they contain in lowering pressure at the lower esophageal sphincter.[42] These should be avoided. No pills or tablets should be given uncrushed. A supplement of water-soluble vitamins is given to ensure that temporary deficiencies owing to a restricted diet do not occur. Two-hourly doses of antacids of 60 mEq to 120 mEq neutralizing-capacity and an evening dose of cimetidine to suppress nocturnal gastric acid secretion, combined with elevation of the head of the bed by 6 to 8 inches will usually bring relief in 2 days to 3 days. In obese subjects it is believed that weight reduction may bring about improvement, but there is no formal study to support this.

Monilial esophagitis is usually, but not always, associated with evidence of thrush in the mouth and fauces. It is treated with oral nystatin. A soft or liquid diet of high protein and caloric content and supplemented with daily vitamin and mineral requirements may be necessary until a response is obtained.

In acute esophagitis caused by ingestion of corrosives, nothing should be given by mouth until endoscopy has been performed with extreme caution to determine the extent of injury. When only minor injury is present, the patient is allowed to eat a soft, bland diet for a few days. If ulceration or hemorrhage is seen, it is recommended that the patient be fed parenterally until the risk of perforation is over, a matter of 10 days to 20 days. Early mechanical dilatation should be done to prevent stricture formation.[14]

Simple esophageal strictures may result from esophagitis or the action of corrosives. Treatment by dilatation by bougie is often successful, but surgery may be essential. If dysphagia has been severe, the patient may be seriously undernourished and require continuous hyperalimentation by fine nasogastric tube or parenteral feeding both before and after surgery. Malignant stricturing of the esophagus is often diagnosed late, and the patient may be severely undernourished. Prior to surgery, tube feeding is sometimes possible; otherwise, the parenteral route should be used. In this way the general state of patients can now be much improved, thereby decreasing surgical risks and permitting more radical procedures.

Achalasia, a neuromuscular disorder of the lower third of the esophagus, behaves similarly to a stricture, but the pain on swallowing food or associated with emotive events is not like heartburn, but rather of a more cramping or spastic nature. Dietary support is similar while mechanical dilatation or surgical myotomy are performed. The goal of treatment is elimination of dysphagia on a normal diet.

PEPTIC ULCER DISEASE

The nutritional status of the patient with ulcer disease has changed twice since the turn of the century. The haggard, underweight individual sometimes displaying specific nutrient deficiencies owing to intermittent blood loss, inadequate dietary intake, and gastric outlet obstruction was displaced by the obese, overnourished patient, prone to myocardial infarction but protected from the complications of pyloric obstruction by earlier surgical intervention. The introduction of effective antisecretory drugs, the use of adequate doses of antacids, the recognition that milk stimulates gastric acid secretion, and modern surgical techniques that do not mutilate the stomach have all transformed the situation and seem likely to reduce morbidity and improve the quality of life.

Dietary management probably does not play any role in the treatment of peptic ulcers. A comparison of a bland with an unrestricted diet in patients with duodenal ulcer showed no difference in healing rates.[10] Patients should be encouraged to eat anything that causes them no upset, to avoid those things that do, and to maintain a steady and desired weight. In spite of such encouragement, white and bland diets may be selected by some patients as a consequence of cultural conditioning. Supplementation with essential nutrients, especially ascorbic acid and other water-soluble vitamins and iron, is then indicated. Late evening snacks stimulating nocturnal acid secretion are discouraged, a definite change in regimen in recent years. Coffee and alcohol, both stimulants of gastric secretion, are often prohibited, although compliance with this is probably poor. For the tea-drinking, teetotal patient this prohibition presents no problem, but for many the total exclusion of either coffee or alcohol may cause real hardship. Reason (there are no experimental data) suggests that a glass of wine with a meal is less of an insult to the gastric mucosa than two martinis before a meal, and that the effect of the wine on acid secretion must be totally eclipsed by the effect of the meal itself. Similarly, a cup of coffee at the end of the meal is not to be equated with continuing coffee consumption between meals. There is no evidence for the long-held belief that citrus juices increase gastric acidity. Intolerance to orange juice (and other foods) certainly occurs, but it is usually associated with symptomatology suggesting peptic esophagitis. A recent study by Isenberg and his colleagues represents the first attempt to quantify the relative stimulatory effects of various beverages on gastric acid secretion. They have shown that Tab, a soft drink, is as effective a gastric secretagogue as coffee, and that milk and beer have a greater stimulatory effect than coffee.[35]

Any rigid exclusion of foodstuffs is poor medical practice in that it ignores individual needs and will probably be disregarded by many patients. The pain of an uncomplicated peptic ulcer is relieved by antacids and buffering foods, and its relief is a definable goal that the patient can understand. But we do not at present have the knowledge to achieve healing of an ulcer by dietary means, and attempting to impose irrational dietary restrictions, instead of encouraging the patient to use his own judgment and experience, is probably an expression of the frustration of ignorance.

The continuing use of antacids in the doses now recommended (80 mEq–160 mEq of neutralizing power every 2 hr) or of the H^+ secretory inhibitor, cimetidine, may have an adverse effect on the absorption of inorganic iron from the diet. Antacids either enhance destruction of thiamin or inhibit its absorption, and aluminum antacids may reduce phosphate absorption. The importance of these and other similar undocumented changes is debatable but should be borne in mind when treating patients with peptic ulcer or peptic esophagitis.

COMPLICATIONS OF PEPTIC ULCER DISEASE

The important complications are bleeding, perforation, and gastric outflow obstruction due to pyloric stenosis. Meulengracht was the first publicly to challenge the 20-year reign of Sippy and to give food by mouth, following a hematemesis, to patients as soon as they felt hungry, thereby converting a 4% to 20% mortality to about 1%. Yet, there is still some reluctance to follow this course, and many patients are fasted unnecessarily after upper GI bleeding.

In the management of perforated peptic ulcer, either by surgical intervention or conservative treatment, depending on the length of time following perforation and the condition of the patient, total parenteral nutrition (TPN) is mandatory. Details of the procedure may be found in Chapter 13. To maintain adequate nutrition in a markedly hypercatabolic state with mere infusions of 5% glucose–saline, to which a vitamin supplement may or may not have been added, is impossible. TPN should be continued until the patient's condition is stable, return from nasogastric suction is minimal, and bowel sounds have returned.

The patient with pyloric obstruction is also supported best by TPN for 3 to 4 days while gastric contents are being aspirated continuously prior to surgery and following surgery, until bowel sounds are restored, and until small amounts of food and drink by mouth are unequivocally tolerated.

Nutritional Management after Gastrointestinal Surgery

As emphasized elsewhere in this text, all types of physical trauma induce a catabolic response in excess of that associated with starvation. Patients undergoing GI surgery are especially vulnerable to acute nutritional insufficiency for the following reasons:

1. Preoperative undernutrition associated with complications of esophageal disease, peptic ulcer, inflammatory bowel disease, cirrhosis, and the like, and resulting in varying degree from reduced intake of food, malabsorption, metabolic disturbance, and nutrient losses from the GI tract
2. What might well be termed *diagnostic starvation* imposed by preoperative, radiologic, and other procedures
3. Prolonged postoperative depression of gastrointestinal functions

Preoperative improvement in nutritional status can now be achieved by TPN. The value of this procedure in terms of reduction in mortality and morbidity, is hard to assess quantitatively. There are serious potential complications of TPN, which decrease in frequency with the development of onsite special TPN teams, the handling of materials for intravenous use by pharmacists or other specially designated personnel, and technical improvements.

Earlier efforts to restore, at least in part, lean body mass and nutritional parameters preoperatively in patients with intractable peptic ulcer and other GI disease are now surpassed with a success seldom possible before. Subjects with severe inflammatory bowel disease, with or without fistula formation, have probably benefitted most from the introduction of effective parenteral feeding before surgery. It is extremely difficult to derive quantitative estimates of benefit, however, and currently we can use as a guide only clinical impression. Major indications are listed below.

Indications for Total Parenteral Nutrition

In selected cases of the following:

1. Obstructive disease of the esophagus
2. Any postoperative state where oral feeding is contraindicated for longer than 4 days
3. Perforated peptic ulcer
4. Small bowel resection
   Inflammatory bowel disease with or without enterocutaneous fistulae
   Celiac sprue
   Sclerodermatous bowel disease
5. Acute pancreatitis
6. Hepatic coma
   Viral hepatitis
   Alcoholic hepatitis

IMMEDIATE POSTOPERATIVE NUTRITIONAL CARE

After gastric or intestinal surgery in most hospitals, TPN is not used in the uncomplicated patient because feeding by mouth is usually restored in 3 days to 7 days postoperatively, as soon as bowel sounds return and the patient feels hungry. Even when trauma to the lower esophagus during truncal vagotomy results in edema (causing dysphagia with substernal pain, which may persist for 10–15 postoperative days), the patient can be encouraged to eat a soft diet, and this is usually successful.

Enthusiasts recommend that when restoration of oral feeding is delayed beyond 3 days to 4 days TPN should be commenced, and others favor full TPN for the first 5 to 6 postoperative days. Lacking convincing data, we have restricted TPN to patients who were clearly malnourished before surgery (especially in Crohn's disease of the small gut and gastroesophageal cancer) and to those in whom confident prediction of continuing absorptive failure and nutrient loss can be made, the best examples being small bowel resection and intestinal bypass procedures.

Wright and Tilson recommend that after resection of small bowel, fluid and nutrient requirements should be supplied entirely by TPN until the postoperative diarrhea has fallen below eight bowel movements or two liters daily fecal output.[50] Feeding small quantities by oral route or by nasogastric tube is then commenced, using a slow continuous drip of an isotonic solution, the osmolarity of which is gradually increased. Carbohydrate is used first and when 50 g to 100 g is absorbed in 24 hr, protein hydrolysates are added, and finally small but increasing amounts of fat. If these cause significant steatorrhea, medium-chain triglycerides, which are more easily absorbed, are substituted.

Hofmann suggested that bile salts, unabsorbed when distal ileum has been resected, pass into the colon and inhibit water absorption, thus adding to the diarrhea. There is evidence now that bile salts stimulate the colonic mucosa to secrete water. Administration of cholestyramine, a bile salt chelating agent, improved the diarrhea in many patients if less than 100 cm of small intestine had been resected.[26] After more extensive resection, cholestyramine may be ineffective and diarrhea is probably due to increased fat content of the stool.

CONTINUING POSTOPERATIVE NUTRITION CARE

One problem amenable to nutritional manipulation in the later stages following gastric surgery is prevention or correction of loss of lean body mass.

Weight loss invariably occurs after total gastrectomy in 5% to 42% of patients after a Billroth I procedure, and more often after Billroth II and similar operations, and it often persists.[18] It is due to diminished food consumption because of early satiety and the various components of *dumping*.[37] This syndrome is characterized by nausea, abdominal bloating, epigastric cramping pains, and diarrhea, together with vasomotor disturbances such as palpitations, sweating, weakness, drowsiness, and dyspnea, 5 min to 90 min after eating. A later phenomenon, sometimes termed *late dumping*, is reactive hypoglycemia, which is equally unpleasant to the patient, and is manifested by sweating, palpitations, lassitude, confusion, and rarely by stupor 90 min to 180 min after ingestion of carbohydrate.

Dumping is due to the too-rapid passage of hyperosmolar gastric contents into the upper part of the small intestine, whereas late dumping is due to the rapid absorption of glucose. The mechanisms involved are not clearly understood. Dumping is thought to be due to some combination of autonomic reflexes stimulated by intestinal disten-

tion, a contraction of blood volume, and release of intestinal vasoactive hormones. Late dumping is due to disturbance of coordination of insulin, glucagon, and possible enteroglucagon release.

Dumping occurs in up to 20% of subjects after partial gastrectomy and in a smaller percentage after truncal vagotomy and pyloroplasty. After highly selective or parietel cell vagotomy, which is becoming the surgical treatment of choice in intractable, uncomplicated duodenal ulcer disease, dumping occurs in only 5% of cases according to Amdrup and Jensen.[2]

The principles of treatment of underweight patients following gastric surgery are persistent encouragement to eat coupled with maneuvers to reduce dumping. Johnson and co-workers showed that the average caloric intake in such underweight subjects was 75% of the requirements for maintaining normal weight.[28] Successful persuasion to eat more food resulted in satisfactory weight gain. Dietary counseling before leaving the hospital is not sufficient; it must be reinforced by subsequent consultations as the patient gradually returns to a fully active life and attempts a normal diet. Frequent small, dry meals that are low in simple carbohydrate reduce dumping and late dumping to a minimum. Fluids should be taken at least 30 min before meals, and milk consumption should be excluded or reduced if diarrhea occurs after its ingestion. This may be due to rapid gastric emptying and inability of intestinal lactase to achieve complete hydrolysis of the lactose load (see Table 21-1).

It is known that gastric emptying is delayed in the recumbent position after gastric surgery and that lying down after meals often improves dumping.[22] In some patients a small oral dose of propantheline bromide 30 min before a meal reduces symptoms, and a high dietary pectin content has been shown to reduce or prevent postprandial hypoglycemia in postgastrectomy subjects.[27] Techniques are being developed to study differential rates of gastric emptying of different components of the same diet simultaneously, and rapid development of knowledge in this area may lead to more effective management.[49]

There is frequently mild steatorrhea after gastric surgery, but the degree of steatorrhea and postoperative weight loss show no correlation.[32] The causes are thought to be incoordination of pancreatic and biliary secretion, bacterial overgrowth causing bile salt deconjugation, sometimes pancreatic disease, and rarely the unmasking of gliadin-sensitive enteropathy. Fortunately the steatorrhea is seldom sufficiently severe to cause symptoms and to require dietary fat restriction. But it persists

TABLE 21-1
Special Diets in Gastrointestinal and Hepatic Disease

Condition	Diet
Peptic ulcer	Avoidance of gastric stimulants
Peptic esophagitis	
Dumping	Small, frequent dry meals, low in simple carbohydrate
	Exclude milk if necessary
Gliadin-sensitive enteropathy (celiac sprue)	α-gliadin exclusion (see Table 21-2 for short-term treatment)
Steatorrhea > 15 g/day if associated with diarrhea (pancreatitis, radiation enteritis, short-bowel)	High carbohydrate and protein
	Limit long-chain triglycerides
	Medium-chain triglycerides
	Supplements of all vitamins
	Low oxalate
Intestinal stricture	Low fiber
	$K^+Ca^{2+}Mg^{2+}$ if necessary
	Extra NaCl in fibrocystic disease in hot weather
Diverticulosis	High fiber
Portacaval encephalopathy	Protein to tolerance
	Lactulose
Alimentary allergy	Exclusion of specific allergens
Alactasia (primary and secondary)	Exclusion of milk
Lactase, sucrase, isomaltase deficiency	Exclusion of specific sugars
Cirrhosis with ascites	High protein
	Low salt (< 1 g/day)

for years and is an important factor in the later development of calcium deficiency and osteomalacia, which occurs in up to 25% of subjects after gastrectomy and shows significant correlation with fecal fat excretion.[17] Whether vitamin D deficiency plays a part in this calcium deficiency is not known. Insufficient concern is given to prophylaxis. If the patient can tolerate milk and milk products, calcium supplementation is probably unnecessary; otherwise, 325 mg calcium lactate four times daily should be taken. A strong case can be made as well for giving 50,000 units (1250 μg) vitamin D$_3$ daily, monitoring urinary calcium in the initial 2 months to 3 months.

Following gastric surgery, patients exhibit a gradual decrease in blood hemoglobin concentration, which is most commonly due to iron deficiency.[3] Factors implicated include reduced dietary iron intake, reduction in total food consumption, choice of diet, reduced iron absorption, stomach gastritis, and recurrent ulcer disease with bleeding. Treatment usually consists of administration of oral inorganic iron, the effectiveness of which is enhanced by giving the iron with 500 mg ascorbic acid or by giving iron parenterally.

Serum vitamin B$_{12}$ concentrations may fall progressively after gastric surgery, but surveys have not shown megaloblastic anemias in more than 4% to 6% of subjects 10 years after surgery. Folic acid deficiency is a relatively rare (1%–2%) cause of anemia. Red blood cell folate and serum vitamin B$_{12}$ assay should be done, and if levels are found to be low, appropriate supplementation should be given, using the intramuscular route for vitamin B$_{12}$ (100 μg/month) and oral folic acid (5 mg–10 mg/day). The serum B$_{12}$ activity of all postgastrectomy patients must be measured at 5 years after the operation.

INTESTINAL MALABSORPTION

A whole range of nutritional deficiencies occurs in diseases of the gastrointestinal tract and liver in which malabsorption of nutrients from the small intestine is a major factor. Malabsorption usually connotes reduced absorption, but some disease states may occur as a consequence of increased absorption of toxic substances. There are many causes of malabsorption, which can best be categorized according to the nature of the defect.

Decreased Absorption:

Acute

1. Nonspecific gastroenteritis due to toxigenic *E. coli* or rotavirus infection
2. Acute pancreatitis

Chronic

1. Disturbed coordination of digestive and absorptive processes (*e.g.*, vagotomy, partial gastrectomy)
2. Bacterial overgrowth in the upper small intestine (*e.g.*, intestinal stricture, duodenal afferent loop syndrome, jejunal diverticulosis)
3. Impaired activity of digestive enzymes or other factors
   Pancreatic (*e.g.*, cystic fibrosis, chronic pancreatitis)
   Brush border (*e.g.*, celiac sprue, tropical sprue, radiation enteritis)
   Biliary secretion (*e.g.*, primary or secondary biliary cirrhosis)
4. Reduction of absorptive surface (*e.g.*, celiac sprue, tropical sprue, small intestinal resection, intestinal bypass, Crohn's disease)
5. Infiltration of intestinal wall (*e.g.*, intestinal lymphoma)
6. Effect of drugs (*e.g.*, alcohol, neomycin)

Increased Absorption:

Hemochromatosis, Wilson's disease

The commonest manifestations of malabsorption are diarrhea, steatorrhea, loss of weight, and evidence of specific nutrient deficiency.

ACUTE MALABSORPTION

Gastroenteritis occurs more frequently in infants and children than in adults, except in special epidemic or pandemic situations, such as cholera. Treatment is directed to causative infecting organisms and fluid and electrolyte replacement, and control should be achieved before deficiency of other nutrients occurs. Therefore, in a previously healthy child or adult there is no indication for other support. In the nutritionally deprived subject, especially in children and when diarrhea persists, parenteral feeding may be lifesaving. In areas of endemic protein deficiency, gastroenteritis may precipitate kwashiorkor and only parenteral protein supplements are effective.

Acute pancreatitis attacks rarely last more than a week. The usual practice is to use a nasogastric tube and suction to remove gastric secretions, to give fluid and electrolytes by peripheral vein, to administer analgesics, and to give nothing by mouth until the pain has completely disappeared. Only in the mildest attack, without nausea or vomiting and with only minimal pain, is the patient given a fat-free diet after an initial 24-hr period of observation. However, patients with severe disease accompanied by complications such as pancreatic ascites, evidence of pseudocyst formation (best detected by computerized tomographic scans), or pancreatic abscess may run a longer course. These patients sometimes require surgery and are likely to be in a significantly catabolic state. In such patients intravenous infusions of amino acids and glucose are now widely used, although their value has not been demonstrated by any controlled trials. Some deplore this approach, on the basis that intravenous amino acids stimulate the pancreas. Lipids are excluded, since it is believed that high circulating lipid concentrations may, through some unknown mechanism induce, and therefore possibly aggravate, pancreatitis. In summary, the value of gastric suction and parenteral feeding has not been well established but would seem to be consistent with what is known of the physiology of pancreatic exocrine secretion and the observed hypercatabolic state that patients with severe acute pancreatitis display.

CHRONIC MALABSORPTION

Malabsorption consequent to gastric surgery has been discussed. Bacterial overgrowth in the upper small intestine may also occur in association with stricture owing to adhesions, inflammatory lesions, scleroderma, diabetic neuropathy, jejunal diverticulosis, and ischemic lesions occurring spontaneously or as a late result of irradiation. Congenital or acquired defects of neuromuscular activity and massive duodenal diverticula are rare causes. Normally the upper small bowel in humans has a sparse bacterial population, which probably does not interfere with the absorption of nutrients. Although the absorptive capacity of the intestine is greater in gnotobiotic (germ-free) than in conventional animals, this is not necessarily applicable to humans, since the species studied have been coprophagous. The major consequences of bacterial overgrowth are malabsorption of fat and vitamin B_{12}. Steatorrhea may be accompanied by failure to absorb fat-soluble vitamins and some mineral elements, such as calcium and magnesium. The steatorrhea is due to deconjugation of bile salts, and the deconjugation in the proximal small bowel can be demonstrated, using ^{14}C-glycine-labeled bile salts and demonstrating abnormally high $^{14}CO_2$ excretion in exhaled air. Conjugated bile salts (glycocholate and taurocholate) are essential for the formation of micelles, which is a prerequisite of long-chain fatty acid absorption. Vitamin B_{12} malabsorption is probably due to bacterial sequestration, with the B_{12} bound to some microorganism and no longer available for absorption in the ileum, a situation similar to that occurring with fish tapeworm (*Diphyllobothrium latum*) infestation.

Treatment of these conditions varies according to the cause. Surgical revisions or excisions may be appropriate and curative. This is not always feasible, since patients with these conditions tend to be advanced in years and frail. They may develop progressive malnutrition with hematologic and neurologic lesions that do not respond to massive doses of all known essential nutrients. Broad-spectrum oral antibiotics may be effective, but frequently the initial beneficial effect is not maintained. However, a long-term minor improvement of a degree consonant with maintenance of fair nutrition may be achieved. Medium-chain triglycerides may be used as a supplement when caloric utilization is seriously impaired and also as a replacement for long-chain dietary triglycerides, since their absorption does not require bile salts. Vitamin B_{12} is given intramuscularly, 100 μg/month. If the above measures fail, complete parenteral feeding should be used in an attempt to reverse severe malnutrition.

Pancreatic Disease

The important causes of pancreatic exocrine deficiency are cystic fibrosis (mucoviscidosis) and chronic pancreatitis.

CYSTIC FIBROSIS

Cystic fibrosis is a generalized disease of all the exocrine glands that is genetically transmitted as an autosomal recessive characteristic with a gene frequency of 1:20. Mucous secretions are abnormally viscous, and secretions of sweat have an abnormally high content of sodium, potassium, and chloride. The pancreas, which is involved in about 80% to 90% of cases, ultimately becomes a small, fibrosed organ as a consequence of atrophy of the exocrine structures following the obstruction of the duct system by plugs of eosinophilic debris. The volume, *p*H, lipase, amylase, trypsinogen, chymotrypsinogen, and carboxypeptidase contents of pancreatic secretion are much reduced, and malabsorption of fat and protein, oligosaccharides, water-soluble and fat-soluble vitamins, and some minerals results. Until the last two decades, most children affected died of the pulmonary effects of the disease, bronchiolar plugging, and obstructive emphysema resulting in bronchopulmonary infections. Significant improvements in respiratory toilet have resulted in survival into adult life of many subjects with this disease. In addition to malabsorption, they may also develop focal biliary and parenchymal cirrhosis as a consequence of intrahepatic cholangiolar plugging, pericholangitis, and unknown factors leading to portal hypertension with its complications.

Treatment of malabsorption, if present, consists of adequate oral supplements of pancreatic extracts, a high-carbohydrate, low-fat diet, all vitamins (if necessary, by injection), and extra sodium chloride, particularly in hot weather (see Table 21-1). Oral supplements of calcium and magnesium may also be required, as determined by estimating blood levels. If growth is not maintained in children with this disease, added calories may be provided by a palatable form of medium-chain triglycerides. These do not require bile salts for their absorption, and about 30% of a given dose is absorbed directly without the action of pancreatic lipase. Amino acid supplements are given with meals in the form of one or another short-chain polypeptide preparation, thus bypassing the need for the enzyme proteolytic activity of normal pancreatic secretion.

CHRONIC PANCREATITIS

Chronic pancreatitis, in which inflammation and scarring of the exocrine glandular tissue of the pancreas occur, has many causes, of which alcohol is the most important in the United States, followed by biliary tract disease. The lesion is functionally similar to that in fibrocystic disease. However, since it is a disease of adults, the nutritional problems are usually less severe. It is apparent, too, that 85% to 90% of the exocrine pancreas must be destroyed before malabsorption occurs.[15] Usually oral supplementation with pancreatic extract (Cotazym, 3–5 tabs with each meal) and vitamin supplementation are adequate. Large doses may be given if steatorrhea is not decreased. Antacids and H^+-inhibitors to reduce gastric acidity may enhance pancreatic enzyme activity. In some patients the extracts are poorly tolerated or less effective and supplements of medium-chain triglycerides and short-chain polypeptide amino acid mixtures should be given, using the patient's weight as a guide.

Failure of absorption of vitamin B_{12} is an uncommon consequence of chronic pancreatitis. It has been suggested that it is caused by a failure of release of vitamin B_{12} from a non-intrinsic-factor vitamin B_{12} binder prior to its binding with intrinsic factor.[1] Treatment is with intramuscular vitamin B_{12} 100 μg monthly.

Diseases of the Small Intestinal Wall

Celiac sprue is a disease of the small intestinal mucosa. The villi of the mucosa, particularly of the proximal jejunum, become atrophic and the lamina propria is infiltrated with inflammatory cells. The brush border is disrupted, and activity of brush border enzymes is impaired. The activity most affected is that of lactase, so that milk intolerance may be a feature of the untreated disease. There is impaired absorption of fat and protein, and the daily fecal fat excretion in the untreated adult may be 60 g or more. Hypoalbuminemia occurs in patients with severe disease and is due to malabsorption and excess loss of protein from the bowel wall (protein-losing enteropathy). It has become rare in recent years. Essential fatty acids, both fat-soluble and water-soluble vitamins, trace elements, and electrolytes, even water, are poorly absorbed. Important deficiencies are of vitamin K, vitamin D, and calcium leading to osteomalacia, and folic acid and possibly pyridoxine and zinc.[5,6,46] Deficiency of vitamin B_{12} occurs in less than half of all patients and is rarely the cause of hematologic or neurologic change. The site of its absorption in the distal part of the small intestine is infrequently affected in celiac sprue.

Since the classic observations of Dicke in the 1940s, it has been repeatedly confirmed that complete exclusion of wheat, rye, and barley gluten from the diet results in recovery of the intestinal mucosa.[13] More recently it has been demonstrated that it is the α-gliadin component of gluten which is the noxious factor, but how it exerts its effect is still uncertain. The aim of management of celiac disease is to encourage the patient to adopt and adhere rigidly to a gluten-free diet. This has not been easy in the past because wheat flour is used widely as an extender in many processed foods. The American Celiac Society provides exhaustive information about gluten content of foods, which should be available to every celiac patient.* Each component of the diet should be carefully evaluated by the dietitian and the patient, who must be made aware that even traces of gluten may inhibit mucosal recovery or precipitate a relapse. The diet should be balanced and should achieve maximal variety. When one member of a family is found to be affected it is often more convenient for the whole family, when eating at home, to adopt a gluten-free regimen.

Before a response to gluten exclusion is achieved, vigorous nutritional support is very often necessary. Untreated patients may be deficient in electrolytes, especially potassium, calcium, and magnesium, in fat-soluble and water-soluble vitamins, in iron, and possibly in trace elements, of which zinc has received much attention. Most patients

*For information, American Celiac Society, 45 Gifford Ave., Jersey City, N.J. 07304 (201-432-1207).

TABLE 21-2
Daily Oral Supplements in Gluten Sensitive Enteropathy Before a Response to Gluten Exclusion is Obtained

Nutrient	Daily Dosage
Potassium chloride	
Calcium gluconate	
Magnesium sulfate	
Vitamin A	25,000–50,000 IU
Vitamin D	30,000 IU
Vitamin K (Mephyton)	10 mg
Vitamin B-complex tablets containing daily requirements of thiamin, riboflavin, and niacin	2–3 tabs
Vitamin B_{12}	100 µg/4 weeks IM
Folic acid	10 mg
Vitamin C	50 mg

respond to oral supplementation (see Table 21-2) and protein supplements, and medium-chain triglycerides can be used. Patients may be intolerant of milk and lactose-containing products until mucosal recovery has occurred and brush-border enzyme activity is restored.

In some children diagnosed late, and in older adults, the degree of malnutrition may be severe; anorexia is a major symptom, and a rather malignant form of malnutrition supervenes. Total parenteral feeding is lifesaving in such patients, in whom oral feeding can be gradually re-introduced. If diarrhea is a major factor, drugs such as loperamide or opium preparations are used until gluten exclusion brings it under control.

TROPICAL SPRUE

This is a malabsorptive disease of tropical or subtropical areas with definite but unexplained geographical distribution. It is endemic but may assume epidemic frequency. The current view is that tropical sprue, subclinical tropical enteropathy, and post-infective malabsorption in the tropics are probably all expressions of population of the upper small bowel with enteropathic coliform organisms. The chronicity of sprue as compared with postinfective malabsorption may be due to a prolonged small bowel transit time in the former, favoring persistence of bacterial flora, which responds to antibiotics. Another theory is that dietary fat plays an important role, long-chain fatty acids having an inhibitory effect on coliforms in the jejunum. This may explain the geographical distribution of the disease as an expression of differences in fats consumed.

Treatment is with oral tetracycline and folic acid and intramuscular vitamin B_{12}. Improvement oc-

curs within 2 weeks to 3 weeks. Folic acid, 5 mg/day, is given for at least 2 years to achieve full restoration of small intestinal structure and function. It is more effective when it is commenced in the early stages of the disease.[31]

RADIATION ENTERITIS

The acute response of the small bowel to doses of radiation above 5000 rads is expressed as nausea, diarrhea, and malabsorption within 10 days to 20 days of treatment. It has become one of the commonest diseases of the wall of the small gut. Supportive treatment includes maintenance of a satisfactory nutritional state. Oral, intragastric hyperalimentation and parenteral feeding both have a place, and choice depends on the patient's nutritional status, the outcome of therapy—which is always for malignant disease—and the duration of symptoms. Systemic steroids may help to reduce diarrhea and malabsorption.

The delayed effects of radiation enteritis may appear months or years later. The acute changes of inhibition of epithelial cell turnover, ulceration of the epithelium, infection, inflammation, and edema are succeeded by ischemic changes of the whole thickness of the bowel wall due to obliterative endarteritis. Fibrosis and stricturing may supervene. The nutritional support of this chronic condition is discussed at the end of the section on small bowel resection.

CROHN'S DISEASE

Changes similar to those found in radiation enteritis occur in the small intestine in Crohn's disease. Inflammation, mucosal and submucosal damage, and subsequent stricturing are associated with diarrhea, malabsorption, and bleeding. The disease has a special predilection for the terminal ileum, though it may involve any part of the gastrointestinal tract. The distal 90 cm of the ileum play an essential role in absorption of vitamin B_{12} and bile salts, both of which undergo enterohepatic recirculation. A deficiency of vitamin B_{12} may contribute a megaloblastic-macrocytic component to an iron deficiency anemia, which commonly occurs in this condition as a consequence of blood loss, inadequate intake, and possibly malabsorption. Careful studies, particularly of children with Crohn's disease, have shown that their failure to grow is due in part to inadequate consumption of food as well as to malabsorption of food.[29] During an active phase of the disease they will be in negative nitrogen imbalance. Anorexia, abdominal cramping pain, and postprandial diarrhea inhibit intake, and it has been well demonstrated that a period of parenteral feeding will reverse the nitrogen imbalance, correct other nutritional deficiencies, and allow the growing child to achieve a reasonable weight and height for age. After 4 weeks to 6 weeks, patients have been fed once more by mouth, sometimes successfully because the underlying disease is less active; however, relapse does occur. A combination of oral and parenteral feeding, particularly in the prepubertal phase of maximal potential growth, may become an important part of treatment. Recently a deficiency of zinc has been demonstrated in some patients with Crohn's disease.[47] In patients who develop skin lesions and growth retardation the serum zinc level should be estimated, or 220 mg zinc sulfate may be given orally bid, on an empirical basis.

In Crohn's disease, low-residue and elemental diets and parenteral feeding have been used in attempts to reduce abdominal pain, the risks of obstruction, and the volume of diarrhea, and to allow healing of enteroenteric and enterocutaneous fistulae. There are no controlled trials to support general application of these diets, however, and uncritical enthusiasm is now on the wane.

Reduction of bulk in the lumen may reduce smooth muscle activity in the bowel, but the concept of "resting the bowel" demands critical appraisal. Relief of pain and reduction in diarrhea certainly occur. Permanent closure of fistulae has not occurred in our experience. It must be rare, if it occurs at all. Complete exclusion of nutrients by mouth does induce changes in the intestinal mucosa. Experiments in dogs have shown some atrophy of small intestinal villous structure when the animal is fed by parenteral route exclusively.[19] The same changes probably occur in humans and may underlie the temporary failure of function with diarrhea on resuming oral feeding. Surgical bypass of segments of bowel affected by Crohn's disease does seem to be associated in some cases with reduction in the inflammatory response in the bowel wall. This has certainly been so in subjects with Crohn's disease of the colon.[30] Our policy in adults is to use TPN only when anorexia, nausea, or vomiting after meals is protracted and a state of nutritional deficiency is likely to ensue, or when diarrhea is uncontrollable. Other aspects of nutritional support in Crohn's disease are described at the end of this section.

Intestinal Bypass

This operation was introduced about 15 years ago for the treatment of gross and life-threatening obesity unresponsive to medical and behavioral management. The usual practice has been to exclude surgically all but 30 cm of proximal small bowel and 10 cm of distal ileum. After surgery, patients behave similarly to those in whom extensive small bowel resection has been performed and must be treated according to the regimen well outlined by Wright and Tilson.[50] Subsequent persisting diarrhea is usual and in a small proportion of patients is impossible to control and sometimes intolerable. The metabolic consequences of this operation are extremely severe and serious, and sometimes lethal nutritional complications have occurred. There are patients in our experience during the past 12 years who have received virtually no proper nutritional assessment after surgery, with the only concern evident in their management being a focus on loss of weight. We have seen irreversible parenchymal hepatic, central nervous, and bone disease, and clinical evidence of deficiency of protein, ascorbate, thiamin, folic acid, vitamin B_{12}, essential fatty acid, and possibly zinc, and hyperoxaluria with urinary calculi. Whether this surgical approach should be used at all is questionable, although it may have been life saving in some very obese patients. The procedure is now being displaced by gastric stapling. If intestinal bypass is done, careful monitoring of the patient at frequent subsequent intervals is essential. Patients who have had intestinal bypass for many years should be screened for hepatic and bone disease.

The pattern of weight loss after bypass, and metabolic studies, make it clear that the major cause of the initial calorie deficit is not malabsorption but anorexia, which in many subjects subsides in 10 months to 18 months.[40] Thus, inadequate intake of essential nutrients and some malabsorption occur together.

SMALL-BOWEL RESECTION

Providing the duodenum, distal ileum, and ileocecal valve are spared, up to 40% of the small intestine may be removed without long-term sequelae. More extensive resection (50% or more, or resection of the distal ileum and ileocecal valve) results in variable malabsorption, the severity of which depends on three factors: (1) the extent of resection, (2) the site of resection, and (3) the presence of retained diseased segments of bowel. Crohn's disease, ischemia due to thrombosis or embolism, trauma, and malignant infiltration are some of the conditions treated by resection. The immediate postoperative management has been described. TPN has clearly diminished morbidity and mortality. Subsequently, appetite returns, and diarrhea occurs only following ingestion of food.

Small meals, low in fat content, should be given every 2 hr to 3 hr. We do not use so-called elemental diets as routine; they are hyperosmolar, increase diarrhea, and are unpalatable, but occasionally they are well tolerated. Long-chain triglycerides are added by degrees but should be restricted to an intake that does not increase steatorrhea, usually in a range of 25 g/day to 75 g/day. Medium-chain triglycerides can be added as a source of energy. Usually 25 g/day to 40 g/day is tolerable; larger amounts cause diarrhea. The cutaneous application of sunflower seed oil has been advocated as a source of essential fatty acid, and if long-chain triglycerides are not well absorbed, this procedure, to which little attention has been given, is very important.

When the patient's bowel has achieved a stable function, some or all of the supplements listed in Table 21-2 will be given according to need as judged by laboratory data, since malabsorption of fat, fat-soluble vitamins, calcium, magnesium, iron, and water-soluble vitamins may persist. Intramuscular vitamin B_{12} must be given, 100 μg every 3 weeks to 4 weeks, if the terminal ileum has been resected. Hyperoxaluria occurs in nearly 75% of subjects with ileal resection. It is believed to be due to calcium being unavailable to form insoluble calcium oxalate in the lumen, since an increased amount forms calcium "soaps" with unabsorbed fat. Free oxalic acid is then absorbed in the colon. Treatment consists of avoidance of oxalate-containing foods, especially many green vegetables, beets, rhubarb, nuts, and chocolate, or in giving calcium lactate or carbonate orally, since the calcium binds oxalate in the lumen. However, calcium compounds theoretically may exert a stimulatory effect on gastric acid secretion, which is often high after small bowel resection, possibly due to reduction of a hormonal inhibitor. Avoidance of dietary oxalate may be preferable. Cholestyramine is useful to control persisting diarrhea by binding bile salts which stimulate water secretion by the colon. Diphenoxylate or loperamide serves to control diarrhea; occasionally opiates, which are most effective, must be used.

TABLE 21-3
Diet in Ulcerative Colitis

Degree of Disorder	Aliments and Nutrients
Mild or moderately severe	High protein; vitamin supplement Exclude cow's milk if history of intolerance or failure to respond to medical treatment Avoid citrus fruits and other laxative foods and beverages. Treat iron deficiency by IM route
Severe	Parenteral fluid replacement and steroids; TPN until controlled

Nonspecific Ulcerative Colitis

In nonspecific ulcerative colitis the role of any special dietary regimen is not established. In the acute phase of a severe attack, including toxic megacolon, oral feeding is suspended and effective intravenous nutrition must be maintained. However, if the patient can tolerate food by mouth, the diet should be designed first to stimulate the individual appetite and second to provide high nutritional value. Protein losses from the diseased colon can be very large. Only well-tolerated foods are given. A history of cow's milk intolerance justifies its exclusion. The intolerance may be a consequence of hypersensitivity to the protein content or of primary or secondary hypolactasia and lactose intolerance. My own practice is to advise milk exclusion in addition for those patients who fail to respond favorably to a proven medical regimen. Where necessary, a soy–protein substitute for cow's milk may be used. As regards supplementation with amino acid diets, my own experience has led me to avoid them. They are unappetizing as well as being hyperosmolar, and since there is no evidence of significantly impaired small intestinal proteolysis in ulcerative colitis there is no rationale for their administration. High-protein intake can be designed around egg or meat protein, with some vegetable proteins included, and if, as sometimes happens, normal dietary fats can be ingested only in limited amounts, useful minor supplementation with medium-chain triglycerides in a palatable form (*e.g.*, mayonnaise and in cooking) is worth testing.

Citrus fruits and other laxative foods and beverages should be excluded during an attack and taken in remissions, if the patient feels seriously deprived, with caution and moderation. The major points of diet in inflammatory large bowel disease are tabulated in Table 21-3.

COLONIC DIVERTICULOSIS

A growing body of evidence has shown that diverticular disease of the colon is better managed by use of diets of high fiber content plus stool bulk producers (bran, psyllium, methyl cellulose, polycarbophil) than by traditional low-residue diets. One trial showed significant reduction in attacks of supervening diverticulitis in subjects ingesting bran regularly.[9] However, a recent rigorous, controlled trial has cast doubt on the symptom-relieving effects of fiber supplementation in diverticulosis, and currently the matter must be regarded as unresolved.[39] Meanwhile, various fiber diets are enthusiastically prescribed. Whether diverticular disease can be prevented by high fiber diets is unproven and rests on inadequate epidemiologic evidence gleaned from African and Asian populations. A long-term prospective trial is required to test this speculation.

Exclusion Diets in Food Intolerance and Gastrointestinal Allergies

Consideration of exclusion diets would alone fill a whole volume. Many patients with irritable bowel syndromes have been committed to a lifetime of rigid and unappetizing diets from which some essential nutrients have in many cases been partly or wholly excluded on the basis of medical superstition and inadequate empirical testing. This should not be interpreted as implying that all exclusion diets are unnecessary.

ENZYME DEFICIENCY STATES

Congenital absence of certain enzyme systems, such as the lactase of the intestinal brush border, may be an indication for the exclusion of a specific sugar. Another example is sucrose-isomaltase deficiency present in infancy. Rarely, intolerance of carbohydrate is due to a congenital and isolated defect in intestinal transport, as in glucose–galactose malabsorption, so that diarrhea occurs when these sugars are ingested. Replacement of dietary glucose and sucrose with fructose results in relief of symptoms.

GASTROINTESTINAL ALLERGIES

Hypersensitivity to foodstuffs has been well documented ever since the observations of Prausnitz and Küstner more than half a century ago.[41] Many patients have alimentary allergic reactions as acute and severe as those of Prausnitz, and these problems may often be at least partly remedied. The nature of the particular allergen or allergens to which the patient is sensitive may be an important determinant of success. Caviar is more easily avoided, at least in Western cultures, than soybean protein or spray-dried skim milk, which seem to be ubiquitous. Heiner has estimated that 0.3% to 0.7% of infants are hypersensitive to cow's milk protein.[24] This may express itself in a failure to thrive, a fretful, flatulent child, or, in extreme cases, in a hemorrhagic colitis with secondary iron deficiency anemia.

Although less severe and less acute, GI and alimentary allergies create greater therapeutic problems. Patients in this group may present in the clinic seriously underweight and overanxious, some-times displaying symptoms and signs of specific nutritional deficiency. They may, by a reductive process, have adopted a diet of overcooked lamb and rice or something similar. They are desperate, but often initially impervious to rational management. Inquiry elicits the fact that their original symptoms may have been only a transient bout of nausea or of diarrhea, sometimes associated, although this was not initially recognized, with some medication, often an oral antibiotic for intercurrent infection. Many subjects believe that they are, for the above or other reasons, allergic to a specific food, or a number of foods. To prove an allergy is usually difficult and often impossible. It is likely that informative tests may shortly become available that are more permissible in this hepatitis-ridden age than the original Prausnitz-Küstner test, which requires transfer of human serum. The addition of suspected allergens to amino acid diets, which are to a large extent allergen-free, for testing on a double blind basis, has in our hands proved disappointing, since these diets are unappetizing and are so poorly tolerated that most test subjects fail to stay on them the required 10 to 14 days.

Earlier claims by Rowe and others that inflammatory bowel diseases, such as nonspecific ulcerative colitis, are an expression of a chronic dietary allergy have never been fully substantiated, although Wright and Truelove found that a cow's milk exclusion diet appeared to result in a significantly reduced relapse rate in about one sixth of a group of patients with ulcerative colitis.[51] In the treatment of patients with nonspecific ulcerative colitis, our policy has been to advise the exclusion of milk and milk products initially only to those who give a history of intolerance to milk at any time from infancy on, and subsequently to the few who fail to respond promptly to conventional modes of medical therapy, before considering surgery.

In managing alimentary allergies the physician must take a thorough, probing history. He should never express skepticism but rather should attempt to gain the patient's confidence and then to design a dietary regimen of addition of foodstuffs one by one. The help of the dietitian is valuable here.

Since 1973 there have been some reports of benefit being derived from oral sodium cromoglycate, which is thought to stabilize cells in the mucosa that release pharmacologically active substances when involved in some immune reactions. Development of this drug or similar ones may be so successful as to obviate wholly the need for identification of suspected allergens and their exclusion. Another approach may develop from studies currently being conducted on the relationship between the time of first presentation of various foods to the weanling infant and subsequent development of hypersensitivity.

Two principles should be kept in mind. As far as it is consonant with achieving and maintaining satisfactory nutrition, the aim should be to devise an attractive diet. Eating is one of life's pleasures, and it outlasts all the others as Brillat–Savarin noted in 1825.[8] Secondly, as with other therapeutic components, diet should be regularly reviewed. The value of the trained dietitian's assistance cannot be exaggerated in achieving these aims, and it is regrettable that their aid is not solicited more by medical practitioners, since they possess the expertise and the opportunity to apply themselves single-mindedly to these matters (see Chaps. 5 and 6).

FLATULENCE

Few if any modern texts on gastroenterology, diet, or nutrition, address the topic of flatulence, although there are many advocates of vegetarian diets, which must comprise beans and pulses in order to achieve adequate protein complementarity. Such diets are unquestionably flatugenic. A pioneer in attempts to bring some understanding into the troublesome topic is Levitt, who has produced lists of foods of variable flatugenicity, based on studies in one individual.[48] Clearly, individual variability exists, and extensive studies are needed. Even now the relationship between the amount of gases produced, their transit, and the variable threshold for symptoms to occur, is imperfectly understood.

GASTROINTESTINAL DISEASE IN THE AGED

The prevalence of gastrointestinal symptoms and diseases increases with age. In patients over 70 years of age carcinoma of the stomach or large bowel, peptic ulcer, and intestinal obstruction due to hernias and colonic diverticular disease constitute the major portion of the 20% of all deaths attributable to GI disease. Such disorders in the older patient require the same modalities of management, including attempts to maintain caloric and nitrogen balance, as in younger patients. More important as special problems of the elderly are anorexia, nausea and vomiting associated with extraintestinal diseases and their treatment, diarrhea, with or without fecal incontinence, and constipation.

Loneliness, lack of motive, and loss of gustatory sensation are major factors in development of malnutrition in the old as a consequence of reduced food intake compounded by exclusion of specific foods resulting from idiosyncracy. Surveys of the aged in the United Kingdom have revealed daily caloric consumption of 1100 Cal to 1500 Cal in 20% to 30% of populations surveyed. These factors play a far more important part in the development of nutritional deficiencies in otherwise relatively healthy elderly people than any possibly impaired digestive or absorptive mechanism associated with age.

When disease of the GI tract supervenes, as a consequence of direct involvement or of the secondary effects of extraintestinal disease, such as heart failure, or of the effects of drugs, such as digitalis, latent malnutrition may be compounded, and overt changes may appear. Older patients should be monitored carefully, and special attention should be paid to their nutrition. Food should be attractively prepared, and the subject encouraged to eat communally, rather than alone. Dentition should be checked and corrected if necessary. A daily supplement of vitamins and minerals should be given to compensate for the deficiencies of a reduced total dietary intake.

A full treatment of the problems of diarrhea and constipation in the aged is outside the range of this chapter (but see Chap. 22). The former may be due to fecal impaction, and this can be discouraged, as can constipation without pseudodiarrhea, by adding bran to the diet. However, stool softeners and laxatives may also be required. Underlying organic causes must be sought when appropriate.

Nutritional Support of Diseases of the Liver and Biliary Tract

Although the liver occupies a focal position in intermediary metabolism, relatively little has been accomplished in specific dietary management of liver disease. Currently, some form of nutritional support or modification is required in the following:

1. Hepatic encephalopathy
2. Ascites as a consequence of cirrhosis
3. Hepatolenticular degeneration (Wilson's disease)
4. Hemochromatosis
5. Chronic biliary obstruction
6. Possibly in viral hepatitis

HEPATIC ENCEPHALOPATHY

In a few patients with massive, fulminant hepatitis and in many patients with cirrhosis in whom a significant degree of portal-systemic shunting occurs, either spontaneously or as a consequence of surgery to relieve portal hypertension, ingestion of protein, or a similar endogenous protein load of blood due to bleeding into the lumen of the gut, may be associated with onset of a metabolic encephalopathy. The patient's consciousness deteriorates and confusion, stupor, or coma supervene. Electroencephalography reveals the slow waves of metabolic brain dysfunction. Asterixis, expressed as flapping tremor of the hands and arms and sometimes "tromboning" of the tongue, is often regarded as pathognomonic of the condition. Precipitating factors other than bleeding, such as analgesics, sedatives, hypokalemia, and azotemia induced by diuretic overdose, may also occur. The encephalopathy in itself is not life threatening, providing a good airway is maintained, but some of the precipitating factors, such as severe bleeding and liver or renal failure may well be.

The cause of the changes of brain activity are usually ascribed to elevated concentrations of ammonium ions in the blood and cerebrospinal fluid, derived from the GI tract and kidneys. If these are reduced, the changes in consciousness are completely reversible. Measures are therefore taken to reduce the production of ammonia or associated nitrogenous products and their absorption from the small bowel and to reduce ammonia production by the kidneys.

In the acute phase, when the patient is in stupor or coma, dietary management is superfluous. Fluid and electrolyte balance are restored parenterally, together with glucose. Urea-splitting organisms are removed from the colon by water enemas, and their growth is inhibited with neomycin retention enemas. Hypokalemia is often present as a consequence of diuretics, diarrhea, vomiting, and renal tubular acidosis. Restoration of normal potassium depresses renal ammonia synthesis.[44] Currently, studies are being made of the value of giving intravenous branched-chain amino acids, concentrations of which are low in chronic liver disease.[20]

When consciousness is regained, feeding by mouth is restored, using a carbohydrate and low-fat diet. Lactulose, a nonabsorbable synthetic disaccharide, is given.[4] This is metabolized by bacteria in the distal ileum and colon to acids that lower the *p*H and trap ammonium ions, preventing their absorption. Proteins are excluded from the diet initially, but as soon as the patient can cooperate and there is no evidence of GI bleeding, dietary protein is added in 20-g increments every 3 days. The aim is to restore nitrogen balance without precipitating intoxication. Intakes above 40 g/day of protein of high biologic value probably provide adequate maintenance. The desirable range of the usual dietary proteins is 60 g/day to 80 g/day. Continuing use of lactulose has made this possible in all but a small number of cirrhotics, without need of neomycin or other broad-spectrum antibiotic. Amino acid content of various proteins may be important, since some amino acids elevate ammonia levels in the blood more than others; (*e.g.,* glutamine, gly-

cine, and histidine). The pattern of release from the intestinal lumen and rates of absorption may also vary. Results of studies using vegetable rather than animal proteins are still indeterminate but are of great interest. Vitamin supplements are given, with the rationale that the patient is likely to be depleted on account of dietary inadequacy. Of these, vitamin K is probably the most important.

CIRRHOTIC ASCITES

Formation of ascites is usually a late stage in the natural history of cirrhosis. The two major causes are portal hypertension and reduced oncotic plasma pressure owing to hypoalbuminemia. The associated disturbances of homeostatis are complex and include redistribution of body water and sodium retention with hyperaldosteronism. Dietary management of the patient at bed rest comprises water and sodium restriction. These are modulated according to urinary output, but sodium intake should be less than 1 g/day. There need be no restriction of protein intake unless encephalopathy supervenes. The low salt requirement is a bar to certain proteins only if a sodium intake of less than 500 mg daily is indicated. Dialyzed milk should be used, the daily meat ration reduced to less than 100 g, with not more than one egg, and green vegetables must be restricted. Some patients tolerate a salt substitute.

WILSON'S DISEASE (HEPATOLENTICULAR DEGENERATION)

Wilson's disease is a rare disease that is an expression of an autosomal recessive trait. The prevalence of heterozygotes is about 0.5%. The homozygote lacks the capacity to excrete copper into the bile. The metal accumulates, especially in the liver, the basal ganglia, and the kidneys as well as in the cornea, producing Kaiser–Fleischer rings. Urinary copper concentrations are elevated, while serum copper and ceruloplasmin levels are usually depressed. The liver is enlarged, contains about five times the normal amount of copper, and may show changes ranging from periportal fibrosis to macronodular cirrhosis. There may be splenomegaly and portal hypertension.

Diagnosis early in the course of the disease and treatment directed to the removal of copper result in significant improvement and even normal life expectancy. The major therapy is the use of D-penicillamine and oral potassium sulfide. Exclusion of copper-containing foods such as shellfish, liver, chocolate, nuts, mushrooms, and broccoli is advocated by many, although not universally. Iron, calcium, and zinc deficiency and even pyridoxine deficiency have been reported in association with long-term D-penicillamine treatment. It has been suggested that the drug be discontinued each week for two days and that copper-free mineral supplements be given.

HEMOCHROMATOSIS

A number of different factors may be responsible for increasing the amounts of iron stored in the liver, including the following: dietary iron overload, cirrhosis from many causes, multiple blood transfusions in dyshematopoietic anemias resistant to treatment with all known hematinics, thalassemia, and, finally, so-called idiopathic hemochromatosis, in which iron overload appears to precede the development of cirrhosis. The disease is familial, and first-degree relatives can be screened by serum iron estimations; the concentration is high in idiopathic hemochromatosis. Dietary control has little place in the disease, other than in the diabetes mellitus which occurs frequently. The basic lesion is faulty regulation of absorption of dietary iron from the intestine, so that avoidance of foods with a high content of iron is recommended. These foods include liver of all species and some wines. Recently, tea drinking has been shown to inhibit the absorption of nonheme iron and may be a useful means of preventing iron overload.[16] The mainstay of treatment is repeated phlebotomy.

CHRONIC BILIARY OBSTRUCTION

Both intrahepatic and extrahepatic biliary obstruction cause cholestasis. In chronic cholestasis steatorrhea, malabsorption of calcium and fat-soluble vitamins occurs. These risks must not be forgotten if obstruction persists for more than 1 week to 2 weeks, and appropriate nutritional supplementation should be provided.

Vitamin K should be given parenterally in daily doses of 10 mg for 3 days if there is any indication of hypoprothrombinemia. In chronic cholestatic disease associated with primary biliary cirrhosis, bile duct carcinoma, or sclerosing cholangitis, daily intake of long-chain triglycerides should be limited to 40 g because they are poorly tolerated, poorly absorbed, and may be a factor in inhibiting calcium absorption. Medium-chain triglycerides are used as a supplement, usually 25 g/day to 40 g/day. They are well absorbed without bile salts and provide a source of energy.[21] They do not provide essential fatty acid. If there is doubt, therefore, about absorption of long-chain fatty acid, sunflower oil inunctions should be used. Vitamin A, 100,000 IU, Vitamin D, 100,000 IU; and Vitamin K₁, 10 mg, are given intramuscularly every 4 weeks. Calcium

gluconate, 6 g/day, should be given by mouth as well as nonfat milk to tolerance. If bone pain occurs, calcium gluconate (15 mg calcium/kg body weight) is given intravenously daily for 1 week. Reversal of osteomalacia has been achieved in primary biliary cirrhosis by oral 25-hydroxyvitamin D.[43] If cholestyramine must be given to control pruritus, the above nutritional regimen may have to be increased, especially the vitamin K. The dose of cholestyramine should be the lowest that provides relief of symptoms.

Copper retention occurs in primary biliary cirrhosis, but evidence that copper depletion is beneficial is still not established.

ACUTE VIRAL HEPATITIS

Comparatively early studies suggest that *ad libitum* consumption of a complete diet, high in fat as well as protein and carbohydrate, by patients suffering from viral hepatitis may shorten the course of the disease.[12] It has not been shown that tube or parenteral feeding in those subjects with viral hepatitis who also have anorexia has significant benefit. When nausea and vomiting occur, parenteral fluids and glucose are given, as in the rare instances of fulminant hepatitis with coma. Trials of TPN or TPN modified in amino acid content might yield useful information for improving current practice.

ALCOHOLIC HEPATITIS

In addition to those diseases of the liver already discussed, one other may deserve mention, namely alcoholic hepatitis. In the past decade, it has been possible to provide nutritional support in the early stages of management for subjects with this disease, many of whom are significantly malnourished. To date, the most persuasive evidence for the value of parenteral nutrient supplementation is the work of Galambos, who has shown that intravenous administration for 28 days of 70–85 g/day amino acids, in the form of Aminosyn or Travasol, to supplement a 3000 Cal diet, may reduce mortality and may be associated with earlier restoration of serum bilirubin concentration to normal.[38]

Diet and Gallstone Formation

From review of the current literature about prevention of formation of gallstones or their dissolution by dietary modifications, there emerges no convincing pattern. Fasting and overnight bile have been shown to be lithogenic, that is, it displays cholesterol supersaturation. One hopeful development is the observation that, in women, low frequency of meals or overnight fasting prolonged by eating no breakfast, is accompanied by a high incidence of gallstones.[11] This makes good sense physiologically, but awaits confirmation.

References

1. Allen RH, Seetharam B, Podell E et al: Effect of proteolytic enzymes on binding of cobalamin to R protein and intrinsic factor. J Clin Invest 61:47, 1978
2. Amdrup E, Jensen H-E, Johnson D, Walker BE et al: Clinical results of parietal cell vagotomy (highly selective vagotomy) two to four years after operation. Ann Surg 180:279, 1974
3. Baird IM, Blackburn EK, Wilson GM: The pathogenesis of anaemia after partial gastrectomy. Q J Med 28:21, 1959
4. Bircher J, Haemmerli UP, Scollo–Lavizzari G: Treatment of chronic portalsystemic encephalopathy with lactulose—Report of six patients and review of the literature. Am J Med 51:148, 1971
5. Bossak ET, Wang CI, Adlersberg D: Clinical aspects of the malabsorption syndrome (idiopathic sprue). Journal of Mt. Sinai Hospital 24:286, 1957
6. Brain MC, Booth CC: The absorption of tritium-labelled pyridoxine HCl in control subjects and in patients with intestinal malabsorption. Gut 5:241, 1964
7. Bray GA: UCLA conference on intestinal bypass operation as a treatment for obesity. Ann Intern Med 85:97, 1976
8. Brillat–Savarin JA: The Physiology of Taste. Charles Monselet (trans). New York, Liveright, 1948
9. Broadribb AJM: Treatment of symptomatic diverticular disease with a high-fibre diet. Lancet 1:664, 1977
10. Buchman E, Kaung VT, Doland K et al: Unrestricted diet in the treatment of duodenal ulcer. Gastroenterology 56:1016, 1969
11. Capron JP, Delamarre J, Herve MA et al: Meal frequency and duration of overnight fast: A role in gall-stone formation? Br Med J 283:1435, 1981
12. Chalmers TC, Eckhardt RD, Reynolds WE et al: The treatment of acute infectious hepatitis: Studies of the effects of diets, rest, and physical reconditioning on the acute course of the disease and on the incidence of relapse and residual abnormalities. J Clin Invest 34:1163, 1955
13. Dicke WK: Therapy of celiac disease. Ned Tijdschr Geneeskd 95:124, 1951
14. DiCostanzo J, Noirclerc M, Jouglard J et al: New therapeutic approach to corrosive burns of the upper gastrointestinal tract. Gut 21:370, 1980
15. DiMagno EP, Go VLW, Summerskill WH: Relations between pancreatic enzyme outputs and malabsorption in severe pancreatic insufficiency. N Engl J Med 288:813, 1973
16. Disler PB, Lynch SR, Charlton RW et al: The effect of tea on iron absorption. Gut 16:193, 1975
17. Eddy RL: Metabolic bone disease after gastrectomy. Am J Med 50:442, 1971
18. Everson TC: Nutrition following total gastrectomy, with particular reference to fat and protein assimilation (abstr). Int Surg 95:209, 1952
19. Feldman EJ, Dowling RH, McNaughton J et al: Effects of oral versus intravenous nutrition on intestinal adaptation after small bowel resection in the dog. Gastroenterology 70:712, 1976
20. Fischer JE, Funovics JM, Aguirre A et al: The role of plasma amino acids in hepatic encephalopathy. Surgery 78:276, 1975
21. Greenberger NJ, Skillman TG: Medium chain triglycerides. Physiological considerations and clinical implications. N Engl J Med 280:1045, 1969
22. Hancock BD, Bowen–Jones E, Dixon R: The effect of posture on the gastric emptying of solid meals in normal subjects and patients after vagotomy. Br J Surg 61:945, 1974
23. Hawkins C: Personal view. Br Med J 4:362, 1970
24. Heiner DC, Wilson JF, Lahey ME: Sensitivity to cow's milk. JAMA 189:563, 1964
25. Hoagland CL, Labby DH, Kunkel HG et al: An analysis of the effect of fat in the diet on recovery in viral hepatitis. Am J Public Health 36:1287, 1946
26. Hofmann AF, Poley JR: Role of bile salt malabsorption in pathogenesis of diarrhea and steatorrhea in patients with ileal resection. Gastroenterology 62:918, 1972
27. Jenkins DJA, Gassull MA, Leeds AR et al: Effect of dietary fiber on complications of gastric surgery: Prevention of postprandial hypoglycemia by pectin. Gastroenterology 72:215, 1977
28. Johnson IDA, Welbourn RD, Acheson K: Gastrectomy and loss of weight. Lancet 1:1242, 1958
29. Kirschner BS, Voinchet O, Rosenberg IH: Growth retardation in inflammatory bowel disease. Gastroenterology 75:504, 1978
30. Kivel RM, Taylor KB, Oberhelman HA Jr: Responses to bypass ileostomy in ulcerative colitis and Crohn's disease of the colon. Lancet 2:632, 1967
31. Klipstein FA: Tropical sprue. In Bockus HL (ed): Gastroenterology, pp 285–305. Philadelphia, WB Saunders, 1974
32. Lawrence W, Vanamee P, Peterson AS: Alterations in fat and nitrogen metabolism after total and subtotal gastrectomy. Surg Gynecol Obstet 110:610, 1960
33. Lieber CS, DeCarli LM, Rubin E: Sequential production of fatty liver, hepatitis and cirrhosis in sub-human primates fed ethanol with adequate diets. Proc Natl Acad Sci 72:437, 1975
34. Martorell R, Yarbrough C, Yarbrough S et al: The impact of ordinary illnesses on the dietary intakes of malnourished children. Am J Clin Nutr 33:345, 1980
35. McArthur K, Hogan D, Isenberg JI: Relative stimulatory effects of commonly ingested beverages on gastric acid secretion in humans. Gastroenterology 83:199, 1982
36. Meulengracht E: Treatment of haematemesis and melaena with food. Acta Med Scand (Suppl) 59:375, 1934
37. Mix CL: "Dumping stomach" following gastrojejunostomy. Surg Clin North Am 2:617, 1922
38. Nasrallah SM, Galambos JT: Amino acid therapy of alcoholic hepatitis. Lancet 2:1276, 1980
39. Ornstein MH, Littlewood ER, Baird IM: Are fibre supplements really necessary in diverticular disease of the colon? A controlled clinical trial. Br Med J 282:1353, 1981
40. Pilkington TRE, Gazet JC, Ang L: Explanations for weight loss after ileojejunal bypass in gross obesity. Br Med J 1:1504, 1976
41. Prausnitz C, Küstner H: Studiérn über die Ueberemphindlickeit. Zentralbl Bakteriol (Orig) 86.160, 1921
42. Price SF, Smithson KW, Castell DO: Food sensitivity in reflux esophagitis. Gastroenterology 75:240, 1978

43. Reed JS, Meredith SC, Nemchausky BA et al: Bone disease or primary biliary cirrhosis: Reversal of osteomalacia with oral 25-hydroxyvitamin D. Gastroenterology 78:512, 1980

44. Shear L, Gabuzda GJ: Potassium deficiency and endogenous ammonium overload from kidney. Am J Clin Nutr 23:614, 1970

45. Sippy BW: Gastric and duodenal ulcer: Medical care by an efficient removal of gastric juice corrosion. JAMA 64:1625, 1915

46. Solomons NW, Rosenberg IH, Sandstead HH: Zinc nutrition in celiac-sprue. Am J Clin Nutr 29:371, 1976

47. Solomons NW, Rosenberg IH, Sandstead HH, et al: Zinc deficiency in Crohn's disease. Digestion 16:87, 1977

48. Sutalf LO, Levitt MD: Follow-up of a flatulent patient. Dig Dis Sci 24:652, 1979

49. Weiner K, Graham LS, Reedy T et al: Simultaneous gastric emptying of two solid foods. Gastroenterology 81:257, 1981

50. Wright HK, Tilson MD: Postoperative Disorders of the Gastrointestinal Tract. New York, Grune & Stratton, 1973

51. Wright R, Truelove SC: A controlled therapeutic trial of various diets in ulcerative colitis. Br Med J 2:138, 1965

22
Geriatrics
Ronald D. T. Cape

"We eat to live rather than live to eat" is an aphorism more relevant to old than to young people, the latter often suggesting that the converse is true by their overindulgence and obesity. Food gathering is a basic biologic exercise protected deep in the skull by an appetite center. In modern advanced nations, this activity has been made easy with a plentiful supply of every nutrient to be found in an array of large and small food-dispensing stores. Civilization is far removed from the situation that prevailed in the days when man had to search for, chase, and catch his food with the aid of primitive tools.

There are exceptions, however, to that general rule. Those who have physical disabilities that impair mobility, economic handicaps that reduce purchasing power, or central nervous system (CNS) problems that reduce appetite and memory, may all experience difficulty in securing an adequate diet. The group of the population in which these three attributes exist to a significant degree is the elderly. For this reason, special attention to their nutritional needs is important. Are these needs identical in quantity and quality to those of persons still at the peak of mature adulthood? Can diet influence longevity or affect the diseases of old age? Is there a significant incidence of undernutrition among our elderly population? How can one assess this, and what can be done to correct the situation where it is demonstrably true?

It is not enough to obtain food. One must prepare, cook, and consume it. This requires knowledge, skill, and equipment. Most homes are furnished with adequate cooking stoves and most

persons can produce reasonable, if not exciting, meals, but many older subjects may have problems chewing food because of loss of teeth. This may reduce the quantity, and will certainly affect the quality, of what is eaten. It is not surprising, therefore, that in the United Kingdom a nutrition survey that examined random samples of elderly people living at home in six areas, showed that malnutrition occurred in 3% of the subjects studied.[15]

Biologic Aging

As one ages, changes occur in the function of all bodily systems and the whole person. The process of development that achieves its peak in the middle twenties continues to produce a constant series of changes, imperceptible from day to day but increasingly more obvious from year to year. The wrinkling of skin, shortening of stature, loss of hair, and change in hair color are all commonly observed phenomena. Throughout the first five or six decades of life, however, there are few obvious changes in general strength or ability to function fully and independently. From the age of sixty onward, however, decremental alterations in function become more obvious. Accompanying these overt variations are concealed changes that affect the body's chemical content and the function of internal systems, such as the urogenital, cardiovascular, or respiratory systems. The general pattern is illustrated in Figure 22-1, with generalized function shown as a band to indicate the variations that occur from person to person, the range widening out with increasing age.

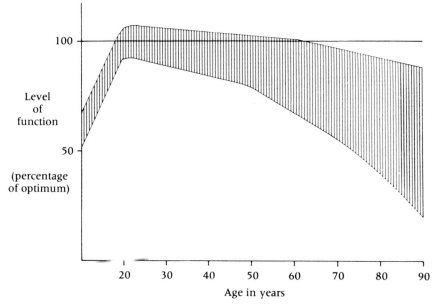

FIG. 22-1 The effect of aging on function—band of optimum function. (From Singhal SK, Sinclair NR, Stiller CR: Developments in Immunology: Aging and Immunity. New York, Elsevier North Holland, 1979)

CHANGES IN MUSCLE

From a nutritional standpoint, these general changes are important, but even more so are the alterations in lean body mass (LBM) which occur concurrently. At maturity, fat-free or LBM of men averages 60 kg, while that of women is less at about 40 kg.[30] These levels are maintained until the mid-forties, beyond which there is a slow decrease that speeds up beyond the age of 65. By the age of 75, average figures for the LBM of men would be 48 kg and for women 36 kg. The muscular male loses proportionately more of this mass and gains more adipose tissue to replace it. This latter increases by approximately the same amount as is lost by muscle. Accompanying these changes, there is an associated but lesser loss of tissue from liver, brain, and kidneys.

BASAL METABOLIC RATE

A number of workers have demonstrated a reduction in basal metabolic rate (BMR) with age, with the change averaging 1.66 Cal/m²/hr/decade. In a recent study from Baltimore, however, in which subjects were studied on a longitudinal basis, the regression on age was only 0.93 Cal/m²/hr/decade. This subject is discussed by Shock, who found that the reason for the apparent reduction in BMR was the replacement of muscle by fat, which maintained or even increased the body's surface area but resulted in less active metabolism.[31] If oxygen consumption is plotted against body water volume in liters, there is no fall in basal metabolism (see Figure 22-2). Thyroid hormone activity, which is the primary regulator of metabolism, is not affected by age. The reduction in metabolically active cells diminishes the amount of energy-producing food that is required by an older person.

Concurrently with the loss of LBM, many subjects will take less exercise and become generally less active, which further diminishes the need for such foods. One can anticipate, therefore, that there would be a significant reduction in caloric intake with age, a fact which proves to be the case.

CARBOHYDRATE METABOLISM

The prevalence of diabetes mellitus increases with age. Many studies agree that the elderly individual is less able to tolerate glucose than is the younger person. The tolerance reduction, that is, the ability to metabolize and use glucose effectively, is a metabolic change that increases throughout life but still varies widely between different individuals. All tests to determine the body's ability to handle glucose confirm this and, in some cases, the deterioration is sufficiently great that by normal standards for younger people half of the elderly would be regarded as diabetic (see Chap. 18).

It is not known why this situation occurs, and it may well be caused by a number of different factors. There is some evidence that the β-cells of the pancreas become less efficient at producing insulin,

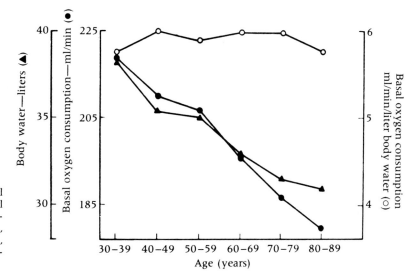

FIG. 22-2 Effect of age on basal metabolism in normal males. ▲, total body water determined as antipyrine space; ●, basal O_2 consumption, ml/min; o, basal O_2 consumption, ml/min/liter body water. (From Gregerman, 1967)

and there may be changes in cellular insulin receptors. The insulin that is produced may be less effective. This phenomenon of aging has been fully described and documented by Andres and Tobin.[2] The alteration in carbohydrate tolerance, however, has to be considered when preparing diets for elderly patients.

DIET AND LONGEVITY

More than 40 years ago, McCay and his co-workers demonstrated that feeding rats a low-calorie diet caused them to live longer.[28] In one such study, 106 rats were divided into two groups of 73 and 33 animals, respectively. The larger group was fed a diet that was rich in protein, minerals, and vitamins, but deficient in calories. The aim of the investigators was to give a diet that would maintain the retarded animals at stationary body weight. The experimental group was then divided into four groups, allowing one group to eat freely after 300, 500, 700 and 1000 days, respectively.

Unfortunately, almost half of the test rats died before the experiment began at 300 days owing to two heating failures in the animal house. The drastic drop in temperature proved too severe for the underweight rats. In spite of this, the survivors went on to live for longer periods than the controls. If the mean survival time of the control animals were taken at 100%, those whose growth was delayed for 300 days had a mean survival of 128%, those delayed until 500 and 700 days, 137%, and those retarded at 1000 days, 146% (see Fig. 22-3).

Not only did the animals live longer, but they remained healthier, with fine hair rather than coarse; they were smaller, but fitter. This aspect of

the influence of diet on prolongation of life was more clearly shown by Berg and Simms.[6] Good, Fernandes, and West have reviewed the influence of nutrition on immunologic aging and disease in studies that have, *inter alia,* confirmed the earlier work cited.[23] These workers gave NZB mice a variety of diets with diminished total food intake. If the animals were fed 10 Cal/day rather than 20, it resulted in a doubling of their life-span. The precise composition of the diet did not affect this result; diets used included normal protein (22%) with low calories, low protein (6%) and low calories, or normal protein and low fat (5%) with low calories. In all cases autoantibody formation was reduced and life-span was increased. Immunologic function deteriorates early in this hybrid strain, with reduced numbers of B-cells and impairment of T-cell responses, excessive proliferation of B-cells and plasma cells but with diminished output of antibody and decreased antibody response to T-dependent antigens. All of these changes were shown to be lessened by reduced calorie diet.[23]

The same researchers described two other experimental situations, each of which confirms the value of a restricted calorie diet. C3H mice are particularly prone to develop mammary carcinoma, with 80% succumbing to this condition. This figure was reduced to 25% on a low-fat, low-calorie diet, with the former restriction being essential in this example. KdKd mice live for only 7 to 9 months before dying from progressive renal disease, but restriction of total calories doubled their life span by preventing this morbidity. Good and his co-workers concluded that their studies supported "the view that development of malignancy, as well as autoimmunity, immunodeficiency disease, and other

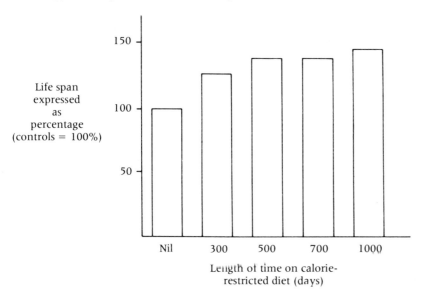

Life span expressed as percentage (controls = 100%)

Length of time on calorie-restricted diet (days)

FIG. 22-3   Mean survival of rats fed a calorie-restricted diet.

diseases of aging, may be significantly influenced by diet."[23]

REDUCED DIET—A STRESS?

The key to an animal's life span lies in its tissues which, no matter how they vary in structure and function, have to be maintained at a mass that is constant relative to the total mass of the body. The rate of function must be geared to the latter's need at any given moment of time. Bullough has shown how the former control is achieved by varying the rate of mitosis in tissues, the cells of which retain this potential.[9] Control is through a chalone, antimitotic messenger agent causing inhibition of cell division; this substance acts only in the presence of epinephrine. The action of chalone–epinephrine complex is reinforced in the presence of glucocorticoid hormone.[9]

Bullough and Lawrence have also confirmed that in mice fed on a restricted diet, life is prolonged and that in such animals, the suprarenal glands became greatly enlarged.[10] They postulated that the reduced diet was a stress factor to the animals and the resultant stimulus to the suprarenals played a significant role in their increased life span. Experimentally, a relative calorie deficiency in an otherwise adequate diet increases life span and health while reducing deterioration of immune function and increasing suprarenal hormonal activity.

SIGNIFICANCE OF DIET RESTRICTION

The significance of these experimental findings for humans is debatable. In the most highly developed countries, obesity is a greater problem than un-

dernutrition, and it is a truism that we all eat more than we need. The reports of very long-lived individuals living in Vilcabamba in rural Ecuador, even if the authenticity of the ages of those individuals over a hundred is questioned, included evidence that their average daily diet consists of only 1200 calories. As general advice, therefore, one would suggest that eating less is likely to lead to improved health and fitness, provided that the diet includes adequate protein, minerals, and vitamins. Having a *little* of what you fancy is a sound principle and perhaps receives support from the experimental work cited.

Nutritional Surveys

LONDON, ENGLAND

In an age when surveys are a popular research tool, a number of reviews of the dietary habits of elderly people living at home have been carried out. Exton–Smith and Stanton, in 1965, reported such an investigation of elderly women living alone in the two north London boroughs of Hornsey and Islington.[16] The average age of the subjects was 76. In choosing these two boroughs, it was hoped to compare the effect of the presumed better living conditions and, therefore, better diet of the Hornsey group but, contrary to expectation, little difference was found between the two. The authors, therefore, studied their subjects as one group.

The mean level of calorie intake was 1890, with a range extending from 1100 to 2900. Between the ages of 70 and 90, there was a reduction in average caloric intake of 20%. The average intake for the group as a whole was 57 g protein/day, but again there was a tendency to a progressive reduction with age which reached 25%. Similar findings were reported for the intake of iron and calcium.

The method used in this study was a meticulous assessment by a trained dietitian of the actual food consumed over a period of a week, following two earlier visits to the subjects to explain the survey and to supply scales, plastic bags for waste, and charts for recording weights of foods. The attention to detail and thoroughness of this particular study is commendable.

It was possible to relate the amount of protein to the number of main meals (defined as containing a serving of meat, fish, cheese, or egg). Twenty-eight percent of the subjects had 14 or more main meals during the week, and these individuals averaged an intake of 462 g protein. On the other hand, 17% had only 7 or fewer main meals, and this group averaged 314 g protein in the week.

Clinical examination of 44 of the 60 subjects, who consented to this, was carried out. Of the 44, 9 were classified as thin, with a skinfold thickness of 5.1 mm; 7 as obese, with a skinfold thickness of 15 mm; and 28 as normal, with an average skinfold thickness of 8.3 mm. The mean body weight of the subjects in the highest age group (51 kg) was 14% less than that of the subjects in their early seventies (59 kg). The percentage reduction in intake of calories and nutrients was similar in the clinically examined group as in the group as a whole. The correlation between diet and health was striking. Only 4 out of 21 subjects with better than average diets did not also enjoy better than average health; 17 of 23 with poor diets also had poor health.

This study was carried out in 1962, and the subjects involved were followed up 7 years later.[32] By that time, 18 of the original group had died; 5, who were unable to be traced, had probably died; 3 had moved from the district; and 7 were in residential or hospital care, which left a total of 27 available for review. Of those who were available, 5 declared themselves unable to participate. Nine of the 22 subjects available for this second study, who represented the elite of the original sample, had reached their late 70s and had done so with little change in their health and degree of physical activity, or in the amount of food that they ate. The remaining 13 consumed less, with a mean decrease in protein intake of 20% and a decrease in calorie intake of 17%. These reductions seen in the longitudinal study were similar to those found in the original cross-sectional one. The authors concluded that those who maintained their health continued to eat well. They were unable to say whether the deterioration in health of the other group caused the reduced intake of food or resulted from it.

SAN MATEO COUNTY, CALIFORNIA

Between 1948 and 1962, a population group in San Mateo County, California was studied on four occasions. The participants in this study included 577 healthy volunteers, none of whom had consulted their physician within the past three months or were following a special diet for any reason. The group included 281 men and 296 women. At the 1962 review, 217 of the original group were known to have died and 70 could not be located. Of those whose addresses were available, 273 out of a possible 290 participated. A comparison of the mean calorie consumption of the different age groups taken from the data cited by Steinkamp, Cohen and Walsh and by Gillum and Morgan is illustrated in Figure 22-4.[21,34]

The former group also reported the intake of protein for the survivors at each stage of the 14-year study, and their results are expressed graphically in Figure 22-5. A feature to note is that there is no consistent pattern with protein as there is with calories. This suggests that the reduction in the latter, as seen in Figure 22-4, is due to less carbohydrate and fat intake, while the protein content of the diet has not been altered greatly with age. The significance of this finding is debatable. It may be that the survivors of the original 577 maintained an adequate protein intake, while those who died did not. Although that is speculation, it is likely that in San Mateo as well as in London, a good diet was associated with good health and vice versa.

GOTHENBURG, SWEDEN

Steen, Isaksson, and Svanborg surveyed the dietary habits of subjects within a population study of "70-year-old people in Gothenburg, Sweden."[33] They assessed the diets of their randomly selected group by two methods, a 24-hour recall and a dietary history. In the first method, subjects were invited to recall their food consumption during the previous 24 hours, assisted by prompting from an observer; the latter asked about the number and distribution of meals and used a classification to assist in this. Foods were divided into seven main groups, which were green vegetables, fruit or berries, potatoes and other starches, milk products, meat, fish or eggs, bread and flour products, and fats or oils used for cooking or spreading on bread. Details of alcohol or other beverages and confectionery or sugar consumed were also included. The dietary history was based on a questionnaire that was constructed for the purpose. A number of cross checks were introduced into this. This data did not include information on wine or liquor consumption but did include beer. Each interview concluded with

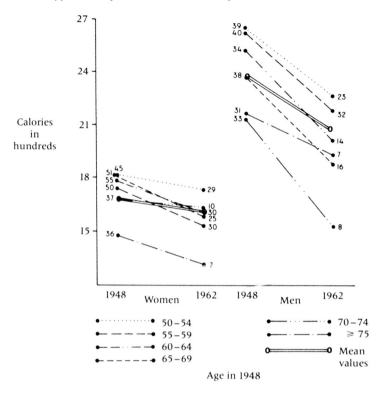

FIG. 22-4   Change in calorie intake over 14 years of subjects of varying ages. Number of subjects at beginning of study are to left of lines and number of survivors after 14 years are on the right. (Compiled from data of Gillum HL, Morgan AF: Nutritional Status of the Aging, J Nutr 55:265–303 (1955); and Steinkamp RC, Cohen NL, Walsh HE: Resurvey of an aging population: Fourteen year follow-up. J Am Diet Assoc 46:103–110, 1965)

questions about alcohol intake to avoid antagonizing the subject at an early stage of the interview with questions that might be mistaken for accusations. In the opinion of the researchers, the dietary history method proved more accurate, and for this reason their results obtained by this method are shown in Table 22-1.

In this table, the mean intakes of the major nutrients are listed from the three studies cited. The 1962 San Mateo study (average ages of 74.5 years for men and 75.5 years for women), the 1970 Gothenburg study (random samples of each sex, aged 70 years) and the 1965 London study (women aged 70–90 years) are compared with dietary al-

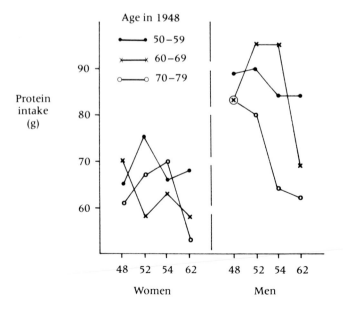

FIG. 22-5   Longitudinal survey of protein intake of 72 women and 68 men. (Data from Steinkamp RC, Cohen NL, Walsh HE: Resurvey of an aging population: Fourteen year follow-up. J Am Diet Assoc 46:103–110, 1965)

TABLE 22-1
Average Daily Consumption of Nutrients Reported in Three Surveys

	Recommended Dietary Allowance (1964)		San Mateo (1962)		London (1965)	Gothenburg (1970)	
	Men	*Women*	*Men*	*Women*	*Women*	*Men*	*Women*
Calories	2200	1600	2075	1605	1890	2344	1928
Protein (g)	70	58	76	62	57	74	63
Calcium (mg)	800	800	800	600	860	1033	927
Iron (mg)	10	10	12	10	9.9	16.5	14.0
Vitamin A (IU)	5000	5000	7961	8065		1505	1357
Ascorbic acid (mg)	70	70	82	90	37.6	82	87
Thiamin (mg)	0.9	0.8	1.1	0.9		1.4	1.2
Riboflavin (mg)	1.3	1.2	1.7	1.4		1.8	1.6

Data from Steinkamp RC, Cohen NL, Walsh HE (1965), Exton–Smith AN, Stanton BR (1965), and Steen B, Isakksson B, Svanborg A (1977)

lowances recommended in 1964 by the American Food and Nutrition Board.[18] These three detailed surveys produced very similar results, which do not suggest that there is a large group of elderly individuals with latent undernutrition. The men of San Mateo were taking a slightly low calorie diet, while their female counterparts had an unsatisfactory intake of calcium. In Gothenburg, both sexes required more vitamin A in their diets, while the women in London were at risk of an inadequate intake of ascorbic acid.

Other large-scale surveys have been carried out in randomly selected population groups in Canada and Scotland, all reaching the same general conclusions. The incidence of significant undernutrition is low, the average consumption lying between 1900 Cal and 2400 Cal for men aged 70 to 79 years and between 1500 Cal and 2000 Cal for women of the same age. Protein intakes are usually 70 g to 85 g for men and 55 g to 65 g for women. There has been little evidence produced of significant lack of vitamins or minerals, although concern has been expressed about calcium and iron, the B vitamins, and ascorbic acid. The known deterioration of renal function has also raised the question of a possible lack of vitamin D metabolites such as dihydroxycholecalciferol.

If the information that has been established by surveys has proved reassuring, it does not exclude the possibility of particular dietary areas in which the elderly may be at risk. To examine this possibility, a number of essential constituents will be reviewed.

Nutrients Important in the Elderly

PROTEIN

The reduction in LBM results in a progressive decrease in total body protein with age. This sub-stance is constantly being synthesized and broken down in the body. With smaller stores of protein, the total turnover is less in elderly people. Attempts have been made to relate protein turnover to a variety of parameters which might enable valid comparisons to be made between old and young subjects.

Uauy, Scrimshaw, and Young have shown that if whole body synthesis and breakdown of protein are related to creatinine excretion as a measure of muscle mass, there is a small but significant difference between the old and young.[36] This indicates more rapid synthesis and breakdown in elderly people. If the process is related to either body cell mass or basal energy expenditure, there is no significant change (see Fig. 22-2). Their results were attributed to the reduced amounts of muscle, as opposed to nonmuscular cellular protein, in the elderly person. Protein from visceral organs turns over at a faster rate than that of muscle. The same authors point out that the consumption of protein per calorie of energy remains relatively constant throughout life, being about 0.12 g to 0.13 g of protein/Cal.

Breakdown of muscle protein can be measured by the excretion of 3-methylhistidine in the urine.[36] It has been shown that 27% of protein breakdown in young subjects is derived from muscles in both men and women, but the proportion in the elderly falls to 20% in men and 16% in women. Measurement of urinary nitrogen excretion after consumption of an essentially protein-free diet indicates a greater loss per kilogram of body cell mass and per milligram of urinary creatinine in elderly subjects than in young ones. The differences are again deemed to be the result of a greater proportion of protein turnover in the elderly being derived from visceral rather than muscular sources.

Yan and Franks have demonstrated that the total intravascular and interstitial albumin is less in old than in young subjects.[39] Intravascular albumin is reduced by 11% and interstitial by about 25%, with the total albumin pool thus being reduced by about 20%. Exton–Smith suggests that this decrease may be due to a decline in the sensitivity of a homeostatic mechanism in the liver which reacts to serum osmotic pressure by adjusting the level of albumin in the plasma.[15] It has been suggested that 10% of the energy requirements should be derived from protein. In Great Britain the Department of Health and Social Services has recommended amounts of protein for old people of between 38 g and 59 g daily on the basis of a consideration of these various factors.

A slight but consistent relationship between intake of protein and the bulk of arm muscle has been reported.[15] No consistent relationship was found, however, between protein intake and serum albumin levels. Low albumin was associated with edema (*e.g.*, 40% of 48 subjects with albumin levels less than 3.5 g/dl had overt edema). In only three of the affected group was the edema considered to be due to hypoalbuminemia. In all the others, factors such as congestive cardiac failure were also implicated. To date, there is no satisfactory evidence pointing to a clear advantage in taking a relatively high protein diet for individuals with a low albumin pool. This possibility, however, is one that deserves careful consideration.

The changes that occur in protein metabolism can thus be seen to follow a pattern established by the increasing loss of muscle during biosenescence, which begins in the fourth decade and speeds up in the seventh and later ones. It is reasonable to postulate that this will result in a reduced need for protein, but it is difficult to arrive at an accurate figure for obligatory demand. For the healthy elderly person, 50 g to 70 g of protein in a diet containing 1800 to 2400 calories can be considered an adequate supply of both this substance and most essential amino acids. There are, of course, conditions which may well increase this quantity, for instance, individuals undergoing surgery, patients with chronic wasting diseases, and others with indolent ulcerations of leg or back that are proving difficult to heal. In all of the surveys cited in the previous section, survivors in longitudinal studies continued to ingest adequate or even quite large quantities of protein. It is not possible at this stage to say whether this protected their health or simply represented the result of a healthy state.

CALCIUM

Calcium absorption diminishes with age in both women and men, the decrease beginning in the sixth decade for the former and the seventh for the latter. While calcium is absorbed by passive ionic diffusion and facilitated diffusion throughout the small intestine, it is likely that the most important mechanism is an active carrier-mediated transport system which operates in the duodenum and proximal jejunum. Bile and bile salts are important as they increase solubility of calcium salts. Bile also contains calcium, which may be preferentially reabsorbed by the intestinal mucosa.

The active transport mechanism appears to be a two-stage one. The first step is a facilitated diffusion transfer from intestinal lumen into the mucosal cell. Thereafter, the substance becomes linked to a specific calcium-binding protein, of which there may be two, and then passes through to the extracellular fluid compartment. A full discussion of current knowledge of this aspect of calcium metabolism is given by Wills.[38] He points out that this active absorption process depends to a considerable extent on the presence of adequate quantities of 1-25 dihydroxycholecalciferol, the metabolite of vitamin D produced by the liver and kidneys (see Chap. 3).

The importance of calcium in the diet of elderly subjects lies in its relation to the inevitable loss of bone that accompanies aging. It has been shown that adequate quantities of calcium (about 1 g/day–1.5 g/day) may preserve postmenopausal women in positive calcium balance.[1] The quantity is less if the calcium is given concurrently with estrogen. From the available evidence, to achieve that level of intake would require some calcium supplementation of the diet. The need for this is debatable, however, as a positive calcium balance *per se* does not guarantee prevention of osteoporosis and its potential consequent fractures.

The presence of phytic or oxalic acids in the diet can interfere with the adequate absorption of calcium by converting it into insoluble salts, or by binding it into a complex. This latter is present in high concentration in whole-meal bread. Many cereals, however, also contain phytase, an enzyme that may largely destroy the acid during the leavening process.

There is a 12% loss of bone tissue in men and a 25% loss in women between the fifth and ninth decades.[19] This appears to represent a true aging phenomenon that occurs concurrently with a loss of muscle tissue already described. According to Garn, populations continue to lose bone irrespective of their calcium intake, and it follows that an inadequate intake of mineral is not the cause of the bone loss.[19] It may have some relevance to it, however, in terms of degree. To sum up, one can only support the consensus that presently exists that a daily intake of 800 mg of calcium, as recommended by the United States Food and Nutrition Board (1980), continues to be reasonable advice for the requirement of this element. Further information on calcium metabolism is included in Chapters 3 and 4.

IRON

There are a large number of studies from different countries describing the prevalence of anemia in old people. Some of the major ones have been quoted by Ehtisham and Cape, who found a significant number of unexplained anemias due to iron deficiency, which were presumed to be caused by lack of iron in the diet.[14] If one reviews the evidence of inadequate intake in randomly selected population groups, there is no suggestion of a widespread lack of iron in diets. The serum ferritin concentration in healthy adults has been measured in over 1000 randomly selected Canadians between the ages of 1 year and 90 years. Valberg and co-workers found no evidence to support the view that iron stores were less adequate in elderly subjects than younger ones on the basis of estimates of serum ferritin.[37] To support their views, they cite data to confirm that a highly significant correlation has been found between serum ferritin concentration and three other indices of body iron status—hemosiderin content of bone marrow, percentage absorption of iron, and size of body iron stores as measured by quantitative phlebotomy.

It has been suggested that both hemoglobin levels and iron stores may be less in elderly subjects. The consensus of evidence from most studies indicates that there is no reason to postulate such age changes. It may be dangerous to do so, because a low hemoglobin or lack of adequate iron stores are almost certainly an indication of morbidity. Appropriate investigation for sites of bleeding, particularly in the alimentary tract, is required. When such investigation is pursued thoroughly, a site of blood loss will be found in 50% to 70% of cases.

There is no need for routine iron supplements as these may serve only to conceal a potentially dangerous clinical state such as the presence of a gastric or colonic neoplasm. A study from Boston has shown that fortification of diet of mildly anemic subjects with iron can result in improved hemoglobin levels, but no satisfactory evidence was produced that adequate investigation of the alimentary tracts of the subjects was carried out.[20] The statement was made by the Boston group that "it is unlikely that the anemia was generally related to occult gastrointestinal bleeding." Evidence of this was found repeatedly, however, in 2 out of 47 volunteers tested daily over a period of 30 days, while 8 others had positive results on more than three occasions. Thus, more than 20% had good evi-

dence of periodic blood loss, and there may well have been others with occasional transient bleeding.

From a physician's viewpoint, therefore, fortification of foods with iron is to be deprecated because it will result in concealment of a potentially valuable clue to the diagnosis of gastrointestinal cancer, which is notoriously symptomless in its early stages. The discovery of a mild anemia on a routine check is a vital pointer to the need for appropriate investigation, with emphasis on excluding gastrointestinal disease. The prevalence of cancer of the colon or rectum increases markedly with age. There are thus two reasons for avoiding such fortification of foods. First, surveys cited previously indicate that there are few, if any, adults lacking adequate iron intake in their diet, and second, there is a danger of masking lethal conditions by unnecessary attempts at overprotection.

ZINC

Zinc deficiency has been linked with altered thymus-dependent immunity, cancer, and other immunodeficiency diseases.[24] A rare disorder among Holstein–Friesian cattle due to an autosomal recessive mutation results in affected calves being unable to absorb zinc. The animals are undergrown, with skin lesions resembling acrodermatitis enteropathica. Elderly individuals with already diminishing immune potential may be susceptible to moderate degrees of zinc deficiency. In cases of indolent ulceration that are slow to heal, a possibility of a deficiency should be borne in mind.

Greger has reported serum zinc levels in 65 volunteers (mean age 75) who were mobile and lived in a state-run institution for the aged in Indiana.[24] During a 10-day period, food intake, taste acuity, height, and weight were documented. Drug and smoking histories were noted and specimens of hair were obtained. Of these, 19% of the men and 53% of the women took nutritional supplements, none of which contained zinc. The mean diet consumed by the 65 subjects contained more than the recommended daily allowance of calories, protein, fat, carbohydrate, vitamin A, ascorbic acid, thiamin, riboflavin, niacin, calcium, and iron but not of magnesium or zinc. The amount of the latter consumed was 8 mg/day by men and 8.6 mg/day by women. The recommended allowance is 15 mg/day for both sexes. Mean hair zinc concentration for men was 176 ± 40 µg/g and for women 170 µg/g. Only 5% of the subjects, all of them women, had levels less than 75 µg/g, which would indicate a deficiency. In this study, evidence was described that subjects' taste acuity was less than that of young adult females, but the findings did not correlate with zinc levels. At present, the precise significance of zinc depletion is not clear, but Greger's study does not suggest that zinc deficiency is common in the elderly.

MAGNESIUM

Greger's study indicated that the mean intake of magnesium daily in 65 subjects was 251 mg for men and 283 mg for women.[24] The recommended allowances are 350 mg and 300 mg, respectively. It is worth noting that mild to moderate magnesium deficiency may occur in elderly individuals, particularly when there is a history of alcoholism. Neuromuscular excitability, seizures, ataxia, tremors, and weakness are all relatively common problems encountered in geriatric medicine. These all may be signs of hypomagnesemia. Without suggesting, however, that all cases will have low serum magnesium levels, it is useful to be aware of the possibility of such a deficiency.

POTASSIUM

Judge and McLeod have suggested that elderly people may take a diet that is deficient in potassium.[26] He based his belief on the fact that low serum potassium levels occur frequently in elderly subjects, many of whom are not taking diuretics. Recent work has shown that, in fact, serum potassium levels may not be a very satisfactory measure of the body's potassium stores. Comparison of serum potassium levels with red blood cell potassium levels under the influence of a variety of diuretics and digoxin, demonstrated that while there were significant rises and falls in the serum level, these did not mirror what was going on in total body potassium, which remained unchanged.[25]

Because of this new evidence, it is perhaps difficult to accept the idea of potassium deficiency occurring as a result of a poor diet. It is likely that we need to review our reliance on serum levels as an adequate indication of potassium stores. The quantity of potassium in the plasma as opposed to the muscles and tissues in general is, of course, very small and, if 95% of the substance is elsewhere, the significance of a slight fall in the serum level is hard to evaluate.

VITAMINS

Much has been written about vitamins and the elderly and it is difficult to present a clear picture of present knowledge. There is evidence that a number of elderly subjects may be deficient in one or more vitamins, but clear-cut severe deficiencies are seldom seen. Methods for estimating levels of the

B vitamins are difficult and not in common routine laboratory use. Brin has pointed out that nutritional diseases do not arise spontaneously or quickly but result "from long periods of depletion during which dietary intake is inadequate to meet the physiological needs of the body."[8] No one can argue with this statement, but, unfortunately, he goes on to suggest that lack of well-being, loss of appetite, and general malaise may be symptomatic of lack of a variety of nutritional substances.

It is of obvious importance to determine the precise symptomatology of mild forms of deficiency states, and it is not helpful to accept complaints such as those mentioned above which may be due to any number of causes. One example that is frequently quoted is the development of a dementia due to deficiency of vitamin B_{12} or folic acid. In more than 20 years of investigating elderly demented patients for remedial causes of their sad state, I have yet to encounter one which either had a definite deficiency or responded to treatment with either of these substances. In 1960, Cape and Shinton examined serum B_{12} levels in an elderly population and did find a group of cases with lower than usual levels between 100 pg/ml and 200 pg/ml. There was no association between mental confusion and these suspect B_{12} levels. The significance of the lower levels has not been explained to date, but the occurrence of megaloblastic anemia or subacute combined degeneration of the cord is unusual until the serum B_{12} level is well below 100 pg/ml.

In Britain, occasional overt cases of scurvy can be seen in old men living alone, usually presenting with either massive ecchymoses into thighs or legs, or more commonly with a widespread petechial eruption on the lower limbs. Such cases do not present to the same extent in North America. Many studies have been carried out on ascorbic acid levels in white blood cells that suggest a relative deficiency of the vitamin. These have all fallen far short of overt scurvy.

Extensive examinations of tongue and mouth were the features of a well-illustrated series of studies from Bromley in Kent on the incidence of vitamin B deficiency.[35] The best evidence of such vitamin B deprivation has occurred in elderly people who are living in an institutional setting. In Bromley, the results of an examination of vitamin C status following 6 months in a hospital were appreciably poorer than the results on admission to the institution. It is not surprising that institutional cooking may well cost the food its vitamin constituents or at least some of them.

As a result of this wealth of literature, the value of which is variable, many physicians and perhaps even more old people have taken to supplementing their diets with a variety of vitamin preparations. In North America, there is little doubt that vitamins are big business, and one has only to walk through a drug store to note the vast numbers of bottles of vitamins running the gamut from A to E. As the evidence of real vitamin deficiency is difficult to evaluate, so the worth of vitamin supplements is highly suspect.

In one recent study, Baker, Frank, and Jaslow have shown in a group of elderly, ambulatory, nursing home residents, whose mean age was 87 years, that one multivitamin pill every day over a period of 3 to 5 months was ineffective in preventing single and multiple deficits of pyridoxin, nicotinamide, vitamin B_{12}, folate, and thiamin. On the other hand, for these same residents, a single intramuscular injection of multivitamins, without any other vitamin supplementation, was successful in replacing these deficits, and 3 months after this single treatment, they were no longer detectable in 89% to 100% of the vitamin-deficient group. This work is very recent and has not as yet been confirmed but would certainly suggest that wholesale oral consumption of multivitamins is a costly exercise in futility.

There is little doubt that the more carefully a survey has been conducted, the less dramatic and more borderline appears to be the evidence of lack of particular nutrients. The very carefully conducted study by Exton–Smith and Stanton, which has already been quoted, gave little evidence that suggested significant vitamin deficiency in the 60 elderly women living on their own whose diet was described.[16] Those who emphasize the risks of potential deficiency and who attribute a variety of nonspecific symptoms, such as loss of appetite, malaise, insomnia, or irritability to lack of vitamins, must produce much more clear-cut evidence to make their case. It is very easy when an appreciable number of elderly people have to exist on a rather poor stipend to blame their ills on poor nutrition. In a later survey, Exton–Smith and Stanton were joined by Windsor and tried to reach some conclusion about those elderly people who were particularly at risk.[17] The results of this study demonstrated unequivocally that the house-bound consumed less food than those who were active. Tables 22-2 and 22-3 are taken from this study and illustrate this point very clearly both in terms of the main meals consumed during the week and the quantity of dietary elements that were included.

In discussing the reasons for individuals becoming house-bound, these workers showed that 80% were suffering from a variety of physical ailments, such as osteoarthritis, chronic obstructive lung disease, arteriosclerotic heart disease, old strokes with hemiplegias, and dementia. The remaining 20% became house-bound because they were terrified of going out and mixing with other people in the streets. They suffered from an old person's form of agoraphobia or a crisis of confidence that made them cling to what they regarded as the safety of their own homes.

The best evidence that is available suggests that fit, elderly people continue to consume a diet that is not only adequate in calories and minerals but also in vitamins. On the other hand, there is every reason to believe that those whose health is not of the best may well consume an inadequate diet that may be deficient in a number of vitamins. Exton–Smith and his co-workers are clear in their belief that it is the deterioration in health that comes first and leads to the change in dietary habits. No

TABLE 22-2
Mean Nutrient Intakes of 70 to 79-Year-Olds

	Men			Women		
	Residential Homes	Active	House-bound	Residential Homes	Active	House-bound
Number of people	8	32	2	6	53	10
Calories	1846	2345	1406	1715	1745	1190
Protein (g)	55.8	87	64	52.4	57.6	38.5
Protein (percent Cal)	12	14.8	18	12	13	13
Fat (g)	80	102	59	76	82	56
Carbohydrates (g)	245	261	160	217	199	137
Calcium (mg)	835	922	944	747	778	634
Iron (mg)	8.6	11.5	8.3	8.3	9.3	5.6
Vitamin C (mg)	30	46	27	39	50	27
Vitamin D (IU)	85	123	73	75	99	68

From Exton–Smith AN, Stanton BR, Windsor ACM: Nutrition of housebound old people. London, King Edward's Hospital Fund of London, 1972.

TABLE 22-3
Mean Nutrient Intakes of Those Over 80 Years in Three Groups

	Men			Women		
	Residential Homes	Active	House-bound	Residential Homes	Active	House-bound
Number of people	6	5	8	17	15	32
Calories	1858	2535	1816	1496	1656	1320
Protein (g)	50.9	70.3	55	46.4	54	42
Protein (percent Cal)	11	11	12	12	13	13
Fat (g)	69	91	87.6	68	77	60
Carbohydrates (g)	274	340	208	187	188	160
Calcium (mg)	920	944	810	688	807	660
Iron (mg)	6.7	11.8	8	7.2	8.2	6
Vitamin C (mg)	16	49	32	37	37	31
Vitamin D (IU)	100	89	83	58	76	47

From Exton–Smith AN, Stanton BR, Windsor ACM: Nutrition of housebound old people. London, King Edward's Hospital Fund of London, 1972.

one, to the best of my knowledge, has to date produced cast-iron evidence indicating that malnourishment occurs for any reason in the elderly other than as secondary to ill health. Malnutrition is, therefore, the result of disease and not its cause.

There are, of course, obvious exceptions to that statement. Those unfortunate elderly people, who seek the solace of alcohol and become addicted to its use, may present with quite gross vitamin and other deficiencies. Again, however, there is the clinical problem, alcoholism, which has produced the situation. The figure often quoted of the number of elderly people who do resort to vitamin supplements is large and probably of the order of 30% to 35%. If, indeed, such attempts at preventive treatment are useless, it is time that the medical profession were appraised of this fact and that physicians stopped prescribing or encouraging their patients to consume vast quantities of useless chemicals. What is needed is a properly controlled experiment (which might have difficulty passing appropriate ethics committees) in which individuals were randomly allocated to two groups on a double-blind basis, the one group consuming satisfactory multivitamin preparations and the other an appropriate placebo. Until such a study is carried out over a period of a number of years, doubts will remain on the validity of the vitamin-deficiency story as far as old people are concerned.

FIBER

During the last ten years, largely owing to the work of Burkett, it has become obvious that the highly civilized North American or European has come a long way from the natural state of his fellow humans who live in the forests, jungles, and plains of Africa.[11] There the major part of the diet is composed of the rough husks of grains, and there is a considerable quantity of fiber consumed with the carbohydrate, fat, and protein of the diet. According to Burkett, the native African has almost never suffered from a number of diseases that are highly prevalent in his so-called more civilized contemporaries in North America. Diverticulosis is a common condition in the elderly American. This is very rarely seen, however, in the native African.

For a satisfactory soft but bulky stool, fiber is essential. Many people are now consuming bran in their breakfast cereal or in soup to provide this fiber, and this is a particularly important constituent of the diet for the elderly person. Burkett claims that diverticulosis could be prevented to a large extent if one were to develop the fiber-diet routine early enough.

Old people are notoriously liable to develop constipation, which may in turn have a rather sinister significance. The constipation–dehydration syndrome is a common situation in the very old person and usually develops as a result of a bad habit and, perhaps, loss of mobility. For the elderly who are becoming a little less able to manage their diet and look after themselves in their own homes, the next stage is often a tendency to reduce intake, particularly of fluid. Lack of bulk and lack of fluid are the two major reasons for the development of a chronic constipation situation. When this occurs, days may go by without a bowel movement, and during this time the stool in the colon will become dryer and harder, leading eventually to fecal impaction. The first symptom of this may well be a spurious diarrhea caused by the dry stool irritating the colonic mucosa, which pours out a watery secretion that carries a little of the surface of the stool mass to the exterior, often as bursts of fecal incontinence. Accompanying these features, the unfortunate sufferer from this condition will often develop mental confusion and can, on occasion, be very difficult to manage. The best method of preventing this is to ensure good bowel function by providing the individual with a high-fiber diet and encouraging a regular habit. Almost everyone will respond to this, provided they are willing to persevere for a few days.

Burkett has also advanced extensive claims that carcinomas of the bowel can be avoided if a high-fiber diet with lots of bulk is consumed over the years. There is no doubt that such gastrointestinal tumors are among the commonest forms of cancer in elderly people, but one suspects that the high-fiber diet routine would need to begin back in the 20s and 30s if it were to have any significant effect in the early 80s.

The effect of increased fiber in the diet is to increase the stool bulk. Fiber from fruit and vegetables alone is less effective than bran in correcting constipation, but in all cases there is an increase in the weight and volume of the stool. The effect of increased fiber on transit time through the bowel is variable. It is likely, however, in individuals who are taking an adequate amount of bran or other fiber, that transit time will be decreased. Other effects of increased fiber in the diet are to increase bile acid excretion and possibly to reduce serum cholesterol and triglyceride levels, but there is as yet no general agreement on the results of studies on this subject.

Increased fiber in the diet has been used to alleviate the symptoms of diverticular disease and irritable bowel syndrome. Although the results are difficult to assess, there does seem to be some beneficial effect in people with diverticulosis. To prevent this condition from developing, it is likely that one needs to begin a high-fiber diet much earlier in life than in the geriatric age group. Energy, fat, nitrogen, and mineral absorption may be decreased with increased fiber intake, but it is unlikely that this would be a significant feature.

In the practical everyday care of elderly patients, there is little doubt that the use of added bran, or other fiber to the diet, improves bowel function, and for this reason alone it is a useful measure to adopt.

ABSORPTION OF NUTRIENTS

Clear evidence of the effect of age on the absorption of nutrients is not available. There are observations that suggest that the absorption of fat, thiamine, glucose, iron, and xylose are all less efficient and slower in the older individual. This may be due to a reduction in cells of the intestinal mucosa, an alteration in their function, or a reduction in the quantities of enzymes produced. Another factor that may affect absorption is the circulation to the gut. In some elderly people this may well be less than adequate, thereby altering absorptive capabilities.

It is well known that there is an increase in relative hypochlorhydria and a reduction in secretion into the stomach in many elderly individuals. This has been suggested as a factor reducing the stomach's resorption capacity. It has to be stated, however, that there is very little hard evidence on the changes in absorption as a result of aging, and a good deal of what has been said must be taken as speculative.

HIATUS HERNIA AND DUODENAL, JEJUNAL, AND COLONIC DIVERTICULOSIS

Hiatus hernia and duodenal, jejunal, and colonic diverticulosis do occur with increasing frequency the older the patient. All will affect the digestive system and clearly may interfere with absorption. Perhaps the most important aspect of hiatus hernia, however, is its association with occasional erosions and iron-deficiency anemias as a result of low-grade oozing or loss of blood. The presence of duodenal diverticuli or diverticuli in the jejunum may result in overgrowth of bacteria and associated malabsorption. In individuals in whom there has been weight loss or inability to gain weight this possibility should be borne in mind, particularly if accompanied by chronic looseness of the bowels. Upper GI series with follow-through may reveal the evidence of diverticuli, and appropriate tests should be undertaken to demonstrate the possibility of bacterial overgrowth which can then be treated with antibiotics.

Colonic diverticuli, undoubtedly the commonest of all in elderly patients, have little effect on the nutritional state of the individual. The possibility that their incidence might be significantly reduced by younger individuals maintaining a fiber-rich diet is one which has already been discussed and needs no further emphasis.

Other intestinal abnormalities that may influence the elderly person's nutritional state are partial gastrectomies or abdominal surgery that has left a blind loop. In both of these situations there may be a tendency to malabsorption, and under such circumstances appropriate adjustment to the diet should be made.

Assessment of Nutritional State of the Elderly Patient

It is now possible, in large population centers, to obtain serum levels of a variety of vitamins and other essential nutrients. On the whole, for many physicians such methods are not quickly available. To determine the nutritional state of one's patient, therefore, demands an evaluation of certain simple, straight-forward parameters.

The history will provide confirmatory evidence of a situation in which there is a possibility of malnutrition. Close friends or relatives of the patient may complain that he or she has not been eating well, and, if one questions specifically, one can make an approximate assessment of the situation. It is wise to inquire about alcoholic intake and any other factor that might have prevented the taking of good meals. Confirmation of the history may be gleaned from the amount of food in the individual's home should a home visit have been made, or one can obtain information on the state of the larder either from relatives or public health nurses. This is the first, most obvious evidence to investigate.

A second clue is the patient's current weight, which can be compared with the last weight recalled by the patient or relatives, although this may relate to years earlier. On close physical examination, the presence of pallor that would suggest

anemia and the recognition of tongue abnormalities or angular cheilosis may point to possible vitamin B deficiencies. Evidence of bleeding in the mouth or petechial spots on the legs may be an indication of an early or mild scurvy. Koilonychia was a common sign of iron deficiency in mothers during the depression years, when the little meat that could be bought was given to the husband, the bread winner, while the mother had to exist on bread and milk. This sign is seen very seldom in the latter part of the 20th century.

Relevant investigations include hemoglobin and white blood cell levels, serum albumin, globulin, iron, and calcium. Most of these measurements are easy to obtain, and this straightforward basic approach offers as much information as is required to establish whether or not there is a chance of a patient's suffering from a deficiency state. In anemic patients with a suggestion of macrocytosis, it would be appropriate to have serum B_{12} and folate levels estimated.

If one wishes to probe more deeply, there are two useful measures of change in the body's composition. The first is the assessment of skin fold thickness and the second the creatinine–height index (CHI). Standard tricep skinfold thickness in men is 12.5 mm and in women 16.5 mm. Arm circumference (see Chap. 10), which should be measured at a point midway between the shoulder and the elbow averages 29.3 cm in men and 28.5 cm in women. These figures are based on the "ideal" man and woman, and one would obviously expect some reduction in them in older people. The CHI is calculated by measuring the actual urinary creatinine excretion in 24 hours, multiplying this by 100, and dividing by the ideal urinary creatinine excretion over the same period. Ideal urinary creatinine values are given in Table 22-4, which has been taken from Blackburn and associates.[7] CHI will be reduced by age in association with the reduction of LBM and account must be taken of this in deciding whether or not a person is malnourished.

TYPES OF MALNUTRITION ENCOUNTERED IN THE ELDERLY

In the first report by the Panel of Nutrition of the Elderly of the Department of Health and Social Security in the United Kingdom, published in 1970, the types of malnutrition that were diagnosed by consultants in 1,367 hospitalized geriatric patients were listed and are shown in Table 22-5.[12] Malnutrition included obesity, in addition to other more generally recognized deficiency states, and it proved to be the most common condition noted in the study. If one examines Table 22-5, the other pre-

TABLE 22-4
Ideal Urinary Creatinine Values

Men*		Women†	
Height (cm)	Ideal Creatinine (mg)	Height (cm)	Ideal Creatinine (mg)
157.5	1288	147.3	830
160	1325	149.9	851
162.6	1359	152.4	875
165.1	1386	154.9	900
167.6	1426	157.5	925
170.2	1467	160	949
172.7	1513	162.6	977
175.3	1555	165.1	1006
177.8	1596	167.6	1044
180.3	1642	170.2	1076
182.9	1691	172.7	1109
185.4	1739	175.3	1141
188	1785	177.8	1174
190.5	1831	180.3	1206
193	1891	182.9	1240

* Creatinine coefficient (men) = 23 mg/kg of ideal body weight
† Creatinine coefficient (women) = 18 mg/kg of ideal body weight
From Blackburn GL, Bistrian BR, Maini BS et al: Nutritional and metabolic assessment of the hospitalized patient. Journal of Parental and Enteral Nutrition 1:11–22, 1977

dominant condition is anemia. There were 94 cases of anemia ascribed to non-nutritional causes, 25 marked anemia, cause unknown, and 35 labeled as nutritional in origin. It is possible that more rigorous investigation might well have revealed causes other than dietary deficiencies in those cases of anemia of unknown cause. If they were excluded along with the cases of obesity and anemia of unknown etiology (a total of 81), the evidence would indicate that malnutrition in the form of deficiencies in the diet occurred in only 44 of the 1,367 patients, an incidence of 3.2%.

The nature of the sample in this study was that all were suffering from significant morbidity, since they were geriatric patients who were being admitted to hospital. If the level of malnutrition in disabled, elderly people is of the order of 3% to 4%, it is surely a reasonable assumption that the general level of nutrition of old people, particularly those living active lives in the community, is likely to be very much less and probably not more than the 1% suggested by Bender.[5] It is important that the expression *subclinical malnutrition* be brought out into the open and defined. There may well be factors in our diets about which we, as yet, know nothing. However, it appears to me that it is an unsatisfactory expression that attempts to compensate for lack of knowledge by postulating a likely, but by no means certain, statement. Until techniques are developed to give us more information about the effect of diet on health and the importance of different constituents of the diet, such an expression should be avoided. It does seem important to adopt an iconoclastic attitude to vague statements about the nutrition of elderly people that are based on impressions or suppositions.

FUTURE NUTRITIONAL DEVELOPMENTS

Nothing that has been written above excludes the possibility that there may be important dietary constituents the nature and function of which have not yet been established. In geriatric medicine one of the most exciting discoveries of the second half of the 1970s was the discovery, which has now been well confirmed, that the brains of persons who have died with senile dementia of Alzheimer type have a highly specific deficiency of acetylcholine transferase activity. This has suggested the hypothesis that failure of cholinergic neurotransmission in the hippocampus and other parts of the brain may be the key disorder in this most disabling of the common diseases of the senium. To date, variable results have been obtained by attempts in both human and animal subjects to replace the missing neurotransmitter. These have included the administration of choline or methionine

TABLE 22-5
Malnutrition Diagnosed by Consultants in 1367 Geriatric Patients

	Total	Men	Women
	1367	542	825
Anemia ascribed to non-nutritional cause	94	40	54
Anemia cause unknown	25	5	20
Nutritional anemia	35	11	24
Obesity and anemia	3	—	3
Obesity	53	13	40
Scurvy	2	1	1
Fracture—osteomalacia	2	—	2
Fracture—osteoporosis	9	3	6
Tongue abnormalities	5	1	4
Other forms of malnutrition	22	7	15

From Bender AE: Malnutrition in the elderly. Update 2:229–236, 1971

on the one hand, or the use of the cholinomimetics, physostigmine, or arecoline, in small doses.

A number of trials in human subjects are included by Glen and Whalley in their edited proceedings of a conference on Alzheimer's disease held in Edinburgh.[22] The results have been variable. There is general agreement that the giving of choline or methionine as a nutritional additive has proved ineffective in a number of trials in which cognitive function has been assessed. On the other hand, Bartus and co-workers have demonstrated significant alteration of behavior in mice by giving supplements of choline in drinking water.[4] Moks and associates have also claimed beneficial memory effects by the use of small doses of the cholinesterase inhibitor, physostigmine, and arecoline.[29]

Much work remains to be done before the place of dietetic manipulation in dementia becomes clear. The prospects are exciting, however, and one must temper the iconoclasm evident in the preceding section with an eagerness to pursue leads in establishing new potentially "essential" substances for the human diet.

DIETETIC ADVICE FOR OLD PEOPLE

"A little of what you fancy" is the soundest advice you can offer to the elderly person about diet. The importance of main meals containing adequate portions of protein should be stressed, and the need to have at least one each day is a useful practical suggestion. In studies of Exton–Smith and his co-workers, this was a good guide to the quantity of protein in the diet.[16] As far as we know at the present time, the precise nature of the protein does not matter. One half to one pint of milk daily is an excellent source of protein, particularly for people with somewhat inadequate teeth. In addition to providing protein, milk is also the main source of calcium, and while the precise influence of the quantity of calcium in the diet on osteoporosis has not been established, most are agreed that it is wise to have between 800 mg and 1000 mg of this substance each day.

With reasonable quantities of meat and plenty of vegetables and fruit, there should be little possibility of inadequate quantities of iron and vitamins, and the available evidence suggests that the essential feature of the diet should be its mixed nature.

One of the other facts that appears to be well documented by surveys is that people tend to continue to eat in the manner to which they have become accustomed. It is wise, therefore, to begin an attempt to evaluate the need for nutritional advice for elderly patients by discovering what is their normal pattern of eating. Attempting to modify that may be a much more effective method of converting this into the good mixed diet that is required than simply providing a diet sheet that bears relatively little relation to the foods that they normally eat.

Finally, a most important consideration about food is that it be enjoyed. If one can introduce diets that are enjoyable and to which people look forward to eating, one will have done much to ensure that the elderly eat properly. Unfortunately, a great many of the elderly may have to eat by themselves, which does not make for much enjoyment. One of the great benefits of luncheon clubs, as opposed to meals-on-wheels services, is that they bring elderly people into contact with their fellows and enable them to eat in a pleasant social atmosphere. This may do more than any other single factor to ensure adequate diets. Attention to what may be regarded as minor details, such as the state of the teeth or the comfort of eating, is also of great importance. It has been said on many occasions that corns or similar small lesions on feet may do more to prevent mobility in old people than anything else. In the same way, uncomfortable or unsatisfactory dentures, lack of teeth, gingivitis, chronic infection, or lack of oral hygiene may ruin the possibility of enjoyable meals and thus do more to create malnutrition than anything else.

As with so many aspects of life in old age, it is likely that the specter of malnutrition has been held up to an excessive degree. All the evidence suggests that the great majority, probably at least 99%, of healthy elderly people living in their own homes do have a perfectly adequate diet in all respects. Equally, those less fortunate persons, who have sustained chronic disabling illnesses of one kind or another and who have become house-bound as a result, or that smaller group of people who have become shut-ins in their own homes because of a crisis of confidence in their ability to get out in the world, constitute the major *at risk* groups. Physicians should make every effort to have such patients visited regularly by public health nurses or, indeed, by themselves, to keep a watch for evidence of inadequate nutrition. This seems to be the major preventive step that can usefully be undertaken.

References

1. Albanese AA, Edelson AH, Lorenze EJ et al: Problems of bone health in elderly. NY State J Med 75:326–336, 1975
2. Andres R, Tobin JD: Endocrine systems. In Finch CE, Hayflick L (eds): Handbook of the Biology of Aging, pp 357–378. New York, Van Nostrand Reinhold, 1977
3. Baker H, Frank O, Jaslow SP: Oral versus intramuscular vitamin supplementation for hypovitaminosis in the elderly. J Am Geriatr Soc 28:42–45, 1980
4. Bartus RD, Dean RL, Goas JA et al: Age-related changes in passive avoidance retention: Modulation with dietary choline. Science 209:301–303, 1980
5. Bender AE: Malnutrition in the elderly. Update 2:229–236, 1971
6. Berg BN, Simms HS: Nutrition and longevity in the rat. II. Longevity and onset of disease with different levels of food intake. J Nutr 71:255–263, 1960
7. Blackburn GL, Bistrian BR, Maini BS et al: Nutritional and metabolic assessment of the hospitalized patient. JPEN 1:11–22, 1977
8. Brin M: Biochemical methods of findings in U.S.A. surveys. In Exton–Smith AN, Scott DL (eds): Vitamins in the Elderly, pp 25–33. Bristol, John Wright & Sons, 1968
9. Bullough WS: Ageing of Mammals. Zeitschrift für Alternforschung 27:247–253, 1973
10. Bullough WS, Lawerence EB: Mitotic control by internal secretion: The role of the chalone–adrenaline complex. Exp Cell Res 33:176–194, 1964
11. Burkett DP: Economic development—not all bonus. Nutrition Today 1:6–13, 1976
12. Department of Health and Social Security, United Kingdom: Reports on Health and Medical Aspects No. 123, First Report by the Panel on Nutrition of the Elderly, H.M.S.O., 1970
13. Cape RDT, Shinton NK: Serum–vitamin B_{12} concentration in the elderly. Gerontol Clin 3:163–172, 1961
14. Ehtisham M, Cape RDT: Protocol for diagnosing and treating anemia. Geriatrics 32:91–99, 1977
15. Exton–Smith AN: Nutritional problems of elderly populations. In Nutrition of the Aged, Proceedings of a Symposium. Calgary, Canada, Nutrition Society of Canada, 1968
16. Exton–Smith AN, Stanton BR: Report of an investigation into the dietary of elderly women living alone. London, King Edward's Hospital Fund for London, 1965
17. Exton–Smith AN, Stanton BR, Windsor ACM: Nutrition of housebound old people. London, King Edward's Hospital Fund of London, 1972
18. Food and Nutritional Board: Recommended dietary allowances, Sixth Revised Edition, pp 114–116. Washington, DC, National Research Council, 1963

19. Garn SM: Bone loss and aging. In Hawkins WW (ed): Nutrition of the aged, pp 73–90. Calgary, Canada, The Nutrition Society of Canada, 1977

20. Gershoff SN, Brusis OA, Nino HV et al: Studies of the elderly in Boston. 1. The effects of iron fortification on moderately anemic people. Am J Clin Nutr 30:226–234, 1977

21. Gillum HL, Morgan AF: Nutritional status of the aging. J Nutr 55:265–303, 1955

22. Glen AIM, Whalley JL (eds): Alzheimer's Disease: Early Recognition of Potentially Reversible Deficits, pp 139–197. London, Churchill-Livingstone, 1979

23. Good RA, Fernandes G, West A: Nutrition, immunologic aging and disease. In Singhal SK, Sinclair NR, Stiller CR (eds): Aging and Immunity, pp 141–163. New York, Elsevier/North Holland, 1977

24. Greger LJ: Dietary intake and nutritional status in regard to zinc of institutionalized aged. J Gerontol 32:549–553, 1977

25. Henschke PJ, Spence DJ, Cape RDT: Diuretics and the institutionalized elderly: A case against routine potassium prescribing. J Am Geriatr Soc 29:145–150, 1981

26. Judge TG, MacLeod CC: Dietary deficiency of potassium in the elderly. Proceedings of the Fifth European Meeting of Clinical Gerontology, p 295. Brussels, 1968

27. Leaf A: Getting old. Sci Am 229:44–54, 1973

28. McCay CM, Maynard LA, Sperling G et al: Retarded growth, life span, ultimate body size and age changes in the albino rat after feeding diets restricted in calories. J Nutr 18:1–13, 1939

29. Moks RC, Davis KL, Tinklenberg JR et al: Choline chloride effects on memory in the elderly. Neurobiology of Aging 1:21–25, 1980

30. Novak LP: Aging, total body potassium, fat free mass and cell mass in males and females between the ages of 18 and 85 years. J Gerontology 27:438–443, 1972

31. Shock NW: System integration. In Finch CE, Hayflick L (eds): Handbook of the Biology of Aging, pp 639–665. New York, Van Nostrand Reinhold, 1977

32. Stanton BR, Exton–Smith AN: A longitudinal study of the dietary of elderly women. London, King Edward's Hospital Fund, 1970

33. Steen B, Isaksson B, Svanborg A: Intake of energy and nutrients and meal habits in 70-year-old males and females in Gothenburg, Sweden. A population study. Acta Med Scand (Suppl) 611:39–86, 1977

34. Steinkamp RC, Cohen NL, Walsh HE: Resurvey of an aging population: Fourteen year follow-up. J Am Diet Assoc 46:103–110, 1965

35. Taylor GF: A clinical survey of elderly people from a nutritional standpoint. In Exton–Smith AN, Scott DL (eds): Vitamins in the Elderly, pp 55–56. Bristol, John Wright & Sons, 1968

36. Uauy R, Scrimshaw NS, Young VR: Human protein metabolism in relation to nutrient needs in the aged. In Hawkins WW (ed): Nutrition of the Aged, pp 53–71. Calgary, Canada, The Nutrition Society of Canada, 1977

37. Valberg LS, Sorbie JS, Ludwig J et al: Serum ferritin and the iron status of Canadians. Can Med Assoc J 114:417–421, 1976

38. Wills MR: Intestinal absorption of calcium. Lancet 1:820–823, 1973

39. Yan SH, Franks JJ: Albumin metabolism in elderly men and women. J Lab Clin Med 72:449–454, 1968

23
Hematology and the Anemias

Victor Herbert

This chapter will be concerned with the *nutritional anemias,* which are defined as those conditions in which the hemoglobin content of the blood is lower than normal as a result of deficiency of one or more essential nutrients.[48] Deficiency of an essential nutrient may arise through inadequate ingestion, inadequate absorption, inadequate utilization, increased excretion, increased requirement, or increased destruction.[30] To delineate a given anemia as nutritional, two criteria must be met: lack of the specific nutrient must produce the anemia, and provision of the nutrient must correct the anemia. By these two criteria, there are only three unequivocal simple nutritional anemias: those due to lack of the mineral, iron, and those due to lack of either vitamin B_{12} or the vitamin, folic acid.

Iron Deficiency

Iron deficiency is one of the most common conditions of humans.[49] Fairbanks and Beutler calculate the prevalence of iron deficiency anemia in the United States to be as high as 25% in infants, 6% in children, 15% in women in the childbearing years, and 30% in pregnant women.[49] They estimate the prevalence of iron deficiency *without anemia* to be as high as 50% in infants, 50% in women in the childbearing years, and 90% in pregnant women. Although the peak incidence of childhood iron deficiency occurs between 6 months and 2 years of age, there is another peak during early adolescence that is associated with the growth spurt. The prevalence of iron deficiency is as high as 10% among high school students from poverty-stricken areas.

The iron-deficient patient is often asymptomatic and hence goes undetected. Even careful questioning may fail to elicit symptoms when anemia is lacking or mild, or has developed slowly. Nevertheless, it is inappropriate to give iron therapy without laboratory testing to demonstrate that iron deficiency exists because there are many anemias that have nothing to do with iron deficiency, and giving iron in some of those instances may produce iron overload or exaggerate an already existing iron overload (such as in thalassemia).[49,50]

Figure 23-1 shows the biochemical and hematologic sequence of events as iron deficiency develops. Normally, the adult has about 2.5 g iron in his circulating hemoglobin. Hemoglobin contains 0.33% iron; thus, every 100 ml of blood (containing 15 g hemoglobin) contains 50 mg iron. In addition to the 2.5 g iron in the circulating hemoglobin, the average American adult man has a store of approximately 1 g (1000 mg) iron in his bone marrow reticuloendothelial cells and other storage sites, and the average American adult woman has a store of approximately 300 mg iron. Since each milligram of ferritin per milliliter of plasma is in equilibrium with approximately 10 mg storage iron, the mean plasma ferritin of the healthy adult man is approximately 100 ± 60 ng/ml ($100 \times 10 = 1000$), and the mean plasma ferritin of the healthy adult woman is approximately 30 ng/ml ($30 \times 10 = 300$).

The normal absorption, metabolic pathways, and

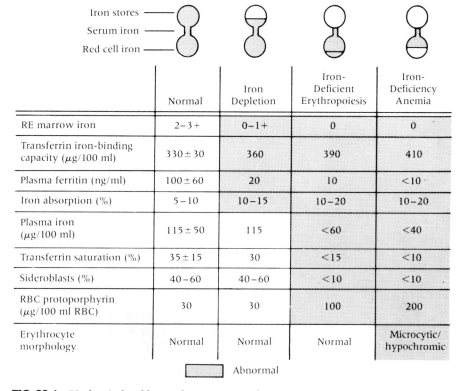

	Normal	Iron Depletion	Iron-Deficient Erythropoiesis	Iron-Deficiency Anemia
RE marrow iron	2–3+	0–1+	0	0
Transferrin iron-binding capacity (μg/100 ml)	330 ± 30	360	390	410
Plasma ferritin (ng/ml)	100 ± 60	20	10	<10
Iron absorption (%)	5–10	10–15	10–20	10–20
Plasma iron (μg/100 ml)	115 ± 50	115	<60	<40
Transferrin saturation (%)	35 ± 15	30	<15	<10
Sideroblasts (%)	40–60	40–60	<10	<10
RBC protoporphyrin (μg/100 ml RBC)	30	30	100	200
Erythrocyte morphology	Normal	Normal	Normal	Microcytic/ hypochromic

▨ Abnormal

FIG. 23-1 Biochemical and hematologic sequence of events as negative iron balance progresses. (Modified from Bothwell TH, Carlton RW, Cook JD, et al (eds): Iron Metabolism in Man. St Louis, Blackwell, 1979)

excretion of iron are indicated in Figure 23-2. The average 70-kg adult has about 750 g circulating hemoglobin containing about 2.5 g iron; 1% of circulating hemoglobin requires 25 mg iron for its formation.

The estimated daily iron requirement is indicated in Table 23-1. As pointed out by the Committee on Dietary Allowances of the Food and Nutrition Board (National Research Council) in the 1980 Recommended Dietary Allowances (RDAs), knowledge of the existence of the two categories of iron in food (heme and nonheme compounds) and of the various dietary factors influencing their absorption makes it possible now to specify absorption rates. The previous estimate of an average 10% absorption of dietary iron can be replaced by the more precise concept that the amounts of heme and nonheme iron in any *particular meal* must be considered separately because of their different availability and susceptibility to influences from other dietary ingredients.[17] Nonheme iron, which includes all the iron of plant products and 60% of the iron in animal tissues, is only about 3% absorbable. An average of 40% of the total iron in all animal tissues, including meat, liver, poultry, and

fish is heme iron and is approximately 23% absorbable. The poor absorption of nonheme iron may be enhanced by two well-defined factors: ascorbic acid and the quantity of animal tissue present in the meal; the animal tissue factor has not yet been isolated in pure form. Nonheme iron absorption is decreased by calcium and phosphate salts, edetate (EDTA), phytates, tannic acid in tea or coffee, and antacids. When the iron status of an individual is compromised, these substances should be avoided. Because of the poor absorbability of vegetable iron, vegetarians run a much greater risk of iron deficiency than do those who eat meat, fish, and poultry. The assumption of 10% absorption of the iron content of food (as obtained from standard food composition tables) is only valid when a diet is balanced (*i.e.,* consists of foods from the four food groups: grains, milk, meats, and fruits and vegetables). Absorption is much lower from a heavily vegetarian diet and substantially greater from a diet high in meat.

Bothwell, Charlton, Cook, and Finch produced a superb book in 1979 entitled *Iron Metabolism in Man* that covers in detail the subjects of prevalence of iron deficiency, dietary iron absorption, food iron

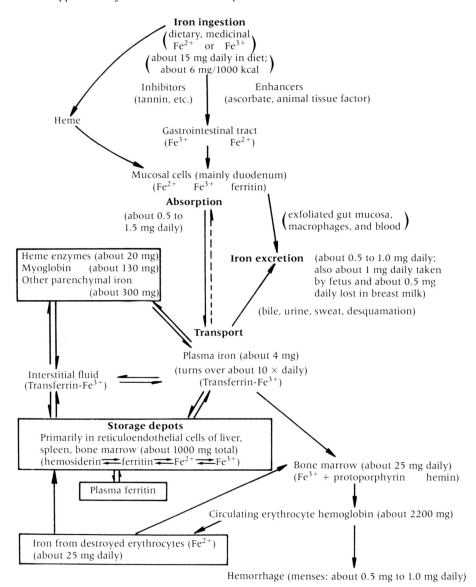

Iron ingestion
$\begin{pmatrix}\text{dietary, medicinal}\\ \text{Fe}^{2+} \quad \text{or} \quad \text{Fe}^{3+}\end{pmatrix}$
$\begin{pmatrix}\text{about 15 mg daily in diet;}\\ \text{about 6 mg/1000 kcal}\end{pmatrix}$

Inhibitors
(tannin, etc.)

Enhancers
(ascorbate, animal tissue factor)

Heme

Gastrointestinal tract
(Fe^{3+} Fe^{2+})

Mucosal cells (mainly duodenum)
(Fe^{2+} Fe^{3+} ferritin)

Absorption
(about 0.5 to
1.5 mg daily)

$\begin{pmatrix}\text{exfoliated gut mucosa,}\\ \text{macrophages, and blood}\end{pmatrix}$

Heme enzymes (about 20 mg)
Myoglobin (about 130 mg)
Other parenchymal iron
(about 300 mg)

Iron excretion (about 0.5 to 1.0 mg daily;
also about 1 mg daily taken
by fetus and about 0.5 mg
daily lost in breast milk)

(bile, urine, sweat, desquamation)

Transport

Plasma iron (about 4 mg)
(turns over about 10 × daily)
(Transferrin-Fe^{3+})

Interstitial fluid
(Transferrin-Fe^{3+})

Storage depots
Primarily in reticuloendothelial cells of liver,
spleen, bone marrow (about 1000 mg total)
(hemosiderin ⇌ ferritin ⇌ Fe^{2+} ⇌ Fe^{3+})

Bone marrow (about 25 mg daily)
(Fe^{3+} + protoporphyrin hemin)

Plasma ferritin

Circulating erythrocyte hemoglobin (about 2200 mg)

Iron from destroyed erythrocytes (Fe^{2+})
(about 25 mg daily)

Hemorrhage (menses: about 0.5 mg to 1.0 mg daily)

FIG. 23-2 Normal absorption, metabolic pathways, and excretion of iron. All amounts are for iron content. The total content of iron in men is about 50 mg/kg and in women about 35 mg/kg of body weight; this difference is due to the fact that women average only about 300 mg of iron in storage depots. Plasma ferritin is normally about 100 ng/ml in men and 30 ng/ml in women. (Modified from Herbert V: Drugs effective in iron deficiency anemia. In Goodman LS, Gilman A (eds): The Pharmacological Basis of Therapeutics, 5th ed., New York, Macmillan, 1975)

fortification, the pathogenesis and treatment of iron deficiency, iron poisoning, the estimation of body-iron stores, and iron overload, including basic concepts, laboratory methods, and more than 2600 references.[2]

The delivery protein in the plasma for iron is transferrin, which will deliver iron to specific receptors on the membranes of red cells and other cells that need iron; the number of receptors in a given cell relates to the requirement of that cell for iron.[1]

The distribution of the approximately 3.5 g total body iron in the average 70-kg adult man has been shown in Figure 23-2. Iron in humans is complexed almost exclusively to the proteins apotransferrin and apoferritin or in heme (hemoglobin, myoglobin, heme-containing enzymes). About two thirds is found in hemoglobin, about one fourth in

TABLE 23-1
Estimated Dietary Iron Requirements

	Absorbed Iron Requirement (mg/day)	Dietary Iron Requirement* (mg/day)
Normal men and nonmenstruating women	0.5–1	5–10
Menstruating women	0.7–2	7–20
Pregnant women	2.0–4.8	20–48†
Adolescents	1.0–2	10–20
Children	0.4–1	4–10
Infants	0.5–1.5	1.5 mg/kg‡

*Assuming 10% absorption.
†This amount of iron cannot be derived from diet and should be met by iron supplementation in the latter half of pregnancy.
‡To a maximum of 15 mg.
(After Council on Foods and Nutrition: Iron Deficiency in the United States. JAMA 203:119–124, 1968)

the body's reserve stores as ferritin and hemosiderin, about 3% in myoglobin, about 0.5% in heme enzymes, and a minute fraction in transferrin, which holds about 0.1% of the total body iron. The stores of iron occur mainly in reticuloendothelial cells, particularly in the liver, spleen, and bone marrow. The storage iron is a reserve derived from the diet and the continuous physiologic destruction of red blood cells, which normally amounts to a little less than 1% of the red cell mass per day, since the normal red cell life span is approximately 120 days.

Iron is tenaciously conserved and is used over and over again, so that it is almost impossible to produce a severe anemia in an adult man by simply limiting iron intake. Iron deficiency in adults occurs almost exclusively from blood loss; in women blood loss is usually from the uterus associated with menses; in men blood loss is usually from the gastrointestinal (GI) tract. The normal body excretion of iron is only 0.5 mg/day to 1 mg/day, from the nail, hair, feces, and urine, mainly as enzyme iron of exfoliated cells, but also from trace losses in bile and cell-free sweat. The main excretory pathway

for iron, as for many minerals, is by way of epithelial cells sloughed from the skin and GI tract, which carry out unneeded iron as ferritin.

The average loss of iron in a normal menstruation, spread evenly over the 28 days of the menstrual cycle, is about 0.5 mg/day to 1 mg/day. The iron "cost" of a normal pregnancy may vary from 440 mg to 1050 mg (see Table 23-2). To calculate the total additional requirement for iron to support pregnancy, in addition to the "cost" of lost iron, one must add iron needed for expansion of the red cell mass. The iron lost in subsequent lactation is compensated by the iron saved from the associated amenorrhea.

Because only about 10% of iron from a balanced diet is absorbed, the amount of iron ingested must be tenfold the daily requirement. The average American diet contains about 6 mg iron/1000 Cal. Therefore, iron intake from dietary sources is borderline for teenage girls and women and may be inadequate for infants and pregnant women.[17] However, a woman with sufficient iron stores to provide for her increase in hemoglobin mass dur-

TABLE 23-2
Iron Requirements for Pregnancy

	Average (mg)	Range (mg)
External iron loss	170	150– 200
Expansion of red blood cell mass	450	200– 600
Fetal iron	270	200– 370
Iron in placenta and cord	90	30– 170
Blood loss at delivery	150	90– 310
Total requirement*	980	580–1340
Cost of pregnancy†	680	440–1050

*Blood loss at delivery not included.
†Expansion of red cell mass not included.
(After Council on Foods and Nutrition, 1968. Courtesy of the Journal of the American Medical Association.)

ing pregnancy, and who also breast-feeds her infant for 6 months, will have her iron needs covered by adequate intake of dietary iron.[14]

Diagnosis of Iron Deficiency

As indicated in Figure 23-1, the first abnormality in iron status is negative iron balance, classified as iron depletion. At this earliest stage in the development of iron deficiency, the iron content of the reticuloendothelial cells in the bone marrow is decreased from the normal 2+ to 3+ to 0 to 1+. This decrease in storage iron is accompanied by a decrease in plasma ferritin, because plasma ferritin is in close equilibrium with storage iron. Thus, of the three most commonly used indirect laboratory measurements for iron deficiency (plasma ferritin, percent saturation of transferrin, and free erythrocyte protoporphyrin, also known as FEP or RBC protoporphyrin), plasma ferritin is the screening test which will pick up the most cases of iron depletion in a population uncomplicated by infection, inflammation, and chronic systemic disease (any one of which will tend to elevate the plasma ferritin level abnormally). Because of the occurrence of these other coincidental disorders, it is generally wise to do two screening tests rather than just one (*i.e.,* also measure percent saturation of transferrin or FEP).

The earliest abnormalities in the development of iron deficiency are (1) loss of bone marrow iron, (2) rise in total iron binding capacity (TIBC) of serum, (3) a fall in plasma ferritin, and (4) a rise in the ability to absorb an administered dose of radioactive iron. At that point anemia is not present, so tests for anemia will not reveal the iron-deficient state.

A population screening study indicated that, with anemia defined as less than 13 g hemoglobin/dl blood for adult men and less than 12 g hemoglobin/dl blood for others: 37% of the iron-deficient subjects were not anemic when the following parameters were used for iron deficiency: transferrin saturation below 15%, red cell protoporphyrin (FEP) above 100 μg/dl packed red cells and serum ferritin

below 12 ng/ml.[15] Serum ferritin correlated least closely with the other parameters in the young men in their study, presumably owing to the presence of infection or chronic inflammatory states, which raises serum ferritin but lowers serum iron and transferrin.

Thomas and co-workers assessed the same indexes in measuring the frequency of iron deficiency anemia in infants.[45] They found that the FEP:hemoglobin ratio gave a better measure of iron deficiency anemia than either serum ferritin or transferrin saturation, especially when there was concomitant acute infection. In lead poisoning and chronic inflammatory states, however, it was hard to make the distinction from iron deficiency by the FEP:hemoglobin ratio.

The only infallible test of uncomplicated iron deficiency anemia is a rise in hemoglobin as a result of iron therapy. Response to treatment is the best test for iron deficiency anemia in adult women.

Testing for iron deficiency *without* anemia requires more laboratory parameters of iron status than testing for iron deficiency *with* anemia, because the anemia itself provides a parameter (response of the low hemoglobin level to iron therapy). Thus, if anemia has already been diagnosed, only percent transferrin saturation or serum ferritin or FEP need be measured; but if one wants to diagnose iron deficiency *prior* to the development of anemia, two of the tests should be done.

Once the diagnosis of anemia is made, the mean corpuscular volume (MCV) should be determined. A low MCV means inadequate hemoglobin synthesis and, statistically, the majority of such cases represent iron deficiency. A minority is due to thalassemia, sideroblastic anemia, lead poisoning, or chronic inflammatory disease (see Table 23-3). Finding a low MCV mandates determination of either transferrin saturation, FEP, or serum ferritin. If the patient is a child in an urban area where lead poisoning is prevalent, the child with a high FEP should be studied further by assay of blood lead or δ-aminolevulinic acid dehydrase.

The final test for iron deficiency anemia will always be the therapeutic trial. Iron therapy should continue for 6 months to ensure replenishment of body iron stores.[23] The laboratory abnormalities should reverse in less than half that time. The reticulocyte count will rise about 3 to 10 days after the start of therapy, but if anemia is mild, the rise may be of such small magnitude that it is difficult to detect. Once iron therapy is instituted, measurement of serum ferritin will no longer reflect the magnitude of iron stores. On the other hand, measurement of serum ferritin will serve to detect the occasional case of iron overload, provided the assay is performed at two dilutions to overcome the *high-dose hook effect* (a curve alteration).[19]

TABLE 23-3
Normal Mean Corpuscular Volume Progressively Increases from Infancy to Adulthood

	Normal Mean Corpuscular Volume (μ^3)
Infant–2 years	70–77
2–6 years	74–81
6–12 years	76–86
Adolescents	78–88
Adults	80–90

Anemia and low MCV by themselves are not adequate to make a diagnosis of iron deficiency, since they also may be present with infection, chronic disease, thalassemia minor, and sometimes in other conditions. If one treats on the basis of these two criteria only, one runs the risk of treating with iron a condition in which excessive iron may be present already. For this same reason, medicinal iron should not be used as a tonic, nor should patients succumb to advertisements to self-medicate with iron without first being tested to determine whether iron deficiency is present.

Iron supplementation in therapeutic doses should be used only following specific diagnosis of iron deficiency, based on appropriate laboratory findings.

Iron deficiency anemia is but the final stage in the progressive depletion of iron stores in the body. Detection of iron depletion may serve as an early warning of an impending anemic state; it may be the first indicator of chronic insidious blood loss. It also aids the physician in evaluating the nutritional status of the patient.

It has been estimated that more than 20 million people in the United States are iron depleted, although fewer than half of these are clinically anemic. On the other hand, more than half of all anemias are due to iron deficiency.

Conversely, patients with non-iron-deficiency anemias may have an iron overload, in which case iron supplementation would be contraindicated. In these cases the measurement of iron stores in the body also provides the physician with important information.

For all these reasons, diagnostic testing for iron deficiency is an important laboratory procedure in the evaluation of the patient, particularly from the nutritional viewpoint. The three best indirect laboratory tests for iron deficiency, using blood samples, are percent saturation of transferrin, serum ferritin, and FEP.[1] While one of these tests may suffice when anemia is present, at least two of these tests are necessary to diagnose early iron deficiency. The least equivocal test is direct, that is, evaluation of the iron content of aspirated bone marrow, obtained by needle biopsy.*

*In our laboratory, we routinely use the following methods:
1. Percent saturation of transferrin, International Committee for Standardization in Hematology (Iron Panel). Recommendations for Measurement of serum iron in human blood. Br J Haematol 38:291–294, 1978; Bothwell TH, Charlton RW, Cook JD et al (eds): Iron Metabolism in Man, pp. 372–375. London, Blackwell Scientific, 1979

2. Serum ferritin. Miles LEM, Lipschitz DA, Beiber CP et al: The measurement of serum ferritin by a 2-site immunoradiometric assay. Anal Biochem 61:209–224, 1974

3. Free erythrocyte protoporphyrin. Langer EE, Haiening RG, Labbe RF et al: Erythrocyte protoporphyrin. Blood 40:112–128, 1972

There are three distinct stages in the progression of iron deficiency (see Fig. 23-1). First, a simple depletion in iron stores occurs. This is followed by iron-deficient erythropoiesis, a state of iron deficiency without clinical anemia. Then, as depletion is allowed to continue, anemia results.

Even at the earliest stage, a fall in bone-marrow iron and a drastic fall in plasma ferritin are evident, whereas the ability to absorb iron begins to rise. At the same time, iron concentration in serum remains within normal range. In iron-deficient erythropoiesis, the second stage, the serum iron becomes affected and shows a descending trend, which may approach 50% of normal, and red blood cell protoporphyrin more than triples. Finally, erythrocytes, which remained normal through the first and second stages, appear microcytic and hypochromic, and a state of frank iron deficiency anemia is reached.

Treatment

Oral ferrous sulfate, least expensive of the iron preparations, is the treatment of choice for iron deficiency. Contrary to many advertisements, GI tolerance to *any* iron preparation is primarily a function of the total amount of soluble elemental iron per dose and of physiologic factors, and is *not* normally a function of the form in which iron is administered. Because absorption of iron is crucially dependent on the dose administered, the largest dose tolerated without side-effects should be given. For most persons, that dose is 300 mg of the hydrated salt of ferrous sulfate, or 200 mg of the dry salt, thrice daily, between meals. The value of spaced daily doses lies in the fact that the absorption rate returns to normal 4 hr following a prior dose. If GI symptoms develop, the dose is given just after meals, and if symptoms persist, the dose is reduced by one third or one half. Some patients will tolerate, and may be given, as much as double the usual dose. When the bone marrow is operating at maximal capacity, in a 70-kg man with iron deficiency anemia less than 100 mg iron/day can be incorporated into hemoglobin. Assuming an average of 25% absorption of iron given as ferrous sulfate, 2 g/day of the hydrated salt (which is 20% iron) provides 100 mg of absorbed iron, which is the maximum usable per day. Administration of larger daily doses is without hematopoietic value.

Duration of oral therapy for iron deficiency anemia should be approximately 6 months, assuming usual therapy (300 mg $FeSO_4 \cdot 7H_2O$, thrice daily) and an initial severe anemia. Such average therapy will result in absorption of about 45 mg iron/day during the first month while the iron deficiency anemia is rapidly improving; about 25 mg/day during the second and third months while the anemia is disappearing but before stores are repleted; and about 5 mg/day to 10 mg/day after the third month when the stores approach repletion. Thus, one can assume absorption of about 1350 mg in the first month, 1500 mg in the next two months, and 225 mg in each of the succeeding 3 months, for a total absorption of about 3500 mg (*i.e.,* repletion of body stores) in 6 months. It is important for the physician to remember not only that iron absorption decreases as anemia diminishes, but also that *the factors originally producing the iron deficiency may persist.* If these factors are not corrected, oral iron therapy must continue until such correction occurs. Failure to heed this admonition will result in relapse owing to persistent negative iron balance.

Iron salts have many incompatibilities and should be prescribed alone, preferably between meals for maximal absorption but just after meals, if necessary, to minimize gastric symptoms. GI absorption of iron is adequate and essentially equal from the following six *ferrous* salts: sulfate, fumarate, gluconate, succinate, glutamate, and lactate. Absorption of iron is lower from ferrous citrate, tartrate, pyrophosphate, cholinisocitrate, and carbonate. Absorption of iron from all *ferric* salts is poor. Reducing agents (*e.g.,* ascorbic acid) and some chelating agents (*e.g.,* succinic acid, sulfur-containing amino acids) may increase absorption of iron from ferrous sulfate, but are not worth the extra cost because of the high efficacy of ferrous sulfate when administered alone. Cobalt is especially undesirable because it may produce a rise in hematocrit by an unknown mechanism, and thus obscure the response to iron; additionally, it may produce various toxic side-effects such as skin rashes, goiter, or angina.[2]

IRON POISONING

All iron preparations are probably equally toxic per unit of soluble iron. Iron poisoning is very rare in adults; it would be very unlikely in adults with ingestion of doses of ferrous sulfate below 5 g. Serious *acute poisoning* in children can result from the ingestion of doses in excess of 1 g.[2] In the United States, prior to child-proof containers, there was an average of at least one death a month from the ingestion by infants and young children of doses of ferrous sulfate in excess of 2 g. Doses of 1 g may be toxic in children. The colored sugar coating of many of the commercially available tablets gives them the appearance of candy. All iron preparations should be labeled, "Caution! Keep out of the reach of children."

Signs and symptoms may occur within 30 min or may be delayed several hours. They are largely those of GI irritation or necrosis, often with nausea, vomiting, and shock; they include pallor or cyanosis, lassitude, drowsiness, hematemesis, diarrhea of green and subsequently tarry stools, and cardiovascular collapse. If death does not occur within 6 hr, there may be a transient period of apparent recovery followed by death in 12 hr to 48 hr. The corrosive injury to the stomach may result in subsequent pyloric stenosis or severe gastric scarring. Hemorrhagic gastroenteritis and hepatic injury are prominent findings at autopsy.

Treatment should begin quickly with the induction of vomiting. Eggs and milk are then fed (to form iron–protein complexes) until it is possible to perform gastric lavage. Within the first hour following ingestion of the iron preparation, the stomach should be lavaged with 1% sodium bicarbonate solution, to convert the iron to a less soluble form. If an iron-chelating drug is available, it should be used for the treatment of both local and systemic effects. The most specific chelating agent for iron is desferrioxamine.

SIDE-EFFECTS OF IRON THERAPY

The patient given iron should be forewarned that conventional oral doses of the iron salts produce constipation in about 10% of cases, diarrhea in about 5%, and nausea and epigastric pain in about 7% (when salts contain the equivalent of 180 mg of ferrous iron per day). These side-effects are primarily a function of the total amount of absorbable iron per dose, and they can be reduced or eliminated by prescribing iron just after meals instead of between meals (food usually reduces absorbability of medicinal iron) or, more reliably, by reducing the dose by one third to one half. Iron medication colors the feces black, and large amounts may interfere with some tests used for detection of occult blood in the stools; the guaiac test occasionally yields false positive results for blood, whereas results with the benzidine test are not as affected by iron medication.

When iron balance is restored to normal (usually after about 6 months, unless factors favoring negative iron balance persist), therapy with iron should be stopped, to avoid iron overload hemosiderosis.

Therapy with Parenteral Iron

Parenteral iron is indicated only when an iron deficiency anemia exists and a trial of oral iron has been ineffective owing to (1) failure to absorb adequate amounts of oral iron (occasional patients with various malabsorption syndromes), (2) inability to tolerate oral iron (some patients with severe regional enteritis or ulcerative colitis), (3) exhausted iron stores in patients with chronic bleeding, in whom the average daily iron lost equals or exceeds the absorption of iron from oral ferrous sulfate, or (4) refusal or inability to take oral iron in necessary dosage (some children and psychiatric and geriatric patients). The fourth problem is sometimes solved by furtive administration of ferrous sulfate syrup or elixir in fruit juice.

The patient who fails to respond to oral iron should be reevaluated, since he may not have an iron deficiency anemia. Bone-marrow stores should be demonstrated to be absent prior to parenteral iron medication, so that conditions (such as infection) that produce anemia partly due to poor utilization of iron can be excluded. In contrast to the safety, efficacy, and low cost of orally administered iron, the metal given by injection is painful, expensive, and sometimes dangerous.

INTRAMUSCULAR PREPARATIONS

Iron-dextran injection, U.S.P. (iron-dextran; Imferon), is a sterile colloidal solution of ferric hydroxide in complex with partially hydrolyzed dextran of low molecular weight, in water for injection; it contains 50 mg elemental iron/ml. The dark brown solution has a pH of 5.2 to 6.5 and is usually provided in 10-ml vials containing 0.5% phenol as a preservative. It should be injected deeply with a 5-cm or 7.5-cm (2-inch or 3-inch), 19-gauge or 20-gauge needle, only into the upper outer quadrant of the buttock and *not* into the arm or other exposed area. (It is absorbed slowly from subcutaneous tissue, and may stain the skin brown for 1 to 2 years; a Z-track injection technique into muscle should be used to avoid leakage back into subcutaneous tissue.) The iron is absorbed by way of the lymphatic drainage from muscle. *Total dosage* to restore hemoglobin and replenish stores may be approximated from the following formula:

$$0.3 \times \text{body weight in lb}$$
$$\times (100 - \text{patient's hemoglobin in g\%}/14.8$$
$$\times 100)$$
$$= \text{mg to be injected.}$$

Each day's dose should ordinarily not exceed 25 mg for infants under 4 kg to 5 kg, 50 mg for children under 9 kg, 100 mg for patients under 50 kg, and 100 mg to 250 mg for others.

INTRAVENOUS PREPARATIONS

Iron-dextran injection, U.S.P., may also be given by intravenous infusion; only the preparation without preservatives (2-ml or 5-ml ampuls) should be used for intravenous administration. To minimize toxic reactions, the initial dose should be 1 or 2 drops over 5 min to determine whether any evidence of anaphylaxis appears. If not, one may then give 500 mg over 5 to 10 min, or total repletion over several hours.[2] The dose should be given slowly (1 min/20 mg–50 mg).

TOXICITY OF PARENTERAL PREPARATIONS

Local side-effects following intramuscular administration of iron include pain at the injection site, skin discoloration, local inflammation with tender inguinal lymphadenopathy, and lower-quadrant abdominal pain. Systemic toxicity occurs in approximately 0.5% to 0.8% of cases, and includes reactions occurring more frequently within 10 min of injection, such as headache, muscle and joint pain, hemolysis due to ionized (unbound) iron, faintness, tachycardia, flushing, sweating, nausea, vomiting, bronchospasm with dyspnea, hypotension, dizziness, and circulatory collapse. These reactions are much more common with intravenous than with intramuscular iron preparations. Reactions that occur more frequently from 30 min to 24 hr after injection include dizziness, syncope, fever, chills, rash, urticaria, constricting chest pain, backache, generalized body aches, encephalopathy with convulsive seizures, generalized lymphadenopathy, and leukemoid reactions. Approximately one fatal case of anaphylactic shock occurs per 4 million doses administered.

Generally, local inflammatory reactions are much less frequent with intravenous than with intramuscular administration of iron. Conversely, shock or cardiac arrest is more frequent (although rare) with intravenous preparations than with intramuscular preparations. As should be obvious, oral iron therapy is preferable to parenteral; *the latter should be used only when clearly indicated by patient status or circumstances.*

Nutritional Anemia Due to Vitamin B$_{12}$ or Folate Deficiency— The Megaloblastic Anemias

The megaloblastic (Greek: *megas* = large, *blaste* = germ) anemias (macro-ovalocytic anemias) are those that are characterized by a common morphology of giantism of every proliferating cell and an underlying common biochemical defect of slowed DNA synthesis per unit time. Classically, the diagnosis of megaloblastic anemia is made when the evaluation reveals anemia (often pancytopenia), and the peripheral blood smear shows the progeny of a megaloblastic bone marrow: macro-ovalocytic red cells, granulocytes the nuclei of which are hypersegmented ("hypersegmented polys"), and giant platelets. Megaloblastic anemia is a single *morphologic* entity but the underlying slowed DNA synthesis may result from a wide variety of causes. The diagnosis of megaloblastic anemia is usually easy, but the differential diagnosis of underlying cause and, therefore, proper therapy rests on determination of the precise etiologic classification into which the patient fits.[4,20]

Pernicious anemia is not a synonym for megaloblastic anemia, but is rather that etiologic subcategory of megaloblastic anemia due to inadequate intrinsic factor secretion of uncertain etiology (see Table 23-4).

ETIOLOGIC CLASSIFICATION AND PATHOGENESIS

In about 95% of cases, megaloblastic anemia proves to be a nutritional anemia (or, more broadly, a pancytopenia) caused by deficiency of vitamin B_{12}, folic acid, or, in some cases, both. Classification falls into one of the six etiologic categories common to all nutritional deficiencies: inadequate ingestion, absorption, or utilization or increased requirement, excretion, or destruction.[30] Table 23-4 presents an etiologic classification of the causes of slowed DNA synthesis and hence of the megaloblastic anemias, and Figures 23-3 and 23-4 present the flow charts of vitamin B_{12} and folate metabolism, respectively, which provide the nutritional, physiologic, and biochemical underpinnings on which most of the etiologic classification rests.

As indicated in Figure 23-3, food vitamin B_{12} is liberated from its bonds by gastric acid and gastric and intestinal enzymes.[1,21] The freed B_{12} (of which there is less when there is no gastric acid) attaches to salivary and gastric B_{12} binders (called "R binders" for their rapid mobility on electrophoresis, and cobalophilins because of their strong affinity for B_{12}) and to intrinsic factor (IF), a glycoprotein (molecular weight about 50,000) secreted by gastric parietal cells. The B_{12}–IF complex dimerizes and passes with B_{12}–R–binder complexes into the ileum, where it adheres to specific brush border receptors for the IF–B_{12} complex in the presence of ionic calcium and a pH of more than 7, at which pH pancreatic proteases degrade R protein and free its B_{12} to become exclusively bound to IF.[3,21,24] The vitamin is absorbed and transported in the blood, attached to the B_{12}–delivery protein, transcobalamin II (TC II), which rapidly delivers it to the liver, hematopoietic system, and other proliferative cells.[18,24] Some of the absorbed B_{12} attaches to the serum B_{12}-binding cobalophilins (also called "R binders"), transcobalamin I (TC I, half-life of 10 days), and transcobalamin III (TC III, half-life 3 min). These B_{12}-binding glycoproteins deliver B_{12}

only to the liver and may be involved in clearing undesired B_{12} analogues from the body.[33] Normally, plasma B_{12}-binding capacity is about one third saturated. Of the unsaturated B_{12}-binding capacity, approximately 90% is TC II, because TC II delivers most of its load of B_{12} within seconds to cells.[33] The liver is the main storage organ for B_{12} in humans, normally containing about 1 μg B_{12} per gram of liver. There is usually a larger enterohepatic circulation than absorption from the diet of the vitamin, and this B_{12} reabsorption explains why vitamin B_{12} deficiency takes decades to develop in vegetarians, but only 1 to 3 years to develop when B_{12} absorption (and therefore reabsorption) is shut off by disease of the stomach, pancreas, or ileum.[21,26]

As indicated in Figure 23-4, food folates are predominately in polyglutamate form.[6,16,30] Prior to absorption, the excess glutamates must be split off by conjugases (gamma-glutamyl carboxypeptidases) present in bile and intestine; this process is variably inhibited by inappropriate pH (optimal pH for conjugase action is 4.6) and by conjugase inhibitors in beans, yeast, and some other foods. Once deconjugated, folate is absorbed primarily across the upper third of the small bowel, mainly as reduced monoglutamate, but partly as the oxidized pteroylglutamic acid (PGA).[16] An *intrinsic factor* in mother's milk may enhance absorption of milk folate by the infant.[9] The absorption of 5-methyl tetrahydrofolate (5-methyl THF) does not appear to be B_{12} dependent, but the uptake and retention of 5-methyl THF by blood cells is B_{12} dependent.[5,46] Dilantin and certain other drugs inhibit folate absorption at step 2 in Figure 23-4.

After absorption, folate is transported, mainly as 5-methyl THF, probably by a carrier protein, to cellular sites of utilization. Vitamin B_{12} appears necessary to get 5-methyl THF across cell walls (or to retain it in the cell once absorbed; step 5 in Fig. 23-4), and this vitamin B_{12}-dependent cell uptake (and cell retention) of folate helps to explain why patients with uncomplicated vitamin B_{12} deficiency have a "pile-up" of folate in serum, resulting in a high serum folate and a low red cell folate.[46] This "folate trap" in vitamin B_{12} deficiency consists in this folate "pile-up" largely owing to inability to convert body folate stores (which are mainly 5-methyl THF), because this conversion (step 6 in Fig. 23-4) is vitamin B_{12} dependent.[10,30,43] Normal total body folate stores are in the range of 5 mg to 10 mg, about half of which is in the liver. There is an enterohepatic circulation of about 100 μg folate daily.[24]

The defective DNA synthesis in B_{12} or folate deficiency is due to inadequate thymidylate synthesis (step 11 in Fig. 23-4). Folate deficiency directly

(*Text continues on p. 398.*)

TABLE 23-4
Etiologic Classification of Megaloblastic Anemias: A Tabular Lexicon

I. *Vitamin B_{12} deficiency* (normal B_{12} body stores last 3 to 6 years after cessation of B_{12} absorption, but 20 to 30 years after cessation of only B_{12} ingestion, because of continuation of reabsorption of the 3 to 6 μg of B_{12} excreted daily in bile):
   A. Inadequate ingestion
      1. Poor diet (lacking microorganisms and animal foods, which are the sole B_{12} sources)
         a. Strict vegetarianism (eating no meat, fowl, seafood, eggs, milk, or any products thereof)
         b. Chronic alcoholism (no B_{12} or folate in hard liquor; folate deficiency occurs first, and is more common, partly because body stores of B_{12} last much longer than those of folate)
         c. Poverty, religious tenets (Hinduism, Seventh-Day Adventism, certain Catholic orders), dietary faddism
   B. Inadequate absorption
      1. Gastric disorder, producing inadequate or absent secretion by gastric parietal cells of intrinsic factor
         a. Addisonian pernicious anemia (PA—that form of B_{12} deficiency disease due to inadequate intrinsic factor secretion of uncertain etiology)
            (1) Hereditary absence of normal intrinsic factor secretion; absent secretion at birth (circulating antibody to intrinsic factor never present; supports theory that antibody only occurs when antigenic stimulus is produced by intrinsic factor, which enters bloodstream from damaged parietal cells and is recognized as foreign by the immunologic surveillance system); rare
            (2) Congenital production of defective intrinsic factor molecule (one published case)
            (3) Autoimmunity-associated gastric atrophy. These patients almost always have nondiagnostic-for-PA circulating parietal cell antibody, which is index only of past or present gastric damage and *not* of amount of intrinsic factor secretion (circulating diagnostic-for-PA antibody to intrinsic factor is always present under age 21; there is a gradual decrease in measurable antibody, so that by age 65 only two thirds of cases present with measurable circulating antibody to intrinsic factor)
               (a) Juvenile pernicious anemia (usually presents between ages 3 and 14)
               (b) Hereditarily determined degenerative gastric atrophy (gradually progressing with increasing age; almost half of all adult PA cases fall in this category)
               (c) Acquired gastric atrophy as the end result of superficial inflammatory gastritis; superficial gastritis with atrophy (almost half of all adult PA cases fall in this category, which includes acquired gastric damage related to iron deficiency, alcohol, etc.)
               (d) Endocrine disorders (hypothyroidism, polyendocrinopathy, etc.) associated with gastric damage
         b. Gastrectomy
            (1) Total
            (2) Subtotal (approximately 20% develop PA within ten years after surgery, associated with atrophy of remaining parietal cells)
               (a) Proximal
               (b) Distal
         c. Lesions that destroy the gastric mucosa (ingested corrosives, linitis plastica, etc.)
         d. Intrinsic factor inhibitor in gastric secretion.
            (1) Antibody to intrinsic factor (in saliva or gastric juice)
               (a) "Blocking" antibody (attaches to intrinsic factor so as to block ability of intrinsic factor to take up B_{12})
               (b) "Binding" antibody (attaches to intrinsic factor at site distal to site of B_{12} attachment)
      2. Small intestinal disorder (affecting ileum, which is the main site of B_{12} absorption)
         a. Gluten-induced enteropathy (childhood and adult celiac disease); idiopathic steatorrhea; nontropical sprue
         b. Tropical sprue (B_{12} is often the first nutrient to be subnormally absorbed and the last to return to normal absorption)
         c. Regional enteritis
         d. Strictures or anastomoses of the small bowel, other "stagnant bowel" syndromes
         e. Intestinal resection
         f. Malignancies and granulomatous lesions involving the small intestine
         g. Other conditions characterized by chronically disturbed intestinal function
         h. Drugs damaging B_{12} absorption
            (1) Para-aminosalicylic acid (PAS) (therapy of tuberculosis)
            (2) Colchicine (therapy of gout)
            (3) Neomycin (antimicrobial)
            (4) Ethanol (societal)
            (5) Metformin (and other biguanide oral antidiabetic agents?)
            (6) Oral contraceptive agents?
         i. Specific malabsorption for vitamin B_{12}
            (1) Due to long-term ingestion of calcium-chelating agents (ionic calcium required for B_{12} absorption)
            (2) Due to inadequately alkaline pH in ileum (Zollinger–Ellison syndrome, pancreatic disease, etc.) (pH > 6 required for B_{12} absorption)
            (3) Unknown causes (lack of intestinal receptors for B_{12}-intrinsic factor complex? absence of "releasing factor"?)
               (a) Congenital (Imerslund–Gräsbeck syndrome; receptors probably functioning)
               (b) Acquired (forme fruste of sprue; receptors absent or nonfunctioning?)
      3. Competition for vitamin B_{12} by intestinal parasites or bacteria
         a. Fish tapeworm (*Diphyllobothrium latum;* decreasing in Finland because of pollution)

b. Bacteria: The blind loop syndrome (B_{12} adsorbing bacteria)
4. Pancreatic disease (normal pancreatic exocrine secretion of trypsin and bicarbonate required for normal B_{12} absorption)
C. Inadequate utilization
  1. Vitamin B_{12} antagonists
    a. Substituted B_{12} amides and anilides (experimental agents)
    b. Cobaloximes (experimental agents)
    c. Anti-B_{12} analogues?
  2. Congenital or acquired enzyme deficiency or deletion
    a. Methylmalonyl-CoA mutase
    b. Methyltetrahydrofolate-homocysteine methyltransferase
    c. B_{12a} reductase
    d. B_{12r} reductase
    e. Deoxyadenosyltransferase
    f. Other enzyme reduction or deletion
  3. Abnormal B_{12}-binding protein in serum, irreversibly binding B_{12} and making it unavailable to tissues
    a. Increased TC I or TC III glycoprotein (myeloproliferative disorders—"granulocyte-related" B_{12} binders)
    b. Increased TC II protein (liver disease; "liver-related" B_{12} binders)
    c. Other abnormal B_{12} binding (a glycoprotein in some hepatoma cases, etc.)
  4. Inadequate serum B_{12}-binding protein (congenital or acquired)
    a. TC II protein (lack produces megaloblastic anemia; it delivers B_{12} to blood cells, as transferrin delivers iron)
    b. TC I glycoprotein (lack not known to produce megaloblastic anemia; it is mainly a storage protein for B_{12}, somewhat akin to ceruloplasmin for copper)
    c. TC III (large amounts produced *in vitro* by granulocytes)
  5. Protein malnutrition?
  6. Malignancy?
  7. Liver disease?
  8. Renal disease?
  9. Thiocyanate intoxication?
D. Increased requirement (normal adult daily requirement from exogenous sources is 0.1 μg)
  1. Hyperthyroidism
  2. Increased hematopoiesis?
  3. Infancy (increased requirement for growth)
  4. Parasitization
    a. By fetus
    b. By malignant tissue?
E. Increased excretion
  1. Inadequate B_{12}-binding protein in serum (inadequate TC II particularly?)
  2. Liver disease (inadequate storage capacity for B_{12})
  3. Renal disease?
F. Increased destruction
  1. By pharmacologic doses of ascorbic acid
II. *Folic acid deficiency* (normal folate body stores will last only 3 to 6 months after cessation of folate ingestion or absorption):

A. Inadequate ingestion
  1. Poor diet (lacking unprocessed fresh, uncooked, or slightly cooked food or fruit juices—folates are heat labile)
    a. Nutritional megaloblastic anemia
      (1) Tropical
      (2) Nontropical
      (3) Scurvy (diets poor in vitamin C are also poor in folate)
    b. Chronic alcoholism with or without cirrhosis
B. Inadequate absorption (affecting upper third of small intestine, which is the main site of folate absorption; since most food folates are in polyglutamate forms, biliary and intestinal gamma glutamyl conjugases are necessary to split off excess glutamates to make folates absorbable)
  1. Malabsorption syndromes
    a. Gluten-induced enteropathy (childhood and adult celiac disease; idiopathic steatorrhea, nontropical sprue; coincident B_{12} malabsorption rare)
    b. Any other chronic functional or structural disorder involving the upper small intestine
      (1) Tropical sprue (coincident B_{12} malabsorption almost invariably present)
      (2) Associated with herpetic and other skin disorders
    c. Drugs
      (1) Diphenylhydantoin (Dilantin—anticonvulsant)
      (2) Primidone (anticonvulsant)
      (3) Barbiturates
      (4) Oral contraceptive agents (?)
      (5) Cycloserine (tuberculosis)
      (6) Ethanol (societal)
      (7) Metformin (diabetes therapy)
      (8) Dietary amino acid excess of glycine or methionine
      (9) Nitrofurantoin? (antimicrobial)
      (10) Glutethimide? (sedative)
      (11) Cholestyramine
      (12) Salicylazosulfapyridine (Azulfidine)
  2. Specific malabsorption for folate
    a. Congenital nonconjugase defects (four cases published)
    b. Acquired nonconjugase defects
    c. Inadequate biliary or intestinal conjugase
    d. Conjugase inhibitors (such as contained in some beans)
  3. Blind loop syndrome (folate-greedy bacteria; more commonly, bacteria make folate and actually raise serum folate level of host)
C. Inadequate utilization (metabolic block)
  1. Folic acid antagonists (dihydrofolate reductase inhibitors)
    a. 4-amino-4-deoxyfolates (*i.e.*, methotrexate) (Chemotherapy, immunosuppression, psoriasis)
    b. 2,4-Diaminopyrimidine
      Pyrimethamine (Malaria, toxoplasmosis)
      Trimethoprim (Antibacterial)
    c. Triamterene (Diuretic)

    d. Diamidine compounds (*Pneumocystis*
      (*i.e.,* pentamidine   *carinii,*
      isothionate)   protozoacidal)

  2. Diphenylhydantoin and possibly other anticonvulsants (possibly block cell uptake or use of folate)

  3. Enzyme deficiency
    a. Congenital
      (1) Formiminotransferase
      (2) Dihydrofolate reductase
      (3) Methyltetrahydrofolate transmethylase
      (4) Other enzymes (some secondarily affect folate)
    b. Acquired
      (1) Liver disease
        (a) Formiminotransferase
        (b) Other enzymes

  4. Vitamin B_{12} deficiency (reduces folate uptake and retention by cells)

  5. Alcohol (both specific and nonspecific damage to folate metabolism)

  6. Ascorbic acid deficiency (increased hematopoiesis associated with bleeding reduces folate stores; may also decrease ability of body to retain folates in their metabolically active reduced state)

  7. Dietary amino acid excess (glycine, methionine)

D. Increased requirement (normal adult daily requirement from exogenous sources is 50 μg)
  1. Parasitization
    a. By fetus (especially in multiple and twin pregnancies)
    b. By malignant tissue (especially lymphoproliferative disorders)
    c. By breast-fed infant
  2. Infancy (increased requirement for growth)
  3. Increased hematopoiesis (hemolytic anemias; chronic blood loss, including scurvy)
  4. Increased metabolic activity (hyperthyroidism, chronic temperature elevations)
  5. Lesch–Nyhan syndrome
  6. Drugs (L-Dopa?)

E. Increased excretion
  1. Vitamin B_{12} deficiency? (? of obligatory excretion of folate in urine and bile; possible inability to reabsorb methylfolate excreted in bile, because B_{12} required for it)
  2. Liver disease?
  3. Kidney dialysis
  4. Chronic exfoliative dermatitis

F. Increased destruction
  1. Oxidant in diet?

III. *Interference with purine ring synthesis and interconversion of purine bases:*
A. Purine antagonists
  1. 6-Mercaptopurine (6-MP)   Chemotherapy, immunosuppression
  2. Thioguanine   Chemotherapy, immunosuppression
  3. Azathioprine   Immunosuppression

B. Enzymatic defects in ability to make purine nucleotide from performed bases
  1. Lesch–Nyhan syndrome (there is an associated increased requirement for folate, which is needed at two steps in the increased *de novo* biosynthesis of purine)

IV. *Interference with pyrimidine synthesis:*
A. Pyrimidine antagonists
  1. 5-Fluorouracil (5-FU)   Chemotherapy
    (blocks thymidylate synthetase)
  2. 6-Azauridine   Chemotherapy, psoriasis

B. Enzymatic defects in ability to make pyrimidine
  1. Hereditary oroticaciduria (not responsive to therapy with vitamin B_{12} or folic acid, but responsive to yeast extract or its active ingredients, uridine or the pyrimidine nucleotides, cytidylic, and uridylic acids)

V. *Inhibition of ribonucleotide reductase (cytidylic to deoxycytidylic acid):*
A. Cytosine arabinoside (inhibits DNA polymerase also)   Chemotherapy, antiviral
B. Hydroxyurea   Chemotherapy, psoriasis
C. Iron deficiency: Iron is required for ribonucleotide reductase, but it is not yet established that lack of iron can produce megaloblastosis; some workers have reported hypersegmented polys in iron deficiency that disappear with iron therapy, but coincident folate deficiency has not yet been excluded fully
D. Procarbazine (depolymerizes DNA)

VI. *Inhibition of protein synthesis:*
A. L-Asparaginase   Chemotherapy

VII. *Mechanism unknown:*
A. Benzene   Solvent
B. Azulfidine   Ulcerative colitis
C. Arsenic   Poison
D. Pyridoxine-responsive megaloblastic anemia (only about 10% of patients with pyridoxine-responsive sideroblastic anemia have megaloblastic morphology)
E. Thiamin-responsive megaloblastic anemia (one case reported)
F. Megaloblastoid anemias (differentiated from megaloblastic anemias by bizarre morphology, including marked polyploidy, few to no orthochromatic megaloblasts, tendency to hyposegmentation, and sometimes karyorrhexis in nucleated red cells)
  1. DiGuglielmo syndrome (erythremic myelosis—a myeloproliferative disorder usually presenting as refractory anemia and eventuating in death from "erythroleukemia" or myelogenous leukemia); preleukemia
  2. Occasional cases of polycythemia vera and other myeloproliferative disorders
  3. Occasional cases of aplastic anemia (which may subsequently develop myeloproliferative disorders)
  4. Occasional cases of miliary tuberculosis (in such cases, the megaloblastoid marrow is often accompanied by monocytosis and leukopenia or leukocytosis)

reduces the amount of 5,10-methylene THF available for thymidylate synthesis, and vitamin B_{12} deficiency reduces production of 5,10-methylene THF by blocking utilization of 5-methyl THF (step 6 in Fig. 23-4) and possibly directing reducing synthesis of thymidylate synthetase.[10,13]

INCIDENCE AND PREVALENCE

Dietary vitamin B_{12} deficiency megaloblastic anemia occurs among strict vegetarians who eat no animal protein, because animal protein is the sole source of the vitamin.[4,30] The ultimate source of B_{12} is microbial synthesis.[4,30] Conversely, this form of anemia rarely occurs among meat eaters because

the vitamin is almost indestructible by cooking or other processing. On the other hand, dietary folate deficiency megaloblastic anemia occurs in about one third of all the pregnant women in the world (*megaloblastic anemia of pregnancy*) despite the fact that folate is found in nearly all natural foods, because folate is heat labile and rapidly destroyed by extensive cooking, especially of finely divided foods such as beans and rice. Any pregnant woman whose daily diet contains neither a fresh or fresh-frozen uncooked fruit or vegetable or fruit juice, nor a fresh lightly cooked vegetable, and whose food is all heated at 100°C for periods in excess of 15 min, can be assumed to have folate deficiency until proved otherwise. Dietary folate deficiency is also

FIG. 23-3 Flow Chart of vitamin B_{12} metabolism. *MDR*, adult minimum daily requirement from exogenous sources to sustain normality.

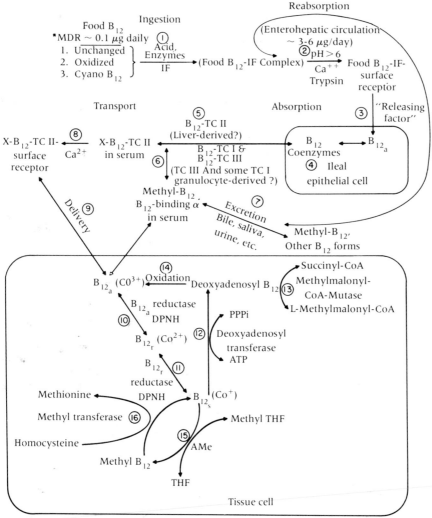

*MDR, Adult minimum daily requirement from exogenous sources to sustain normality.

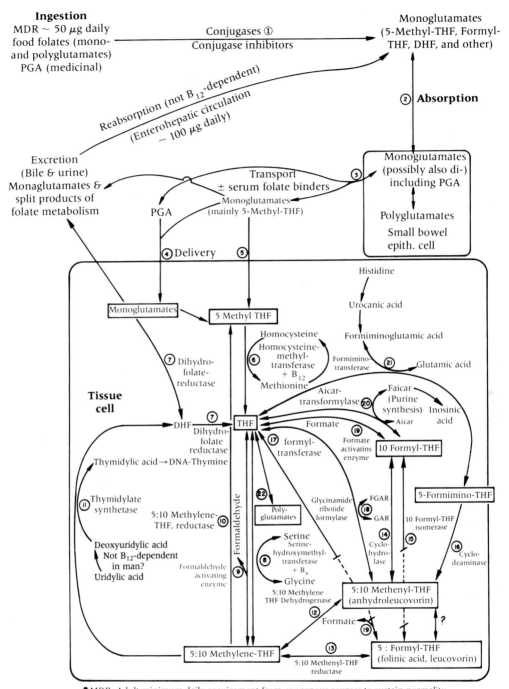

Ingestion
MDR ~ 50 μg daily
food folates (mono-
and polyglutamates)
PGA (medicinal)

Conjugases ①
Conjugase inhibitors

Monoglutamates
(5-Methyl-THF, Formyl-
THF, DHF, and other)

② **Absorption**

Reabsorption (not B₁₂-dependent)
(Enterohepatic circulation
~ 100 μg daily)

Excretion
(Bile & urine)
Monaglutamates &
split products of
folate metabolism

Transport
± serum folate binders
Monoglutamates
(mainly 5-Methyl-THF)

③

Monoglutamates
(possibly also di-)
including PGA

Polyglutamates
Small bowel
epith. cell

PGA

④ Delivery   ⑤

**Tissue
cell**

Monoglutamates

5 Methyl THF

Histidine

Urocanic acid

Formiminoglutamic acid

⑦ Dihydro-
folate-
reductase

Homocysteine

Homocysteine-
methyl-
transferase
+ B₁₂

Methionine

Formimino-
transferase

㉑   Glutamic acid

Aicar-
transformylase ⑳

Faicar
(Purine
synthesis) Inosinic
acid

DHF

⑦
Dihydro-
folate
reductase

THF

Formate

Aicar

Thymidylic acid→DNA-Thymine

⑰ formyl-
transferase

⑲
Formate
activatins
enzyme

10 Formyl-THF

⑪ Thymidylate
synthetase

㉒

Poly-
glutamates

Glycinamide
ribotide
formylase

FGAR

⑱
GAR

5-Formimino-THF

10 Formyl-THF
isomerase

5:10 Methylene-
THF, reductase ⑩

⑭
Cyclo-
hydro-
lase

⑮

⑯Cyclo-
deaminase

Deoxyuridylic acid
Not B₁₂-dependent
in man?
Uridylic acid

Formaldehyde
activating
enzyme

Serine
Serine-
hydroxymethyl-
transferase
+ B₆

⑧

Glycine

5:10 Methenyl-THF
(anhydroleucovorin)

⑨
Formaldehyde

5:10 Methylene
THF Dehydrogenase

⑫
Formate

⑲

?

5:10 Methylene-THF

⑬

5:10 Methenyl-THF
reductase

5 : Formyl-THF
(folinic acid, leucovorin)

*MDR, Adult minimum daily requirement from exogenous sources to sustain normality.

FIG. 23-4 Flow chart of folate metabolism. *MDR,* adult minimum daily requirement from exogenous sources to sustain normality.

present in over 90% of hard-liquor alcoholics, a majority of wine and beer alcoholics, and about half of narcotics addicts, because these groups tend to spend little money on solid food.[6]

Pernicious anemia (megaloblastic anemia caused by inadequate secretion of gastric IF) is age related, with an approximate incidence of 1 per million persons at ages 6 months to 1 year, 1 per 10,000 at ages 1 year to 10 years, 1 per 5,000 at ages 30 years to 40 years, and a progressive increase in frequency thereafter so that the incidence is approximately 1 per 200 persons at ages 60 years to 70 years. Age of onset of pernicious anemia is earlier when there are immune disorders present, other than just circulating antibody to IF, which is a diagnostic test when present (as is the case in two thirds of patients with pernicious anemia).[4,30]

Megaloblastosis caused by subnormal intestinal absorption of vitamin B_{12} (often with associated folate deficiency) is almost always present in active tropical sprue, which is a presumed infectious disease of unknown causative agent endemic in the Caribbean and Southeast Asia. It has been studied most in Puerto Ricans, Haitians, Vietnamese, Pakistanis, and Indians, but is also found in other nationals from these two geographic regions. A person born in an endemic sprue region who gets sprue may have remissions and exacerbations of the disease throughout life; recurrences are seen in such persons even after they have lived in a temperate zone and have been apparently without symptoms for up to 20 years. We speculate that this may relate to reinfection by means of close association with conationals. For this reason, when a person born in Puerto Rico develops megaloblastic anemia in the continental United States, he should be considered to have tropical sprue until proved otherwise. Subnormal absorption of vitamin B_{12} is also present in a majority of persons with chronic pancreatic disease.[3,21]

HEMATOLOGIC AND OTHER PATHOLOGY

The pathology of megaloblastic anemia is generated by slowed DNA synthesis per unit time, and this is observed in all proliferating cells.[1,4,26,49] Normally, cells capable of reproducing themselves are in the resting state (*i.e.*, 1 unit of DNA) most of the time. When they reproduce, they do so by rapidly doubling their DNA, dividing, and returning to the resting state. Thus, at any instant, 100 such normal cells may contain 101 units of DNA (99 cells with 1 unit each plus 1 cell which is about to divide and has rapidly doubled its DNA to do so). Unlike normal cells, at any given instant few megaloblastic cells are resting, because nearly all are engaged in a slowed attempt to complete the dou-

bling of their DNA, with frequent arrest in the S (synthesis) phase and lesser arrest in other phases. Thus, the amount of DNA observed per megaloblastic cell may be about 1.8 units, so that instead of the hypothetical 101 units of DNA per 100 normoblastic cells, there may be about 180 units of DNA per 100 megaloblastic cells. This largely explains the apparent anomaly that megaloblastic cells are seen under the microscope to have larger than normal nuclei with *increased DNA content* and yet to have biochemically *defective DNA synthesis.* Megaloblasts have an even larger cytoplasm than nucleus, as compared with normal cells, because, although their synthesis of DNA is impaired, their ability to synthesize RNA is usually relatively unimpeded. This disparity, or *nuclear-cytoplasmic dissociation* or *asynchrony,* as it is variously termed, is reflected in the finely particulate nuclear chromatin ("young nucleus," or nucleus with retarded maturation) of the erythroid megaloblasts at all stages of their development, even at the orthochromatic stage when hemoglobin is clearly visible in the cytoplasm ("old cytoplasm"), easily differentiating them from orthochromatic normoblasts with their coarsely clumped "old" nuclear chromatin.

Another striking feature of megaloblastic hematopoiesis is the megaloblastic myelopoiesis, manifested most dramatically by the presence of many giant metamyelocytes, the increased DNA of which is eventually packaged in an increased number of lobes in the mature neutrophil.

The evolutionary biochemical and hematologic sequence in development of folate deficiency is indicated in Figure 23-5; the sequence of development of vitamin B_{12} deficiency is similar, but is measured in years rather than months.

When there is concomitant iron deficiency, as is often the case in pregnancy, various malabsorption syndromes, and alcoholism, and in about one third of cases of pernicious anemia, the bone marrow erythroid megaloblastosis and peripheral blood macrocytic "overcolored" erythrocytes may be masked by the countervailing tendency of iron deficiency to produce microblasts and hypochromic microcytic erythrocytes. The result may be "intermediate megaloblasts" (cells halfway between megaloblasts and normoblasts) in the bone marrow, and in the peripheral blood both red cell forms may be present ("dimorphic anemia"), or, more frequently, the picture will be that of the more severe deficiency. The myeloid megaloblastosis in the bone marrow and the hypersegmented polymorphonuclear leukocytes ("hypersegmented polys") in the peripheral blood are not masked by iron deficiency, and they provide the morphologic key to the coincident existence of less severe vitamin

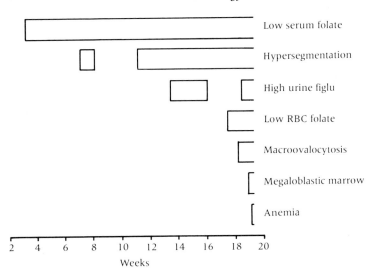

FIG. 23-5 Biochemical and hematologic sequence of events with progressive negative folate balance.

B_{12} or folate deficiency even in the presence of more severe iron deficiency.[27]

Thus, hypersegmentation can be a crucial clue to covert folate deficiency despite normal serum and red cell folate levels in many patients with seemingly uncomplicated iron deficiency.[12,27] Such patients have abnormal lymphocyte *dU* (deoxyuridine) *suppression* tests (the suppression by nonradioactive deoxyuridine of the incorporation into a cell's DNA of subsequently added radioactive thymidine, Fig. 23-4). After 3 weeks to 6 weeks of treatment with iron alone, their normoblastic erythroid bone marrow converts to megaloblastic.[12] Hypersegmented polys are sought by either the simple *rule of fives* (*i.e.*, if more than 5 of 100 neutrophils have 5 or more lobes, hypersegmentation is present) or the more elaborate *lobe average* (*i.e.*, the number of lobes in 100 polys is counted and divided by 100; whereas the normal lobe average is 3.2 ± 0.15, hypersegmentation is present if the lobe average is greater than 3.5). Normally 20% to 40% of polys have two lobes, 40% to 50% have three lobes, and 15% to 20% have four lobes. A substantial increase in percentage with four or more lobes means megaloblastosis, congenital hypersegmentation, or chronic renal disease. Congenital hypersegmentation is present in 1% of Caucasians. As Figure 23-5 indicates, in incipient megaloblastic anemia, hypersegmentation is present prior to the appearance of an obviously megaloblastic bone marrow or anemia. When the peripheral blood smears of all new patients are screened on a routine basis for hypersegmentation, one third of those presenting such are subsequently proved to have early vitamin B_{12} or folate deficiency, with low serum vitamin level but no anemia and no clinical suspicion of the diagnosis. The alternative *20% rule* (*i.e.*, if less than 20% of 100 neutrophils have two or less lobes, hypersegmentation is present) is particularly useful in early megaloblastosis when there are few or no polys with more than five lobes.[4,12,26,39]

In the megaloblastic anemias there is ineffective erythropoiesis, with a hemolytic component and an iron overload pathologic picture. The increased intramedullary fetal death rate is recognized by the frequent finding of up to 25% reticulocytes among the bone-marrow erythrons but 1% or less in the peripheral blood, the high serum lactate dehydrogenase, the modestly elevated serum bilirubin, and the low serum haptoglobin. Ineffective utilization of iron results in increased saturation of the iron-binding capacity of transferrin and increased iron stores. This is so prominent that when a patient exhibits megaloblastic anemia and normal rather than elevated serum and bone-marrow iron, often with an elevated total iron-binding capacity, one must suspect iron deficiency, and should repeat the measurements of serum and bone-marrow iron a month after vitamin therapy to determine whether overt iron deficiency has now been unmasked.[12,27]

Megaloblastosis with underlying defective DNA synthesis is present in all proliferating cells, particularly marked in rapidly turning over cells such as those of the alimentary tract and vagina. This defective DNA synthesis results in a variable degree of atrophy in epithelial cells of the tongue, stomach, and small intestine. It is this atrophy that produces secondary failure of gastric IF secretion in one third of patients with tropical sprue, secondary failure of intestinal absorption of vitamin B_{12} in about half of patients with primary failure of IF secretion, and a variety of other vicious cycles whereby vitamin B_{12} deficiency results in secondary decreased absorption of folate (and B_{12}), and folate deficiency results in secondary decreased absorption of vitamin B_{12} (and folate). These secondary malabsorption phenomena disappear after a variable period of vitamin therapy.[21]

In addition to the defective DNA synthesis common to all megaloblastic anemias, there is a defect in ability to synthesize myelin that is present only in vitamin B_{12} deficiency. This results in the insidious development of demyelinating vitamin B_{12} deficiency neuropathy, often beginning in peripheral nerves and progressing to involve the posterior and lateral columns of the spinal cord (variously called subacute combined degeneration, combined systems disease, posterolateral sclerosis, and funicular degeneration) and the cerebrum ("megaloblastic madness").[34] Irish workers have prevented this defect in monkeys with methionine.[43,44] Recently, the question has been raised as to whether B_{12} analogues could play a role in nerve damage development.[31,37]

CLINICAL MANIFESTATIONS

Infrequently, the patient with megaloblastic anemia exhibits bleeding caused by thrombocytopenia or infection caused by the leukopenia, but usually one or more of the symptoms of gradually developing and slowly progressing anemia is present: easy fatigability, weakness, tiredness, shortness of breath, occasional faintness (particularly on suddenly rising from a recumbent or sitting position), headache, palpitations, and syncope. Before such symptoms are brushed off as neurotic, as such symptoms frequently are, laboratory testing for anemia should be carried out, consisting at the least of determination of hematocrit or hemoglobin and examination of peripheral blood smear morphology for macro-ovalocytic or hypersegmented neutrophils.

If the patient has vitamin B_{12} deficiency and a good diet supplying adequate folate to mask the hematologic picture substantially, he may have no anemia and only slight morphologic evidence of megaloblastosis, and may present as a neurologic or neuropsychiatric problem. Paresthesias, especially numbness and tingling in the hands and feet, and diminished vibration or position sense may be present, with loss of perception of 256 vibrations per second (vps) and loss of position sense in the index toes preceded by many months loss of perception of 128 vps as well as loss of position sense in the great toes. Examination with a 256-vps tuning fork may reveal complete loss of vibration sense from toes to iliac crests bilaterally before any loss of perception of vibration of a 128-vps tuning fork.

The classic neurologic disorder associated with vitamin B_{12} deficiency is combined system disease (subacute combined degeneration). Usually slow and insidious in onset, it is characterized by degeneration of the dorsal and lateral columns of the spinal cord, with paresthesias of the hands and feet, ataxia of the legs with variable spasticity and weakness, and eventual paraplegia. The classic symptoms are symmetrical paresthesias (numbness, tingling, burning) in feet or hands, followed by unsteadiness of gait associated with loss of position sense, manifested by inability to detect passive movements of the great toes. Prior to the appearance of deficits in the great toes, there may be inability to detect passive movements of the index toes. Knee and ankle jerks may be diminished or lost, or the knee jerks may be increased; extensor plantar responses (indicating damage to the spinal cord) commonly occur. Mental changes are variable; they may include paranoid ideation and depression, and may be sufficiently severe to mimic paranoid schizophrenia or senility. British workers have referred to this phenomenon as "megaloblastic madness." Ataxic paraplegia similar to that resulting from vitamin B_{12} deficiency results from any kind of damage to the dorsal or lateral columns of the spinal cord, as may occur with multiple sclerosis or chronic meningeal syphilis.[34]

Subjective neurologic dysfunction, such as irritability, forgetfulness, and sleeplessness, occurs not only with vitamin B_{12} deficiency but even more frequently with folate deficiency. Such subjective stigmata are of limited differential diagnostic value in separating the two vitamin deficiency states; when caused by folate deficiency, these stigmata disappear dramatically within 24 hr of the start of folate therapy.[8]

Occasionally, a chronic alcoholic with megaloblastic anemia caused by folate deficiency is erroneously diagnosed as having vitamin B_{12} deficiency because he has neurologic damage, including impaired position and vibration sense. However, associated thiamin deficiency in the alcoholic produces peripheral neuropathy mimicking that caused by vitamin B_{12} deficiency. Confusion may also arise in patients with folate deficiency and diabetes mellitus, because diabetic neuropathy may also mimic the neuropathy resulting from vitamin B_{12} deficiency.[34]

The skin may have a lemon-yellow cast owing to the combination of pallor from anemia and low-grade icterus from the hemolytic component of the disorder. The classic pernicious anemia patient still appears as described by Addison in 1855:

The countenance gets pale, the whites of the eyes become pearly, *the general frame flabby rather than wasted;* the pulse is perhaps large but remarkably soft and compressible, and occasionally with a slight jerk, especially under the slightest excitement. There is an increasing indisposition to exertion with an uncomfortable feeling of faintness or breathlessness on attempting it; the heart is readily made to palpitate; the whole surface presents a blanched, smooth, and waxy appearance: the lips, gums and tongue seem bloodless; *the flabbiness of the solids increases;* the appetite fails, extreme languor and faintness supervene, breathlessness and palpitation being produced by the most trifling exertion or emotion; some slight edema is probably perceived about the ankles. The debility becomes extreme; the patient can no longer arise from his bed; *the mind occasionally wanders;* he falls into a prostrate and half torpid state, and at length expires. *Nevertheless, to the very last, and after a sickness of perhaps several months' duration, the bulkiness of the general frame and the obesity often present a most striking contrast to the failure and exhaustion observable in every other respect.*[20,35]

The parts of Addison's classic description which do *not* fit folic acid deficiency have been italicized. In folate deficiency, emaciation is more common than flabbiness, and diarrhea is more common than the constipation often seen in vitamin B_{12} deficiency.

About one third of patients with megaloblastic anemia have splenomegaly, but this may be observable only on abdominal radiography, because the spleen exceeds two to three times normal size in fewer than 10% of cases. Moderate hepatomegaly also may be present.

A smooth or sore tongue is frequent, owing to megaloblastosis of the cells of the papillary surface. Almost 10% of patients have hyperpigmentation, often most marked in the palmar creases, but occasionally in bizarre patterns such as occur with Addison's disease, sometimes with vitiligo. Occasionally, low-grade fever is present.

LABORATORY FINDINGS AND DIFFERENTIAL DIAGNOSIS

Primary laboratory findings include macro-ovalocytic anemia, leukopenia (with "hypersegmented polys"), thrombocytopenia (with giant platelets), and megaloblastic bone marrow. Hypersegmented nuclei are seen not only in neutrophils, but also basophils and eosinophils. Reticulocyte count below 1% is common with vitamin B_{12} deficiency, but 1.5% to 8% is common with folate deficiency. *Secondary* findings include reduced haptoglobin, hyperbilirubinemia, increased fecal stercobilin, elevated serum lactate dehydrogenase, formiminoglutamic aciduria (found not only in primary folate deficiency but also in primary vitamin B_{12} deficiency and primary liver disease), high serum iron and high saturation of transferrin, loss of gastric acid and abnormal liver function, and intestinal

absorption tests showing various degrees of malabsorption. Megaloblasts are usually present in the buffy coat of centrifuged peripheral blood.

An elevated mean corpuscular volume (MCV) does not mean megaloblastosis unless the red cells are *oval* as well as large. About one quarter of patients with an elevated MCV have large red cells caused by hypothyroidism, hypoplastic anemia, hemolytic anemia, sideroblastic anemia, neoplasia, liver disease, or other conditions producing large, but not oval, red cells.[4,26]

A serum B_{12} level below 100 pg/ml is essentially diagnostic for primary vitamin B_{12} deficiency and *both* a serum folate of less than 3 ng/ml and a red cell folate below 150 ng/ml are diagnostic for primary folate deficiency. Low serum folate simply means negative folate balance, so it may occur long before tissue folate depletion and may simply mean that the patient has eaten poorly for several weeks. Low red cell folate occurs also in primary vitamin B_{12} deficiency, because B_{12} is necessary to keep methylfolate in red cells. One caveat obtains: when the serum levels of both vitamins are low, the primary deficiency may be of just one, with resultant intestinal megaloblastosis producing malabsorption and therefore secondary deficiency of the other. For example, in megaloblastic anemia of pregnancy, both vitamin levels may be low, but Mollin and others have shown that treatment with only folic acid results in gradual rise to normal of the serum B_{12} level.[4] Normal red cell folate may be present despite folate deficiency owing to a lag in replacing normal with low folate red cells as pregnancy develops, because of the presence of high folate cells (reticulocytes or transfused cells), or because of iron deficiency.[4,12]

Methylmalonic aciduria occurs only in vitamin B_{12} deficiency and not in folate deficiency.[42]

Absence of IF in the gastric juice on *in vitro* assay is essentially diagnostic for pernicious anemia. Primary intestinal malabsorption of B_{12} or folate deficiency may produce secondary loss of IF secretion; this secretion will return to normal after vitamin therapy.[21] Gastric juice *p*H greater than 5 and viscid rather than watery character, plus a volume of less than 25 ml in the 45 min after histamine or histalog stimulation, all suggest pernicious anemia. Generally, as pernicious anemia develops, acid is lost first, then pepsin, then IF. Exceptions occur, with loss of IF first.

In vivo tests for detection of vitamin B_{12} malabsorption involve feeding 0.5 μg to 2 μg of the vitamin, labeled with ^{56}Co (half-life, 77 days), ^{57}Co (half-life, 270 days), ^{58}Co (half-life, 71 days), or ^{60}Co (half-life, 5.26 years), and measuring the amount absorbed by detecting the amount of radioactivity in either stool, urine, blood, liver, or whole body.[21] The test is divided into three stages:

1. Feed radio-B_{12} alone. Subnormal absorption means gastric or ileal dysfunction. It need not be done if *in vitro* radioassay for IF is carried out.

2. Feed radio-B_{12} plus IF concentrate. Subnormal absorption means ileal dysfunction, but does not rule out concomitant gastric dysfunction.

3. Only done if second stage is subnormal: feed antibiotic (or antihelmintic) for appropriate period, then feed radio-B_{12}. A normal result means that the patient had blind loop syndrome (or fish tapeworm). When pancreatic dysfunction is suspected, the third stage consists in feeding the radio-B_{12} with added bicarbonate or pancreatin or both. When drug-induced B_{12} malabsorption is suspected, the third-stage test is carried out after withdrawal of the offending agent.

Every patient in whom tests reveal gastric or intestinal malabsorption of B_{12} that is not due to a clear single cause should have the tests repeated after therapy with B_{12}, or after therapy with folic acid, if deficiency of folic acid is present.[21] Vitamin B_{12} deficiency is a vicious-cycle disease (as is folic acid deficiency); severe deficiency of either B_{12} or folic acid may produce a variable degree of gastric or intestinal damage, and therefore may itself produce a variable degree of secondary reduction of gastric secretion of IF or ileal ability to absorb B_{12} (or intestinal ability to absorb folate). This secondary malabsorption of B_{12} or folate is corrected by therapy.

Repetition of tests after therapy will establish which damage was secondary (*i.e.,* a result of deficiency of B_{12} or folic acid) and which was primary (*i.e.,* a lesion not produced by deficiency of B_{12} or folate). The B_{12} deficiency of a patient with regional enteritis may produce secondary gastric damage that may reduce IF secretion; this secondary gastric damage may be corrected by B_{12} therapy. Conversely, the B_{12} deficiency of a patient with pernicious anemia may produce secondary ileal damage and resultant malabsorption of a test dose of B_{12} fed with IF. This secondary ileal damage may be corrected by B_{12} therapy. Additionally, the B_{12} deficiency of either patient may increase the malabsorption owing to his primary lesion.

Circulating antibody to IF is present in two thirds of patients with pernicious anemia and, when found, is essentially diagnostic.[4,22,26] Less than 10% saturation of serum vitamin B_{12}-binding capacity is also essentially diagnostic.[22,33]

The deoxyuridine (dU) suppression test on bone marrow cells aspirated from the patient is diagnostic for folate deficiency if a deficit in deoxyuridine suppression of subsequently added radioactive iododeoxyuridine incorporation into DNA is found, and is corrected *in vitro* by methylfolate; it is diagnostic for vitamin B_{12} deficiency, if corrected by B_{12} but not by methylfolate.[10–13,22] This "therapeutic trial in a test tube" is the laboratory equivalent of the classical clinical trial described below. Because circulating mature lymphocytes are impervious to vitamin B_{12} and folic acid, the dU suppression test on lymphocytes can reveal a past deficiency of vitamin B_{12} or folic acid up to two months after the start of vitamin therapy.[11] The test can also reveal occult folate deficiency in patients with dominant iron deficiency, as can measurement of lymphocyte folate level.[7,12]

THERAPY

Therapeutic trial is diagnostic for vitamin B_{12} or folate deficiency. Such trial is carried out by giving the patient a diet devoid of foods high in folate, such as fresh uncooked or fresh-frozen fruits and vegetables, fruit juices, nuts or other uncooked foods, and liver. After 10 days on such a diet, and while continuing the diet, the patient is then treated with 1 μg/day vitamin B_{12} parenterally if vitamin B_{12} deficiency is suspected, and with 50 μg/day to 100 μg/day folic acid parenterally if folic acid deficiency is suspected. Unless hematopoiesis is suppressed by infection, uremia, chloramphenicol, alcohol, or some other chronic systemic disease or drug, approximately 3 days after the start of therapy, reticulocytosis will appear and will reach a peak at approximately 7 days (range: 5–12 days) after the start of daily vitamin therapy. The lower the initial red count, the higher the reticulocyte peak will be. The hemoglobin will gradually rise, and by approximately 7 days after the start of therapy the white cell and platelet counts will rise to normal. The platelet count will usually, and the white count will in 10% of cases, exceed normal before falling back into normal range. It is important that the therapeutic trial vitamin dose not be larger than the aforementioned, to avoid nonspecific response (see Fig. 23-6).

Immediate therapy is advisable in patients with megaloblastosis accompanied by anemia so severe as to be associated with dyspnea, congestive failure, and occasionally angina. Such symptoms, when found, usually occur in association with a hematocrit below 15%. Rapid and dramatic relief of these symptoms may be obtained by administration of packed cells into one arm, accompanied by withdrawal of a slightly lesser quantity of whole blood from the contralateral arm. Venous pressure should be monitored, and only that amount of whole blood removed that is necessary to prevent elevation of the venous pressure. Packed cells may be given at the rate of 1 unit/5 min by interposing a three-way

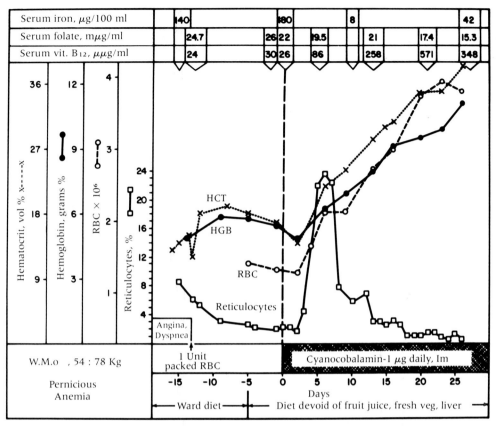

Serum iron, μg/100 ml	140		180	8			42
Serum folate, mμg/ml	24.7		26	22	19.5	21	17.4	15.3
Serum vit. B$_{12}$, $\mu\mu$g/ml	24		30	26	86	258	571	348

W.M.o , 54 : 78 Kg

Pernicious Anemia

1 Unit packed RBC

Cyanocobalamin-1 μg daily, Im

Ward diet — Diet devoid of fruit juice, fresh veg, liver

Angina, Dyspnea

FIG. 23-6 Therapeutic trial with 1 μg of vitamin B$_{12}$ daily. Note the "spontaneous" reticulocytosis present on admission (more frequent in folate deficiency), the termination of angina and dyspnea by a single unit of packed red blood cells (*RBC*), the initial high serum and folate, and their fall on vitamin B$_{12}$ therapy.

stopcock and a 50-ml syringe between the bottle or bag of packed cells and the vein, drawing the packed cells from the source into the syringe and injecting into the vein. By using the three-way stopcock, one can monitor venous pressure and draw off whole blood as required. In this procedure, packed cells with a hematocrit of approximately 80 are going into one arm, while whole blood with a hematocrit of less than 15 is coming out the same or the other arm. There is, therefore, no dangerous sudden rise in circulating blood volume to induce the irreversible congestive failure so dreaded when chronically anemic patients are given packed cells or whole blood in the conventional manner.

Immediate therapy with vitamin B$_{12}$ or folate is advisable in patients with severe infection, coma, severe disorientation, marked neurologic damage, severe liver disease, uremia, or other markedly debilitating illness complicating the deficiency of vitamin B$_{12}$ or folate. When one of these reasons makes immediate vitamin therapy necessary before estab-

lishing the etiologic diagnosis, such therapy should be given intramuscularly with a minimum of 30 μg (1 ml) of vitamin B$_{12}$ (cyanocobalamin) and 1 mg (1 ml) of folic (pteroyglutamic) acid followed by 1 tablet (1 mg) of folic acid by mouth daily for a week and a minimum of 30 μg of vitamin B$_{12}$ by intramuscular injection daily for a week. The fall in serum potassium in the first week after commencing therapy is rarely of clinical significance and does not require therapy. There is a slow increase in whole body potassium with treatment, which parallels the increase in red cell mass. In England, hydroxocobalamin rather than cyanocobalamin is the pharmaceutical of choice, but we are unconvinced of any real superiority over cyanocobalamin.[4,24]

After a week of therapy to carry the patient from the critical state to a state of well-being, all vitamin therapy should be stopped, if necessary, to make an etiologic diagnosis. However, with a combination of foresight and laboratory facilities, blood will have been obtained from the patient immediately on admission and prior to treatment, and diagnosis of vitamin B_{12} or folate deficiency will have been made from determination of the serum and erythrocyte levels of these vitamins, supplemented by the various tests that may be performed even when the patient is being treated. Initial therapy for inadequate absorption of vitamin B_{12} is 30 μg monthly. This quantity is not adequate to sustain complete normality and allows morphologic damage of moderate degree to persist; therefore, a monthly injection of 100 μg of cyanocobalamin is preferable, because it will sustain in complete remission all patients with uncomplicated vitamin B_{12} deficiency.

Monthly maintenance therapy must be carried out for life in the patient whose inadequate absorption of B_{12} is due to lack of IF secretion or to a noncorrectable structural or functional lesion of the ileum. Although there is no evidence that greater or more frequent therapy has any value, it has become general practice to give patients with neurologic damage 250 μg or more of vitamin B_{12} once or twice weekly for several months, followed by similar doses once or twice monthly for another year. Neurologic damage resulting from vitamin B_{12} deficiency, when of a behavioral nature such as paranoia, may improve very rapidly (even within 24 hr) after the start of therapy. Objectively ascertainable neurologic damage, such as loss of position or vibration sense, improves more slowly, and ability to perceive 128 vps may return before ability to perceive 256 vps. Likewise, ability to perceive motion of the great toes may return before ability to perceive passive motion of index toes. *Any neurologic damage which has not been corrected at the end of approximately one and a half years may be considered to be irreversible.* Neurologic damage caused by vitamin B_{12} deficiency begins as inability to make myelin, followed by gradual deterioration of the axon, followed by deterioration of the nerve head. This process occurs very slowly and is reversible until the nerve head deteriorates.

Oral therapy with large doses of vitamin B_{12} (500 μg/day–1000 μg/day) is reliable only when the patient does not have vitamin B_{12} malabsorption. It is unreliable in pernicious anemia and intestinal malabsorption syndromes. Daily injections in excess of 30 μg have no therapeutic advantage, although it is possible that larger daily doses may result in slightly more rapid repletion of body stores. However, the percentage of the injected doses of vitamin B_{12} excreted in the urine rises logarithmically as the quantity of cyanocobalamin injected rises above 30 μg/day.

The most frequent complications of vitamin B_{12} deficiency, particularly that caused by pernicious anemia, are infections, especially of the genitourinary tract, and variable degrees of congestive failure. These should be managed appropriately. Since the incidence of carcinoma of the stomach in patients with pernicious anemia is approximately threefold higher than chance, this entity should be looked for at yearly intervals.

In patients with chronic pancreatic disease, the mechanism may not be operative and may be enhanced by feeding sodium bicarbonate, pancreatin, or trypsin.[3,21] Pancreatic proteolytic enzymes free B_{12} from R proteins so that the B_{12} can bind to IF.[12] Bicarbonate raises intestinal pH so that IF can better compete with R proteins for B_{12}.

Initial therapy with doses of pteroylglutamic acid larger than 0.1 mg/day is desirable when the folate deficiency state is complicated by conditions that may suppress hematopoiesis (infection, uremia, tumor; active inflammatory lesions such as rheumatoid arthritis, ulcerative colitis, or hepatitis; hypermetabolic states; states of increased hematopoiesis such as occur with hemolytic anemia or protracted blood loss). Therapy should then consist of 0.5 mg to 1 mg pteroylglutamic acid daily.

There is no evidence that doses greater than 1 mg/day have greater advantage. Hematologic improvement should be followed by obtaining a blood count and reticulocyte count just prior to the start of therapy and a reticulocyte count about every 2 to 3 days from then until the reticulocyte peak has passed, plus a hemoglobin or hematocrit determination at weekly intervals for the first month and then every 2 weeks for the next month or two. If hematologic recovery does not follow the expected response pattern, either the diagnosis is wrong or complications suppressing hematopoiesis are present.

All patients with megaloblastic anemia should be evaluated for iron deficiency. Approximately one third of patients with vitamin B_{12} deficiency and approximately one half of patients with folate deficiency also have iron deficiency. In a large percentage of such patients, when the megaloblastic anemia is dominant, it is impossible to diagnose coexisting iron deficiency. This is because megaloblastic anemia produces a pathologic picture akin to iron overload: ineffective erythropoiesis resulting in "piling up" in the tissues of iron from the missing hemoglobin; elevation of transferrin saturation and serum ferritin; and low free erythrocyte protoporphyrin. Only after the vitamin deficiency has been adequately treated and stored iron has been incorporated into new hemoglobin is it possible to determine the true iron status. Every patient with megaloblastic anemia, even if previously evaluated for iron deficiency, should be evaluated for iron deficiency a second time approximately one month after the start of vitamin therapy. This will uncover a substantial number of patients with iron deficiency whose laboratory tests prior to vitamin therapy conveyed an impression of normal iron status.[26,27]

All patients with iron deficiency should be evaluated for hidden megaloblastic anemia.[12,27] When a patient has severe vitamin deficiency and less severe iron deficiency, only the vitamin deficiency may be demonstrable when the patient first presents. The patient with severe megaloblastic anemia should have the laboratory findings of iron overload, and if those laboratory findings indicate normal iron instead, then iron deficiency probably exists. It is also the case that a patient having severe iron deficiency often has a less severe folate deficiency or B_{12} deficiency. This condition which is not recognized because the peripheral blood picture is that of hypochromic anemia owing to the dominant iron deficiency, rather than the dimorphic anemia of combined iron deficiency and megaloblastosis. The only clue to the coexistence of a less severe vitamin deficiency anemia superimposed on a more severe iron deficiency will be neutrophil hypersegmentation.[12] This hypersegmentation tends to be subtle rather than blatant. The normal neutrophil *lobe average* is 3.2. ± 1.5, whereas in severe iron deficiency with less severe folate deficiency, the *lobe average* may be only 3.6 or 3.7.[12] With severe megaloblastic anemia and a hemoglobin of one-third normal, there may be sufficient iron for the one-third normal hemoglobin, but not enough iron for the patient to rise to a normal red cell mass (*i.e.,* there is true iron deficiency, meaning that there is not enough iron to reach normality). In severe iron deficiency, serum and red cell folate may be normal but there may not be enough folate in the patient's body to allow the red cell mass to return completely to normal on iron therapy. Before the iron deficiency has been treated, the coincident folate or B_{12} deficiency should be suspected if there is neutrophil hypersegmentation, and can be proved by dU suppression test on the peripheral blood lymphocytes or by lymphocyte folate assay.[7,12] Al-

ternatively, the patient may be treated with just iron for a month, after which repeat bone-marrow examination will demonstrate the megaloblastosis previously hidden by the iron deficiency.[12]

Table 23-5 shows why it is necessary to measure serum and red cell folate as well as serum B_{12} level if one wishes to separate the four clinical situations: normality, vitamin B_{12} deficiency, folate deficiency, and deficiency of both vitamins.

As indicated in Table 23-5, low serum folate is diagnostic for current negative folate balance only and not for folate deficiency.[4] The level may be low in many people whose tissue folate content and metabolism are normal but who simply had poor appetite for several weeks. It is this fact that explains why two thirds of patients in acute-care hospitals have low serum folate levels. Their red cell and other tissue folate are usually normal, and their serum folate will return to normal without folic acid treatment as they regain their appetite.

A caveat regarding serum vitamin B_{12} assay is that one should follow one's clinical judgment when it conflicts with the laboratory report. There may be megaloblastic anemia due to vitamin B_{12} deficiency, and yet the serum vitamin B_{12} level may be normal if the patient has a liver disorder or a myeloproliferative disorder releasing into the plasma binding proteins which hold vitamin B_{12} (and sometimes folic acid) in the serum without delivering these vitamins to deprived tissues.[33] Additionally, the serum contains not only "true vitamin B_{12}" (metabolically active for humans) but also analogues of vitamin B_{12} that may be inactive for humans or even, in some cases, act as anti-B_{12} molecules.[28,29,36,37] With occasional exceptions, "true" B_{12} is measured by microbiologic assay or by radioassay with either pure IF or IF concentrate that has been "spiked" with nonradioactive analogue to "tie-up" its non-IF B_{12} binders, which are capable of binding analogues of B_{12}, thus leaving available only the IF portion, which can bind only true cobalamins.[33,36] Radioassays using serum not adequately pretreated to destroy endogenous B_{12} binders and endogenous antibody to IF may give erroneously high results in patients with perni-

TABLE 23-5
Clinical Distinctions Defined by Measurement of Serum B_{12}, and Serum and Red Cell Folate

Clinical Situation	Serum Vitamin B_{12}	Serum Folate	Red Cell Folate
Normal	Normal	Normal or low	Normal
Vitamin B_{12} deficiency	Low	Normal or high	Low
Folic acid deficiency	Normal	Low	Low
Deficiency of both B_{12} and folic acid	Low	Low	Low

cious anemia and erroneously low results in patients with increased endogenous B_{12} binders.[22] Radioassays of either true cobalamins or total serum corrinoids appear equally accurate for separating normal from vitamin B_{12}-deficiency, provided the cutoff point below which deficiency is suggested is accurately set.[28a]

Other Nutrients and Anemia

Copper deficiency without general malnutrition has not been shown to cause anemia. Patients with Menkes' disease, an inherited disorder affecting copper transport, have no hematologic abnormalities. However, infants depleted of copper and other nutrients by diarrhea superimposed on a copper-deficient milk diet, patients following intestinal bypass surgery, and patients on long term parenteral alimentation do get a copper-responsive anemia, leukopenia, and thrombopenia.[15]

Pyridoxine deficiency has not been demonstrated to produce anemia. However, about one sixth of patients with sideroblastic anemia ("sideroachrestic" anemia) improve to a variable degree when given 50 mg/day to 200 mg/day of pyridoxine hydrochloride. Response is evaluated by quantitating reticulocytes at the end of the first week or by findings of a later increase in the concentration of hemoglobin.[32] Rarely, pyridoxal phosphate works after pyridoxine fails. Patients whose erythrocytes show only moderate variations in size and shape and moderate hypochromicity may have a hemoglobin rise to within the range of normal, whereas those with erythrocytes that show extreme variation in size and shape and marked hypochromicity may show a response only to about half normal. The fundamental biochemical lesion in the pyridoxine-responsive patient is unknown.

Riboflavin deficiency by itself does not produce anemia, although restriction of dietary riboflavin plus administration of the riboflavin antagonist, galactoflavin, will produce a pure red cell anemia correctable by 10 mg/day riboflavin.[38]

Protein–calorie malnutrition produces a sharp fall in lean body mass, resulting in a lower oxygen need, causing reduced erythropoietin production and therefore a physiologic (rather than pathologic) anemia. The lower circulating hemoglobin is adequate to supply the reduced oxygen need of the reduced quantity of tissue.[25,47]

A hemolytic anemia occurs in premature infants who receive large amounts of potentially oxidant agents, usually iron, together with large doses of polyunsaturated fatty acids (PUFA), along with inadequate vitamin E to metabolize the PUFA. This hemolysis responds to oral vitamin E antioxidant action but will respond just as well to formula alteration with a reduction in the dose of iron and PUFA. This anemia is not, therefore, a simple nutritional anemia owing to vitamin E deficiency, but rather one resulting from oxidant action compounded by an adverse alteration in the PUFA:vitamin E ratio.

References

1. Babior BN (ed): Cobalamin: Biochemistry and Pathophysiology. New York, John Wiley & Sons, 1975
2. Bothwell TH, Charlton RW, Cook JD et al (eds): Iron Metabolism in Man. London, Blackwell, 1979
3. Brugge WR, Goff JS, Allen NC et al: Development of a dual label Schilling test for pancreatic exocrine function based on the differential absorption of cobalamin bound to intrinsic factor and R protein. Gastroenterology 78: 937–949, 1980
4. Chanarin I: The Megaloblastic Anemias. St Louis, CV Mosby, 1979
5. Colman N, Bernstein LH, Herbert V: Preferential absorption of methyltetrahydrofolate (MTHF) over folic acid (PGA) in pernicious anemia (PA). Clin Res 23:576A, 1975
6. Colman N, Herbert V: Dietary assessments with special emphasis on prevention of folate deficiency. In Botez MI, Reynolds EH (eds): Folic Acid in Neurology, Psychiatry and Internal Medicine, pp 63–74. New York, Raven Press, 1979
7. Colman N, Herbert V: Abnormal lymphocyte deoxyuridine suppression test: A reliable indicator of decreased lymphocyte folate levels. Am J Hematol 8:169–174, 1980
8. Colman N, Herbert V: Folate metabolism in brain. In Kumar S (ed): Biochemistry of Brain, pp 103–125. New York, Pergamon Press, 1980
9. Colman N, Hettiarachchy NS, Herbert V: Detection of a milk factor that facilitates folate uptake by intestinal cells. Science 211:1427–1429, 1981
10. Das KC, Herbert V: Vitamin B_{12}–folate interrelations. Clin Haematol 5:697–725, 1976
11. Das KC, Herbert V: The lymphocyte as a marker of past nutritional status: Persistence of abnormal lymphocyte deoxyuridine (dU) suppression test and chromosomes in patients with past deficiency of folate and vitamin B_{12}. Br J Haematol 38:219–233, 1978
12. Das KC, Herbert V, Colman N et al: Unmasking covert folate deficiency in iron-deficient subjects with neutrophil hypersegmentation: dU suppression tests on lymphocytes and bone marrow. Br J Haematol 39:357–375, 1978
13. Das KC, Manusselis C, Herbert V: *In vitro* DNA synthesis by bone marrow cells and PHA-stimulated lymphocytes. Suppression by nonradioactive thymidine of the incorporation of ^{3}H-deoxyuridine into DNA: Enhancement of incorporation when inadequate vitamin B_{12} or folate is corrected. Br J Haematol 44:61–63, 1980
14. FAO/WHO Expert Group: Requirements of Ascorbic Acid, Vitamin D, Vitamin B_{12}, Folate and Iron. World Health Organization Technical Report. Geneva, World Health Organization, 1970
15. Finch CA: Drugs effective in iron deficiency and other hypochromic anemias. In Gilman AG, Goodman LS, Gilman A (eds): The Pharmacological Basis of Therapeutics, 6th ed, pp 1315–1330. New York, Macmillan, 1980

16. Food and Nutrition Board, National Research Council: Folic Acid: Biochemistry and Physiology in Relation to Human Nutrition Requirement. Washington, DC, National Academy of Sciences, 1977
17. Food and Nutrition Board, National Research Council: Recommended Dietary Allowances, 9th ed. Washington, DC, National Academy of Sciences, 1980
18. Glass GBJ: Gastric intrinsic factor and other vitamin B_{12} binders. Biochemistry, physiology and relation to vitamin B_{12} metabolism. New York, Georg Thieme Verlag and Intercontinental Medical Book Corp, 1974
19. Green R, Saab GA, Crosby WH: "Normal" serum ferritin—another caution: Reply. Blood 51:765–766, 1978
20. Herbert V: The nutritional anemias of childhood—folate, B_{12}: The megaloblastic anemias. In Suskind RM (ed): Textbook of Pediatric Nutrition, pp 133–144. New York, Raven Press, 1981
21. Herbert V: Detection of malabsorption of vitamin B_{12} due to gastric or intestinal dysfunction. Sem Nuclear Med 2:220, 1972
22. Herbert V: B_{12} and folate deficiency. In Rothfeld B (ed): Nuclear Medicine *In Vitro*, pp 69–84. Philadelphia, Lippincott, 1974
23. Herbert V: Drugs effective in iron-deficiency and other hypochromic anemias. In Goodman LS, Gilman A (eds): The Pharmacological Basis of Therapeutics, 5th ed, pp 1309–1323. New York, Macmillan, 1975
24. Herbert V: Drugs effective in megaloblastic anemias. In Goodman LS, Gilman A (eds): The Pharmacological Basis of Therapeutics, 5th ed, pp 1324–1349. New York, Macmillan, 1975
25. Herbert V: Blood in hypothyroidism. In Werner SC, Ingbar SH (eds): The Thyroid, 4th ed, pp 773–778. New York, Harper & Row, 1978
26. Herbert V: The megaloblastic anemias. In Beeson PB, McDermott W, Wyngaarden JB (eds): Cecil Textbook of Medicine, 15th ed, pp 1719–1729. Philadelphia, WB Saunders, 1979
27. Herbert V: The nutritional anemias. Hosp Pract 15, No. 3:65–89, 1980
28. Herbert V: Vitamin B_{12}. Am J Clin Nutr 34:971–972, 1981
28a. Herbert V: Megaloblastic anemia with two nutrient deficiencies: Two cases. Med Grand Rounds 1, No. 4, 1982
29. Herbert V, Colman N: Evidence humans may use some analogues of B_{12} as cobalamins (B_{12}): Pure intrinsic factor (IF) radioassay may "diagnose" clinical B_{12} deficiency when it does not exist. Clin Res 29, No. 2:571A, 1981
30. Herbert V, Colman N, Jacob E: Folic acid and vitamin B_{12}. In Goodhart RS, Shils ME (eds): Modern Nutrition in Health and Disease, 6th ed, pp 229–259. Philadelphia, Lea & Febiger, 1980
31. Herbert V, Drivas G, Foscaldi R et al: Multivitamin/mineral food supplements containing vitamin B_{12} may also contain analogs of vitamin B_{12}. New Engl J Med 307:255–256, 1982
32. Hillman RS: Vitamin B_{12}, folic acid and the treatment of megaloblastic anemias. In Gilman AG, Goodman LS, Gilman A (eds): The Pharmacological Basis of Therapeutics, 6th ed, pp 1331–1346. New York, Macmillan, 1980
33. Jacob E, Baker SJ, Herbert V: Vitamin B_{12}-binding proteins. Physiol Rev 60:918–960, 1980
34. Jacob E, Herbert V: Vitamin B_{12} and the nervous system. In Kumar S (ed): Biochemistry of Brain, pp 103–128. New York, Pergamon Press, 1980
35. Kass L: Pernicious Anemia. Philadelphia, WB Saunders, 1976
36. Kolhouse JF, Kondo H, Allen NC et al: Cobalamin analogues are present in human plasma and can mask cobalamin deficiency because current radioisotope dilution assays are not specific for true cobalamin. N Engl J Med 299:785–792, 1978
37. Kondo H, Osborne ML, Kolhouse JF et al: Nitrous oxide has multiple deleterious effects on cobalamin metabolism and causes decreases in activities of both mammalian cobalamin-dependent enzymes in rats. J Clin Invest 67:1270–1283, 1981
38. Lane M, Alfrey CP, Megel CE et al: The rapid induction of human riboflavin deficiency with galactoflavin. J Clin Invest 43:357–373, 1964
39. Lindenbaum J, Nath B: Megaloblastic anemia and neutrophil hypersegmentation. Br J Haematol 44:511–513, 1980
40. Longo DL, Herbert V: Radioassay for serum and red cell folate. J Lab Clin Med 87:138–151, 1976
41. Poncz M, Colman N, Herbert V et al: Therapy of congenital folate malabsorption. J Pediatr 98:76–79, 1981
42. Rosenberg LE: Disorders of propionate, methylmalonate and cobalamin metabolism. In Stanbury JB, Wyngaarden JB, Fredrickson DS (eds): The Metabolic Basis of Inherited Disease, 4th ed, p 411. New York, McGraw–Hill, 1978
43. Scott JM, Weir DG: The methyl folate trap: A physiological response in man to prevent methyl group deficiency in kwashiorkor (methionine deficiency) and an explanation for folic-acid-induced exacerbation of subacute combined degeneration in pernicious anemia. Lancet 2:337–340, 1981
44. Scott JM, Dinn JJ, Wilson P et al: Pathogenesis of subacute combined degeneration: A result of methyl group deficiency. Lancet 2:334–337, 1981
45. Thomas WJ, Koenig HM, Lightsey AL et al: Free erythrocyte protoporphyrin: Hemoglobin ratios, serum ferritin and transferrin saturation levels during treatment of infants with iron-deficiency anemia. Blood 49:455–462, 1977
46. Tisman G, Herbert V: B_{12} dependence of cell uptake of serum folate: An explanation for high serum folate and cell folate depletion in B_{12} deficiency. Blood 41:465–469, 1973
47. Viteri FE, Alvarado J, Luthringer DG et al: Hematological changes in protein calorie malnutrition. Vitam Horm 26:573, 1968
48. WHO Scientific Group on Nutritional Anemias. WHO Technical Report Series 405:1, 1968
49. Williams WJ, Beutler E, Erslev AJ et al (eds): Hematology, 2nd ed. New York, McGraw–Hill, 1977
50. Wintrobe MM, Lee GR, Boggs DR et al (eds): Clinical Hematology. Philadelphia, Lea & Febiger, 1975

24
Immunology
Robert M. Suskind

It is estimated that roughly 100 million children under 5 years of age currently are moderately or severely malnourished. Malnutrition, it must be remembered, is a problem of the developed as well as the developing world. Although primary protein–calorie malnutrition (PCM) is not commonly seen in hospitals in the United States, physicians are becoming increasingly aware of the existence of such malnutrition, which may be secondary to other disease states such as renal, hepatic, or cardiopulmonary disease (see Chap. 9). Such secondary nutritional deficits must also be considered when evaluating the nutritional status of children throughout the world. In this chapter we will focus on children, as a particularly vulnerable fraction of human populations.

Classification of Protein–Calorie Malnutrition

WEIGHT AND HEIGHT CRITERIA

Gomez and colleagues, in 1955, were among the first to define malnutrition in terms of deficits in weight-for-age.[27] Using local standards, they defined first, second, and third degree malnutrition in terms of 75% to 90% of weight-for-age, 60% to 75% of weight-for-age, and less than 60% of weight-for-age, respectively. Over time, Gomez's classification has been modified. Instead of using local standards as a basis for comparison, internationally accepted standards derived from the mean weights and heights of healthy children from North America or Europe are used. Inasmuch as there is little or no evidence that genetic differences affect growth

potential during the early years of life, the norms of developed countries are considered applicable to any community where malnutrition is presented.

Height-for-age and weight-for-height, however, are often more useful tools for defining an individual's nutritional status than is weight-for-age, which does not take into consideration the height deficit caused by chronic malnutrition. The child who has a decreased weight-for-height is wasted or *acutely* malnourished, while the child who has a decreased height-for-age is stunted or *chronically* malnourished. Waterlow has developed criteria for grading children in terms of acute and chronic malnutrition. Children who are 80% to 90%, 70% to 80%, and less than 70% of *weight-for-height* are classified as having evidence of acute malnutrition, grades one, two, and three, respectively. Children who are 90% to 95%, 85% to 90%, and less than 85% of *height-for-age* are classified as having evidence of chronic malnutrition or stunting, grades one, two, and three, respectively. Studies from several developing countries have shown that both wasting and stunting are commonly seen in children between the ages of 1 year and 2 years. By 3 years or 4 years of age, children who may still be underweight for age are largely stunted rather than wasted. In other words, they have stopped growing linearly but are of normal weight-for-height.

MARASMUS AND KWASHIORKOR

The severely malnourished child with marasmus or kwashiorkor has an increased morbidity and mortality secondary to his response infection. Chil-

410

dren develop marasmus as a result of severe deprivation of both protein and calories. They clinically present with growth retardation, weight loss, muscular atrophy, and loss of subcutaneous tissue. Children develop kwashiorkor as a result of acute protein loss or deprivation. Their contrasting clinical picture is characterized by edema, skin lesions, hair changes, apathy, anorexia, an enlarged fatty liver, and decreased serum total protein. These children have abundant subcutaneous fat, recover rapidly on a high-protein diet, and are generally older than those with marasmus. Serum proteins, including transferrin, albumin, lipase, amylase, esterase, and others, are significantly depressed in children with kwashiorkor. Children with marasmus–kwashiorkor have clinical and biochemical parameters somewhere between those with marasmus and those with kwashiorkor.

Children with primary and secondary PCM have nutrient deficits of protein and calories, as well as vitamins and minerals. Their nutrient status is often further confused by superimposed infection (see Chap. 26). Deficiencies of such nutrients as iron, folate, pyridoxine, vitamin A, protein, and calories have been associated with alterations in the immune response. However, in discussing changes in the malnourished child's immune parameters, one cannot unambiguously associate these with any specific nutrient deficiency. One can only initially document the changes in the immune response, and then determine whether the changes are indeed reversible with improved nutrient intake.

Infection and Malnutrition

It is well accepted that the malnourished child is more in jeopardy from the consequences of infection, and that infection is a major stress factor in the increased morbidity and mortality associated with PCM. Infection is itself often a major factor in precipitating acute nutritional deficiencies. The mechanisms by which infection worsens nutritional status include a reduced appetite, a cultural tendency for solid foods to be withheld, especially those of animal origin, increased urinary nitrogen losses, and decreased nitrogen absorption when infection involves the gastrointestinal (GI) tract.

A child's weight gain during the first 4 to 6 months more or less follows the Harvard Standard. Thereafter, the child in the developing world more frequently experiences recurrent infections that result in a plateauing of his weight and height. During the period when there is no significant weight gain, there is usually no increase in height, and the child's weight-for-height remains unchanged. However, with the recurrent acute infections and actual weight loss, a decrease in weight-for-height results and

signifies a worsening of the child's nutritional status.

It is now realized that even the mildest infectious diseases lead to increased urinary nitrogen excretion. The increased nitrogen excretion results mainly from increased mobilization of amino acids from peripheral muscle for gluconeogenesis in the liver, with deamination and the excretion of nitrogen in the form of urea. Unless the loss of nitrogen is compensated by increased dietary intake, depletion will occur and precipitate a kwashiorkorlike syndrome (see Chaps. 11 and 26).

Malnutrition and the Immune Response

Clinical observations suggest that the malnourished individual's immune system may respond to infection differently from that of the well-nourished individual. An organism that may be relatively harmless to the well-nourished child may give rise to a severe or even fatal infection in the malnourished child. When localized infection spreads in a child with PCM, it does so with the development of gangrene and not suppuration.[52] Children with PCM also tend to develop gram-negative septicemia.[41] Several host defenses have been implicated as being affected in the malnourished child. These include (1) the cell-mediated immune (CMI) response, (2) the humoral immune response, (3) the phagocytic and killing function of leukocytes, and (4) the complement system.

THE CELL-MEDIATED IMMUNE RESPONSE

HISTOLOGICAL CHANGES

Jackson was the first to call attention to the lymphoid atrophy associated with severe PCM.[29] He noted at autopsy that children with kwashiorkor had atrophied thymus glands represented by only a few strands of tissue. In addition to atrophy of the thymus, lymph nodes, and tonsils, the spleen appeared to be smaller in malnourished children.[38] Mugerwa found that the thymus weights from ten children who had died of kwashiorkor were significantly less than those from a control group of patients.[38] Histologically, the malnourished thymuses had marked depletion of all small lymphocytes and consisted principally of reticular and epithelial tissue. There were only a few, poorly formed Hassall's corpuscles and no distinction between cortex and medulla. In addition, Mugerwa noted similar changes in peripheral lymph nodes. Not only were abdominal lymph nodes decreased in number, but they also showed evidence of a reduced follicular size as well as depletion of the paracortical areas. Lymphoid follicles were significantly smaller in the appendix and spleen of the malnourished children than of the well-nourished controls. In addition, lymphoid follicles from the malnourished often lacked the normal cuff of small lymphocytes.

Smythe and co-workers, who examined 47 children dying of kwashiorkor and 29 dying of marasmus, noted that the thymuses were abnormal in all of the kwashiorkor cases and in 92% of the cases of marasmus.[52] Douglas and Schopfer also described marked atrophy of the malnourished thymus, which contained very few typical Hassall's corpuscles.[18] Smythe and co-workers also noted significant changes in the spleen weight of the marasmic cases, finding that the spleens weighed only 70% of the control weights, while the spleens of the children with kwashiorkor weighed only 54% of the controls.[52] Histologically, there was marked reduction in germinal center activity in 90% of the cases of kwashiorkor and in 78% of the cases of marasmus. Seventy percent of the cases with kwashiorkor also demonstrated depletion of the lymphocytes in the paracortical and periarteriolar areas, both of which are thymus dependent. Chandra and Smythe and colleagues demonstrated decreased adenoid and tonsillar tissue in children with PCM.[7,52] In addition, Smythe and colleagues observed a significant reduction in the size of the Peyer's patches in the appendix.[52]

A number of investigators have demonstrated moderate lymphopenia in children with PCM.[7] Chandra found that 50 of 90 malnourished children had total lymphocyte counts of less than 2500/mm³.[7] Douglas and Schopfer, who also reported peripheral lymphopenia, described an increased number of "plasmacytes" as identified by electron microscopy in the peripheral blood.[18] Occasional lymphoblasts were also described. Inasmuch as the peripheral lymphocytes responded to the pokeweed mitogen, which is characteristic of B cells, one might conclude that the unusual findings in the peripheral blood may be due to the presence of activated B cells. One might conclude from the information to date that PCM may have a differential effect on subpopulations of lymphocytes, as suggested by the findings of at least partial preservation of the thymus-independent or B cell areas as well as the finding of normal plasma cell numbers in the lymph nodes and spleen. One might, therefore, conclude that based on those studies alone the cellular immune function would be more severely affected than humoral function in patients with PCM.

The etiology of the changes in the lymphoid tissue is not clearly understood. It is obvious that cell division and proliferation are severely restricted. The concentrations of certain hormones, such as thyroxine, epinephrine, and steroids, which are all capable of having significant effects on lymphocytes and lymphoid tissue, are all altered in PCM (see Chap. 20).

IN VIVO CELL-MEDIATED IMMUNE CHANGES

In 1958 Jayalakshami and Gopalan were the first to note that the percentage of positive tuberculin skin tests was significantly lower in children with PCM than in a control population.[30] They were also the first to suggest that nutritional rehabilitation could lead to a repair of a defective skin test response. Harland and Brown found that children whose weight-for-age was less than 80% of standard had significantly smaller tuberculin skin reactions following BCG immunization than did well-nourished controls.[28] Lloyd also noted that only 11 of 51 children (22%) admitted to the Kampala Hospital in Uganda with severe malnutrition and active tuberculosis were tuberculin skin-test positive as measured by Heaf test.[36] However, this defect appeared to be relative. When 40 of the children who were negative were rechallenged with 100 TU of old tuberculin, 18 subsequently had positive skin tests.

Subsequently, there have been several reports describing a defective delayed cutaneous hypersensitivity (DCH) response when children with PCM were challenged with a battery of recall antigens, including Tricophyton, streptokinase–streptodornase, diphtheria, *Candida albicans,* and PPD.[21] Geefhuysen and co-workers demonstrated a significantly impaired DCH response to diphtheria and *Candida* in children with varying degrees of kwashiorkor. After 21 days of nutritional support, positive responses were obtained in all 10 children when challenged with *Candida* skin testing and in 12 who had been tested with diphtheria antigen. Work and colleagues found a significantly depressed DCH reaction to *Candida* in children with kwashiorkor, with the greatest impairment found in those who were most severely malnourished.[56] He also noted a reduced skin-test response in undernourished children with growth retardation, but with normal serum albumin concentrations. Chandra has reported that the majority of Nigerian adults with pulmonary tuberculosis and evidence of malnutrition have negative skin-test responses to 5 TU of PPD, with the size of the induration correlating significantly with serum transferrin and albumin levels.[13] Investigators have noted improved subcutaneous hypersensitivity responses after nutritional repair.[7]

Some investigators have also demonstrated significant impairment of the primary DCH response in children with PCM. Chandra noted that only 22% of patients with PCM converted after BCG vaccination as compared to 72% of controls.[7] Sinha and co-workers noted a decreased tuberculin response after BCG in children whose weight-for-age was less than 60% of standard.[50] Keilman and colleagues noted that a group of nonhospitalized clinically normal children who had decreased body weight-for-age had impaired BCG tuberculin sensitivity when immunized as malnourished children.[33] This deficit improved after nutritional repair. Smith and co-workers found significant impairment of both the inflammatory response and recall challenge to dinitrochlorobenzene in children with PCM, with marasmic patients responding less than those with marasmus–kwashiorkor.[51] Work and colleagues noted a correlation between the severity of the PCM and depression of the dinitrochlorobenzene reactivity, with significant improvement occurring in response after the initiation of nutritional therapy.[57]

To evaluate the inflammatory response in children with PCM, 2 mg dinitrofluorobenzene (DNFB) was applied to the forearms of 30 children on admission to the hospital.[22] Five additional children were studied on hospital day 15, and 8 were studied on day 56 (see Table 24-1). The presence or absence of erythema and induration was determined 2 days after application of DNFB. Of children studied with DNFB on admission, only 4 of 30 (13%) had positive inflammatory responses, with 6 of 8 (75%) of children on day 56 having positive responses ($p < 0.01$). The results of this initial study indicated that the children with PCM were unable to develop a normal inflammatory response, whereas nutritionally recovered children were able to respond.

Next, the ability to sensitize PCM patients with 2 mg DNFB was evaluated. Ten children sensitized with DNFB on day 1 and all of the children sensitized on days 15 and 56 were rechallenged on day 72 with 100 μg DNFB (see Table 24-2). Of those sensitized on admission only 2 (20%) recalled the initial sensitization while 7 (87%) of the 8 children sensitized on day 56 recalled the challenge on day 72 ($p < 0.05$). The results of this study suggest that most children with severe PCM have circulating lymphocytes that cannot be sensitized. However, noncomitted lymphocytes that *can* be sensitized are regenerated with nutritional repair.

Most children with severe PCM are not able to recall prior sensitization to a foreign antigen. However, because of the depressed inflammatory response, it is difficult to determine whether the decreased skin-test reactivity is secondary to a depressed recall phenomenon or to the depressed inflammatory response itself.

In summary, most studies to date have demonstrated that varying degrees of malnutrition impair

TABLE 24-1
Cutaneous Inflammatory Response to 2 mg Dinitrofluorobenzene (DNFB)

Day Tested	Number of Patients	Skin Response	
		Positive	Negative
1	30	4 (13%)*	26
15	5	3 (60%)	2
56	8	6 (75%)*	2

*Significantly different ($\chi^2 = 9.4$; $p < 0.01$)

From Edelman R, Suskind R, Olsen RE et al: Mechanisms of defective delayed cutaneous hypersensitivity in children with protein–calorie malnutrition. Lancet 1:506–508, 1973

the DCH response. However, with nutritional rehabilitation the defects in DCH are readily reversible.

IN VITRO T-CELL RESPONSES

Peripheral T-cell Numbers. Several reports have documented decreased peripheral blood T cells in children with PCM.[4] T cells may be identified operationally by their ability to bind spontaneously to sheep red blood cells (SRBC), forming a rosette. Chandra was the first to describe the profound depression in peripheral T-cell levels in Indian children with PCM.[8] He found a significant correlation between the degree of weight deficit and depressed T-cell levels. With nutritional rehabilitation, the mean level increased from 23% to 60% with the control level being 71%. Ferguson and colleagues found a similar depression in T-cell levels in Ghanaian children with marasmus or kwashiorkor.[25] The admission T-cell level rose from 16.6% to normal levels within 7 to 17 days after the starting of a high-protein, high-carbohydrate diet.

Kulapongs and co-workers likewise found that the severe T-cell depression returned to normal within 29 days of initiation of nutritional therapy

TABLE 24-2
Attempt to Sensitize PCM Patients Against 2 mg Dinitrofluorobenzene (DNFB)

Day of Sensitizing Dose Application	Number of Patients	Skin-test Response*	
		Positive	Negative
1	10	2†	8
15	5	1	4
56	8	7†	1

*Skin test dose of 100 g DNFB applied on day 70 and read on day 72

†Significantly different ($\chi^2 = 4.7$; $p < 0.05$)

From Edelman R, Suskind R, Olson RE et al: Mechanisms of defective delayed cutaneous hypersensitivity in children with protein–calorie malnutrition. Lancet 1:506–508, 1973

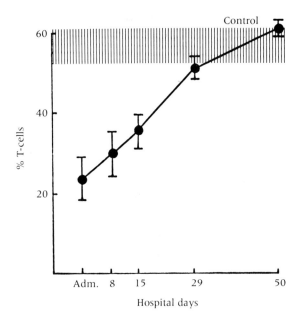

FIG. 24-1 Percentage of T-cells in children with protein–calorie malnutrition (PCM) on admission and throughout recovery (mean ± SEM). (From Kulapongs P, Suskind RM, Vithayasai V, et al: *In vitro* cell-mediated immune response in Thai children with protein–calorie malnutrition. In Suskind RM (ed): Malnutrition and The Immune Response, pp 99–104, New York, Raven Press, 1977)

(Fig. 24-1).[35] Although Schopfer and Douglas found no significant difference in the percentage of T cells in children with PCM as compared to controls, the absolute number of T cells in the malnourished children was significantly depressed.[44] While most reports indicate that depression of T-cell number is the rule rather than the exception, Drenick and colleagues found that, when healthy adults were starved for ten or more days, there was no effect on T-cell concentration or functional activity.[20] Chandra reported that in addition to the depressed T lymphocytes and normal B cells in children with PCM that the relative proportion of "null" cells, the function of which is unknown, was significantly increased as they are in clinical disorders associated with depressed cellular immunity, such as leprosy, cancer, and primary immunodeficiency syndromes.[11] *Null cells*, which are defined as lymphocytes that do not carry conventional surface markers of T or B cells, have an unknown functional significance. The reduction in T-cell numbers in malnourished children may be secondary to thymic atrophy and a decreased circulating thymocin level, a quantitative defect in T-lymphocyte function, or a simple redistribution of T and B cells. Smythe and co-workers have reported significant increases in C-reactive protein in over 40 patients

with PCM.[52] Mortensen and co-workers recently noted that C-reactive protein selectively binds to human T lymphocytes, thus inhibiting their ability to form erythrocyte (E) rosettes and to respond to allogenic cells *in vitro*.[37]

Lymphocyte Transformation. Isolated lymphocytes when incubated with plant lectins, known as mitogens, or antigens such as tetanus toxoid, undergo blast transformation and synthesize DNA prior to division. Response to these mitogens may be assessed by determining the percent blast-cell transformation or by determining the incorporation of tritiated thymidine into DNA. Most investigators have found a significant impairment in phytohemagglutinin (PHA)-induced lymphocyte transformation correlating well with simultaneous tests of delayed cutaneous sensitivity.[7]

Kulapongs and colleagues also described decreased thymidine uptake and blast-cell transformation of isolated lymphocytes stimulated with PHA (see Figs. 24-2 and 24-3).[35] With two weeks of the nutritional therapy, lymphocytes from the formerly malnourished children were responding normally to mitogenic stimulation.

FIG. 24-2 Thymidine incorporation of PHA-stimulated lymphocytes. Stimulation index = Counts/min PHA-stimulated cells × counts/min unstimulated cells (mean ± SEM). (From Kulapongs P, Suskind RM, Vithayasai V, et al: *In vitro* cell-mediated immune response in Thai children with protein–calorie malnutrition. In Suskind RM (ed): Malnutrition and The Immune Response, pp 99–104, New York, Raven Press, 1977)

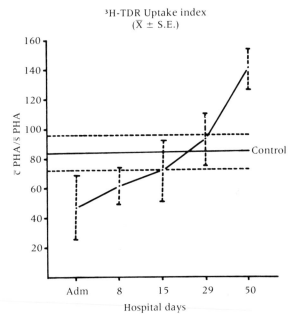

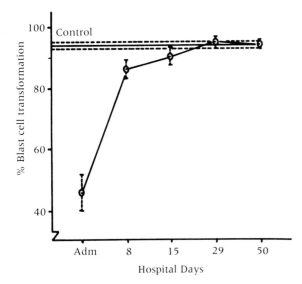

FIG. 24-3 Percentage of blast cell transformation of PHA-stimulated lymphocytes (mean ± SEM). (From Kulapongs P, Suskind RM, Vithayasai V, et al: *In vitro* cell-mediated immune response in Thai children with protein–calorie malnutrition. In Suskind RM (ed): Malnutrition and The Immune Response, pp 99–104, New York, Raven Press, 1977)

Not all workers, however, have found an impaired T-cell response in malnourished children. Work and colleagues found a depressed PHA response in only the most severely malnourished children.[56]

Lymphokine Production. When lymphocytes are stimulated *in vivo* or *in vitro*, they normally produce a wide variety of substances that mediate the responses of the cellular immune response. To date there is only one report of lymphokine production in malnourished children; Schlesinger and colleagues found that interferon production was significantly reduced in cultures from marasmic infants as compared to control cultures.[43] Decreased lymphokine production has also been noted in animals with PCM.

SUMMARY

Thus, a significant body of clinical and laboratory data suggests that the malnourished child has a reduced capacity to mount a cellular immune response to a variety of infectious agents. Fortunately for the host, the depression of this system lasts only as long as the nutritional deprivation. It should be pointed out, however, that in the clinical studies to date it has been impossible to determine which factors interacting with the immune response are responsible for the depressed *in vivo* and *in vitro* CMI response.

THE HUMORAL IMMUNE RESPONSE

There is a large body of information dealing with humoral immunity in PCM. Investigators have determined immunoglobulin levels and specific antibody responses. The results, however, have often been conflicting and confusing. Major reasons for the lack of consistency have been primarily the lack of control over such variables as the presence of concomitant infection, the duration and severity of malnutrition, the dose and type of antigen used, the presence of other nutrient deficiencies, and the effect of nutritional intervention on the response. In spite of the conflicting data, several of the observations regarding humoral immunity in malnourished patients are pertinent. Investigators assessing the humoral immune system have measured the five classes of immunoglobulin (IgG, IgM, IgA, IgD, IgE), the number of B lymphocytes, and the antibody response to specific antigenic stimuli.

IMMUNOGLOBULIN LEVELS

Although decreased serum albumin is characteristically found in children with kwashiorkor, total gamma globulin is usually normal or increased. Cohen and Hansen, who evaluated albumin and gamma globulin metabolism in kwashiorkor, found that the albumin anabolic and catabolic rates, as well as the total albumin pool, were significantly reduced.[15] In contrast to albumin metabolism, distribution and turnover of gamma globulin were unaffected in the malnourished child. In the severely infected malnourished child the rate of synthesis of gamma globulin was three times that of noninfected patients, while the catabolic rate for gamma globulin was unchanged. It is obvious that the increased gamma-globulin synthesis does confer some survival advantage to the host.

The serum immunoglobulin level generally reflects past infections and other antigenic experiences of the host. The vast majority of studies have found that the five classes of serum immunoglobulins are either normal when compared to control values or increased. Work and colleagues found increased immunoglobulin levels in the malnourished patients whom he studied, as did Chandra, who studied 90 children with PCM.[7,56] Other studies have correlated either normal or elevated levels of different immunoglobulins with the severity of the disease or with the age of the patients.[23] Some investigators, however, have not found the severity of the deficiency state to be a factor in determining the immunoglobulin levels.[55] One study reported by Kielmann and colleagues revealed normal IgM and IgG levels with decreased IgA levels in children with mild undernutrition.[33] For an extensive study of all five immunoglobulins in marasmus and kwashiorkor see the article by Suskind and co-workers.[53]

SERUM B CELLS

The bursa cell, or B lymphocyte, is responsible for immunoglobulin production. The competency of the B-lymphocyte system is determined by enumerating the number of B lymphocytes that can be identified by the presence of one of five major classes of immunoglobulin on the surface membrane, the presence of membrane receptors for the C3 component of complement, and the receptors for the *Fc* portion of the *aggregated IgG*. To date, only a few clinical studies have been undertaken in which peripheral B-cell levels have been evaluated in children with PCM. No studies to date have evaluated tissue B-cell changes in PCM. Thus Bang and colleagues found increased levels of B cells in malnourished children, but attributed this to concomitant infection.[4] Schopfer and Douglas studied noninfected children with kwashiorkor and found that, although there was no significant difference in the percentage of circulating B cells between the malnourished patients (8.3%) and the controls (14.6%), the absolute number of B cells was significantly decreased.[44]

SERUM ANTIBODY RESPONSE

Antibody response to antigens such as yellow fever vaccine, influenza vaccine, and typhoid vaccine have been shown to be impaired in malnourished children, while the antibody response to other antigens such as Keyhole limpet hemocyanin, lipopolysaccharide, measles, polio virus, tetanus, and diphtheria toxoid appears to be adequate.[6,31] Malnourished children also respond normally to smallpox immunization.[6] In some studies, lack of specific nutrients such as pyridoxine and pantothenic acid has been implicated in the suppression of the antibody response.[3] It has not been determined which of the specific nutrient deficiencies in the malnourished child is responsible for the depressed response. The presence of associated infection may suppress antibody synthesis.[31] Interpretation of the data is very difficult in most studies because of lack of information on several critical variables, such as dose of the antigen, its route of delivery, the severity of the malnutrition, the presence of infection, differences in nutritional therapy, and the status of liver function.

Suskind and co-workers studied antibody response in malnourished children to typhoid antigen.[53] Children with PCM who were immunized on admission showed essentially no increase in antibody titer in the first week, during which they received 100 Cal and 1 g protein/kg. The nutritionally recovered children, who were receiving 175 Cal and 4 g protein/kg, showed a significant increase in antibody activity over the preimmunization level within a week after immunization (p < 0.05).

The response to an antigenic stimulus constitutes a more sensitive and reliable evaluation of the humoral immune system than does the level of circulating immunoglobulins. When the malnourished child's nutritional state improves, his antibody response to some antigenic stimuli also improves.

SECRETORY ANTIBODY RESPONSE

Secretory antibodies, which protect the mucosal surfaces, may be the first immunological defense encountered by a parasite. This system of immunoglobulins is widely distributed throughout the body and is found in secretions of the bronchopulmonary and intestinal mucosa, the lacrimal glands, salivary glands, and breast secretions. Although IgE and IgA may both be present in the secretions of these organs, the major antibody is secretory IgA which consists of a dimer of IgA molecules bound tightly together by a nonimmunoglobulin glycoprotein, the so-called secretory component. Immunocompetent plasma cells and lymphocytes in the submucosa secrete IgA, which combines with the secretory component elaborated at the mucosa surfaces and is itself synthesized by epithelial cells. Secretory IgA has been shown to demonstrate antibody activity against bacteria, viruses, food antigens, and bacterial toxins. Abnormalities of secretory IgA have been reported in children with PCM.

Chandra demonstrated that malnourished children respond to immunization with live attenuated measles or polio virus with significantly lower levels of secretory IgA than do controls.[9] The mechanism by which secretory IgA production is decreased in PCM is unclear. It is unlikely that the decreased levels result from an impairment of local protein synthesis or local proteolysis because other proteins, such as IgE and albumin lysozymes, are reported in normal concentrations. Chandra excluded reabsorption of secretory IgA through the mucous membrane by showing that the reaction between the patient's serum and antiserum to the secretory component was negative.[13] The most likely explanation for the decreased secretory IgA is a selective depression of IgA synthesis in the submucosa or a reduction in the synthesis of the secretory component by epithelial cells or both.[13] This hypothesis is consistent with the pathological finding in PCM of a loss of intestinal epithelial cells with mucosal thickening in association with atrophy of such GI-associated lymphoid tissue as the appendix, Peyer's patches, and the tonsils.[52] The consequences of a reduced secretory IgA are not known.

POLYMORPHONUCLEAR LEUKOCYTE

Although polymorphonuclear leukocyte function has been extensively studied in malnourished children, the results have not always been clear. The results of the studies have often been contradictory because of the poorly defined patient population which was inadequately nutritionally assessed and which was not well defined in terms of the presence or lack of superimposed infection. Several more specific phases of phagocyte function have been studied in the malnourished child, including mobilization, chemotaxis, phagocytosis or ingestion of particles, postphagocytic function including phagocytic vacuole formation, and specific metabolic changes leading to intracellular killing of the microorganism.

MOBILIZATION

Chandra and colleagues were among the first to evaluate as a functional parameter the mobilization of polymorphonuclear leukocytes from marginal bone marrow and other pools.[12] They demonstrated that with epinephrine, which leads to splenic constriction and release of leukocytes from other sites, there was a normal increase in peripheral blood leukocytes in untreated children with PCM. In addition, they found that with the administration of *Pseudomonas* polysaccharide the neutrophilia which normally occurs as a result of the administration of this polysaccharide did not occur in children with PCM, suggesting inadequate marrow reserves of polymorphonuclear leukocytes.

CHEMOTAXIS AND
THE INFLAMMATORY RESPONSE

Chemotaxis, the ability of the polymorphonuclear leukocyte to migrate toward an external stimulus, is of fundamental importance to a normal inflammatory response. This inflammatory response should result in localization of invading pathogens and activation of systems in order to deal with infecting organisms. One might expect that children with kwashiorkor, who have superficial pyogenic infections and who are unable to develop suppurative lesions, would have a depressed polymorphonuclear leukocyte response. Freyre, who studied the inflammatory response in 33 uninfected Peruvian children with PCM, found that these chil-

dren had a normal polymorphonuclear leukocyte response.[26] However, there was a significant depression in the macrophage response in these same malnourished children. This is a pattern which is similar to that seen in neonates and was found in children with kwashiorkor as well as those with marasmus.

PHAGOCYTOSIS

Most studies to date have found that phagocytosis by the polymorphonuclear leukocyte using a variety of particles is not significantly affected in malnourished children.

Macrophages are the phagocytes that provide primary defense against facultative intracellular organisms such as *Salmonella typhimurium*, *Brucella*, and *Mycobacterium* tuberculosis. In addition, they play an important role in antigen recognition and processing, with subsequent interaction with T and B cells to initiate cellular and humoral antibody responses. Indeed, very few studies have been done in human populations looking at macrophage function because of the large quantity of cells required. Animal studies have demonstrated a rather normal macrophage function in PCM.

POSTPHAGOCYTIC EVENTS

Although information is scarce, electron micrograph (EM) studies of phagocytes have revealed no qualitative difference between those from malnourished and control children with regard to vacuole formation after the phagocytosis of *C. albicans*, *E. coli* or *Staphylococcus aureus* or after the ingestion of several microbial species in protein-deficient rats.[32]

Intracellular Killing. As indicated above, studies evaluating chemotaxis and phagocytosis have indicated relatively normal polymorphonuclear leukocyte function with regard to these two activities in PCM. There is, however, conflicting evidence regarding the intracellular killing function of polymorphonuclear leukocytes (PMNs) in these circumstances. A number of investigators have reported normal intracellular killing by the phagocytes of malnourished children.[5] Arbeter and co-workers noted that the intracellular killing activity was unaffected in children and adults with PCM unless iron deficiency was also found.[1] Seth and Chandra noted an inefficient killing of phagocytosed bacteria by PMNs from patients with PCM, as did Douglas and Schopfer who found impaired bacterial killing activity of PMNs isolated from malnourished children when incubated with *S. aureus*, *E. coli*, and *C. albicans*.[17,19]

BIOCHEMISTRY OF THE PHAGOCYTE

METABOLITES

Glycolysis is the major metabolic pathway that provides energy for the polymorphonuclear leukocyte to phagocytize particles. Yoshida and co-workers found that PMNs from severely malnourished children had decreased levels of lactate, pyruvate, and oxaloacetate in addition to a decrease pyruvate kinase, which is the rate-limiting enzyme in glycolysis.[57] Only lactate was diminished in patients with mild to moderate PCM. Likewise, they found that the total adenine nucleotide content was significantly decreased owing to a decrease in ATP with the ratio of ATP to AMP/ADP being significantly decreased in the severely malnourished group. They also found other metabolites to be normal, including phosphoenolypyruvate, malate, and alpha-ketoglutarate.[57] The relevance of these findings with regard to phagocytic function remains unclear, for although certain metabolites and enzymes are indeed depressed in the glycolytic pathway, phagocytosis has ultimately been characterized as being relatively normal in the malnourished host.[17]

ENZYME ACTIVITIES

Pineda and co-workers found that in normal children who were either protein or calorie deprived for short periods of time, changes in enzyme activities were detectable in their polymorphonuclear leukocytes.[42] Low-protein diets resulted in increases in fumarase, isocitrate, and malate dehydrogenases and aspartate and alanine amino transferases. On the other hand, decreased calorie intake caused depression of the same enzymes within three days. Again, the relevance of these findings is unclear. Douglas and Schopfer noted increased hexose monophosphate shunt activity in the polymorphonuclear leukocytes from children with kwashiorkor. Although the hexose monophosphate shunt was elevated, activity increased normally during phagocytosis, suggesting preservation of normal metabolic activity. Other key enzymes in the polymorphonuclear leukocyte are myeloperoxidase and NADPH oxidase. Douglas and Schopfer found normal resting NADPH and NADH oxidases in the polymorphonuclear leukocytes from children with kwashiorkor, while Selvaraj and Bhat found decreased granule-bound NADPH oxidase activity and a failure to increase with phagocytic stimulation.[19,46,47] Activity of these enzymes returned to normal with the intake of a high-protein, high-calorie diet. When investigators looked at myeloperoxidase in peripheral PMNs from children with kwashiorkor and marasmus, they found

normal levels.[2,45] Lysosomal enzymes that have been measured, including alkaline and acid phosphatase, have been found to be normal, increased, or decreased in PCM patients when compared to controls.[2,40,54] Acid cathepsin, another lysosomal enzyme involved in digestion of vacuole contents, has been reported to be normal in children with kwashiorkor and decreased in white cells from marasmic patients as well as from protein-deficient monkeys.[2,24,33]

FUNCTIONAL BIOCHEMISTRY

Several investigators have examined nitroblue tetrazolium (NBT) as a measure of intraneutrophilic metabolic function. Results of the qualitative and quantitative NBT tests have differed. Kendall and associates found a significant reduction in the percentage of formazan-positive cells in malnourished children.[34] Likewise, Shousha and Kanel found a markedly depressed percentage of formazan-positive cells despite the presence of infection in each of the undernourished subjects he studied.[49] There appeared to be a significant correlation between the percentage of cells reducing NBT, the total serum protein, serum albumin, and hemoglobin levels. On the other hand, Wolfsdorf and Nolan found a significantly increased percentage of NBT-positive PMNs in infants with PCM whether or not they were infected.[55]

In contrast to the qualitative NBT tests, Bhuyan and colleagues found that the resting quantitative NBT reduction test was normal in children with PCM.[5] Chandra had similar findings, noting that even though quantitative NBT reduction in resting PMNs from children with PCM was increased, maximum production of formazan after phagocytosis was comparable with controls.[14] Avila and associates also found increased NBT reduction in children with marasmus and kwashiorkor.[2] The above results suggest that the PMNs from malnourished children had been stimulated *in vivo* either by infection, bacterial pathogens, bacterial products, or immune complexes.

The final functional parameter, which has been studied by Schopfer and Schopfer, was the incorporation *in vitro* of I^{131} into precipitable protein after phagocytosis.[45] They found that the kinetics of iodination in PMNs from noninfected children with PCM resulted in a significantly lower iodination of protein that correlated closely with reduced killing activity against *C. albicans*, *S. aureus*, and *E. coli*.

Thus, the weight of evidence suggests that the increased consequences of infection in malnourished children may be due, at least in part, to somewhat depressed polymorphonuclear leukocyte function. Although the studies are conflicting, a series of small defects, including delayed chemotaxis, slightly depressed bactericidal activity, and mildly abnormal metabolic functions, seems to point to a somewhat defective polymorphonuclear leukocyte in a few selected malnourished children. In addition, there appears to be increased resting activity of the hexose monophosphate shunt with impaired activation during phagocytosis and decreased iodination during particle ingestion. Obviously, additional studies in well-controlled patient groups are required to define fully the abnormalities in phagocytic function in PCM.

COMPLEMENT SYSTEM

Several investigators have found that the complement system in children with PCM is adversely affected. Indeed, it may be the depressed complement system that is responsible for the decreased inflammatory response and the nature of serious gram-negative sepsis found in malnourished children.

Smythe and colleagues found that the majority of children with PCM had significantly reduced total hemolytic complement levels.[52] The finding of C3 and C4 components on the surface of red cells in many patients also suggested activation of the complement system. Chandra found significantly decreased serum C3 levels in undernourished infants who had deficits in height and weight-for-age.[7] Other investigators have also noted decreased C3 and C4 levels in malnourished children.[16,39] Chandra found that the mean total hemolytic activity and C3 levels were significantly decreased in young children with PCM, with the reductions being most pronounced in those children with overt infections.[10] Chandra also found evidence of complement activation in reporting an altered C3 level as well as the presence of immunoconglutinin, which is an antibody for activated or converted C3 or C4 in several malnourished patients.[10]

Studies indicate that the malnourished host, whether primarily or secondarily malnourished, is at risk of developing secondary infections. The increased susceptibility of the host to infection is now more clearly understood because of investigations of the various immune parameters that have been undertaken during the past ten years. It has been clearly demonstrated that the cell-mediated immune system, whether studied *in vivo* or *in vitro*, is severely depressed in the undernourished host. It is not yet clear to what degree nutrients and superimposed infection are responsible for this depressed system. Although circulating immunoglobulins are elevated in PCM, the ability of the malnourished child to respond to certain antigenic stimuli is compromised by the child's nutritional status. Small defects in the polymorphonuclear

leukocyte in terms of chemotaxis, intracellular killing, and metabolic responses may indeed be responsible for a mildly defective polymorphonuclear leukocyte in selected patients. On the other hand, the complement system has been clearly demonstrated to be compromised in the malnourished host. One cannot say whether the deficiency in one system or another is responsible for the increased host susceptibility. It is most likely a summation of the various immune deficits that causes the malnourished host to be at greater risk of developing serious, overwhelming infections leading in turn to his becoming even more malnourished as a result of the superimposed infection.

References

1. Arbeter A, Echeverri L, Franco D et al: Nutrition and infection. Fed Proc 30:1421–1422, 1971
2. Avila JL, Velaquez–Avila G, Correa C et al: Leukocyte enzyme differences between the clinical forms of malnutrition. Clin Chim Acta 49:5–10, 1973
3. Axelrod AE: Immune processes in vitamin deficiency states. Am J Clin Nutr 24:265–271, 1971
4. Bang BG, Mahalanabis D, Mukherjee KL et al: T and B lymphocyte rosetting in undernourished children. Proc Soc Exp Biol Med 149:199–203, 1975
5. Bhuyan UN, Mohapatra LN, Ramalingaswami V: Phagocytosis, bactericidal activity and nitroblue tetrazolium reduction by the rabbit neutrophil in protein malnutrition. Indian J Med Res 62:42–51, 1974
6. Brown RE, Katz M: Failure of antibody production to yellow fever vaccine in children with kwashiorkor. Trop Geogr Med 18:125–218, 1966
7. Chandra RK: Immunocompetence in undernutrition. J Pediatr 81:1194–1200, 1972
8. Chandra RK: Rosette-forming T lymphocytes and cell-mediated immunity in malnutrition. Br Med J 3:608–609, 1974
9. Chandra RK: Reduced serum and secretory antibody response to live attenuated measles and poliovirus vaccines in malnourished children. Br Med J 2:583–585, 1975
10. Chandra RK: Serum complement and immunoconglutinin in malnutrition. Arch Dis Child 50:225–229, 1975
11. Chandra RK: Lymphocyte subpopulations in human malnutrition: Cytotoxic and suppressor cells. Pediatrics 59:423–427, 1977
12. Chandra RK, Chandra S, Ghal OP: Chemotaxis, random mobility and mobilization of polymorphonuclear leukocytes in malnutrition. J Clin Pathol 29:224–227, 1976
13. Chandra RK, Newberne PM: Nutrition, immunity and infection. New York, Plenum, 1977
14. Chandra RK, Seth V, Chandra S et al: Polymorphonuclear leukocyte function in the malnourished Indian children. In Suskind RM (ed): Malnutrition and the Immune Response, pp 259–264. New York, Raven Press, 1977
15. Cohen S, Hanssen JDL: Metabolism of albumin and gamma globulin in kwashiorkor. Clin Sci 23:351–359, 1962
16. Coovadia HM, Parent MA, Loening WEK et al: An evaluation of factors associated with the depression of immunity in malnutrition and in measles. Am J Clin Nutr 27:665–669, 1974

17. Douglas SD, Schopfer K: Phagocyte function in protein–calorie malnutrition. Clin Exp Immunol 17:121–128, 1974
18. Douglas SD, Schopfer K: *In vitro* studies of lymphocytes from children with kwashiorkor. Clin Immunol Immunopathol 5:21–30, 1976
19. Douglas SD, Schopfer K: The phagocyte in protein–calorie malnutrition—a review. In Suskind RM (ed): Malnutrition and the Immune Response, pp 231–244. New York, Raven Press, 1977
20. Drenick EJ, Alvarez LC: Neutropenia in prolonged fasting. Am J Clin Nutr 24:859–863, 1971
21. Edelman R: Cell-mediated immune response in protein–calorie malnutrition—a review. In Suskind RM (ed): Malnutrition and the Immune Response, pp 47–75. New York, Raven Press, 1977
22. Edelman R, Suskind R, Olson RE et al: Mechanisms of defective delayed cutaneous hypersensitivity in children with protein–calorie malnutrition. Lancet 1:506–508, 1973
23. El–Gholmy A, Helmy O, Hashish S et al: A study of immunoglobulins in kwashiorkor. J Trop Med Hyg 73:192–195, 1970
24. Felsenfeld O, Gyr K: Polymorphonuclear leukocytes in protein deficiency. Am J Clin Nutr 30:1393–1397, 1977
25. Ferguson AC, Lawlor CJ Jr, Neumann C et al: Transient cellular immunodeficiencies in malnutrition. Fed Proc 34:227, 1975
26. Freyre EA, Chabes A, Poemape O et al: Abnormal Rebuck skin window response in kwashiorkor. J Pediatr 82:523–526, 1973
27. Gomez F, Galavan R, Cravioto J et al: Malnutrition in infancy and childhood with special reference to kwashiorkor. Adv Pediatr 7:131–169, 1955
28. Harland PS, Brown RE: Tuberculin sensitivity following B.C.B. vacciniation in undernourished children. East Afr Med J 42:233–238, 1965
29. Jackson CM: The Effects of Inanition and Malnutrition Upon Growth and Structure, p 285. Philadelphia, Blakiston, 1925
30. Jayalakshmi VT, Gopalan C: Nutrition and tuberculosis. I. An epidemiologic study. Indian J Med Res 46:87–92, 1958
31. Jose DG, Welch JS, Doherty RL: Humoral and cellular immune responses to streptococci, influenza and other antigens in Australian aboriginal children. Aust Paediatr J 6:192–202, 1970
32. Kabat EA, Mayer MM: Experimental Immunochemistry, p 133. Springfield, IL, Charles C Thomas, 1961
33. Keilmann AA, Uberoi IS, Chandra RK et al: The effect of nutritional status on immune capacity and immune responses in preschool children in a rural community in India. Bull WHO 54:477–483, 1976
34. Kendall AC, Nolan R: Polymorphonuclear leukocyte activity in malnourished children. Cent Afr J Med 18:73–76, 1972
35. Kulapongs P, Suskind RM, Vithayasai V et al: *In vitro* cell-mediated immune response in Thai children with protein–calorie malnutrition. In Suskind RM (ed): Malnutrition and the Immune Response, pp 99–104. New York, Raven Press, 1977
36. Lloyd AVC: Tuberculin test in children with malnutrition. Br Med J 3:529–531, 1968
37. Mortensen RF, Osmand AP, Gewurz H: Effects of C-reactive protein on the lymphoid system. I. Binding to thymus-dependent lymphocytes and alteration of their functions. J Exp Med 141:821–839, 1975
38. Mugerwa JW: The lymphoreticular system in kwashiorkor. J Pathol 105:105–109, 1971
39. Munson D, Franco D, Arbeter A et al: Serum levels of immunoglobulins, cell-mediated immunity, and phagocytosis in protein–calorie malnutrition. Am J Clin Nutr 27:625–628, 1974
40. Palmblad J: Fasting (acute energy deprivation) in man: Effect on polymorphonuclear granulocyte functions, plasma iron and serum transferrin. Scand J Haematol 17:217–226, 1976
41. Phillips I, Wharton B: Acute bacterial infection in kwashiorkor and marasmus. Br Med J 1:407, 1968
42. Pineda O, Viteri F, Braham JE: Leukocyte enzyme adaption to low protein–calorie diets. Fed Proc 30:231, 1971
43. Schlesinger L, Oldbaum A, Grez L et al: Cell-mediated immune studies in marasmic children from Chile: Delayed hypersensitivity, lymphocyte transformation, and interferon production. In Suskind RM (ed): Malnutrition and the Immune Response, pp 91–98. New York, Raven Press, 1977
44. Schopfer K, Douglas SD: *In vitro* studies of lymphocytes from children with kwashiorkor. Clin Immunol Immunopathol 5:21–30, 1976
45. Schopfer KS, Schopfer D: Neutrophil function in children with kwashiorkor. J Lab Clin Med 88:450–461, 1976
46. Selvaraj RJ, Bhat KS: Metabolic and bacterial activities of leukocytes in protein–calorie malnutrition. Am J Clin Nutr 25:166–174, 1972
47. Selvaraj RJ, Bhat KS: Phagocytosis and leukocyte enzymes in protein–calorie malnutrition. Biochem J 127:255–259, 1972
48. Seth V, Chandra RK: Opsonic activity, phagocytosis, and bactericidal capacity of polymorphs in undernutrition. Arch Dis Child 47:282–284, 1972
49. Shousha S, Kamel K: Nitroblue tetrazolium test in children with kwashiorkor with a comment on the use of latex particles in the test. J Clin Pathol 25:494–497, 1972
50. Sinha DP, Bang FB: Protein and calorie malnutrition, cell-mediated immunity, and B.C.G. vaccination in children from rural West Bengal. Lancet 2:531–534, 1976
51. Smith NJ, Khadroui S, Lopez V et al: Cellular immune response in Tunisian children with severe infantile malnutrition. In Suskind RM (ed): Malnutrition and the Immune Response, pp 105–110. New York, Raven Press, 1977
52. Smythe PM, Brereton–Stiles GG, Grace HJ et al: Thymolymphatic deficiency and depression of cell-mediated immunity in protein–calorie malnutrition. Lancet 2:939–943, 1971
53. Suskind RM, Sirisinha S, Edelman R et al: Immunoglobulins and antibody response in Thai children with protein–calorie malnutrition. In Suskind RM (ed): Malnutrition and the Immune Response, p 185. New York, Raven Press, 1977
54. Trakatellis AC, Axelrod AE: Effect of pyridoxine deficiency on nucleic acid metabolism in the rat. Biochem J 95:344–349, 1965
55. Wolfsdorf J, Nolan R: Leukocyte function in protein deficiency states. S Afr Med J 48:528–530, 1974
56. Work TH, Ifekwunige A, Jelliffe D et al: Tropical problems in nutrition. Ann Intern Med 79:701–711, 1973
57. Yoshida T, Metcoff J, Frenk S et al: Intermediary metabolites and adenine nucleotides in leukocytes of children with PCM. Nature 214:525–526, 1967

25
Inborn Errors
of Metabolism

George K. Summer
Dianne M. Frazier

In 1902 Garrod postulated a genetic basis for human biochemical individuality and introduced the concept of Mendelian inherited monogenic "inborn errors of metabolism."[29] It was not until almost 50 years later, however, that his genetotrophic concept was fully appreciated as the basis of biochemical individuality, and programs for early detection, diagnosis, and treatment of inherited disorders of amino acid and carbohydrate metabolism were initiated.[57]

Although inborn errors of metabolism are rather rare, the rate of discovery of these disorders has increased dramatically over the past two decades, and enthusiastic study of them has paid significant dividends in modern pediatrics. Recent investigations have brought a realization of the aggregate importance of inherited disease in child health and have contributed in large measure to a better understanding of the value of screening and of the concept of biochemical individuality and genetic heterogeneity. Perhaps the greatest dividend from these studies, however, has been in the development of successful treatment.[52]

Ideal treatment of inborn errors of metabolism would restore directly the normal genotype, but research in this area has not yet led to a significant number of successful clinical applications, and therapy for the most part is now limited to modification of the biochemical environment in an attempt to offset the impact of these disorders and reduce their burden on the individual and society.[57]

Nutritional methods of therapeutic intervention have been applied to many inborn errors of metabolism. Success is varied with the disease in question and the ease with which dietary modifications can be achieved by three basic modes of treatment: (1) prevention of (toxic) accumulation of substrate and its metabolites, (2) replacement of (deficient) product or its derivatives, and (3) amplification of catalytic activity of the deficient (mutant) enzyme by cofactor (coenzyme) supplementation. Timing of intervention by any of the foregoing methods of treatment is of great importance, and it is for this reason that genetic screening has become such a critical factor in detection of persons at risk with incipient inherited diseases. At least 50 monogenic disorders are candidates for treatment by substrate restriction or product replacement, and over a dozen may also be vitamin responsive.[52,56]

This chapter presents an overview of the dietary treatment of certain inborn errors of metabolism that should be of practical importance in management of patients with these disorders. Phenylketonuria and galactosemia will be covered in more detail as classical examples of inborn errors of amino acid and carbohydrate metabolism amenable to dietary therapy because these diseases meet the following general criteria for practical application of dietary management of single-gene disorders: (1) the untreated disease must be harmful; (2) dietary treatment must abate the ill effects; (3) the proposed treatment should not be harmful to the patient or to others who may inadvertently adopt it; and (4) facilities must be adequate to ensure confirmation of diagnosis and suitable biochemical monitoring of the course of treatment.[37,47,52]

Inborn Errors of Amino Acid Metabolism

PHENYLKETONURIA

The best-known example of disorders treated by dietary substrate restriction is phenylketonuria, an autosomal recessive condition with an incidence of between 1:15,000 and 1:20,000.[45] The primary defect in classical phenylketonuria, a lack of phenylalanine hydroxylase in liver, results in an inability to convert the essential amino acid phenylalanine to tyrosine. This leads to accumulation in blood and urine of phenylalanine and its metabolites, phenylpyruvic, phenyllactic, phenylacetic, o-hydroxyphenylacetic acids, and the glutamine conjugate of phenylacetic acid, phenylacetylglutamine. These relationships are shown in Figure 25-1. If affected children go untreated, a very high percentage develop brain damage and severe mental retardation, and most patients show a significant loss of myelin at postmortem examination.

Phenylketonuria is of special interest for two reasons. First, diets low in phenylalanine have been developed and extensively used which will prevent accumulation of phenylalanine and its metabolites. Second, many countries now have successful screening programs for this disorder that ensure early detection and prompt dietary treatment.[52] In spite of the fact that a low phenylalanine diet was introduced 27 years ago, the effectiveness and long-term results of dietary therapy for phenylketonuria

are still under investigation.[9,10] However, it is clear that studies thus far on significant numbers of patients strongly suggest that adequate dietary treatment begun early in life can greatly ameliorate the development of the expected mental defect.

DETECTION

Approximately 1% of all patients in institutions for the mentally retarded have been diagnosed as having phenylketonuria, indicating that the threat posed by this disorder is significant if cases are not detected and treated promptly early in the newborn period. Screening programs initiated in the 1950s and early 1960s were dependent upon ferric chloride and dinitrophenylhydrazine testing of urine for phenylpyruvic acid at the age of 2 weeks to 6 weeks, but these tests alone proved to be unreliable for detection of phenylketonuria. Phenylpyruvic acid is easily oxidized on exposure to air to phenylacetic acid, which will not give positive reactions with the test reagents. It has been noted also that the phenylketonuric infant often does not excrete phenylpyruvic acid in the urine, even though the level of phenylalanine in the blood is high. In treated cases, phenylpyruvic acid seldom appears in the urine unless the plasma phenylalanine level is 15 mg/dl or more. Therefore, the use of urine tests in monitoring or controlling dietary treatment may mean that the plasma phenylalanine is maintained at an undesirably high level. Because of these problems, it is now accepted practice to do a blood test for elevated amounts of phenylalanine using

FIG. 25-1 Intermediates in the metabolism of phenylalanine and tyrosine.

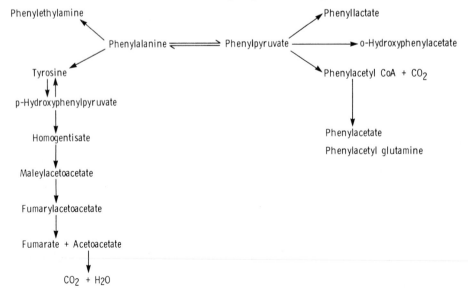

the technique of whole blood spotted on filter paper for screening and for monitoring dietary treatment.[33,36,45]

In phenylketonuria, plasma phenylalanine rises from a normal of 2 mg/dl to 4 mg/dl at birth to 20 mg/dl or higher by the end of the first 2 weeks of life. This marked hyperphenylalaninemia persists if treatment is not instituted promptly at this stage. Serum tyrosine may be normal or low. Phenylalanine concentration above 4 mg/dl in whole blood spotted on filter paper obtained within the first 2 days to 3 days of life requires a repeat determination within the first 2 weeks and ideally follow-up testing and studies to confirm the diagnosis in suspected cases before the end of the second or third week of life. In 1966, almost 90% of the 3.5 million live births in this country were screened for phenylketonuria. This preventive health measure detected 222 infants with the disorder. Today, 47 of the 50 states and all provinces of Canada have effective programs for screening newborn infants for phenylketonuria and a number of other genetic and metabolic disorders, which include between 90% and 95% of all live births in the two countries.[67]

DIET THERAPY

Principles, Objectives, and Strategies. The immediate objective of nutritional management of phenylketonuria is to reduce the level of phenylalanine in the blood by limiting intake of this amino acid. Thereafter, adjustments must be made in intake to maintain a blood level of phenylalanine that ensures normal growth (see Chap. 14) and development without production of abnormal metabolites that usually appear when this amino acid is in excess. In addition to providing adequate nourishment, the diet should also permit development of good eating habits.

When large-scale screening programs were begun 15 to 20 years ago, it was clear that no one knew what a desirable blood phenylalanine level should be in phenylketonuria. With experience, it was found that the phenylalanine requirement varied widely from patient to patient, particularly in the transient hyperphenylalaninemic states and atypical forms of the disorder. Also, with a restricted diet there was always a risk of producing phenylalanine deficiency and protein malnutrition. As a result, the initial approach to dietary management, which focused on keeping the phenylalanine blood level in the normal range at 2 mg/dl to 4 mg/dl, has been changed so that one now attempts to modify the dietary intake of protein to keep the blood phenylalanine between 5 mg/dl to 10 mg/dl. Experience has shown that frequent alterations must be made in the infant's diet in order to meet rapidly changing requirements for adequate growth and development. Treatment of patients with a low phenylalanine diet requires continual biochemical monitoring of blood and urine, and, therefore, it should not be attempted without the assistance of a reliable laboratory from which test results can be obtained promptly.

Effectiveness and Feasibility. The first report of the effect of a low phenylalanine diet in phenylketonuria was published in 1953 by Bickel, Gerrard, and Hickmans.[9] The patient was a 2-year-old mentally retarded girl who was given a formula derived from a casein hydrolysate from which phenylalanine and tyrosine had been removed by activated acid-washed charcoal. Tyrosine, tryptophan, and cystine were re-added to the preparation in suitable amounts. The patient lost weight, and the biochemical abnormalities disappeared in blood and urine over a 4- to 6-week period after instituting the diet low in phenylalanine; however, subsequently, presumably as a result of tissue breakdown, the biochemical abnormalities returned to some extent, along with a generalized aminoaciduria. Phenylalanine was then added in small amounts in the form of whole milk (0.3 g to 0.5 g phenylalanine, sufficient for normal weight gain) with greatly improved biochemical findings. Over a 10-month period, there was gradual improvement in the child's mental state. She learned to crawl, stand, and climb on chairs; her eyes became brighter and her hair grew darker, and she no longer cried continuously and banged her head.

While this patient had already suffered significant irreparable brain damage by 2 years of age, the experience with this case illustrates the problem that can occur with too low an intake of phenylalanine, and the limiting effect that this may have on the synthesis of body proteins. It is important to recognize that brain damage can occur as a result of phenylalanine deficiency, and it has been postulated that this effect may well explain why "optimally" treated phenylketonuric children still show a significantly lower intelligence quotient than their unaffected siblings in some studies. The effect of dietary treatment initiated at different times after birth on intellectual development in classical phenylketonuria is shown in Table 25-1 using sib–sib comparisons.[56]

It has been stated that treatment of classical phenylketonuria consists of an intake of phenylalanine high enough to meet the nutritional needs of a growing child without exceeding his limited capacity to utilize it. This balance can be achieved by considering blood or serum phenylalanine levels and urinary excretion of phenylalanine and its metabolites, including o-hydroxyphenylacetic acid, in relation to phenylalanine intake. During periods of phenylalanine deficiency, excessive intake of

TABLE 25-1
Effect of Dietary Treatment of Classical Phenylketonuria

Type of Patient	Number	Average Age at Onset of Treatment	IQ (Mean ± SD)	Age at Testing (Years)
A. *Treatment beginning at*				
0–2 mo	35	0.8 mo	89.9 ± 13.3	2⅓
2–6 mo	6	3.7 mo	64.5 ± 18.4	4½
6–12 mo	19	9.4 mo	57.5 ± 17.2	5
12–24 mo	24	18.9 mo	54.2 ± 16.8	5½
B. *Sib–sib comparison*				
(1) Early treatment (<2 mo)	10	0.6 mo	92.2	2⅚
(2) Late treatment (>2 mo)	10	11.7 mo	53.0†	5½
C. *Early-treated patients*				
(1) Without complication	10	13.4 days	100.4	1⁷⁄₁₂
(2) With complications*	18	15.7 days	87.2‡	2⁵⁄₁₂
(3) Delayed treatment (6th–8th wk)	7	55.8 days	80.6†	2⅚

*Complications include undertreatment; overtreatment resulting in growth failure and low concentrations of phenylalanine in plasma; obstetrical complications at birth.
†Significantly different from B (1), p = <0.01.
‡Significantly different from C (1), p = <0.05.
From Scriver CR, Katz L, Clow C: Phenylketonuria and Diet. Can Med Assoc J 98:124–5, 1968

phenylalanine, or febrile illnesses, characteristic changes occur in the relationship between intake of phenylalanine and the biochemical parameters in blood and urine, and interpretation of these changes is the basis upon which dietary alterations are made. Blood or serum phenylalanine measurements at frequent intervals are necessary for checking effective adjustments in the diet. Urinary phenylalanine and o-hydroxyphenylacetic acid excretions provide a continuing measure of the ability or inability of patients to eliminate excess phenylalanine; increase of phenylalanine in urine is frequently the first sign of an approaching illness. Urinary o-hydroxyphenylacetic acid is not detected at serum phenylalanine levels of 2 mg/dl to 7 mg/dl, and its presence is a signal that the capacity of the child to utilize or eliminate phenylalanine has been exceeded and that serum or blood phenylalanine has increased to an undesirable level.[6,56]

The ideal treatment program should consist of the following elements:

1. Early prescription (ideally before one month and not later than two months) of a diet restricted only in its phenylalanine content and otherwise meeting accepted nutritional requirements
2. Precise and frequent monitoring, using microtechniques, of the serum or blood phenylalanine levels and urinary phenylalanine metabolite excretion products, to maintain phenylalanine in blood within a reasonable range (5 mg/dl–10 mg/dl)
3. Prompt dietary alteration based on monitoring of blood phenylalanine level and urinary phenylalanine excretion products, and information routinely supplied by the parents, especially during periods of rapid growth and febrile illnesses
4. Establishment of individual dietary requirements based on monitoring biochemical results rather than standard requirement tables
5. Creation of the most normal eating atmosphere possible under an unusually restrictive regimen[62]

Formulating Dietary Prescriptions. During the first 6 months of life, infants usually receive most of their nutrient requirements from synthetic formulas or breast milk. The dietary management of many inborn errors of metabolism, which usually requires restriction of a particular amino acid or carbohydrate, is relatively easy during this period with semisynthetic products, many of which are commercially available. These preparations are made from hydrolysates of a protein such as casein, or amino-acid mixtures to which other required nutrients are added to simulate a standard infant formula. The requirements for the other nutrients—calories, fat, carbohydrates, minerals, and vitamins—are usually met by adding special formulations to the preparation or by supplementation with milk or natural foods of known composition.

Dietary requirements of the infant with phenylketonuria are largely supplied by special low-phenylalanine, balanced milk-substitute formulas such as Lofenalac (0.08 g phenylalanine/100 g) or PKU–aid (Albumaid–XP), the composition of which is shown in Table 25-2.[65] Product 3229-A, which

TABLE 25-2
Approximate Nutritive Composition of Special Dietary Products*

Nutrient	Lofenalac (MJ)†	PKU-Aid (MS)†	Low-methionine Isomil (RL)†	Phenyl-Free (MJ)†	3200-AB (MJ)†	MSUD-Aid (MS)†	MSUD Diet Powder (MJ)†	Methionaid (MS)†	3200-K (MJ)†	Histi-naid (MS)†	80056 (MJ)†
Calories	460	240	516	406	460	248	476	242	518	240	445
Protein (g)	15	60	12.5	20.3	15	64.4	8.2	63.1	15.8	61.2	0
Fat (g)	18	0	28.1	6.8	18	0	20.1	0	28	0	20.4
CHO (g)	60	0	57.0	66	60	0	63.7	0	51.1	0	65.3
L-AMINO ACIDS (g)											
Essential											
Isoleucine	0.75	2.6	0.56	1.10	0.86	0	0	2.4	0.76	2.5	0
Leucine	1.41	6.1	1.02	1.73	1.76	0	0	32	1.31	3.8	0
Lysine	1.57	6.1	0.77	1.89	1.91	7.1	0.8	6.0	0.98	5.8	0
Methionine	0.45	1.5	0.14	0.63	0.56	1.9	0.25	0.2	0.18	1.6	0
Phenylalanine	0.08	<0.07	0.6	0	0.08	3.8	0.55	4.3	0.86	2.2	0
Threonine	0.77	4.8	0.51	0.94	0.65	3.3	0.55	3.2	0.59	3.1	0
Tryptophan	0.19	0.9	0.12	0.28	0.20	1.2	0.20	0.9	0.18	1.1	0
Valine	1.20	4.6	0.52	1.26	1.38	0	0	3.2	0.80	3.1	0
Histidine	0.39	1.8	0.28	0.47	0.40	2.7	0.25	2.8	0.38	0	0
Nonessential											
Arginine	0.34	3.1	0.83	0.69	0.39	5.1	0.50	4.4	1.08	4.6	0
Alanine	0.64	4.1	0.53	NL	0.76	7.1	0.45	5.6	0.68	5.9	0
Aspartate	1.34	8.1	1.29	5.20	1.60	12.1	1.14	9.5	1.94	10.6	0
Cystine	0.025	1.5	0.15	0.35	0.042	2.1	0.25	3.7	0.107	1.8	0
Glutamate	3.78	9.3	2.48	1.88	4.31	13.3	2.09	11.0	3.12	12.3	0
Glycine	0.35	3.1	0.52	3.35	0.40	3.9	0.60	4.3	0.67	5.9	0
Proline	1.13	3.6	0.6	NL	1.13	2.3	0.90	1.6	0.77	1.9	0
Serine	1.02	4.8	0.68	NL	1.09	2.4	0.60	1.7	0.81	1.9	0
Tyrosine	0.81	6.0	0.40	0.93	<0.04	3.8	0.65	4.3	0.55	4.5	0
Glutamine	NL†	NL	NL	4.75	NL	NL	NL	NL	NL	NL	0
VITAMINS											
Vitamin A (IU)	1,151	0	2,200	2,030	1,151	0	1,190	0	1,296	0	1,308
Vitamin D (IU)	288	0	340	406	288	0	297	0	324	0	327
Vitamin E (IU)	7.2	0	12	10	7.2	0	7	0	8.0	0	8
Vitamin C (mg)	37	0	60	53	37	0	39	0	42	0	41
Thiamine (μg)	360	2,000	0.5	609	360	2,000	370	2,000	360	2,000	409
Riboflavin (μg)	430	2,000	0.6	1,015	430	2,000	450	2,000	490	2,000	491
Vitamin B_6 (μg)	290	2,000	0.5	508	290	2,000	300	2,000	290	2,000	327
Vitamin B_{12} (μg)	1.4	20	35	2.5	1.4	20	1.5	20	1.6	20	16.4
Niacin (μg)	5,800	25,000	9	8,122	5,800	25,000	5,900	25,000	6,500	25,000	6,545
Folic acid (μg)	72	400	0.12	102	72	400	74	400	81	400	82
Pantothenic acid (μg)	2,200	20,000	7	3,046	2,200	20,000	2,200	20,000	2,400	20,000	2,454
Choline (mg)	61	0	94	86	61	0	63	0	69	0	69
Biotin (μg)	36	600	0.13	30	36	600	40	600	36	600	41
Vitamin K (μg)	72	0	0.12	102	72	0	74	0	81	0	82
Inositol (mg)	22	0	0	30	22	250	22	100	24	100	25
MINERALS											
Calcium (mg)	432	2,500	650	609	432	2,500	491	2,500	486	700	491
Phosphorus (mg)	324	1,500	440	457	324	1,500	268	1,500	324	1,500	270
Magnesium (mg)	51	300	40	71	50	300	52	300	49	80	57
Iron (mg)	8.6	25	10	12	8.6	50	9	50	10	4	10
Iodine (μg)	32	150	120	46	32	150	33	150	36	60	37
Copper (μg)	430	2,500	500	609	430	2,500	400	2,500	500	500	491
Manganese (mg)	0.7	3.5	0	1	0.7	3.5	0.7	3.5	0.8	0.5	0.8
Zinc (mg)	2.9	15	4	4.1	2.9	15	3	15	4	0.9	3.3
Sodium (mEq)	9	61	10.4	11	9	61	9.7	61	9	34	2.8
Potassium (mEq)	12	66	10.4	18	12	66	8.6	66	11.4	19	7.9
Chloride (mEq)	9	80	12.7	14	9	80	10.5	80	9	NL	3.5

*Per 100 g of powder. In these formulas, protein = nitrogen in grams × 6.25.

†MJ = Mead Johnson Company; RL = Ross Laboratories; MS = Milner Scientific; NL = not listed.

From American Academy of Pediatrics, Committee on Nutrition (ed): Pediatric Nutrition Handbook, pp 224–225. Evanston, IL, 1979. Copyright American Academy of Pediatrics, 1979.

is currently undergoing clinical trials, is another preparation designed for a child 2 years of age or older. These preparations are supplemented by sufficient cow's milk or regular infant formula to meet the patient's minimum requirement of phenylalanine, which may vary in the range of 20 mg/kg/day to 100 mg/kg/day or more, since Lofenalac alone and the other preparations do not. Palatability is not a significant problem when Lofenalac is administered by bottle to infants. As low-protein solid foods are introduced into the diet, the cow's milk component is adjusted to maintain just sufficient phenylalanine intake to keep the phenylalanine level within the prescribed limits and to ensure normal growth and development in the individual patient. When a child is well established on a low-protein solid food regimen, the Lofenalac is gradually replaced by an increase in intake of low-protein foods and addition of the phenylalanine-free protein supplement. Thus, a definitive diet consists of three equally important components: (1) a basic allowance of low-protein foods, which provide the bulk of calories, such as fruit, vegetables, wheat or corn starch, pure sugars, and fats; (2) phenylalanine-free protein supplements to provide the other essential (as well as nonessential) amino acids required for normal growth and development; and (3) complete vitamin and mineral supplements (Product 80056) shown in Table 25-2, which replace those usually supplied by meat, fish, poultry, milk, and eggs.[65]

Meal Planning. Low-phenylalanine diets require expert nutritional guidance regardless of the protein source. As the child grows older, clinicians characteristically report increasing difficulty in meeting dietary protein recommendations, since the product initially used was designed primarily for infant feeding, and, accordingly, had a high fat and carbohydrate content compared to protein content. The need to continue low-phenylalanine dietary treatment during adolescent growth years has prompted workers in the field to seek a low-phenylalanine protein source that is relatively high in protein in comparison to fat and carbohydrate. This led to the development of Albumaid–XP (PKU–aid), shown in Table 25-2, prepared from beef protein by acid hydrolysis. This product contains amino acids equivalent to approximately 40% by weight, carbohydrate 50%, with the remainder consisting of fat, vitamins, minerals, and moisture. Lofenalac has been recommended for use in the hungry child with a large appetite and Albumaid–XP for the picky eater; combinations of the two can be used to adjust protein and phenylalanine prescriptions to the volume of food a child will take. During periods when appetites change, but protein needs remain

constant, the flexibility offered by a high-protein product (Albumaid–XP) and a high-carbohydrate–fat product (Lofenalac) can be invaluable in maintaining an adequate regimen for treatment of phenylketonuria.[7]

The composition of solid foods and the quantity ingested must be strictly regulated to keep the amino acid content of the diet under control and to ensure provision of other nutritional requirements. Total nutritional intake, including micronutrient composition, should be known and monitored daily to be certain the child is receiving a nutritionally adequate diet.

Typical phenylalanine-restricted diets for infants and children of different ages are shown in Table 25-3.[1] It is important to be aware of the phenylalanine, protein, and caloric content of the serving lists of vegetables, fruits, breads, and cereals used for phenylalanine-restricted diets (see Table 25-4 and Table 25-5). This is done usually by including suitable exchanges from the basic food groups in the diet so that 15 mg or 30 mg phenylalanine is provided per serving.[1,2]

In the past, most children with phenylketonuria were cared for in institutions for the retarded; however, today most cases are cared for in the home, requiring broader community services to assist the family with medical, nursing, psychological, and nutritional problems associated with this condition. Parental education is essential. Parents need more intensive assistance by the nutritionist and other professionals in the following areas: menu planning, food preparation, particularly the mixing of Lofenalac by itself and with other preparations, excessive hunger and other feeding problems, provision of an inexpensive, low-phenylalanine bread that is palatable, greater knowledge of child growth and development, discipline, and instruction of the child regarding the nature of the disorder and the foods that he or she cannot eat. The nutritionist should give greater assistance with menu planning, food preparation, and development of recipes (particularly one for bread). When assistance is given in these areas, perhaps fewer children will be perpetually hungry or craving food or having other feeding problems.

POSSIBLE NUTRITIONAL RISKS

It has been recognized that treatment phenylketonuria by dietary restriction of phenylalanine without adequate monitoring of patients has produced rather profound malnutrition during the first year of life, in some cases manifested by anorexia, listlessness, deficient growth, anemia, hypoproteinemia, and x-ray bone changes of osteoporosis. The possibility has been raised that mental retar-

TABLE 25-3
Phenylalanine-Restricted Diets for Infants and Children

Age	1 Mo	8 Mo	2 Yr	4 Yr
Weight, lb	8	18	26	36
Diet prescription				
Phenylalanine, mg	160–176	324–360	416–468	360–576
Protein, g	14–16	27	32	40
Energy, Cal	440	810	1300	1700
Lofenalac, measures*	10	18	19	23
Water to make	24 oz	32 oz	24 oz	24 oz
Milk as necessary	1½ oz	1 oz	—	—
Vegetables, servings	—	2	4	4
Fruits, servings	1	1	4	4
Breads, servings	—	3	5	4
Fats, servings	—	—	1	1
Desserts,† servings	—	—	—	1
Free foods‡	—	—	As desired	As desired
Nutritive values				
Phenylalanine, mg	172	325	417	447
Protein, g	16.8	30.4	33.1	40.6
Energy, Cal	540	944	1302	1724

*One measure = 1 tablespoon

†Special recipes are required for desserts.

‡If free foods are given in excessive amounts, child may not consume proper amounts of other foods.

From Acosta PB: Nutritional aspects of phenylketonuria. In The Clinical Team Looks at Phenylketonuria, p 52. Washington, DC, Children's Bureau, Department of Health, Education, and Welfare, 1964

dation in a number of cases has been produced by early malnutrition from too vigorous application of dietary therapy, and a few deaths have been reported.[34] It has been suggested further that more liberal diets would prevent malnutrition and that, despite moderate elevation of phenylalanine levels in blood, ultimate intellectual function would be improved. More recently, in most treatment programs, an attempt has been made to maintain the level of phenylalanine in the range of 5 mg/dl to 10 mg/dl. During the first year of life, this can be accomplished by approximately 50 mg to 100 mg phenylalanine/kg/24 hr in the diet. It is very important, therefore, as a primary preventive measure, to monitor the phenylalanine levels in serum once or twice weekly during the first 6 months to 12 months of life, and also to watch for evidence of malnutrition by monitoring serum protein and hemoglobin levels, height and weight, and, if necessary, x-rays of bone.[34]

The second important preventive measure is to teach the mother to calculate the child's intake of phenylalanine at the end of each day. It should be noted that the sick child might on occasion have a normal or high blood level of phenylalanine, yet the patient might be dietarily deficient in phenylalanine. If there is a deficiency because of anorexia,

illness, or any other cause, it must be corrected. This is usually done by administration of appropriate amounts of cow's milk, which contains approximately 50 mg phenylalanine/30 ml.

TREATMENT OF PREGNANT AND PHENYLKETONURIC WOMEN

The success of neonatal screening for phenylketonuria means that an increasing number of healthy and intelligent women with phenylketonuria are now reaching childbearing age and will create a new therapeutic problem for physicians and obstetricians in the next decade. Children of untreated phenylketonuric women have a significantly higher mortality and morbidity than the average child.[43] When the fetus is exposed to a hyperphenylalaninemic environment generated by the homozygous phenylketonuric mother, profound mental retardation and congenital anomalies are likely results. This undesirable outcome is accompanied by an unfavorable transplacental gradient of phenylalanine, which provides the fetus with about 1.7 times the already elevated phenylalanine concentrations in maternal blood.[57]

It appears that in women with phenylketonuria who wish to bear children a strict low-phenylala-

TABLE 25-4
Serving List for Phenylalanine-Restricted Diet

Food	Amount	Food	Amount
VEGETABLES—15 mg phenylalanine per serving		Cantaloupe, diced	½ cup*
Asparagus	1 stalk	Dates, dried	2
Beans, green, cooked	3 tbsp	Fruit cocktail, canned	2 tbsp
junior	2 tbsp	Grapefruit sections or juice	⅓ cup
strained	2 tbsp	Grapes, green, seedless	20 medium
Beets, cooked	3 tbsp	Grape juice	⅓ cup
strained	2 tbsp	Guava, raw	⅓ medium
Cabbage, raw, shredded	4 tbsp	Lemon or lime juice	3 tbsp
Carrots, raw	½ large	frozen, diluted	½ cup
canned	4 tbsp	Mango	½ small
junior	3 tbsp	Orange	1 medium*
strained	3 tbsp	Papaya, cubed	¼ cup
Cauliflower	2 tbsp	juice	½ cup
Celery, raw, 5-in stalks	2 stalks	Peach, raw	1 medium+
Cucumber, raw	⅓ medium	canned in syrup	1½ halves
Lettuce, head	2 leaves	junior	7 tbsp
Mushrooms, cooked	2 tbsp	strained	5 tbsp
Okra, pod, cooked	1 pod	Pear, raw	1⅓ med.*
Onion, green	2 medium	canned in syrup	3 halves
mature	¼ medium	junior	10 tbsp
Parsley	2 sprigs	strained	10 tbsp
Pumpkin, cooked	2 tbsp	Pear–pineapple, junior and strained	7 tbsp
Radish	3 small	Pineapple, raw	⅓ cup
Spinach, cooked	1 tbsp	canned in syrup	1½ small can
creamed, junior, and strained	2 tbsp		
Squash, summer, cooked	4 tbsp	juice	½ cup
Squash, winter, cooked	2 tbsp	Plums, canned	1 medium
junior	6 tbsp	with tapioca, junior	7 tbsp
strained	3 tbsp	with tapioca, strained	5 tbsp
Tomato, raw	¼ small	Popsicle with fruit juice	2 medium
canned	2 tbsp	Prunes, dried	2 large*
juice	2 tbsp	juice	⅓ cup
Turnip	4 tbsp	strained	3 tbsp
Yam or sweet potato, strained	2 tbsp	Raisins, dried	2 tbsp*
		Strawberries	3 large
FRUITS—15 mg phenylalanine per serving		Tangerine	⅔ small
Apple, raw	2 medium	Watermelon	⅓ cup
Apricots, canned	2 halves		
dried, halves	4 large	BREADS AND CEREALS—30 mg phenylalanine per serving	
juice	¼ cup	Barley cereal, Gerber's dry	2 tbsp
Apricot–applesauce,		Biscuit*	1 small
junior	10 tbsp	Cereal food, Gerber's dry	2 tbsp
strained	10 tbsp	Corn, cooked	2 tbsp
Avocado	2 tbsp	Cornflakes	⅓ cup
Banana, 6-in long	½*	Crackers, Barnum animal	6

*Special recipes required.
Data from Acosta PB: Nutritional aspects of phenylketonuria. In The Clinical Team Looks at Phenylketonuria, p 40. Washington DC, Children's Bureau, Department of Health, Education, and Welfare, 1964; and Miller GT, Williams VR, Moschette DS: Phenylalanine content of fruit. J Am Diet Assoc 46:43, 1965

nine diet should be instituted before conception, and even then a normal outcome cannot be guaranteed. In maternal phenylketonuria, fetal damage leading to reduced brain growth, microcephaly, and cardiac malformations probably occurs within a few weeks of conception. The small number of good results of dietary treatment in both early and late pregnancy encourages one to believe that early treatment (before conception) in well-motivated, intelligent women with the disease who had been on diets since childhood may allow the fetus to develop normally. Nevertheless, the alternatives of contraception and sterilization must be put clearly to any woman with phenylketonuria who is considering marriage and motherhood. If dietary treatment is to be carried out, it should, whenever pos-

TABLE 25-5
Phenylalanine, Protein, and Caloric Content of Serving Lists Used in Phenylalanine–Restricted Diets

	Phenylalanine mg	*Protein*	*Kilocalories*
Lofenalac, 1 measure (1 tablespoon)	7.5	1.5	43
Vegetables	15	0.3	5
Fruits	15	0.2	80
Breads	30	0.5	20
Fats	5	0.1	45
Desserts (special recipes required)	30	2.0	270
Free foods	0	0.0	Varies
Milk (per ounce)	55	1.1	20

Acosta PB: Nutritional aspects of phenylketonuria. In The Clinical Team Looks at Phenylketonuria, p 40. Washington, DC, Children's Bureau, Department of Health, Education, and Welfare, 1964

sible, start before conception and aim at keeping the plasma phenylalanine around 8 mg/dl. Pueschel and co-workers have compared the composition of the preparations Lofenalac and Product 3229 to nutritional requirements of the pregnant woman.[55] These basic formulas, when used in conjunction with appropriate food exchanges, should provide a reasonable variety in the diet and better toleration of the low-phenylalanine regimen during pregnancy.[43,55,59]

Whether it is possible to nourish the pregnant human woman safely with a low-phenylalanine diet, or whether the intrauterine environment will respond to such manipulation to prevent the fetal effects of maternal phenylketonuria is, as yet, an unmet challenge for nutritional research. The need for such knowledge is pressing. Approximately half of today's phenylketonuric patients who benefit from postnatal dietary therapy are women. They will be potential candidates in a few years for nutritional therapy during pregnancy should they desire to bear children.[55,57]

TREATMENT OF VARIANT FORMS

It is now recognized that about 50% of children with phenylketonuria have the classic disease caused by deficiency of phenylalanine hydroxylase, and most of the other half have a transient form which appears to subside with time. There are also variant or atypical forms that have been discovered recently in which phenylalanine hydroxylase activity is normal and in which other defects in this complex enzyme system have been found.[51,66] A deficiency of dihydropteridine reductase has recently been shown to produce phenylketonuria, and a deficiency of biopterin, the essential cofactor in the hydroxylation of phenylalanine and other aromatic amino acids, also causes hyperphenylalaninemia and a clinical condition indistinguishable from classical phenylketonuria.[39,40] Dihydropteridine

reductase is an essential component of the hydroxylation systems for phenylalanine, tryptophan, and tyrosine. This enzyme is required to maintain the pteridine cofactor (biopterin) in the reduced state (quinonoid dihydrobiopterin → tetrahydrobiopterin) so that hydroxylation of the aromatic amino acids will occur according to the illustrative reactions involving phenylalanine shown in Figure 25-2.

Hydroxylation of tryptophan and tyrosine is involved with the synthesis of the neutrotransmitters serotonin, dopamine, and noradrenalin. It has been postulated that interference with the synthesis of these biologic amines is the basis of the neurologic deterioration in some of the recently discovered atypical forms of phenylketonuria. Dietary restriction of phenylalanine and correction of the elevated serum phenylalanine levels in these patients does not correct the hydroxylation defect, and it appears that adversely affected neurotransmitter synthesis and neurologic deterioration continue. Experience at a number of medical centers suggests that the incidence of these newly discovered atypical forms of phenylketonuria is about 2% to 5% of the hyperphenylalaninemic cases detected by screening programs. The clinical significance of these recent findings is that one cannot be certain that a newly diagnosed infant with phenylketonuria will be normal even with dietary restriction of phenylalanine. Studies are now proceeding to determine if administration of dopamine and serotonin precursors, L-3,4-dihydroxyphenylalanine and 5-hydroxytryptophan (5-HTP), or pharmacologic doses of the pteridine cofactor, tetrahydrobiopterin, will correct the biochemical defects and prevent the brain damage and neurologic deterioration manifested by several of the newly described atypical forms of phenylketonuria.[66]

Carbidopa, a peripheral L-aromatic amino acid decarboxylase inhibitor, has also been given to some patients with dihydropteridine reductase (DHPR)

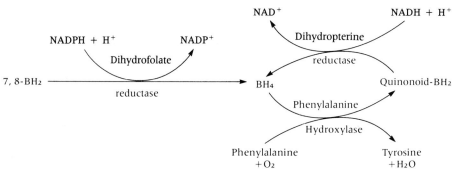

FIG. 25-2 The phenylalanine hydroxylation system. *B* is the symbol for biopterin.

deficiency in an attempt to decrease the conversion outside the brain of 5-HTP to serotonin and L-dopa to dopamine. In one patient with DHPR deficiency, when treatment was initiated with 5-HTP and carbidopa, the frequency of seizures immediately decreased from daily episodes to 8 or 9 per month.[11] L-Dopa, which was initiated two months after the onset of 5-HTP and carbidopa treatment, was associated with a decrease in irritability and dystonia and improvement in fine motor function. Another atypical form of phenylketonuria with normal phenylalanine hydroxylase and dihydropteridine reductase activities in liver has responded to oral administration of L-sepiapterin by dramatic lowering of the blood phenylalanine level. L-sepiapterin is a precursor in the synthesis of biopterin, and it has been postulated that these patients, who excrete large quantities of neopterin in the urine, have a deficiency of dihydrobiopterin synthetase, an enzyme that is thought to convert dihydroneopterin to sepiapterin. The latter is then converted to dihydrobiopterin by the action of sepiapterin reductase.[50]

It is clear, therefore, that dietary restriction of phenylalanine, while important in treatment of classical phenylketonuria, must not be considered the only therapeutic approach to management of hyperphenylalaninemic conditions. Detection, diagnostic confirmation, and treatment of phenylketonuria, in view of newly discovered atypical forms of the disorder, must be considered in a completely different light.

DISCONTINUATION OF TREATMENT

Although there is general agreement on the value of early treatment of children with phenylketonuria, still to be determined is the optimal time and method, if any, for discontinuing the low-phenylalanine dietary treatment and the best management thereafter. The principal concerns about termination of diet therapy have included lessening of general well-being, adverse behavioral changes, decrease in functional intellectual capacity, and subsequent pregnancies in phenylketonuric women.

It is apparent now that a number of clinicians who manage phenylketonuric patients are taking a very conservative position on discontinuation of the low-phenylalanine diet. Recent reports following termination of the diet indicate that patients show significant decreases in IQ (by as much as 10 points), hyperactivity, short attention span, drowsiness, and increased irritability.[5,12,60]

It is clear that long-term results of early dietary treatment in phenylketonuric patients are closely related to the age of starting treatment during the first 3 months of life, to the quality of dietary control, and to the duration of treatment. Dietary treatment, even when initiated several years after birth, has some beneficial effect on intellectual development in classical phenylketonuria, as shown in Figure 25-3.[10]

Neurologic disturbances have been reported in a large majority of phenylketonuric patients, and an abnormal electroencephalogram is the most frequent finding. Severe neurologic dysfunction characterized by motor signs, abnormal gait, hypotonia, hyperkinetic behavior, and seizures have been observed most frequently in the most retarded patients.[53] Progressive motor dysfunction has been shown to occur in the second and third decade in a number of patients, which raises the question of the appropriateness of discontinuing the diet at a young age (5–6 years), especially in view of the fact that the cause of brain damage in this disorder is still unknown.[53]

More data are needed to decide whether at a particular age intellectual deterioration is to be expected when a normal or relaxed diet is introduced. However, at this time available evidence suggests that introduction of a completely normal diet before the age of 8 years leads to intellectual deterioration in many, but not all, patients. Normal mental development and good school performance in milder hyperphenylalaninemic variants with a mean treatment time of 3.5 years suggests that the dietary therapy can be shorter than in classical phenylketonuria.[13]

OTHER INHERITED AMINO ACID DISORDERS

Inborn errors of metabolism have been discovered that affect utilization of seven out of nine essential amino acids and a number of nonessential ones. When compared to the incidence of phenylketonuria, most of these conditions are quite rare. However, it was a natural consequence that success of dietary treatment in phenylketonuria would lead to use of restricted diets in a number of these disorders. Over the past 10 to 15 years, dietary restriction, generally of specific amino acids or of protein, has been used with varying degrees of success in the treatment of maple syrup urine disease, tyrosinosis, valinemia, isovaleric acidemia, β-methylcrotonylglycinuria, propionic acidemia, an isoleucine-related type of ketotic hyperglycinemia, methylmalonic acidemia, nonketotic hyperglycinemia, hyperprolinemia, citrullinemia, argininosuccinic aciduria, hyperammonemia types I and II, hyperargininemia, cystathioninuria, homocystinuria, histidinemia, cystinuria, cystinosis, hyperlysinemia, saccharipinuria, and ornithinemia.[38] Unfortunately, the composition of many of these diets for optimum management is still unknown, and treatment of the patients still forms a challenge to the physician, biochemist, and nutritionist. In many of these disorders there is wide variation in severity of symptoms, and less severe forms of the metabolic disturbances may easily escape notice. This means that more effective programs for early detection should be instituted for diagnosis and treatment of these incipient disorders.[38]

Other inborn errors of metabolism (or transport) of vitamins lead to clinical syndromes that may resemble a vitamin deficiency or may mimic or even present as an inborn error of amino-acid metabolism. Defects in utilization of vitamin B_{12} and folic acid provide examples. Seven inherited disorders of vitamin B_{12} metabolism have been described; three of these defects can be ascribed to impaired intestinal transport; two, to defective plasma transport; and two, to lack of synthesis of the coenzyme. The defects in intestinal transport respond to parenteral (but not oral) administration of physiologic amounts of vitamin B_{12} (1 μg/day–5 μg/day). The plasma transport defects, which are related to almost complete deficiency of vitamin B_{12}-binding globulin proteins, TC II and TC I, respond to huge doses of B_{12} parenterally (500 μg every other day). Of the two coenzyme synthesis defects, one ap-

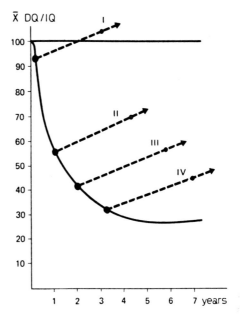

FIG. 25-3 Mental development of 61 phenylketonuric patients in relation to start of therapy. ----- treated cases; ———— untreated cases and normal (upper line); ● first DQ/IQ; ● last DQ/IQ. *I,* start of therapy in first 3 months; *II,* start of therapy between 4th and 12th month; *III,* start of therapy between 13th and 36th month; *IV,* start of therapy between 37th and 80th month. The developmental quotient *(DQ)* = maturity age/chronologic age × 100; the intelligence quotient *(IQ)* = mental age/chronologic age × 100. The developmental quotient is a clinical estimate of maturity based on assessment of the overall behavioral development. The intelligence quotient is derived primarily from comparative scores on intelligence tests. (Bickel H, Schmidt H, Schürrle L: Dietary treatment of inborn errors of amino acid and carbohydrate metabolism. Bibl Nutr Dieta 18:181, 1973)

pears to affect the intermediary metabolism of hydroxocobalamin and leads to decreased synthesis of 5'-deoxyadenosylcobalamin. This leads to a severe, often fatal, form of methylmalonic aciduria because lack of 5'-deoxyadenosylcobalamin impairs methylmalonyl mutase activity secondarily. In this disorder of coenzyme formation, parenteral administration of 500 μg to 1000 μg vitamin B_{12} has resulted in sustained biochemical and clinical improvement. Another defect in coenzyme formation results in decreased conversion of vitamin B_{12} to both 5'-deoxyadenosylcobalamin and methylcobalamin. The latter compound is a cofactor for the transferase enzyme that converts homocysteine to methionine. Deficiency of both 5'-deoxyadenosylcobalamin and methylcobalamin produces clinical and biochemical features of methylmalonic aciduria combined with an unusual type of homocystinuria. In most cases of vitamin B_{12} deficiency, one also observes a megaloblastic bone marrow, macrocytic anemia, neurologic dysfunction, and reduced levels of B_{12} in blood and tissues.[38]

Five inherited disorders of folic acid metabolism have been reported, with one involving impairment of intestinal transport, while four are concerned with coenzyme formation or interconversions. The intestinal absorptive defect is not well defined, but the other four are due to deficiencies of formiminotransferase, cyclohydrolase, dihydrofolate reductase, and N^5,N^{10}-methylenetetrahydrofolate reductase. Most patients with mutations affecting folate transport and coenzyme synthesis suffer from major central nervous system dysfunctions, including mental retardation, psychotic behavior, seizures, and cerebral cortical atrophy. Folate deficiency also results in hematopoietic dysfunction manifested by megaloblastic anemia, hypersegmented polymorphonuclear leukocytes, and thrombocytopenia. While no other reproducible clinical manifestations have emerged, it is noteworthy that there is an increased requirement for folate *in vivo* in most of the inherited folate disorders by up to 1000 times normal in some cases (10 mg/day). Unfortunately, while the anemia appears to be corrected by large folate doses, none of the patients reported thus far have been treated early enough to determine if their central nervous system defects can be prevented by appropriate folate supplements.[38]

Considerable experience has now been obtained in use of special diets for treatment of maple syrup urine disease, hereditary tyrosinemia, histidinemia, and some forms of homocystinuria. The composition of these preparations is shown in Table 25-2; they contain either an extremely low amount of the implicated amino acid or carbohydrate or are free of them.[65] Again, these conditions require careful monitoring of the treatment, and this is usually done by determining the concentration of the offending substrate in blood at frequent intervals to ensure that it is present in adequate amounts to sustain normal growth and development, but not elevated to the extent that toxic symptoms develop. Within the past few years the Federal Food and Drug Administration (FDA) has changed its policy regarding use of these preparations for inherited disorders. Instead of classifying these dietary products as drugs, the FDA has ruled that the preparations are "foods for special dietary use," a category that does not require an investigational new drug application for use. This ruling by the FDA means that the preparations will be more readily available for treatment of patients, and the food industry may be encouraged to develop new products for treating other genetic and metabolic disorders.[65]

MAPLE SYRUP URINE DISEASE

The metabolic block in maple syrup urine disease involves a deficiency of the enzymes responsible for decarboxylation of the three branched-chain amino acids, leucine, isoleucine, and valine, resulting in accumulation of their keto acids—a condition that can lead to rapid development of brain damage and even death within the first weeks or months of life. The treatment requires restriction in one or more of the three branched-chain amino acids, and two products are available for this purpose. MSUD-AID* is a synthetic mixture of L-amino acids lacking leucine, isoleucine, and valine. The product also contains minerals and water-soluble vitamins (see Table 25-2). Supplementary fat-soluble vitamins and calories are needed from carbohydrate and fat to meet nutritional requirements, and additional protein should be added to the diet to supply the minimal amount of the branched-chain amino acids needed for the individual patient. Natural foods of known composition can be used in older children to meet nutritional requirements and to provide variety in the diet. Several other dietary preparations which lack the branched-chain amino acids are available commercially (GIBCO amino-acid mixes and Product 80056 from Grand Island Biological Company, Grand Island, New York and Meade Johnson Company, Evansville, Indiana, respectively). With appropriate supplements for additional calories, minerals, and fat-soluble vitamins, including milk, these preparations can provide a complete diet for infants with branched-chain aminoacidopathies.

As with phenylketonuria, the objective of the dietary approach to treatment of maple syrup urine disease is to keep the blood level of the three branched-chain amino acids as normal as possible while permitting satisfactory growth and development. In the individual patient this is rather difficult to achieve despite meticulous monitoring of the amino acid(s) by quantitative chromatographic techniques. Success of treatment is usually dependent upon timely intervention early in life and close monitoring of dietary treatment.[10,65]

HEREDITARY TYROSINEMIA

The primary defect in this disorder is still unknown, although the original description of the disease pointed to a hereditary enzyme deficiency of p-hydroxyphenylpyruvic acid oxidase associated

---

*Manufactured by Milner Scientific and Medical Research Company, Liverpool, England; available also from Ross Laboratories, Columbus, Ohio.

with severe liver cirrhosis and proximal renal tubular damage that produces a generalized aminoaciduria. There is general agreement that dietary restriction of phenylalanine and tyrosine ameliorates the acute stage of the illness, and for this reason Product 3200-AB, a hydrolysate low in phenylalanine and tyrosine, has been used in the first month of life to manage patients with this disorder. This preparation is manufactured by Meade Johnson Company, Evansville, Indiana, and is similar to Lofenalac (see Table 25-2) and meets the necessary standards for a complete food for infants when milk is added to provide sufficient phenylalanine and tyrosine for normal growth and development.[10,65]

HISTIDINEMIA

The pathophysiology of histidinemia, especially with respect to effects on brain development and metabolism, is unclear and therefore not well defined. The enzyme histidine ammonia lyase has been shown to be deficient in this disorder, thereby blocking conversion of histidine to urocanic acid. While definitive studies are lacking, it appears that some patients with this condition may develop mild to moderate brain damage during early childhood. In some cases a low-protein diet with natural foods can ameliorate the histidinemia; however, this approach runs the risk of over restriction of all amino acids and may lead to significant growth retardation and protein malnutrition. It should be noted that protein or histidine restriction may be unnecessary because the degree and duration of histidinemia in many cases may be short-lived. However, if one elects to use selective restriction of histidine as an approach, Histinaid, a powdered L-amino acid mixture devoid of histidine, is available (Milner Scientific and Medical Research Company, Liverpool, England) but other foods must be added to provide calories, fat-soluble vitamins, and essential fatty acids (see Table 25-2). Close biochemical and clinical monitoring of the patient is required when restriction of protein or histidine is used as a form of treatment intervention.[10,65]

HOMOCYSTINURIA

In the classical form of homocystinuria, deficiency of cystathionine synthetase prevents normal condensation of homocysteine and serine to cystathionine. Homocysteine and its precursor methionine accumulate in the body fluids. At least two forms of homocystinuria have been recognized, one of which is amenable to pyridoxine treatment; the other requires a diet supplemented with cysteine and restricted in methionine. It has been postulated that pyridoxine may be acting to stabilize a mutant cystathionine synthetase apoenzyme rather than to enhance its ability to bind coenzyme. The activity increases because more holoenzyme is present, not because the specific activity of each enzyme molecule is increased. Several products are available commercially for dietary management of this disorder. Product 3200-K from Meade Johnson Company is a soybean formula low in methionine (see Table 25-2) that provides a sufficient amount of this amino acid for most children. However, sufficient amounts of cysteine must be provided for normal protein synthesis because this amino acid has become essential as a result of the genetic mutation. Methionade is another preparation available from Milner Scientific and Medical Research Company, Liverpool, England, which is free of methionine, but otherwise contains an adequate amount of L-amino acids, water-soluble vitamins, and minerals. Additional carbohydrate and fat must be added to provide for fat-soluble vitamins and additional calories to meet necessary growth requirements. Another preparation is low-methionine Isomil from Ross Laboratories, Columbus, Ohio, a product low in methionine and cysteine, which contains sufficient carbohydrates, fat, protein, minerals, and vitamins to meet normal infant formula standards. This preparation meets only the minimum requirements for sulfur-containing amino acids, and care should be taken to supplement the dietary preparation in accordance with the nutritional requirements of the individual patient for normal growth and development.[10,65]

Inborn Errors of Carbohydrate Metabolism

TRANSFERASE-DEFICIENCY GALACTOSEMIA

Transferase-deficiency galactosemia is an autosomal recessive disorder of carbohydrate metabolism with an overall incidence of about 1:65,000.[46,58] It falls into the category of disorders treated by substrate or precursor restriction.

Classical galactosemia is caused by a deficiency of galactose-1-PO_4 uridyl transferase, an enzyme necessary for the body's utilization of exogenous galactose. This carbohydrate is an important functional constituent of glycolipids, glycoproteins, and mucopolysaccharides, and the major source of it is derived from lactose, the disaccharide in milk and milk products. A major portion of the total caloric intake is derived from galactose in milk-fed infants. This is made possible by the reaction sequence that converts lactose to glucose shown in Figure 25-4.

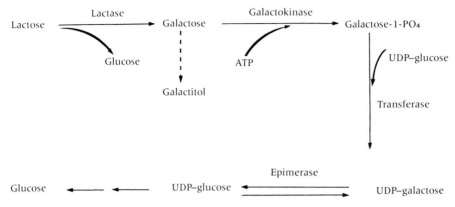

FIG. 25-4   Conversion of lactose to glucose via galactose-1-PO_4 uridyl transferase.

When a deficiency of galactose-1-PO_4 uridyl transferase (or, transferase) exists, galactose is unavailable as an energy source, and the metabolites galactitol and galactose-1-PO_4 increase to toxic levels, thereby interfering with normal metabolic processes. The untreated newborn infant with transferase-deficiency galactosemia may show nausea, vomiting, aminoaciduria, galactosuria, hepatosplenomegaly, cirrhosis, and failure to thrive, and death may ensue within the first weeks of life. If the infant survives the neonatal period without treatment, he will most likely manifest liver damage, cataracts, and mental retardation. If a galactose-restricted diet is instituted early in the neonatal period, the severe clinical symptoms can either be avoided or ameliorated.

DETECTION

Many neonatal screening programs include tests for detection of galactosemia. A variety of methods, using samples of either cord or whole blood and analyzing for the presence of galactose-1-PO_4 uridyl transferase or one of its reaction products, are employed.[26,46,58] When results of tests show a deficiency of transferase in the red blood cells, dietary therapy can be instituted before clinical symptoms are apparent. More often, however, the affected infant shows early symptoms and signs (*i.e.,* vomiting, diarrhea, and reducing substances in the urine) very soon after the first milk feedings are begun. In some cases, an infant may display clinical symptoms and signs of classical galactosemia, including cataracts, before the first milk feeding, because of high concentrations of galactose *in utero.* This may occur because the heterozygous mother has half-normal enzyme activity and the fetus has little or no enzyme activity. As a result, galactose-1-PO_4 and other minor metabolites could increase to toxic levels when the mother's dietary galactose is increased during pregnancy. In some rare cases the correct diagnosis is never made, but the infant still survives the neonatal period. In these cases, the infant is thought to have a milk intolerance of a more common etiology, such as intestinal lactase deficiency or a malabsorption syndrome. Several different formulas are tried until one is found that the infant can tolerate, and this preparation is often low in galactose. Upon recognition of the clinical manifestations of galactosemia by the physician, it is important that use of all milk-based formulas be suspended until a definitive diagnosis can be made.

DIET THERAPY

Principles, Objectives, and Strategies. The galactose-restricted diet for the newborn infant makes use of a milk-free proprietary formula. Nutramigen (Mead Johnson Laboratories, Evansville, Indiana) is the most often recommended formula in the United States. Like other proprietary formulas, it is based on a casein hydrolysate and can provide the complete nutrient, vitamin, and mineral requirements for the infant. It compares favorably in nutritional value with cow's milk for the older child. Prosobee (Mead Johnson Laboratories, Evansville, Indiana) and Isomil (Ross Laboratories, Columbus, Ohio) are also suitable for use. These formulas are prepared from an isolate of soy protein and have a low oligosaccharide content (some of which may be galactose). Growth and development of galactosemic children on galactose-restricted diets using proprietary formulas as a base compare favorably with their age-matched controls.

As solid foods are introduced into the infant's diet, care should be taken to eliminate all foods that contain milk or milk products, lactose, or galactose. A list of foods that can be included and excluded (and other products that contain lactose

TABLE 25-6
Foods Allowed and Prohibited on Galactose-Restricted Diet

Type of Food	Foods Allowed	Foods Prohibited
Milk and milk products	Isomil, Nutramigen, Prosobee, meat base formulas, nondairy creamers without lactose	Breast milk, milk from any animal source in any form, lactose cream, butter, cheese, yogurt, ice cream, ice milk, sherbert
Meat	Plain meats, fish, poultry, eggs	Organ meats (*i.e.,* pancreas, liver, brain) Creamed, processed, breaded meats Poultry or eggs which may contain milk products or lactose
Breads and cereals	Any breads that do not contain lactose, casein, or milk products; home-made cakes, pies, cookies made from acceptable ingredients; macaroni, spaghetti, noodles, rice; cooked or dry cereals without milk products, lactose, or casein	Prepared mixes (*i.e.,* muffins, biscuits, waffles, pancakes, cookies, and cakes) Most brands of enriched white bread
Fruits and vegetables	All fresh, canned, or frozen that are processed without lactose, casein, or milk products Legumes except in infants with diarrhea*	Any vegetable creamed, breaded, buttered, or processed with lactose, casein, or milk products
Fats	Margarines and dressings that do not contain milk, milk solids, or lactose; oils, shortenings, bacon lard, nuts, nut butters, olives	Margarines and dressings containing milk or milk products, butter, cream, cream cheese
Soups	Clear soups, vegetable soups, cream soups made with milk substitutes listed	Cream soups, chowders, commercially prepared soups with lactose
Miscellaneous	Unbuttered popcorn, marshmallows, sugar corn syrup, molasses, honey, fruits, gelatin, fruit-flavored corn-starch pudding made with water, carbonated beverages, instant coffee, unsweetened cocoa, unsweetened cooking chocolate, pure spices, punch base without lactose	Caramels, toffee, and most candies, milk chocolate, pre-sweetened punch base with lactose, medicines compounded with lactose,† seasoning mixes, sugar substitutes made with lactose

*See Gitzelmann R, Auricchio S: The handling of soya alpha-galactosides by a normal and a galactosemic child. Pediatrics 36:231, 1965
†Sugar-free liquid preparations are listed in American Druggist 171, No. 10:51, 1975

that may be intentionally or unintentionally ingested) is shown in Table 25-6. The exclusions for a galactose-restricted diet are much more stringent than for a lactose-restricted diet for persons with lactose intolerance. Note, for example, the exclusion of organ meats which have high concentrations of galactose-containing complex carbohydrates.[32]

There is some disagreement among physicians and biochemists as to whether beans and legumes and soybean-based formulas should be eliminated from the diet. Their original inclusion in the restricted list is due to the fact that the cell wall contains various α-galactosides, notably stachyose and raffinose, which contain galactose. However, Gitzelmann and co-workers determined that the normal intestinal disaccharidases were not capable of releasing galactose from these disaccharides.[32] However, they did find that the intestinal bacterial flora of the lower bowel can hydrolyze the disaccharides to some extent. Since the lower bowel does not absorb the free sugars, this would have little effect on blood galactose levels. Gitzelmann considers soybean formulas safe for galactosemic

infants with the possible exception that when diarrhea occurs, the lower bowel flora may colonize the upper bowel and hydrolyze the galactose-containing disaccharides, thereby releasing free galactose which may be absorbed by the small intestinal mucosa.[32]

Effectiveness and Feasibility. Close clinical and biochemical monitoring of the galactosemic patient should be done at daily, weekly, or biweekly intervals after the diagnosis is made and during the period of adjustment to the galactose-restricted diet. Blood galactose-1-PO_4 levels should be monitored at regular 3-month intervals in galactosemic infants up to 2 years of age who are progressing satisfactorily, and at 6-month intervals during childhood. More frequent determinations of galactose-1-PO_4 may be required during illness and when any milk-containing foods are introduced.[20,25,41] An empirical upper limit of 3 mg/dl galactose-1-PO_4 is accepted as safe for galactosemics on a galactose-restricted diet.[19] However, it should be recognized that some clinical manifestations such as mental retardation and cataracts may exist even when the diet is carefully followed, owing to either *in utero* damage, late introduction of galactose restriction, or individual genetic differences that might require an even lower galactose intake. Galactose is not an essential sugar, since it can be synthesized endogenously from glucose; hence, there is no lower limit on the daily requirement of galactose similar to the essential amino acid, phenylalanine, in phenylketonuria. Therefore, the physician and dietitian must search for possible additional sources of galactose in the diet of a patient who appears to be under adequate dietary control but still manifests clinical symptoms and signs of galactosemia. Under these circumstances, more frequent monitoring of the galactose-1-PO_4 level and stricter dietary surveillance and restriction may be required.

Follow-up of patients at frequent intervals should include physical examination to check for hepatomegaly, observation by slit-lamp for cataracts, growth measurements, nutrition evaluation for adequacy for the diet and possible ingestion of galactose, and, in addition, an annual psychological evaluation.[64]

Complicating Conditions. Nutramigen is usually readily accepted by most young infants. However, when it is introduced to an older child who may have escaped early diagnosis and treatment, there may be poor acceptance. Careful dietary counseling of both patient and parents should be undertaken. The mother can be instructed in ways to flavor the milk-substitute or to add the dry milk-substitute powder during preparation of other foods to increase protein content *in lieu* of the cow's milk eliminated from the diet.

Regardless of the age when treatment is begun, the child should be taught to understand the need for eliminating galactose from the diet and should be told what foods to avoid. However, it is important in dietary management that the child should not be made to feel abnormal. Several studies have linked socio-emotional abnormalities in galactosemic children to parental zeal in "protecting" the galactosemic child from galactose, thereby adversely affecting the child's self-image and social maturity.[22,30,42,44]

The question of whether galactose restriction should be a life-time treatment has been under debate for many years.[35] Careful studies have shown that no enzymes capable of metabolizing galactose appear later in the development of galactosemic individuals.[8] It is likely that older or adult galactosemics appear to tolerate galactose because in these patients the sugar constitutes a proportionately smaller percentage of the total caloric intake. With respect to the problem of mental retardation, some workers feel that once full brain growth has been reached, in about 6 years, the diet could be relaxed.

However, the problems of galactose-induced cataracts and hepatic damage can be a life-long threat. Thus, it appears that restriction of galactose should be maintained indefinitely. However, many physicians ease the restriction when older children have difficulty maintaining the diet. This relaxation of dietary restriction of galactose usually means introducing food prepared with small amounts of milk such as bread, sauces, and prepared mixes with lactose but not milk as a beverage or in ice cream.

Another group for whom galactose restriction should be instituted is the pregnant woman who is either heterozygous or homozygous for galactosemia.[63] To prevent any possible *in utero* damage to the fetus, galactose should be eliminated from the diet, either prior to conception in a planned pregnancy or as early in the pregnancy as possible. The mother's blood should be monitored for galactose-1-PO_4 levels on a monthly basis. Like the older child, the pregnant woman may find the proprietary formula unpalatable. However, an attempt should be made either to include a galactose-free milk-substitute formula into the diet or to provide the equivalent amount of protein, calcium, and vitamins D and A from other food sources. The pregnant woman should also restrict her alcohol intake, as ethanol depresses the liver's utilization of carbohydrates.

There are other inborn errors of metabolism that interfere with utilization of galactose. These include galactokinase deficiency, epimerase deficiency, and variants of the galactose-1-PO_4 uridyl transferase enzyme which lead to somewhat less than complete deficiency of the enzyme.[3,14,15,18,31] Although the individual with galactokinase deficiency does not show clinical complications as severe as the transferase-deficient patient, dietary restriction of galactose is recommended. Few patients have been discovered with epimerase deficiency, but since galactose becomes an essential sugar when the conversion of UDP glucose to UDP galactose is blocked (see Fig. 25-4), it is important to recognize that complete galactose restriction in patients with this disorder would be contraindicated.[31] Patients with variant forms of galactose-1-PO_4 uridyl transferase can often tolerate an unrestricted diet, but if the activity of the variant enzyme falls below 25% of normal, some patients may show clinical signs of classical galactosemia and must moderate their intake of galactose.[27] For these reasons a definitive diagnosis based on enzymatic analysis, and, in some cases, on a galactose loading study, is imperative for successful treatment.

Restriction of galactose from the diet of a galactosemic patient can bring about dramatic clinical improvement, and it can also be a life-saving measure. When the diet is instituted early and patients are followed carefully and monitored both

TABLE 25-7
The Glycogen Storage Diseases

Disease (type)	Enzyme Defect	Clinical Symptoms
Von Gierke's I	Liver and kidney glucose-6-phosphatase	Hepatomegaly, severe hypoglycemia, ketosis, hyperuricemia, hyperlipidemia and bleeding
Pompe's II	Lysosomal α1,4-glucosidase (or acid maltase)	Cardiac hypertrophy, skeletal muscle dysfunction, CNS deterioration (Death may occur before age 2.)[49]
Cori's III	Muscle and liver amylo-1,6-glucosidase (debranching)	Similar to but milder in symptoms than Type I; some muscle weakness
Andersen's IV	Liver amylo-1,4-1,6-transglucosylase (branching)	Cirrhosis of the liver; splenomegaly (Death due to liver failure may occur before age 2.)
McArdle's V	Muscle phosphorylase	Severe muscle cramps when performing strenuous exercise; usually appears first in young adulthood
Hers' VI	Liver phosphorylase	Similar symptoms to but a milder course than Type I
VII	Muscle phosphofructokinase	Similar to Type V
VIII	Liver phosphorylase kinase	Mild hepatomegaly, mild hypoglycemia, expressed fully only in males

chemically and by physical examination, this approach to treatment can prevent or almost completely ameliorate the clinical symptoms and signs of the disorder.

CHARACTERISTICS OF THE GLYCOGEN-STORAGE DISEASES

The group of inborn errors of carbohydrate metabolism shown in Table 25-7, which affect either the structure or amount of stored glycogen in various organs, is collectively known as the glycogen-storage diseases (GSD). At least eight different enzymatic defects have been discovered, which form the etiologic basis for these disorders. All have been shown to be genetically transmitted in an autosomal recessive manner except for type VIII, liver phosphorylase kinase deficiency, which is sex-linked and occurs only in males. Because there is a similarity in symptoms between some of the types, definitive diagnosis is based on glucose loading studies, epinephrine and glucagon tolerance tests, enzymatic assay of tissue from affected organs, and glycogen analysis.

Dietary treatment is effective in reducing the metabolic symptoms of hypoglycemia, acidosis, ketosis, hyperlipidemia, and hyperuricemia. Dietary intervention strategies have been most effec-

tive with Types I, III, and VI, and these will be described in more detail.

TYPE I GLYCOGEN-STORAGE DISEASE

The patient with glucose-6-phosphatase deficiency is incapable of sustaining a normal blood glucose level and consequently suffers from severe hypoglycemia. The effect appears to be most pronounced in early childhood. In severe cases, feedings on a 3-hr to 4-hr schedule are necessary.

A diet with meals having a carbohydrate:fat:protein ratio of 70–75:15–20:10% of total Cal and with high carbohydrate snacks has been recommended by Fernandes.[21] Throughout early childhood, milk, fruits, and cane sugar should be restricted because the galactose and fructose are converted to glycogen and lactic acid and can result in excess glycogen storage and acidosis. The carbohydrate sources should be glucose and starch, and bicarbonate should be given, if needed, to control acidosis. Meals high in either total calories or total proteins or fats should be avoided to prevent glycogen or lipid deposits. In some cases, severe hyperlipidemia can be successfully treated by medium-chain triglycerides. Severe hypoglycemia may lessen with age, and attempts can be made to lower the carbohydrate and raise the fat intake (as medium-chain triglycerides) in the diet. This would be especially true of patients who appear to have a carbohydrate-induced lipogenesis. Because of the hyperlipidemia and the possible vascular sequelae in later life, the dietary fats should have a high polyunsaturated to saturated ratio.

Evaluation of dietary intervention includes clinical appraisal of growth and development and frequent monitoring of blood sugar, lactate, free fatty acids, and urinary ketones. Blood chemistries should be followed closely during periods of illness or stress, and careful meal planning and subsequent dietary evaluation should be done to ascertain that adequate levels of calcium, vitamins A, C, and D, and fiber are ingested in view of the milk and fruit restrictions.

In general, as patients approach adolescence they are able to withstand the nighttime fast and can usually handle a less frequent eating schedule. Postadolescents may suffer from acute gouty arthritis, gouty nephropathy, and tophi owing to hyperuricemia. One of the possible mechanisms for overproduction of uric acid may be related to an abnormally high glucose-6-phosphate to ribose conversion without the phosphatase. Excess ribose could be converted to purines and then to uric acid. Although allopurinol has been shown to be effective in treating elevated serum urate in patients with Type I glycogen-storage disease, there is no direct dietary therapy to prevent uric acid production from excess ribose. However, it appears that lactate competitively inhibits renal tubular secretion of uric acid, and early dietary measures (*i.e.*, restricting the type of dietary carbohydrate) directed at curbing hyperlactic aciduria may lessen the consequences of later urate overproduction.

Portacaval transpositions or shunts, to deliver glucose-rich blood to the tissues before it reaches the liver, have been performed on at least 20 Type I patients.[61] Folkman and colleagues have improved on this form of treatment by long-term intravenous hyperalimentation prior to surgery.*[23]

TYPE III GLYCOGEN-STORAGE DISEASE

Deficiency of amylo-1,6-glucosidase prevents complete hydrolysis and utilization of stored glycogen. Therefore, dietary management in patients with Type III glycogenosis is directed toward preventing

*However, the surgical approach has now been replaced by continuous nocturnal feedings of a high carbohydrate mixture through a small intragastric tube. Marked improvement in growth and biochemical abnormalities as well as reduction in liver size have been noted using this approach. More recent innovations include use of corn starch in patients over 2 to 3 years of age (when amylase levels are normal) in an average dosage of 1.7 g/kg every 6 hr which now appears to obviate continuous nocturnal feedings (J. B. Sidbury, Jr., personal communication, 1982).

hypoglycemia and excess glycogen storage. Recommendations are similar to those for Type I in terms of frequency of meals in early childhood, restriction of carbohydrates containing fructose and galactose, and control of fat intake to prevent hyperlipidemia and acidosis. However, patients with Type III have a functioning gluconeogenic pathway and can maintain blood glucose levels from protein sources. Therefore, dietary recommendations include having a high-protein, high-carbohydrate meal at night to sustain blood glucose levels during the overnight fast. However, night feedings and, in some cases, continuous nocturnal intragastric feedings are recommended during infancy and childhood during periods of stress or illness.

The recommended ratio of carbohydrate, fat, and protein is 50:30–35:15–20% of total Cal.

TYPE VI GLYCOGEN-STORAGE DISEASE

Patients who have liver phosphorylase deficiency make up the largest proportion of those affected by glycogen-storage disease. Clinical symptoms are qualitatively similar to those with Type III, but they are milder and are sometimes manifested only after fasting. This may be due to the fact that the majority of the Type VI patients studied have some residual phosphorylase activity, allowing a variable degree of glycogenolytic function. Dietary intervention is not necessary on a continual basis for all patients with liver phosphorylase deficiency. However, if any of the symptoms of hypoglycemia, hyperlipidemia, acidosis, or ketosis should become apparent, especially during infancy or illness, the dietary recommendations given for Type III would be appropriate.

HEREDITARY FRUCTOSE INTOLERANCE

Hereditary fructose intolerance (HFI) is a rare inborn error of carbohydrate metabolism, which is caused by a deficiency of the enzyme fructose-1-PO_4 aldolase. The disorder was first described in 1956, and appears to be inherited in an autosomal recessive manner.[16] The enzymatic defect causes an increase of fructose-1-PO_4 as shown in the following sequence of reactions:

$$Fructokinase \xrightarrow{\text{Fructose}} Fructose\text{-}1\text{-}PO_4$$

$$Fructose\text{-}1\text{-}PO_4 \xleftrightarrow{\text{F-1-}PO_4 \text{ Aldolase}} Glyceraldehyde + Dihydroxyacetone\text{-}PO_4$$

It is believed that excess fructose-1-PO_4 competitively inhibits fructose-1,6-diPO_4 aldolase, an enzyme catalyzing crucial steps in both glycogenesis and gluconeogenesis.

The symptoms of HFI depend on the extent of the enzyme defect and the age of the individual. The infant, upon ingesting fructose-containing foods, may display some or all of the following symptoms and signs: failure to thrive, vomiting, hepatomegaly, jaundice, hypoglycemia, coma, and convulsions. Persons surviving infancy without treatment often demonstrate liver damage, proteinuria, and generalized aminoaciduria. Removal of fructose (levulose), fructose-containing sugars, sucrose and invert sugar, and sorbitol from the diet is usually very effective treatment for HFI patients.

Diagnosis of the disorder is often made by taking a careful diet history, which usually shows a close correlation between introduction of fruits, fruit juices, or infant formulas containing added sucrose and the onset of clinical symptoms. Older children and adults often show an aversion to sweets and, as a result, have fewer dental caries. An intravenous fructose tolerance test (preferable to an oral load which usually induces vomiting and nausea) is used to confirm the diagnosis. Froesch recommends giving 0.25 g/kg body weight fructose intravenously.[28] Blood glucose should fall to within the range of 20 mg/dl to 30 mg/dl in less than an hour, after which it will slowly return to normal. Inorganic phosphate levels will also fall. The tolerance test should be done only under conditions in which hypoglycemia can be treated immediately by intravenous glucose, if necessary. A definitive diagnosis includes measurement of liver aldolase activity from a liver biopsy to rule out a deficiency of the enzyme fructose-1,6-diphosphatase. A deficiency of the latter enzyme would give a similar profile after a fructose loading test (unlike the aldolase deficiency, it does not cause gastrointestinal disturbances after fructose ingestion, but does cause hypoglycemia and lactic acidosis after stress, fasting, or infection.)[4] In the acutely ill neonate, a tentative diagnosis is established on the basis of the clinical symptoms and analysis of fructose in the urine. The infant may then be placed on a fructose-free formula even before the definitive enzyme assays are done on liver biopsy. However, with the severely intoxicated neonate it may be necessary to rehydrate first with a slow glucose and electrolyte infusion.

The fructose-restricted diet must be continued throughout life. In the older child or adult this poses no problem because they soon learn that fructose-containing foods make them ill. Lists of foods by brand name, permitted or prohibited on a fructose-free diet, are available.[28] Infant feeding is a little more difficult because the limited diet of an infant traditionally contains fruit juices and many products sweetened with sucrose. Table 25-8 contains a list of foods that are acceptable for the infant who must have a sucrose–fructose-restricted diet. Meeting the carbohydrate requirement in the diet poses no problem for the HFI patient, since there are no restrictions on starches, glucose, and lactose. The patient should receive a vitamin C supplement because the restrictions on fruits and vegetables make the diet deficient in this vitamin.

General Considerations

EDUCATION OF PHYSICIANS, PARENTS, AND THE PATIENT

Special diets used in the treatment of inborn errors of metabolism may well affect the quality of family life. It is clear that food plays an important part in daily living, more than merely supplying amino acids, carbohydrates, fats, vitamins, and minerals. Studies have indicated that 13 out of 27 families with phenylketonuric children on dietary treatment had serious social and psychological problems.[48] Therefore, in order for a treatment program for inborn errors of metabolism to be successful, close cooperation is required between parents, physician, dietitian, and biochemist to maintain satisfactory biochemical control and achieve adequate growth and development.

Successful treatment of the child with an inborn error of metabolism is enhanced by improvement of the emotional stability of the family unit. Parents of these children are usually completely unprepared to cope with the problem of retardation. For example, much of the repression, denial, and guilt shown by parents of phenylketonuric children appears to be displaced or expressed as an unrealistic attitude toward the problem of dietary control, including its cost, preparation, and quality of maintenance. This negative attitude often carries over in presentation of the diet to the child.

Inasmuch as no objective criteria are available at present on which to base a decision regarding diet termination in many of the inborn errors of metabolism, it is evident that more preparatory discussion should be conducted with the family prior to diet discontinuation. In this respect, increased support to the parents and age-appropriate educational efforts directed to the child should reduce undue anxiety and avoid unnecessary conflict situations. The social worker, nutritionist, nurse, and physician all have important roles in the process of fostering a healthy parent–child relationship during the period of diet discontinuation or relaxation.[54]

Perhaps one of the most important aspects of education of physicians, parents, and patient is in providing sufficient information to guard against phenylalanine deficiency. It should be emphasized

TABLE 25-8
Sucrose-Fructose-Free Diet for Infants

Food Groups	Foods to Include	Foods to Avoid
Milk and other formulas*	Human milk; cow's milk; evaporated milk formula with glucose or lactose as added carbohydrate; Similac, Enfamil, SMA, or other nonsoy formulas; CHO–Free is allowable	All soy formulas; Nutramigen, Premature, Probana formula (Mead–Johnson)
Other fluids	Glucose water	Gelatin or Karo water
Fruits, juices	None	All
Cereals, cookies, teething rings	Gerber's Oatmeal or Rice Cereal (dry variety); saltines; Old London Melba Toast	All
Vegetables	Gerber's Creamed Spinach; Heinz Creamed Spinach	All others
Meat, egg yolks	Beef, chicken, turkey, lamb, pork, egg yolks (all brands); Gerber's Ham	Other brand names of strained ham; egg yolks and bacon; meat and chicken sticks
Dinner and soups	None	All
Desserts	None except specially prepared egg custards, tapioca puddings, cornstarch puddings using glucose as sweetener	All commercially prepared strained desserts

*Corn syrup (Karo brand by Best Foods) does contain added sugar, so it cannot be used as a fluid for the infant. Pure glucose powder mixed with water must be used instead. (From Hack S: Hereditary Fructose Intolerance. In Palmer S, Ekvall S (eds.) (illus): Pediatric Nutrition in Developmental Disorders, pp 252–254. Courtesy of Charles C Thomas, Publisher, Springfield Il, 1978)

in this respect that regular and frequent testing of blood and urine is required. In addition, it is particularly important that successfully treated phenylketonuric women be apprised of the risk involved as they reach the child-bearing age. These individuals must be made aware that should they become pregnant, the low-phenylalanine diet must be reinstituted, and that preferably the diet should be begun before conception and continued throughout pregnancy. It is important that the prospective parents understand that there is widespread damage to the fetus by high levels of phenylalanine in the maternal blood. Experience has shown that reinstituting the low-phenylalanine diet presents a number of psychological problems in some cases.

RESPONSIBILITY FOR MANAGING DIETARY TREATMENT

Dietary management of phenylketonuria and other inborn errors of metabolism and their careful biochemical control require considerable experience with the diseases. For optimal results patients should be managed in circumstances in which full supportive facilities are available. It is recommended that these children should be cared for by a team (or special regional advisory center), including clinical and biochemical staff in addition to a dietitian, psychologist, and social worker who would share in management of the case with the family physician or local pediatrician.[24,68]

Responsibility for treatment may fall around development of the crisis situations involving one or more of the following critical findings in affected children: (1) excessively high or low blood concentration of an offending substrate, (2) growth failure, and (3) suspected or documented developmental delay. These situations usually develop as the result of the inability of a given family to accomplish a successful transition from one developmental stage to another in administration of a restricted diet. Families must make a considerable adjustment in their life-styles to accommodate the presence of a child with a chronic, potentially handicapping condition. At the same time, families have differing abilities to cope effectively with this stressful condition.

Treatment programs for dealing with phenylketonuria and other inborn errors of metabolism can be divided into the following three mutually dependent areas: close medical supervision, dietary management, and biochemical control:

1. Medical supervision includes periodic evaluations by a pediatrician or family physician, routine neurologic examinations, x-rays, and hematologic and other laboratory tests needed to assess nutritional status.
2. Dietary management in phenylketonuria, for example, consists of prescribing and maintaining a formula that will provide protein in the form of a low-phenylalanine protein substitute, sufficient calories from the protein substitute and other sources, and phenylalanine in amounts sufficient for normal growth and development. Nutritional information in the form of diet records kept by the parents is needed for adequate management.
3. Biochemical control is usually achieved in most inborn errors of metabolism by periodic measurement of the offending substrate in whole

blood, serum, or urine. On the basis of the biochemical data and dietary information supplied by the parents and nutritionist, adjustments in the diet can be made to maintain appropriate levels of protein, carbohydrate, and other nutrients in serum. Periodic psychological evaluation, using standardized intelligence tests, associated with appraisals of the child's growth and mental development measures the overall results produced by the treatment.[17]

If signs of family disequilibrium and crisis occur without being recognized, and if no intervention takes place, the family may become unable to mobilize their energies to cope with potential crisis situations. The long-term outcome and success of the treatment program may be placed in jeopardy, and the child may be damaged either physically or mentally or both.

By providing support and guidance to the family through the stresses imposed by the diagnosis of an inborn error of metabolism and its treatment, it is possible to avert, or at least to minimize, crises that may be harmful to the patient.[17]

SUMMARY

Dietary treatment of inborn errors of metabolism offers a challenging opportunity for altering the biochemical environment of patients with a number of human genetic disorders, with the prospect of preventing severe developmental disabilities and reducing the burden on the affected individual and on society. It is clear that successful programs for early detection, diagnostic confirmation, and treatment of inherited disorders require a regionalized team effort by physicians, biochemists, geneticists, public health agencies, nutritionists, nurses, psychologists, and social workers in cooperation with the food industry in providing therapeutic regimens for many genetic and metabolic diseases. There is a pressing need for more effective coordination of efforts in dietary management of many different inborn errors of metabolism, and prospective studies should be instituted to provide a more rational basis for evaluating therapeutic efficacy of dietary treatment.

References

1. Acosta PB: Nutritional aspects of phenylketonuria. In The Clinical Team Looks at Phenylketonuria (revised), p 52. Washington, DC, Children's Bureau, Department of Health, Education and Welfare, 1964
2. Acosta PB: Nutritional aspects of phenylketonuria. In The Clinical Team Looks at Phenylketonuria (revised), p 40. Washington, DC, Department of Health, Education and Welfare, 1964
3. Applegarth DA, Donnell GN, Mullinger M et al: Study of a family with Los Angeles, Duarte and classical galactosemia variants of gal-1-PUT. Biochem Med 15:206–211, 1976
4. Baker L, Winegrad AI: Fasting hypoglycemia and metabolic acidosis associated with deficiency of hepatic fructose-1,6-diphosphatase activity. Lancet 2:13–16, 1970
5. Beckner AS, Centerwall WR, Holt L: Effects of rapid increase of phenylalanine intake in older PKU children. J Am Diet Assoc 69.2:148–151, 1976
6. Berry HK, Umbarger B, Sutherland BS: Procedures for monitoring the low-phenylalanine diet in treatment of phenylketonuria. J Pediatr 67, No. 4:609–616, 1965
7. Berry HK, Sutherland BS, Hunt MM et al: Treatment of children with phenylketonuria using a phenylalanine-free protein hydrolysate (Albumaid XP). Am J Clin Nutr 29, No. 4:351–357, 1976
8. Beutler E: "Galactose dehydrogenase," "nothing dehydrogenase" and alcohol dehydrogenase: Interrelation. Science 156:1516–1517, 1967
9. Bickel H, Gerrard J, Hickmans EM: Influence of phenylalanine intake on phenylketonuria. Lancet 2:812–813, 1953
10. Bickel H, Schmidt H, Schürrle L: Dietary treatment of inborn errors of amino acid and carbohydrate metabolism. Bibl Nutr Dieta 18:181–201, 1973
11. Brewster TG, Moskowitz MA, Kaufman S et al: Dihydropteridine reductase deficiency associated with severe neurologic disease and mild hyperphenylalaninemia. Pediatrics 63:94–99, 1979
12. Brown ES, Warner R: Mental development of phenylketonuric children on or off diet after the age of six. Psychol Med 6, No. 2:287–296, 1976
13. Cabalska B, Duczynska N, Borzymowska J et al: Termination of dietary treatment in phenylketonuria. Eur J Pediatr 126, No. 4:253–262, 1977
14. Chacko CM, Christian JC, Nadler HL: Unstable gal-1-PUT: A new variant of galactosemia. J Pediatr 78:454–460, 1971
15. Chacko CM, Wappner RS, Brandt IK et al: The Chicago variant of clinical galactosemia. Hum Genet 37:261–270, 1977
16. Chambers RA, Pratt RTC: Idiosyncrasy to fructose. Lancet 2:340, 1956
17. Cox AW, Engstron BS, Berry HK et al: Children with phenylketonuria: Crisis prevention or crisis intervention. Matern Child Nurs J 3, No. 3:157–168, 1974
18. deBruyn CHMM, Oei TL, Monnens LAH et al: An unusual form of galactosemia: Studies on erythrocytes and hair roots. Clin Genet 13:8–16, 1978
19. Donnell GN, Bergren WR, Perry G et al: Galactose-1-phosphate in galactosemia. Pediatrics 31:802–810, 1963
20. Donnell GN, Koch R, Bergren WR: Observations of management of galactosemic patients. In Hsia D Y–Y (ed): Galactosemia, pp 247–268. Springfield, IL, Charles C Thomas, 1969
21. Fernandes J: Hepatic glycogen storage diseases. In Raine DN (ed): The Treatment of Inherited Metabolic Disease, pp 115–150. New York, American Elsevier, 1974
22. Fishler K, Donnell GN, Bergren WR et al: Intellectual and personality development in children with galactosemia. Pediatrics 50:412–419, 1972
23. Folkman J, Philippart A, Tze WJ et al: Portacaval shunt for glycogen storage disease: Value of prolonged intravenous hyperalimentation before surgery. Surgery 72:306–314, 1972
24. Francis DE: Therapeutic special diets. Practitioner 212 (Spec No): 545–551, 1974

25. Frazier DM, Cozart WS, Summer GK: Analysis of galactose-1-PO$_4$ and galactose in blood by a new microfluorometric method. Biochem Med 20:344–352, 1978

26. Frazier DM, Summer GK: Automated fluorometric micromethod for detection of transferase-deficiency galactosemia. J Lab Clin Med 83:334–352, 1974

27. Frazier DM, Frazier JR, Summer GK: Behavioral effects of dietary galactose in galactosemia heterozygotes. FASEB Abstracts 34:930, 1975

28. Froesch ER: Hereditary fructose intolerance and fructose-1,6-diphosphatase deficiency. In Raine DN (ed): The Treatment of Inherited Metabolic Disease, p 155. New York, American Elsevier, 1974

29. Garrod AE: The inborn errors of metabolism. Lancet 2:1–7, 73–79, 142–148, 1908

30. Gershen JA: Galactosemia: A psycho-social perspective. Ment Retard 13:20, 1975

31. Gitzelmann R: Deficiency of uridine diphosphate galactose-4-epimerase in blood cells of an apparently healthy infant. Helv Paediatr Acta 27:125–130, 1972

32. Gitzelmann R, Auricchio S: The handling of soya alpha-galactosides by a normal and a galactosemic child. Pediatrics 36:231–235, 1965

33. Guthrie R, Susi A: A simple phenylalanine method for detecting phenylketonuria in large populations of newborn infants. Pediatrics 32:338–343, 1963

34. Hanley WB, Linsao L, Davidson W et al: Malnutrition with early treatment of phenylketonuria. Pediatr Res 4.4:318–327, 1970

35. Herman RH: Galactosemia. Am J Clin Nutr 21:923, 1968

36. Hill JB, Summer GK, Pender MW et al: An automated procedure for blood phenylalanine. Clin Chem 11:541–546, 1965

37. Holtzman NA: Dietary treatment of inborn errors of metabolism. Annu Rev Med 21:335–356, 1970

38. Jonxis JHP: The nutritional significance of inborn errors of amino acid metabolism. Second European Nutrition Conference, Munich, 1976. Zollner M, Wolfram G, Keller CH (eds): Nutr Metab 21:33–48, 1977

39. Kaufman S, Berlow S, Summer GK et al: Hyperphenylalaninemia due to a deficiency of biopterin. N Engl J Med 299:673–679, 1978

40. Kaufman S, Holtzman NA, Milstien S et al: Phenylketonuria due to a deficiency of dihydropteridine reductase. N Engl J Med 293:785–790, 1975

41. Kirkman HN, Lanier DC, Clemons EH et al: Estimation of Gal-1-PO$_4$ in blood spotted on filter paper. J Lab Clin Med 88:515–519, 1978

42. Komrower GM, Lee DH: Long-term follow-up of galactosemia. Arch Dis Child 45:367–373, 1970

43. Komrower GM, Sardharwalla IB, Coutts JM et al: Management of maternal phenylketonuria: An emerging clinical problem. Br Med J 1, No. 6175:1383–1387, 1979

44. Lee DH: Psychological aspects of galactosemia. J Ment Defic Res 16:173–190, 1972

45. Levy HL: Genetic screening for inborn errors of metabolism. In Harris H, Hirschhorn K (eds): Advances in Human Genetics, Vol. 4, pp 1–104. New York, Plenum Press, 1973

46. Levy HL, Hammersen G: Newborn screening for galactosemia and other galactose metabolic defects. J Pediatr 92:871–877, 1978

47. Lowe CU: Nutritional management in hereditary metabolic disease. Pediatrics 40:289–304, 1967

48. McBean MS, Stephenson JB: Treatment of classical phenylketonuria. Arch Dis Child 43:1–7, 1968

49. Martin JJ, deBarsy T, Van Hoff F et al: Pompe's disease: An inborn lysosomal disorder with storage of glycogen. Acta Neuropathol 23:229–744, 1973

50. Niederwieser A, Curtius HCR, Bettoni O et al: Atypical phenylketonuria caused by 7,8-dihydrobiopterin synthetase deficiency. Lancet 1:131–133, 1979

51. Niederwieser A, Curtius HCH, Viscontini M et al: Phenylketonuria variations. Lancet 1:550, 1979

52. O'Brien D: Dietary management of inborn errors of amino acid metabolism. Postgrad Med 65, No. 4:133–138, 1979

53. Pedersen HE, Birket–Smith E: Neurological abnormalities in phenylketonuria. Acta Neurol Scand 50, No. 5:588–598, 1974

54. Pueschel SM, Yeatman S, Hum C: Discontinuing the phenylalanine-restricted diet in young children with PKU. Psychosocial aspects. J Am Diet Assoc 70, No. 5:506–509, 1977

55. Pueschel SM, Hum C, Andrews M: Nutritional management of the female with phenylketonuria during pregnancy. Am J Clin Nutr 30, No. 7:1153–1161, 1977

56. Scriver CR, Katz L, Clow C: Phenylketonuria and diet. Can Med Assoc J 98, No. 2:124–125, 1968

57. Scriver CR: Realized and potential neutralization of mutant genes in man by nutritional selection. Fed Proc 35, No. 11:2286–2290, 1976

58. Shih VE, Levy HL, Karolkewicz V et al: Galactosemia screening of newborns in Massachusetts. N Engl J Med 284:753–755, 1971

59. Smith I, Erdohazi M, Macartney FJ et al: Fetal damage despite low-phenylalanine diet after conception in a phenylketonuric woman. Lancet 1, No. 8106:17–19, 1979

60. Smith I, Lobascher ME, Stevenson JE et al: Effect of stopping low-phenylalanine diet on intellectual progress of children with phenylketonuria. Br Med J 2, No. 6139:723–726, 1978

61. Starzl TE, Marchioro TL, Sexton AW et al: The effect of portacaval transposition on carbohydrate metabolism: Experimental and clinical observations. Surgery 57:687–697, 1965

62. Sutherland BS, Umbarger B, Berry HK: The clinical management of phenylketonuria. GP 35, No. 5:93–98, 1967

63. Tedesco TA, Morrow G, Mellman WJ: Normal pregnancy and childbirth in a galactosemic woman. J Pediatr 81:1159–1161, 1972

64. Wenz E, Michell M: Galactosemia. In Palmer S, Ekvall S (eds): Pediatric Nutrition in Developmental Disorders, pp 256–260. Springfield, IL, Charles C Thomas, 1978

65. American Academy of Pediatrics. Committee on Nutrition (ed): Pediatric Nutrition Handbook, pp 224–225. Evanston, Ill, 1979

66. Editorial. The growing problems of phenylketonuria. Lancet 1, No. 8131:1381–1383, 1979

67. Genetic Screening, pp 97–102. Programs, Principles and Research, Division of Medical Sciences, National Research Council, National Academy of Sciences, 1975

68. Results of dietary control in phenylketonuria. Med J Aust 2, No. 14:613–614, 1970

26
Infectious Diseases
William R. Beisel

A generalized infectious illness causes widespread metabolic responses in the host and in addition leads to nutritional deficiencies. Localized infections may also result in metabolic and nutritional derangements if the accompanying inflammatory response is of sufficient magnitude and severity.

During the first decades of this century, the medical management of infectious illnesses consisted solely of symptomatic therapy. Much importance was placed on dietary aspects of treatment. However, the close attention given to nutritional management diminished with the advent of the antibiotic era. As various new antimicrobial agents were recognized, the nutritional or dietary aspects of therapy were either neglected or relegated to an occasional role.[7]

Observations in humans and in a variety of animal species indicate that deficiencies of isolated nutrients or generalized forms of protein–energy malnutrition may result in an impairment of host defensive mechanisms.[1,9,15] On the other hand, infectious illnesses produce losses of body constituents that can lead to nutritional deficiencies. Thus, there is a tendency for a sequence of infection and malnutrition to develop into a synergistic cycle, with each new infection causing more profound nutritional deficits. These can, in turn, predispose the host to secondary infections. Such a vicious cycle occurs most often in young children in underdeveloped nations and helps to account for their high mortality rates.[9]

During an infection, some nutrients are lost from the body because of negative body balances.[1,5] Other nutrients are lost functionally because of metabolic and biochemical responses to hormonal stimuli.[1] As detailed below, functional forms of nutrient loss include increased utilization, diversion from normal pathways of metabolism, or sequestration within body pools or depots in a manner that renders them temporarily unavailable for utilization.

To help develop a comprehensive nutritional plan for assisting in the therapy of infectious diseases, this chapter reviews underlying biochemical, metabolic, and hormonal mechanisms that account for the loss of body nutrients. By understanding these mechanisms and predicting their onset, magnitude, and duration, the thoughtful clinician should be able to anticipate probable nutritional deficits. This should help in planning appropriate measures for supportive care. In infectious diseases for which specific antimicrobial therapy is neither available nor effective, the clinician is faced with an even more important need to use nutritional measures as a key aspect of supportive management.

Forms of Nutrient Loss During Infection

NEGATIVE BODY BALANCES (ABSOLUTE LOSSES)

Studies in volunteers have documented the changes in body balances of many nutrients during the course of bacterial, viral, or rickettsial diseases.[5] Information has been obtained concerning the time of onset, magnitude, and sequential patterns of response during the prodromal and early febrile periods of acute infectious illnesses. Although these

The views of the authors do not purport to reflect the positions of the Department of the Army or the Department of Defense.

prospective studies include only a small variety of brief uncomplicated infections, such information can assist in the interpretation of data derived during infections of overwhelming severity or of a chronic protracted nature.

STEREOTYPIC PATTERNS OF ABSOLUTE LOSS

The most conspicuous nutritional consequence of infectious illness is an absolute loss of body constituents. This is shown clinically by loss of body weight and muscle tone and a progressive wastage of muscle mass and body fat. These losses are associated with negative body balances of the principal intracellular elements, including nitrogen, potassium, magnesium, inorganic phosphorus, zinc, and sulfur.[5] Losses of nitrogen serve as a prototype for losses of the other intracellular components.

Negative nitrogen balances do not begin during the incubation period of an infection or even during the first day of fever. However, once a febrile response is fully established, body balances become negative. Measured losses of nitrogen and other intracellular elements then exceed their respective intake values. As an acute infection persists, additional daily losses lead to a progressive depletion in body content of many elements. A self-limited mild viral illness induces losses of about 20 g nitrogen; if promptly treated, generalized tularemia may cause losses of 40 g to 60 g; and untreated malaria can produce losses of 80 g to 100 g. Losses of other intracellular elements are proportional to those of nitrogen.

Absolute nutrient wastage during hypercatabolic illness produces changes that overshadow other metabolic responses of the body. These catabolic losses are qualitatively similar during febrile illnesses caused by many different microorganisms. They represent a consistent stereotyped host response to illnesses of relatively short duration. Not all elements follow the pattern of cumulative wastage seen with the principal intracellular elements. Although losses of sodium and chloride occur at the onset of a febrile infection, hormonal mechanisms quickly come into play to cause urinary retention of salt during the febrile phase of acute infections. The body then tends to retain water as well as salt.

Thus, body composition during a severe generalized infection is altered by a combination of factors, including increased metabolic needs of body cells, a lessening of dietary intake, complex endocrine responses, an overall wastage of most body nutrients, and retention of salt and water. In portraying this situation during septic starvation, Moore and colleagues comment that "the body cell mass quickly melts away into a hypotonic ocean of extracellular fluid."[11]

FACTORS CONTRIBUTING TO NEGATIVE BALANCES

Fever. Even though fever may support the function of body defensive mechanisms, fever is a major factor in initiating body nutrient losses. Such losses are provoked equally by infectious fevers or the induction of fever by means of bacterial endotoxin or a hot, humid environment.[2] For each degree centigrade elevation of body temperature, basal metabolic rates increase by 11% to 13%. In addition, fever produces other direct losses through sweat. The magnitude of catabolic loss appears to be proportional to the severity and duration of fever. However, a protracted fever causes smaller losses as the body becomes severely depleted. The catabolic losses resulting from a short illness may require several weeks for correction.[2,5]

Anorexia. Like fever, anorexia may also be a defensive measure during some infections. However, the anorexia experienced by most patients during an infection contributes to body deficits. Anorexia leads to a diminution in the consumption of foods and a reduced intake of calories, protein, vitamins, and other nutrients. If food intake is restricted to a comparable degree in a noninfected normal subject, metabolic processes readjust rapidly, endogenous nitrogen sources are conserved, greater amounts of energy are derived from fat depots, and the body diminishes its rates of loss of vital nutrients. In simple starvation, nitrogen-sparing responses are initiated which reduce losses to 3 g/day to 4 g/day. Such responses do not generally occur in the presence of fever. Indeed, some febrile patients actually increase nitrogen losses through the urine to above-normal values despite the anorexia and diminished intake of food. Should diarrhea or vomiting develop, additional losses occur through the intestinal tract. This combination of events leads to a measurable net loss of a large variety of nutrients during periods of acute infection.

Endocrine Responses. Hormonal responses during infection are generally of limited duration and magnitude.

ADRENAL HORMONES. An increased secretion of adrenal glucocorticoid hormones begins with, or shortly before, the onset of fever. Increases in daily rates of cortisol production may reach values two to five times normal. Plasma cortisol loses its circadian periodicity and generally maintains concentrations near, or slightly above, usual peak morning values. The increase in glucocorticoid secretion is accompanied by smaller increases in the output of adrenal ketosteroids and pregnanetriol. These

ACTH-mediated adrenocorticoid responses do not persist beyond the onset of recovery. If an infection becomes subacute or chronic, the urinary excretion of adrenal steroids generally falls below normal.

The onset of septic shock or the progression of infectious illness to an agonal stage is often accompanied by steadily increasing plasma cortisol concentrations. High values result from a functional failure of hepatic enzyme systems that normally metabolize steroids. On the other hand, hemorrhage into the adrenal gland during bacterial sepsis or hemorrhagic viral diseases may cause glucocorticoid production to cease. If this occurs, cortisol and mineralocorticoid replacement therapy becomes an acute necessity.

Changes in aldosterone secretion do not coincide with those of cortisol. Increased production of aldosterone becomes evident only after fever has begun, and abates gradually in early convalescence. The increase in aldosterone secretion contributes to renal salt retention during acute infections. In addition, a tendency for excessive body water to accumulate during many severe infections has been attributed to inappropriate secretion of antidiuretic hormone.

THYROID HORMONES. Changes in thyroid hormone economy are best evaluated in relation to the stage of an infectious process. A biphasic pattern of thyroid response seems evident. An accelerated disappearance rates of T_4 and T_3 from plasma occurs during early stages of infection. Changes in serum T_3 values may be accompanied by reciprocal changes in reverse T_3, and the binding of thyroid hormones to serum proteins may be altered. These early changes suggest increased utilization, deiodination of thyroid hormones, or both, by peripheral tissues during fever and periods of increased phagocytic activity. A sluggish response of the pituitary–thyroid axis helps to account for the initially depressed T_3 and T_4 values, but eventually the thyroid is activated. Thus, during early convalescence, hormonal values may increase, and the rate of T_4 disappearance may decrease. These latter observations are in keeping with an eventual overshoot in thyroid gland activity in response to the earlier acceleration of hormone degradation. Further, thyroid glands from patients with overwhelming infections show histologic changes typical of increased secretory activity.

GLUCOREGULATORY HORMONES. Hormones that influence carbohydrate metabolism are intimately involved in host responses during febrile illnesses. Fasting plasma concentrations of glucose, insulin, glucagon, cortisol, and even growth hormone tend to be increased.[13] The hepatic production and release of glucose is accelerated as a consequence.

If carbohydrate tolerance is measured by means of a glucose load during early fever, the insulin responses and glucose disappearance rates show changes resembling those of maturity-onset diabetes. Elevated fasting glucagon values decline appropriately after intravenous glucose test loads, but growth hormone secretion seems to undergo an acute paradoxical stimulation.[13] Catecholamine values are also increased during some infections, especially those accompanied by hypotension.

These combined hormonal responses initiate molecular mechanisms to release glucose from stored hepatic glycogen and to increase rates of gluconeogenesis from available substrates. An increased flux of gluconeogenic amino acids, such as alanine, from muscle to plasma to liver supports this activity. The increase in hepatic gluconeogenesis may cause fasting hyperglycemia of 120 mg/dl to 150 mg/dl despite an increased rate of glucose utilization by body cells. Newly produced glucose appears to serve as the principal fuel used by body cells for the extra energy requirements of fever. However, during overwhelming sepsis in newborns and in patients with severe liver damage, such as that due to viral hepatitis or yellow fever, glycogen reserves in liver and skeletal muscles become depleted and hypoglycemia may result. No specific enzyme failure has been identified in any biochemical pathway that could account for an agonal breakdown in carbohydrate synthesis without hepatocellular necrosis.

Other consequences of the unusual hormonal ratios seen during infection include a partial to complete inhibition of hepatic ketone production and a slowed release of free fatty acids from storage depots.

Duration of Illness. If a febrile illness is of brief duration, negative balances are quickly reversed and the body begins to retain depleted nutrients. To reconstitute normal body composition, a patient generally develops positive balances for depleted nutrients in early convalescence. The magnitude and duration of positive balances appear to be determined by the type and quantity of dietary intake, as well as by the extent of cumulative deficits incurred during illness. For most uncomplicated minor illnesses, deficits are reconstituted within a period of several weeks in a manner similar to convalescent patterns of recovery after trauma. Recovery of depleted body stores may be assisted by a transient hyperphagic increase in appetite during convalescence. In some children, this is sufficient to permit "catch-up" growth, but a series of infections may cause severe growth retardation in young children.[1,9]

Should an acute infectious process become chronic, daily nitrogen balances gradually become less negative each day. Thus, as day-by-day losses diminish, a chronically ill patient begins to return to a new equilibrium state, although at a wasted, cachectic level. The body can generally reconstitute such chronic losses if protracted infections are treated successfully.

Severity of Illness. As a general rule, severe infectious illnesses produce greater nutritional insults than do mild ones. However, an overwhelmingly severe infection that leads to death in a matter of hours or days may run its course before an appreciable wasting of body tissue has a chance to occur.

Localization of Infection. The generalized stereotypic metabolic response to infection may be altered by processes that are localized in certain organs. For example, marked losses of fluid and electrolytes complicate diarrhea, important metabolic functions of the liver may be lost during hepatitis, and impaired pulmonary gas exchange and losses through sputum may occur in pneumonia.

FUNCTIONAL FORMS OF NUTRIENT LOSS

In addition to direct losses of body nutrients, metabolic and biochemical host responses produce several functional forms of nutrient loss.[1] Functional losses are defined as the within-body losses due to metabolic or pathophysiologic responses. They include overutilization, diversion, or sequestration of nutrients. In facing the challenge of an acute febrile illness, the body utilizes muscle protein, endogenous fuels, and other nutrients in an apparently inefficient and wasteful manner. On the other hand, the redirected metabolism may contribute to host defensive mechanisms. Nevertheless, these functional forms of loss add to the nutritional requirements of the body and must be considered when planning comprehensive therapy for infection.

OVERUTILIZATION OF NUTRIENTS

Overutilization of body nutrients is one example of functional wastage. Increased cellular needs for body fuel can virtually deplete carbohydrate stores during severe sepsis or endotoxemia. However, during uncomplicated infections, amino acids and other substrates for gluconeogenic activity are metabolized in sizable quantities. The presence of fever has long been known to increase the metabolic rate of body tissues. An accelerated utilization of metabolized fuel by cells throughout the body is accompanied by accelerated rates of hepatic synthesis of cholesterol and triglycerides, degradation of liver and muscle glycogen, and the accelerated utilization of amino acids for glucose production.

An increased utilization of vitamins must also be anticipated. Severe infections in humans may precipitate clinically apparent vitamin deficiency states, for instance, scurvy, beriberi, pellagra, or vitamin A deficiencies. Vitamin losses through urine during infection do not seem to account for such instances of overt vitamin deficiency. Of 14 vitamins studied during experimentally induced sandfly fever in volunteers, only riboflavin showed an increased rate of urinary loss.[3] Thus, a depletion of vitamin stores in the tissues during infectious illnesses or the decline in blood concentrations of several vitamins can be ascribed to accelerated utilization of vitamins by body tissues rather than to measurable excretory losses.

DIVERSION OF NUTRIENTS

The second form of functional wastage involves the diversion of nutrients from their usual metabolic pathways. The infectious process stimulates a marked increase in the rate of uptake of plasma amino acids by the liver. In addition to their enhanced hepatic utilization for gluconeogenesis, the exaggerated movement of amino acids into the liver is followed by rapid incorporation into newly synthesized acute-phase reactant plasma proteins. These proteins include α_1-antitrypsin, seromucoid, haptoglobin, ceruloplasmin, C-reactive protein, and others. Although these proteins appear to modulate inflammatory and immunologic responses, their synthesis has a high cost in terms of amino acid and energy expenditures.

Some of the amino acids that enter the liver in excess are used for incorporation into newly synthesized hepatic enzymes, some are diverted for metallothionein formation, and some enter normal metabolic pathways, but in excess amounts. An example of the last is the accelerated metabolism of tryptophan by means of the kynurenin pathway during many infections, especially typhoid fever.[1] A variety of metabolic products of tryptophan are then excreted in excess and lost from the body as urinary diazo reactants.

SEQUESTRATION OF NUTRIENTS

Another form of nutrient wastage during infection is represented by the temporary sequestration of nutrients in relatively inaccessible forms.[1,4] For example, an increased movement of iron from plasma to liver is a characteristic host response in many infectious diseases, especially those accompanied by a prominent inflammatory response. Iron in the form of hemosiderin or ferritin then accumulates in hepatic storage depots. Sequestered iron is not readily reused for the formation of hemoglobin as long as the infection persists. This sequestration eventually leads to the "anemia of infection," which resembles iron deficiency anemia in its peripheral red blood cell and serum iron values. Unlike iron deficiency anemia, however, supplies of iron accumulate in body stores during infection, and total serum iron-binding capacity tends to decrease rather than to increase.

The combination of low serum iron values with increased concentrations of unsaturated transferrin appears to have some protective value for the host.[1] Because ferric iron is extremely insoluble in body fluids, many bacteria synthesize siderophores to acquire the iron they need to proliferate. The siderophores have association constants high enough to compete successfully with saturated transferrin for iron.[1] However, the increased concentration of unsaturated transferrin in an infected host makes it difficult for bacteria to acquire sufficient iron to carry out their normal metabolic functions, to achieve logarithmic growth patterns, or to produce certain toxic products.[1,4]

Zinc is also sequestered within the liver. After an increased flux into liver, the zinc is sequestered within hepatic cells by newly synthesized metallothioneins, and serum zinc values decline.

Sodium can also become sequestered in various body cells during severe illness, especially in infections accompanied by marked acidosis.

CELLULAR NEEDS

An infectious illness is accompanied by hypermetabolism and accelerated utilization of cellular energy. A sudden increase of energy expenditure occurs whenever a phagocyte is activated. A burst of glycolytic energy production develops when neutrophils begin to take up and kill invading bacteria or other microorganisms. Other body cells need to be supplied with energy from circulating metabolic fuels to perform their infection-stimulated functions.

To meet the added demands for cellular energy, the body utilizes its molecular machinery for producing glucose. This process involves increased secretion of hormones such as glucagon, the adrenal glucocorticoids, and the catecholamines; these hormones combine to induce two related patterns of response within the liver. The enzymes that control the release of glucose from glycogen stores are activated. In addition, the rate of production of glucose is accelerated, utilizing gluconeogenic amino acids, lactate, pyruvate, and glycerol as substrates.

Well-controlled, insulin-dependent diabetic patients who develop an acute infection are likely to develop hyperglycemia with glycosuria. It has long been taught that these diabetic patients need additional amounts of insulin if they develop an infection. Infection-induced hyperglycemia has tra-

ditionally been thought to represent an impairment of the ability of insulin to act on peripheral body cells. This is accompanied during infection by great increases in both production rates and body pool sizes of glucose, with accelerated glucose turnover within the enlarged pools. The body appears willing to sacrifice scarce amino acids and other nutrient precursors to provide cells with more than adequate concentrations of glucose during periods of acute febrile illness. This response begins within several hours of the onset of fever.[13]

In addition to producing additional amounts of glucose during infection, the liver also speeds up its synthesis of both cholesterol and fatty acids from acetate and other precursors. Excess triglycerides are formed within the liver; these either accumulate in lipid droplets within hepatic cells or are secreted into the plasma.[1]

SUMMARY OF NUTRITIONAL CHANGES

Even the least complicated generalized infections stimulate a wide variety of metabolic and nutritional responses. These result in expenditures or losses of essential body nutrients. Loss of body weight is the combined result of fever-induced hypermetabolism, impaired appetite, and complex series of hormonal and physiologic responses that lead to absolute losses of body nitrogen, potassium, magnesium, zinc, and sulfur. There are increased expenditures of calories, vitamins, and amino acids. Host defensive mechanisms require increased formation of new cells, such as those of the phagocytic and lymphoid series, the synthesis of intracellular enzymes, hormones, other products, and new serum proteins, including the acute-phase reactants, specific antibodies, complement, interferon, and fibrinogen.

Approaches to nutritional therapy should be based on the metabolic responses known to occur during an infection. The absolute loss of body nutrients can be reduced during an infectious illness and should be corrected early in convalescence. Excessive nutrient requirements can be reduced by therapeutic measures to diminish the febrile response and to eliminate invading microorganisms.

General Management of Infectious Disease Problems

INCIDENCE OF INFECTIOUS DISEASES

Infectious diseases occur at every age and in all population groups. Infection-related problems also play a secondary or complicating role in other varieties of medical, surgical, or pediatric illness. Infectious disease problems are of greatest importance at the extreme ends of the normal human life span. Although no age group is free of infectious diseases, middle-aged persons generally have the lowest incidence of serious infections.

Contrary to the hopes and expectations that accompanied the advent of the antibiotic era, infectious diseases have not been eliminated from the medical scene, even in the most advanced societies. Also, although advances in medical and surgical technology have generally increased life expectancy, they have sometimes introduced nutritional debilities, immunologic defects, and other iatrogenic factors that break down natural host defensive mechanisms. As a result, the older classic infectious diseases have been replaced in major hospital centers by an increased incidence of opportunistic infections. This unanticipated consequence of medical progress has forced practitioners of all medical specialty fields to face new varieties of infections caused by bacteria, fungi, viruses, or parasites not previously thought to be widely pathogenic or of more than incidental concern.

General improvements in sanitation and vigorous programs of preventive medicine and public health have shown that it is possible to control or virtually eliminate many of the epidemic or endemic infectious diseases of previous years. Smallpox may never be seen again. Development of safe and effective vaccines has gone far toward controlling such epidemic diseases as diphtheria, pertussis, measles, and poliomyelitis. The incidence of tuberculosis and enteric bacterial, parasitic, and venereal diseases has been minimized in the highly industrialized nations. Although these advances have lessened the danger from common communicable killers of previous generations, infectious diseases continue to cause death and debility in modern societies. Further, infectious diseases account each year for more deaths on a global scale than any other form of illness.

Thus, despite the availability of many antibiotic, public health, and immunoprophylactic measures, infectious diseases are likely to remain a continuing and serious health problem. In addition to the growing incidence of opportunistic infections in advanced medical centers, the reemergence in some localities of venereal diseases, malaria, and poliomyelitis shows how easily an apparently well-controlled situation can be reversed unless prophylactic and public health measures are pursued with continuing diligence.

Of major concern is the well-recognized synergistic cycle that relates infectious disease to malnutrition. The prevalence of malnutrition and infection continues to produce high childhood-mortality rates in underdeveloped nations, especially those with tropical and subtropical climates. This problem will remain unsolved in the presence of world population growth and a continuing failure to produce or distribute sufficient food for all people.[9]

THERAPEUTIC MODALITIES

The obvious aim of therapy is to control and eliminate invading microorganisms before serious illness or lasting complications can occur. The first line of medical management is to identify the causative agent—if this is possible—and to define effective chemotherapeutic or immunotherapeutic approaches.

Proper antimicrobial management involves the selection of the drug and dosage schedules most likely to produce complete and rapid control of the infection without causing untoward secondary effects. Exact identification of the infecting microorganism and its range of sensitivity is valuable if these can be obtained. However, if the severity and course of an infection require that therapeutic decisions be made without such information, judgments must be based on a careful evaluation of the available clinical and laboratory findings.

Some infections require the use of active or passive immunotherapeutic procedures rather than antimicrobial drugs, and some must still be managed without such benefits.

Nutritional modalities of therapy are usually, and most appropriately, classified among the secondary forms of general supportive therapy. Nevertheless, this support can be of benefit to patients receiving specific antimicrobial therapy. For infectious diseases that lack specific therapy, nutritional support is of even greater importance. Nutritional therapy is especially useful in patients with viral illnesses or in individuals with preexisting nutritional deficiencies. In rare instances, such as fulminant cholera or hepatitis-associated hypoglycemia, rapid correction of life-threatening physiologic or biochemical imbalances can be achieved only through the administration of an essential nutrient such as water, glucose, or electrolytes. Under such conditions, emergency replacement therapy, a form of nutritional management, must be given first priority.

Nutritional Modalities of Therapy

DIRECT NEEDS

There are relatively few instances in clinical medicine in which nutritional modalities of therapy are of specific direct importance in managing an immediate life-threatening problem. However, these situations must be recognized quickly and treated effectively when they occur. Perhaps the best example of such an emergency requirement is the need to correct the massive loss of body fluids and electrolytes that occurs during fulminant diarrhea. In patients with cholera or severe *Escherichia coli* enterotoxemia, intestinal losses of water, sodium, chloride, and other nutrients can lead quickly to hypovolemic shock and death.

Other forms of acute nutritional imbalance may occur in infections that damage key body cells and precipitate secondary depletions of body nutrients or an accumulation of toxic metabolites. If of sufficient severity, infectious hepatitis may produce hypoglycemia or hepatic failure. Severe hypoglycemia is also a common danger in neonatal infants with sepsis. Life-threatening hypoglycemic shock can be suspected through clinical signs, diagnosed by blood glucose analysis, and corrected with glucose infusions. In contrast to the infection-induced depletion of an essential body nutrient such as glucose, the accumulation of potentially toxic metabolic products can occur in patients with liver failure of infectious origin. This can be managed as outlined in Chapter 21.

SECONDARY AND SUPPORTIVE MODALITIES

Supportive nutritional therapy is based on the anticipated loss of nutrients during an infectious illness. The practitioner should actively seek to prevent or lessen the harmful consequences of nutritional wastages. Supportive therapy should be initiated concurrently with antimicrobial measures.

FEVER

Catabolic losses in a patient with an infectious process generally do not begin until after the onset of the febrile phase of illness. Thereafter, the duration and severity of fever influence the magnitude of both absolute and functional losses. Lessening of fever by antipyretic drugs or by direct physical methods serves to reduce the nutritional needs for the excessive energy production required by the presence of fever. Control of fever also reduces dermal losses of nutrients through sweat.

When fever is not controlled, its impact must be taken into account when calculating daily caloric and protein needs.

ANOREXIA

A major nutritional problem associated with acute infectious illness is the presence of anorexia. This is often compounded by overt nausea and vomiting. It then becomes almost impossible for a patient to maintain a normal oral intake of fluids, calories, protein, and other nutrients. This problem can not be solved by ordering a properly calculated dietary intake to be delivered to the bedside or by instructing a sick patient to eat the quantities and varieties of foods calculated to meet nutritional needs. Kindly and purposeful encouragement by an attentive nursing staff or family is similarly ineffective in many instances. However, a sick patient should be offered soft or liquid foods of high nutrient and caloric value. When marked anorexia and nausea severely restrict food intake, anticipated deficits should be minimized by using the parenteral route.

ESTIMATION OF CALORIC NEEDS

The caloric needs of a patient with an infectious illness should include the normal recommended daily dietary allowance plus extra amounts needed because of fever. Daily requirements can be derived from standard table values (see Appendix Table A-1), and the added needs can be calculated according to the amount of fever (7% increase for each °F of elevation).

Thus, a 35-year-old-man weighing 70 kg, who ordinarily requires an energy intake of 2700 Cal (Appendix Table A-1), with a body temperature 3°F above normal, would require 2700 Cal, plus 3 × 7% of 2700 Cal. This amounts to 2700 plus 567 Cal, or 3267 Cal/day. Alternatively a febrile adult could be given 30 Cal/kg/day to 40 Cal/kg/day, a child, 100 Cal/kg/day to 150 Cal/kg/day, and an infant, 200 Cal/kg/day.[1]

Caloric adequacy during an acute illness can also be determined by changes in body weight. Body weight changes during infection should be evaluated with the knowledge that weight loss may be masked by the tendency for febrile patients to retain salt and water. Water retention of one or more kilograms may occur during a febrile illness and obscure equivalent losses in tissue mass. The true extent of body loss may not become apparent until after the fever, when postfebrile diuresis causes excessive fluid to be excreted. If caloric intake has not kept pace with body needs during an illness, deficits should be made up as early as possible in the convalescent period.

PROTEIN REQUIREMENTS

Every host defensive mechanism is ultimately dependent on the protein-synthesizing capabilities of individual cells. Nevertheless, the body will sacrifice amino acids through functional diversions to provide for total caloric needs. Thus, the protein requirements of a febrile patient will depend in part on the daily availability of caloric energy.

If energy intake is inadequate, amino acids derived from dietary protein or existing body pools are diverted to meet energy needs rather than for incorporation into the structure of new proteins or for metabolic uses unique for each amino acid. Because metabolic energy must be expended to deaminize amino acids for carbohydrate synthesis, the use of amino acids for calorigenesis is doubly wasteful.

In the presence of fever, the body fails to initiate the metabolic adjustments used to conserve body nitrogen during periods of simple starvation. Nevertheless, it is possible to reduce excessive losses of body nitrogen in febrile patients by increasing the intake of total calories. Although the extra energy needs should be met preferably by adding nonnitrogenous sources of calories to the daily nutrient intake, the body should not be forced to depend on endogenous tissue protein for its amino acid requirements.

Exact protein requirements have not been determined during periods of fever. However, a consensus holds that the desirable nitrogen intake should be 1.5 g/kg/day for febrile adults and 3 g/kg/day for febrile children.[1] The nitrogen source should include a balanced supply of essential amino acids.

Several simple methods are available for estimating protein requirements. Urea nitrogen assays can be performed by most clinical laboratories on 24-hr urine specimens. A daily urea nitrogen excretion value plus 4 g (2 g for nonurea nitrogen in urine and 2 g for stool nitrogen) provide a reasonable estimate of nitrogen loss. If this value is compared with an estimate of nitrogen intake based on table values, a rough idea of nitrogen balance can be obtained. Measurements of serum albumin concentration, skin-fold thickness, and midarm muscle circumference are also of value in determining the adequacy of protein intake, especially in patients whose illness is protracted.

ACID–BASE STABILIZATION

Infectious diseases cause a variety of changes in acid–base equilibrium. Different pathogenic mechanisms may allow metabolic acidosis, metabolic alkalosis, respiratory alkalosis, or respiratory acidosis to develop singly or in complex physiologic derangements. The clinician must be aware of these possibilities to determine if corrective therapy is required during illness, or replacement therapy during convalescence.

Respiratory Effects.   The pathophysiologic course of an infectious process or its complications may cause complex respiration-induced changes in acid–base equilibrium. Fever is typically accompanied by increased cardiac and respiratory rates.

Fever-induced hyperventilation leads to an increased rate of gas exchange within the lungs and causes an exaggerated loss of dissolved carbon dioxide from the blood. This produces uncompensated respiratory alkalosis during periods of rising fever. Respiratory alkalosis may persist as long as tachypnea exists in the presence of a free exchange of pulmonary gases. Rarely, however, is respiratory alkalosis sufficient to produce carpopedal spasm or to require therapy.

On the other hand, if pulmonary consolidation prevents adequate gas exchange, hypoxia and respiratory acidosis are observed. Impaired gaseous exchange is also a problem in botulism, poliomyelitis, or tetanus, diseases which impair neuromuscular components of pulmonary function. Under these conditions, oxygen becomes a nutrient that must be supplied.

Metabolic Effects.   Metabolic factors influence acid–base equilibrium if an infectious process becomes chronic or severe. In high fever or prolonged illness, the generation of lactic acid and other metabolic products exceeds the capacity of the body to dispose of them. If the quantity of acid metabolites is sufficiently great, metabolic acidosis begins to emerge. If bacterial sepsis produces hypotension and vascular stasis, impaired oxygen transport leads to cellular hypoxia, exaggerated formation of lactic acid, and a further increase in the severity of metabolic acidosis.

Diarrheal diseases can produce two different additional varieties of acid–base imbalance. Since the lower small bowel and proximal colon contain intraluminal bicarbonate concentrations almost double those of plasma, massive diarrhea causes large losses of bicarbonate from the body. This loss of bicarbonate can lead acutely to metabolic acidosis, and can be treated by adding bicarbonate or lactate to replacement fluid infusions. Bicarbonate should be replaced until the urine pH becomes alkaline.

In severe or chronic diarrheas, large amounts of potassium are also lost. If these losses are great, vacuolar degeneration of body cells may be observed histologically, especially in the renal tubules. A massive loss of body potassium will also produce severe metabolic alkalosis, which can persist for many months unless treated. The development of hypokalemic nephropathy and metabolic alkalosis can be prevented by replacement therapy with potassium. This essential nutrient can be provided by using commercial solutions to provide 20 mEq to 35 mEq of potassium per liter. During severe diarrhea, the massive losses of potassium can be treated by potassium-containing maintenance fluids given primarily to compensate for continuing losses of water. Residual or chronic deficits should be corrected with high-potassium foods during the convalescent period.

ELECTROLYTE AND WATER REQUIREMENTS

An infectious process may lead to death from fluid imbalances ranging from severe overload to severe dehydration. Direct losses of salt and water occur in diseases accompanied by severe or protracted diarrhea, vomiting, or marked diaphoresis. Without such direct losses, the body usually retains fluid and electrolytes. With severe illness, sodium may accumulate within poorly functioning cells; hyponatremia is then seen, despite a normal total body content of sodium. Water retention due to inappropriate antidiuretic hormone secretion will increase the severity of hyponatremia. Appropriate therapy in the latter types of salt and water derangements requires a restriction of fluid and electrolyte intake. Thus, a patient with infectious illness may have an emergency need for electrolyte replacement or may, on the other hand, be seriously harmed by fluid and electrolyte administration. An understanding of the pathophysiologic mechanisms leading to deranged fluid and electrolyte balance is therefore necessary when deciding on the proper therapeutic measures.

Sodium Wastage. The losses of body water and electrolytes during Asiatic cholera provide insight into the conceptual approaches required for planning optimal therapy for exaggerated forms of acute diarrhea. In massive diarrhea, the watery stools are virtually iso-osmotic with plasma. Because stool losses are iso-osmotic, water does not move from body cells to maintain the extracellular volume, and an immediate threat to life emerges owing to depletion of circulatory volume and consequent shock.

Losses of body water and electrolytes in equivalent iso-osmotic amounts lead to extracellular dehydration without appreciable changes in the concentrations of plasma sodium in relation to plasma water. However, the extent of body dehydration can be assessed by clinical signs, together with high hematocrit values and increased concentrations of total plasma proteins in relationship to plasma water. This type of dehydration increases the specific gravity of both whole blood and plasma. Because plasma proteins may undergo a two-fold increase in concentration during severe cholera, measured sodium and chloride concentrations may appear to be diminished, if they are calculated and expressed conventionally on the basis of whole plasma values. To be physiologically accurate and therapeutically meaningful, electrolyte concentrations of such dehydrated patients must be recalculated to reflect the high protein concentration and diminished amount of water present in the plasma.

Iso-osmotic dehydration owing to massive diarrhea must therefore be corrected by the use of iso-tonic replacement fluids.[6] Emergency fluids are given rapidly to correct shock and acidosis and to return hematocrit and plasma protein concentrations to normal. After initial rehydration, homeostasis is maintained by infusing solutions at a rate to match measured hourly stool volume losses. Potassium deficiency can be made up by mouth or by potassium-containing fluids.

Severely dehydrated hypotensive cholera patients may have pulmonary rales when first examined or may develop acute pulmonary edema during rehydration.[6] If due to severe coexisting acidosis, this cardiopulmonary problem should be managed by the use of bicarbonate- or lactate-containing resuscitation fluids.

Sodium Retention and Sequestration. Dehydration is not usually a problem in generalized infectious diseases that do not include diarrhea or massive vomiting. Rather, the onset of fever is accompanied by increased secretion of aldosterone and antidiuretic hormone. Acting in concert on distal renal tubular cells, these hormones cause the kidneys to retain both salt and water. Sodium and chloride may virtually disappear from the urine, and urine volume may be sharply reduced.

If the secretion of antidiuretic hormone persists in an inappropriate fashion, body water is retained even in the presence of declining plasma concentrations of both sodium and chloride. Because of the retention of salt and water in many infectious illnesses, it is generally unwise to administer saline in intravenous solutions. Further, if chronic metabolic acidosis develops, variable amounts of sodium may accumulate within body cells. The sequestration of sodium within body cells is evidence of severe illness and is not easily reversed. The unwise administration of saline in an attempt to correct depressed serum sodium concentrations in such patients may have serious consequences, such as cerebral edema in children with meningoencephalitis.

Severe hyponatremia that cannot be explained by direct sodium losses should be managed by restricting salt and water intake until after the infectious process is controlled and serum sodium concentration begins to increase. This type of problem is most common in the aged, or in children with central nervous system infections, Rocky Mountain spotted fever, or other severe generalized infections. Daily fluid intake should be severely restricted. Body weight, urinary specific gravity and volume, and serum and urine values for sodium and osmolality should be measured each day; central venous pressures may need to be followed in some patients. When urinary specific gravity begins to decline and the daily urine volume increases, fluid intake can be liberalized.

MINERAL AND TRACE ELEMENT REQUIREMENTS

Little direct information is available about the need to employ minerals or trace elements as therapeutic agents.[4] For the present, the wisest course of action would seem to demand that natural foodstuffs be given—if possible—in adequate quantities during illness, and certainly during early convalescence, in an effort to correct or restore any infection-induced mineral or trace element imbalance or deficit.

Magnesium. Magnesium concentrations in serum may decline somewhat during the course of a generalized infection, as the result of a dilutional phenomenon associated with the retention of body water. In addition, metabolic balance studies in volunteers with relatively mild infections demonstrate negative balances of magnesium.[5] These occur in close proportion to negative balances of nitrogen. Since potassium is also lost in generally proportional amounts, it can be postulated that these nitrogen-equivalent losses are derived from cellular pools. No data are available concerning the use of magnesium supplements in infectious illnesses, but they may be needed if there is a prolonged negative balance of this element, as during surgical complications that induce major losses of magnesium from intestinal drainage or burned surfaces.

Calcium. Calcium concentrations in plasma may undergo a dilutional decline, but otherwise calcium metabolism does not seem to be influenced significantly by most infectious illnesses. However, body balances of calcium and other bone minerals do become negative if an infectious disease causes body immobilization or paralysis. Calcium accumulates in devitalized tissues, and the tendency for granulomatous tubercular lesions to become calcified is well known. Although a high calcium intake was employed in the preantibiotic management of tuberculosis, there is little to suggest that this mineral was of importance in arresting the disease. On the other hand, tuberculous patients may develop a sarcoidosislike hypersensitivity to vitamin D; if this occurs, vitamin D and calcium intakes must both be carefully controlled to avoid hypercalcemia.

Phosphorus. Inorganic phosphate metabolism shows a complex variety of changes in different infectious illnesses. Unusually low serum concentrations of inorganic phosphate have been reported in patients with gram-negative sepsis and in Reye's syndrome. Reduced serum phosphate concentrations may serve as a possible diagnostic indicator of sepsis. Serum phosphate values also decline rapidly, but transiently, during the early stages of fever, apparently as a secondary manifestation of respiratory alkalosis. Hypophosphatemia during an acute rise in body temperature is accompanied by the virtual disappearance of phosphate from urine and sweat. These changes occur too rapidly to be accounted for by parathyroid gland responses.

In volunteers with experimentally induced infections, body balances of phosphorus become negative.[5] Like the negative body balances of potassium and magnesium, phosphate losses parallel quite closely the magnitude and timing of nitrogen losses.

The participation of organic phosphates in many aspects of intermediary metabolism is well recognized. Organic phosphate moieties and high-energy phosphate bonds undoubtedly contribute at the cellular level to host responses to infection. Infection-related changes also occur in the activities of phosphatase enzymes contained in many body cells and in serum. It is not known how these changes influence the outcome of an infection, and there is no direct evidence that the administration of phosphate as a single nutrient would be of clinical significance.

Iron. Iron metabolism is markedly altered by infection. Many bacterial and viral infections, as well as malaria, cause red blood cell destruction. In addition, the concentrations of iron decline rapidly in serum at the onset of an infectious illness. This change appears to be due to a flux of iron from serum to liver. There, the iron becomes sequestered in cellular stores of hemosiderin and ferritin. The initial acute decline in serum iron occurs without appreciable changes in serum iron-binding capacity. As a result, the quantity of unsaturated transferrin is increased in serum during the initial stages of infection. If an infectious process becomes chronic, serum iron values remain low and iron-binding capacity begins to decline slowly. The iron sequestered in tissue stores represents a form of functional wastage, inasmuch as the iron seems to be trapped and unavailable for reutilization in the synthesis of hemoglobin for new red blood cells. This infection-induced sequestration of iron, together with a tendency for red blood cell survival to be shorter, can give rise to the so-called anemia of infection.

During chronic infections, the administration of iron by either oral or parenteral routes is ineffective in reversing the anemia of infection. If parenteral iron therapy is given while an infectious process remains active, administered iron also becomes sequestered in storage forms. Liver extract, the folates, and vitamin B_{12} are similarly without value.

Further, if parenteral iron therapy is used in children with kwashiorkor or protein–energy malnutrition, it can have disastrous consequences. The additional therapeutic iron serves to saturate the low serum iron-binding capacity common in protein-malnourished children. The presence of saturated transferrin in serum makes iron available to aerobic and facultative bacterial pathogens that may then proliferate rapidly to overwhelm the already impaired host defensive mechanisms of the malnourished child. Thus, if total serum iron-binding capacity is depressed in a malnourished child, iron therapy is actually contraindicated until protein repletion therapy has increased serum iron-binding capacity to normal values.

Copper.   Concentrations of copper in serum usually show an increase during infectious processes. The increase is secondary to accelerated hepatic synthesis and release of ceruloplasmin, the principal copper-binding protein. This response appears to have potential value with respect to host defensive mechanisms. Serum copper and ceruloplasmin values remain elevated for a week or more during early convalescence.

Zinc.   Zinc metabolism is also altered during acute infectious illnesses. Like iron, serum zinc moves rapidly from serum into the liver during the early stages of most infectious illnesses, but the depression of serum zinc values is not usually as great as that of iron. Unlike iron, however, a zinc-binding metallothionein protein must be synthesized rapidly within hepatic cells in order to sequester the zinc. It is postulated that this extremely rapid adaptive process is of positive value in terms of host survival. In addition, as illness progresses, zinc balances can become negative as a result of diminished dietary intake of the metal along with increased losses in urine, feces, and sweat.

VITAMIN REQUIREMENTS

Ever since the discovery of vitamins, research efforts and clinical trials have been used to test the attractive hypothesis that the ability of a host to resist infection is related to vitamin nutrition. Acute infections are followed in some instances by the onset of classic vitamin A deficiency, beriberi, pellagra, or scurvy.[14] Such complications generally occurred in patients whose antecedent nutritional status was either unknown or poor. Blood concentrations of several vitamins, such as A, B_6, or C, may decline during acute bacterial and viral illnesses, malaria, or chronic tuberculosis. Depressed concentrations of several vitamins in blood or tissues have also been reported in a variety of experimental infections in laboratory animals.[14]

In contrast, when healthy volunteers were given normal recommended daily amounts of vitamins throughout the course of a mild viral illness, relatively little change was seen in either the urinary excretion or blood concentrations of most vitamins.[3] However, an increased excretion of urinary riboflavin in these subjects began coincidentally with the onset of fever. The losses of riboflavin increased in magnitude during the early convalescent period and could be explained by the negative nitrogen balance.

Despite the paucity of detailed information concerning the rate of utilization or metabolic fate of vitamins in body stores during an infectious process, there can be no doubt that the metabolic actions of many vitamins are required to activate various host responses. The adrenal content of vitamin C is depleted during active steroidogenesis. The group-B vitamins, vitamin C, and folate all contribute to the adequacy of phagocytic activity by host cells. A number of vitamins, including A, B_1, riboflavin, niacinamide, B_6, B_{12}, E, and folate, contribute to maintaining the complex immune functions of B and T lymphocytes and macrophages. The antioxidant activity of vitamin E may help protect cellular lysosomes in leprosy. Absorption of B_{12} is impaired by competition from fish tapeworms within the gut of infested patients, and the absorption of fat-soluble vitamins, folate, and B_{12} may also be impaired transiently in patients with enteric infections or parasitic infestations.

The antimicrobial drugs can also influence vitamin metabolism. Isoniazid, for example, has been thought to induce peripheral neuropathy in some tuberculous patients by causing a deficiency of vitamin B_6. Pyridoxine supplementation has therefore been suggested for patients taking isoniazid. On the other hand, patients with tuberculosis may become overly sensitive to the normal action of vitamin D and become hypercalcemic, as in sarcoidosis.

Normal quantities of vitamins and other nutrients help to maintain host resistance at optimal levels. A mounting body of evidence suggests that many individual nutrients are essential for maintaining the normal function of host immune responses. In contrast, deficiencies, excesses, or imbalances of single nutrients may be harmful. Some immunological benefit has been shown in animal studies involving modest increases of dietary vitamin E and selenium. However, no evidence is yet available to show that megavitamin therapy benefits humans by improving resistance against the invasion and proliferation of infectious microorganisms. Nevertheless, this prophylactic or therapeutic concept continues to intrigue both lay and scientifically trained individuals. Arguments have been widely publicized concerning the possible prophylactic value of taking vitamin C in massive doses. In contrast, the carefully prepared statement of the American Academy of Pediatrics Committee on Drugs points out that there is no acceptable scientific evidence that ascorbic acid prevents the common upper respiratory viral infections.[8]

Based on evidence presently available, practicing physicians should employ vitamins in normally recommended doses throughout the course of an infectious illness or, at most, should increase doses onefold or twofold to cover the possibility that vitamins may be metabolized (or excreted) in increased amounts during hypermetabolic states. The scientific evidence needed to justify megavitamin therapy in the treatment or prevention of infectious illnesses does not exist.

NEW ALIMENTATION TECHNIQUES DURING INFECTION

Techniques developed to meet the unusually large nutritional requirements of severely burned or traumatized patients now allow surgeons to provide the total daily caloric requirements despite the presence of hypermetabolic states. The technique of total parenteral nutrition (TPN) is described in other chapters (see Chaps. 13 and 14). Another technique for supplying nutrients involves using a constant-drip gavage of a chemically defined diet. Gavage is accomplished through thin-walled nasogastric catheters; the procedure has been termed *enteral hyperalimentation.* Balanced free amino acid and carbohydrate mixtures, when given at proper concentrations and rates, can be fully absorbed in the upper intestine with a minimum of digestive work, and gavage can therefore be used in patients with lower intestinal lesions. Either technique carries certain risks that must be balanced against potential benefits.

In patients whose nutritional stores have been depleted by severe disease or a complex surgical problem, secondary sepsis is a relatively common complication. It is generally difficult, if not impossible to control or eliminate the septic process in such patients, even with the most vigorous utilization of normally appropriate and effective antibiotics. In contrast, when total parenteral alimentation is used to provide adequate nutritional support, many patients become free of fever, clear their blood and tissues of the invading microorganisms, and heal their surgical lesions.[1]

The correction of nutritional deficiencies in patients with severe septic complications appears to permit host defensive mechanisms to regain their functional adequacy. It is therefore reasonable to consider the possible usefulness of total parenteral nutritional support for overwhelming infections of a primary nature. Because of the technical need to infuse hypertonic solutions by means of chronically implanted central venous catheters, the process is not without danger. Microorganisms can gain access to the body through or around the catheters, and thrombus formation can be initiated within central veins. Early experiences with techniques of TPN were frequently complicated by bacterial or fungal contamination of the catheter, infusion solutions, or catheter entry sites. In addition, hyperosmolality caused by the infused nutrients can produce an osmotic diuresis with dehydration and, further, may cause impaired function of phagocytic cells. Hypertonic glucose concentrations may also disturb phagocytic functions. Severe hypophosphatemia can develop in patients receiving TPN; this has been shown to reduce leukocytic ATP content and to produce a marked depression in chemotactic, phagocytic, and bactericidal activities of granulocytes. Fluid overload must also be avoided. The potential value of enteral hyperalimentation must also be weighed on the basis of its potential dangers, which include induction of diarrhea, regurgitation, aspiration, changes in gut flora, and hyperosmolar dehydration.

Despite the potential dangers of these newer forms of nutritional therapy, patients with severe gram-negative bacterial sepsis or long-standing infectious processes may benefit from their use. Life-threatening septic processes resulting from opportunistic microorganisms can often be eliminated if appropriate antimicrobial therapy is supplemented by vigorous nutritional measures. Such demonstrations are highly instructive, for they point out the value of nutritional therapy in an unequivocal manner. On the other hand, this form of nutritional support has not been adequately studied in life-threatening acute viral infections, and the dangers could outweigh any potential advantages. If the acute stages of a short-term hypercatabolic infectious process make it impossible to maintain an adequate daily intake of energy and other nutrients, the resulting losses should be made up quickly in the early convalescent period when the problems of fever and anorexia have disappeared.

POSTILLNESS NUTRITIONAL ADJUSTMENTS

Infection-induced changes in the nutritional status of a subject, including the long-term depletion of body nutrients, are potentially reversible conditions. The full restitution of nutritional deficits that result from even a mild, self-limited infection of relatively brief duration may require several weeks of convalescence. The prolonged periods required for reconstituting body pools of essential nutrients following an infection resemble the prolonged periods of convalescence necessary after severe trauma or operative procedures. Thus, careful attention must be paid to the maintenance of optimal nutrient intakes during convalescence from an infection.[1,7,9]

With the cessation of fever and anorexia, the early convalescent period represents a "nutritional window" that should be used to replace lost body nutrients. Some patients develop hyperphagia for several days, making the replacement of nutrients an easy task. In nutritionally depleted children, the nutritional aim should be to obtain catch-up growth, with the mother having a key role for achieving this objective.[1,9,15] Good medical practice requires that patients be instructed about the need for maintaining a nutritional program that will allow for the reconstitution of measured or suspected losses.

Although nutritional therapy during convalescence should aim to correct deficits incurred during an infection, the temporary presence of these deficits can predispose a patient to secondary infections or weaken his resistance against an invasion by other virulent microorganisms. Body nutrient stores and the functional capabilities of host defensive mechanisms are at their lowest points in the days immediately after fever has abated. This problem is greatest in infants and small children whose nutritional requirements for growth are superimposed on nutritional needs for the maintenance of body homeostasis or for the reconstitution of nutrient stores after an infection. Thus, in the growing child, an infection often creates nutritional deficits that lead to new problems with secondary infections. Such synergistic cycles are the rule rather than the exception in children who suffer from preexisting deficits of protein, calories, or both.[1,9] Nutritional therapy in early convalescence may be life saving by reversing the cycle of infection, further malnutrition, and reinfection.

Strategies for Prevention

NON-NUTRITIONAL

Non-nutritional approaches have been highly effective in lowering the incidence of many diseases, including the historic scourges of mankind. For example, the widespread use of vaccines has been of major importance in helping to control or prevent infectious diseases, especially those of viral origin. The development of toxoids has been of further help in blocking the toxicity of such diseases as diphtheria and tetanus. Improvements in sanitation and various environmental measures have gone far to eliminate water-borne and food-borne infectious diseases and virtually to eradicate arthropod-borne infections, such as yellow fever and malaria, in the highly developed nations. A combination of effective antibiotic therapy and case-finding measures to identify carriers has helped to reduce the incidence of tuberculosis and the venereal diseases. Although none of these measures can prevent infectious diseases entirely, their implementation has proven to be of inestimable value in changing the patterns of disease incidence within the past century.

NUTRITIONAL

Evidence derived from laboratory studies, clinical observations, and field investigations suggests that the ability of the human or animal host to resist infection reaches optimal levels when host nutritional status is adequate and there are no overt or borderline nutritional deficiencies. Chronic malnutrition predisposes the infants and children in many parts of the world to life-threatening infections.[9] This problem is also seen in the elderly and in hospitalized patients suffering from severe medical or surgical illnesses.[7]

On the other hand, an overabundance of some nutrients may be harmful and may, in fact, increase host susceptibility to infection. Obesity causes an increase in susceptibility to many infections in humans and laboratory animals.[12] If excesses of minerals, trace elements, or vitamins reach toxic levels, the host's ability to defend against certain microbial invaders is impaired. Thus, body nutrient stores should be adequate, but not excessive, if all aspects of normal host defensive mechanisms are to function optimally.

EVIDENCE OF INTERACTION

An impaired nutritional status generally lessens the ability of host defensive mechanisms to prevent infectious illnesses. This type of interaction is best exemplified by impairments in host immune mechanisms that may accompany various forms of malnutrition.[15] Impaired immunologic functions are seen most commonly in children with nutritional deficits of proteins, calories, or both, but they also occur in adults who develop acute nutritional losses as a result of serious disease or surgical procedures. Impaired immune function has also been recognized in individuals with deficiencies of single vitamins (A, B_6, B_{12}, folate) or other nutrients (iron, zinc).

The increased incidence and severity of infectious diseases in malnourished individuals can best be explained by functional inadequacies of both immunologic and nonspecific systems of host defense. Subtle to marked derangements develop in virtually every facet of immunologic function that has been studied in patients with nutritional inadequacies.

The immunologic abnormalities owing to malnutrition can usually be corrected by nutritional therapy, but animal studies suggest that some residual immunodeficiency may persist.

The ability to synthesize new proteins from amino acid precursors is a key necessity for producing either cellular or humoral immunity. Protein synthesis is also a basic requirement for maintaining nonspecific host defensive mechanisms, including the formation of phagocytic cells, as well as their ability to mobilize and function. In protein–energy malnutrition, competition appears to exist among tissues that need amino acids for growth, maintenance of body homeostasis, diverse subcellular activities, and immunogenesis. With such nutritional deprivations, body systems are unable to function optimally, and even a mild infection can stimulate an excessive body demand for scarce nutrients.

The cellular uptake of free amino acids is governed by their intracellular and extracellular concentrations as well as by hormonal and metabolic influences on amino-acid receptor sites of cell surface membranes. The body does not appear to possess a centralized control mechanism or specific priority system to distribute individual amino acids equitably among various body cells. In a malnourished individual, the lack of a priority-defining mechanism seems to work to the detriment of cells of the lymphoid system, which are responsible for immunogenesis and immunocompetence. Lymphoid cells must therefore compete with cells hungry for amino acid, such as those of muscle and liver, or with cells needed for tissue growth and repair.

A deprivation of body protein, with or without a coexisting deficit in energy intake, will lead to widespread anatomic abnormalities of lymphoid tissues. These anatomic changes include thymic and tonsillar atrophy, generalized lymphoid hypoplasia, and a reduction in the number of circulating blood lymphocytes. Similar anatomic changes also may occur when malnutrition involves certain single essential micronutrients.

Malnourished individuals may show a depressed antibody response after immunization with widely used vaccines. Some of the differences in response during malnutrition may be related to the antigenic nature and potency of a vaccine. It has been found that children with kwashiorkor who respond normally to a live polio vaccine may show a depressed antibody response to a live yellow fever vaccine. Children with kwashiorkor also show an impaired

ability of their lymphocytes to respond to the mitogenic actions of phytohemagglutinin. Deficient persons may fail to generate a delayed dermal hypersensitivity reaction against skin-test antigens to which they were previously sensitized. Malnutrition also leads to impaired phagocytic activity or bactericidal capability of peripheral blood neutrophils and to diminished concentrations of most components of the complement system in serum.

Final Evaluation

Approaches to the nutritional management of infectious disease problems can be summarized in a series of guidelines and therapeutic steps in most clinical situations.

Body defensive mechanisms that prevent or minimize infectious illnesses seem to function best when a patient is in normal nutritional balance. Deficits or excesses of nutrients may predispose to an increased risk of infection or to an infection of increased severity.

Although nutritional management during the therapy of most infections falls into the realm of secondary or supportive care, on rare occasions immediate correction of a nutritional abnormality may be of life-saving importance. It should then take precedence in the management of the illness. These emergency situations generally involve the correction of severe fluid and electrolyte or acid–base abnormalities. Severe hypoglycemia or anoxia must also be corrected without delay.

In most nonviral infections the selection of an appropriate antimicrobial drug and dosage schedule, or a combination of drugs should form the major bulwark of therapy. In a previously healthy person, the nutritional management of infection should aim at preventing or lessening the absolute and functional forms of anticipated nutrient losses. Control of fever will lessen the ultimate severity and duration of nutrient wastage and can thus be categorized as a preventive measure in nutritional management. In addition to the control of fever, efforts should be made to supply adequate amounts of key nutrients to meet body needs during the illness.

Maintenance of an adequate caloric intake is the most important single need. Adequate, but not excessive, intakes of protein (or other amino acid sources) and vitamins are important secondary goals. Adequate nutritional therapy may require the use of parenteral infusions to meet the caloric needs of patient with protracted illnesses. In patients who are already severely malnourished, the use of parenteral nutrients may make it possible to control and eliminate septic processes that cannot be managed by antibiotics alone. The administration of specific minerals or trace elements is not generally required during an acute, brief infectious illness.

Nutritional deficiencies begin to develop in infections of even short duration and become clinically important if febrile patients are unable to consume dietary nutrients for more than a few days. Should an infectious process become chronic, it will be accompanied by a more complex variety of nutritional inadequacies, some of which are difficult to correct until the infectious process can be controlled or eliminated.

Because of their nutritional deficits, patients who recover from an acute infectious illness face greater than normal danger from occurrence of secondary infections during early convalescence. This danger can be lessened by vigorous attempts to repair or to correct nutritional deficits suffered during the acute phases of illness.

Finally, in patients with overt preexisting nutritional defects, corrective nutritional therapy should lead to a reversal of abnormal host defensive functions and lessen the danger from superimposed new infections.

References

1. Beisel WR, Blackburn GL, Feigin RD et al: Symposium on impact of infection on nutritional status of the host. Am J Clin Nutr 30:1202–1371, 1439–1566, 1977
2. Beisel WR, Goldman RF, Joy RJT: Metabolic balance studies during induced hyperthermia in man. J Appl Physiol 24:1–10, 1968
3. Beisel WR, Herman YF, Sauberlich HE et al: Experimentally induced sandfly fever and vitamin metabolism in man. Am J Clin Nutr 25:1165–1173, 1972
4. Beisel WR, Pekarek RS, Wannemacher RW Jr: The impact of infectious disease on trace-element metabolism of the host. In Hoekstra WG, Suttie JW, Ganther HE et al (eds): Trace Element Metabolism in Animals—2, pp 217–240. Baltimore, University Park Press, 1974
5. Beisel WR, Sawyer WD, Ryll ED et al: Metabolic effects of intracellular infection in man. Ann Intern Med 67:744–779, 1967
6. Benenson AS: Cholera. In Mudd S (ed): Infectious Agents and Host Reactions, pp 285–302. Philadelphia, WB Saunders, 1970
7. Butterworth CE Jr: Malnutrition in the hospital. JAMA 230:879, 1974
8. Committee on Drugs, American Academy of Pediatrics: Vitamin C and the common cold. Nutr Rev 32(Suppl):39–40, 1974
9. Keusch GT, Katz M (eds): Effective interventions to reduce infection in malnourished populations. Am J Clin Nutr 31:2035–2126, 2202–2356, 1978
10. Long CL, Spencer JL, Kinney JM et al: Carbohydrate metabolism in man: Effect of elective operations and major injury. J Appl Physiol 31:110–116, 1971
11. Moore FD, Olesen KH, McMurrey JD et al: The Body Cell Mass and Its Supporting Environment, pp 224–277. Philadelphia, WB Saunders, 1963
12. Newberne PM, Young VR, Gravlee JF: Effects of caloric intake and infection on some aspects of protein metabolism in dogs. Br J Exp Pathol 50:172–180, 1969
13. Rayfield EJ, Curnow RT, George DT et al: Impaired carbohydrate metabolism during a mild viral illness. N Engl J Med 298:618–621, 1973
14. Scrimshaw NS, Taylor CE, Gordon JE: Interactions of Nutrition and Infection. (WHO Monograph Series No. 57.) Geneva, World Health Organization, 1968
15. Suskind RM (ed): Malnutrition and the Immune Response. New York, Raven Press, 1977

27
Neurologic Disease
Pierre M. Dreyfus

The nervous system, both the central nervous system (CNS) and peripheral nervous system (PNS), can be affected by improper or inadequate nutrition. The most common nutritional disorders of the nervous system are caused by a deficiency of essential nutrients and vitamins, as a consequence of chronic alcoholism, debilitating diseases of the gastrointestinal (GI) tract, food faddism, poverty, and ignorance.[17] Nutritional depletion can also occur in the presence of an adequate diet when the body, including the nervous system, is under stress. Prime examples of such stress conditions are chronic infection, endocrine imbalance, and overwhelming psychiatric disease.[2] The adult nervous system is generally more resistant to altered nutrition than is the developing and actively myelinating nervous system, which seems particularly sensitive to protein–calorie undernutrition. The immature nervous system is also vulnerable to a number of genetic errors of metabolism that may respond favorably to nutritional manipulation. Vitamin utilization or conversion to active coenzyme forms may be either faulty or incomplete as a result of such genetic errors.[14] It is generally accepted that the nervous system is dependent on most, if not all, of the water-soluble vitamins for its normal development and for the subsequent maintenance of its function. Under normal dietary circumstances, taking into consideration the patient's age and medical status, the recommended minimal daily allowance of vitamins adequately protects the integrity of the nervous system. With very few exceptions, the use of massive daily doses of vitamins does not hasten or enhance the regeneration of diseased structures, nor

does it improve their function. Protein–calorie malnutrition (PCM), a serious and ever-present problem in a large segment of the infant population in most developing countries of the world, has deleterious effects on the ultimate physical and psychological development of the afflicted subjects. Whereas much is known about the nutritional, biochemical, and metabolic aspects of the problem, information on psychosocial and environmental factors that may further complicate the effects of PCM remains inadequate.

In general, knowledge concerning the effects of malnutrition or vitamin deficiencies on the nervous system has been derived from experiments conducted on animals using synthetic diets and contrived circumstances that produce results that bear little or no resemblance to the naturally occurring diseases in man. Although useful data have been obtained, some of which find direct application to humans, the wholesale extrapolation of experimental results gleaned from animals to the complex problems of human nutrition is totally unwarranted.

Unfortunately, the scientific basis of nutrition continues to be obscured by clever commercialism, fads, frauds, and cults, all of which contribute heavily to the improper use of nutrients or vitamins in the management of patients afflicted with neurologic disease. In this chapter, the diseases of the nervous system that are known to have a nutritional etiology will be reviewed briefly, and a practical approach to their dietary management will be outlined. An attempt will be made to separate fact from fiction by discussing common neurologic disorders in which the use of vitamins or special diets has no proven scientific validity.

Neurologic Diseases of Nutritional Etiology

In the developed nations of the world, a majority of nutritional disorders of the nervous system are the result of chronic alcoholism and undernutrition. It has been shown that during periods of heavy drinking, the absorption of vitamins, their intestinal transport, tissue storage, utilization, and conversion to metabolically active forms is sharply curtailed, while the need for vitamins and essential nutrients increases.[2] In addition to causing abnormal vitamin metabolism, chronic alcoholism may have profound effects on mineral, carbohydrate, protein, and lipid metabolism. The majority of nutritional disorders of the nervous system, although most commonly associated with chronic alcoholism, have also been encountered in malnourished, debilitated, nonalcoholic individuals suffering from various illnesses, such as malabsorption syndromes, renal disease, and neoplasia. Actually, alcohol-engendered nutritional syndromes of the nervous system are relatively rare, considering the size of the chronic alcoholic population and the magnitude of the sociologic, physiologic, and general medical problems caused by chronic alcoholism. It is estimated that nutritional disorders comprise only approximately 1% to 3% of the alcohol-related neurologic diseases requiring hospitalization. The various alcoholic nutritional syndromes may present separately in relatively pure form, but more frequently they occur together in varying combinations, some decidedly more prevalent than others.[16] It is not known why under seemingly identical circumstances one nutritionally depleted patient develops one or several neurologic complications while another seems to emerge essentially unscathed. The chronic alcoholic patient not infrequently exhibits symptoms and signs of withdrawal that may in part mask those attributable to nutritional depletion. The relatively frequent coexistence of these two alcoholic complications should be kept in mind when therapeutic measures are instituted. It is particularly important to remember that in patients who are marginally depleted, a full-blown nutritional syndrome can be precipitated by the parenteral administration of large amounts of a mixture of dextrose and water that does not contain vitamins; calorie-rich fluids tend to deplete inadequate vitamin stores further. When treating alcohol withdrawal with parenteral fluids, adequate doses of all of the B vitamins should always be administered, despite the fact that withdrawal symptoms are not caused by vitamin deficiency (see Chap. 15).

WERNICKE–KORSAKOFF SYNDROME

CLINICAL ASPECTS

Wernicke–Korsakoff syndrome is probably the most common alcoholic nutritional complication affecting the CNS. Contrary to common belief, the Wernicke–Korsakoff syndrome is not restricted to the alcoholic population but is also encountered in patients who suffer from severe nutritional depletion unrelated to drinking.[10] In order of frequency, the most common presenting symptoms are mental confusion that soon gives way to a characteristic disorder of memory (faulty immediate recall and recent memory) and confabulation, ataxia (primarily of stance and gait), abnormal ocular motility (ophthalmoplegia followed by nystagmus), and peripheral neuropathy. The correct diagnosis may be obscured when symptoms and signs of abstinence (*e.g.*, delirium tremens and hallucinosis) are superimposed on those of Wernicke–Korsakoff syndrome. Careful clinical studies have clearly demonstrated that a specific deficiency of thiamin (vitamin B_1) plays a central role in the pathogenesis of this disorder.[15] Since the disturbance of immediate recall and recent memory associated with Korsakoff syndrome may become irreversible, this condition requires prompt recognition and therapeutic intervention. The improvement of neurologic signs can be closely correlated with levels of activity of blood transketolase (a thiamin-dependent enzyme), which are reduced prior to thiamin administration and revert toward normal with clinical improvement.[3,4]

TREATMENT

An initial dose of 50 mg to 100 mg of thiamin hydrochloride, either intravenously or intramuscularly, usually results in reversal of ocular paralysis within a matter of 2 hr to 5 hr and prevents the advent of a severe disturbance in memory. The administration of thiamin by the IV route should proceed with caution since severe idiosyncratic reactions resulting in acquired sensitivity to the vitamin and even sudden death have been reported.[19] The use of oral thiamin preparations should be avoided during the acute phase of the illness because the vitamin may be absorbed in an erratic and unpredictable manner. Initial thiamin treatment should be followed by the regular administration of thiamin (25 mg–30 mg, 3 times/day IM or PO) and a well-balanced diet. In the presence of significant liver disease, thiamin (coenzyme) therapy alone may not bring about the expected rapid response. The combination of undernutrition and liver disease can result in significant protein (apoenzyme) depletion. In such instances, the prolonged administration of a nutritious and vitamin-supplemented diet is essential in order to bring about apoenzyme replenishment.

NUTRITIONAL NEUROPATHY

CLINICAL ASPECTS

Nutritional neuropathy, the most common of all the nutritional diseases of the nervous system, may occur in a variety of clinical settings. Although it is most frequently encountered in malnourished, chronic, alcoholic patients, it may complicate a number of other systemic illnesses in which malnutrition is an important feature, such as those resulting from malabsorption syndromes and food faddism. Typically, the neuropathy is symmetric, distal, areflexic, mixed motor, and sensory, affecting legs more than arms. Occasionally it involves the peripheral autonomic nervous system.[11] The malnourished patient may complain of severe burning, shooting, lightning, or "electric" types of pain in the feet, but no clear-cut clinical signs of neuropathy can be elicited. This particular neuropathic disorder, generally known as the *burning feet syndrome*, is believed to be due mainly to a lack of pantothenic acid. Neuropathy caused by a deficiency of pyridoxal phosphate, the active vitamin B_6 cofactor, may develop in the course of isonicotinic acid hydrazine (INH) therapy for tuberculosis. The drug has been found to interfere with the phosphorylation of pyridoxine.

TREATMENT

The common form of nutritional polyneuropathy is most probably caused by a deficiency of a combination of B vitamins. Therefore, therapy for this disorder should include a minimum of 25 mg thiamin, 75 mg niacin, 5 mg riboflavin, 5 mg pyridoxine, and 5 μg vitamin B_{12}, all taken three times daily. When nutritional polyneuropathy is caused by GI malabsorption, vitamins should be administered by the parenteral route. Recovery from nutritional polyneuropathy is notoriously slow, requiring a period of several months to a year; prolonged and continuous dietary treatment and physiotherapeutic maneuvers are consequently of the utmost importance. Patients afflicted with the burning feet syndrome should receive pantothenic acid (10 mg–20 mg/day), whereas those being treated with isoniazid (INH) should have the benefit of pyridoxine (100 mg–200 mg/day).

NUTRITIONAL AMBLYOPIA

CLINICAL ASPECTS

Nutritional amblyopia, also known as tobacco–alcohol amblyopia or nutritional retrobulbar neuropathy, is a remarkably uniform and stereotyped visual disturbance in which bilaterally symmetric central, cecocentral, or paracentral scotomata of varying sizes can be elicited.[5] Although the syndrome most frequently afflicts those persons habituated to alcohol or, occasionally, to tobacco, who neglect their nutrition, it has been encountered in undernourished populations all over the world during periods of famine and among civilian and military prisoners of war who have had no access to alcohol or tobacco. Occasionally, a similar syndrome may present as a complication of pernicious anemia as well as other vitamin B_{12} deficiency states.[9]

TREATMENT

Nutritional amblyopia is readily reversible, provided that the patient receives the benefit of oral or parenteral B vitamins and improved nutrition. Improvement occurs despite continued drinking or smoking, the degree and speed of recovery being largely dependent on the severity of the amblyopia and its duration before therapy was initiated. As yet, the specific nutrient the absence of which is responsible for the syndrome has not been identified, hence all of the B vitamins should be included in the treatment of this disorder.[15]

PELLAGRA

CLINICAL ASPECTS

The neurologic manifestations of pellagra, that is, mental symptoms (confusion, delusion, disorientation, and hallucinations), spasticity, ataxia, and, occasionally, peripheral neuropathy, have become increasingly rare in the developed world as a consequence of education about nutrition, the enrichment of flour, and the practice of vitamin self-medication. In the United States, pellagra was once most prevalent among impoverished and chronic alcoholic individuals.[5] Today, sporadic cases are encountered in severely malnourished patients and food faddists.

TREATMENT

Since a deficiency of nicotinic acid (niacin) or its precursor, tryptophan, is responsible for the disease, these must be included in the diet. The patient's diet should contain 500 mg to 1000 mg of tryptophan and 10 mg to 20 mg of niacin each day.

VITAMIN B₁₂ DEFICIENCY

CLINICAL ASPECTS

Vitamin B_{12} deficiency is caused by insufficient absorption of this vitamin by the GI tract, as may occur in pernicious anemia, tapeworm infestation, malabsorption syndromes, GI surgery, and, occasionally, vegetarianism. A deficiency of this vitamin may cause subacute degeneration of the spinal cord, optic nerves, cerebral white matter, and peripheral nerves.

Progressive symmetric paresthesias of feet and hands, weakness, spasticity, and ataxia of legs, occasional confusion and dementia, and sometimes bilaterally failing vision constitute the main neurologic symptoms of vitamin B_{12} deficiency. Diminution or loss of position and vibratory senses (blunting of pain, temperature, and tactile sensations over the distal parts of the legs) and hyperactive knee jerks without ankle jerks are the main neurologic findings.

Both vitamin B_{12} and folic acid deficiency have been implicated in the etiology of rare cases of dementia without other neurologic manifestations in elderly patients. Clinical reports indicate definite improvement following the administration of the appropriate vitamin. It is now well established that patients receiving anticonvulsant medications, particularly diphenylhydantoin, may develop folic acid deficiency. Conversely, the administration of folic acid has been found to significantly reduce the blood levels of these drugs. Presumably the vitamin and the drug compete for intestinal absorption.

TREATMENT

Since the early neurologic manifestations of vitamin B_{12} deficiency are rapidly and completely reversible, prompt initiation of therapy is of the utmost importance. In patients with pernicious anemia, the greatest degree of improvement is achieved when treatment takes place within 3 months of the onset of symptoms, although variable degrees of amelioration can be obtained after longer untreated periods (6 months–12 months). In the first 2 weeks, IM injections of 50 μg/day cyanocobalamin or an equivalent amount of liver USP should be administered. During the next 2 months, 100 μg IM every month should be administered to prevent a relapse, such as that which might be caused by the metabolic stress induced by systemic illness or surgery. The administration of oral vitamin preparations containing folic acid

must be avoided in patients suffering from an anemia of unknown etiology since, in unsuspected instances of pernicious anemia, folic acid, while reversing the anemia, fails to improve and may in fact precipitate neurologic complications of the disease.

Elderly, demented patients whose vitamin B_{12} or folic acid serum levels have been found to be reduced to significantly low levels (below 50% of normal) should receive doses of the appropriate vitamin to bring serum levels to within normal limits.

A significant degree of folic acid deficiency can occur as a consequence of anticonvulsant therapy with drugs such as diphenylhydantoin, phenobarbital, and primidone.[7] The relationship between the metabolism of these drugs and that of folic acid is poorly understood. It seems reasonable to measure the serum folate levels of patients treated with these anticonvulsant agents, particularly in the presence of anemia. Since the administration of folic acid may result in decreased blood levels of anticonvulsant drugs, the latter should be monitored and the dose of either vitamin or drug adjusted accordingly.[7]

VITAMIN E DEFICIENT STATES

Vitamin E and its use in health and disease continue to be the subject of considerable controversy. Experimentally induced deficiency of the vitamin in animals has resulted in a dystrophic process of voluntary muscles, pathologic changes in the spinal cord, and the deposit of a pigment usually associated with aging in muscles and nerve cells. The persistent inability to absorb fats is the most likely mechanism by which human subjects become deficient in this fat-soluble vitamin, yet clinical signs and symptoms of deficiency cannot be readily identified.

In children, the most common underlying causes of deficiency are malabsorption syndromes such as occur as the result of cystic fibrosis and biliary atresia. In adults, sprue and chronic pancreatitis have been the most frequent offenders. On occasion, a progressive myelopathy thought to be caused by a deficiency of vitamin E has been reported in both children and adults. In such circumstances supplemental vitamin E, perhaps as much as 500 IU/day to 1000 IU/day, appears to be indicated.

Recently it has been suggested that the administration of a mixture of 2 g vitamin E, 200 mg butylated hydroxytoluene, 1 g L-methionine, and 0.5 g vitamin C has a beneficial effect on the course of Batten's disease.[20] This disease, a juvenile form of amaurotic familial idiocy, is characterized by progressive visual disturbance, seizures, and neurologic impairment.

TABLE 27-1
Vitamin-responsive Diseases

Vitamin	Disease
Thiamin (vitamin B_1)	Pyruvic decarboxylase deficiency Maple syrup urine disease
Pyridoxine (vitamin B_6)	Neonatal convulsions Homocystinuria Cystathionuria
Cobalamin (vitamin B_{12})	Methylmalonic aciduria Homocystinuria
Folic acid	Homocystinuria
Nicotinamide	Hartnup disease

Adapted from Rosenberg LE: Vitamin-responsive inherited diseases affecting the nervous system. In Plum F (ed): Brain Dysfunction in Metabolic Disorders, 263–272. New York, Raven Press, 1974

The administration of the vitamin may also be useful in the treatment of infantile neuroaxonal dystrophy, a rare disorder of the nervous system of early childhood characterized by progressive spasticity, seizures, blindness, and mental deterioration.

In all of the above-mentioned neurologic diseases, vitamin E appears to act as a nonspecific antioxidant, and as such it appears to prevent the peroxidation of polyunsaturated fatty acids, the product of which is highly damaging to nerve cells.

VITAMIN-RESPONSIVE DISEASES

During the past decade, a number of genetically determined diseases, referred to as vitamin-responsive or vitamin-dependent states, in which either a vitamin-dependent enzymatic step or a reaction involved in the conversion of a vitamin to its active form is faulty, have been identified.[14] In these disorders the basic biochemical defect involves either the structure of the apoenzyme, its coenzyme binding sites, or some aspect of coenzyme synthesis, although blood vitamin levels are normal when measured. Some of these diseases may affect the nervous system, with symptoms ranging from mental retardation, psychosis, and convulsive seizures to ataxia, spasticity, and peripheral neuropathy (see Table 27-1). As their name implies, these diseases are responsive to the appropriate vitamin, showing marked improvement of neurologic symptoms after treatment with doses far exceeding the minimal daily nutritional requirement.

Neurologic Diseases of Questionable Nutritional Etiology

While cerebellar degeneration, central pontine myelinolysis, and Marchiafava–Bignami disease are often encountered in chronic alcoholic patients, they have been thought to be caused in part by malnutrition and have been diagnosed in patients with no history of alcoholism.

Cerebellar cortical degeneration, better known as alcoholic degeneration, is a syndrome characterized primarily by progressive unsteadiness of stance and gait, with relative sparing of arms and cranial nerves and demonstrable ataxia of trunk and legs.[5] The disease has also been reported in malnourished individuals who allegedly did not drink. Improved nutrition and the administration of B vitamins may result in some degree of amelioration of ataxia. Depending upon the severity of the illness, abstinence alone may be equally effective. It is conceivable that alcohol or some of its metabolites superimposed upon malnutrition may have a damaging effect on parts of the cerebellum.

Central pontine myelinolysis, a rare disorder originally described in alcoholic patients, has also been seen in abstemious individuals, young and old, who are afflicted with neoplasia, chronic renal disease, hepatic insufficiency, or a variety of infectious disorders. Although the etiology of central pontine myelinolysis remains essentially unknown, it has been shown that in many patients the disease follows a period of severe hyponatremia.[13] The symptoms are progressive quadriparesis leading to quadriplegia, dysphasia, emotional lability, decerebrate posture, respiratory paralysis, coma, and eventually death, all of which indicate a spreading pontine lesion. These symptoms may be associated with poor nutritional status, but a casual relationship is not evident. It appears more likely that a significant abnormality of electrolytes and water metabolism is the major contributing factor to the genesis of the disease. Supportive therapy may tide the patient over the worst part of the illness while spontaneous recovery takes place.

Marchiafava–Bignami disease, about which very little is known, also affects nonalcoholic patients. The neurologic symptoms and signs include disturbance of language, gait, and motor skills; seizures; incontinence; rooting; grasping; sucking; delayed initiation of action; tremulousness of hands; and dysarthria. The clinical description in the literature and the pathologic attributes suggest either a nutritional or toxic etiology. No specific treatment is recommended.[5]

Neurologic Diseases of Non-Nutritional Etiology

Despite recent advances in the field of neurology, the etiology and pathophysiology of a large number of diseases of the nervous system continue to be poorly understood. Therefore, it has been impossible to devise rational therapy for many of these disorders. Lack of knowledge, frustration on the part of the patient and the physician, and the desire to try any essentially harmless "shotgun" therapeutic measure have led to the irrational and scientifically unsound use of vitamins and special diets in the treatment of neurologic disorders of obscure nature. The popularity of prescribing large doses of B vitamins as therapy for neuropathies, peripheral nerve injuries, neuralgias, and demyelinating diseases stems from the fact that experimentally induced deficiencies of these vitamins in animals frequently result in lesions of the PNS and CNS that can be reversed, totally or in part, depending upon the time of vitamin administration. In most instances, the lesions, in their most advanced stages, show demyelination and destruction of nerve fibers, a frequent occurrence in many neurologic disorders. This observation has led to the erroneous belief that the treatment of diseases characterized by demyelination or destruction of nerve fibers with vitamins, in doses far exceeding their nutritional value, will either hasten their improvement or protect the involved structures from further damage.

Thiamin (vitamin B_1), also known in the past as *aneurin* (an abbreviation for antineuritic factor), has been administered in increasingly large quantities since it was first synthesized in 1936. It appears to be reasonably well established that the diphosphoric and triphosphoric esters of thiamin are involved in the function of excitable membranes, where these esters are presumably situated.[6] Thus, they are presumed to regulate the sodium influx and efflux through axonal and other membranes of peripheral nerves. This function of thiamin, which is independent of its function as a coenzyme or nutrient, fails in severe states of deficiency and may actually be responsible for most of the neurologic manifestations, particularly those that respond rapidly and dramatically to a single dose of thiamin, such as ophthalmoplegia in Wernicke's disease. Recently it has been demonstrated that thiamin and its active phosphoric esters are not related to the myelin sheath in either the CNS or the PNS. Based on these observations, thiamin appears to have no effect on reparative processes of nerve fibers, such as remyelination. It seems rather unlikely that large doses of thiamin are useful in the management of trigeminal and postherapetic neuralgia and various forms of neuritis. The vitamin should be reserved for the treatment of neuropathy seen in states of severe malnutrition or undernutrition.

The same can be said for the use of vitamin B_{12}, which does not appear to influence the metabolism of brain, spinal cord, and peripheral nerves that are not deprived of the vitamin. The literature contains reports suggesting that B vitamins are useful in the treatment of migraine and Meniere's disease, but at the present time there appears to be no scientific basis for this assertion. Since neurologic diseases, such as trigeminal and postherpetic neuralgia, Meniere's disease, and certain types of peripheral nerve disorders are self-limiting and tend to improve spontaneously, it is most difficult to assess the value of thiamin therapy in an objective manner. The administration of vitamins is undoubtedly responsible for a significant placebo effect, which helps the physician in the management of patients afflicted with essentially incurable or self-limited diseases. Although large oral doses of B vitamins tend to be harmless, their repeated parenteral administration may result in symptoms and signs of hypersensitivity; anaphylactic reactions and sudden death have been reported, and other toxic manifestations are possible.[19]

Nutritional therapy using vitamins or other substances has been advocated for a number of neurologic diseases of unknown etiology. Although supplemental B vitamins may improve the well-being of patients afflicted with multiple sclerosis, they do not influence the course of the disease. A low-fat diet has been recommended as an effective means of reducing the incidence of exacerbations in patients with known multiple sclerosis. To date, however, it has not been possible to evaluate objectively the efficacy of this mode of treatment.

Epidemiologic studies relating multiple sclerosis to nutritional factors have revealed a possible correlation between the incidence of the disease and the total fat intake and percentage of calories of animal origin consumed. Multiple sclerosis tends to be more prevalent in countries where the use of animal fat is high. Whether the restriction of dairy products and other foods high in the content of animal fats is useful in the management of multiple sclerosis cannot be ascertained from available data.[1]

It has been suggested recently that the administration of the unsaturated fatty acids, linoleic or arachidonic, may reduce the number and the severity of multiple sclerosis attacks.[8] This is based on the observations that multiple sclerotic brain and spinal cord are relatively deficient in the content of unsaturated fatty acids and that linoleic and arachidonic acid strongly inhibit the lymphocyte–antigen interaction, a cellular mechanism that may be responsible for demyelination. It is believed that during attacks of multiple sclerosis, sensitized lymphocytes interact with myelin components in the affected parts of the nervous system. Whether the prolonged ingestion of unsaturated fatty acids, such as linoleic acid, which is contained in safflower oil, has any effect on the course of multiple sclerosis remains to be demonstrated.

A nutritional approach to the management of chronic neurologic diseases affecting intellectual function (*e.g.*, dementia or mental retardation) has been advocated by therapeutic enthusiasts who believe that certain vitamins, substances, or foods can enhance the metabolic activity of the brain or raise the patient's IQ. Vitamin B_6, which is an essential cofactor for biochemical reactions involved in the synthesis of biogenic amines (serotonin and dopamine) and the inhibitory substance γ-aminobutyric acid, found uniquely in the brain, has been used in large doses and indiscriminately in children afflicted with a variety of diseases characterized by seizures and mental retardation. Similarly, glutamic acid, the precursor of γ-aminobutyric acid, has been administered to both demented adults and mentally retarded children. Except for specific instances where a pyridoxine-dependent metabolic block (such as occurs in homocystinuria, cysinuria, and xanthurinic aciduria) or pyridoxine-responsive seizures of the neonate can be demonstrated, the use of large doses of the vitamin seems to be inappropriate, and the claimed therapeutic success cannot be evaluated by objective means. Contrary to popular belief, it is doubtful that so-called "brain foods" (fish heads, squeezed calves brains, and certain vegetable juices) have any influence on the chemical composition of the nervous system, its metabolism, or its function.

Finally, some neurologic diseases, such as Parkinson's disease, which does not have a nutritional etiology, respond favorably to a combination of specific therapy and dietary manipulation. Parkinson's disease, a degenerative disorder of the nervous system characterized by symptoms of rigidity, bradykinesia, and tremor, can be treated with some degree of success by the administration of the amino acid levodopa (1-dihydroxyphenylalanine), which upon entry into the appropriate nerve cells of the affected parts of the brain is converted to the deficient catecholamine, dopamine. The majority of ingested levodopa is converted to dopamine in the nerve cells located in peripheral ganglia, and only about 1% of the amino acid is made available to the brain. The enzymatic reaction that converts levodopa to dopamine, a vitamin B_6 (pyridoxine)-dependent decarboxylase, can be stimulated by excessive amounts of the vitamin. It has been observed that the beneficial effects of levodopa on the neurologic symptoms of the disease may be markedly reduced when supplemental vitamin preparations containing pyridoxine are added to the daily dose of levodopa. Therefore, vitamin preparations containing pyridoxine should be avoided. In addition, it has been demonstrated that amino acids contained in the diet tend to compete with the absorption of levodopa. Consequently, it is recommended that the daily protein intake of the patient receiving levodopa be kept in the vicinity of 0.5 g protein/kg/day and that the medication not be ingested together with foods rich in amino acids, such as milk or cheese.[12]

SUMMARY

Scientific knowledge gathered to date about nutrition as it pertains to the etiology or treatment of diseases of the nervous system is relatively meager when one considers recent advances in the fields of biochemistry and nutrition. If, indeed, nutrition has a wider application to the management of neurologic disorders than has been recognized heretofore, more sensitive and critical techniques for assessing the nutritional status of the nervous system and evaluating treatment are required before rational methods of therapy can be devised.

References

1. Alter M, Yamour M: Multiple sclerosis prevalence and nutritional factors. Trans Am Neurol Assoc 98:253–254, 1973
2. Baker H, Frank O: Vitamin status in metabolic upsets. In Bourne G (ed): World Review of Nutrition and Dietetics, Vol 9, pp 124–160. London, Pittman, 1968
3. Brin M: Erythrocyte transketolase in early thiamin deficiency. Ann NY Acad Sci 98:528, 1962
4. Dreyfus PM: Clinical application of blood transketolase determinations. N Engl J Med 267:596, 1962
5. Dreyfus PM: Diseases of the nervous system in chronic alcoholics. In Kissin B, Begleiter H (eds): The Biology of Alcoholism, Vol 3, pp 265–290. New York, Plenum Press, 1974
6. Dreyfus PM, Geel SE: Vitamin and nutritional deficiencies. In Siegel GJ (ed): Basic Neurochemistry, pp 605–626. Boston, Little, Brown, 1976
7. Dreyfus PM: Nutritional disorders of the nervous system. In Hodges RE (ed): Nutrition in Metabolic and Clinical Applications, pp 53–81. New York, Plenum Press, 1979
8. Field EJ: Multiple sclerosis: Treatment and prophylaxis. J R Soc Med 72:487–488, 1979

9. Lerman S, Feldmahn AL: Centrocecal scotoma as a presenting sign in pernicious anemia. Arch Ophthalmol 65:381–385, 1961
10. Lopez RI, Collins GH: Wernicke's encephalopathy: A complication of chronic hemodialysis. Arch Neurol 18:248–259, 1968
11. Mayer RF, Garcia–Mullen R: Peripheral nerve and muscle disorders associated with alcoholism. In Kissin B, Begleiter H (eds): The Biology of Alcoholism, Vol 2, pp 29–65. New York, Plenum Press, 1972
12. Mena I, Cotzias GC: Protein intake and treatment of Parkinson's disease with levodopa. N Engl J Med 292:181–184, 1975
13. Messert B, Orrison WW, Hawkins MJ et al: Central pontine myelinolysis: Considerations on etiology, diagnosis and treatment. Neurology 29:147–160, 1979
14. Rosenberg LE: Vitamin-responsive inherited diseases affecting the nervous system. In Plum F (ed): Brain Dysfunction in Metabolic Disorders, pp 263–272. New York, Raven Press, 1974
15. Victor M, Mancall EL, Dreyfus PM: Deficiency amblyopia in the alcoholic patient. Arch Ophthalmol 64:1–33, 1960
16. Victor M: The effects of nutritional deficiency on the nervous system: A comparison with the effects of carcinoma. In Brain L, Norris FH (eds): The Remote Effects of Cancer on the Nervous System, pp 134–161. New York, Grune & Stratton, 1965
17. Victor M, Adams RD: On the etiology of the alcoholic neurologic diseases with special reference to the role of nutrition. Am J Clin Nutr 9:379–397, 1961
18. Victor M, Adams RD, Collins GH: The Wernicke–Korsakoff's Syndrome. Philadelphia, FA David, 1971
19. Weigand CG: Reactions attributed to administration of thiamin chloride. Geriatrics 5:274–279, 1950
20. Zeeman W: Studies in the neuronal ceroid–lipofuscinoses. J Neuropathol Exp Neurol 33:1–12, 1974

28
Obesity

George A. Bray

Obesity is a common problem in all affluent societies. The estimated number of overweight people in the United States varies from 10 to 50 million. Using 20% above desirable weight as an index of obesity, recent prevalence data for this country show that 24% of women and 14% of men from 18 years to 74 years of age are overweight.

Thus, at least 16.3 million American women and 8.5 million American men are significantly overweight. The importance of these data lies in the associated medical and social risks and the current social setting which says that "thin is in."

How Obesity Is Measured

Before discussing obesity in detail, the subject must be defined. *Overweight* is an increase of body weight above some arbitrary standard usually defined in relation to height. To be *obese*, on the other hand, means to have an abnormally high proportion of body fat. In order to determine whether a person is obese or simply overweight owing to increased lean body mass (*i.e.,* athletes), one needs techniques and standards for quantitating body fatness.

Measurement of body composition by analysis of individual cadavers has been performed several times in this century.[4] Water was the major component; fat and protein each accounted for about 15% of the body weight. Since direct analysis cannot be performed under normal circumstances, investigators have turned their attention to indirect methods for measuring body fat.

Superficial analysis of fatness is done by self-examination or through examination by another person. Increased bulging of skinfolds or excessive roundness in most instances suggests increased fatness. Although such observations provide a good individual guide, they are not quantitative. One solution to this problem is the assignment of body types using photographs taken in the nude. With this technique, called somatotyping, the degree of endomorphy (roundness), mesomorphy (muscularity), and ectomorphy (leanness) can be given numerical values.[4]

Anthropomorphic measurements are among the most widely used techniques and involve determination of height and weight; determination of various body circumferences or diameters (waist, chest, or hip circumferences; distances between the iliac crests; greater trochanters or acromioclavicular joints); and measurements of skinfold thickness. However, the most widely used indices for determining the degree of overweight are based on body weight in relation to height. The tables of desirable weight provided by the Metropolitan Life Insurance Company have received the widest use. In these tables, *desirable weight* is defined as that weight at which the lowest mortality rate occurred among individuals taking out life insurance policies. The table of desirable body weights is divided into three subgroups based on *frame size*. Unfortunately, there is no suitable criteria to determine frame size. For this reason we prefer the Fogarty modification of their table shown in Table 28-1. This gives a single median weight for each height and a range of acceptable body weights that encompasses the three frame sizes of the Metropolitan table.

TABLE 28-1
Guidelines for Body Weight
Metric

Height* (m)	Men Weight (kg)* Average	Men Weight (kg)* Acceptable Weight		Women Weight (kg)* Average	Women Weight (kg)* Acceptable Weight	
1.45				46	42	53
1.48				46.5	42	54
1.50				47	43	55
1.52				48.5	44	57
1.54				49.5	44	58
1.56				50.4	45	58
1.58	55.8	51	64	51.3	46	59
1.60	57.6	52	65	52.6	48	61
1.62	58.6	53	66	54	49	62
1.64	59.6	54	67	55.4	50	64
1.66	60.6	55	69	56.8	51	65
1.68	61.7	56	71	58.1	52	66
1.70	63.5	58	73	60	53	67
1.72	65	59	74	61.3	55	69
1.74	66.5	60	75	62.6	56	70
1.76	68	62	77	64	58	72
1.78	69.4	64	79	65.3	59	74
1.80	71	65	80			
1.82	72.6	66	82			
1.84	74.2	67	84			
1.86	75.8	69	86			
1.88	77.6	71	88			
1.90	79.3	73	90			
1.92	81	75	93			

Guidelines for Body Weight
English

Height* Ft	Height* In	Men Weight (lb)* Average	Men Weight (lb)* Acceptable Weight		Women Weight (lb)* Average	Women Weight (lb)* Acceptable Weight	
4	10				102	92	119
4	11				104	94	122
5	0				107	96	125
5	1				110	99	128
5	2	123	112	141	113	102	131
5	3	127	115	144	116	105	134
5	4	130	118	148	120	108	138
5	5	133	121	152	123	111	142
5	6	136	124	156	128	114	146
5	7	140	128	161	132	118	150
5	8	145	132	166	136	122	154
5	9	149	136	170	140	126	158
5	10	153	140	174	144	130	163
5	11	158	144	179	148	134	168
6	0	162	148	184	152	138	173
6	1	166	152	189			
6	2	171	156	194			
6	3	176	160	199			
6	4	181	164	204			

*Height without shoes, weight without clothes
Adapted from the recommendations of the Fogarty Center Conference 1973.

The degree of overweight can be expressed in several ways. Relative weight uses the ratio or percentage of actual weight to desirable weight. A man who is 5 feet, 10 inches tall and weighs 180 pounds would have a relative weight of 1.17 ($\frac{180}{153} = 1.17$) or 17% above desirable weight. Weight and height can also be related by various ratios such as W/H; W/H^2 (body mass index); and $H/\sqrt[3]{W}$ (ponderal index). None measures body fat very well, since the correlation of these indexes with body fat measured from body density (see below) is between 0.7 and 0.8.[4] The body mass index (W/H^2) has the best correlation with body fat and is thus preferred. A nomogram for obtaining body mass index using metric units for height and weight is shown in Figure 28-1.[7] Other body measurements have been added to improve the assessment of body fat. Steinkamp and co-workers and Behnke and Wilmore have both provided equations which estimate body fatness with a fair degree of accu-

racy.[1,39] However, they require a number of different measurements that must be taken by skilled observers.

From a practical point of view, the most widely used criterion for obesity is based on the thickness of skinfolds. Skinfold thickness from four separate sites (usually biceps, triceps, subscapular, and suprailiac area) has been shown to provide a reliable estimate of obesity.[16] One difficulty with this method is that body fat increases with age even when the sum of the skinfolds remains constant. This implies that the accumulation of fat with age occurs in large part at sites other than the four included in this study.

The thickness of the triceps skinfold was used to estimate obesity in the Ten State Nutrition Survey conducted by the United States Public Health Service. Obesity in adults was defined as "a fatfold measurement greater than the 85th percentile of measurements for young white adults" (18.6 mm

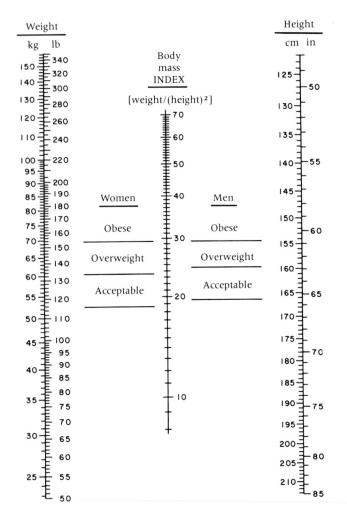

FIG. 28-1 Nomogram for determining body mass index. To use this nomogram, place a ruler or other straight edge between the body weight in kilograms or pounds located on the left-hand line and the height in centimeters or inches located on the right-hand column. The body mass index is read from the middle of the scale and is in metric units. (© G. A. Bray, 1978. Used with permission)

for males and 25.1 mm for females). The subscapular skinfold appears to provide a much better index of fatness than the triceps skinfold and is thus to be preferred. Waist circumference, particularly in males, may be better than either of the two skinfolds. Use of ultrasound to measure the thickness of subcutaneous fat has also been used and may find wide application in the future.

In summary, body fat can be estimated in many ways, but the most accurate methods are densitometry or isotopic dilution techniques, which, however, have technical requirements not usually available. From the practical point of view, methods involving measurement of height and weight, preferably expressed as the body mass index (W/H^2), or the use of the subscapular skinfold, or the circumference, at the waist would appear to be the best approaches to determining who is overweight and of those, who is obese.

DEFINING THE OBESE

A number of factors influence body fat, including age, sex, and physical activity. At birth the human body contains about 12% fat, a content which is higher than in most other animals.[4] In the newborn period, body fat rises rapidly to reach a peak of about 25% by 6 months and then declines over the next 10 years to 18%. At puberty there is a significant increase in the percentage of fat in females. In males, on the other hand, there is a small, but significant, drop in body fat with puberty. By the age of 18 years, men have approximately 15% to 18% body fat and women, 20% to 25%. Fat increases in both sexes after puberty, and during adult life rises to between 30% and 40% of body weight.[18]

The composition of the body is also influenced by the level of physical activity. During physical training, body fat decreases and lean tissue increases. After training ends, however, this process is reversed. These shifts between body fat and lean tissue can occur without any change in body weight. If regular activity is maintained throughout adult life, the increase in body fat, which usually occurs even when body weight is stable, can be prevented.

The prevalence of overweight or obesity depends upon the criteria that are used to define obesity. The massively obese are readily recognized, and it is clear that body weight is skewed toward the heavy side. That is, the median or most frequent weight is less than the mean or average weight. Using 20% above desirable weight as the criterion, 14% of American men aged 20 years to 74 years are overweight; the comparable figure for women is 24%. A breakdown by age and a comparison of figures obtained in 1960 to 1962 and again in 1971 to 1974 are shown in Table 28-2.[8] The Health and Nutrition Examination Survey (HANES), using skinfold measurements, obtained similar, although not identical, data.[8] More women than men are obese and the frequency of overweight increases in older age groups of both sexes. After 55 years to 65 years there is a decline in the percentage of the population that is overweight. Rural populations may be more overweight than urban populations.

Racial differences in body weight may exist, but it is often difficult to separate racial from environmental factors. Socioeconomic conditions, however, clearly play an important role in the development of obesity. Excess body weight is 7 to 12 times more frequent in women from lower social classes than in women from the upper social classes.[2]

TABLE 28-2
Prevalence of Overweight

| | *Percent of Population Deviating by 20% or More from Desirable Weight** | | | |
| | *Men* | | *Women* | |
Age	*1960–62*	*1971–74*	*1960–62*	*1971–74*
20–74	14.5%	14%	25.1%	23.8%
20–24	9.6	7.4	9.1	9.6
25–34	13.3	13.6	14.8	17.1
35–44	14.9	17	23.2	24.3
45–54	16.7	15.8	28.9	27.8
55–64	15.8	15.1	38.6	34.7
65–74	14.6	13.4	38.8	31.5

*Estimated from regression equation of weight on height for men and women ages 20–29 years, obtained from HANES I. National Center for Health Statistics. Abraham S, Johnson CL: Overweight Adults 20–74 Years of Age: United States, 1971–74. Vital and Health Statistics. Advance Data No. 51. Hyattsville, Public Health Service, DHEW. In preparation.

Among men, social class has a significant, but much smaller, relationship to overweight. Cultural background also seems to affect the development of obesity. Individuals from Eastern Europe living in the United States have a higher frequency of obesity than those who originated in Western Europe. Recent immigrants to the United States have a higher frequency of obesity than do fourth generation Americans from the same heritage.

CHARACTERISTICS OF OBESITY

Obesity can influence many aspects of life, and its effects will be examined here in detail.

HEALTH CONSEQUENCES OF OBESITY

Life insurance statistics published in 1979, as well as those assembled earlier, showed that excess weight was associated with a higher mortality rate. This effect is shown in Figure 28-2, which plots relative mortality for various deviations from average weight. The minimal mortality for both men and women occurs among individuals 10% below average weight. Deviations in body weight above and below this are associated with an increase in mortality. The effect on life expectancy of small deviations in weight, however, is small. Based on the 1979 data, a deviation of 10% above average weight is accompanied by an 11% decrease in life expectancy in men and a 7% decrease in women; if 20% above average weight, the risk of excess mortality rises to 20% for men and 10% for women.[8]

Hypertension, gallbladder disease, and diabetes mellitus are the most prevalent in overweight individuals and are the leading causes of excess mortality. An increased risk of kidney stones and certain types of cancer (*e.g.*, endometrial cancer) may also exist.

The insurance companies have also provided retrospective data that suggest that weight reduction may prolong life.[4] In both men and women who successfully lose and maintain a lower weight, mortality was reduced to within the normal limits based on sex and age. The increases in body fat increases cholesterol turnover and the concentration of cholesterol in bile, thus predisposing to gallstones.[4] Increased stores of fat also require more blood to be circulated for supply of substrates, and this may increase cardiac output and blood pressure. Finally, it is known that obesity increases insulin secretion, and in susceptible people this may lead to diabetes mellitus.

These findings by the insurance industry have served as a major stimulus for further study of the influence of body weight on life expectancy.

In addition to its possible effects on mortality, obesity has a number of effects on the function of various organ systems. Obesity increases the work of the heart, and the heart enlarges with a rise in body weight. The cardiac output, stroke volume, and blood volume also increase. These effects on cardiovascular function are reversible with weight loss. The relation of hypertension to obesity has been widely recognized.[6,33] Blood pressure measured with a standard blood pressure cuff may be higher

FIG. 28-2 Relation of excess mortality to body weight. The excess mortality of insured individuals in relation to the mortality ratio of normal-weight individuals (= 100) is plotted against the body mass index (weight/height²).

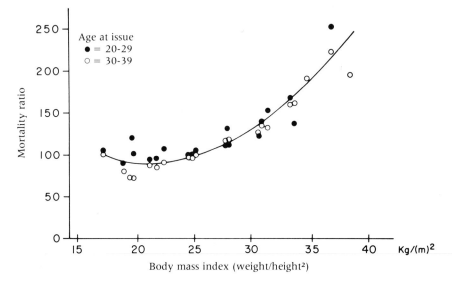

Body mass index (weight/height²)

or lower than values obtained by direct intra-arterial measurement. The major source of error occurs when the bladder of the blood pressure cuff does not encircle 75% or more of the arm. A wider cuff will not improve the reading unless it is also longer. Unless the arm is very large, however, the error in measurement of blood pressure is probably small and not consistently skewed in one direction or the other. The relationship between obesity and blood pressure is thus usually not an artifact of measurement. After weight loss, blood pressure is significantly reduced in over 50% of the patients, and thus may be an important mode of treatment of some forms of hypertension.[4,33]

Pulmonary function is impaired by obesity.[4] With moderate degrees of obesity, a number of changes in pulmonary function can be detected. With gross obesity, however, some individuals develop a syndrome of severe alveolar hypoventilation, called the *pickwickian syndrome,* after Joe, the fat boy in Dickens' novel *The Pickwick Papers.* This syndrome is characterized by obesity, hypoventilation, somnolence, and cyanosis. The alveolar hypoventilation may be associated with pulmonary hypertension. This syndrome often represents a medical emergency, and such patients may require vigorous respiratory therapy to preserve life.[34]

Endocrine function is also modified by obesity. Glucose tolerance is frequently impaired in obesity. Plasma insulin in the fasting state, and after glucose, is increased in obesity whether or not glucose tolerance is impaired. The rise in fasting insulin occurs in normal subjects who gain weight under observation.[38] The mechanism by which an increase in body fat increases the demand for insulin is unknown. The rise in serum insulin is associated with resistance to insulin. The insulin resistance appears to result from both a reduction in insulin receptors on the cell membrane and decreased intracellular effects of insulin.

Like the cardiac and pulmonary changes in obesity, the hyperinsulinemia and glucose intolerance can be reversed by weight loss. These data, and information from studies of experimental animals, suggest that by a mechanism as yet unknown obesity can alter pancreatic function. In susceptible individuals this may in turn lead to the development of clinical diabetes mellitus. Support for this concept has come from epidemiologic data, which show a high correlation between relative body weight and the frequency of diabetes in numerous populations.[6] Where obesity is uncommon, the incidence of diabetes mellitus is low. The precipitation of diabetes by obesity occurs if the secretory capacity of the pancreas is impaired by genetic or environmental factors. The detrimental effect of obesity in adult-onset diabetes mellitus can be reversed by weight loss.

Abnormalities in the reproductive system in obesity include low levels of sex hormone binding globulin in men and abnormal menstrual cycles in women.[20,24] A return of menstrual regularity is usually observed with weight loss.[4] Whether obesity changes fertility, however, is unknown. Pregnancy augments weight gain. Twenty-four months from the onset of pregnancy, a woman will be, on the average, 5 lb to 7 lb (2.3 kg–3.2 kg) heavier than if she had not been pregnant.[4]

Obesity also impairs the release of growth hormone from the pituitary. Insulin-induced hypoglycemia, the infusion of arginine, administration of L-dopa, and sleep will all normally produce a rise in growth hormone. In the obese adult none of these stimuli produces a normal rise in growth hormone. The impaired response of growth hormone returns to normal with weight loss.[4] Moreover, when subjects of normal weight overeat to gain weight, the responsiveness of growth hormone is reduced.[38] Thus, the blunted output of growth hormone in obesity appears to be the result of overnutrition.

Obesity increases the secretion of adrenal steroids from the adrenal cortex and the excretion of 17-hydroxycorticosteroids in the urine rises.[4] Circulating levels of cortisol, however, do not change. The concentration of triiodothyronine shows a small, but significant, positive correlation with overweight, but other parameters of thyroid function do not appear to be influenced by obesity. Both total calorie intake and the fraction taken as carbohydrate can influence the metabolism of thyroxine; with starvation the concentration of 3, 5, 3'-triiodothyronine (T3) falls and 3, 3', 5' triiodothyronine increases. With overfeeding calories or carbohydrates, this metabolic process is reversed.

How Obesity Develops

An increase in body fat reflects an increase in total stored calories. Excess fat occurs because there is an imbalance between ingested calories and the calories that are utilized for energy. The constancy of body weight in adult humans and animals suggests that the body regulates its storage of calories within narrow limits. Given free access to food, this implies that some components of total stored calories are recognized by the body. Support for this hypothesis has come from several studies. Forced feeding by stomach tube in animals and by conscious overeating in humans causes body weight to rise.[38] After the tube feeding stops, or when human volunteers cease stuffing themselves, body weight falls and approximates its initial level. Conversely, starvation produces weight loss. When food is again available, eating resumes, and body weight in both humans and animals rises to the prestarvation level. Second, hypothalamic hyperphagia (the increased food intake that follows bilateral injury of the ventromedial region of the hypothalamus) in one rat in a parabiotic pair leads to loss of body fat in its parabiotic mate.[14] However, as pointed out by Garrow, body weight of many individuals shows considerable variation during life, suggesting that the control mechanisms are relatively complex and not highly sensitive to stored energy.[19]

Several prospective studies have examined the relation between obesity and various diseases.[27,28] The Framingham Study, conducted on more than 5,000 residents of this New England town, showed that an increased relative weight was associated with a significant increase in sudden death and angina pectoris but was not associated with an increase in the frequency of myocardial infarction.[27] Since most sudden deaths are probably of cardiovascular origin, one might interpret the Framingham data as supporting the association of obesity with fatal cardiac events. However, if other risk factors, such as hypertension and high cholesterol, were considered, obesity, or more properly overweight, in and of itself seemed to be less significant. In another prospective study of risk factors and cardiovascular disease, excess relative weight was associated with a small, but significant, increase in mortality, particularly in men under 40 years of age (see Fig. 28-2). A third study measured relative weight and skinfold thickness. Over 11,000 subjects from six countries were included.[28] Increased skinfold thickness and overweight were both associated with increased deaths. Careful analysis of the data showed that the association of overweight or obesity with increased mortality was due to the high correlation of body weight with increased blood pressure. In subgroups where the blood pressure was similar, there was no independent effect of obesity on the mortality from cardiovascular disease. These data indicate that obesity and overweight may be important clues to those at risk for cardiovascular disease, but that obesity may not be a major independent risk factor in cardiovascular disease.

Integrating mechanisms for the regulation of calories in the body include both central and peripheral components. The central components involve the hypothalamus, as well as the amygdala, cortex, and thalamus. The long-term regulation appears to be centered in the ventromedial hypothalamus. After bilateral destruction of the ventromedial hypothalamus, there is a constellation of changes which include hyperphagia, abnormal estrus cycles, and rage.[14] The increased food intake is followed by a rise in body weight, and obesity develops. The way in which the ventromedial hypothalamus modu-

lates caloric balance is unknown, but appears to involve fiber tracts traversing the ventromedial hypothalamus.[14]

Short-term regulation of meal-eating and food-seeking behavior appears to be integrated in the lateral hypothalamus. Destructive lesions in this region of the brain decrease food intake, and total aphagia may result.[14] Conversely, electrical stimulation of the lateral hypothalamus increases food intake.[14] Inhibition of food intake by the hungry animal occurs when isoproterenol, a beta-adrenergic drug, is injected into the lateral hypothalamus. Application of norepinephrine to the ventromedial hypothalamus will stimulate food intake in the satiated rat, an effect which is blocked by phentolamine, an alpha-adrenergic blocking drug. These data suggested that adrenergic receptors in the medial and lateral hypothalamus may play a role in the modulation of food-seeking activity.[14]

Both neural and humoral factors may participate in the termination of a meal. Since stored calories are derived from fat, carbohydrate, and protein, it is likely that circulating levels of amino acids, glucose, fatty acids, and glycerol may play a role in signaling the quantity of stored calories. Glucose has received the most attention because it is carefully regulated in the body. The administration of glucose intraperitoneally reduces food intake, but its intravenous administration does not. Blockade of intracellular glucose utilization after injecting 2-deoxyglucose enhances food intake. In all likelihood, however, glucose utilization represents only one component of the metabolic mix that is recognized by the body as an index of stored calories.[9] Amino acids, when deficient or when in excess, can also decrease food intake.[4] The available evidence suggests that the depression of food intake resulting from distortion of the amino-acid composition of the diet is sensed in areas of the nervous system other than the hypothalamus. Fatty acids and glycerol may also play a role in the control of food intake. Glycerol is a particularly interesting molecule in this regard. It is released from adipose tissue during the hydrolysis of triglyceride but is not reused by this tissue. This glycerol enters the circulation and is metabolized by liver and, to a small extent, by muscle. Its rate of release from adipose tissue could thus signal the rate of hydrolysis of lipid and, indirectly, the total quantity of lipid stored. Recent experiments show that parenteral administration of glycerol will reduce food intake and body weight.[46]

Hormones may also serve in the short-term control of food intake. Injections of insulin will increase hunger and food intake and, if continued, obesity will develop.[4] A possible mechanism for the long-term regulation of body weight involving insulin has recently been proposed by Woods and Porte.[47] They proposed that the hypothalamus may respond to insulin concentration in the cerebrospinal fluid. Glucagon has an effect opposite that of insulin and decreases food intake. Injections of small doses of cholecystokinin will also suppress food intake in rats and in humans.

In addition to these internal signals that regulate food-seeking behavior, most animals, including humans, receive cues about food from sight, smell, and taste. Environmental cues may play a major role in controlling human food intake, particularly in the obese. The data of Schachter and his colleagues have suggested that environmental cues may be more important in controlling food intake in the obese than are internal cues.[36] External factors, such as the time of day, the availability of food, the intensity of lighting, and the tastiness of the food have all been shown to modulate eating.

Over 90% of the body energy is stored as triglyceride in adipose tissue. Protein and glycogen provide important but smaller quantities of energy.[4] Adipose tissue has two principal functions: (1) the synthesis and storage of fatty acids, and (2) mobilization of fatty acids as a source of fuel.[11,33]

The growth of adipose tissue in the early period of life occurs by an increase in the size of fat cells, as well as by an increase in the number of adipocytes in each depot that stores fat.[3] The multiplication of fat cells continues throughout the growing years and appears to terminate in adolescence. Current evidence suggests that after puberty fat is stored primarily by increasing the size of adipocytes that already exist with little or no change in total number. When obesity develops in the early years of life, almost all of the persons have *hypercellular* obesity. Adult-onset obesity is thus usually *hypertrophic* in type, whereas childhood-onset obesity is most commonly *hyperplastic* obesity.

The anatomic difference between hypertrophic and hypercellular obesity is important because the life expectancy of the fat cell is very long. Fat cells differentiate from stem cells of mesenchymal origin, which do not contain fat and do not appear to divide thereafter. It has been shown by studies on experimental animals that the half-life of a fat cell appears to be very long.[23] Thus, with changes in body fat, the size of the individual adipocyte varies with its store of triglyceride, but there is little or no change in the total number of fat cells. Even marked and prolonged weight loss apparently does not decrease the number of fat cells. Patients with hypercellular obesity thus have a lifelong increase in the total mass of fat cells. In people with an increased total number of adipocytes, weight loss occurs by shrinkage of these fat cells but without a change in total number.

Energy expenditure is the other component in the balance between energy as food intake and stored calories.[4,19] Basal energy expenditure is involved in the transport of ions across cell membranes for protein synthesis and for the repair and function of smooth muscle. In the normal adult, basal metabolism consumes about 800 Cal/M^2/24 hr to 900 Cal/M^2/24 hr. The rate of basal metabolism (BMR) is lower in females than males and declines with age. The decline in BMR with age is due in part to increasing fat depots. Individuals who maintain a regular program of physical activity may not show an increase of fat with age, and BMR may show only a very small decline.

Energy is also used for muscular contraction. The efficiency of muscular work is about 30% and shows no difference between lean and obese subjects.[44] Energy expenditure rises following the ingestion of a meal. This is called the *thermic effect* of food (formerly called *specific dynamic action* of food). This is reflected by a rise in oxygen utilization. It is produced by all foods, but protein appears to have the greatest effect.[19] The thermic effect of food itself dissipates about 10% of the ingested calories when a mixed diet is eaten.

CAUSATIVE FACTORS IN THE DEVELOPMENT OF OBESITY

From data on experimental animals, it is clear that obesity, or a susceptibility to the development of obesity, can be genetically transmitted.[14] This inheritance may occur by dominant or recessive modalities or may be polygenic. In the appearance of human corpulence, genetic factors manifest themselves in two ways. First, there is a group of rare diseases in which evidence indicates that genetic factors are of prime importance.[4] Second, there is a genetic substrate upon which environmental factors interact in the development of obesity.[4] Clearcut evidence of genetically transmitted obesity has been documented in the Laurence-Moon-Bardet-Biedl syndrome (LMBB), an entity consisting of retinal degeneration, polydactylism, mental retardation, and obesity. Other examples are Alstrom's syndrome and the Morgagni-Stewart-Morel syndrome.[4]

The importance of genetic factors in obesity is illustrated in the studies on body weight of twins and in the studies on family patterns among the obese. Among pairs of identical twins reared in the same environment the mean difference in body weight between the 50 pairs of twins reared in the same environment was 4 lb. In only three pairs was the difference in body weight greater than 12 lb. Among 19 pairs of identical twins reared in separate environments, however, the deviation in body weight averaged 9.9 lb. This latter difference was similar to that found among 52 pairs of fraternal twins raised in a similar environment. The effect of environment is shown again by comparing the correlation coefficients for the 50 pairs of twins reared in the same environment (r = 0.973) with the correlation coefficient for the 19 pairs of identical twins reared separately (r = 0.886).

Another approach that demonstrates the importance of genetic factors has been presented by Withers who examined the correlations between body weights of adopted children and their natural and foster parents. The correlations in body weight between mother and father and an adopted child were very low. In contrast, there were higher correlations between the weight of a father and his natural child and between the weight of a mother and her natural child. Further, among obese individuals more than 80% had one or both parents who were obese. In only a small percentage were both parents recorded as having a normal body weight. Thus, genetic factors play an important role in the development of obesity either by environmentally independent direct transmission, or by providing the biochemical and physiologic mechanisms on which environmental factors potentially can operate.

There are two classifications of obesity. These are based on the anatomic characteristics of the adipose tissue in relation to the age of onset and on etiologic factors.

The anatomic classification is based on the number of adipocytes. The work of Hirsch and Bjorntorp showed that the number of adipocytes in the body could be estimated by determining the size of fat cells from several subcutaneous sites and simultaneously estimating total body fat.[3,23] In normal adults the upper limit is approximately 4 × 10^{10} fat cells. In many of the obese whose problem began in childhood, the number of adipocytes may be increased twofold to fourfold. People with increased numbers of fat cells are classified as having hypercellular obesity. This kind of obesity is to be distinguished from other forms of obesity in which the total number of adipocytes remain normal, but the size of individual fat cells is increased. In general, all obesity is associated with an increase in the size of adipocytes, but only selected forms have an increase in the total number of such fat cells.

There are a number of etiologic factors in obesity. The genetically transmitted forms of obesity were described above.[4] Endocrine alterations, although rare, are a second category of causative factors for obesity. The increase in fat observed with human endocrine diseases is usually limited. Hyperinsulinism produced by islet cell tumors or by injection of excess quantities of insulin can produce increased food intake and increased fat storage, but the magnitude of this effect is small. A somewhat more substantial obesity is observed with the increased cortisol secretion that occurs in Cushing's syndrome and also with hypothyroidism. Finally, aberrations in the distribution of body fat are also observed with hypogonadism.

Physical inactivity plays an important role in the development of obesity in humans and in the experimental animal. Gross obesity in rats can be produced by severe restriction of activity. In the modern affluent society, energy-sparing devices reduce energy expenditure and may enhance the tendency to caloric accumulation. As we increase our affluence, the caloric requirements for maintenance of body weight probably decline.

The composition of the diet is another etiologic category. This is particularly prominent in experimental animals but may also play a role in the development of human obesity. When rodents are exposed to a high-fat diet, most strains are unable to appropriately regulate calories and ingest more calories than are needed for weight maintenance. The rest are accumulated as fat, and the animals become grossly obese. Whether the rising fat consumption observed in most Western nations and the increase in corpulence in these societies are manifestations of a similar phenomenon is less clear.

Hypothalamic obesity is a rare syndrome in humans but can be produced regularly in animals by injury to the ventromedial region of the hypothalamus.[14] This region is responsible for integrating information about the caloric stores in the body. When the ventromedial hypothalamus is damaged, hyperphagia develops, and obesity follows. The increased secretion of insulin observed in this syndrome may be one pathogenetic link in its development. The connection between the ventromedial hypothalamus and the insulin secretion appears to be through the vagus and sympathetic nerves. Transection of the vagi prevents the hyperphagia and obesity that occur after injury to the ventromedial nuclei.

Hypothalamic obesity has been reported in human subjects under a variety of circumstances.[10] The major factors producing hypothalamic damage are trauma, malignancy, and inflammatory disease involving the hypothalamus. Three groups of findings accompany the syndrome. The first is related to changes in intracranial pressure, such as headache and diminished vision owing to papilledema. The second group of symptoms is a manifestation of endocrine alterations and includes amenorrhea, impotence, diabetes insipidus, and thyroid or adrenal insufficiency. The third group of symptoms is a variety of neurologic and psychological derangements including convulsions, coma, somnolence, hypothermia, or hyperthermia. Treatment of the syndrome requires treating the underlying disease and giving appropriate endocrine support.

Treatment for Obesity

Although vanity is a major reason why individuals seek help to lose weight, other reasons, particularly the potential risk for developing other diseases, may be more cogent. In our society, in which an excess of weight is socially undesirable, particularly in women, the search for successful treatments is never ending, and in the process may lead to exposure to undue or inappropriate risk. Medical complications or diseases associated with obesity are a second reason why people seek treatment for this problem and represent a particularly important motivational factor for middle-aged men. At the time of his first heart attack, the overweight man who is advised to reduce his body weight finds that the pounds just seem to "melt off." Weight reduction is also indicated for persons with diabetes mellitus, those suffering from osteoarthritis or hypertriglyceridemia, and those with hypertension and cerebral or peripheral vascular insufficiency.

Whatever the reason for seeking help for obesity, a high degree of motivation is needed to achieve and to maintain weight loss with any form of therapy. The rate of relapse (*i.e.,* regaining weight that has previously been lost) is high.[42,45]

EVALUATION OF THE OBESE PATIENT

When an overweight patient seeks medical attention for his problem, a minimum standard of evaluation is needed. The first important decision is whether the individual is sufficiently overweight to require or justify treatment. Although it is difficult to assign any medically significant risks to small degrees of deviation from desirable weight levels, it must nevertheless be an appropriate goal for the physician to recommend maintenance of desirable or optimal body weight. Since the risks from being 10% to 20% overweight are small, however, the therapies used must also carry minimal risk to the individual.

In evaluating any overweight individual it is appropriate to obtain the following pieces of information:

1. Anthropometric measurements, including the following: (1) height, (2) weight, (3) circumference of the waist, and (4) (if equipment is available) measurements of skinfold, with preference for the subscapular area, followed by additional measurements of the biceps, triceps, and iliac fat fold. (Appropriate formulas or tables for assessing degrees of fatness with these measures are provided elsewhere.)[4]

2. Functional status of an overweight individual including a listing of those complications that are known to be most frequently associated with overweight. (1) Diabetes mellitus should be evaluated by summing of glucose concentration in fasting 1-, 2-, and 3-hr samples of blood after an oral glucose tolerance test with 50 g to 100 g of glucose.[12] (2) Blood pressure should be taken, preferably in both arms. (3) Serum triglycerides, uric acid, and cholesterol would be reasonable measurements. As auxiliary measurements, the presence of gallstones by ultrasonography and the determination of cardiovascular fitness with a treadmill should be considered. An algorithm for evaluating the obese patient is presented in Figure 28-3. It summarizes the series of measurements that can be made and their interpretation.

3. A nomogram for determining body mass index from height and weight is shown in Figure 28-1. The body mass index has a better correlation with body fat than other relationships between height and weight.[7]

There are a number of modalities that can be used for treatment of overweight patients.[2] Undoubtedly, the safest and most appropriate is the use of diet. The use of pharmacologic agents as adjuncts to diet in the restoration of energy balance may help reduce caloric intake. Finally, under selected conditions, certain surgical procedures may be considered. Each of these approaches to therapy will be dealt with below.

DIET AND NUTRITION

The goal of all dietary treatment is to redress the caloric imbalance by reducing caloric intake, increasing energy expenditure, or both.[7] To do this requires first an assessment of caloric requirements. This can be done in one of two ways. The first is to determine the patient's age and, from Table 28-2, which shows median caloric intake as a function of age, to obtain some estimate of the average need, and then to reduce intake below that level. A second and more accurate approach is based on a nomogram developed at the Mayo Clinic and reproduced in Figure 28-4. From this nomogram for estimating energy expenditure, it is possible to arrive at a more precise assessment of energy requirements for a particular person. Use of Figure 28-4 involves measuring height and weight, determining age, and estimating the relative level of

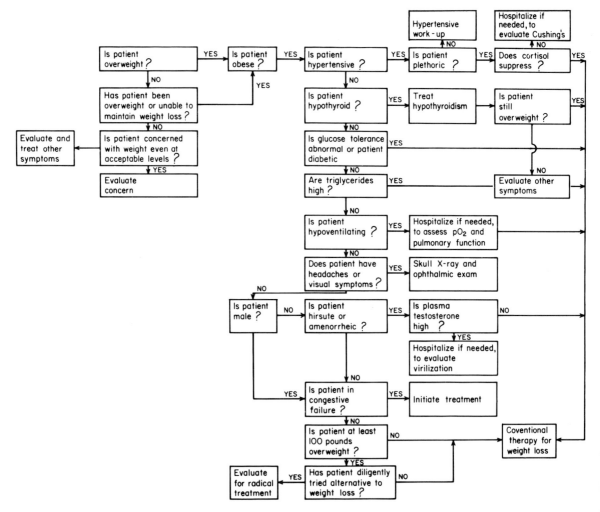

FIG. 28-3 An algorithm for use in evaluating an obese patient. (© G. A. Bray, 1979. Used with permission)

physical activity. Energy expenditure fluctuates with a number of factors, including physical activity, environmental temperature, hormonal status, and age.[4]

After assessing caloric requirements, the next goal is to provide a diet which has a reasonable caloric deficit. A maximal caloric deficit can be produced by total starvation, a technique which was once widely applied in the treatment of obesity.[4] For most people, however, it is not appropriate to restrict caloric intake this severely. If a caloric deficit of 500 Cal/day is maintained for 7 days, 3500 Cal must be provided from body energy stores to maintain energy supplies. Since 1 lb of fat tissue contains approximately 3500 Cal, a caloric deficit of 500 Cal/day will produce the loss of 1 lb of fat tissue each week.

STARVATION

Without doubt, the fastest way to lose body weight is by total starvation.[15] In this process, as with any other diet, there are two phases of weight loss. The first phase is rapid and primarily reflects the loss of fluids as the body adjusts to using its stored fat depots. After 24 hr to 48 hr, glycogen stores and the associated water are depleted. Gluconeogenesis from proteins is at a maximum at this time. After the first week to 3 weeks of starvation, the rate of weight loss falls below 1 lb/day, reflecting loss of both body fat and protein. With less severe caloric restriction most patients become distressed by the slowness of weight loss that occurs after the excess of fluids and readily mobilized body tissues have been depleted. This frustration is compounded by

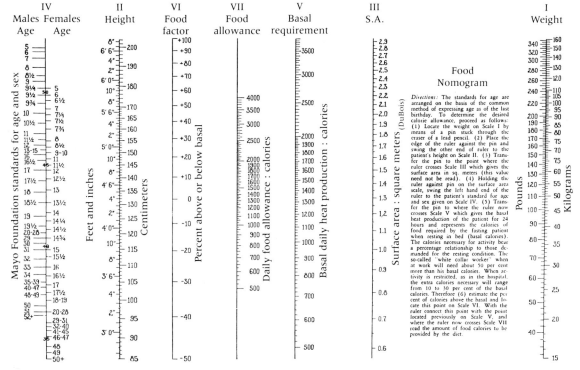

FIG. 28-4 Nomogram for estimating caloric needs. The use of this nomogram is described in the printed inset under Food Nomogram. (© Mayo Clinic. Used with permission)

the decrease in caloric expenditure that occurs during adaptation to caloric restriction.

VERY LOW CALORIE DIETS

Total fasting, although the most effective form of rapid weight loss, is now rarely used other than in the hospital. The reason for this is that fluid depletion enhances the risk of hypotension and the undue loss of protein. In an effort to prevent the losses of body protein, diets with protein supplements have been provided to individuals who are otherwise on a program of fasting. These diets reduce the loss of nitrogen from normal levels of 14 g/day to a value less than 5 g/day (equivalent to more than 30 g/day protein). However, there is no satisfactory evidence that the loss of protein is completely stopped by this technique. These very low calorie diets provide from 240 Cal/day to 500 Cal/day, predominantly as protein. In addition, supplements of electrolytes, including potassium, and micronutrients and vitamins, including folate, pyridoxine, and thiamin, are usually given. In the recent past the use of a proteolytic digest of collagen was widespread until a series of more than 16 deaths among women adhering to this program was reported. The

Center for Disease Control in Atlanta has now released the data on the 16 women treated with liquid-protein diets who died, and for whom no other adequate explanation for their death was available. These women ranged in age from 23 years to 51 years and when autopsy data was available, abnormalities of the myocardium with premorbid evidence of cardiac arrhythmias existed. Because of this unfortunate experience with very low calorie–protein diets, it would appear judicious for programs, regardless of the source of protein, to remain under investigative conditions, since the possibility exists that any form of protein diet without adequate carbohydrate or fat might produce the same untoward reactions.

CONVENTIONAL DIETS

The remaining dietary approaches to the treatment of obesity can be divided into two categories: those diets that are balanced and those that would be considered generally unbalanced.[2] Balanced diets are those in which calories have been restricted, but no single food or food substance predominates. The unbalanced diets are those in which one food substance or one type of food predominates. In this latter group are the low-carbohydrate diets and the many other diets identified by special names, such as the grapefruit diet, the banana diet, the ice cream diet, the candy diet, and so forth. The unbalanced diet has one major disadvantage of monotony, which results when certain classes of food are eliminated. Moreover, these diets may well be unhealthy if continued for a prolonged period.

When eating fewer calories than usual, it may be difficult to achieve an adequate intake of all needed nutrients. We have taken two approaches in attempting to provide useful information for our patients to help them determine their level of energy intake and their nutrient intake. The first approach involves training our patients to *count calories*. To do this, we provide each patient with a *monitor* for recording their calories (see Fig. 28-5). These monitors are printed on index cards that are handy to carry. On this monitor patients are instructed to write down each food they eat, the amount of that food using weight, volume, or portion size, and the calorie value of liquid and solid foods as obtained from a calorie guide. At the end of 7 days the patients add up their liquid and solid calories for each of the 7 days and record the values on the analysis form. Once patients have become accustomed to this procedure of counting calories, some of them like it so much that they use it as a primary technique for controlling and monitoring their weight loss; others, however, find it very difficult to count calories. Recently we have developed a glass calibrated to show the caloric values of various beverages as an additional technique for continuous monitoring and feedback about the energy content of liquids. The markings on the glass were drawn to provide an estimate of the caloric value for given foods and beverages (see Fig. 28-6). Each time a liquid is poured into the calorie glass, the caloric value is immediately visible. This

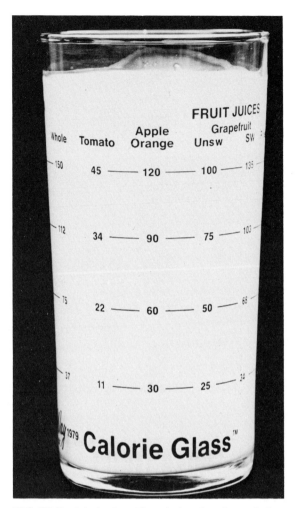

FIG. 28-6 Calorie glass. The calorie values for equivalent amounts of fruit juices are shown.

FIG. 28-5 Daily calorie monitor. The food eaten is recorded on the left, and the calories in that item of food are recorded under the liquid (things that are drunk from a glass or cup) and under the solid (eaten with a fork) category. (© G. A. Bray, 1976. Used with permission)

Daily Calorie Monitor		Calories	© BRAY 1976
Food Eaten	Day	Liquid	Solid

provides a continuous feedback about the caloric value of foods or liquids that are being ingested. For example, skim milk has about two thirds the calories of whole milk, and this difference is registered whenever milk is poured into the glass. Caloric values for various juices are also provided, showing that tomato juice is much lower in calories than most other juices.

Because of the difficulty we have had in getting patients to count calories carefully and faithfully, we have approached the problem of helping individuals to achieve lower calorie intake with good nutrition by other techniques. The first of these is to use the information that is published on the nutrition label of food packages. A sample of such a nutrition label is shown in Figure 28-7. A typical nutrition label shows the serving size and the number of servings per container. Below this infor-

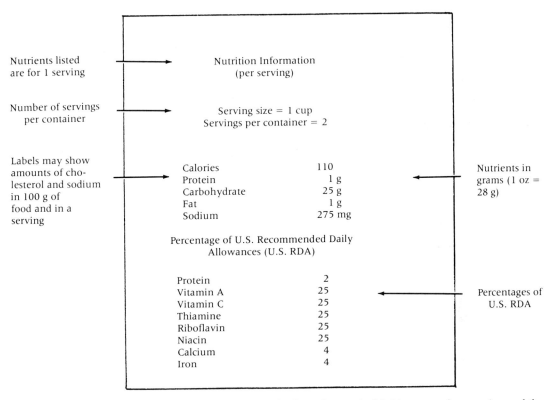

Nutrients listed are for 1 serving

Number of servings per container

Labels may show amounts of cholesterol and sodium in 100 g of food and in a serving

Nutrition Information
(per serving)

Serving size = 1 cup
Servings per container = 2

Calories	110
Protein	1 g
Carbohydrate	25 g
Fat	1 g
Sodium	275 mg

Percentage of U.S. Recommended Daily
Allowances (U.S. RDA)

Protein	2
Vitamin A	25
Vitamin C	25
Thiamine	25
Riboflavin	25
Niacin	25
Calcium	4
Iron	4

Nutrients in grams (1 oz = 28 g)

Percentages of U.S. RDA

FIG. 28-7 Nutrition label. The nutritional information on the label is expressed per serving, and the serving size is indicated (1 cup in this case). The values for calories, protein, carbohydrate, fat, and sodium are also indicated along with the percentage of certain of the vitamins and minerals.

mation are the most important facts for the person who is counting calories, that is, the number of calories in a serving from that container. We use the information about protein, carbohydrate, and fat to show that one can calculate the number of calories from proteins, carbohydrates, and fat by using calorie values of 4, 4, and 9, respectively.

A significant number of foods have relatively low caloric value, and many of them add flavor and taste to other foods. For this reason, we also provide our patients with a list of foods that they can eat in any amount they choose:

Coffee, without sugar, cream, or milk
Tea, without sugar, cream, or milk
Clear broth
Bouillon
Consomme
Lemon
Gelatin (unsweetened)
Pepper
Spices and seasonings
Vinegar
Vegetables:
    Asparagus

Broccoli
Cabbage
Cauliflower
Celery
Cucumber
Greens (beet, chard, dandelion, kale)
Lettuce
Mushrooms
Peppers
Radishes
Sauerkraut
Spinach
Watercress

The final approach which we use with our patients is to help them plan their own diet. This is done with the modification of the four food group system to which fats have been added and in which the fruits and vegetables as well as the bread and cereals have been subdivided. A listing of unit servings is provided in a form of a calorie exchange list (see Table 28-3). With this list patients can meet certain minimal nutrient levels of intake as well as keep calories in control by making calorie exchanges within each of the groupings shown. With

TABLE 28-3
Diet Planning Worksheet

Time of Day	Number of Caloric-Unit Servings in Each Group						
	Milk 2 Unit-Servings	Meat 4 unit-Servings	Fruit 2 Unit-Servings	Vegetables 2 Unit-Servings	Bread 2 Unit-Servings	Cereals 1 Unit-Serving	Fat 1 Unit-Serving
A.M.	☐	☐	☐			☐	
Noon	☐			☐	☐		
P.M.	☐	☐☐		☐	☐		☐
			☐				
Total calories in each group	200	300	100	200	150	100	75

Total calories in this diet plan 1125. The boxes under each heading are the servings. They can be moved from meal to meal, and some variations can be made from day to day and yet provide an overall balance among the various food groups.

Milk serving = 100 Cal; Meat serving = 75 Cal;
Fruit serving = 50 Cal; Vegetable serving = 100 Cal;
Bread serving = 75 Cal; Cereal serving = 100 Cal;
Fat serving = 75 Cal;
(© 1982 George A. Bray, M.D.)

the diet planned as in Table 28-3, the total calories would be 1125. It could be lowered by reducing the amounts of food in any category, and reasonable control of nutrition could be achieved by varying these changes in one category or another from day to day. This has proven to be a useful way of combining calorie exchanges with a sensible approach to nutrition.

BEHAVIORAL ASPECTS OF TREATMENT

For many patients the use of calorie counting, education about food groups, and the use of nutritional contents of foods is not a sufficient and satisfactory technique to help them lose weight. For this reason, we have adopted a variety of behavioral techniques. The basic principles of these behavioral approaches can be summarized under the "ABCs" of eating. The *A* stands for *Antecedent*. If one looks at eating as the response to events in the environment, then the antecedent events which trigger eating are of major importance. Eating might be triggered by passing a pizza parlor, or entering the home after working, or by turning on the television set. Whatever the antecedents may be, it is important for the obese person and his therapist to come to grips with them. The *B* in the *Behavior* of eating is the rate and frequency with which an individual eats, that is, the actual act of eating. In addition to monitoring the antecedents, we also teach our patients to monitor their eating behavior. Finally, the *C* represents the *Consequence* of the eating, the feelings an individual has about it, and more important, the procedures that a person can use to provide rewards for changing the pattern of behavior.

The practical approach to eating behavior used in our clinic has been developed over a period of several years. Like most investigators in this field, we began with the classic experiments of Stuart and Davis, Stunkard, and Jordan and colleagues.[26,40,41] These investigators used a single monitoring sheet contained in a notebook which the subjects were instructed to carry with them, and in which they wrote the day, date, time, food eaten, and a variety of factors about that eating situation, including the place, associated activities, their mood, and hunger associated with that eating event. When I tried this procedure myself, I found it impossible to carry out for more than a few days. Gradually, we evolved a stepwise approach to this analysis using index cards. In the first step, the patients are instructed to identify the foods that they eat and two antecedents, the associated activity and place where they eat (see Fig. 28-8). At the end of a week of this monitoring the patients analyze the results. After completing this analysis, they have some estimate of the events and places that are associated with eating. We then make suggestions for changes that they can make based on this analysis. For example, if eating occurs primarily when watching television, we suggest that they avoid eating while watching television. We then use the technique of stimulus control to help them to modify their eating. (By stimulus control, we mean reducing the number of places or times at which they eat.) This can be done by confining the act of eating to a single place and concentrating on the act of eating itself, rather than watching television. Distracting events of other types are also to be avoided. For many individuals the very act of writing down what they eat and observing themselves eating in this fashion is a unique and valuable experience that in and of itself initiates changes in eating behavior.

During the next week, we have patients monitor the same events of associated activity and place of eating, but ask them in addition to note whether they are eating a meal or a snack. A snack is defined as a single item or two, while a meal consists of three or more items consumed at the same time. When they return after a week of monitoring their associated activity and place, they have a much better feeling about whether they have been able to achieve some element of stimulus control. Moreover, they are beginning the analysis of eating itself by counting the frequency of eating and the rate at which they eat. This is done by counting the number of meals during each hour. The peak frequency of meals and the rate of eating are both counted. We again encourage patients to make some change in the number of meals or in the frequency with which food is eaten. During the ensuing week they make more notes and return to repeat the analysis and to observe their progress.

As a third exercise, we have them record their hunger at the time of eating and the taste of the food they ate. The purpose of this exercise is to have each subject spend time judging the flavor of food and deciding whether they were hungry when they began eating. The goal of this exercise is to decrease the amount of eating at times when they are not hungry and to become more discriminating by eating only foods they really like. After coming to grips with taste and hunger, we encourage them to try to eliminate some of those events when they were eating without being hungry and to avoid eating those foods which do not taste good. For many overweight patients this analysis of the ABCs of eating has been of great value in helping their ability to control eating. For some, these approaches are much more effective than counting calories, while for others, counting calories is a much more rewarding approach.

EXERCISE AND PHYSICAL ACTIVITY IN TREATMENT

Another approach to losing weight is to increase energy expenditure. Over the past 70 years, a voluminous medical literature has accumulated concerning metabolic requirements of human beings. These can be divided into the following three components: a requirement for basal metabolism, one for heat losses owing to thermic effects of food, and

FIG. 28-8 Monitor card for recording associated activities and place where food is eaten.

a third for the energy needed for physical activity. Basal metabolic needs are slightly lower for women than for men, but in general they are approximately 1000 Cal/day/M^2. Heat losses resulting from the thermic effects of food are small and not more than 10% of the caloric value of the ingested foods. The energy needed for physical activity obviously depends on the degree of activity. Since basal metabolism is not subject to significant changes and thermic effects are small, the only part of expenditure that is amenable to significant manipulation is physical activity.

Table 28-4 summarizes levels of physical activity (adapted from the Recommended Dietary Allowances, Appendix Table A-1). The lowest level of activity is slightly less than 0.8 Cal/min. Thus, if an individual sleeps for 24 hr, fewer than 1400 calories will be expended. Reclining increases this level from 0.8 Cal/min to approximately 1.4 Cal/min. Very light activity (*i.e.,* the level at which people spend much of their time) consumes between 1.5 Cal/min and 2 Cal/min. Light activity increases this to 2 Cal to 3.5 Cal/min, while moderate activity ranges from 3.5 Cal/min to 7 Cal/min and heavy activity from 7.5 Cal/min upward. Few people spend much of their time involved in physical activity of this latter level. Since physical activity can be a useful way of expending extra energy, we have spent a considerable amount of time attempting to devise effective ways of helping people to monitor their physical activity. The monitor shown in Figure 28-9 is used to record activity on an hour-to-hour basis. The activity level in each hour was scored as the highest activity the individual achieved during that hour using the analysis shown in Table 28-4. These monitors were used twice. During the first week subjects scored an activity level as the highest level during each time interval, and during the next week they used a value for a level maintained for at least 45 min out of the hour. At the

TABLE 28-4
Analysis of Activity

Level	Examples of Activities	
0	*Sleeping:* 0.8–1.2 Cal/min	
1	*Reclining:* 1–1.4 Cal/min	(Watching television, reading quietly)
2	*Very light:* 1.5–2 Cal/min	(Seated or standing activities such as painters, cab and truck drivers, laboratory workers, typists, musicians, stitchers, office workers)
		Office workers, most professional workers, homemakers with mechanical aids such as dishwashers
3	*Light:* 2–3.5 Cal/min	(Walking on level at 2.5–3 mph, tailors, pressors, garage work, electrician, carpentry, restaurant trades, cannery workers, manual clothes washing, shopping with light load, golf, sailing, table tennis, volleyball)
		Most light industry workers, students, building workers except for heavy laborers, many farmers, homemakers without mechanical appliances, department store workers
4	*Moderate:* 3.5–7 Cal/min	(Walking 3.5–4 mph, plasterers, gardeners, scrubbing floors, stockroom with loading and stacking heavy loads, shopping with a heavy load, bicycling, skiing, tennis and dancing)
		Some agricultural workers, unskilled laborers, forestry workers (except lumberjacks), soldiers, miners, steelworkers, dancers, athletes
5	*Heavy:* 7–12 Cal/min	(Walking uphill with a load, lumberjacks, pick and shovel work, basketball, swimming, climbing, football)
		Lumberjacks, blacksmiths, rickshaw–pullers, construction workers

(© George A. Bray, M.D.)

		© George A. Bray 1977			
Day		Activity Monitor			
Hour	Activity Level	Hour	Activity Level	Hour	Activity Level
12–1AM		8–9		4–5	
1–2		9–10		5–6	
2–3		10–11		6–7	
3–4		11–12		7–8	
4–5		12–1PM		8–9	
5–6		1–2		9–10	
6–7		2–3		10–11	
7–8		3–4		11–12	

FIG. 28-9 Activity monitor. This form is used for recording on an hourly basis the maximal (or minimal) activity during that hour using the levels obtained from the Recommended Dietary Allowances, in Table 28-4.

end of two weeks they had an assessment of their range of energy expenditure.

As a final exercise we review the minutes of walking required to expend the calories in various foods (see Table 28-5). When these records and the analysis were completed, our patients had obtained some understanding of nutrition, exercise, and the behavioral features of eating, and were able to achieve considerable degrees of weight loss by these techniques alone. Indeed, during the 10 weeks of this program many patients achieved weight losses of over 20 lb.

DRUGS IN THE TREATMENT OF OBESITY

The drugs that have been used to treat obesity fall into several categories. The two most important are those that act on the central nervous system to suppress appetite (the amphetamines and related drugs) and the calorigenic agents, of which thyroid hormone is the most important clinical example. A third group of drugs consists of those agents postulated to increase fat mobilization. A fourth group of drugs acts at the level of intestinal absorption or, like cholecystokinin and glucagon, may be released by food intake and may act to reduce further ingestion of food. Finally, there are drugs for treating specific complications of obesity. For a discussion of the mechanism of the action of these drugs, the reader is referred elsewhere.[4,37]

APPETITE-SUPPRESSING DRUGS

The clinically useful appetite-suppressing drugs are listed in Table 28-6. All of them can increase locomotor activity and stimulate the central nervous system, but the relative potency differs greatly. Amphetamine and methamphetamine are the most potent, while fenfluramine hydrochloride is the least

TABLE 28-5
Minutes of Walking to Burn the Calories in Various Foods

		Weight		
	Calories	*120 (lb) min*	*160 (lb) min*	*200 (lb) min*
Apple (1)	75	21	17	14
Apple Pie	330	91	75	62
Beer (12 oz)	170	47	38	31
Blueberries (cup)	84	23	19	16
Beef steak	300	83	68	57
Bologna (1 slice)	116	32	26	22
Biscuit (1)	130	36	30	24
Bread (1)	65	18	15	12
Broccoli (cup)	50	14	12	10
Cola (8 oz.)	100	28	23	19
Cereal cooked (cup)	165	46	38	31
Cheese (1 oz)	100	28	23	19
Chocolate cake	150	42	34	28
Egg	100	28	23	19
Flounder (4 oz)	78	22	18	15
Frankfurter	124	34	28	23
Hamburger and bun	400	111	91	76
Milk (whole) (8 oz)	166	46	38	31
Orange	106	29	24	20
Potato (baked)	100	28	23	19
Salmon steak	200	56	46	38
Strawberries (1 cup)	54	15	12	10

(© George A. Bray, M.D.)

potent. The latter drug is both a stimulant and depressant. In experimental animals benzphetamine hydrochloride and d-amphetamine produce the greatest increase in spontaneous activity. Fenfluramine and chlorphentermine hydrochloride on the other hand have almost no effect on locomotor activity. The appetite-suppressant effect of these drugs in monkeys is greater for amphetamine and methamphetamine than for the other drugs, which on a molar basis are only a third to a tenth as active.

Cardiovascular effects are frequently observed when these drugs are used. An increase in heart rate and an increase in blood pressure are the most common responses. Some of these drugs also produce metabolic effects. Amphetamine, methamphetamine, phenmetrazine hydrochloride, and fenfluramine increase the concentration of free fatty

TABLE 28-6
Appetite-Suppressing Drugs Used in the Treatment of Obesity

Schedule*	Generic Name	Trade Names
II	d,1-Amphetamine	Benzedrine and others
	Methamphetamine	Desoxyn and others
	Phenmetrazine	Preludin
III	Phendimetrazine	Plegine
	Benzphetamine	Didrec
	Chlorphenteramine	Pre-Safe
	Chlortermine	Voranil
	Mazindol	Sanorex
IV	Diethylpropion	Tenuate, Tepanil
	Phentermine	Ionamin (resin), Fastin
	Fenfluramine	Pondimin

*Assigned by the Drug Enforcement Agency

acids or glycerol in the plasma. Fenfluramine seems to act like insulin at the adipocyte receptor, inhibiting lipolysis and increasing glucose utilization by the fat cell. Of the appetite-suppressing drugs, only mazindol appears to be without effect on lipid metabolism, indicating a different mechanism of action from that of the other drugs listed in Table 28-6.

In evaluating the clinical usefulness of these drugs two questions need to be answered: (1) Are they effective? and (2) Are they safe?

Effectiveness.   The Food and Drug Administration (FDA) recently evaluated 105 drug applications submitted for marketing these drugs. The applications contain over 200 controlled studies of which about 160 trials compared placebo and active drug. The data analyzed by the FDA contained 4543 patients on active drugs and 3182 patients on placebo.[37] In this group, the dropout rate was approximately 18.5% for the patients on placebo and 24% for patients with active drug in studies lasting 3 weeks, 4 weeks, or 6 weeks. At the end of the study period, whatever that duration might be (3, 4, 6, 8, 12, 20 weeks, or more), equal numbers of patients receiving placebo and active drug were retained (49% for placebo versus 47.9% for active drug). The weight loss averaged 0.56 lb/week more for patients receiving active drugs than for patients receiving placebos.

FIG. 28-10   Weight loss during treatment with an appetite suppressant. Weight loss is more rapid in the patients treated with the active drug. (M ± S.E. − mean ± standard error).

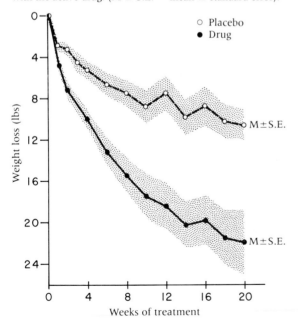

These same data can be examined diagrammatically by looking at the weight loss in pounds per week for patients on a placebo and those on an active drug (Fig. 28-10). It is clear that the patients receiving the placebo in this study lost weight, but the patients receiving the active drug lost significantly more weight. Thus, the effectiveness of amphetaminelike drugs is significantly greater than that of placebo. Analysis of the data from the studies, which compared two active drugs, revealed no significant differences between any of the drugs in Table 28-6. Thus, in clinically effective doses, there is little to choose between these compounds in terms of effectiveness for weight loss or the duration over which this weight loss could be induced.

The long-term effectiveness of these drugs, however, has never been established. The longest trials in which effective numbers of patients were retained in the placebo and drug treatment groups was 50 weeks. In most studies, however, the dropout rate was too high after 16 to 20 weeks to allow effective evaluation. The data on studies of up to 20 weeks suggest the possibility that these drugs might retain their ability to reset the internal control systems that regulate body fat at a lower level for a prolonged period of time.

Safety.   The safety of these agents has also been the subject of considerable discussion. The possibility of enhanced mortality in patients receiving diet pills was brought forcefully to public attention in 1967. The agents incriminated were usually amphetamine, thyroid, diuretics, and laxatives. In some patients, it would appear that potassium deficiency and the ensuing hypokalemia may have been a major factor leading to death. However, one review of deaths using amphetamines and thyroid in "reasonable doses" could find no evidence for increased mortality. An equally serious problem is the potential for development of tolerance and the possibility of drug abuse. Indeed, it is the problem of habituation and addiction that has led to the current reassessment of value of these drugs in the treatment of obesity. Drug abuse has been reported for amphetamine, methamphetamine, and phenmetrazine. Claims of drug abuse for other members of this class are less frequent.

In addition to the potential for abuse, there are a number of side-effects.[4] The two most prominent are insomnia and dry mouth The other effects occur in small numbers with the exception of depression and diarrhea, which occur mainly with fenfluramine.

From the previous discussion, it is clear that these agents can be effective as adjuncts in the treatment of obesity. Their usefulness depends on employing them as part of a total program for treatment of obesity. Several rules would appear to be applicable to their use. First, the drug abuse potential is higher for those compounds in Schedule II (Table 28-6), and it would thus appear more reasonable to select a preparation classified in Schedule III or IV in which drug abuse potential is less. Some of these drugs have been used with apparent effectiveness in children and in pregnancy. Fenfluramine, chlorphentermine, and diethylpropion hydrochloride, for example, produce no statistically significant reduction in linear growth velocity of children treated over a period of one year. For the present, however, it would be wise not to use these drugs in pregnant women.

Among the group of compounds listed in Table 28-6, the last three appear to merit initial consideration in the treatment of obesity. Diethylpropion may be the first choice, with phentermine, fenfluramine, and mazindol in second place. Among patients with a history of depression or mental illness, mazindol and diethylpropion would merit first choice; fenfluramine should probably not be used. Among diabetics, fenfluramine may be the drug of choice. Among hypertensive patients, mazindol or diethylpropion appear to merit first consideration. The potential of intermittent or interrupted courses of therapy should be kept in mind. Interrupted courses of therapy lasting for 3 weeks to 6 weeks with discontinuation for a period half or more the length of the original period of treatment have been reported. Because of the tendency in some patients to postdrug depression, intermittent therapy with fenfluramine is inadvisable.

GASTROINTESTINAL HORMONES

Cholecystokinin and its synthetic terminal octapeptide have been demonstrated to decrease food intake in both rats and monkeys. On the basis of these observations, cholecystokinin was proposed as the short feedback loop for appetite suppression. Studies in humans, however, have been variable. Both intravenous infusions of cholecystokinin and bolus injections of the synthetic octapeptide subcutaneously or intravenously prior to eating failed to reduce food intake in humans in spite of the development of GI side-effects. However, when infusion was begun 12 min after the start of the meal, a small reduction in food intake was observed.

CALORIGENIC DRUGS

Thyroid Hormones. Weight loss in obese patients treated with triiodothyronine or with thyroxine is more rapid than with a placebo. In one study, doses of each hormone were gradually increased to tolerance. The patients receiving either thyroid preparation lost weight steadily, but the patients with placebo did not. The mechanism for this enhanced weight loss during treatment with thyroid hormones resides in two effects: (1) increased oxygen consumption and (2) increased protein catabolism. Within the first days after hormone administration, there is increased excretion of nitrogen with onset of a negative or increased negative nitrogen balance. This effect persists for at least 30 days, although it reaches its peak within the first 10 days. Whether nitrogen balance returns to normal after long-term treatment with small doses of thyroid hormone is not known. Two recent studies have shown that the loss of nitrogen can be prevented. In one of these, anabolic steroids and growth hormone were used to prevent the loss of nitrogen induced by treatment with triiodothyronine.[13] Prevention of the negative nitrogen balance with these drugs did not reduce the consumption of oxygen. Thus, under these conditions, all of the incremental calories were coming from the catabolism of fat. In the other report, the loss of nitrogen was prevented by increasing the dietary intake of protein. The effects of 180 mg and 540 mg of desiccated thyroid on nitrogen balance were examined in four patients on a 600-Cal or 1200-Cal diet. The rate of weight loss was comparable using 180 mg thyroid with a 600-Cal intake or a 1200-Cal diet and 540 mg thyroid. The nitrogen balance was maintained in both groups, but the authors felt that the patients were happier on the higher dose of thyroid.

Approximately two thirds of the increment in oxygen used during T_3 administration is related to the catabolism of fat and the remaining one third is related to the catabolism of protein. In terms of weight loss, however, more than two thirds of the increment is due to breakdown of lean body mass. As the initial burst of protein catabolism subsides, weight loss declines.

A potentially dangerous side-effect of thyroid hormone is the change in chronotropic and inotropic properties of cardiac muscle. Although the mechanism for these effects is not known, it is clear that treatment with thyroid hormones will increase the mass of the heart in experimental animals, and probably in humans as well. Since obesity itself increases the work of the heart as well as its size, the added cardiac load imposed by treatment with thyroid hormones could be detrimental. Indeed, the deleterious cardiac effects of D-thyroxine (a pharmacologic isomer of the naturally occurring L-thyroxine) observed when D-thyroxine is used to lower serum lipids in patients with atherosclerosis have led to its withdrawal from the trial of agents used in a coronary drug project. This project dealt with patients who had already had a myocardial infarct, and hence the conclusions may not apply to normal people.

Finally, any beneficial effect of treatment with thyroid hormone must be evaluated in terms of long-term weight loss as compared to other modes of treatment which do not use thyroid hormones. From the data in the literature, an average of 25% of patients treated with diet alone will maintain a weight loss of more than 20 lb at the end of one year. Two reports have followed-up patients previously treated with T_3 initiated in low doses and increased stepwise. In one study the patients were started on treatment in the hospital. When they were reevaluated two years later, 12% had maintained a weight loss of 20 lb or more, and 6% had maintained a loss of more than 40 lb; only one of 199 patients had approached ideal weight.[4] This outcome was no better than that achieved with diet alone. A similar conclusion was reached in another study where 55 patients were treated in two groups. Four of 28 in one group had maintained a 40 lb weight loss one year later. Although one can look at these data as an indictment of all forms of therapy in obesity, there is a positive side. By the use of techniques of nutritional modification, manipulation of eating habits, and patterns of exercise, weight can, indeed, be lowered in a significant number of patients by sympathetic clinical management without use of drugs.

DRUGS POSTULATED TO INCREASE FAT MOBILIZATION

Human Chorionic Gonadotropin.   Human chorionic gonadotropin (HCG) is formed by the placenta of some mammals. It is released into the serum and is excreted in the urine during pregnancy. The blood concentrations or urinary levels can be used as a diagnostic test for the presence of pregnancy and for some forms of abnormal pregnancy. The biological functions of HCG are similar to those of luteinizing hormone (LH) secreted by the pituitary. During pregnancy, HCG functions to maintain the corpus luteum, which produces the steroidal hormones, including progesterone. The chemical preparations of HCG that are sold are impure and contain minute amounts of a number of other substances in addition to HCG. The drug has been approved for treatment of menstrual dysfunction and use in threatened abortion but has not been approved for treatment of obesity.

The safety of HCG at the doses that are used for treatment of obesity has rarely been questioned. The major question is whether this agent is effective as a treatment for obesity. A number of clinical trials have been performed to answer this question. Most of the studies were randomized double-blind trials. A review of the published studies provided little support for the concept that HCG is an effective agent in the treatment of obesity.[22] Few would contest however, that adhering to a 500-Cal diet for 40 days would be expected to produce a weight loss approximating .5 lb/day (200 g) or more. In summary, then, injections of HCG have not been shown to be associated with a greater weight loss than placebo in obese patients eating a 500-Cal/day diet.[22] It is worth noting that the placebo-treated patients in this and other studies with HCG or placebo injections have rates of weight loss exceeding the results from almost all other studies using either behavioral, dietary, or pharmacologic techniques.[45]

Surgery in Treatment of Obesity

Two considerations provide the rationale for surgery as a treatment for obesity.[5,17] First, the success of most conservative methods for treating obese patients has a low yield; and second, the risks of morbidity and mortality in the grossly obese, as has been discussed earlier, are substantial.

The indications for surgical intervention has been defined in many papers.[5] Most operations should be reserved for patients who are substantially overweight (*i.e.,* more than 50 kg [110 lbs] above desirable weight), although this may not apply to jaw wiring. Patients with such complications as diabetes mellitus, hypertension, pulmonary alveolar hypoventilation (the pickwickian syndrome), and serious orthopedic problems may qualify at a somewhat lower weight limit because these problems are likely to be ameliorated by weight loss. There is a feeling that intestinal operations on patients who are over 50 years of age may be more hazardous because of the increased difficulties in adjusting to the consequences of these surgical procedures. Patients should have faithfully tried other means of losing weight and failed on more than one occasion before being accepted for high-risk surgery. Some authors have suggested that a stable adult life-style and emotional stability are desirable, but this contention is not supported by psychiatrists who have dealt with these patients.

INTESTINAL BYPASS

Several major operative procedures are now in use. There are two major types of intestinal bypass. In one operation the end of the distal segment of the jejunum is attached to the side of the ileum near the ileocecal valve (end-to-side or Payne operation). The other operation anastomoses the distal end of the jejunum to the end of the ileum and drains the defunctionalized bowel into the colon with an ileocolonic anastomosis (end-to-end or Scott operation).[17] These operations are presented sche-

End to side   End to end

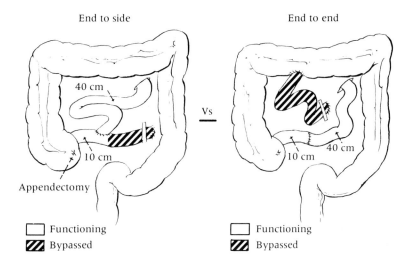

Vs

40 cm

10 cm

Appendectomy

40 cm

10 cm

FIG. 28-11 Operations for jejuno-ileal bypass.

☐ Functioning
▧ Bypassed

☐ Functioning
▧ Bypassed

matically in Figure 28-11. Recently, a modification has been introduced in which the upper end of the defunctionalized intestine is anastomosed to the gallbladder. This reduces the diarrhea.

Weight loss after intestinal bypass seems to occur for two main reasons: (1) a decrease in food intake and (2) malabsorption of ingested calories. The reduction in food intake can account for most of the weight loss observed in patients who have had an intestinal bypass. Malabsorption also occurs after intestinal bypass surgery. There is a decrease in the intestinal absorption of fat, nitrogen, carbohydrate, vitamins, and minerals (inorganic molecules). The loss of calories in the stools rises from 131 Cal/day preoperatively to a maximum of 593 Cal/day postoperatively, and this produces a small increase in the rate of weight loss. (A net deficit of 450 Cal/day in the stool accounts for a weight loss of 58 g adipose tissue/day.)

Intestinal adaptation has been measured by histological and physiological methods. There is increased turnover of cells in the intestinal crypts. The decline in absorption of vitamin B_{12}, D-xylose, and oxalate immediately after surgery is followed by a gradual increase in absorption. Bile-acid metabolism is also altered. Initially, bile becomes more lithogenic, but lithogenicity gradually returns to normal, usually within 6 months after surgery. The loss of bile acids in the stool may contribute to the diarrhea in these patients. The adaptation of intestinal function may account for the decline in the diarrhea and slowing of weight loss as the months pass after surgery.

The benefits of an intestinal bypass procedure can be summarized under three headings. First, there is weight loss that is usually permanent. The second benefit of this operative procedure is an improvement in psychosocial function. Major adjustments may be required of the patient during the postoperative period, and these commonly have emotional repercussions. The patients usually show greater self-confidence and self-esteem, and this changed mood may become a source of friction with spouses or parents. However, this surgery may also serve to break the vicious cycle of unrelieved ineffectiveness, guilt, and resignation, and may facilitate new hopes and new constructive adjustments in these patients. Improvement in risk factors for cardiovascular diseases is a third benefit of intestinal bypass surgery. There is a decrease in blood pressure, a decline in insulin requirements, and a decrease in serum cholesterol and triglycerides.

The list of complications following this operation has grown steadily longer. It now includes not only those problems associated with the surgery itself, but a growing list of medical complications resulting from the altered anatomy produced by this surgery.

The overall mortality following surgery is approximately 2.8% for the series of 6518 patients in the literature (see Quaade).[31] This figure varies from no deaths in smaller series to over 11% in other series. In addition to operative mortality, there are many other surgical complications including pulmonary embolism, serious wound infection, GI hemorrhage, renal failure, and pancreatitis.

All patients who have had a jejunoileostomy develop diarrhea. In the early postoperative period, liquid stools may range from 8/day to 20/day or more and may produce rectal irritation and associated hemorrhoidal pain. There is a gradual decline in the frequency and severity of this problem. By 6 weeks following surgery stools usually range between 4/day and 15/day, and by 6 months this figure usually has decreased to between 2/day and 6/day. The diarrhea can be controlled by one of several methods, including bulk, or fiber in the diet, laxatives such as psyllium seed extracts which absorb water, the use of calcium salts (calcium carbonate), or the use of diphenoxylate (Lomotil).

Malnutrition of variable degree occurs in all patients and is produced by the malabsorption of many nutrients. Hypoproteinemia may be profound in some patients, and serum albumin declines in all. In our patients this decline was approximately 20% from preoperative levels. There is also increased fecal excretion of nitrogen and impaired absorption of amino acids from the intestine. Malnutrition also is manifested by vitamin deficiencies. The absorption of vitamin B_{12} is uniformly impaired, and plasma concentrations decline. Plasma levels of vitamin A and vitamin E also are reduced, and night blindness may be a problem in these individuals.

Another manifestation of malnutrition and malabsorption is the loss of electrolytes in the stools. Potassium loss is particularly prominent and may be associated with profound hypokalemia and symptoms of weakness. If diarrhea is severe, losses of calcium and occasionally magnesium also can be significant, and tetany has been reported in a number of patients. Excretion of fecal fat also increases and may account in part for the increased loss of calcium, which is complexed with fatty acids in the stools.

Malabsorption of carbohydrates has been demonstrated by the decreased absorption of D-xylose. Segmental absorption of glucose also may diminish. There now is convincing evidence that these early problems with malabsorption and its associated malnutrition eventually lead to intestinal adaptation with increased absorptive capacity in the remaining intestinal segment. There also is an increase in the length of the colon as the quantity of undigested foods entering this organ rises.

Pregnancy in the first year following intestinal bypass surgery is frequently associated with an exacerbation of the problems of malnutrition. The presence of a fetus with its demands on the mother can lead to the precipitation of nutritional deficiencies that might not have surfaced otherwise.

Liver disease is one of the most perplexing postoperative complications. The majority of obese patients have abnormal liver function preoperatively, and most get worse postoperatively. However, only a small number of them go on to develop cirrhosis and progressive liver failure. Tests of liver function, such as the serum transaminase and alkaline phosphatase, rise in the early postoperative period and have not proven useful as a guide to the severity of the liver problem. Liver biopsies have shown that between 1 month and 6 months after surgery, fat is frequently increased. There also may be a deterioration in the histologic appearance of the liver. However, this usually improves slowly, but it is uncommon for liver histology to return to nor-

mal. A number of hypotheses have been proposed for the development of liver disease, including the following: (1) protein deficiency, (2) deficiency of choline, (3) inadequate absorption of the essential amino acids, (4) formation and absorption of excess quantities of lithocholic acid, (5) endogenous formation of ethanol, (6) deficiency of vitamin E, and (7) formation of toxic bacterial products. Recent evidence has provided support for the latter hypothesis. When bypass patients are treated with metronidazole, an antibiotic which is primarily active against anaerobic microorganisms, the development of liver abnormalities can be prevented.

Two syndromes of bacterial overgrowth have been described. The first of these has been called pseudo-obstructive megacolon. It presents clinically with intermittent abdominal swelling and distention and usually has its onset one or more years after the bypass. The intestine can distend so much that abdominal girth may increase 7.5 cm to 12 cm (3 in–5 in) in a matter of an hour. Air fluid levels may be detected on x-ray film, with a picture of obstruction that is relieved by intubation or with the passage of gas and stool rectally. This syndrome appears to be related to anaerobic organisms in the small intestine and colon, and temporary relief may be produced by antibiotics effective against the anaerobic organisms. A second syndrome, so-called *bypass enteropathy*, consists of fever, abdominal pain, and bacterial growth in the intestinal segment. This appears to be a less common problem than that associated with pseudo-obstruction.

Urinary calculi have been reported with a frequency varying between 0.3% and 30%. The mechanism for the increased stone formation appears to reside in the increased absorption of oxalates. Following intestinal bypass surgery, increased amounts of fatty acids are complexed with calcium and excreted in the stool. Thus, calcium that would normally be available in the intestine to bind oxalate is complexed with fatty acids, and more oxalate is in the soluble form in which it can be absorbed. There are now several techniques for increasing oxalate loss in the stool, thereby decreasing its absorption. Among these are the administration of calcium, the use of a low-fat diet, and administration of antacids, particularly the aluminum oxide variety. This, accompanied with an increased urine volume, can serve as satisfactory techniques for diminishing the likelihood of developing oxalate stones. Unfortunately, some patients develop intrarenal deposits of oxalate, and renal impairment may result.

ARTHRITIS

Polyarthritis with migratory arthralgia has been described in up to 6% of patients with bypass. These symptoms are usually associated with pain, but only rarely does joint swelling and effusion occur. Fingers, knees, and ankles may be involved. Rheumatoid factor, antinuclear factor, and lupus erythematosus (LE) cells have not been detected. In one recent study, however, cryoprotein complexes against *E. coli* and *B. fragilis* were found in the circulation of three patients with intestinal bypass. These antigens may serve as the basis for an inflammatory response in the synovium of the joint.

Reanastomosis and restoration of intestinal continuity is done for many reasons in fewer than 10% of patients. Severe liver disease, inability to live with the intestinal bypass, and inability to solve the problems of pseudo-obstructive megacolon included the reasons for reanastomosis.

As the number of patients having an intestinal bypass has increased, the enthusiasm for this procedure as a treatment for obesity has declined somewhat. The mortality from this form of therapy far exceeds that of all other forms of treatment of obesity, including diet pills, treatments with thyroid hormone, "shots," and other medications. Whether the prolongation of life after this operation is significant has not been clearly established. However, it does appear from the careful psychiatric studies that the quality of life for the obese bypass patient is improved. It is, therefore, our opinion that intestinal bypass surgery is justified for some of the grossly obese persons who are severely impaired in their social or medical function.

GASTRIC BYPASS

Several gastric operations provide a second surgical approach to obesity. These procedures, like the intestinal bypass described above, involve rearrangement of the GI tract. Two approaches have been used. The first transects the stomach a short distance below the esophagus, connects the smaller upper pouch to the jejunum, and closes off the larger gastric pouch, which drains normally into the duodenum. The size of the upper gastric pouch is designed to approximate 50 ml to 60 ml. When it is filled with food, the patient feels full and cannot eat more. The second surgical approach to preparing a small upper gastric pouch is called a gastroplasty. In this operation, a small channel is constructed between a small upper and large lower gastric segment.[30]

The gastric bypass for obesity shares some of the problems of intestinal bypass surgery but is free of a number of the metabolic complications. Mortality from gastric bypass ranges in the neighborhood of 3% but varies from one institution to another. Following this form of surgery, the patient may need reoperation for the various problems that can arise from marginal ulcers and obstruction. There is also the problem of estimating the size of the pouch that has been constructed.

The metabolic problems, which have plagued the intestinal bypass operations, do not appear to occur after gastric bypass. Thus, liver failure, oxalate renal stones, problems with bacterial overgrowth in the defunctionalized bowel, and malabsorption and malnutrition do not appear. The long-term problems of the gastric bypass, however, await more complete studies.

VAGOTOMY

Vagotomy is the most recent surgical procedure that has been tried for patients with obesity. In experimental animals with obesity following injury to the ventromedial hypothalamus, a subdiaphragmatic vagotomy has been found to reverse obesity. This experimental observation suggested the possibility that vagotomy might work in human obesity. A small group of patients having this procedure has now been studied with promising results. The first three patients all lost weight at the rate of 10 kg/month for the first few months after surgery. In a larger series of ten patients from the same clinic, nine out of the ten had a successful loss of weight. The surgeon reported that the patients did not experience hunger during the postoperative period. These findings open the door to a new surgical approach to obesity.[29]

JAW WIRING

Preventing a patient from ingesting solid food by occluding the teeth with wires can facilitate weight loss. This technique utilizes the methods developed for treating patients with broken jaws. When the wires are in place, the patients can only ingest liquid foods. With this procedure there has been successful weight loss during the time when the jaws are wired shut. However, weight is usually regained after the wires are removed. In one clinic, jaw wiring is performed as an initial way of helping patients lose weight before a surgical bypass is performed. This combination of surgical modalities in treatment of obesity has potential merit.[32]

References

1. Behnke AR, Wilmore JH: Evaluation and Regulation of Body Build and Composition. International Research Monograph Series in Physical Education. Englewood Cliffs, Prentice–Hall, 1974
2. Berland T: Diets '79. Everything you should know about the diets making news. Consumer Guide Magazine Health Quarterly, 223, 1979
3. Bjorntorp B: The fat cell: A clinical view. In Recent Advances in Obesity Research: II. Proceedings of the 2nd International Congress on Obesity. London, Newman Publishing, 1978

4. Bray GA: The Obese Patient. Major Problems in Internal Medicine, Vol 9. Philadelphia, W B Saunders, 1976
5. Bray GA: Surgical treatment of obesity: A review of our experience and an analysis of published reports. Int J Obes 1:331, 1977
6. Bray GA: To treat or not to treat—that is the question? In Recent Advances in Obesity Research: II. Proceedings of the 2nd International Congress on Obesity. London, Newman Publishing, 1978
7. Bray GA: Definition, measurement, and classification of the syndromes of obesity. Int J Obes 2:99, 1978
8. Bray, GA (ed): Obesity in America. Washington, DC, DHEW (NIH) No. 79–359, 1979
9. Bray GA, Campfield LA: Metabolic factors in the control of energy stores. Metabolism 24:99, 1975
10. Bray GA, Gallagher TF, Jr: Manifestations of hypothalamic obesity in man: A comprehensive investigation of eight patients and a review of the literature. Medicine 54:301, 1975
11. Bray GA, Glennon JA, Salans LB et al: Metabolism of glycerol phosphate and pyruvate by human adipose tissue in spontaneous and experimental obesity: Effects of dietary composition and adipose cell size. Metabolism 26:739, 1977
12. Bray GA, Jordan HA, Sims EAH: Evaluation of the obese patient. I. An algorithm. JAMA 235:2008, 1976
13. Bray GA, Raben MS, Londono J et al: Effects of triiodothyronine, growth hormone and anabolic steroids on nitrogen excretion and oxygen consumption of obese patients. J Clin Endocrinol Metab 33:293, 1971
14. Bray GA, York DA: Hypothalamic and genetic obesity in experimental animals: An autonomic and endocrine hypothesis. Physiol Rev 59:719, 1979
15. Drenick E, Johnson D: Weight reduction by fasting and semistarvation in morbid obesity: Long-term follow-up. Int J Obes 2(2):123, 1978
16. Durnin JVGA, Womersley J: Body fat assessed from total body density and its estimation from skinfold thickness: Measurements of 481 men and women aged from 16–72. Br J Nutr 32:77, 1974
17. Faloon WS (ed): Symposium on Jejunoileostomy for obesity. Am J Clin Nutr 30:1 (Jan), 1977
18. Forbes GB, Reina JC: Adult lean body mass declines with age: Some longitudinal observations. Metabolism 19:653, 1970
19. Garrow JS: Energy balance and obesity in man. Amsterdam, Elsevier/North Holland Biomedical Press, 1978
20. Glass AR, Swerdloff RS, Bray GA et al: Low serum testosterone and sex-hormone-binding globulin in massively obese men. J Clin Endocrinol Metab 45:1211, 1977
21. Goldblatt PB, Moore ME, Stunkard AJ: Social factors in obesity. JAMA 192:1039, 1965
22. Greenway FL, Bray GA: Human chorionic gonadotropin (HCG) in the treatment of obesity: A critical assessment of the Simeon's method. West J Med 127:461, 1977
23. Hirsch J, Batchelor B: Adipose tissue cellularity in human obesity. Clin Endocrinol Metab 5:299, 1976
24. Hosseinian AH, Kim MH, Rosenfield RL: Obesity and oligomenorrhea are associated with hyperandrogenism independent of hirsutism. J Clin Endocrinol Metab 42:765, 1976
25. Jolliffe N: Reduce and stay reduced on the prudent diet. New York, Simon & Schuster, 1963
26. Jordan HA, Levitz L, Kimbrell G: Eating is OK! A radical approach to successful weight loss. The behavioral-control diet explained in full (edited by Steve Gelman). New York, Rawson Associated Publishers, 1976
27. Kannel WB, Gordon T: The physiological and medical concomitants of obesity: The Framingham Study. In Bray GA (ed): Obesity in America. DHEW (NIH) Publ No 79–359, 1979
28. Keys A: Overweight and the risk of heart attack and sudden death. In Obesity in Perspective. Proceedings of the Fogarty Center Conference on Obesity. Washington, DC, Government Printing Office, 1975
29. Kral JG: Vagotomy for treatment of severe obesity. Lancet 1:307 (Feb) 1978
30. Mason EE, Printen KJ, Blommers TJ et al: Gastric bypass for obesity after ten years experience. Int J Obes 2:197, 1978
31. Quaade F: Intestinal bypass for severe obesity, a randomized trial. A report from the Danish Obesity Group. In Bray GR (ed): Recent Advances in Obesity Research: II, pp 385–390. London, Newman Publishing Chap 39:385, 1977
32. Rodgers S, Goss A, Goldney R et al: Jaw wiring treatment of obesity. Lancet 1:1221, 1977
33. Reisen E, Abel R, Modan M et al: Effect of weight loss without salt restriction on the reduction of blood pressure. N Engl J Med 298:1, 1978
34. Rochester DF, Enson Y: Current concepts in the pathogenesis of obesity. Hypoventilation syndrome: Mechanical and circulatory factors. Am J Med 57:402, 1974
35. Salans LB, Bray GA, Cushman SW et al: Glucose metabolism and the response to insulin by humans in spontaneous and experimental obesity: Effects of dietary composition and adipose cell size. J Clin Invest 53:848, 1974
36. Schacter S, Rodin J: Obese Humans and Rats. Washington, DC, Erlbaum/Halsted, 1974
37. Scoville BA: Review of amphetamine-like drugs by the food and drug administration. In Obesity in Perspective, Vol 2, Part 2. US Government Printing Office, 1976
38. Sims EAH, Danforth EH, Jr, Horton ES et al: Endocrine and metabolic effects of experimental obesity in man. Recent Prog Horm Res 29:457, 1973
39. Steinkamp RC, Cohen NL, Siri WE et al: Measures of body fat and related factors in normal adults. I. J Chronic Dis 18:1279, 1965
40. Stuart RB, Davis B: Slim chance in a fat world: Behavioral control of obesity. Champaign, Research Press, 1972
41. Stunkard AJ: New therapies for the eating disorders. Arch Gen Psychiatry 26:391, 1972
42. Stunkard AJ, McLaren–Hume M: The results of treatment for obesity. Arch Intern Med 103:79, 1959
43. Sullivan AC, Comai K: Pharmacological treatment of obesity. Int J Obes 167, 1978
44. Whipp BJ, Bray GA, Koyal SN et al: Exercise energetics and respiratory control in man following acute and chronic elevation of caloric intake. In Bray GA (ed): Obesity in Perspective, Fogarty International Center Series on Preventive Med. Section II, Chap 20, Vol 2, Part 2. Washington, DC, US Government Printing Office, 1976
45. Wing RR, Jeffrey RW: Outpatient treatments of obesity: A comparison of methodology and clinical results. Int J Obes, 1979
46. Wirtshafter D, Davis JD: Body weight: Reduction by long-term glycerol treatment. Science 198:1271, 1977
47. Woods S, Porte D, Jr: Central nervous system, pancreatic hormones, feeding and obesity. Adv Metab Disord 9:283, 1978

29
Obstetrics and Gynecology
Roy M. Pitkin

The discipline of obstetrics/gynecology is that branch of medicine concerned with reproduction; obstetrics refers to pregnancy, its antecedents, and its sequelae, and gynecology deals with diseases of the female reproductive system. In addition, the obstetrician/gynecologist, by virtue of being considered the "woman's doctor," is responsible for primary health care for a substantial proportion of the female population.

Reproductive medicine includes a number of areas with profound nutritional implications. Some of these are common to other medical specialities, whereas others are unique to the discipline. This chapter reviews three specific areas in the latter group—pregnancy, lactation, and sex hormone therapy. Each area is considered separately, with emphasis on altered nutrient needs, and each section concludes with a brief summary statement of clinical implications.

Nutritional Support During Pregnancy

Throughout much of recorded history, nutrition has been regarded as representing an important influence on the course and outcome of pregnancy. Several recent reviews have summarized contemporary concepts about this relationship.[2,30,33,36]

During the course of gestation the maternal organism undergoes a remarkable series of physiologic adjustments in order to provide for fetal growth and development and at the same time preserve maternal homeostasis. Concomitantly, the fetus exchanges materials with its mother across the placenta and modifies its own development by its maturing regulatory processes. The resultant physiologic system is complex, integrated, and intricate, as well as being dynamic in the sense of constantly changing throughout the course of pregnancy. Many aspects of the process are either nutritional in nature or have obvious implications for nutrition.

ENERGY, WEIGHT, AND WEIGHT GAIN

ENERGY REQUIREMENTS

In the mature nonpregnant person, energy sources are required to maintain basic metabolic processes and provide for physical activity. Pregnancy imposes additional energy needs for growth of the fetoplacental unit and added maternal tissues, as well as for support of increases in maternal metabolism. The total energy cost attributable to pregnancy, calculated from the amounts of protein and fat accumulated by mother and fetus and the addition to metabolism incurred by these additions, averages approximately 75,000 Cal.[20] Caloric expenditure is not evenly distributed throughout pregnancy, nor does it parallel fetal growth. Instead, it is minimal during early pregnancy, increases sharply during the first trimester, and remains essentially constant throughout the remainder of gestation. During the second trimester, the extra caloric cost is due primarily to maternal factors (expansion of blood volume, growth of uterus and breasts, and accumulation of storage fat), whereas during the third trimester it is related mainly to growth of the fetus and placenta.

491

Since caloric expenditure is relatively constant, throughout the last three quarters of gestation, the added daily increment necessary for pregnancy can be estimated by dividing the total cumulative caloric cost of pregnancy by its duration. Thus, the Recommended Dietary Allowances (RDA) of the Food and Nutrition Board (see Appendix Table A-1) contain an added allowance of 300 Cal/day throughout pregnancy. The Food and Agriculture Organization–World Health Organization recommends an additional 150 Cal/day during the first trimester and 350 Cal/day during the last two trimesters. These values represent, in effect, the amount required by pregnancy and do not take into account such variables as ambient temperature, physical activity, or growth requirements unrelated to gestation (*e.g.,* as in the adolescent).

WEIGHT GAIN

The amount of normal or optimal weight gain during pregnancy has been the subject of much speculation. Little if any reliable information exists to provide a basis for judging normality nor, indeed, is it clear that a specific value for weight gain is optimal for all individuals. Data regarding average gain, which may or may not be optimal, have been calculated and, in spite of methodologic discrepancies such as differing dietary advice and variable methods of determining baseline weight, these show a remarkable degree of consistency. From an extensive review of the literature in 1944, Chesley found the average to be 11 kg (24 pounds).[8] This value is identical to that reported more than 25 years later by the Committee on Maternal Nutrition of the National Research Council and is at the midpoint of the 10 kg to 12 kg stated by the Committee on Nutrition of the American College of Obstetricians and Gynecologists.[30,36] A slightly larger amount, 12.5 kg, is suggested by Hytten and Leitch for healthy primigravids eating without restriction. The slight difference may be due to age, since younger women tend to gain somewhat more weight than older women, or it may reflect a somewhat more lenient British attitude toward weight gain during pregnancy.[20]

It should be emphasized that these data refer to *average,* as opposed to *optimal,* gain, and the level associated with best overall outcome for mother and infant is not entirely certain. Nevertheless, current opinion holds that the lowest frequency of obstetric complications seems to occur with gains around these mean values, and it therefore appears likely that average and optimal levels are similar.

Virtually all available data relate to total weight gain during gestation, a figure of limited clinical value because it is unknown until pregnancy is completed. Of much greater interest would be the pattern by which weight accumulates throughout gestation. Unfortunately, information about outcome with various patterns of gain is limited. The customary pattern consists of minimal gain (1 kg–2 kg) during the first trimester and a progressive accumulation thereafter to term. Although the maximal rate occurs during the second trimester, for practical purposes the rate of gain may be considered linear from approximately 10 weeks until term, averaging 0.35 kg/week to 0.4 kg/week. These relationships are expressed in Figure 29-1, which also illustrates the components of gain. It is apparent from a consideration of Figure 29-1 that most of the accumulation during the second trimester is related to the maternal compartment and that most gain during the third involves the fetal compartment. At term, the mother accounts for slightly more than half, and the fetus slightly less than half, of the total cumulative gain.

RELATIONSHIP TO BIRTH WEIGHT

A number of studies in experimental animals have examined the relationship between maternal dietary restriction and fetal development. In general, experiments involving rodents have found substantial effects on size of the fetus and growth of various organs, notably that of the brain.[49] However, caution must be exercised in applying these observations in species in which total fetal weight at term amounts to as much as 30% of maternal weight to the human situation with a single fetus representing only 5% or so of maternal weight.

Although there remain many unresolved questions regarding the influence of pregnancy nutrition on fetal development in the human, the relationship between weight gain during pregnancy and birth weight of the infant seems reasonably clear. Virtually all major studies have documented a significant positive correlation between total maternal gain and birth weight, with weight gain ranking second only to duration of pregnancy as a determinant of infant weight.[3,14,32,40,42] Maternal prepregnant weight is also related to birth weight, usually ranking behind, though occasionally ahead of, weight gain during pregnancy.

Certain "natural experiments" in human malnutrition have indicated a clear effect on birth weight. Two particularly well-studied episodes occurred during World War II during the siege of Leningrad in 1942 and the famine in western Holland during the winter of 1944 to 1945. Both were characterized by severe protein–calorie malnutrition (PCM), and pregnancies during the period of deprivation produced infants with significantly lower mean birth weights than those recorded before and

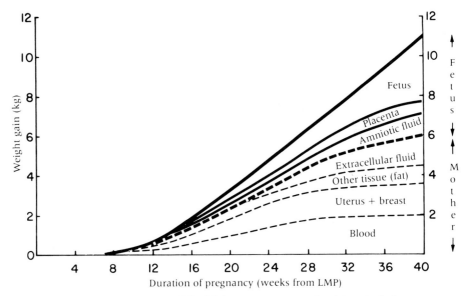

FIG. 29-1 Average maternal weight gain during pregnancy.

after the famine. In Holland birth weight fell by an average of 250 g; in Russia the drop was twice as great. The difference between the Dutch and Russian experiences may have related to differing quality of nutritional status prior to the famine as well as to the severity of deprivation.

Confirmatory evidence has been provided by several nutritional intervention studies conducted in various areas of the world. In these investigations, provision of protein–calorie supplements to women of known or presumed deficient nutritional status have generally resulted in some degree of increase in birth weight. The magnitude of augmentation observed has varied; in developing countries mean birth weight increases of as much as 200 g or 250 g have been reported, but in populations from developed nations the effects appear to be quite modest.[46]

In spite of the reasonably well-documented relationship between pregnancy weight gain and birth weight, many questions regarding the influence of maternal nutrition on the fetus remain unresolved. Weight gain is at best a crude index of nutrition, providing little information on nutrients other than energy, and birth weight is a similarly gross index of fetal development.

DEVIATIONS IN WEIGHT AND WEIGHT GAIN

Deviations from usual values for either prepregnant weight or weight gain during pregnancy are relatively common. Although standard definitions are lacking, the following are suggested as reasonable guidelines:

1. Underweight—prepregnant weight 10% or more below ideal weight for height (see Appendix Table A-16)
2. Overweight—prepregnant weight 20% or more above ideal weight for height (see Table A-16)
3. Inadequate gain—gain of 1 kg or less per month in the second or third trimester
4. Excessive gain—gain of 3 kg or more per month

The hazards presented by the underweight obstetric patient generally have not been appreciated. The likelihood of a low-birth-weight infant is increased substantially. Higgins has shown that both intensive dietary counseling and supplemental feeding of underweight patients increase mean birth weight. Increased risk of preeclampsia with low prepregnancy weight has also been found in some studies.

The obese woman entering pregnancy faces increased risk of several complications, notably hypertensive disorders and diabetes mellitus, which have adverse effects on pregnancy outcome. Some have advocated restriction of weight gain in such patients so that they conclude pregnancy with a net loss. However, the advisability of such a course seems questionable on several grounds. First, severe dietary restriction to limit calories may also result in displacement of other nutrients from the diet. Second, optimal protein utilization in pregnancy apparently requires a minimum of approximately 30 Cal/kg/day. Finally, severe dietary restriction results in catabolism of fat stores, which in turn produces ketonemia. This consideration may be particularly important in view of data suggesting that women with acetonuria during pregnancy (presumably as a result of starvation) have children who score less well on IQ tests at age 4 compared with children of nonacetonuric women.[9]

The patient with inadequate gain during pregnancy presents an increased risk of delivering a low-birth-weight infant. She should be followed closely and receive careful dietary counseling in an effort to bring her weight gain to normal.

Excessive weight gain during pregnancy has long been thought to be associated with several obstetric complications. The past several generations of American physicians have been taught that excessive weight gain leads to preeclampsia and that dietary restriction, particularly caloric restriction, protects against its development. Moreover, the definition of excessive weight gain has often been considerably more stringent than that proposed here.

Until relatively recently, total weight gain as low as 7.26 kg (16 lb) has been advocated. Undoubtedly, much of the confusion surrounding the relationship between weight gain and preeclampsia results from failure to differentiate between weight due to actual tissue accumulation and weight due to fluid retention. Since edema is one of the signs of preeclampsia, any group of edematous patients will contain a somewhat larger proportion of gravidas with preeclampsia, as well as greater mean total weight gain, than will a group of nonedematous pregnant women. However, traditional concepts notwithstanding, the evidence fails to support a relationship between caloric intake (as reflected in weight gain) and preeclampsia.[30] Energy intake above normal requirements during pregnancy results in increased fat deposition, and this increase, if not lost after delivery, may contribute to obesity. To prevent initiation of this chain of events, some limitations of excessive gain may

be desirable. The aim of such management should be to bring the rate of gain near the normal, rather than to markedly restrict gain.

PROTEIN

REQUIREMENTS

A need for additional protein during pregnancy is a clear *a priori*. Amino acids derived from dietary protein are required in increased amounts for protein synthesis essential in growth of the uterus and breasts, expansion of the maternal extracellular fluids, and development of the fetus and placenta.

The magnitude of the increased protein need of gestation may be estimated in two ways, theoretical and experimental, and the values derived differ considerably with the method used. The theoretical approach utilizes the quantities of protein (calculated from measured nitrogen contents) in the maternal and fetal compartments. From a consideration of representative values (Table 29-1) it is apparent that total protein accumulation during term pregnancy amounts to slightly less than 1 kg. This level of protein accretion amounts to 3.4 g/day over the whole of pregnancy, or to 0.8 g/day, 4.4 g/day, and 7.2 g/day in the first, second, and third trimesters, respectively. Correcting the values for individual variability, efficiency of conversion of dietary to tissue protein, and biologic quality of food protein leads to recommended additional protein intakes of 11 g/day to 15 g/day (0.19 g/kg/day–0.26 g/kg/day) throughout the last half of pregnancy.

Another method of estimating protein requirements involves nitrogen balance studies, in which intake and losses are carefully measured over a range of protein intakes to determine the level required to maintain the subject in nitrogen equilib-

TABLE 29–1
Cumulative Protein Increment in Maternal and Fetal Compartments*

	Cumulative incremental protein content (g)		
	End of first trimester	*End of second trimester*	*End of third trimester*
Blood proteins	10	100	135
Uterus	30	90	166
Breast	12	65	81
(Maternal subtotal)	(52)	(255)	(382)
Fetus	1	150	440
Placenta	3	55	100
Amniotic fluid	0	2	3
(Fetal subtotal)	(4)	(207)	(543)
	56	462	925

*Hytten FE, Leitch I: The Physiology of Human Pregnancy, 2nd ed. Oxford, Blackwell Scientific Publications, 1971

rium. Such studies have, in general, led to estimations of protein requirements some two to three times those estimated theoretically.

The reason for this discrepancy between estimates based on theoretical and experimental methods is unclear. Impaired efficiency of protein metabolism during gestation seems unlikely on evolutionary grounds. Nitrogen storage in maternal nonreproductive tissues may be responsible, although evidence from studies in lower animals is lacking. Finally, the discrepancy may reflect either methodologic problems or a systematic tendency on the part of balance studies to overestimate requirements. In view of the uncertainty involved, particularly that surrounding protein storage with gestation, the prevailing philosophy at present is to tentatively accept the higher value. Thus, the current RDA is 30 g/day during pregnancy in addition to the allowance for the nonpregnant woman, making the total protein allowance 1.3 g/kg/day in the mature gravida, 1.5 g/kg/day in the pregnant adolescent aged 15 years to 18 years, and 1.7 g/kg/day in the girl under 15 years of age.

The total serum protein concentration falls during pregnancy, a pattern due largely to albumin which declines fairly rapidly during the first trimester and somewhat more slowly during the second trimester, reaching a nadir of approximately 30% below nonpregnant levels during the third trimester. Globulins behave somewhat differently, with α globulins rising minimally, β rising more substantially, and γ globulins changing little, if any. While the explanation of these changes is obscure, they reflect normal physiologic adjustments, and dietary protein deficiency is almost certainly not a significant factor.

PROTEIN–ENERGY INTERRELATIONSHIPS

The inextricable metabolic relationships between protein and energy make it impossible to differentiate between these two nutrients with respect to estimating requirements or defining effects on pregnancy outcome. It has been demonstrated repeatedly that energy intake correlates strongly with measured nitrogen retention when protein intake is held constant. Thus, it must be kept in mind that optimal protein utilization in pregnancy presupposes adequacy of energy sources.

Confirmation of these relationships is provided by the results of a recent nutritional intervention study conducted in rural Guatemala.[25] The investigation was designed to assess the differential effects of energy and protein supplementation in a population with generally inadequate diets. With 20,000 Cal or more supplemented throughout pregnancy, the incidence of low birth weight was halved, irrespective of the nature of the supplement. In other words, the augmentation of birth weight was similar with carbohydrate and protein supplements.

EFFECT ON PREGNANCY OUTCOME

A number of studies in rats have demonstrated that protein-restricted diets during gestation characteristically produce serious consequences in the offspring. Intrauterine growth, both of the whole organism and of individual organs, is impaired. Restriction of cellular growth in the brain may have a functional correlate in findings that liveborn pups of these pregnancies subsequently exhibit impaired learning and behavioral aberrations. Provocative as such observations may be, their relevance to the human is problematic in view of the great differences between the two species with respect to length of gestation, number of offspring, proportion of litter weight to maternal weight, and state of maturity of the young at birth.

Zlatnik recently reviewed reported studies of the effect of dietary protein on birth weight in the human and, in noting conflicting results, judged that all were subject to criticism on methodological grounds.[50] Among the potentially confounding variables identified were failure to take into account preconception weight or pregnancy weight gain, conscious or unconscious manipulation of the diet, selection bias on the basis of volunteer populations or other factors, and the inherent subjectivity of data based on dietary surveys. The reviewer concluded that the evidence "does not clearly define the importance of diet in general or protein in particular as related to human pregnancy outcome."[50]

A potential relationship between dietary protein and preeclampsia has long been a subject of speculation. Fifty or more years ago it was widely believed that the disease resulted from high intakes of protein. Gradually, the concept evolved that low intakes led to limitation of plasma volume expansion and in turn to pregnancy-induced hypertension. To be sure, a number of retrospective studies have indicated a general association between low protein intake (determined by dietary history) and preeclampsia, but any cause and effect relationship is far from clear because of such confounding variables as socioeconomic status, race, marital status, age, and parity.

In spite of the many uncertainties surrounding the influence of dietary protein on the course and outcome of pregnancy, protein is generally regarded as a particularly important nutrient for the pregnant woman. Physicians and nutritionists typically advise ample protein intake, particularly from animal sources, during gestation. In many instances intakes above even the most generous estimates of requirements are advocated. Though the value of such an approach has never been demonstrated, the prevailing philosophy seems to be that it is harmless and possibly may be helpful. Concern about this practice has been raised by the recent observations in one of the nutritional intervention studies alluded to previously.[41] Among poor women in Harlem, those given in a protein-rich supplement exhibited significantly *increased* perinatal mortality, primarily due to an increased frequency of premature labor. Although this association is not yet confirmed and its significance is uncertain at present, it should be regarded as indicating some degree of caution about the routine advice of giving high-protein diets to pregnant women.

IRON

BLOOD VOLUME

The changes in maternal blood volume accompanying pregnancy represent a fundamental physiologic adjustment. Plasma volume begins to increase during the first few weeks after conception and continues to expand at a relatively rapid rate until the early third trimester, when the rate slows and then ceases altogether. Although it was previously believed that the plasma volume actually declines in late pregnancy, it now appears that the terminal "fall" is actually an artifact resulting from measurement in the supine position with attendant vena caval obstruction by the pregnant uterus. Thus, maximal plasma volume is reached at 34 weeks to 36 weeks, at which point the incremental increase amounts to an average of 1350 ml above the nonpregnant mean of 2600 ml, an increase of 50%. Erythrocyte volume also increases during pregnancy, but both the pattern and magnitude differ from that of plasma. The pattern is much more nearly linear, beginning at early pregnancy and increasing progressively to term. Erythrocyte volumes rise an average total of 250 ml over the average nonpregnant value of 1400 ml, a factor of less than 20%. However, in patients taking supplemental iron throughout pregnancy, erythrocyte volume increases by 400 ml.

Figure 29-2 illustrates the relative increases in plasma and erythrocyte volumes. Early in pregnancy more plasma than erythrocytes is being added to the circulation; late in pregnancy the opposite is true. From a consideration of these relationships, it would be predicted that erythrocyte count, hemoglobin concentration, and hematocrit will all

decline progressively during pregnancy to a nadir in the late second or early third trimester and thereafter increase slightly. Exactly these changes (see Fig. 29-2) have been described in a number of studies.

REQUIREMENTS

The extent of augmented erythropoiesis during pregnancy depends in part on the amount of iron available. Without supplemental iron, erythrocyte volume increases by 250 ml, but if iron supplements are given, red cell mass increases by an average of 400 ml. Therefore, if adequate iron is available to the bone marrow, an average of 500 mg elemental iron will be utilized in the pregnancy-related maternal erythropoiesis. To this must be added the amount of iron present in the fetus and placenta—200 mg to 400 mg. Blood shed with parturition is another mechanism of iron loss, but this may be disregarded in calculating the iron requirements of pregnancy, since the augmented blood volume more than compensates for it. In the interests of accuracy, the amount of iron "saved" by the amenorrhea of pregnancy, estimated at 120 mg, should be subtracted. Thus, the total iron requirements of pregnancy amount to 600 mg to 800 mg of elemental iron.

Dietary surveys indicate that the usual mixed diet provides approximately 6 mg elemental iron/1000 Cal. Absorption in healthy subjects amounts to approximately 10% of dietary iron. Although some evidence indicates a somewhat enhanced degree of absorption at times of physiologic need, including pregnancy, it is unlikely that diet can provide more than 2 mg/day to 3 mg/day elemental iron, an amount little more than that lost in sweat, urine, and feces. Quite clearly, dietary iron is generally inadequate to meet the requirements of pregnancy.

Iron stored in the reticuloendothelial cells of the bone marrow is potentially available for meeting pregnancy demands. By using histochemical evaluation of marrow stores during quantitative phlebotomy, Scott and Pritchard estimated that the storage iron of presumably healthy nulligravid American women averages 300 mg. Moreover, approximately a third of these subjects had no demonstrable storage iron. These observations indicate that iron stores are usually inadequate for the demands of pregnancy.

Considerations such as these suggest that during her reproductive years a woman is in a precarious state with respect to iron sufficiency. For whatever reasons—repetitive menstrual blood loss, previous pregnancies, or a relative lack of androgenic hormones—her iron stores are minimal. When she

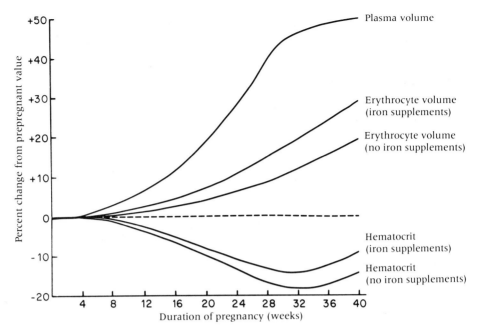

FIG. 29-2 Changes in maternal blood during pregnancy.

conceives, the marked increase in plasma volume, coupled with fetal transfer, results in a falling hemoglobin concentration.

The fetus appears to be an effective parasite in extracting iron from its mother regardless of the state of maternal iron sufficiency. Thus, the hemoglobin level of infants born to pregnant women with iron deficiency anemia is typically normal and recent studies of plasma ferritin levels indicate that this index of storage iron in the newborn is unaffected by maternal iron status.[21]

SUPPLEMENTATION

Because dietary and storage iron is often inadequate to meet the iron demands of pregnancy, routine iron supplementation of virtually all gravidas is advocated by many authorities. Consistent with this view is the observation noted above that the augmented erythrocyte volume is nearly twice as great in patients given supplemental iron as in unsupplemented patients. Moreover, numerous studies have demonstrated that the decline in hemoglobin concentration and hematocrit in pregnancy may be ameliorated, though not entirely prevented, by iron supplementation. In several studies of pregnant women at or near term, mean hemoglobin concentrations were 12.3 g/100 ml with supplementation (78 mg/day–200 mg/day during at least the last trimester) and 11.1 g/100 ml without; hemoglobin levels below 11 g/100 ml were

virtually eliminated by iron supplements.[38] Similarly, the fall in serum iron concentration in pregnancy is minimized by iron prophylaxis.

The reasoning that a declining hemoglobin concentration during pregnancy without iron supplementation represents iron deficiency anemia is not universally accepted. A contrary view, particularly prevalent in Britain, questions the use of nonpregnant standards to define normality during pregnancy and suggests that the maintenance of hemoglobin concentration and total hemoglobin mass with iron supplementation is a *pharmacologic effect*, as opposed to the presumably *physiologic decline* exhibited by unsupplemented patients. The possibility that routine iron supplementation may actually be undesirable has been suggested recently by observations that erythrocyte macrocytosis is induced.[47]

An obvious implication of this controversy is the practical question of whether patients should routinely receive iron supplements during pregnancy. It is perhaps, as Hytten and Leitch suggest, more a matter of philosophy than of science.[20] In any event, the preponderance of opinion, particularly among clinicians and particularly in the United States, favors routine supplementation.[30,36] Levels of supplementation as low as 12 mg/day fail to affect the fall in hemoglobin concentration and hematocrit, but those of 30 mg/day or more result in normal values at term.[38] Somewhat larger amounts may be necessary to protect maternal stores.[13] Therefore, the recommended amount of supplementation is 30 mg/day to 60 mg/day elemental iron.[30,36]

Elemental iron contents of common supplemental preparations are listed in Table 29-2.

FOLACIN

REQUIREMENTS

Considerable evidence reviewed in detail by Kitay indicates that folate requirements are substantially increased during pregnancy. Among the factors potentially responsible are impaired absorption, defective utilization, and increased demand. Impaired absorption may be a factor in some patients, particularly those with recurrent megaloblastic anemia in repetitive pregnancies, but a pregnancy-specific characteristic interfering with folate absorption does not seem likely. Defects in utilization or metabolism of folacin may be related to the increased levels of sex steroid hormones, as suggested by a possible increased incidence of folate deficiency in oral contraceptive users (a highly controversial subject to be considered in detail in a subsequent section). However, it appears that increased demand represents the most important factor. Because folate acts as an essential coenzyme in purine and pyrimidine metabolism, needs for the vitamin are especially high with rapid tissue growth. Thus, the augmented maternal erythropoiesis of pregnancy and the growth and development of the fetus and placenta all account for substantially increased folacin needs.

The precise magnitude of folacin requirements during gestation is unknown. The RDA is 800 µg/day, which represents a doubling of the allowance for the nonpregnant woman. It may be that needs more than double with gestation and if so, the difference between requirement and allowance (*i.e.,* the "safety factor") is narrower in the gravid than in the nongravid patient.

Certain clinical conditions increase folacin requirements further. The patient with multiple pregnancy has more than one fetus, (usually) more than one placenta, and additional augmentation in her blood volume. Chronic hemolytic anemia involves abnormally high rates of maternal erythro-

TABLE 29–2
Elemental Iron Content of Supplements

Preparation	Iron (%)
Ferrous fumarate	32.5
Ferrous sulfate (exsiccated)	30.0
Ferrous sulfate (nonexsiccated)	20.0
Ferrous gluconate	11.0

TABLE 29–3
Morphologic and Biochemical Effects of Folate Deprivation*

Time (weeks)	Event
3	Low serum folate (< 3 ng/ml)
7	Neutrophil hypersegmentation
14	Elevated foriminoglutamic acid excretion
18	Low erythrocyte folate (< 20 ng/ml)
19	Megaloblastic marrow
20	Anemia

*Data from Herbert V: Trans Assoc Phys 75:307, 1962

poiesis and, therefore, increased folacin needs. The anticonvulsant drug diphenylhydantoin interferes with folate metabolism in such a way as to increase requirements.

EFFECT OF DEFICIENCY

The biochemical and morphologic sequelae of experimental folate deficiency are listed in Table 29-3. The developmental sequence is probably unaltered during pregnancy, but some evidence suggests that temporal relationships may be accelerated.

The incidence of folate deficiency varies widely throughout the world, presumably as a result of varying dietary intake. Moreover, the incidence depends directly on the diagnostic criteria employed. In its most severe form—anemia—it is relatively uncommon in contemporary American practice. At the opposite extreme, low serum folate levels (less than 3 ng/ml) are observed in 20% to 25% of otherwise normal pregnancies.

Although the relationship between folate deficiency and megaloblastic anemia is clearly established, the clinical significance of preanemic folate deficiency remains problematic. Early reports involving mainly retrospective approaches correlated various parameters (elevated formiminoglutamic acid excretion after a test dose of histidine, megaloblastic erythropoiesis, and low serum or erythrocyte folate levels) in nonanemic patients with a variety of pregnancy complications including abruptio placentae and other antepartum bleeding, spontaneous abortion, fetal malformation, and preeclampsia. Other studies, however, have failed to indicate a relationship between folate deficiency and any of these complications of reproduction. Thus, the role of folate deficiency in the causation of pregnancy wastage is controversial. However, the preponderance of opinion appears to suggest that folate deficiency is probably not associated with any complication other than maternal anemia. The fetus seems to be a highly efficient parasite for folate, just as it is for iron, and infants born to women with megaloblastic anemia of pregnancy typically have normal hemoglobin indexes.

SUPPLEMENTATION

In view of evidence summarized above indicating substantially increased folacin needs during pregnancy, coupled with dietary survey data suggesting that usual diets are marginal in folate content, some authorities advocate entire folacin supplementation of all pregnant women. Others question this practice on the basis of cost–benefit consideration. Without question, folacin supplements will prevent megaloblastic anemia in a pregnant population, but the occurrence of this complication, at least among middle and upper socioeconomic classes in developed nations, is quite unusual. Thus, routine supplementation to such populations generally have been without demonstrable effect, although some increase in birth weight has been noted in developing nations.[16]

The maternal serum folate level normally declines during gestation, an effect minimized by folacin supplements. Whether the maintenance of vitamin levels in the serum is a desirable end in itself is controversial. Moreover, as summarized previously, the clinical significance of preanemic folate deficiency is open to question. For these reasons, opinion is divided on the question of routine folacin supplementation, with one point of view advocating it in all patients and the other reserving it for those in whom dietary history reveals the likelihood of inadequate intake, those with multiple pregnancy or chronic hemolytic anemia, or those taking anticonvulsant drugs. Certainly if vitamins are to be given at all, there is more reason to supplement folate than any other. However, it should be kept in mind that prescription of folacin, or for that matter of any other vitamin supplement, is but a minor part of efforts to improve maternal nutrition. It is more important to recognize inappropriate dietary habits and to assist the patient in correcting them.

The recommended level of supplementation is 400 μg/day, although supplemental preparations designed for use in pregnancy typically contain somewhat higher levels (*e.g.,* 1 mg).

WATER-SOLUBLE VITAMINS

The blood levels of water soluble vitamins generally decline during pregnancy. Thus, an increased proportion of pregnant women will exhibit low or deficient values when judged by standards for nonpregnant women. Whether these findings represent actual deficiency states or whether they reflect normal physiologic adjustments (*e.g.,* increasing plasma volume) is uncertain. In support of the latter point of view are findings that supplementation does not usually alter blood vitamin levels in pregnant women. A second generalization applicable to water-soluble vitamins is that fetal levels regularly exceed those in the mother, often by a factor of two or three, presumably reflecting active transport across the placenta. To provide for fetal transfer, some degree of increased maternal intake is obviously needed.

ASCORBIC ACID

Maternal plasma ascorbic acid levels generally decline by about one half during the course of pregnancy, and cord levels are usually twice maternal levels. Little is known about the possible clinical significance of these findings, although associations of vitamin C deficiency with premature rupture of the membranes and preeclampsia have been suggested in individual (and unconfirmed) reports.

The RDA for vitamin C during pregnancy is increased by 20 mg from the 60-mg allowance for the nonpregnant adult woman.

Vitamin C in greatly excessive doses possesses a theoretical potential for fetal damage. Certain anecdotal reports in the human, and a single animal study, suggest that this practice might lead to scurvy in the infant some time after birth, presumably as a result of over-stimulation of metabolic systems by long-term high maternal levels magnified by a placental concentrating capacity throughout intrauterine life.

VITAMIN B$_6$

It has long been recognized that pregnancy is associated with laboratory findings that, at least in the nonpregnant woman, are considered as evidence of vitamin B$_6$ deficiency. Urinary xanthurenic acid excretion following a test dose of tryptophan—the classic laboratory test for B$_6$ deficiency—increases progressively throughout gestation and by term is 15 times that in nonpregnant women. Similarly, blood levels of the vitamin fall progressively during pregnancy. Supplementation with pyridoxine in amounts of 6 mg/day to 10 mg/day is associated with normalization of both blood levels and xanthurenic acid excretion.[10,29]

Whether these changes actually reflect a deficiency state or merely represent normal physiologic adjustments is controversial. From a review of published data, Rose and Braidman suggest that the modification of tryptophan metabolism in pregnancy is due primarily to estrogenic stimulation of corticosteroid production with resultant increased levels of tryptophan oxygenase. Late in pregnancy, however, these same authors feel that a true deficiency state is superimposed, presumably owing to fetal uptake of the vitamin.

A number of clinical correlates potentially related to vitamin B_6 in pregnancy have been raised. Hypertensive disorders of pregnancy have been noted to be associated with elevated xanthurenic acid excretion, low placental pyridoxine values, and low pyridoxal phosphate levels in maternal and cord blood.[6] These observations notwithstanding, vitamin B_6 deficiency is not widely believed to be the cause of toxemia of pregnancy. A prospective double-blind trial failed to identify any difference in outcome with pyridoxine supplementation.

Considerable interest has centered recently on a possible association with gestational diabetes mellitus. Xanthurenic acid inactivates insulin *in vitro*, and if a similar effect occurs *in vivo*, pyridoxine treatment might correct impaired carbohydrate tolerance. Beneficial effects of pyridoxine, usually given in pharmacologic doses of 100 mg/day to 200 mg/day, have been reported in some, but not all, studies.[11,34,43]

Among other suggested clinical correlates of vitamin B_6 deficiency during gestation are maternal dental caries and atherosclerosis development in the offspring. By contrast, pyridoxine supplements did not prevent postpartum depression.

The clinical significance of these observations on vitamin B_6 metabolism in pregnancy (both normal and abnormal) is far from clear. Although the laboratory data suggest a deficiency state, it is rather difficult on intuitive grounds alone to accept that dietary inadequacy of any nutrient could be both so widespread and yet lacking in clear-cut clinical correlations. Current dietary allowances appear to reflect this uncertainty. For example, the RDA for vitamin B_6 is 2 mg/day for adults and 0.5 mg/day additionally for pregnancy, an amount far below that necessary to "normalize" biochemical studies in the pregnant woman. Presumably this means that the biochemical "aberrations" are viewed as normal physiology rather than indicators of deficiency. In view of evidence that vitamin B_6 requirements seem to be increased with high-protein diets, there is probably some reason for a modest increase in B_6 intake in pregnancy.

OTHERS

Studies of urinary excretion of thiamin, blood thiamin levels, and erythrocyte transketolase activity all indicate that thiamin requirements increase with gestation.[19] The RDA is increased by 0.4 mg during pregnancy.

A decrease in urinary excretion of riboflavin and increasing erythrocyte glutathione reductase activation test results during pregnancy are considered as indicating increased riboflavin needs. The RDA is increased by 0.3 mg during gestation.

Little is known of niacin needs in pregnancy. However, since requirements for this nutrient relate closely to energy intake, an additional allowance of 2 niacin equivalents is recommended during gestation to account for the increased caloric intake of the gravida.

Increased vitamin B_{12} is needed in pregnancy to provide for fetal transfer and to support increased maternal erythropoiesis. The RDA is increased by 1 μg during gestation.

Blood levels and urinary excretion of pantothenic acid have been observed to be low in pregnant teenagers consuming an average daily intake of 4.7 mg, leading to the recommendation that 5 mg/day to 10 mg/day be provided in supplemental form.[12]

FAT-SOLUBLE VITAMINS

Blood levels of fat-soluble vitamins generally tend to increase during gestation in accordance with the hyperlipemic tendency of pregnancy. In the case of vitamin A, an increase in mid-pregnancy and a decline near term have been described but other factors such as season, age, parity, and social class seem to influence vitamin A nutriture as well.[17] The RDA for vitamin A during pregnancy is increased by 200 retinol equivalents (1000 IU).

The placental permeability of vitamin A is limited, and cord blood levels typically are less than maternal. Nevertheless, the possibility of fetal toxicity with overdosage exists, as evidenced by several reports of fetal malformation with maternal ingestions of 10 or more times the RDA.[4,44]

CALCIUM AND VITAMIN D

REQUIREMENTS

Calcium metabolism during pregnancy and the perinatal period has recently been reviewed in detail.[35] Almost all of the additional calcium required during pregnancy involves that used by the fetus. The term fetus contains an average of 27.4 g calcium, the placenta variable amounts up to 1 g, and the augmented maternal tissue and fluids approximately 1 g, so the total pregnancy requirement, in round numbers, is 30 g. Since most of this need occurs in late pregnancy coincident with calcification of the fetal skeleton, the daily increment averages 300 mg during the third trimester. Attempts to estimate requirements by calcium-balance studies have yielded somewhat higher levels of retention than would be anticipated on the basis of a total accumulation of 30 g. This discrepancy may simply reflect the notorious difficulties in performing precise balance studies, or it may result from storage in the maternal skeleton. The evidence from animal experiments regarding maternal calcium storage during pregnancy is conflicting but seems to favor the hypothesis that some storage in excess of fetal needs occurs, an event reasonable teleologically in anticipation of the greatly increased requirements of lactation.

The current RDA for calcium in pregnancy is 1200 mg, an increase of 400 mg over the allowance for the nonpregnant adult. This would seem to provide adequate amounts, particularly considering the adaptive ability to increase absorption and decrease excretion at times of need, as during pregnancy. Because it is virtually impossible to meet these requirements with natural foods other than dairy products (see Appendix Table A-26), milk is considered by many to be highly desirable for the pregnant woman. The 1200-mg/day allowance for pregnancy is precisely that contained in 1 quart of milk. Individuals who do not consume milk or milk products will require calcium supplementation.

The importance of vitamin D in calcium metabolism has long been recognized. It facilitates calcium absorption and also plays a regulatory role in bone metabolism. Balance studies have documented its important role in promoting positive calcium balance in the pregnant woman. At least one of its metabolites, 25-hydroxyvitamin D, crosses the placenta quite freely. For all of these reasons, vitamin D needs seem to be increased during gestation. The RDA for vitamin D is increased by 5 ng (200 IU) in the pregnant woman.

METABOLISM

Calcium absorption increases during pregnancy, and urinary excretion tends to fall. The serum concentration of total calcium declines in parallel with the fall in serum albumin, but the ionic level falls only slightly, maintained at the lower end of the normal range by increasing output of maternal parathyroid hormone.[37]

Calcium ions are actively transported from mother to fetus against a concentration gradient, and the resultant relative hypercalcemia in the fetus is thought to suppress fetal parathyroid hormone and increase fetal calcitonin, producing a situation favoring fetal bone growth.

Maternal blood levels of 25-hydroxyvitamin D appear to be influenced by a number of variables, particularly diet and exposure to ultraviolet light, but probably not by pregnancy *per se*. Recent evidence indicates, however, that levels of the more active metabolite, 1,25-dihydroxyvitamin D, are increased substantially during gestation.[23,45] Whereas fetal levels of 25-hydroxyvitamin D correlate closely with maternal values, levels of the 1,25-metabolite are low in the fetus, presumably reflecting poor placental transfer and a lack of the renal enzyme 1-hydroxylase.

CLINICAL IMPLICATIONS

A possible relationship between calcium and leg cramps in pregnancy aroused considerable interest several years ago in the hypothesis that cramps result from a relative hypocalcemia owing to dietary phosphate ingestion. According to this theory, leg cramps could be prevented or relieved by several measures, singly or in combination, including curtailment of milk intake (since milk contains relatively large amounts of phosphate), supplementation with nonphosphate salts of calcium, and regular ingestion of aluminum hydroxide antacids (to form insoluble aluminum phosphate salts in the gut). Although some studies appeared to confirm this theory, others failed to find a correlation between leg cramps and ingestion of dairy products or any type of calcium supplement. Thus, the relationship between milk, calcium, phosphate, and leg cramps remains controversial.

Several recent studies have suggested a possible relationship between maternal deficiency of calcium or (particularly) vitamin D intake and the complication of early neonatal hypocalcemia. Lower serum calcium levels during the first two days of life have been associated with deficient maternal milk and vitamin D intake and lack of exposure to sunlight.[5] A seasonal distribution of neonatal hypocalcemia, with peak incidence when late pregnancy coincides with times of least sunlight, has been described.[39] Vitamin D and at least one of its active metabolites (25-hydroxyvitamin D) apparently cross the placenta freely, producing similar levels in mother and fetus, and low levels are found in at least some hypocalcemic infants. An implication of these observations is that maternal vitamin D deficiency may be an etiologic factor in some cases of neonatal hypocalcemia.

SODIUM

METABOLISM

Sodium metabolism in pregnancy has recently been reviewed in detail by Lindheimer and Katz and by Lindberg.[27,28] Glomerular filtration increases by as much as 50% in early pregnancy and is maintained at this level until term, resulting in an additional filtered sodium load of 5,000 mEq/day to 10,000 mEq/day. Additional natriuretic effects result from progesterone and posture. Changes of this magnitude quite clearly require a compensatory mechanism to promote tubular reabsorption and to preserve maternal homeostasis. The nature of these compensatory mechanisms is not entirely clear, but a major one appears to be increased activity of the renin-angiotensin-aldosterone system. Plasma renin activity is substantially elevated during normal pregnancy, as is renin substrate. As a result, large amounts of angiotensin are formed. However, the pressor effect of angiotensin in normal pregnancy is markedly attenuated, apparently because of inactivation in the maternal plasma, and its principal physiologic effect appears to be stimulation of aldosterone, which in turn promotes sodium reabsorption to prevent sodium loss.

EDEMA

Edema is one of the signs of preeclampsia, and abundant evidence indicates that the preeclamptic patient retains sodium abnormally. It is also seen in a large proportion of otherwise normal patients. This benign edema of normal pregnancy usually occurs late in gestation and may be either generalized or dependent in distribution. The cause of the generalized form is obscure, but among the possibilities are alterations in ground substance under estrogen influence, decrease in plasma osmotic pressure owing to hypoalbuminemia, and an overcompensation of the physiologic mechanisms promoting sodium retention. Dependent edema, on the other hand, is most likely due to mechanical causes such as obstruction of the pelvic veins by the enlarging uterus.

CLINICAL IMPLICATIONS

Few topics in obstetrics excite as much interest and controversy as that of the relationship between sodium and toxemia. According to the older and more traditional view, pregnancy is characterized by insidious sodium retention, which increases vascular reactivity and may lead to arteriolar vasospasm with resultant development of preeclampsia. An obvious implication of this reasoning is that sodium intake should be restricted and diuretics used freely to promote sodium excretion. The more modern theory, based on evidence that pregnancy resembles a salt-wasting state, holds that inadequate sodium intake in the face of excessive losses leads to hypovolemia and in turn to compensatory vasospasm.[28] According to this theory, sodium intake should be increased in pregnancy.

Which of the two views is correct cannot be determined with certainty. However, it does seem clear that no convincing rationale supports a compelling indication for sodium restriction in normal pregnancy. On the other hand, it must be acknowledged that sodium restriction has been practiced widely and there is no overwhelming clinical evidence of its harm. In view of this uncertainty, the most reasonable course at present seems to be to neither restrict nor increase sodium intake, to advise patients to salt their foods to taste, and to rely on the physiologic mechanisms at the renal tubular level to ensure that sodium balance is maintained.

With respect to agents that promote sodium excretion, the evidence is considerably clearer. Thiazide diuretics, in spite of early suggestions to the contrary, are of no benefit in prevention of preeclampsia. Maternal complications with thiazide treatment include electrolyte imbalance, hyperglycemia, hyperuricemia, and pancreatitis, and perinatal complications include hyponatremia and thrombocytopenia. Therefore, since they do no good and may do harm, they have no place in normal pregnancy.

TRACE ELEMENTS

Trace elements are involved in a number of biochemical processes. However, relatively little is known of their role in reproduction. Zinc is of special interest because of the teratogenic influence of zinc deficiency in animals and perhaps in humans. Zinc levels in plasma and hair decline during gestation.[18] The RDA for zinc is increased by 5 mg for the pregnant woman.

Because iodine deficiency goiter is more frequent in women than in men, in order to provide for placental transfer, the RDA for iodine is increased by 25 mg for the pregnant woman, an amount provided amply by iodization of salt.

Plasma copper levels are consistently elevated during gestation, presumably reflecting estrogen-induced ceruloplasmin synthesis.[18]

SUMMARY

Pregnancy is characterized by increased needs for nearly all nutrients. Energy requirements increase by approximately 300 Cal/day, representing an addition of 15% to nonpregnant needs. Caloric intake should be sufficient to support a weight gain of 0.35 kg/wk to 0.4 kg/week through the last two thirds of pregnancy. An additional 30 g protein/day appears advisable. Iron is a unique nutrient in that the amounts required during pregnancy are greater than those that can be provided by diet. Thus, for practical purposes every pregnant woman should receive iron supplements. Folate supplementation is considered optional, and prescription of other vitamins and minerals is probably neither helpful nor harmful. Sodium represents an essential nutrient, and there is no valid reason for its restriction in normal pregnancy.

Nutritional Support During Lactation

Throughout nearly all of history, nutrition of the human infant has depended entirely on breast-feeding. Beginning a half century or so ago, coincident with the development of infant formulas, the frequency of breast-feeding declined markedly in developed nations. This pervasive trend seems to have been reversed over the past decade, and current data indicate that half or more of newborn infants in the U.S. are fed, partially or completely, human milk. The return to widespread breast-feeding is particularly prevalent among members of the upper social and educational strata, precisely those classes that initiated the trend away from the practice two generations earlier. It is motivated by both physiologic and psychological benefits known or presumed to accompany breast-feeding.

In view of the importance of lactation in human biology, both historically and in contemporary society, nutritional support of the process continues to be a major concern.[15]

ENERGY

The additional energy requirements of lactation are proportional to the quantity of milk produced. Since human breast milk has a caloric content of approximately 70 Cal/100 ml and the efficiency of conversion of maternal energy to milk energy is at least 80%, approximately 90 Cal is required for production of 100 ml milk. Thus, 850 ml milk, a reasonable approximation of the average amount produced each day during established lactation, requires nearly 800 Cal.

The current RDA for energy in the lactating reference woman is 500 Cal in addition to the basic allowance. During pregnancy, an average of 3 kg fat are stored, and this may be mobilized postpartum to provide an additional 300 Cal/day for 3 months. Energy intake should be increased above 500 Cal/day if lactation continues beyond 3 months, if maternal weight is below the ideal weight for height, if pregnancy weight gain was less than 12 kg, or if more than one infant is being nursed.

The amount and source of energy intake have some influence on milk composition. With caloric restriction, the fatty acid composition of human milk resembles that of depot fat, reflecting mobilization of fat stores. Increased energy intake as carbohydrate results in increased levels of lauric

and myristic acids, whereas a diet high in polyunsaturated fat content yields milk with increased levels of polyunsaturated fats.

PROTEIN

The protein content of human milk tends to decline during the course of lactation; a reasonable average value is 1 g/dl. Thus, assuming an efficiency of conversion of dietary protein to milk protein of 70% and an average daily production of 850 ml, the amount needed in the maternal diet approximates 12 g/day. The RDA of 20 g additional protein during lactation provides for individual variation.

Protein levels in milk do not appear to be reduced by a maternal diet low in protein or poor in biologic quality. However, recent data suggest that the content of two essential amino acids, lysine and methionine, are lower in milk from women with diets deficient in protein, which may imply a reduction in nutritional quality.

CALCIUM

Calcium output in milk amounts to an average of 250 mg/day to 300 mg/day. The current RDA for calcium in lactation is 1200 mg/day, which represents an increase of 400 mg over the nonpregnant, nonlactating allowance. Considering the adaptive ability to increase absorption and decrease urinary excretion at times of need, this should represent an adequate amount unless milk production is extraordinarily high.

The calcium content of milk appears to be maintained in spite of markedly deficient intake, a phenomenon probably related to the availability of a relatively huge reservoir of calcium stored in the skeleton. Recent studies using the technique of scanning transmission suggest that lactating women mobilize approximately 2% of skeletal calcium over 100 days of nursing.

VITAMINS

Levels of water-soluble vitamins in milk generally correlate closely with blood levels, which in turn reflect dietary intake. Thus, it is possible to influence milk composition by maternal diet. Ingestion of large doses of water-soluble vitamins, as occurs with supplements, produces transient, but significant, elevation in milk levels. At the other extreme, deficient maternal intake can result in deficiencies in the infant, as evidenced by reports of beriberi in infants nursed by women with the disease.

By contrast, the amounts of the fat-soluble vitamins A, D, and E in milk are independent of blood levels and thus unrelated to dietary intake. Although levels of vitamins A and E in human milk are appreciable, the vitamin D content is low, and rickets has been observed occasionally in breast-fed infants. Vitamin D sulfate, a water-soluble form, has been demonstrated recently in appreciable quantities in human milk, but its biologic significance is not yet clear, and most authorities advocate vitamin D supplementation of the breast-fed infant.[24]

OTHER NUTRIENTS

Concentrations of trace elements in human milk are generally low and are unrelated to maternal intake. Iron supplementation of all puerperal women, whether lactating or not, is advised for 2 months to 3 months postpartum in order to replenish maternal stores depleted during pregnancy. Although iron saturation of lactoferrin *in vitro* seems to decrease the antimicrobial properties of this milk constituent, clinical studies have not indicated that any such adverse effect accompanies maternal supplementation. Since maternal iron administration does not influence milk iron levels, many pediatricians advocate routine iron supplementation of the breast-fed infant as well, in order to prevent the otherwise common occurrence of iron deficiency anemia during infancy.

Fluoride levels in milk are unrelated to maternal intake and, in order to provide protection against dental caries, some authorities advocate fluoride supplementation of the infant consuming only breast milk.

The sodium content of human milk correlates quite closely to maternal sodium intake.

SUMMARY

Whereas severe and chronic maternal malnutrition can adversely affect lactation performance, quantitative and qualitative aspects of milk production seem to be maintained surprisingly well across a relatively wide range of maternal diets. Certain parameters of lactation, such as quantity and protein and calcium content, appear to be relatively independent of maternal nutritional status. Others, such as amino acid, fatty acid, and water-soluble vitamin composition, may vary with maternal intake.

Compared with the nonpregnant woman, the nursing mother should have substantially more energy, protein, and calcium, as well as modest increases of most other nutrients. She should receive nutritional counseling using the guidelines provided by the Recommended Dietary Allowances. Maternal iron supplementation is advisable, and

vitamin supplements are a reasonable option. The breast-fed infant should receive supplemental iron, vitamin D, and perhaps fluoride.

Nutritional Support During Hormonal Therapy

Considerable recent interest has centered on the nutritional implications of treatment with sex steroid hormones. This interest is based on the widespread use of oral contraceptives coupled with evidence, principally of a biochemical nature, suggesting that needs for certain nutrients appear to be altered by ingestion of these agents. Oral contraceptives typically consist of a combination of a synthetic estrogen (ethinyl estradiol or mestranol) and any of several synthetic progestogens. Generally, metabolism in women taking oral contraceptives is similar in many respects to that in pregnant women. There are, however, some differences in both degree and kind of change observed.

The effects of oral contraceptives on vitamin and mineral needs and on laboratory tests have recently been reviewed.[31,48] Almost all published observations relate to oral contraceptives, and the extent to which they apply to natural hormones (such as estrogen treatment of the postmenopausal woman) is conjectural.

VITAMIN B₆

Increased urinary xanthurenic acid excretion after a test dose of tryptophan, the classic laboratory finding of vitamin B_6 deficiency, is consistently observed in women taking oral contraceptives, an effect apparently related to the estrogenic component, since it occurs in men taking estrogen. As noted previously, similar effects are found in normal pregnancy, but the level of B_6 supplementation required to normalize the results is greater in oral contraceptive users than in gravid women. For example, supplements of 30 mg pyridoxine hydrochloride (25 mg vitamin B_6) are necessary to consistently suppress xanthurenic acid excretion in patients taking oral contraceptives compared with 10 mg pyridoxine hydrochloride (8.2 mg vitamin B_6) in pregnant women. These values represent 12 times and 4 times, respectively, the RDA for vitamin B_6 in the nonpregnant adult female.

Although the association of rather marked metabolic changes in various indexes of vitamin B_6 metabolism in oral contraceptive users has been documented, the current thinking seems to be that these effects are of doubtful clinical significance.[7,26] A possible exception is the relation with mental depression. In a recent report of 22 depressed women taking oral contraceptives, half exhibited biochemical evidence of B$_6$ deficiency, and all of these responded to supplemental pyridoxine given in a double-blind, cross-over study design.[1]

Although some authorities have advocated routine pyridoxine supplementation of oral contraceptive users, the question remains controversial. At the present time, however, it at least seems reasonable to consider B$_6$ deficiency in the differential diagnosis of patients taking estrogen who exhibit depression.

FOLACIN

A number of investigations have found low serum or erythrocyte folate levels, in up to 50% of oral contraceptive users, but at least an equal number of studies have not found any such association. Even when serum levels are low, the more important erythrocyte values seem to be unaffected.

Folate-responsive megaloblastic anemia has been reported in occasional patients taking oral contraceptives, but the incidence appears to be quite low. Again, the question of routine supplementation is controversial, with some authorities advocating it and others regarding it as unnecessary.[38]

The basis for any change in folate metabolism during oral contraceptive administration is thought to be reduced absorption by interference with absorption of the polyglutamates, the principal food form of folate. However, the concept of folate malabsorption is not accepted by all authorities.

OTHER NUTRIENTS

Several observations suggest that vitamin C needs may be higher in oral contraceptive users. Estrogen appears to increase the rate of ascorbic acid breakdown, apparently by raising levels of ceruloplasmin, a known catalyst of ascorbic acid oxidation. Plasma, platelet, and leukocyte levels of ascorbic acid are lower in patients taking oral contraceptives than in normal pregnant and nonpregnant women.

Low serum vitamin B$_{12}$ levels have been found in approximately half of women taking oral contraceptives. However, Schilling tests and methylmalonate excretion have been reported to be normal, and the effect appears to reflect lowered binding-protein levels, so it seems doubtful that a deficiency state is responsible. At the very least, however, serum B$_{12}$ levels in oral contraceptive users need to be interpreted with caution.

Biochemical findings suggesting mild deficiencies of thiamin and riboflavin have been described in oral contraceptive users; their significance is uncertain.

Serum iron levels and iron-binding capacity are increased moderately in oral contraceptive users, effects apparently related to the progestational component. Menstrual bleeding is reduced in both duration and quantity with oral contraceptives, suggesting that iron requirements may be somewhat lower than in normal nonpregnant women. Absorption of iron, copper, and zinc do not seem to be affected by hormonal contraceptives.[22]

SUMMARY

Treatment with sex steroid hormones induces metabolic changes suggesting increased needs for several nutrients, particularly vitamin B$_6$ and folate. The significance of these observations is unclear at present. Hopefully, the situation will be clarified with further study.

References

1. Adams PW, Rose DP, Folkard J et al: Effect of pyridoxine hydrochloride (vitamin B$_6$) upon depression associated with oral contraception. Lancet 1:897, 1973
2. Anderson GD: Nutrition in pregnancy—1978. South Med J 72:1304, 1979
3. Bergner L, Susser MW: Low birth weight and prenatal nutrition: An interpretive review. Pediatrics 46:946, 1970
4. Bernhardt IR, Dorsey DJ: Hypervitaminosis A and congenital renal anomalies in a human infant. Obstet Gynecol 43:750, 1974
5. Brooke OG, Brown IRF, Bone CDM et al: Vitamin D supplements in pregnant Asian women: Effects on calcium status and fetal growth. Br Med J 1:751, 1980
6. Brophy MH, Siiteri PK: Pyridoxal phosphate and hypertensive disorders of pregnancy. Am J Obstet Gynecol 121:1075, 1975
7. Brown RR, Rose DP, Leklem JE et al: Urinary 4-pyridoxic acid, plasma pyridoxal phosphate, and erythrocyte aminotransferase levels in oral contraceptive users receiving controlled intakes of vitamin B$_6$. Am J Clin Nutr 28:10, 1975
8. Chesley LC: Weight changes and water balance in normal and toxic pregnancy. Am J Obstet Gynecol 48:565, 1944
9. Churchill JA, Berendes HW: Intelligence of children whose mothers had acetonuria during pregnancy. In Perinatal Factors Affecting Human Development. Washington DC, Pan American Health Organization, 185:30–35, 1969
10. Cleary RE, Lumeng L, Li T–K: Maternal and fetal plasma levels of pyridoxal phosphate at term: Adequacy of vitamin B$_6$ supplementation during pregnancy. Am J Obstet Gynecol 121:25, 1975
11. Coelingh Bennick HJT, Schreurs WHP: Improvement of oral glucose tolerance in gestational diabetes by pyridoxine. Br Med J 3:13, 1975
12. Cohenour SH, Calloway DH: Blood, urine, and dietary pantothenic acid levels of pregnant teenagers. Am J Clin Nutr 25:512, 1972
13. DeLeeuw NKM, Lowenstein L, Hsieh Y: Iron deficiency and hydremia in normal pregnancy. Medicine 45:291, 1966

14. Eastman NJ, Jackson E: Weight relationships in pregnancy. I. The bearing of maternal weight gain and prepregnancy weight on birth weight in full term pregnancies. Obstet Gynecol Surv 23:1002, 1968

15. Filer LJ: Maternal nutrition in lactation. Clin Perinatol 2:353, 1975

16. Fletcher J, Garr A, Fellingham FR et al: The value of folic acid supplements in pregnancy. Br J Obstet Gynaecol 78:781, 1971

17. Gal I, Parkinson CE: Effects of nutrition and other factors on pregnant women's serum vitamin A levels. Am J Clin Nutr 27:688, 1974

18. Hambidge KM, Droegemueller W: Changes in plasma and hair concentrations of zinc, copper, chromium, and manganese during pregnancy. Obstet Gynecol Surv 44:666, 1974

19. Heller S, Salkeld RM, Korner WF: Vitamin B_1 status in pregnancy. Am J Clin Nutr 27:1221, 1974

20. Hytten FE, Leitch I: The Physiology of Human Pregnancy, 2nd ed. Oxford, Blackwell Scientific, 1971

21. Kelly AM, MacDonald DJ, McDougall AN: Observations on maternal and fetal ferritin concentrations at term. Br J Obstet Gynaecol 85:338, 1978

22. King JC, Raynolds WL, Margen S: Absorption of stable isotopes of iron, copper, and zinc during oral contraceptive use. Am J Clin Nutr 31:1198, 1978

23. Kumar R, Cohen WR, Silva P et al: Elevated 1,25-dihydroxyvitamin D plasma levels in normal human pregnancy and lactation. J Clin Invest 63:342, 1979

24. Lakdawala DR, Widdowson EM: Vitamin D in human milk. Lancet 1:167, 1977

25. Lechtig A, Habicht JP, Delgago H et al: Effect of food supplementation during pregnancy on birth weight. Pediatrics 56:508, 1975

26. Leklem JE, Linkswiler HM, Brown RR et al: Metabolism of methionine in oral contraceptive users and control women receiving controlled intakes of vitamin B_6. Am J Clin Nutr 30:1122, 1977

27. Lindberg BS: Salt, diuretics, and pregnancy. Gynecol Obstet Invest 10:145, 1979

28. Lindheimer MD, Katz AI: Sodium and diuretics in pregnancy. N Engl J Med 288:891, 1973

29. Lumeng L, Cleary RE, Wagner R et al: Adequacy of vitamin B_6 supplementation during pregnancy: A prospective study. Am J Clin Nutr 29:1376, 1976

30. Maternal Nutrition and the Course of Pregnancy: Summary Report. Washington DC, Committee on Maternal Nutrition, Food and Nutrition Board, National Academy of Sciences, 1970

31. Miale JB, Kent JW: The effects of oral contraceptives on the results of laboratory tests. Am J Obstet Gynecol 120:264, 1974

32. Niswander K, Jackson EC: Physical characteristics of the gravida and their association with birth weight and perinatal death. Am J Obstet Gynecol 119:306, 1974

33. Osofsky HJ: Relationships between nutrition during pregnancy and subsequent infant and child development. Obstet Gynecol Surv 30:227, 1975

34. Perkins RP: Failure of pyridoxine to improve glucose tolerance in gestational diabetes mellitus. Obstet Gynecol 50:370, 1977

35. Pitkin RM: Calcium metabolism in pregnancy: A review. Am J Obstet Gynecol 121:724, 1975

36. Pitkin RM, Kaminetzky HA, Newton M et al: Maternal nutrition: A selective review of clinical topics. Obstet Gynecol 40:773, 1972

37. Pitkin RM, Reynolds WA, Williams GA et al: Calcium metabolism in pregnancy: A longitudinal study. Am J Obstet Gynecol 133:781, 1979

38. Pritchard JA: Anemias complicating pregnancy and the puerperium. In: Maternal Nutrition and the Course of Pregnancy, pp 74–109. Committee on Maternal Nutrition, Food and Nutrition Board, National Academy of Sciences. Washington, DC, 1970

39. Roberts SA, Cohen MD, Forfar JO: Antenatal factors associated with neonatal hypocalcaemic convulsions. Lancet 2:809, 1973

40. Rosso P, Luke B: The influence of maternal weight gain on the incidence of fetal growth retardation. Am J Clin Nutr 31:696, 1978

41. Rush D, Stein Z, Susser H: A randomized controlled trial of prenatal nutritional supplementation in New York City. Pediatrics 65:683, 1980

42. Simpson JW, Lawless RW, Mitchell AC: Responsibility of the obstetrician to the fetus: II. Influence of prepregnancy weight and pregnancy weight gain on birthweight. Obstet Gynecol 45:481, 1975

43. Spellacy WN, Buhi WC, Birk SA: Vitamin B_6 treatment of gestational diabetes mellitus. Studies of blood glucose and plasma insulin. Am J Obstet Gynecol 127:599, 1977

44. Stange L, Carlstrom K, Eriksson M: Hypervitaminosis A in early human pregnancy and malformations of the central nervous system. Acta Obstet Gynecol Scand 57:289, 1978

45. Steichen JJ, Tsang RC, Gratton TL et al: Vitamin D homeostasis in the perinatal period: 1,25-dihydroxyvitamin D in maternal, cord, and neonatal blood. N Engl J Med 302:315, 1980

46. Stein Z, Susser M, Rush D: Prenatal nutrition and birth weight: Experiments and quasi-experiments in the past decade. J Reprod Med 21:287, 1978

47. Taylor DJ, Lind T: Haematological changes during normal pregnancy: Iron induced macrocytosis. Br J Obstet Gynaecol 83:760, 1976

48. Theurer RC: Effect of oral contraceptive agents on vitamin and mineral needs: A review. J Reprod Med 8:13, 1972

49. Winick M, Brasel JA, Velasio EG: Effects of prenatal nutrition upon pregnancy risk. Clin Obstet Gynecol 16:172, 1973

50. Zlatnik FJ: Dietary protein and human pregnancy performance. J Reprod Med 22:193, 1979

30
Ophthalmology

Edward K. Wong, Jr.
Irving H. Leopold
Michael T. Nakamura

The importance of nutrition to the visual system has been documented by an accumulation of clinical and laboratory reports. It is the purpose of this chapter to delineate nutritional aspects of ophthalmologic practice and to describe recent research trends in this field.

Various deficiency states may result in localized or generalized pathologic changes in the eye. A summary of the etiologic role of some commonly accepted deficiency states follows:

1. Conjunctiva
   Vitamin A—Xerosis: loss of goblet cells, Bitot's spots, and pigmentatary changes
   Pyridoxine—"Conjunctivitis"
   Vitamin C—Subconjunctival hemorrhages
2. Cornea
   Vitamin A—Localized changes due to drying
   Riboflavin—Circumcorneal vascularization
   Vitamin D—Band keratopathy in hypercalcemia
3. Vitreous
   Vitamin C—Vitreous hemorrhages
4. Retina
   Vitamin A—Punctate changes and nyctalopia
   Thiamin—Maculopathy
   Niacin, nicotinic acid, and nicotinamide—Maculopathy
   Vitamin B_{12}—Nerve fiber hemorhages and nerve fiber infarcts
   Vitamin E—Maculopathy
   Zinc—Retinitis pigmentosa?
5. Optic Nerve
   Thiamin—Optic neuropathy
   Niacin (nicotinic acid) and nicotinamide—Optic neuropathy

Vitamin B_{12}—Optic neuropathy
Zinc—Optic neuropathy?

Vitamin Deficient States

VITAMIN A

Vitamin A deficiency causes a substitution of keratinizing cells for other epithelial cells. Specifically, the ocular changes consist of a metaplasia of the corneal and conjunctival epithelium, frequently followed by corneal infection. Vitamin A plays a role in the stabilization of lysosomal membranes and also in the synthesis of visual pigments.

Vitamin A (retinol), in the biosynthesis of the visual pigments, is oxidized to retinal, which is an active component of the photosensitive pigment in both rods and cones. Rhodopsin is composed of 11-*cis* retinal bound to the protein moiety (opsin). Light isomerizes the 11-*cis* retinal to an unstable all-*trans* retinal configuration, which is then released from the protein moiety (Fig. 30-1). This reaction is associated with the initiation of the visual impulse (Fig. 30-2).

Ocular manifestations of a vitamin A deficiency include the following: nyctalopia (night blindness), xerophthalmia (dry eyes), hyperkeratoses of hair follicles, and pigmentary changes of the conjunctiva.

NYCTALOPIA

Nyctalopia, or night blindness, is usually seen as a late symptom of vitamin A deficiency, and it is at-

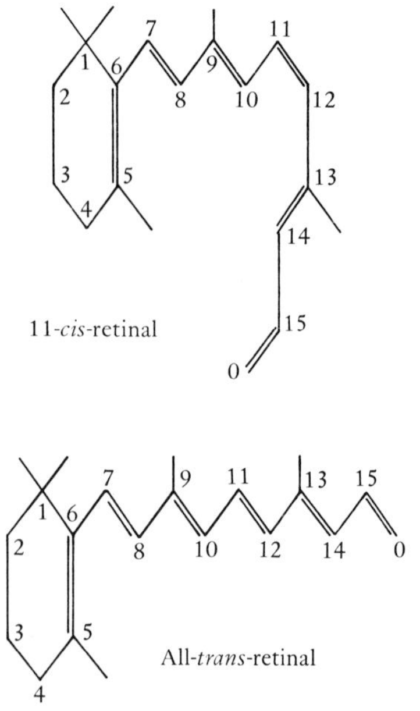

FIG. 30-1. Structures of 11-*cis*-retinal and all-*trans*-retinal.

tributed to the lack of rhodopsin in retinal rod cells. Frequently, vitamin A levels must be quite low before any visual symptoms are noted. Structural and functional changes can be found in the posterior pole. Rods are affected more than cones, and in severe deficiencies, disruption of the rod outer segments can be seen. Since primarily the rods are affected, night acuity is lost, but photopic or cone vision needed for central vision is essentially normal. Carter–Dawson and co-workers reported on regional differences in the rate of photoreceptor cell degeneration of rat retinas.[9] A central-peripheral gradient of photoreceptor cell degeneration was observed.

ELECTRORETINOGRAPHIC CHANGES

The electroretinogram (ERG) has been found to be completely extinguished when the vitamin A deficiency leads clinically to nyctalopia. The ERG is a technique for measuring retinal changes in electrical potential in response to a light stimulus (Fig. 30-3). The dark-adapted tracing (scotopic ERG) represents rod functioning. As in other conditions that cause rod dysfunction, such as retinitis pigmentosa, there is a dampening or extinction of the ERG tracing. In cases diagnosed early, this symptom has been reported to respond quite well to oral doses of vitamin A, whereas advanced cases may remain refractory to treatment. In patients with abetalipoproteinemia, the electroretinographic

changes may be reversed with high doses of vitamin A. There are few encouraging studies available concerning the therapy of retinitis pigmentosa.[8] Chatzinoff and colleagues reported no benefit from therapy with 11-*cis* retinal vitamin A after a double-blind study.[10] Rodger suggests that in retinitis pigmentosa vitamin A appears to delay the shrinkage of the visual field until middle age.[39]

The role of vitamin A in retinal diseases is confusing, but it is well known that vitamin A deficiency causes retinal outer segment dysfunction, possibly due to a decrease in visual pigments. Animal studies have shown anatomic disruption of outer segments in the macular and peripheral retinal in monkeys after vitamin A (and E) deficient diets.

Night blindness may be the result of a congenital or hereditary process and can be seen in the pigmentary degenerative diseases. Dietary deficiencies and liver and intestinal diseases may all be associated with a form of night blindness. Hepatic disease, such as cirrhosis, can alter the retinol transport by damaging the endoplasmic reticulum, thus disrupting its ability to synthesize retinol-binding protein (RBP).

Diseases of the pancreas and hyperparathyroidism may also account for a relative vitamin A deficiency in retinal receptors. Patients with gastrointestinal (GI) problems, for example, sprue, liver disease, and cystic fibrosis of the pancreas, have been described with nyctalopia, probably secondary to poor vitamin A absorption. A dietary deficiency of zinc may also limit the amount of zinc metalloenzyme (NADP retinoldehydrogenase), thereby preventing the conversion of retinol to retinal.

Night blindness has been described in the third trimester of pregnancy; this symptom disappeared postpartum.

ANTERIOR SEGMENT CHANGES

Xerophthalmia and Bitot's spots have long been considered pathognomonic for decreased vitamin A levels. Studies have shown that xerosis can occur in association with nyctalopia as a manifestation of the deficiency state, but the symptom of nutritional xerosis *per se* is more frequently a manifestation of multiple factors.[37] Sullivan and co-workers demonstrated the return of conjunctival goblet cells in alcoholics with dry eye syndrome after treatment with oral vitamin A.[43] In contrast, Sommer and co-workers did not believe the return of mucus-producing goblet cells explained the corneal lesion improvement he observed with vitamin A.[42] The reappearance of the goblet cells lagged long after the corneal improvement was observed.

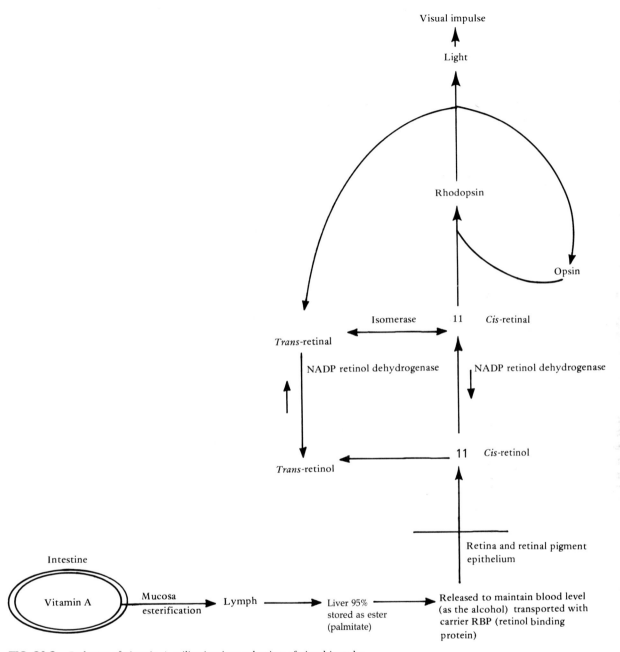

FIG. 30-2. Pathway of vitamin A utilization in production of visual impulse

Although Bitot's spots have similarly been found to be a manifestation of a poor nutritional state that may have little relationship to vitamin A levels, some investigators feel that in infants the presence of the foamy white conjunctival changes is diagnostic of vitamin A deficiency.

Vitamin A deficiency during the neonatal period has been found to be associated with choroidal colobomata, retinal folds, and vitreous fibroplasia in rabbits. Lamba reported a case of congenital microphthalmos and colombomata associated with maternal vitamin A deficiency in humans.[29]

THERAPEUTIC USES

It has been suggested that in patients deficient in vitamin A, one large dose of vitamin A may be employed (200,000 IU, or 60 mg, retinyl palmitate

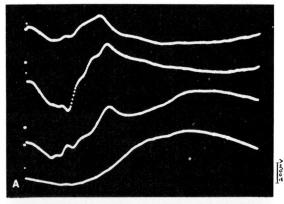

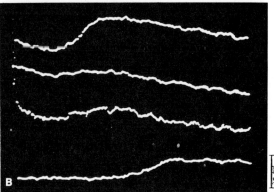

FIG. 30-3. Electroretinograms. (*A*) Normal. (*B*) Nearly extinguished. The four traces in each set show averaged responses to four different stimulus conditions: *Upper trace*—white stimuli, photopic adaptation state; *second trace*—white stimuli, scotopic adaptation state; *third trace*—red stimuli, scotopic adaptation state; and *bottom trace*—blue stimuli, scotopic adaptation state. Duration of each trace is 128 msec. The traces in *B* are shown at 16 times higher amplification than those in *A*. Amplitudes of β-waves were normal in *A*, ranging between 150 and 350 μv. These amplitudes in *B* were between 2 and 10 μv; the photopic response (*upper traces*) was about 10% of normal, and the scotopic responses (*other traces*) were about 1% of normal.

in oil). However, studies have shown that in situations where protein deficiency has existed, vitamin A serum levels are difficult to maintain. This is attributed to a deficit of the retinol-binding proteins and is manifested as a 1-day to 4-day delay in clinical response to exogenous vitamin A treatment. The topical application of 0.1% retinoic acid in conjunction with systemic vitamin A has been suggested to expedite corneal healing in xerophthalmia. Topical retinoic acid, unlike retinyl palmitate, does not require prior deesterification and may not require conjugation with specific carrier proteins.

Many other uncontrolled studies in the literature report topical use of vitamin A for superficial cor-

neal diseases. It has been reported that vitamin A speeds healing time and helps to reduce scar density. Beneficial effects on the healing of corneal abrasions and in the treatment of herpetic lesions of the cornea have also been reported. Schmidtke, however, concluded that therapy with topical vitamin A is of dubious value.[41] Nelkin and Nelkin reported a significant degree of inhibition of corneal neovascularization in a controlled experiment using vitamin A palmitate in rabbits.[35]

B VITAMINS

The B-complex vitamins are a group of water-soluble factors that are nutritionally interrelated. The administration of one component of the B complex may cause the depletion of other B factors. Since the precise etiologies of many ostensible deficiency states are uncertain, therapy with all B-complex factors will allow for the most satisfactory results. Some authors, for instance, believe that peripheral neuritis is due to thiamin deficiency, while others believe that a lack of riboflavin is responsible. Heffley and Williams share the latter view.[27] In their study on galactose-induced cataracts in rats they suggest that therapy should not be limited to the use of one agent (*e.g.*, just a vitamin) when dealing with a putative dietary deficiency.

Nutritional amblyopia demonstrates the classic syndrome of blurred visual acuity with a central or centrocecal scotoma. The exact etiology remains unknown; however, B-complex factors have been implicated, with particular emphasis placed on thiamin and riboflavin.

The *nutritional amblyopia* is believed by some to be manifested as the visual changes obtained in pernicious anemia and tobacco–alcohol amblyopia. In 1969, Foulds, Chisholm, and co-workers stated that the optic neuropathy of tobacco–alcohol amblyopia is the same as that of pernicious anemia.[19,20] Since then, additional theories concerning the etiology have included the detoxification of cyanide in optic nerve tissue. Ayanru reported on the tropical amblyopia syndrome observed in Nigerians living on a diet of cassava, which is a source of cyanide.[3] Foulds and colleagues also described two patients with pernicious anemia who developed optic neuropathy while undergoing therapy with cyanocobalamin and did not improve until placed on hydroxycobalamin therapy.[20] Therapy of this syndrome should be with the hydroxycobalamin form of vitamin B$_{12}$.

The B-complex factors have been suggested as therapy for some of the toxic amblyopias, but few studies are available on the therapy of these conditions. Thiamin is reportedly of no value in altering the severity of tryparsamide amblyopia.

THIAMIN DEFICIENCY

Beriberi. The ocular symptoms of beriberi can be divided into three categories: (1) conjunctival and corneal changes, (2) optic nerve involvement, and (3) ocular muscle paresis.

Animal studies have demonstrated conjunctival changes characterized by dryness and anemia. In humans, few references have been made to corneal epithelial changes. In 1946, Bloom and colleagues described in American war prisoners nutritional amblyopia characterized by central or centrocecal scotomata and later pallor of the optic nerve head resulting in defective vision.[6] Maculae were normal in the majority of cases. With thiamin treatment in the early stages, the syndrome was relieved. Asregadoo made the observation that a thiamin deficiency disease may cause atrophy of endocrine glands and hypertrophy of the adrenals.[2] An increase of endogenous corticosteroids may occur, which can have the pharmacologic effect of increasing the intraocular pressure. In his study, Asregadoo observed a correlation between chronic open angle glaucoma and decreased serum levels of thiamin.

Wernicke's encephalopathy. This syndrome is characterized by delirium, stupor, ataxia, and external ophthalmoplegia. This condition is seen not only in the severely deprived but in alcoholics as well, resulting from an insufficient dietary intake of thiamin. Pathologic focal areas of hemorrhage and gliosis can be found in the brain stem. Nystagmus may be a presenting symptom. Dramatic improvement in ocular motility has been observed hours after a small dose of thiamin, and less dramatic improvement was seen in ataxia and mental changes.

Retinopathy. The usual pathologic findings in beriberi are effusions of the pericardium, pleura, and peritoneum. It has been suggested that a central retinitis with serous changes could also be caused by thiamin deficiency. Therapy of serious retinopathy has been suggested, but controlled studies are lacking.

Hoyt reported that two patients placed on carbohydrate-restricted diets for several months developed optic nerve dysfunction related to an accompanying insufficiency of thiamin consumption.[28]

NIACIN DEFICIENCY

Pellagra. Classically, the symptoms of pellagra include diarrhea, dermatitis, and dementia. However, it is not absolutely clear, in humans, whether the pellagra syndrome is due to a single deficiency or to a combination of factors (see Chap. 12).

Pellagra is not an extremely rare condition and many of the patients are alcoholics.

Reports of ocular involvement with retrobulbar neuritis are quite similar to retrobulbar neuritis cases of other nutritional etiologies.[33]

Mather studied 61 cases of pellagra and described a maculopathy with loss of normal yellow reflex in about 50% and frank pigment migration in 32%.[32] Some improvement was seen following therapy in cases diagnosed early.

Nicotinic acid and nicotinamide. Nicotinic acid and nicotinamide are necessary for the formation of several coenzymes used in tissue metabolism. These cofactors are vital to many enzyme systems. One of these, the alcohol dehydrogenase system, is required in the early steps of rhodopsin synthesis, and therefore a deficiency of these substances could, theoretically, be expected to give symptoms of nyctalopia.

Harris reported a case of development of a paracentral scotoma in an individual taking 6000 mg nicotinic acid/day.[25] The scotoma disappeared on discontinuing the drug.

Systemic nicotinic acid may accelerate the rate of corneal healing and may cause a decrease in corneal scar density.

Nicotinic acid will cause a vasodilatation of certain blood vessels of the skin associated with flushing and a burning sensation. As a vasodilator, its use has been advocated by some in central retinal vascular occlusion resulting from spasm. Balucco–Gabriel reported "noticeable" retinal vascular dilatation using a combination of nicotinic acid, *m*-inositol, and callicrein systemically.[4]

Macular degenerative changes from a variety of causes have been treated with a varied number of vitamin and vasodilating agent combinations. Very few of the studies on these agents are controlled and interpretation of the results is difficult.

Riboflavin. Riboflavin deficiency is felt to be relatively common in humans (see Chap. 12). Classically, a cheilosis or fissuring of the skin of the angle of the mouth is seen. Ocular manifestations of the deficiency state include conjunctival irritation with the development of circumcorneal vascularization. Abnormal pigmentation of the iris may also be seen. Rosacea keratitis appears to be clinically quite similar to riboflavin deficiency. Conflicting reports are available on the efficacy of therapy of rosacea keratitis with riboflavin. There are reports that suggest regression of corneal neovascularization from nutritional deficiency with B-complex therapy.

Pyridoxine B_6. The signs of pyridoxine deficiency include a seborrheic dermatitis, conjunctivitis, a pellagra-like dermatitis, and a polyneuritis (see Chap. 12). In adults, deficiencies are rarely due to insufficient diet, but rather result from use of such drugs as hydralazine, isoniazide, and penicillamine. In patients with Wilson's disease, the optic neuritis observed is thought to be secondary to the administration of penicillamine and its subsequent antagonism of pyridoxine.

Experimental animals raised on a B_6-deficient diet were noted to have a high incidence of angular blepharoconjunctivitis that was responsive to therapy with pyridoxine.

VITAMIN B_{12}

Pale conjunctiva is a general manifestation of an anemic state. Severe anemia *per se* can present with the interesting ophthalmic finding of papilledema, similar to that seen after acute blood loss and in microcytic anemias. It is felt that the severe anemia causes anoxia with edema sufficient to raise intracranial pressure.

The megaloblastic anemia associated with vitamin B_{12} deficiency has several inconstant ocular findings. Flame-shaped hemorrhages are often seen in the nerve fiber layer in the posterior pole. These have also been described with white centers, the so-called Roth's spots. Their etiology is uncertain but may be related to the decreased number of defective platelets. The severe anemic states that develop can also produce a mild chronic retinal edema. The disc may appear pale, but this may be due to the anemia.

If hypotension is present, or if the anemia is severe enough, retinal anoxia can manifest itself as fluffy white, superficial, retinal exudates, the so-called cotton-wool spots. These are actually infarcts in the nerve fiber layer.

Vitamin B_{12} deficiency can cause retrobulbar neuritis that is virtually identical in clinical manifestation to that of tobacco–alcohol amblyopia.[19,20] The prognosis for visual recovery is said to be good if treatment is started early and optic atrophy is not present. As noted above, the best treatment of this condition is probably with hydroxycobalamin.

Suggestions have been made for the use of vitamin B_{12} in the treatment of retinoblastomas. These suggestions are based on reports of the use of vitamin B_{12} in the therapy of neuroblastomas. However, support has not been found for the use of B_{12} in either condition.

FOLIC ACID AND FOLINIC ACID

The therapy of ocular toxoplasmosis includes the use of the folic acid antagonist Daraprim. Oral doses of 10 mg to 15 mg folinic acid can be given every several days to prevent the symptoms of folic acid deficiency. The rationale for this therapy is that humans can utilize the folinic acid, whereas the Toxoplasma organisms cannot.

VITAMIN C

Scurvy is a disease characterized predominantly by hemorrhagic manifestations, such as perifollicular hemorrhages, petechiae, ecchymoses, bleeding gums, and bone pain with subperiosteal hemorrhages. The ocular changes are similarly centered about hemorrhagic changes. Lid ecchymoses, subconjunctival, vitreous, and retinal hemorrhages, proptosis secondary to orbital bleeding, and gaze palsies with subdural hematomas are findings seen with vitamin C deficiency. Scurvy frequently appears with anemia and a mild degree of scleral icterus. The anemia may be due to a frequently associated folate deficiency or to blood loss.

Nyctalopia has, as well, been associated with scurvy. This is probably secondary to an accompanying vitamin A deficiency.

Vitamin C has been suggested as playing a role in such conditions as recurrent vitreous hemorrhages, retinal hemorrhages in diabetes, and cataracts. Little support has been found for these suggestions.

In normal individuals the vitamin C content of the aqueous humor is ten times that of serum. It is felt that the ciliary body is the source of this ascorbate level. The exact physio-pharmacologic role of vitamin C in the eye has yet to be elucidated.

Goldberg has suggested that a high concentration of ascorbic acid in the anterior chamber of guinea pigs may be accompanied by significantly more sickling of hemoglobin sickle cell erythrocytes.[22] This increase may possibly result in the further reduction of vascular perfusion to the ocular tissue. Since acetazolamide raises the concentration of aqueous humor ascorbate, it should be used with discretion when treating hyphema and secondary glaucoma caused by sickled cells.

Attempts have been made to treat glaucoma with vitamin C. It has been given by intravenous (IV) infusion by itself in the form of 20% sodium ascorbate, and in combination with other osmotic agents. Studies have shown that it is an effective osmotic agent for decreasing intraocular pressure. Vitamin C has also been administered orally as a 20% solution in high doses (0.5 g/kg body weight in one dose), and indeed, a significant decrease in intraocular pressure was recorded.[44] Most of the patients were reported to tolerate the dose easily after the first several days of diarrhea, nausea, and vomiting had passed.

Linner obtained an average decrease of 2 mm Hg in ocular pressure after the daily administration of 2 g vitamin C orally.[31] There was no change in the outflow facility, and the decrease in pressure was attributed to a decrease in the rate of aqueous formation. Fishbein and Goodstein showed that oral doses of 4.5 g to 5 g vitamin C/day did not significantly alter the control of the intraocular pressure in patients already on maximal medical glaucoma therapy.[18]

Gnadinger and co-workers applied topically a 10% solution of ascorbic acid over 3 days, and noted no significant changes in ocular outflow or tension.[21] Esila and colleagues noted no change in pressure in normal rabbit eyes after subconjunctival ascorbate.[16]

It has been stated that scurvy causes poor wound healing due to defective collagen formation. Parenteral ascorbate was administered to rabbits in which perilimbal alkali burning reduced aqueous humor ascorbate levels one half to one third normal. Aqueous humor ascorbate levels were elevated and breaking wound strength was enhanced when compared to controls. The National Eye Institute is supporting a clinical trial of vitamin C in treating severe, caustic eye burns. Twelve clinical centers are studying ascorbic acid versus a placebo over a 3-year period.[24a,37a]

An additional use of vitamin C is to acidify the urine and to increase the rate of excretion of such drugs as chloroquine after retinal toxic doses.

VITAMIN D

A discussion of the pathophysiology of vitamin D can be found in other sections (see Chap. 3). Past literature suggests that there may be some improvement in keratoconus with vitamin D therapy.

Calcification of Bowman's membrane of the cornea, the so-called band keratopathy (see Fig. 30-4) has been noted, with most conditions associated with an increase in serum calcium, including hypervitaminosis D.

VITAMIN E

Tocopherol is an antioxidant system protecting the unsaturated bonds of unstable lipoprotein membranes from lipid peroxidation. The result of peroxidative cleavage would be the destruction of cell structure and function accompanied by the release of cellular enzymes capable of damaging the surrounding tissues.

Ocular manifestations resulting from a dietary deficiency of vitamin E have long been in question. Several animal studies involving diurnal and nocturnal animals have shown neurologic and macular changes.

Multiple ocular changes have been observed in vitamin E deficient adult rats presenting with keratoconus, paralysis, progressive exophthalmos, opacification and neovascularization of the cornea, and iridocyclitis with formation of secondary cataracts.

It has been suggested that alpha-tocopherol ace-

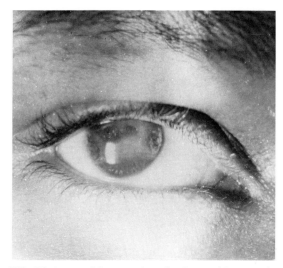

FIG. 30-4. Band keratopathy. The dense white near the limbus represents calcium deposition in Bowman's layer of the cornea.

tate may decrease the incidence of retrolental fibroplasia. Research suggests that excessive oxygen therapy is not solely responsible for retrolental fibroplasia, and renewed interest is being focused on a 1949 study that suggested that vitamin E is effective in treating retrolental fibroplasia.[36] Vitamin E may be capable of reducing the severity of neovascularization of the retina and vitreous humor.

The National Eye Institute is presently conducting a study with premature infants treated with alpha-tocopherol in an attempt to reduce the incidence and severity of retrolental fibroplasia.[23] Robison and colleagues suggest that normal levels of vitamin E serve to protect the photoreceptor membrane from oxidation damage and retard the accumulation of their remnants and other products of lipid breakdown in the pigment epithelium.[38]

DeHoff and co-workers found no effect on the progression of diabetic retinopathy using oral alpha-tocopherol acetate.[12] However, Trevithick hypothesizes that vitamin E may be able to reduce precataractous formation of globules resulting from increased blood glucose levels.[24] In rats in which diabetes was chemically induced, treatment with 35 times the normal dietary level of vitamin E resulted in no cataract formations. Devi and colleagues studied the metabolism of nucleic acid and protein in cataracts of rabbits on diets deficient in vitamin E and demonstrated that DNA polymerase activity is increased.[15]

Hayes showed that in monkeys a deficiency of vitamin E can result in retinal damage similar to that caused by vitamin A deprivation.[26] The hypothesis is forwarded that vitamin E may protect the retina from peroxidase destruction.

Bunce and Hess have demonstrated a relationship between a deficiency of tryptophan and vitamin E in the maternal diet and the formation in infant rats of a central nuclear opacity involving the embryonal protein at the center of the lens.[7]

Calories, Protein and Minerals, Carbohydrates, and Fats

Much has been written in recent years on the etiology, natural history, and therapy of diabetic retinopathy (see Chap. 18). It has been suggested that a decrease in serum lipids in a diabetic patient may be associated with a decrease in retinal exudates.

Yeung and Harris described an animal model that suggests that fatty material and cholesterol may pass through the retina into the subretinal space from the vitreous cavity.[49]

Meyerson and Schneider followed 13 patients with diabetic retinopathy who were treated with low-fat diets; no definite trends were noted in the course of the diabetic retinopathy.[33] Adnitt and colleagues, in a prospective study, showed that the progression of retinopathy appeared to be unrelated to mean blood sugar levels.[1]

Galactosemia is a disease caused by deficiency of galactose 1-phosphate uridyl transferase. The accumulation of dulcitol in the lens can cause cataracts. A quite similar picture can arise from a galactokinase deficiency. Monteleone reports that early dietary galactose control has prevented the appearance of cataracts in a newborn galactokinase-deficient homozygote.[34]

PROTEINS

As mentioned throughout the text, vitamin deficiency can be the result of poor absorption or transport, as a reflection of protein deficiency. Ocular involvement is one of the most common and serious complications of protein–calorie malnutrition in young children. These are largely due to concomitant vitamin A deficiency. Several inborn errors of metabolism with amino-aciduria-related diseases have ocular features as part of the symptomatology. In cystinosis, crystals of cystine may be found in the conjunctiva and sometimes in the cornea. Cataracts have been recorded in nearly half of the cases of Toni-Fanconi syndrome.

MINERALS

Few definite relationships have been shown between mineral metabolism and ocular findings. A zonular cataract has been reported with the hypocalcemia of tetany. Waldbott reported optic neuritis associated with possible fluoride toxicity.[46]

DeRosa reported trophic changes associated with a deep and superficial vascularization in magnesium-deficient rats.[14]

ZINC

In 1977, Bastek and colleagues studied trace metals in a family with sex-linked retinitis pigmentosa.[5] In their study they used six controls, five carriers, and five patients with clinically definite retinitis pigmentosa. They studied ERG, EOG, dark adaptation, and visual fields for the diagnostic workup. In fasting early morning samples plasma zinc levels were found to be significantly higher (p < 0.05, t-test) in the carrier group than in either the control group or the retinitis pigmentosa group. The ratios of plasma zinc to copper in the latter group were significantly lower than those in the carrier group or in the control group (p < 0.01, t-test).

The interest in zinc and copper in studying tapetal-retinal degeneration is based on numerous animal experiments. In 1963 Vogel and Kaiser examined the tapetum lucidum in the beagle after giving high doses of ethambutol.[45] A single dose of 1600 mg/kg resulted in the loss of the brilliant purple blue color of the tapetum lucidum within 2 hr to 3 hr; at 5 hr the tapetum was achromatic. By the seventh day, with no further drugs, the animal had complete return of color and brilliance. In 1966 Buyske and colleagues showed that ethambutol administered to laboratory animals resulted in a drop in zinc concentration within the eye and other organs of the body.[8] In 1971 Figueroa and co-workers measured zinc in the tapetum lucidum of the dog eye after ethambutol administration and found lowered zinc content.[17] A control study was done using dithizone, a known potent chelator of zinc. This also resulted in decoloration and a drop in tapetal zinc content. A return of the tapetal coloration paralleled the return of zinc to normal levels.

In 1978 Leopold proposed an association between various types of optic neuropathy and low zinc levels.[30] He hypothesized that toxic optic neuropathies are due to a long list of various drugs, many of which are metal chelators. Some of these medications include the following: diodoquin, ethambutol, penicillamine, isoniazid, nialamide, isocarboxazid, and iproniazid. In 1975 Saraux reported on 40 patients with optic neuritis.[40] He measured serum levels of zinc and found that of 11 patients with lower than normal levels 7 had tobacco–alcohol optic nerutitis, 3 had optic neuropathy associated with isoniazid and ethambutol, and 1 exhibited disulfiram optic neuritis. Delacoux and colleagues in 1978 studied tuberculosis patients before and after ethambutol treatment.[13] Twelve of 72 patients developed visual dysfunction during therapy. The data suggest a correlation between plasma zinc levels before therapy and the incidence of visual dysfunction following ethambutol. Patients with pretreatment plasma zinc levels greater than 95 μg/dl sustained no damage, while all patients with less than 70 μg/dl developed visual dysfunction.

In 1980 our laboratory first reported the significant association (p < 0.0001) between low levels of plasma zinc and multiple sclerosis (MS), a major cause of demyelination of the optic nerve. We have repeated this study, and with new groups of controls and new groups of patients with MS, the results are similarly convincing.[47,48] If these early attempts at understanding the role of trace metals in optic neuropathy prove fruitful, we may soon have a better understanding of the pathophysiology of optic neuritis and optic neuropathy. A possible mechanism may be the dysfunction in a zinc-dependent enzyme system responsible for the maintenance of normal myelin. Future studies will test the soundness of this hypothesis.

References

1. Adnitt PI, Taylor E: Progression of diabetic retinopathy: Relationship to blood sugar. Lancet 1:652–654, 1970
2. Asregadoo E: Blood levels of thiamine and ascorbic acid in chronic open-angle glaucoma. Ann Ophthalmol 11:1095–1100, 1979
3. Ayanru J: The tropical amblyopia syndrome (or tropical nutritional amblyopia) in the Mid-western state of Nigeria. Afr J Med Med Sci 5:41–48, 1976
4. Balacco–Gabrieli C: Preliminary note on the action of nicotinic acid, *m*-inositol, and callicrein on retinal vessels of normal young people. Arch Otorhinolaryngol 68:385–388, 1964
5. Bastek J, Bogden J, Cinotti A, et al: Trace metals in a family with sex-linked retinitis pigmentosa. Adv Exp Med Biol 77:43–50, 1977
6. Bloom SM, Merz EH, Taylor WW: Nutritional amblyopia in American prisoners of war liberated from the Japanese. Am J Ophthalmol 29:1248–1257, 1946
7. Bunce G, Hess J: Lenticular opacities in young rats as a consequence of maternal diets low in tryptophan and/or vitamin E. J Nutr 106, No. 2:222–9, February, 1976
8. Buyske DA, Sterling W, Peets E: Pharmacological and biochemical studies on ethambutol in laboratory animals. Ann NY Acad Sci 135:711, 1966
9. Carter–Dawson L, Kuwabara T, O'Brien PJ et al: Structural and biochemical changes in vitamin A deficient rat retinas. Invest Ophthalmol Vis Sci 18:437–446, May, 1979
10. Chatzinoff A, Nelson E, Stahl N et al: Eleven-*cis* vitamin A in treatment of retinitis pigmentosa. Arch Ophthalmol 80:417–419, 1968
11. Cirrhosis, abnormal dark adaptation and vitamin A. Nutr Rev 37, No. 3:73–75, March, 1979
12. DeHoff JB, Ozazewski J: Alpha tocopherol to treat diabetic retinopathy. Am J Ophthalmol 37:581–582, 1954
13. Delacoux E, Moreau Y, Godefroy A et al: Prévention de la toxicité oculaire de l'ethambutol: Interêt de la zincémie et de l'analyse du sens chromatique. J Fr Ophthalmol 1, No. 3:191–196, 1978
14. DeRosa L, DeConcilius U: Ocular changes during the course of magnesium-free diet. Arch Otorhinolaryngol 67:313–317, 1963
15. Devi A, Raina PL, Singh A: Abnormal protein and nucleic acid metabolism as a cause of cataract formation induced by nutritional deficiency in rabbits. Br J Ophthalmol 49:271–275, 1965
16. Esila R, Tenhunen T, Tuovenen E: The effect of ascorbic acid on the intraocular pressure and the aqueous humor of the rabbit eye. Acta Ophthalmol 44:631–636,1966
17. Figueroa R, Weiss H, Smith, JCJ, et al: The effect of ethambutol on the ocular zinc concentration in dogs. Am Rev Respair Dis 104:592, 1971
18. Fishbein SL, Goodstein S: The pressure lowering effect of ascorbic acid. Ann Ophthalmol 4:487–491, 1972
19. Foulds W, Chisholm IA, Bronte–Steward J et al: Vitamin B_{12} absorption in tobacco amblyopia. Br J Ophthalmol 53:393–397, 1969
20. Foulds WS, Chisholm IA, Stewart JB et al: The optic neuropathy of pernicious anemia. Arch Ophthalmol 82:427–432, 1969
21. Gnadinger M, Willome J: The influence of topically applied ascorbinic acid on the normal intraocular tension. Klin Monatsbl Augenheilkd 153:352–356,1968
22. Goldberg M: Sickled erythrocytes, hyphema, and secondary glaucoma. Ophthalmic Surg 10:70–77, 1979
23. Gunby P: Trial of vitamin E therapy for retrolental fibroplasia. JAMA 243:1021, 1980
24. Gundi P: Another use for Vitamin E. JAMA 243:1025, 1980
24a.Gundi P: Vitamin C may enhance healing of caustic corneal burns. JAMA 243:623, 1980
25. Harris JL: Toxic amblyopia associated with administration of nicotinic acid. Am J Ophthalmol 55:133–134, 1963
26. Hayes KC: Retinal degeneration in monkeys induced by deficiencies of vitamin E or A. Invest Ophthalmol Vis Sci 13:499–510, 1974
27. Heffley J, Williams R: The nutritional teamwork approach: Prevention and regression of cataracts in rats. Proc Natl Acad Sci USA 71:4164–4168, 1974
28. Hoyt CS: Low carbohydrate diet optic neuropathy. Med J Aust 1:65–66, 1979
29. Lamba PA, Sood NN: Congenital microphthalmos and colobomata in maternal vitamin A deficiency. J Pediatr Ophthalmol Strabismus 5:115–117, 1968
30. Leopold IH: Zinc deficiency and visual impairment. Am J Ophthalmol V85:871, 1978
31. Linner E: The pressure lowering effect of ascorbic acid in ocular hypertension. Acta Ophthalmol 47:685–689, 1969
32. Mather SP: Maculopathy in pellagra. Br J Ophthalmol 53:350–351, 1969
33. Meyerson L, Schneider T: Diabetic retinopathy: Its treatment with a low fat diet; a classification. Med Proc 9:452–459, 1963
34. Monteleone JA, Beutler E, Monteleone DL: Cataracts. galactosuria, and hypergalactosemia due to galactokinase deficiency in a child. Am J Med 50:403–405, 1971
35. Nelken E, Nelken D: Inhibition of corneal neovasculariziation by vitamin B palmitate. Isr J Med Sci 1:243, 1965

36. Owens WC, Owens EU: Retrolental fibroplasia in premature infants II. Studies on the prophylaxis of the disease: The use of alpha tocopherol acetate. Am J Ophthalmol 32:1631, 1949

37. Pirie A: Effect of vitamin A deficiency on the cornea. Trans Ophthalmol Soc UK 98:357–360, 1978

37a. Pfister RR, Hays SA, Paterson CA: The influence of parenteral ascorbate on the strength of corneal wounds. Invest Ophthalmol Vis Sci 21:80–86, 1981

38. Robison WG, Kuwabara T, Bier J: Vitamin deficiency and the retina: Photoreceptor and pigment epithelial changes. Invest Ophthalmol Vis Sci 18:683–690, 1979

39. Rodger FC: Further study of the relation of vitamin A to retinal degeneration. Trans Ophthalmol Soc UK 98:128–133, 1978

40. Saraux H, Bechetoille A, Nour B et al: La baisse du taux du zinc sérique dans certaines névrites optiques toxiques. Ann d'oculist. Paris 208 No 1: 29–31, 1975

41. Schmidtke RL: Hypovitaminosis A in ophthalmology. Arch Ophthalmol 37:653–667, 1947

42. Sommer A, Emran N, Tamba T: Vitamin A-responsive punctate keratopathy in xerophthalmia. Am J Ophthalmol 87:330–333, 1979

43. Sullivan WR, McCulley JP, Dohlman CH: Return of goblet cells after vitamin A therapy in xerosis of the conjunctiva. Am J Ophthalmol 75:720–725, 1973

44. Virno M, Bucci MG, Pecori–Giraldi J et al: Oral treatment of glaucoma with vitamin C. Eye Ear Nose Throat Monthly 46:1502–1508, 1967

45. Vogel AW, Kaiser JA: Ethambutol-induced transient change and reconstitution in vivo of the tapetum lucidum color in the dog. Exp Mol Pathol 2 (Suppl 2): 136, 1963

46. Waldbott GL: Fluoride and optic neuritis. Br Med J 5414:945, 1964

47. Wong EK, et al: Zinc tolerance test in multiple sclerosis. *In preparation*

48. Wong EK, Enomoto H, Leopold IH et al: Plasma zinc levels in multiple sclerosis. Med and Ped Ophthalmol 4:3–8, 1980

49. Yeung JW, Harris G: Coat's disease: A study of cholesterol transport in the eye. Can J Ophthalmol 11:61–68, 1978

31
Oral Health

James H. Shaw
Edward A. Sweeney

The mouth, its component structures, and their diseases are of special interest in any thorough discussion of nutrition. The mouth is the normal point of entry of all food and drink into the body, the sensory zone where the unpleasant and uncomfortable are detected for rejection and the pleasurable and wholesome are savored, and the buffer zone where the particle size is reduced by mastication, food is blended with saliva, and its temperature is moderated so that an appropriate bolus can be swallowed comfortably. Any condition that causes discomfort or otherwise interferes with the oral handling of food has the potential to cause changes in food choices or the amount of food consumed and thereby to affect the nutritional status of the individual.

The several functions listed above require various specialized structures that are uniquely designed to fulfill their roles. For the purposes of this chapter, these structures will be grouped into three major headings: the soft tissues, the teeth, and the supporting tissues for the teeth. In each of these headings, the nature of the structures and the relation of nutrition to these structures and to their characteristic diseases will be described briefly. The emphasis will be placed in large part on the prevention of disease, with sufficient description of the etiology and the mechanisms involved in prevention to allow an understanding of the rationale. In addition, information will be included on the treatment of existing diseases of nutritional origin.

The reasons for emphasis on prevention are obvious in view of the 13.3 billion dollar cost of dental care in 1978 in the United States and the tragic realization that only about one third of the needs for dental care are being met.[24] This figure represents 7.9% of total health-care expenditures and a sizeable increase over the 10.02 billion dollars for 1977. In addition, for all practical purposes, treatment of all dental diseases, if they continue to occur at their present prevalence, seems to be impossible for the entire population from the standpoint of both economics and manpower. Of the two major disease problems in the mouth, it is clear that with the application of all available resources, dental caries could be essentially eliminated and the periodontal diseases materially reduced.

Application of preventive measures for both of these diseases requires a combination of optimally effective community action and strong personal motivation. Individuals need to be educated, not only about the "how" of prevention but also about the importance of prevention. The prevalent fatalistic attitude about the inevitability of oral diseases and tooth loss needs to be overcome so that the average person will want to maintain the natural dentition throughout life. Even the loss of the first permanent molar on the side of the mouth used preferentially for chewing causes a 33% reduction in masticatory efficiency.[59] It is important for everyone to recognize the functional inadequacy of even the best-designed and best-maintained prosthetic replacements. Ideal dentures at the time the patient becomes accustomed to them are only about 30% as efficient in mastication as the natural dentition.[54] This efficiency decreases further as the tissues supporting the dentures change with time.

517

Denture wearers have the tendency to be as negligent in having their dentures relined or replaced periodically as they were in practicing the oral hygiene that would have helped to retain their teeth. Denture wearers tend to avoid meats, raw vegetables, sandwiches, and salads.[60]

Soft Tissues

THE NORMAL TISSUES

The intraoral soft tissues are subjected to a variety of forces—thermal, chemical, and mechanical—and seem uniquely adapted to withstand a wide intensity of these forces.[19] In many ways these soft tissues are transitional tissue forms between the external dermal varieties and the internal gastrointestinal (GI) types. The transition begins at the opening into the GI tract where the vermilion border of the lips marks the loss of the thick keratinizing epithelium characteristic of skin and the beginning of a thin squamous epithelium, which allows the redness of subjacent blood vessels to show through. The lips are largely devoid of glands on their outer aspect, which explains their proneness to become dry. On their inner aspect, the lips and cheeks have a true nonkeratinizing mucosa with hundreds of minor salivary glands of the purely mucous type. These minor mucous glands are widely distributed throughout the oral mucosa and are simple glands, each opening directly to the mucosal surface. They provide upwards of 15% of the total secretions of the mouth and may be of special significance because their openings are in direct contact with the teeth's surfaces. The mucosa lines the entire oral cavity with the exception of a few areas where mechanical forces are highest and where a keratinizing epithelium provides the necessary protection. These areas are on the hard palate, the dorsum of the tongue, and the gingivae (gums), which surround the teeth. The metabolic activity of the mucosa is very rapid, with rapid cell division in the basal layer and sloughing of the external cells, resulting in a complete turnover in 3 days to 5 days.[12] The gingivae will be considered later, since these tissues and their subjacent supporting connecting tissue and bone are so intimately involved in the periodontal diseases.

The tongue is generally divided topographically into an anterior two thirds, the body, which is innervated by the lingual branch of the trigeminal nerve, and a posterior third, the base, which is innervated by the glossopharyngeal nerve. The anterior two thirds is covered by many fine papillae (filiform) composed of a connective tissue core and keratinized epithelium. At the apex of each papilla, the epithelium forms tufts. Fungiform papillae are found interspersed between the filiform papillae and

appear red because of a rich vascular bed. Their appearance becomes more marked when the filiform papillae are denuded or when the tongue becomes swollen due to disease or nutritional deficiency. Atrophy of the filiform papillae reveals the fungiform papillae, the red appearance of which gives the tongue the classic strawberry appearance.

The circumvallate papillae are found in the U-shaped demarcation between the anterior and posterior lingual segments. Each is surrounded by a moatlike depression into the base of which the secretion of small serous glands (Ebner's glands) is released. The inner walls of the moat contain numerous taste buds, each of which is comprised of a peeled orangelike arrangement of cells opening into the trough or oral cavity. While the majority of taste buds are found on the lateral walls of the foliate and circumvallate papillae and on the dorsal surfaces of the fungiform papillae of the tongue, some also have been found in the oropharynx, pharynx, and palate.

The secretions of the salivary glands—both major (parotid, submaxillary, and sublingual) and minor—moisten the oral environment. Saliva aids in mastication and deglutition, lubricates soft tissues as they move over each other and the teeth, and provides both inorganic ions, which facilitate remineralization of the teeth and reduce the potential for demineralization, and organic compounds, some of which are antimicrobial.

The major salivary glands are encapsulated paired secretory structures, and they provide most of the secretion that creates the moist environment, keeping the surfaces of the structure of the oral cavity healthy and lubricated. The secretions of the glands are predominantly of three kinds: serous, mucous, and mixed. The parotid glands represent the first type and the sublingual glands the second (a few serous acini are present). The submaxillary glands represent a mixed secretory type in which serous demilunes are found in association with mucous acini. The grapelike clusters of acini formed by either the serous or mucous cells drain into a series of ducts of increasing size and finally enter the oral cavity through a single excretory duct. The duct of the parotid glands exits in a papilla on the oral mucosa adjacent to the buccal surface of the maxillary first molar. The duct of the submaxillary gland usually joins with that of the sublingual and exits on the frenum of the tongue near the lingual surfaces of the lower incisor teeth.[51]

Abnormalities of Oral Soft Tissues

Abnormalities of nutrition affect the oral soft tissues in a variety of ways. Most deficiencies result in similar oral signs and symptoms such as pain, erythema, and atrophy of tissues with infection superimposed. Since oral tissues have remarkably rapid rates of turnover, in the order of 3 days to 5 days, it is not surprising that the first signs of nutritional deficiency frequently are in the oral cavity.[16] The cells of the lingual epithelium seem to be among the more rapidly dividing, and this structure is usually the first to be affected, with the commissural areas of the lips next, in terms of sequential onset of clinical signs.

In addition to the tongue, other oral signs of vitamin B-complex and iron deficiencies generally involve atrophic changes of the lips and mucosa due to a failure of cell replacement for the cells normally lost to cell turnover. Superimposed on this atrophy, especially at the corners of the mouth, is local infection of cracked epithelial surfaces by pyogenic microorganisms, resulting in scarring or granulomatous changes if prolonged (see Fig. 31-1).[50]

Changes of tongue architecture usually involve an initial loss of the filiform papillae, resulting in a pebbled appearance and a more intense red color than normal. Redness without overt infection is due to the loss or thinning of the keratinized cells on the tongue surface, which normally prevent the bright redness of the richly vascular lingual connective tissue from shining through. The tongue becomes redder to the degree of their loss. As filiform papillae are lost, the fungiform papillae can be seen more clearly and may be inflamed sufficiently to give the surface of the tongue the appearance of a strawberry. With more chronic deficiencies, the fungiform papillae are lost and a smooth red tongue with an atrophic epithelium results (see Fig. 31-2). Obviously, as taste buds are lost on the fungiform and foliate papillae, and probably elsewhere, aberrations of taste acuity can result owing to the loss of taste receptors. However, few experimental data have been reported on the effects of nutritional deficiency on taste acuity and our knowledge is largely anecdotal.

Little is known about the effect of nutrition on salivary glands in humans except for the reported swellings of the parotid gland associated with deficiencies of niacin, thiamin, and vitamin A.[7] Since these conditions are rarely found as pure deficiencies and usually occur as part of a generalized malnutrition, it is difficult to pinpoint specific associations. Parotid swellings have been reported, however, in almost epidemic proportion in groups of prisoners of war, in concentration camp inhabitants, and in kwashiorkor victims during the period of realimentation.[43] Similar findings have been reported in groups of alcoholics. It is unclear why these gland enlargements occur, but there may be an endocrine or neurologic basis.

Niacin deficiency seems to have the most widespread oral effect, since most oral tissues become

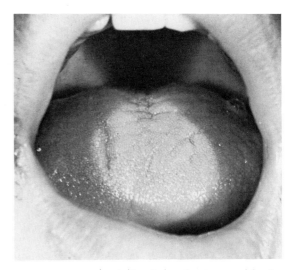

FIG. 31-1. Angular cheilitis due to vitamin B-complex deficiency. (Courtesy Dr. G. Shklar)

involved. The initial symptom is that of pain, described as a burning sensation throughout the oral cavity. The tongue then becomes reddened and swollen at the tip and lateral margins. This eventually progresses to involve the whole dorsal surface. Hyperemia persists while atrophic changes involving loss of the filiform and fungiform papillae eventually result in a smooth, shiny, bright red tongue. The oral mucosa in like manner becomes reddened, and the epithelium separates in some areas, leaving raw patches that are rapidly infected and covered with a fibrinous membrane. The gingivae also follow the same course, with loss of epithelium and with an infection that closely resem-

FIG. 31-2. Atrophic glossitis due to vitamin B-complex deficiency. (Courtesy of Dr. G. Shklar)

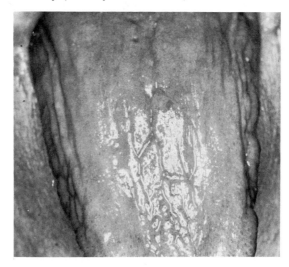

bles that found in acute necrotizing ulcerative gingivitis.[16] The commissures of the lips initially are pale and macerated, but fissuring occurs that radiates in a fanlike manner—outward on the skin and inward onto the buccal mucosa—and may leave permanent scars, even with replacement therapy.

In riboflavin deficiency, the cheilitis described for niacin is a prominent initial part of the clinical signs, as are changes seen on the tongue, where atrophy of the filiform papillae and swelling of the tongue emphasize the fungiform papillae, giving the tongue a granular appearance.[16] Vascular proliferation, dilitation, and perhaps stasis in some cases give the tongue a magenta color.

Pyridoxine deficiency has been described as producing a scalding pain of the tongue followed by a redness and swelling of the tip of the tongue and progressing through the various stages of atrophy to a smooth, somewhat purplish, tongue. The buccal mucosa is also reddened and may develop small, shallow ulcers, which have also been noted on the palate. Replacement therapy results in the rapid improvement of signs and symptoms except for the accompanying cheilitis, which may take 4 days to 5 days to improve.[53]

The oral signs seen in folic acid and B$_{12}$ deficiencies appear quite similar except that burning tongue pain may precede physical signs of B$_{12}$ deficiency. The tongue signs involve reddening of the tip with atrophy of the papillae and the formation of small ulcers. This progresses posteriorly, eventually leading to complete atrophy of the surface architecture of the tongue, giving a smooth, shiny appearance that may be red or pale, depending on the degree of anemia. Loss of epithelium affects the other tissues of the oral cavity in a like manner, producing painful ulcerations of the buccal mucosa and palatal and gingival epithelia, as well as cheilitis.

Iron deficiency produces changes similar to those of deficiencies of the B-complex group, but the prominent sign is pallor and swelling of the tongue, with some pain. The subsequent atrophic changes progress from a patchy denudation of papillae to a smooth, reddened tongue. It is interesting that the three predominant signs of pain, lingual papillary atrophy, and cheilitis were found together only about 15% of the time. Some suggestion that iron deficiency may impair pyridoxine metabolism is found in the fact that pyridoxine supplementation improved the lingual signs of iron deficiency.[28]

In summary, the oral signs of deficiencies of the B-complex vitamins and iron bear marked similarities and display a wide variation in the ways in which an individual may reflect any or all of the classical signs. Indeed, since single deficiencies of these vitamins are generally not seen, and since all

are involved in the regulation of cellular metabolism, it should not be surprising that multiple deficiencies might exist in the same individual or that the relatively greater lack of one vitamin might influence the expression of lack of others producing similar gross clinical appearances.

Since severe protein malnutrition interferes with normal cellular replacement and function and rarely occurs without multiple nutritional or vitamin deficiencies, the oral signs associated with protein deficiency resemble those previously described, among which atrophy of the epithelium with subsequent infection and ulceration are predominant.

Vitamin A deficiency has been described as affecting the oral mucosa, but the reports are at such odds that little credence can be placed on them. If there is any oral effect, it seems minimal and perhaps due to diminished salivary gland function.

Recently, reports have implicated low levels of zinc stores in dialysis patients, with aberrations of taste.[5] However, another recent double-blind study of zinc supplementation in some 106 patients with taste and smell dysfunctions due to a variety of causes did not indicate any clear benefit of zinc supplements.[25] More work is needed in this area to establish if specific subgroups of persons with these sensory dysfunctions might respond to zinc supplementation.

Teeth

COMPONENTS OF TEETH

The teeth are unique structures composed of four distinct tissues: enamel, dentin, cementum, and pulp (see Fig. 31-3).[10,20] The primary function of the teeth is to reduce the particle size of food while it is being blended with saliva, so that it can be swallowed comfortably. The teeth also contribute in important ways to an individual's appearance and to the ability to articulate sounds.

ENAMEL

The enamel, the hardest, densest, and most highly mineralized tissue of the body, is the superficial cap over each tooth and is the only part of the tooth in a disease-free mouth that is exposed to the microorganisms, saliva, and food residues in the oral environment. The physical and chemical characteristics of the enamel enable it to be relatively resistant to the physical and chemical stresses of the oral cavity and to be the first line of defense of the tooth against this difficult environment. The enamel is sufficiently hard and yet resilient enough to wear away sufficiently slowly during normal mastication to last throughout a lifetime, unless the

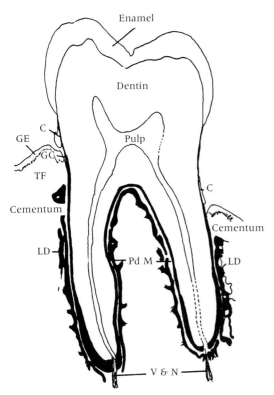

FIG. 31-3. Diagram of a mesiodistal section of a mandibular molar tooth. Normally the gingival epithelium (*GE*) is in close apposition to the neck of the tooth, and the crest of the gingiva is adjacent to the lower margin of the enamel. This case demonstrates formation of calculus (*C*) on the cementum with recession of the gingiva, interruption of the barrier maintained against microorganisms by the gingiva and the transverse fibers (*TF*), absorption of lamina dura (*LD*), and destruction of some of the periodontal membrane (*PdM*) in the fashion typical of periodontitis. *V* and *N*, vessels and nerves supplying the pulp. (Shaw JH: Nutrition in relation to dental medicine. In Goodhart RS, Shils ME, (eds): Modern Nurition in Health and Disease, 6th ed, Philadelphia, Lea & Febiger, 1980)

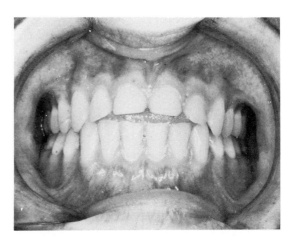

FIG. 31-4. Erosion of dental enamel due to repeated self-induced vomiting. The maxillary anterior four teeth are reduced in size in all dimensions due to the loss of enamel. (Courtesy E. A. Sweeney)

diet has been excessively abrasive. The inorganic components of saliva are present in sufficient concentrations, including supersaturation with calcium phosphates, that the hydroxyapatite in enamel does not dissolve in saliva, but minor demineralized areas may be remineralized with ions from the saliva. The mineral of the enamel is vulnerable to high H^+ concentrations so that direct and prolonged contact of enamel surfaces with acidic solutions, such as in the sucking of citrus fruits, the sipping of carbonated beverages, or the regurgitation of gastric contents, results in conspicuous demineralization and loss of structure (see Fig. 31-4).

DENTIN

Dentin is the major component of the tooth. It is much softer than enamel owing to its lower hydroxyapatite concentration and, therefore, is much less resistant to masticatory forces than enamel. Like enamel, dentin has no haversian canal systems and contains no cells. Throughout life the interface between dentin and the pulp is lined with a single layer of dentin-forming cells, called *odontoblasts,* unless the pulp is obliterated by secondary dentin formation. As long as the odontoblasts are viable, they have long organic processes that stretch through the dentin to its border with enamel or cementum.

While a limited exchange of inorganic elements occurs continually between the dentin and blood and between enamel and saliva, neither enamel nor dentin has any reparative potential beyond simple remineralization of discrete areas and deposition of secondary dentin in the pulp chamber. In this regard, enamel and dentin are completely unlike bone, in which haversian canal remodeling is continually occurring and in which fracture is responded to by callus formation and mineralization. Thus, any mechanical damage or loss of structure owing to dental caries cannot be repaired or replaced by any natural process; to prevent continuing progression of a lesion and the ultimate loss of the tooth, professional action is essential.

PULP

The body of the pulp occupies a confined area within the crown of the tooth, with a small portion extending through a canal in each root. The pulp is a highly vascular connective tissue with an artery, vein, and nerve in each root canal. The pulp is the portion of the tooth that reacts to stimuli by pain. Since the pulp is confined within this nonyielding space in the tooth, any inflammation due to infection that would cause swelling elsewhere in the body is especially painful and is only relieved by opening the pulp cavity to permit drainage and reduction of pressure.

CEMENTUM

The roots of the teeth are covered by a thin layer of a bonelike tissue, called *cementum,* in which the collagenous bundles of the periodontium are attached and anchored. Thus, cementum serves as the transitional structure between the tooth and the supporting structures.

DENTAL CARIES—TOOTH DECAY

Dental caries is a chronic disease with a multifactorial etiology that occurs with almost as high a prevalence as the common cold among the populations of industrialized countries.[44] In contrast, the people in developing countries have had much less dental caries; however, with the trend toward adoption of the dietary habits of the industrialized world, the prevalence and severity of dental caries are increasing rapidly in developing nations.

The carious lesion is initiated as demineralization just below the surface of the enamel at an interface with microbial plaque. *Demineralization* results from an interaction between the acidic metabolic products of the microorganisms in the plaque and the inorganic components of the tooth. The critical pH at which demineralization occurs is not known precisely; the consensus is that demineralization routinely occurs when the pH is decreased below 5.5, although demineralization may occur more slowly above that pH.

Invariably, the carious lesion begins on the external surfaces of the tooth and progresses toward the pulp. In young individuals, the lesions begin almost exclusively on the enamel; approximately three quarters of all lesions occur in the pits and fissures of the occlusal surfaces. In older individuals, in whom root surfaces have been exposed by periodontal disease, carious lesions (root caries) may be initiated on the bonelike cementum covering the root dentin.

Demineralization in the early carious lesion is intermittent, occurring when the microorganisms of the plaque are metabolizing rapidly, as a result of food availability, and being stationary when the microbial metabolism is quiescent between snacks or meals. During these quiescent periods, remineralization of superficial enamel lesions may occur under favorable conditions if only demineralization has occurred and if the surface integrity of the enamel has not been altered grossly. The rate of progression of a carious lesion is dependent on the balance between intervals of active demineralization, quiescence, and remineralization, which is determined by food availability to the microorganisms in the adjacent plaque. The balance further depends on the resistance of the tooth to the carious process, the composition, quality, and quantity of saliva, plaque formation, microbial composition of the plaque, the frequency, duration of availability, and composition of food to support the metabolism of plaque microorganisms, and the frequency and quality of oral hygiene. Current methods for diagnosis of carious lesions *in vivo* are sufficiently insensitive that the typical lesion has been progressing for several months before it it is clinically recognizable.

Once a carious lesion has been firmly established, with loss of surface integrity, unless its progression is interrupted by surgical removal of the decayed material and replacement by an inert restoration, or by a striking change in food or oral hygiene practices, the lesion will continue to progress centripetally through the enamel and dentin until the pulp is infected. Even then, up to a certain point, the pulp may be removed surgically and replaced in an endodontic procedure and the crown of the tooth restored appropriately. However, without adequate treatment, carious lesions progress until the remainder of the tooth has to be extracted.

Unlike many infectious diseases, dental caries does not elicit a sufficient immunologic response to limit the spread of the lesions in the first tooth or teeth to be attacked or to prevent the infection of additional sites on the same teeth or teeth that erupt into the mouth later.

ETIOLOGY

The interrelated causes of dental caries can be grouped into three general categories: microbial agents, host, and environment.[44] In order for carious lesions to occur, three conditions must be met simultaneously: (1) caries-producing microorganisms must be present in sufficient numbers on tooth surfaces, (2) the host and his teeth must be prone to develop carious lesions, and (3) foods with caries-producing potential must be consumed in a caries-conducive way. Unless all three parameters are fulfilled simultaneously, as indicated in the three interlocking circles in Figure 31-5, carious lesions cannot occur. The number of carious lesions and the rapidity of their progression are closely and directly correlated to the total tendency for caries initiation and development exerted by the three parameters. These facts need to be fully exploited in the application of preventive methods by seeking to reduce the caries-producing potential in each of these three major parameters.

Considerable success has been achieved in the application of preventive measures in the industrialized nations. In a recent symposium, epidemiologic data were presented from nine countries, indicating substantial decreases in caries prevalence and increases in the percentage of caries-free children during the past 20 years.[24a] It is not known whether these benefits will increase, plateau, or regress. Obviously, continuing emphasis must be placed on caries prevention in order to maintain these highly desirable changes. Unfortunately, in the developing countries, major increases in caries prevalence are occurring.

Microbial Agents. The mouth routinely has a rich and diverse resident microbial flora. The humidity and temperature of the mouth and the passage of all nutrients through it periodically provide ideal circumstances for the propagation and metabolism of many types of microorganisms. Since the environment varies widely in such different ecological niches as on the coronal surfaces of the tooth, on the root surfaces, in deep carious lesions, on the tongue, in the gingival crevice between the gingiva and the tooth, and in saliva, wide variations in the species and distribution of microorganisms are observed in these various niches.[22]

In order to form plaque and establish a carious lesion, appropriate microorganisms must be able to colonize, multiply, and metabolize on the enamel of the smooth buccal and lingual surfaces of the crowns, in the pits and fissures of the occlusal surfaces, in the approximal space between two adjacent teeth, and on the cementum of tooth surfaces that have been exposed by periodontal disease. Colonization of the smooth buccal and lingual surfaces can be expected to be more difficult than in the pits and fissures of the occlusal surfaces. Since the smooth surfaces are rubbed by the tongue and the cheeks and are bathed extensively by saliva, colonization has to be a relatively active and vigorous process. Colonization of a pit or fissure is more passive and may be aided by mastication, since the environment of such an area is relatively stagnant and inaccessible to saliva. The microorganisms that cause dental caries on the smooth and approximal surfaces and in the pits and fissures produce acid during their metabolism and are aciduric, being able to continue to metabolize at low *p*H values. They metabolize particularly rapidly when carbohydrates are readily available in their surroundings. Carious lesions do not occur in ex-

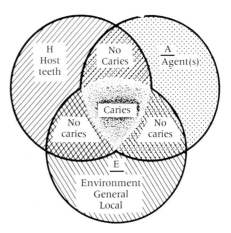

FIG. 31-5. Diagram of the etiologic interrelationship between cariogenic agent(s) (*A*), the host and his teeth (*H*), and the general environment in which the individual lives and the local environment around the teeth (*E*). A comparable relationship exists between agent, host, and environment for the periodontal diseases. (Modified from Keyes PH, Jordan HV: Factors influencing the initiation, transmission, and inhibition of dental caries. In Sognnaes RF (ed): Mechanisms of Hard Tissue Destruction, Washington DC, American Association for the Advancement of Science, 1963)

perimental animals that are fed no dietary carbohydrates.[45]

Numerous species of oral microorganisms have many of these characteristics.[23] *Lactobacillus acidophilus* for many years was suspected to be the most likely caries-producing microorganism. More recently, *Streptococcus mutans* has received special attention. The latter microorganism is either not present in the human oral cavity before teeth erupt or at least is not present in sufficient concentrations to be detected by available methods. However, soon after the primary teeth erupt, *S. mutans* can be detected on their crowns. From serotypic examination, the strain present appears to have been transferred from the mouth of the mother or other adult who is the primary provider of care. *S. mutans* is also of interest because it has the ability to form from sucrose an extracellular polymer of glucose, called *mutans*, which enables the microorganism to adhere to the enamel surface. This factor may be of special importance in the colonization of the smooth surfaces but is probably of less importance in pits and fissures where microorganisms and food are trapped. This microorganism is also identifiable, although often at low concentrations, in most active carious lesions. However, dental plaque and carious lesions contain complex mixtures of microorganisms and rarely, if ever, contain only one or two species of microorganisms. *L. acidophilus* does not have the ability to produce an extracellular polymer or to colonize smooth surfaces. However, high concentrations of the latter organism are present in well-established carious lesions.

The absolute demonstration of a specific microorganism as the causative agent of caries in humans by complete fulfillment of Koch's postualtes is essentially impossible because of the diverse flora that are always present in the oral cavity and on the teeth.

Host.   The factors influencing dental caries in the etiologic parameter associated with the individual and his teeth may be divided into two groups: (1) those associated with the genetic constitution of the individual, and (2) those nongenetic factors associated with the development of the teeth.

GENETIC DETERMINANTS

In human populations, the evidence for truly genetic determinants of caries proneness appears to be weak or nonexistent. The striking difference between the low dental caries prevalence in the people of the countries of the developing world and the high prevalence in the nations of the industrialized world was thought to be possible evidence of genetically determined resistance among some races. Early evidence, from Eskimos in Greenland did not support this premise.[40] Those groups in remote areas continued to have a low dental caries prevalence. However, those to whom the sugars and refined flours and confections of the "outside" world became available at trading posts soon had striking increases in dental caries. Similar information is now available for groups who moved from a developing country to an industrialized nation. As dietary habits changed, their incidence of caries increased dramatically. Likewise, as the economic resources of some developing nations increased, they adopted the use of sugars and various foods and confections of the developed countries and showed a rapid increase in caries.[6]

Thus, if any truly genetic influences on the caries susceptibility of human populations exist, they appear to be weak and easily overwhelmed by cariogenic flora or oral environmental exposure to and frequent use of foods with high caries potential. The exact nature of some possible genetic influences is somewhat ill defined and has been suggested as attributable to tooth structure and the morphology of the pits and fissures of the occlusal surfaces. Several investigators sought evidence for genetic determinants through the study of twins. In general, twins tend to have more similar dental caries experiences to each other than to their siblings. A possible explanation for this could be that their identical ages and more similar environments resulted in more similar situations of infection, diet,

and instruction about health than siblings born a year or more apart could possibly have had. In one study, this time difference was reduced by comparing the caries prevalence in monozygotic and dizygotic twins; it was found that monozygotic twins of either sex had significantly more similar caries experiences than the dizygotic twins of the same sex.[29]

DEVELOPMENTAL INFLUENCES ON THE HOST

The best known example of an influence on the developing teeth concerns the ingestion of fluoride and the resultant increased resistance to tooth decay.[31] However, other nutrients relatively early in the history of the science of experimental nutrition were shown to be related to the development of teeth. The classical studies of Wolbach and Howe in the 1920s demonstrated the need for adequate vitamin A to maintain the integrity of the ameloblasts, which are the enamel-forming cells, and to enable them to form normal enamel and the need for adequate vitamin C to maintain the integrity of the dentin-forming cells, called odontoblasts, and to form normal dentin.[57,58] In the same era, Mellanby demonstrated the inadequate mineralization of the organic matrix of enamel and dentin during vitamin D deficiency, with enamel hypoplasia in prolonged, severe deficiencies.[33] Other investigators demonstrated the adverse influence of calcium or phosphorus deficiencies or of grossly unbalanced calcium: phosphorus ratios on the mineralization of developing teeth. These deficiencies exerted comparable influences on the developing dental structures as the same deficiency exerted on comparable structures elsewhere in the body.

Sufficiently severe nutrient deficiencies to cause the gross and histologic abnormalities produced in the above animal model systems are not likely to occur in human populations in developed countries. Indeed, the evidence to support even the possible role of inadequate mineralization of tooth structure owing to vitamin D, calcium, or phosphorus inadequacy or imbalance as an agent in the etiology of human dental caries is insufficient to clearly establish a causative relationship. However, the fact that numerous nutrients have been so clearly identified as necessary for normal tooth development is again an indication of the need to have a well-balanced, varied diet throughout the period of tooth development.

Another nutritional area of concern during tooth development in experimental models suggests that the dietary composition may not only influence the teeth but also the development and ultimate functional capability of the salivary glands and the quality of their secretions. Borderline protein deficiency during tooth development in rats results in delayed eruption, smaller teeth, and higher caries susceptibility; in addition, the salivary glands are smaller and produce less saliva, which is altered in protein composition.[34,47] Since any condition in humans or experimental animals that causes major reductions in salivary flow causes increases in dental caries incidence, it is particularly important that the salivary glands not be impaired during their development or postdevelopmentally. The question may also be raised whether the development of the rat's immune system has been delayed with reductions in the concentration of secretory IgA in saliva. The interwoven nature of the etiologic parameters of dental caries is particularly evident in such studies as those on the relationship of borderline protein deficiency to the development and maintenance of teeth in rats.

No clear relationship of protein–calorie malnutrition in children in developing countries to an increased susceptibility to dental caries has been demonstrated. In part, this may be because their overall dietary habits and the resulting oral environment are not conducive to high dental caries experience. However, the rapidity with which dental caries experience increases when sugars and sugar-containing foods become available in developing countries suggests that the teeth in these populations are highly susceptible to dental caries and will have high caries activity when the caries-producing challenge is increased. Russell has drawn attention to a paradox in that numerous examples were observed in developing countries of much higher dental caries experiences in the primary teeth than in the permanent teeth.[42] Sweeney and colleagues have pointed out the possibility that the particularly common linear hypoplasia of the anterior teeth in developing countries may be, at least in part, of nutritional origin, and that these areas are highly susceptible to carious lesions.[49] Carious lesions in these hypoplastic areas may explain in part the higher incidence of caries in the deciduous than in the permanent teeth that Russell described.

FLUORIDE

As early as the turn of this century, a developmental error resulting in teeth with chalky white mottled areas was described in Italy.[18] Similar descriptions were provided in Colorado Springs in 1916 by MacKay, who recognized that the problem was related to the drinking-water supply.[32] Children who grew up in Colorado Springs had mottled teeth; those children whose teeth developed and erupted before they moved to Colorado Springs or who lived just outside the water distribution system of Colorado Springs did not have mottled teeth. In 1931, excessive fluoride during tooth development was identified as the cause of mottled enamel; the Colorado Springs water supply contained about 2.5 ppm flouride.[48] The enamel abnormality was described thereafter as chronic endemic dental fluorosis. Where this condition was sufficiently severe as to be esthetically disfiguring, the level of fluoride in the water supply needed to be reduced.

MacKay reported in his early studies that mottled teeth were more resistant to dental caries than normal teeth.[32] However, primary attention was given to how to prevent esthetically undesirable mottling. The importance of MacKay's observation about dental caries was not recognized until the late 1930s and early 1940s. At that time Dean recognized a correlation between the levels of fluoride in the water supply and the dental caries experience of the children in a series of midwestern communities where mottled enamel was not a problem (see Fig. 31-6).[13] The optimal fluoride concentration for the environmental region was 1 ppm to 1.2 ppm fluoride, at which level the 12-year-old to 14-year-old children who had grown up in the community had approximately 60% less caries than in nearby communities where the fluoride concentration was 0.1 ppm or less. As demonstrated by this figure, a good dose response was observed. The benefit was much higher for the anterior teeth than for the posterior teeth and for lesions occurring on

FIG. 31-6. The lifetime dental caries experience for the permanent teeth of 7257 children 12 to 14 years old from 21 cities and 4 states is plotted against the fluoride concentration of the communal water supply. (Dean HT, Arnold FA Jr, Elvove E: Domestic water and dental caries V. Additional studies of the relation of fluoride domestic waters to dental caries experience in 4,425 white children aged 12 to 14 years of 13 cities in 4 states. US Public Health Reports 57:1155-1179, 1942)

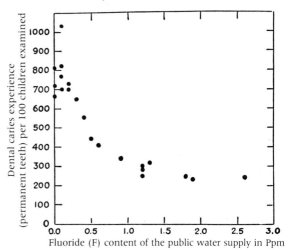

the smooth buccal and lingual surfaces than in the pits and fissures of the occlusal surfaces. The reductions in dental caries have been shown to continue at least into middle age.

While most data on the benefits of fluoride during tooth development on dental caries experience are expressed in terms of the number of decayed, missing, and filled teeth per child, it is important to emphasize that the size of the individual carious lesion and the rate of its progression are also reduced. Tooth loss is also greatly reduced, especially for particularly vulnerable teeth such as the first permanent molar. These reductions in disease manifestation resulted in greatly reduced figures for the annual cost of delivering total dental care to each child.[35]

The observations of dental benefit from the optimal use of fluoride naturally contained in public water supplies, not only in childhood but also in adult life, led to intensive and extensive investigations of whether the ingestion of a water supply containing 1.0 ppm fluoride throughout life in a temperate region was safe in every way.[2] The first concern was about mottled enamel. The most sensitive cells in the body to the toxic manifestations of excess fluoride are the ameloblasts; in the presence of excess fluoride, their function is altered, affecting the enamel formed during the period of excess. The severity of mottled enamel varies in relation to the degree of fluoride excess, ranging from that detectable only by the most careful clin-

ical examination to the grossly visible and esthetically undesirable. Dean assigned grades from 0 to 4 to denote the range from normal to severe and plotted both dental caries experience and degree of mottling against the fluoride concentration of communal water supplies, as shown in Fig. 31-7. The optimal dental caries benefit was obtained at around 1.0 ppm fluoride in the drinking water, whereas mottling did not become a problem until the fluoride concentration was in excess of 2.0 ppm.

Many studies in laboratory animals and in human subjects, as well as epidemiologic surveys, were conducted on varied aspects of metabolism and disease entities. Studies continue to be conducted with increasing refinement on selected topics. The composite body of information satisfied, and continues to satisfy, many national and international organizations that evaluated the evidence, such as the National Research Council–National Academy of Sciences, the National Institutes of Health, the World Health Organization, the American Medical Association, and the American Dental Association.

Safety was sufficiently evident by 1945 that three trial communities—Newburgh, New York; Grand Rapids, Michigan; and Brantford, Ontario—began to add sufficient fluoride in their water-processing facilities to increase the fluoride concentration to 1.0 ppm to 1.2 ppm. Figure 31-8 represents the decrease in dental caries experience among the children of Grand Rapids, Michigan after 9 years of fluoridation. The permanent teeth of the chil-

FIG. 31-7. The relationships between the number of decayed, missing, and filled teeth (*dotted line*) and Dean's index for the severity of chronic endemic dental fluorosis (*solid line*) are plotted against the fluoride concentration of the public water supply expressed on a logarithmic scale. (Hodge HC, Smith FA: Some public health aspects of water fluoridation. In Shaw JH (ed): Fluoridation as a Public Health Measure. Washington, DC, American Association for the Advancement of Science, 1954

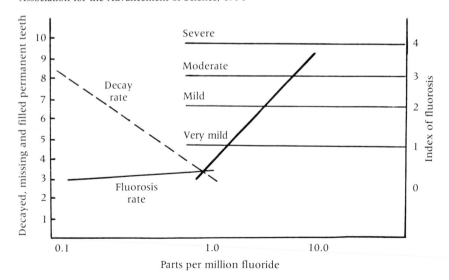

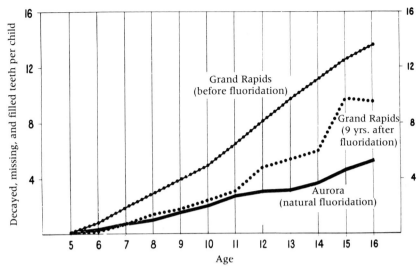

FIG. 31-8. A comparison of the number of decayed, missing, and filled permanent teeth of children 5 to 16 years old in Aurora, Illinois, where the water contains 1.2 ppm fluoride, in Grand Rapids before fluoridation of the public water supply was initiated, and in Grand Rapids nine years after fluoridation of the public water supply was begun. (Dean HT, Arnold FA Jr, Elvove E: Domestic water and dental caries. V. Additional studies of the relation of fluoride domestic waters to dental caries experience in 4,425 white children aged 12 to 14 years of 13 cities in 4 states, US Public Health Reports 57:1155–1179, 1942)

dren 5 years to 11 years of age were formed during optimal fluoride ingestion. Their dental caries experience was remarkably similar to that in a typical community with fluoride naturally present in the drinking water. Likewise, their dental caries experience was strikingly different from children in Grand Rapids of the same ages before fluoridation was initiated. However, for the children 12 years to 16 years of age, the dental caries experience lies midway between that for children in Grand Rapids prefluoridation and that for children of the same ages from a natural fluoride community. The explanation for this difference between these younger and older groups is related to the time when teeth are developing and erupt. The incisors and first permanent molars in the older groups were largely mineralized before fluoridation began, whereas major portions of their canines, premolars, and second permanent molars were mineralized after fluoridation was initiated. Thus within the same mouths, the beneficial effect of fluoridation is shown with prefluoridation, high caries teeth adjacent to postfluoridation, low caries teeth. This demonstration of the developmental influence of the fluoride is important to stress. Undoubtedly the local influence of fluoride in food, water, and saliva on the surface of erupting teeth is important; however, the incorporation of increased fluoride into the crystal lattice of enamel and dentin during development is essential for maximal benefits. The cost

effectiveness of community water fluoridation is clearly higher than for any other preventive measures.

Fluoridation of public water supplies has been and continues to be accompanied by opposition from a small, vocal and aggressive minority that becomes evident in any community whenever fluoridation of a water supply is being considered. The opposition has varied in its emphasis from time to time through such areas as violation of individual rights to allegations of increased Down's syndrome, allergy, or cancer. No amount of laboratory, clinical, or epidemiologic research has been adequate to satisfy the opponents. Possibly the most serious reason for concern about the scientific objectivity of the opponents of fluoridation is provided by their objection that dental benefits of water fluoridation has not been satisfactorily demonstrated.

At present in the United States about 110 million (half of the population) live in communities where the water naturally contains about the correct amount of fluoride or the water is fluoridated at an optimal level. One half or more of the remaining Americans live in small communities or in rural areas with their own wells, making water fluoridation economically unfeasible or impractical. In some rural communities, the water supply in consolidated schools has been fluoridated. Since children are only present for about one third of any day and for about one half of the days in any year, the level of fluoride in the water needs to be appreciably higher than in the water supply for the entire community, usually 5.0 ppm. Under these circumstances, reductions in dental caries experience have been reported in the neighborhood of 40%. The cost per child is approximately tenfold higher for school fluoridation than the per capita figure for community fluoridation.

An additional systemic route for provision of fluoride is by a pharmaceutical preparation provided daily from infancy until tooth development has ceased. This procedure is approximately as effective as water fluoridation when it is followed systematically. However, the prolonged provision daily results in very low levels of compliance except in the most conscientious and health-oriented families. The appropriate levels of administration are shown in Table 31-1. This procedure is also much more expensive than water fluoridation because of the need to purchase on prescription a pharmaceutical preparation.

Nonsystemic procedures to obtain partial benefits of fluoride through application to the outer surfaces of erupted teeth fall into three general categories: (1) fluoridated toothpaste is the least effective and requires regular and thorough use by the individual; (2) application of a concentrated solution to cleaned tooth surfaces by the dentist or hygienist under careful conditions annually or more frequently is intermediate in effectiveness, but most expensive owing to the professional time involved; and (3) rinsing under supervision in school with a 0.02% fluoride solution on a weekly basis is the most effective and intermediate in cost.

ENVIRONMENT

Environmental relationships to dental caries can be divided into two general groups: (1) the impact of the general environment on the community and family in which the individual develops and lives, and (2) the oral environment, particularly on and around the tooth surfaces.

Community and Familial Environment. Numerous components of the general environment influence the prevalence and severity of dental caries among the individuals who grow up and live in a community. Some of these factors influence all individuals in a community, while others are specifically related to familial relationships.

Fluoride availability has undoubtedly the best-known, and most striking, community-wide relationship to the dental caries incidence of a population. Although the fluoride effect operates through systemic mechanisms, as described in the preceding section on the host, fluoride is an environmental variable. Another example concerns the generally lower dental caries experience in developing countries compared to the industrialized nations. The reasons for the lower caries experience in the developing countries probably include less food available, resulting in little or no eating between meals, less use of sugar and sugar-containing foods, and the use of a greater percentage of relatively unrefined foods, including such items as unrefined salt, which often has an elevated fluoride level.

The degree of availability and type of professional dental care in the community is another environmental variable. In general, the easy availability of restorative care probably does not reduce the total amount of dental caries but, rather, influences whether an early lesion is restored or, instead, is allowed to progress until the tooth is destroyed and must be extracted. However, where the available professional care is provided on a preventive basis rather than on simply a restorative basis, the prevalence of dental caries can be materially reduced.

TABLE 31-1
Recommended Fluoride (F) Supplementation

Water supply F concentration (ppm)	Desirable fluoride supplementation for various age groups (mg/day)				
	(0–6 mo)	(6–18 mo)	(18–36 mo)	(3–6 yr)	(>6 yr)
<0.2	0*	0.25	0.50	0.75	1
0.2–0.4	0*	0*	0.25	0.50	0.75
0.4–0.6	0*	0*	0	0.25	0.50
0.6–0.8	0*	0*	0	0	0.25
>0.8	0*	0*	0	0	0†

From Wei SHY, Fomon SJ, Anderson TA: Nutrition and dental health. In Sweeney EA (ed): The Food That Stays: An Update on Nutrition, Diet, Sugar, and Caries. New York, MEDCOM, 1977

*0.25 for totally breast-fed infants.

†In this age group, the hazard of fluorosis is low, and some additional protection will probably be afforded by fluoride supplementation. However, fluoride supplementation is not desirable when the drinking water provides more than 1.1 ppm.

Familial influences encompass a wide variety of parameters, which include the following: (1) supervision and instruction by word and example about nutritional needs and how they can be best fulfilled, not only to nourish the individual adequately but also to maintain optimal oral health; (2) concern about general and oral health and the level of education about this area; and (3) economic resources to purchase appropriate food and health care. The attitudes within the family about undesirable between-meal snacks, the provision of a fluoride supplement when water fluoridation is lacking, oral hygiene, and periodic dental care probably are the most important familial factors in determining whether the individual is typical of, or diverges from, the general baseline of caries prevalence of the community.

Oral Environment. The quality and caries-producing capabilities of the oral environment are largely determined by the community and family environment described in the preceding paragraphs and by peer-group pressures.[36] Caries-producing microorganisms do not metabolize rapidly enough without the frequent presence of carbohydrates in the diet to reduce the *p*H at the plaque–tooth surface interface sufficiently to demineralize tooth substance. However, when carbohydrates are available in the mouth in forms that diffuse into the plaque, the microorganisms metabolize rapidly, and the *p*H decreases sufficiently to demineralize tooth substances. The *p*H does not return to a near-neutral resting value until the available carbohydrates have been neutralized by the reaction with tooth minerals or by the buffers of saliva. Sugars that are in solution or that dissolve readily from foods and confections have the greatest potential to penetrate the plaque and become available to the microorganisms. However, these readily dissolved forms are probably diluted relatively rapidly by saliva, and acids produced from them are neutralized by the buffers in saliva. They may have a more transient influence on the *p*H in plaque than sugars and sugar–starch mixtures in various foods and confections that adhere to tooth surfaces for prolonged periods. In these situations, not only are the sugars metabolized but also the starch is hydrolyzed to some extent to glucose by salivary amylase and becomes available for metabolism by plaque microorganisms. Various hard candies, lozenges, and gum that are customarily held in the mouth for prolonged periods also release their sugar relatively slowly, thereby making the sugar available for a long period for utilization by oral microorganisms. A given weight of sugar made available slowly can be expected to be more

harmful than the same weight of sugar in solution consumed in a brief interval. The frequency of eating potentially caries-producing food items, coupled with the length of time that each item is in the mouth and on tooth surfaces, is the major determinant of how cariogenic the local environment will be.

Apart from the generalities in the preceding paragraph, no information is available on more specific values for the cariogenic potentials of specific foods or confectionary items. Clearly the preference for between-meal snacks should be for fruits, vegetables, nuts, and cheese rather than for candy, cake, lozenges, soft drinks, and gum. The total amount of carbohydrate and even the total amount of sugars consumed in a given period of time are not nearly as important as the frequency of cariogenic food consumption and the length of time that food is in the mouth. Otherwise, the populations of many developing countries where the starches from a staple grain such as corn, rice, or wheat provide 80% or more of the calories could be expected to have a very high prevalence of dental caries. However, their low caries prevalence suggests that the high-starch foods *per se* are not cariogenic. However, when sugar and foods containing sugar are introduced into these cultures, the caries experience increases quickly and strikingly.[6]

The question of whether sucrose is uniquely cariogenic in humans has not been resolved. Many studies in experimental animals indicate that the monosaccharides and disaccharides do not differ appreciably in their caries-producing abilities. However, in assay situations where caries production is uniquely attributable to *S. mutans* as the only or the overwhelming organism present, and where smooth surface lesions predominate, sucrose appears to be more cariogenic than the monosaccharides or other disaccharides. However, this finding has not been substantiated in animal assays or human populations where a mixed population of microorganisms was present or for lesions in the pits and fissures of the occlusal surfaces.

Sucrose is the predominant sugar in the human diet and for that reason alone may be the principal contributor to dental caries (see Table 31-2). However, currently no evidence is available to indicate that major replacement of sucrose by other monosaccharides or disaccharides will reduce the incidence of dental caries to any striking degree in test situations in humans. Once plaque has formed or a lesion has been initiated in a restricted area, its resident microorganisms, including *S. mutans,* are capable of catabolizing the available monosaccharides and disaccharides.

TABLE 31-2
Calculated Average per Capita Consumption of Various Carbohydrates (g/day and lb/yr) per Year

	1910–1913		1960		1974	
	daily (g)	*annual* (lb)	*daily* (g)	*annual* (lb)	*daily* (g)	*annual* (lb)
Starch	342	275.5	188	151.5	179	144.2
Sugars						
Sucrose	101	81.3	121	97.5	123	99.1
Corn sweeteners	8	6.4	19	15.3	33	26.6
Lactose	21	16.9	25	20.1	23	18.5
Glucose	6	4.8	11	8.9	12	9.7
Fructose	6	4.8	4	3.2	3	2.4
Maltose	2	1.6	4	3.2	4	3.2
Others	12	9.7	5	4.0	3	2.4
Total Sugars	156	125.5	189	152.2	200	161.9
Total Carbohydrate	498	401.0	377	303.7	379	306.1
Percent of Sugars	31.5		50.0		52.6	

Compiled from USDA/ARS 1972 data and sugar statistics (USDA), and from Cantor SM. Patterns of use of sweeteners. In Shaw JH, Roussos GG (eds): Sweeteners and Dental Caries. Arlington, VA, Information Retrieval Inc., 1978

ENAMEL HYPOPLASIA

Enamel hypoplasia is manifested in a failure of enamel matrix formation and a subsequent lack of mineralization. The clinical appearance of the hypoplastic areas ranges from simple pits on those teeth undergoing matrix formation at the time of the insult to deep circular indentations around the crowns. In extreme cases in which the insult may have lasted for months, a major portion of the enamel may be lacking. One of the more frequent forms of hypoplasia is the circular or linear variety,

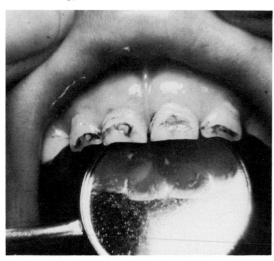

FIG. 31-9. Linear hypoplasia of primary incisors. The time of the hypoplasia corresponds to the natal period. (Courtesy E. A. Sweeney)

where those portions of the enamel that formed both before and after the insult are normal (see Fig. 31-9).

The basic problem in all instances may be nutritional in nature, at least at the cellular level. For instance, while enamel hypoplasia may reflect in kymographic form the exacerbations of the nephrotic syndrome, the cause may be due to either the excessive proteinuria disturbing the availability of amino acid precursors of the enamel matrix, a diminution of plasma carrier proteins for vitamin A or D, or an abnormal mineral balance. The same or similar mechanisms may cause the enamel hypoplasias associated with febrile episodes, especially those due to exanthematous diseases.

Classically, it is stated that a deficiency of vitamin A can result in arrested enamel matrix formation and hypoplasia, but the human cases described for this deficiency are ones in which multiple nutritional deficiencies and other systemic diseases were present simultaneously.[15] While the external manifestation is enamel hypoplasia, milder disturbances of matrix formation are frequently seen in the dentin in the form of interglobular dentin that was forming during the same developmental period.

Enamel hypoplasia is infrequently seen in the permanent teeth of normal human populations from areas in which protein–calorie malnutrition or vitamin A deficiency is endemic. However, in the primary teeth of children in these areas a high incidence (20%–80%) of linear hypoplasia of the primary incisors occurs in portions of the teeth formed in the neonatal period.[49] This form of hypoplasia is also seen in a number of premature infants.[41]

The similarity in findings has led to the speculation that the reported low serum levels of vitamin A with high neonatal infection rates in the former group and inadequate release of liver stores of vitamin A owing to liver immaturity in the latter, may have some common relation with the production of the lesion in these two groups. Certainly in all full-term infants, there is an arrest of enamel formation called the neonatal line, but the arrest is so brief it can usually only be seen microscopically. In some premature infants and in a large number of children from developing nations, this period of arrest seems prolonged and severe, resulting in a macroscopic defect.

Hypomineralization of enamel can also lead to enamel that is more susceptible to decay or, in the case of hypophosphatemia, to a failure of secondary (reparative) dentin formation. This results in wide dentinal tubules, which allow for easy bacterial ingress once the enamel is penetrated.[3] In children affected with this genetic disorder, multiple periapical infections of the mandibular primary incisor teeth occur even without decay, resulting from incisal attrition of the enamel and subsequent bacterial migration along the open dentinal tubules into the pulp chamber.

Periodontal (Supporting) Tissues

THE COMPONENTS OF THE PERIODONTIUM

The oral tissues concerned with anchoring the teeth in the jaws are collectively referred to as the periodontium, and consist of the gingiva, periodontal membrane, alveolar bone, and cementum.

The gingiva (see Fig. 31-10) is a keratinized squamous epithelium that surrounds the neck of the tooth, covers the alveolar bone, and merges with the oral mucosa in the vestibule. It is divided into a fixed and a free gingiva. The free gingiva, including the interdental gingiva, acts as a transition zone between the gingiva fixed to the underlying connective tissue and the tooth surface.[56]

The gingival sulcus is a moatlike depression between the free gingiva and the neck of the tooth. At the base of this sulcus, the junctional epithelium anchors the gingiva to the enamel in a quite fragile manner. The inner walls of the sulcus coronal to the junctional epithelium merge with the keratinized epithelium of the outer aspects of the gingiva. The connective tissue core of the gingival papilla contains numerous collagen fibers that anchor the gingivae to the cementum of the tooth and the surrounding bone (see Fig. 31-11). Other collagenous fibers run in a circular manner around the tooth and function much in the manner of a purse

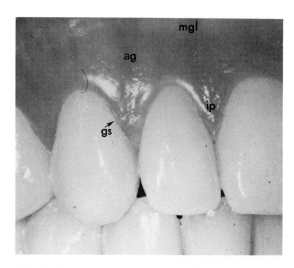

FIG. 31-10. Normal gingiva. *ag,* attached gingiva; *gs,* gingival sulcus; *ip,* interdental papilla; *mgl,* mucogingival line. (Williams RC, Zager NI: The periodontium. In Shaw JH, Sweeney EA, Cappuccino CC, et al (eds): Textbook of Oral Biology, Philadelphia, W B Saunders, 1978)

string in adapting the free gingiva to the neck of the tooth.

Beneath the overlying gingivae of both jaws is the spongy alveolar bone. Compact bone forms the plates of the buccal and lingual vestibules and is continuous with the lining of the alveolus in which the tooth sits, at which point it is called the *lamina dura.*

Between the lamina dura and the cementum of the tooth root lies the periodontal membrane, a dense ligamentous structure consisting predominantly of collagen but with some elastin in association with blood vessels. The collagenous bundles are found in four general arrangements. Crestal fibers run from the tooth and insert onto the crest of the interseptal bone. Apical fibers are found at the apex of the root of the tooth and insert in a fanlike manner into the bone at the base of the tooth socket. The largest numbers of fibers are the horizontal fibers, running from the bone to cementum, and the oblique fibers, which insert at a higher level onto the bone than the cementum in a slinglike arrangement. Interspersed with the collagen bundles are fibroblasts, and along the tooth surface are cementoblasts. Along the bony surfaces are found osteoblasts and occasional osteoclasts. Running throughout the ligament are blood vessels and nerves. The latter provide the proprioceptive information that allows the individual to acutely sense the presence of even a tiny grain of sand between the teeth as they occlude. Many nutritive blood vessels penetrate the lamina dura of the alveolar bone. The periodontal ligament functions as

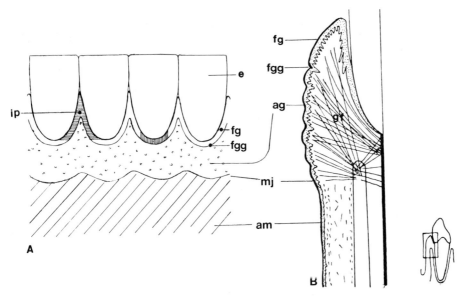

FIG. 31-11. *(A)* Gingival topography. *(B)* Mesiodistal gingiva showing fiber groups, *ag,* attached gingiva; *am,* alveolar mucosa; *e,* enamel; *fg,* free gingiva; *fgg,* free gingival groove; *gf,* gingival fibers; *ip,* interdental papilla; *mj,* mucogingival junction. (Williams RC, Zager NI: The periodontium. In Shaw JH, Sweeney EA, Cappuccino CC et al (eds): Textbook of Oral Biology, Philadelphia, W B Saunders, 1978)

a very efficient shock absorber, which spreads out the forces of mastication rather than having them concentrated at the apexes of the teeth.

PERIODONTAL DISEASES

The etiology of diseases of the periodontium is similar to that of dental caries.[37] The causes of these diseases are multifactorial and involve various permutations of host, environment, and microbial agents interacting to produce tissue destruction. Unlike dental caries, the specific relationships between the various factors are poorly worked out and in certain instances are unknown.

When examining the oral cavity at any age, great care should be taken to identify local and systemic factors that may predispose to the periodontal diseases because physical factors, such as improperly placed or broken dental restorations, promote the impaction of foodstuffs between and around the teeth and may traumatize adjacent tissues. Likewise, excessive or abnormal occlusive forces over time may promote bone loss like any other orthopaedic situation in which abnormal pressure is exerted on bone. The patient's medical status should be clearly defined in terms of endocrine, metabolic, pharmacologic, and psychological problems, since aberrations of any of these parameters may aggravate existing periodontal disease. Indeed, the rapid cellular turnover of the oral tissues reflects metabolic deficiencies of an otherwise subclinical nature

before gross manifestations of deficiency are evident. In the aged or debilitated patient, nutritional deficiency should be suggested when acute soft tissue or periodontal lesions develop or when existing chronic lesions suddenly assume a more aggressive acute form.

Most oral and periodontal lesions have a partial microbiologic etiology, but the degree of the host resistance is due in great part to tissue tone and integrity, and if these are compromised by nutritional inadequacy or systemic metabolic aberration, oral symptoms may result.

GINGIVITIS

Gingivitis is an inflammation of the gingivae and can assume a variety of forms depending on the etiology and chronicity of the problems.

Simple Gingivitis. By far, the most common form of gingivitis is due to the accumulation of bacterial plaque around the cervical areas of the teeth and is characterized by edema, erythema, and easily provoked hemorrage. However, even before these gross signs are apparent, consistent histologic changes occur within as short a period as 2 days to 4 days after the cessation of normal plaque removal by brushing and flossing.[38] Initially, the lesion occurs in the gingival sulcus and involves the junctional epithelium and the most coronal part of the connective tissue. The blood vessels of the gingivae become enlarged and large numbers of polymorphonuclear leukocytes migrate into the junctional epithelium and the gingival sulcus. As much as 15% of the gingival collagen disappears, and the space created is occupied by inflammatory cells and edema fluid. The lesions seem to be a response to plaque-derived substances, which stimulate chemotaxis.

This histologic picture changes rapidly, and by 7 days the dense cellular infiltrate is composed chiefly of lymphoid cells. Within the reaction site, collagen losses may approximate upwards of 60% of the collagen fibers and the cellular morphology of fibroblasts is greatly altered. The appearance of the pathologic aberrations and cellular infiltrate have led to the suggestion that cellular hypersensitivity plays an important role in the early gingival lesion.[27]

If the early gingival lesion does not improve and persists for another 2 weeks to 3 weeks, plasma cells are observed in deeper connective tissues, and the sulcular epithelium may proliferate and migrate into the affected connective tissue and along the root. Antigen–antibody complexes are found around blood vessels that have also undergone marked proliferation. If this picture is maintained over time, fibrosis and scarring of the gingivae can occur, with alteration of gross architecture.

Acute Necrotizing Ulcerative Gingivitis. In addition to the common form of gingivitis associated with poor oral hygiene, another acute form has a different epidemiologic picture. Acute necrotizing ulcerative gingivitis (ANUG, Vincent's infection, trench mouth) occurs as a rapidly acquired acute infection, usually accompanied by fever, malaise, regional lymphadenopathy, a distinctive fetid mouth odor, and exquisitely painful, edematous and erythematous gingivae (see Fig. 31-12). The inderdental gingival papillae undergo gangrenous necrosis leading to cuplike lesions between the teeth, with loss of the triangular-shaped papillae. Not all papillae are equally affected. The onset is usually quite rapid, in the order of 24 hr. The disease is believed to be fusospirochetal in origin, since, unlike other periodontal diseases in which bacteria are rarely seen within the gingival tissues, unusual spirochetal forms can be found deep in the tissue itself. Large collections of fusiform bacteria can be found more coronally. There is no simple explanation, however, why the disease should be initiated, since the same or similar organisms can be found in most mouths. Some factors have been associated with onset of the disease, including the advent of an emotionally stressful event. It is not known whether activation of the stress mechanism alone or a combination of inadequate dietary in-

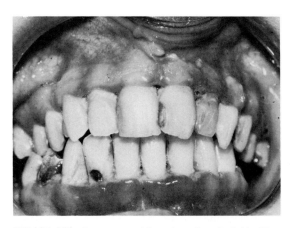

FIG. 31-12. Acute necrotizing ulcerative gingivitis. Note the erythema, edema, and necrotic interdental papillae, especially in the mandible. (Courtesy Dr. R. Williams)

take and lack of oral hygiene accompanying such stressful periods is responsible.

ANUG responds well to antibiotics and to local measures, including scaling and removal of plaque deposits, eating a bland diet, and maintaining adequate fluid intake. The patient should be instructed to avoid spicy or acidic foods until healing has progressed in order to avoid pain. Ingestion of easily swallowed high-protein sources, such as eggnog and other dairy products as well as soybean-containing supplements (e.g., Metrecal), should be encouraged. If the normal architecture of the interdental papillae has been greatly altered, however, surgical recontouring of the remaining gingivae may be necessary to restore a healthy gingival contour that will not impact food and that can be cleaned by the usual oral hygiene measures.

Noma. Nutritional aberration seems to play a major role in the form of ANUG known as noma, which occurs primarily in severely malnourished children in various parts of the world. This rapidly destructive gangrenous lesion of the tissues of the face and jaws appears to involve the same microorganisms as ANUG, and the initial lesion likewise appears to be in the gingivae.[52] The susceptible person is usually severely malnourished, frequently with a history of an antecedent exanthematous or viral disease that has debilitated him. The lesion is, like the more local gingival lesion of ANUG, exquisitely sensitive to penicillin and, like ANUG, the infection can be halted within 24 hr. to 48 hr. However, the rapidity of progression often leads to large disfiguring lesions of the cheeks, lips, and bone, and is frequently fatal if untreated immediately. It seems likely that the decreased host resistance to infection permits the wide dissemination of a lesion that in the healthy person is limited to the gingivae alone. Nomalike lesions have been known to occur in some patients whose immune systems have been severely impaired by chemotherapy.

Hypertrophic Gingivitis. A third form of gingivitis is characterized by hypertrophy, primarily as a result of the abnormal accumulation of cells and cellular products in the gingivae. These hypertrophic conditions may have a marked inflammatory component superimposed upon the basic condition, as in certain leukemias known to show gingival infiltration, particularly the monocytic and acute lymphocytic varieties. By far the most common cause, however, is the hypertrophy associated with the ingestion of phenytoin (Dilantin), which may produce a marked fibrous hypertrophy of the gingivae that, in extreme cases, can cover the occlusal surfaces of the posterior teeth and interfere with mastication. When hypertrophy of this extent is present, the painful impingement of the gingivae may be sufficient to alter normal eating habits and may necessitate the surgical removal of the hypertrophic gingivae. Some evidence suggests that the basic problem in this condition results from a reduced turnover of collagen in the face of normal synthesis and that the hypertrophy will occur to a minor degree in most patients who are on therapeutic dosages of the drug. It seems quite clear, however, that the hypertrophy that is grossly evident and clinically significant can be minimized if scrupulous oral hygiene is practiced before hypertorphy is evident. Surgical treatment of the problem without the assurance of subsequent meticulous oral hygiene postsurgically is doomed to failure. The basic cellular mechanism of this defect is not known.[39]

Vitamin C and Scurvy. Perhaps the clearest relationship between a specific nutrient deficiency and gingival disease is that of vitamin C and scorbutic gingivitis (see Fig. 31-13). The process is seen intraorally as grossly edematous and erythematous gingivae with a marked propensity for spontaneous hemorrhage into tissue and the oral cavity. The failure of normal collagen synthesis results in friable capillaries and loss of the periodontal ligament, and, if prolonged, eventual loss of the tooth. The gingivitis is limited to those areas of the jaws that contain erupted teeth. The disease is relatively rare in adults in developed nations because of the multiplicity of sources of ascorbic acid. However, it is seen occasionally in the infant who, for whatever reason, is not receiving foods, juices, or supplements containing adequate amounts of vitamin C.

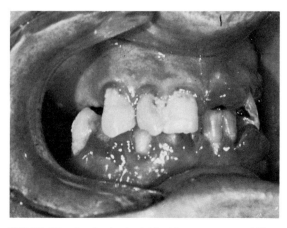

FIG. 31-13. Scorbutic gingivitis. (Courtesy Dr. G. Shklar)

PERIODONTITIS

In simple gingivitis, the inflamed state may be maintained for many years. Most lesions of an established nature do not progress to an active state leading to pocket formation, alveolar bone loss, and destruction of the periodontal ligament—the so-called full-blown *periodontitis*. When this does occur, however, the bony destruction and collagen loss closely resemble that of long-term chronic inflammatory diseases of connective tissue, such as rheumatoid arthritis.[37]

Why the gingival lesion of an established type progresses in some persons to periodontitis is unknown, and it is impossible to predict which lesions will progress and which will not. Perhaps the person needs to acquire certain microorganisms not usually found in normal plaque in order to progress from the gingival lesion to the aggressive periodontal lesion, or perhaps other factors of the host or environment must be altered. If the established gingival inflammatory lesion is transformed into aggressive lesions and is unchecked by local measures of oral hygiene, it may eventually lead to the loss of sufficient bony support and ligamentous attachment to cause exfoliation of teeth.

Little is known of the predisposing systemic or nutritional factors that may influence the initiation or progression of the aggressive periodontal lesion. Various suggestions have implicated poor calcium and phosphorus balances and distorted calcium to phosphorus ratios, lack of vitamins C and D, as well as certain endocrinopathies. Certainly vitamins C and D and calcium play a role in adequate bone formation, and vitamin C is important in the maintenance of normal collagen formation of the periodontal ligament, gingival fibers, and vascular integrity. Suggestions that the B-complex vitamins may play a role in periodontitis rest almost exclusively on animal experiments in which gangrenous lesions were produced in monkey gingivae.[11] However, such lesions do not closely resemble the usual form of periodontal disease. Indeed, such lesions are probably more indicative of the general susceptibility of oral tissues to infection in the face of a generalized or specific nutritional deficiency, as in the case of noma.

Diabetes is known to predispose to severe periodontal disease, but the mechanism is believed to rest more with the microangiopathy associated with diabetes rather than with any more generalized mechanism, and probably represents a special case.[8]

No specific cure is known for periodontitis. The disease can be arrested or significantly slowed in most patients by the institution of vigorous oral hygiene measures and the elimination of local factors. The latter, such as defective or poorly constructed dental restorations or the presence of gingival or bony pockets that have formed as a result of disease and that can no longer be cleaned by normal oral hygiene procedures, may have contributed to the initiation of inflammation.

Nutritional implications in periodontitis relate to the desirability of providing a well-balanced diet rather than to any specific nutritional items. The diet should contain foods that require vigorous chewing rather than those that require little, if any, chewing. Failure of bony stimulation owing to lack of vigorous mastication has been shown to lead to atrophy of alveolar bone, just as it has been shown to occur in other bones as a result of inactivity.

Nutritional support during periodontal therapy is indicated, particularly in relation to periodontal surgery. However, the need for grossly elevated intakes of specific nutrients, such as vitamins and minerals, has never been shown in any clinical trial, and is anecdotal and unsubstantiated.

PERIODONTOSIS (ACUTE JUVENILE PERIODONTITIS)

While rarely does periodontitis become manifest much before the onset of maturity, an unusual form of periodontal destruction is found in the young that is characterized by massive bone loss in the face of minimal gingival inflammation. This syndrome has been called periodontosis, or juvenile periodontitis. The disease is probably not a single entity, since certain systemic abnormalities, such as cyclic neutropenia, other diseases characterized by defective white cells, and certain genetic diseases, such as palmar-plantar hyperkeratosis (Papillon–Lefèvre syndrome), can mimic the observed bone loss. In some children, however, no discernible impairment of host defenses can be ascertained, yet large bony pockets are found in which reside a number of organisms of a highly unusual nature, mostly gram-negative anerobes. The disease is frequently self-limiting or may severely affect only a few teeth. The disease would not appear to have a nutritional component, since the children seem well nourished, and since the process does not seem to involve gingival inflammation and dental plaque. Even the local effects of dietary sugars in the promotion of dental plaque do not seem to be a particularly strong factor.

PRACTICAL CONSIDERATIONS

The health professional is frequently confronted with oral conditions that directly or indirectly have a significant nutritional component or that must be differentiated from disease states that mimic nutritional inadequacy.

DENTAL STAINING

A frequent concern to parents is abnormal color of their children's teeth. A major type of extrinsic (surface) staining is caused by ingestion of iron supplements by persons with inadequate oral hygiene. In these cases, dental plaque is not completely removed around the necks of the teeth. The plaque bacteria form hydrogen sulfide during their normal metabolism, which reacts with the ferrous ion of the supplement and forms black ferric sulfide in the plaque. Adequate oral hygiene practices keep dental plaque from accumulating in the cervical areas and will usually prevent the recurrence of this black-brown stain. Usually, extrinsic stains can be removed easily with a dental scaler and, therefore, pose no problem. However, the intrinsic stains caused by the incorporation of pigmented substances, such as tetracycline, into developing tooth structure cannot be removed.

"BOTTLE BABY SYNDROME"

Certain pediatric feeding practices have recently been recognized as contributing to a particularly vexing, rampant form of dental caries in the young child (12 months–24 months).[14] Decay involves primarily the smooth surfaces of the maxillary incisors and the first primary molars in both arches, but not the mandibular incisors (see Fig. 31-14). The feeding history of the child almost invariably reveals that the child is put to bed each night and often for daytime naps with a nursing bottle with milk, formula, or fruit juice. As the child falls asleep, salivary function and swallowing are practically abolished. The sugars in the milk or formula are fermented to acids, which dissolve tooth structure without the dilution and buffering capacity of sa-

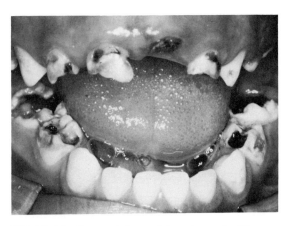

FIG. 31-14. Rampant decay of the primary dentition associated with the prolonged use of a nursing bottle at nighttime (Courtesy E. A. Sweeney)

liva or the oral clearance resulting from swallowing. When acidic substances such as fruit juices are provided, the effect may even be additive since the sugar fermentation process can still proceed and the hydrogen ions of the acidic juices are added to those produced from the sugars. It is believed that the position of the tongue protects the lower incisor teeth from this particularly devastating decay.

Dentists feel that as soon as the child has begun to be weaned and learned to drink from a glass, at about the age of 8 months to 10 months, the bottle should not be provided when the child is put to bed. If for psychological reasons this is not practical, the bottle should contain nothing acidic or fermentable. Water would be the most desirable substance.

This condition has recently been reported in breast-fed infants, many of whom have been breast-fed on demand for in excess of a year and one half and some for as long as 2 years to 3 years.[21] This finding has engendered anxieties in parents who practice and advocate this kind of feeding and believe that the psychological benefits outweigh any contraindications. However, parents should be aware that the child falling asleep with a mouthful of milk, whether human or bovine, is at risk. The question has been raised as to why, in developing nations where prolonged breast-feeding is perhaps the most common practice, such decay has not been reported. In fact, similar decay is quite common in many population groups that have been examined, but it takes a somewhat different pattern. In developed nations, the thinnest enamel occurs at the neck of the incisor tooth where the initial lesions of "bottle" decay are usually found. However, as described earlier, in infants in developing countries, frequently a hypoplastic line is present in the enamel corresponding to the neonatal line, which is the thinnest enamel surface in these children. The described decay tends to be initiated on this line half way up the crown of the tooth and not at the cervical area (see Fig. 31-15). This decay, then, may be analogous to "bottle" decay in general etiology, but it differs somewhat in the anatomic site.[49]

This discussion should not in any way be construed to suggest that normal breast-feeding is deleterious, but rather that prolonged feeding, particularly just before sleep at night or at daytime naps, may have serious dental consequences in decay, pain, and infection for some children.

RAMPANT DECAY OF THE PERMANENT DENTITION

While the rampant decay associated with the prolonged use of the nocturnal nursing bottle has a simple solution for prevention or arrest once the process and its cause have been recognized, rampant decay of the permanent dentition occurring from the age of 6 years through the late teens is a more perplexing problem. It may occur even in the face of adequate fluoride intake if the cariogenic insult is severe enough. If salivary function is not obviously impaired, the cause for such decay is almost invariably found in the dietary pattern of the child, since even a cursory glance at the food habits reveals a multiplicity of exposures to sugar-containing foods throughout the day and evening, often coupled with poor oral hygiene. The problem is to provide for the caloric needs of the active, growing child and to satisfy the psychosocial needs associated with snacking and peer activities, but at the same time to reduce the number of exposures and

FIG. 31-15. Small carious lesions developing on a linear hypoplastic defect on the primary central incisors of a Guatemalan child who has been breastfed for a prolonged period. (Courtesy E. A. Sweeney)

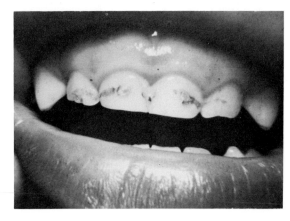

the total duration of exposure to sugar-containing foods. As has been discussed, this is best accomplished not by attempting an across-the-board proscription of all sweets, but instead, by a thoughtful substitution of suitable snack foods and counseling on the appropriate consumption of foods containing sugar.

For example, banning sugar-containing soft drinks is not usually possible, but the child can be counseled to substitute non-sugar-containing drinks. An equally important injunction is to reduce to a minimum the time taken to consume a sugar-containing beverage. The soft drink sipped repeatedly over a 30-min to 45-min period is much more likely to be harmful than the same amount consumed in 2 min to 5 min.

Between-meal snacking patterns should aim to eliminate the sugar-containing candy bar or hard candy that is slowly cleared and to substitute socially acceptable items such as pizza, nuts, popcorn, potato chips, and, whenever possible, fruit and crisp vegetables. The consumption of sugar-containing cakes, candies, and other items should be restricted to mealtimes, when their cariogenic impact seems to be reduced.

Scrupulous oral hygiene practices must be instituted as well as the daily use of self-applied topical fluoride treatments, either with gels or rinses. The use of fluoridated toothpastes should be encouraged for all children.

RAMPANT DECAY DUE TO INADEQUATE SALIVARY FUNCTION

Another serious form of rampant dental decay is found in persons who lack adequate salivary function, usually as a result of therapeutic radiation to the head and neck for malignancy (see Fig. 31-16),

FIG. 31-16. Rampant decay subsequent to therapeutic radiation to the head and neck with consequent reduced salivary function. (Courtesy E. A. Sweeney)

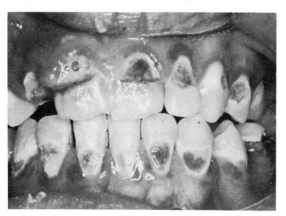

surgical removal of major salivary glands, or systemic disease such as Sjögren's syndrome. Because of the lack of saliva, rampant caries, particularly involving the smooth surfaces of the neck of the teeth, can be seen in as short a period as 30 days.[17] If intensive prophylactic measures are not instituted, loss of most tooth structure will occur within 1 year to 2 years. For such patients, the daily use of self-applied fluoride-containing gels or rinses, coupled with intensive dietary restriction of cariogenic foods to mealtimes, has been successful in reducing this massive decay to a minimum. Obviously, for the older patient with this problem, osteoradionecrosis of the jaws subsequent to dental abscess can be life-threatening. These measures of topical fluoride application and fermentable carbohydrate restriction are imperative.

While therapeutic radiation of the head and neck is the most common cause for the sudden loss of salivary function, significant losses of function over a more prolonged period can be experienced by those suffering from Sjögren's syndrome, which is believed to be autoimmune in nature and may have rheumatoid arthritis as an accompanying component. The dryness due to decreased or absent gland function is also found in the eyes and may result in a keratoconjunctivitis. These patients and any others with pronounced loss of function owing to surgical extirpation or any other cause require the same aggressive management as the postradiation patient if the dentition is to be maintained.

FLUORIDE SUPPLEMENTS

Where community water fluoridation is not possible, either because of local political decisions or the lack of an appropriate water supply, the benefits of systemic fluoride can be achieved through fluoride supplements prescribed by the physician or dentist. The use of such supplements in a community rarely results in the preventive effectiveness of water fluoridation because of poor patient compliance over the minimal period of 10 years to 12 years necessary for optimal caries reduction.

As a result of certain clinical studies on the effectiveness of these supplements, changes in the intake schedule have recently been introduced to reduce somewhat the fluoride exposure of children less than two years of age. These changes have come about as the result of observing increased numbers of children who exhibit very mild dental fluorosis of those portions of permanent teeth undergoing development between birth and age two, particularly the incisors and first molars.[1] The fluoride history of these children usually revealed a high level of parental compliance in administering fluoride supplements of 0.5 mg fluoride daily from birth through age two in areas where water contained less than 0.3 ppm fluoride. For this reason, the newer recommended doses for various ages and water fluoride content are given in Table 31-1.

Notably, no fluoride is recommended for children less than 6 months of age unless they are totally breast-fed, since there tends to be a relatively wide variation in body masses of children below 6 months of age and little development of permanent teeth. From 6 months to 2 years of age, 0.25 mg fluoride is recommended daily for children in communities where the water supplies contain less than 0.3 ppm fluoride. The fluoride level of the supplement is increased to 0.5 mg at 2 years of age and to 1.0 mg fluoride from 3 years of age upward.

When communal water fluoridation is lacking but the natural level of fluoride is high enough not to warrant supplementation until an older age (*i.e.,* communal water fluoride contents from 0.3 to 0.7 ppm), frequently the physician is faced with a child being breast-fed for periods longer than the 6 months of age when fluoride supplements should be started. If the child is not drinking significant amounts of supplemental water, or juices made from concentrates to which water is added, or eating food prepared with fluoridated water, the physician is justified in continuing the 0.25 mg fluoride supplement. This amount is adequate until the child is sufficiently weaned to be consuming reasonable amounts of fluoride-containing water and foodstuffs or the regular fluoride supplement level as determined by age and community water fluoride content. After the age of 3 years, dental fluorosis of the incisors is unlikely to be a significant problem from supplemental or water-borne fluoride intakes of 1.0 to 1.5 mg per day because body mass is great enough to render minor variations in fluoride intake harmless. However, if one were to err on the safe side prior to that age, the lower level of fluoride intake should be preferred, since the incisor teeth are usually visible in the normal situations of talking and smiling. Other minor sources of fluoride usually include toothpastes and other family uses of fluoride-containing water.

POST–ORAL SURGICAL NUTRITION

On occasion, the physician is faced with a patient who, for a variety of reasons, is unable to take food into the oral cavity or to masticate it properly. Jaw fractures, surgery, or burns are common reasons. In such cases, the short-term use of the highly nutritious liquid products commonly used as aids in weight control can be advantageous even if the jaws have been wired together, as in the case of

intermaxillary fixation for fractured mandibles or surgically repositioned jaws. In addition, a wide variety of taste experiences can be provided in most homes by placing the normal family diet into a blender with sufficient amounts of liquid in the form of milk or juices. Individual foods or groups of foods can be comminuted into a puree or semi-liquid state, which can then be taken through the lips and passed along the buccal vestibule of the cheek to enter the oropharynx posterior to the last molars. Adequate space is available in this area. In other situations, if the patient is unable to drink the supplement, it can be placed in a glass cleft palate feeder and delivered by tube to the base of the tongue and then swallowed. The need to avoid negative nitrogen balance by supplying large amounts of quality protein and adequate calories to the postsurgical or trauma patient is obvious and must be a major emphasis in the recuperative care of such patients.

CHEWING ABILITY AND NUTRITION

As the person ages and teeth are lost owing to dental caries or periodontal diseases, the normal stops of the molar teeth are lost and the lower jaw is allowed to overclose (loss of vertical dimension). This is most evident in those persons who are fully edentulous where, without artificial dentures, the "Popeye" appearance is readily seen. A further cause for overclosure occurs with the loss of alveolar bone (residual ridge resorption) resulting from the wearing of full dentures, which brings about overclosure when the dentures are in occlusion. Poorly fitted dentures frequently cause patients to remove one or more of them, also resulting in overclosure. However, less severe overclosure may also occur with loss of the posterior teeth alone, which results in abnormal forces being exerted that in turn can move the anterior teeth forward and cause overclosure of the mandible and straining of the ligaments of the temporomandibular joint.

In all the above examples, the result is that, to a greater or lesser degree, the commissures of the mouth are not stretched apart from each other, but rather overlap, and are continuously wetted by the adjacent inner surface of the lip. Frequently, one finds a chronic cheilosis owing to the continuous maceration in seemingly healthy individuals.

When natural teeth are missing, or when dentures are inadequate to allow comfortable mastication, there is always an inherent danger that food selection will be directed toward foods that need little or no mastication. This diet would not ordinarily be expected to be nutritionally complete, since meats and vegetables and fruits would be avoided. A further complication is that frequently those with seriously reduced vertical dimension are also in a low socioeconomic group, which not only prohibits the acquisition of adequate dental care, but also militates against the purchase, storage, and consumption of an adequate diet.

Summary and Conclusions

The role of nutrition in the prevention of oral diseases can be summarized as follows:

1. A nutritious and varied diet is needed throughout life, with special emphasis on an adequate diet in childhood, when the teeth are developing, and at times of extra stress, such as during wound healing. A systemic supplement of fluoride, either from the community or school water supply or by a proprietary product, is of great importance for the development of caries-resistant teeth.
2. For optimal oral health, the use of sugar-containing foods and confections that are retained in the mouth and on the tooth surfaces should be kept to a minimum between meals. Snacks such as fruits, vegetables, nuts, cheese, and sugar-free drinks are preferable. Sugar intake should be kept down as much as practical and limited to during meals instead of between meals.
3. Since the levels of dental caries and periodontal disease are to a large extent related to the individual's motivation, good oral hygiene practices are of paramount importance to supplement the benefits that are obtainable by following the above recommendations. Oral hygiene includes thorough brushing with a fluoride dentifrice and careful flossing, and possibly a fluoride rinse as well.
4. Professional oral care must be obtained as often as is indicated by the level of disease susceptibility. When caries susceptibility is high, topical fluoride applications will be a component of the care provided. Unless professional care is provided when needed, the only limitation to the spread of dental caries and periodontal disease is the loss of the tooth or teeth.

References

1. Aasenden R, Peebles TC: Effects of fluoride supplementation from birth on human deciduous and permanent teeth. Arch Oral Biol 19:321–326, 1974
2. Adler P, Armstrong WD, Bell ME et al: Fluorides and Human Health. Geneva, World Health Organization, 1970
3. Archard HO, Witkop CJ: Hereditary hypophosphatemia (vitamin D-resistant rickets) presenting primary dental manifestations. Oral Surg 22:184–193, 1966
4. Arnold FA Jr, Dean HT, Jay P et al: Effect of fluoridated public water supplies on dental caries experience. Tenth year of the Grand Rapids–Muskegon study. US Public Health Reports 71:652–658, 1956
5. Atkin–Thor E, Goddard BW, O'Nion J et al: Hypogeusia and zinc depletion in chronic dialysis patients. Am J Clin Nutr 31:1948–1951, 1978
6. Barmes DE: Epidemiology of dental disease. J Clin Periodontol 4 (Suppl) 5:80–93, 1977
7. Buchner A, Sreebny LM: Enlargement of salivary glands. Oral Surg 34:209–222, 1972
8. Campbell MJA: Epidemiology of periodontal disease in the diabetic and the nondiabetic. Aust Dent J 17:274–278, 1972
9. Cantor SM: Patterns of use of sweeteners. In Shaw JH, Roussos GG (eds): Sweeteners and Dental Caries, pp 111–129. Arlington, Information Retrieval, 1978
10. Cappuccino CC, Sheehan RF: The biology of the dental pulp. In Shaw JH, Sweeney EA, Cappuccino CC et al (eds): Textbook of Oral Biology, pp 226–254. Philadelphia, W B Saunders, 1978
11. Chapman OD, Harris AE: Oral lesions associated with dietary deficiencies in monkeys. J Infect Dis 69:7–17, 1941
12. Cutright DE, Bauer H: Cell renewal in the oral mucosa and skin of the rat. I. Turnover time. Oral Surg 23:249–259, 1967
13. Dean HT, Arnold FA Jr, Elvove E: Domestic water and dental caries. V. Additional studies of the relation of fluoride domestic waters to dental caries experience in 4,425 white children aged 12 to 14 years of 13 cities in 4 states. US Public Health Reports 57:1155–1179, 1942
14. Dilley GJ, Dilley DH, Machen JB: Prolonged nursing habit: A profile of patients and their families. J Dentistry for Children 47:102–108, 1980
15. Dinnerman M: Vitamin A deficiency in unerupted teeth of infants. Oral Surg 4:1024–1038, 1951
16. Dreizen S: Oral indications of the deficiency states. Postgrad Med 49:97–102, 1971
17. Dreizen S, Brown LR, Daily TE et al: Prevention of xerostomia-related dental caries in irradiated cancer patients. J Dent Res 56:99–104, 1977
18. Eager JM: Denti di Chiaie (Chiaie teeth). US Public Health Reports 16:2576–2577, 1901
19. Feldman R, Szabo G: Comparative microanatomy of skin and oral mucosa. In Shaw JH, Sweeney EA, Cappuccino CC et al (eds): Textbook of Oral Biology. Philadelphia, W B Saunders, 1978
20. Garant PR: Microanatomy of the oral mineralized tissues. In Shaw JH, Sweeney EA, Cappuccino CC et al: (eds): Textbook of Oral Biology. Philadelphia, W B Saunders, 1978
21. Gardner DE, Norwood JR, Eisenson JE: At-will breast feeding and dental caries: Four case reports. J Dentistry for Children 44:186–191, 1977
22. Gibbons RJ, van Houte J: Oral bacterial ecology. In Shaw JH, Sweeney EA, Cappuccino CC et al (eds): Textbook of Oral Biology, pp 684–705. Philadelphia, W B Saunders, 1968
23. Gibbons RJ, van Houte J: Cariology B—Bacteriology of dental caries. In Shaw JH, Sweeney EA, Cappuccino CC et al (eds): Textbook of Oral Biology, pp 975–991. Philadelphia, W B Saunders, 1968
24. Gibson RM: National health expenditures, 1978. Health Care Financing Review 1:1–36, 1979
24a. Glass RL: The first international conference on the declining prevalence of dental caries. J Dent Res 61:1304–1383, 1982

25. Henkin RF, Schecter PJ, Friedewald WT et al: A double blind study of the effect of zinc sulfate on taste and smell dysfunction. Am J Med Sci 272:285–299, 1976

26. Hodge HC, Smith FA: Some public health aspects of water fluoridation. In Shaw JH (ed): Fluoridation as a Public Health Measure, pp 79–109. Washington, DC, American Association for the Advancement of Science, 1954

27. Horton JE, Oppenheim JJ, Mergenhagen SE: A role for cell-mediated immunity in the pathogenesis of periodontal disease. J Periodontol 45:351–360, 1974

28. Jacobs A, Cavill I. The oral lesions of iron deficiency anaemia: Pyridoxine and riboflavin status. Br J Haematol 14:291–295, 1968

29. Kent RL Jr, Moorrees CFA: Associations in interproximal caries prevalence from a longitudinal twin study. Abstract #526. Proceedings of the International Association of Dental Research, 1979

30. Keyes PH, Jordan HV: Factors influencing the initiation, transmission, and inhibition of dental caries. In Sognnaes RF (ed): Mechanisms of Hard Tissue Destruction, pp 261–283. Washington DC, American Association for the Advancement of Science, Publication #75, 1963

31. McClure FJ: Water Fluoridation. The Search and the Victory. Bethesda, National Institute for Dental Research, NIH, 1970

32. McKay FS, Black GV: Mottled teeth: An endemic developmental imperfection of the teeth heretofore unknown in the literature of dentistry. Dental Cosmos 58:129–156, 1916

33. Mellanby M: An experimental study of the influence of diet on teeth formation. Lancet 2:767–770, 1918

34. Menaker L, Navia JM: Effect of undernutrition during the prenatal period on caries development in the rat. III. Effects of undernutrition on biochemical parameters in the developing submandibular salivary gland. J Dent Res 52:688–691, 1973

35. Newbrun E: Cost-effectiveness and practicality features in the systemic use of fluorides; Gish CW: Reaction to Dr. Newbrun's paper. In The Relative Efficiency of Methods of Caries Prevention in Dental Public Health, pp 27–54. Proceedings of a workshop at the University of Michigan, June 5–8, 1978

36. Newbrun E: Cariology. Chap 4, Substrate: Diet and caries, pp 76–96. Chap 5, In Sugar, Sugar Substitutes, and Noncaloric Sweetening Agents, pp 97–128. Baltimore, Williams & Wilkins, 1978

37. Page RC, Schroeder HE: Pathogenesis of inflammatory periodontal disease. Lab Invest 34:235–249, 1976

38. Payne WA, Page RC, Ogilvie AL, et al: Histopathologic features of the initial and early stages of experimental gingivitis in man. J Periodont Res 10:51–64, 1975

39. Pihlstrom BL, Carlson JF, Smith QT et al: Prevention of phenytoin associated gingival enlargement. A 15-month longitudinal study. J Periodontol 51:311–317, 1980

40. Rosebury T, Waugh LM: Dental caries among Eskimos of the Kuskokwim area of Alaska. I. Clinical and bacteriologic findings. Am J Dis Child 57:871–893, 1939

41. Rosensweig KA, Sahar M: Enamel hypoplasia and dental caries in the primary dentition of prematuri. Br Dent J 113:279–280, 1962

42. Russell AL: World epidemiology and oral health. In Kreshover SJ, McClure FJ (eds): Environmental Variables in Oral Disease, pp 21–39. Washington, DC, American Association for the Advancement of Science, Publication #21, 1966

43. Sandstead HR, Koehn CJ, Sessions SM: Enlargement of the parotid gland in malnutrition. Am J Clin Nutr 3:198–214, 1955

44. Shaw JH: Cariology A—Definition, epidemiology, and etiology of dental caries, pp 955–974. In Shaw JH, Sweeney EA, Cappuccino CC et al (eds): Textbook of Oral Biology. Philadelphia, W B Saunders, 1978

45. Shaw JH, Sweeney EA: The effect of carbohydrate-free and carbohydrate-low diets on the incidence of dental caries in white rats. J Nutr 53:151–162, 1954

46. Shaw JH: Nutrition in relation to dental medicine. In Goodhart RS, Shils ME (eds): Modern Nutrition in Health and Disease, 6th ed, pp 852–891. Philadelphia, Lea & Febiger, 1980

47. Shaw JH, Griffiths D: Dental abnormalities in rats attributable to protein deficiency during reproduction. J Nutr 80:123–141, 1963

48. Smith MC, Lantz EM, Smith HV: The cause of mottled enamel, a defect of human teeth. University of Arizona Agricultural Experimental Station Bulletin, No. 32:1931

49. Sweeney EA, Saffir AJ, de Leon R: Linear hypoplasia of deciduous incisor teeth in malnourished children. Am J Clin Nutr 24:29–31, 1971

50. Sydenstricker VP, Kelly AR, Weaver JW: Ariboflavinosis with special reference to the ocular manifestations. South Med J 34:165–170, 1941

51. Tandler B: Salivary glands and the secretory process. In Shaw JH, Sweeney EA, Cappuccino CC et al (eds): Textbook of Oral Biology. Philadelphia, W B Saunders, 1978

52. Tempest MN: Cancrum oris. Br J Surg 53:949–969, 1966

53. Vilter RW, Mueller JF, Glazer HS et al: The effect of vitamin B_6 deficiency induced by desoxypyridoxine in human beings. J Lab Clin Med 42:335–357, 1953

54. Vinton P, Manly RS: Masticatory efficiency during the period of adjustment to dentures. J Prosthet Dent 4:477–480, 1955

55. Wei SHY, Fomon SJ, Anderson TA: Nutrition and dental health. In Sweeney EA (ed): The Food That Stays: An Update on Nutrition, Diet, Sugar, and Caries, pp 16–21. New York, MEDCOM 1977

56. Williams RC, Zager NI: The periodontium. In Shaw JH, Sweeney EA, Cappuccino CC et al (eds): Textbook of Oral Biology, pp 255–276. Philadelphia, W B Saunders, 1978

57. Wolbach SB, Howe PR: The effect of the scorbutic state upon the production and maintenance of intercellular substances. Proc Soc Exp Biol Med 22:400–402, 1925

58. Wolbach SB, Howe PR: Tissue changes following deprivation of fat soluble A vitamin. J Exp Med 42:753–777, 1925

59. Yurkstas AA: The effect of missing teeth on masticatory performance. J Prosthet Dent 4:120–123, 1954

60. Yurkstas AA, Emerson WH: Dietary selections of persons with natural and artificial teeth. J Prosthet Dent 14:695–697, 1964

32
Pediatrics

Lewis A. Barness

Good nutrition of infants and children is an investment in the future. Poor nutrition at this developmental stage can be devastating, sometimes leading to permanent damage. Studies on brain development suggest that the earlier the deficiency, the longer-lasting the effects.[19] Reserves of the young child, particularly those of calories and vitamins, are smaller per unit weight than in the nongrowing adult. Some of the degenerative diseases may be imprinted or prevented by early nutritional habits.[6]

Normal Feedings

THE NORMAL TERM INFANT

Although infants have been successfully nourished with human milk, attempts to develop breast milk substitutes have included the use of milk of easily available mammals as well as of broths of some cereals. With early attempts at formula feedings, as many as 95% of infants fed animal milks died in the first 2 weeks of life. Not until the major constituents of milk were chemically analyzed in the late nineteenth century was it recognized that the milk of other species contained too much protein for the human infant. Protein intoxication caused diarrhea, fever, severe dehydration, hyperelectrolytemia, and death.

Animal milks, the caloric densities of which are similar to that of human milk, were diluted with water, and sugar was added in sufficient quantity to make the formula isocaloric with that of human milk (see Table 32-1). Infants grew when fed these formulas, and mortality was lowered to approximately 50%, which is similar to the present mortality rate of artificially fed infants in developing countries and is related to bacterial contamination or incorrect preparation of formulas.

With the development of electric refrigeration and less-contaminated water, death from "summer diarrhea" decreased, and infant mortality decreased to a level similar to that of breast-fed infants. Formulas are now fortified with vitamins D and C, iron, and other nutrients, decreasing the incidence of rickets, scurvy, and iron deficiency anemia.

Advantages of breast-feeding persist, including a lower incidence of tetany, infection, dehydration, and allergy; formulas have been modified to even more closely approximate human milk, at least in major constituents. Breast-feeding remains the preferred food for human infants, but mothers who choose to feed their infants with formulas should not be made to feel guilty. Those formulas that most closely simulate human milk (see Table 32-2) should be used.

Investigators and formula manufacturers are continually trying to more closely duplicate human milk. Some of the alterations in formula composition require sophisticated technology (see Table 32-3). Some are termed *simulated human milk.* Protein content is approximately 1% in human milk and has been provided at approximately 1.5% in simulated human milk formulas. Numerous clinical and balance studies have indicated the adequacy or superiority of this quantity of protein for infants.[14] In several commercial formulas, the lactoprotein: casein ratio, approximately 2:9 in cow's

TABLE 32-1
Representative Evaporated Milk Formulas*

	1–3 days	Cal	4–10 days	Cal	10 days	Cal
Evaporated milk	6 oz	240	7 oz	280	13 oz	520
Sugar	1 tbsp	60	1 oz	120	3 tbsp	180
Water	14 oz		14 oz		17 oz	
	20 oz	300	21 oz	400	30 oz	700
Cal/oz		15		19		23
Cal/dl		50		65		78

*Formula is fed every 4 hr. Total volume is divided into six bottles. Total volume is regulated by infant.

milk, has been altered to approach that of human milk, that is, 6:4. The higher cystine content of lactoproteins may be beneficial to the infant.

Infants fed lactose, the major carbohydrate in human milk, develop a stool flora similar to those fed human milk and apparently absorb calcium from the formula better and excrete less phenolic substances in the urine than those fed formulas containing mixed sugars.[3] Lactose is the sole sugar added to many infant formulas.

Whereas the fat of human milk contains approximately 8% polyunsaturated fatty acids, mainly linoleate, cow's milk fat contains approximately 1% linoleate. The simulated human milks have thus included polyunsaturated fatty acids obtained from mixtures of vegetable oils, which are more easily absorbed by the infant. In addition, some consider the polyunsaturated fats given to infants to be a deterrent to later atherosclerosis.[2]

Since the mineral content of human milk is considerably lower than that of other mammalian milks, cow's milk is diluted to lower the mineral content. In certain formulas, the mineral content has been further lowered to approach that of human milk. A theoretic advantage of the dilution of minerals is that the infant may be imprinted so that in later life he will not ingest high salt-containing foods. Although evidence is tenuous that high salt intake may be related to the development of hypertension in humans, voluntary low salt intake appears harmless and may prove to be beneficial. A more easily observed difference is that in hot climates, infants are less likely to become dehydrated when consuming formulas with lowered mineral content.

During the first few days, the infant begun on breast-feeding receives colostrum, which contains slightly fewer calories, more protein, and more ash than mature human milk. Colostrum also contains antibodies that may be significant to the infant. Since infants are not believed to absorb antibodies through the intestinal wall, IgG antibodies may be important in inactivating bacteria or viruses in the intestinal tract so that they cannot proliferate and cause disease. Mature milk contains antibodies that may function in a similar manner. In addition, IgA antibodies may serve as a barrier to absorption of harmful substances.

For the first week, the breast-fed infant should be nursed on both breasts at each feeding and should not be offered supplements. After the first week, the infant should be nursed on alternate breasts at each feeding. Frequent nursing stimulates milk production. He may then be offered 30 ml to 60 ml water twice daily, and supplements of vitamin D should begin. Some breast-fed infants develop jaundice, possibly owing to insufficient ingestion of water (which is corrected by water supplementation) or to factors believed to be progesterone derivatives. Substituting formula for breast for 1 day to 2 days followed by resumption of nursing, usually suffices to obviate the hyperbilirubinemia. Weight gain should be regular and continuous.

Infants fed simulated human milk formulas can be fed directly on undiluted formula, 67 Cal/dl. Water may be offered between feedings. These formulas usually contain sufficient vitamins to meet daily needs when the infant consumes 800 ml to 1000 ml/day.

Infants begun on an evaporated or whole milk formula should be given a more dilute formula containing approximately 40 Cal/dl the first week to avoid protein intoxication and water insufficiency. These infants should also receive vitamin supplements if vitamins are not included in the formula.

From observations of breast-fed and formula-fed infants, the following standards for infant nutrition have been developed. The growing full-term infant requires approximately 100 cal/kg/day to 120 Cal/kg/day to grow during most of the first year. Beginning at about 6 months, this requirement probably decreases to 80 Cal to 100 Cal. Infants less than 1 year require 150 ml/kg day to 200 ml/kg/day water. This satisfies insensible water loss, growth, and waste through urine and stools. For the first 6 weeks to 5 months of life, these requirements are completely met by breast-feeding or for-

TABLE 32-2
Approximate Composition of Colostrum, Human, and Cow's Milk

Constituent	Human		Colostrum		Cow	
Water (g/100 g)	88		87		88	
Protein (g/100 g)	1.1		2.7		3.3	
Casein		0.4		1.2		2.7
Lactalbumin		0.4				0.4
Lactoglobulin		0.2		1.5		0.2
Fat (g/100 g)	3.8		2.9		3.8	
% polyunsaturated		8.0		7.0		2.0
Lactose (g/100 g)	7.0		5.3		4.8	
Ash	0.2		0.5		0.8	
Calcium mg/100 g		34		30		117
Phosphorus mg/100 g		15		15		92
Sodium mEq/liter		7		18		22
Potassium mEq/liter		13		74		35
Chloride mEq/liter		11		80		29
Magnesium mg/100 g		4		4		12
Sulfur mg/100 g		14		22		30
Chromium μg/liter		0		0		10
Manganese μg/liter		10		tr		30
Copper μg/liter		400		600		300
Zinc mg/liter		4		6		4
Iodine μg/liter		30		120		47
Selenium μg/liter		30				30
Iron mg/liter		0.5		0.1		0.5
Amino acids (mg/100 ml)						
Histidine	22		—		95	
Leucine	68		—		228	
Isoleucine	100		—		350	
Lysine	73		—		277	
Methionine	25		—		88	
Phenylalanine	48		—		172	
Threonine	50		—		164	
Tryptophan	18		—		49	
Valine	70		—		245	
Arginine	45		—		129	
Alanine	35		—		75	
Aspartic acid	116		—		166	
Cystine	22		—		32	
Glutamic acid	230		—		680	
Glycine	0		—		11	
Proline	80		—		250	
Serine	69		—		160	
Tyrosine	61		—		179	
Vitamins/liter						
Vitamin A (IU)	1898		—		1025	
Thiamin (μg)	160		—		440	
Riboflavin (μg)	360		—		1750	
Niacin (μg)	1470		—		940	
Pyridoxine (μg)	100		—		640	
Pantothenate (mg)	2		—		3	
Folacin (μg)	52		—		55	
B_{12} (μg)	0.3		—		4	
Vitamin C (mg)	43		—		11	
Vitamin D (IU)	22		—		14	
Vitamin E (mg)	2		—		0.4	
Vitamin K (μg)	15		—		60	

Adapted from Fomon SJ: Infant Nutrition, 2nd ed. Philadelphia, WB Saunders, 1974; Macy IG, Kelly HJ, Sloan RE: The Composition of Milks. 1953, NAS–NRC publ 254

TABLE 32-3
Approximate Composition of Some Commercially Prepared Simulated Human Milk Formulas

Components	Enfamil* Similac†	SMA‡	PM 60/40*
Protein	Nonfat cow milk	Demineralized whey and nonfat cow milk	Demineralized whey and nonfat cow milk
Fat	Vegetable oils	Vegetable oils and oleo oil	Vegetable oils
Added carbohydrate	Lactose or corn syrup solids	Lactose	Lactose
Major Constituents (g/100 ml)			
Protein	1.5–1.6	1.5	1.6
Lactoproteins %	18	60	60
Casein %	82	40	40
Fat	3.6–3.7	3.6	3.5
Linoleic acid %	24–43	13	35
Lactose	7.0–7.1	0.3	0.2
Minerals	0.3–0.4		
Minerals (per liter)			
Calcium (mg)	550–600	445	350
Phosphorus (mg)	440–455	330	180
Sodium (mEq)	11–17	7	160
Potassium (mEq)	16–28	14	580
Chloride (mEq)	12–24	10	460
Magnesium (mg)	40–48	53	42
Sulfur (mg)	130–160	145	—
Copper (mg)	0.4–0.6	0.4	0.4
Zinc (mg)	2.0–4.2	3.2	—
Iodine (μg)	40–69	69	0.04
Iron (mg)	trace–1.5	12.7	2.6
Vitamins (per liter)			
Vitamin A (IU)	1700–2500	2650	2500
Thiamin (μg)	400–650	710	650
Riboflavin (μg)	600–1000	1060	1000
Niacin (mg)	7–8.5	7	7
Pyridoxine (μg)	320–400	423	300
Pantothenate (mg)	2.1–3.2	2.1	3
Folacin (μg)	50–100	32	50
Vitamin B_{12} (μg)	1.5–2.0	1.1	1.5
Vitamin C (mg)	55	58	55
Vitamin D (IU)	400–423	423	400
Vitamin E (IU)	8.5–12.7	9.5	9

*Mead Johnson
†Ross laboratories
‡Wyeth laboratories

mula-feeding, or a combination of these. Infants appear to be satisfied and to grow and gain well on an approximate 4-hr feeding schedule. The infant is fed approximately six times in 24 hr for the first month of life. The very early morning feeding can be eliminated at about 1 month of age. The infant can be fed four times daily beginning at about 5 months of age. The requirements for vitamins and minerals should be satisfied by either formula or breast-feeding supplemented with additional vitamins, following the general recommendation listed in Appendix Table A-1. Mineral intake that provides adequate growth is calculated in Table 32-4. Neither type of feeding alone contains sufficient iron or fluoride. Requirements for iron are listed in Appendix Table A-1; 0.25 mg fluoride should be given daily in those areas where the water is not fluoridated.

More iron than that recommended, 10 mg/day to 15 mg/day, should be avoided because excess iron intake is associated with hemosiderosis. More important for the young child, excess iron may also saturate the iron-carrying proteins, such as transferrin. Iron deficiency anemia is associated with decreased resistance, and iron excess, with decreased free transferrin, is also associated with decreased resistance to bacterial and viral infections (see Chap. 26).[18]

TABLE 32-4
Required Mineral Intake for Adequate Growth*

	Normal intake	
Mineral	(per liter milk/day)	(per kg body weight/day)
Sodium (mEq)	7	1.1
Potassium (mEq)	13	2.1
Chloride (mEq)	11	1.9
Calcium (mg)	340	58
Phosphorus (mg)	140	23
Magnesium (mg)	40	7

*Calculated by assuming ingestion of 1000 ml milk by normal growing 6-kg infant (166 ml/kg)

Other trace minerals, particularly zinc and copper, may be important in the development of the nervous system. Chromium, manganese, silicon, and even aluminum have been reported to influence beneficially coronary heart disease whereas cadmium, cobalt, and lead may be toxic to the heart, blood vessels, and kidneys.[12] Iodine is necessary for proper thyroid function in the growing child but is apparently present in necessary quantities in most areas (see Chap. 20).

The protein requirement of growing infants is approximately 1.5 g/kg/day to 2.5 g/kg/day and the protein, carbohydrate, and fat distribution of calories is satisfied with the approximation of 10% protein, 45% carbohydrate, and 45% fat, a distribution similar to that found in human milk (see Table 32-2).

THE OLDER CHILD

Beginning at about 4 months to 6 months of age, solid foods may be introduced into the diet. Earlier addition of solid foods is not generally recommended. The extrusion reflex, which causes the infant to spit when solids are placed on the anterior third of the tongue, diminishes and disappears at 6 weeks to 3 months. Intestinal amylase, necessary for the digestion of starches, may not reach adequate levels until several months after birth. Furthermore, some mothers mix solids with milk or formula, providing a relatively high-caloric density food. A sample feeding regimen for the first year is as follows:

1st month: Nurse approximately every 4 hr
10 days: Add multivitamins
1 month: Eliminate 2 AM feeding
4 months to 6 months: Add 1 tbsp to 2 tbsp rice cereal, 10 AM, 6 PM
5 months to 7 months: Add fruit, 1 oz to 2 oz jar, 2 PM (*e.g.,* apples, pears, peaches)
6 months to 8 months: Add meats, 1 oz to 2 oz jar, 2 PM (*e.g.,* beef, lamb, liver)

7 months to 9 months: Add vegetables, 1 oz to 2 oz jar, 2PM (*e.g.,* peas, beans, carrots) Also, omit 10 PM feeding
8 months to 10 months: Add egg yolks
8 months to 10 months: Add cottage cheese, Zweibach
8 months to 10 months: Wean to cup. Change infant foods to chopped foods
1 year: Table foods

Ordinarily, the least allergenic foods should be introduced first. The first food given is usually a cereal; rice cereal, which is probably the least allergenic of the cereals, is offered twice daily, usually in the morning and the evening. A month later, other foods are introduced. Foods such as apples, pears, and peaches in a mashed form are given, followed at 6 months by meats, such as beef, lamb, and liver; at 7 months by vegetables, such as peas, beans, and carrots; and at 8 months by egg yolk. Early ingestion of these foods tend to prevent complete reliance on either human milk or formula, which are less fortified with iron and can lead to overingestion of milk and subsequent iron deficiency. Prolonged excessive milk ingestion or delayed weaning or both may be responsible for increased caries. Chewy foods can be introduced at about 7 months of age. The child should be weaned from the breast or the bottle beginning at about 9 months to 12 months, and at this time the child can be given table foods rather than specially prepared baby foods.

As the child ages, the caloric requirements increase (see Appendix Table A-1). A convenient formula for the caloric requirements between the ages of 1 year and 10 years is:

$$\text{Cal required} = 1000 + 100 \times \text{age in years}$$

Distribution of foods eaten for a balanced diet should consist of the major food groups. These include two or more servings from the meat group, four or more servings from the vegetable group, four or more of the bread and cereal, and two of the milk group. The meat group consists of meats, fish, poultry, or eggs, with dried beans, peas, and nuts as alternates. The vegetable and fruit group includes dark green or yellow vegetables, citrus fruits, and tomatoes. The bread and cereal group includes enriched or whole grain cereals. The milk group includes cheese, ice cream, and other milk derived foods. Such a diet when given to provide sufficient calories also provides a suitable distribution of calories as protein, carbohydrate, and fat, and further provides adequate minerals and vitamins. Additional water must be provided. After the age of 1 year water requirements can be estimated by the child's thirst.

During adolescence, there may be an increase both of caloric and nutrient needs similar to that listed in the recommended dietary daily allowance table (see Appendix Table A-1). These needs are met by selecting from the four basic food groups. The increased nitrogen requirement of the pubertal growth spurt is proportional to the increased caloric requirement. Children consuming less than 0.5 g protein/kg/day during the phase of increased pubertal growth may develop decreased resistance to infection.

In general, nutritional needs for vitamins, minerals, water, protein, carbohydrate, and fat are met if caloric needs can be met. Certain children become food faddists or go on food binges. As long as these are short-lived, or the child does not restrict himself to one food, deficiencies do not develop. However, children should be encouraged to take a varied diet. Even such common foods as milk should not be used as a major single source of calories at any age except during the first 5 months of life. Restriction of milk intake to approximately 500 ml/day (350 Cal) usually suffices to encourage a child to take a varied diet.

Special Feedings

Certain states in infants and children require special dietary considerations.

THE LOW-BIRTH-WEIGHT INFANT

Proper nutrition of the low-birth-weight infant requires excellent nursing arts as well as attention to nutritional principles, since the proper feeding of these rapidly growing patients must be considered in flux. The high morbidity and mortality presently attributed to anoxia and birth trauma may be reduced by earlier and more adequate nutrition. The water requirement is more variable than that of the term infant. The amino acids leucine, isoleucine, valine, lysine, phenylalanine, methionine, threo-nine, and tryptophan are essential for all infants, but histidine, tyrosine, and perhaps cystine and taurine are also required by the premature infant.[17] Glucose metabolism is complex; premature infants develop hypoglycemia easily and when treated develop hyperglycemia and glucose intolerance. Premature infants absorb fat poorly.

Several principles appear to be reasonably sound. Low-birth-weight infants should not have liquid or food withheld longer than necessary. Early glucose-containing feedings decrease the incidence of hypoglycemia in low-birth-weight infants and also decrease the incidence of what is presumed to be physiologic jaundice.

Infants weighing less than 1500 g can be fed by gavage with a nasogastric tube as soon as the temperature and respiratory rate become normal, usually within 3 hr to 6 hr. Larger infants can be started directly on nipple feedings. Volume of initial feedings should be regulated to the infant's ability to empty his stomach. The first feeding should consist of distilled water, since a mixture of glucose and water is injurious to the lungs if aspirated. After the first feeding, 2 ml to 4 ml 5% glucose and water can be put down the tube and slowly increased in volume over 3-hr to 24-hr intervals. The volume of subsequent feedings is largely regulated by the infant. The complications of aspiration make it extremely important not to overfeed the baby. For the small infant, feedings given every 3 hr to 4 hr seem adequate. If the baby is sluggish, takes little at one feeding, and becomes active and alert shortly after eating, he may be refed at shorter intervals.

With the attainment of caloric intakes of 110 Cal/kg/day to 130 Cal/kg/day, most low-birth-weight infants will achieve a satisfactory rate of growth (see Table 32-5). If gain is unsatisfactory, a higher caloric intake may be offered, but at the present time, no major advantage seems to accrue to the baby from feeding formulas containing more than 67 Cal/dl. In some nurseries, it has become commonplace to feed formulas of 81 Cal/dl to 91 Cal/

TABLE 32-5
Energy Expenditures of Premature Infants

Item	Caloric requirements (Cal/kg/day)
Resting	50
Intermittent activity	15
Occasional cold stress	10
Specific dynamic action	8
Fecal loss of calories	12
Growth allowance	25
Total	120

dl. These formulas produce infants who gain faster than those fed the more dilute formula, but they may decrease water reserves and may be otherwise harmful. These formulas contain a higher osmotic load, a possible cause of necrotizing enterocolitis of sick premature infants.

The protein requirement of rapidly growing infants is not precisely defined, but 3 g protein/kg/day supports growth at rates similar to that of higher protein intake, and intakes greater than 6 g/kg/day are associated with increased morbidity and mortality of premature infants.[14]

The carbohydrate of choice for premature infants cannot be specified with certainty, but seems to be similar to that for full-term infants, both in quality and quantity.

Fat absorption in low-birth-weight infants is relatively poor, perhaps owing to inadequate bile formation or anatomically decreased villi. Unsaturated fats have been found to be absorbed more easily than saturated fats. Formulas containing medium-chain triglycerides have been found to be absorbed even better than other formulas, especially in those infants with obvious steatorrhea. Fats serve to lower the osmolar load of the formula, and formulas containing 40% to 50% of the calories as fat seem satisfactory.[5]

Although linoleic acid is absorbed more easily than saturated fatty acids by the premature infant and therefore leads to less steatorrhea and more efficient calorie utilization, administration of formulas containing linoleic acid and iron has been associated with the development of a vitamin E-responsive anemia in the premature infant.[13,15]

The optimal mineral content of the formula has not been established. Because of the rapid growth and deposition of minerals in the low-birth-weight infant, the mineral allowance suggested for the term infant is considered the minimum.

Daily oral supplements of vitamins A, C, and D, all of the B vitamins, and perhaps vitamin E are recommended. A single injection of 1 mg vitamin K at birth suffices to prevent hemorrhagic disease of the newborn.

The water requirement of the low-birth-weight infant has been estimated to be approximately 150 ml/kg/day to 200 ml/kg/day. This is similar to that of the term infant. Premature infants should consume this volume of formula by approximately the 6th day to the 7th day of life. This requirement is usually reached if the formula is diluted to 67 Cal/dl.

Some low-birth-weight infants gain poorly or not at all when taking oral feedings. Some have anatomic anomalies that restrict oral or tube feedings, and total or partial parenteral nutrition should be offered these infants, but total parenteral nutrition or gastrostomy feedings should not be adopted as a routine feeding mode (see Chap. 14).

COLIC

Colic describes a symptom complex. The infant is irritable, draws up his legs, appears to have abdominal pain, cries, and develops a distended abdomen. Many causes have been suggested, including underfeeding, overfeeding, parental overconcern or underconcern, abnormal hormones, and food allergy. Symptoms usually begin before 3 months of age and disappear within 2 months to 3 months.

Careful estimate of food intake and correction of feeding volume and density may relieve symptoms. If the baby is formula-fed, one must ascertain that the formula is constituted properly. If the baby is constipated, suitable measures should be taken for correction. Physical examination may reveal rectal fissure, hernia, glaucoma, hair in the eye, or other abnormalities that may cause similar symptoms. Feeding technique should be observed while the mother feeds the infant.

If no cause is found, the formula may be changed to a soybean or meat-base formula. Drugs, including sedatives, are ineffective.

CONSTIPATION

Constipation consists of hard stools. The normal number of stools may vary from one every 2 days to 3 days to eight stools daily, without being either constipation or diarrhea. Breast-fed infants are rarely constipated.

Constipation early in life may be due to inadequate water, carbohydrate, or caloric intake; vomiting; excess water loss; gastrointestinal anomalies, such as megacolon, rectal fissure, or tight anal sphincter; or metabolic abnormalities, such as hypothyroidism. A history of food and water intake should be obtained. Physical examination should include examination of the rectum and rectal sphincter.

Anomalies should be corrected. Diet should be corrected for water and caloric intake. Increasing carbohydrate and water may correct the condition. Suppositories and enemas should be used only rarely and then not more than one or two times.

In the older infant, increasing bulk or fiber in the diet may aid in correcting constipation. Fruit juice, such as prune juice, may help temporarily. Chronic constipation may be a sign of a behavioral disorder and may be associated with fecal soiling, abdominal pain, and enuresis. Treatment of the bowel disorder with mineral oil, 10 ml twice daily for up to 6 months, may correct both the behavior problem and the constipation.

VOMITING AND DIARRHEA

Vomiting may be due to overfeeding, improper feeding, gastroenteritis, or anatomic or metabolic abnormalities. Vomiting should be distinguished from regurgitation (a normal phenomenon of infants) and rumination (an abnormal psychological manifestation) or gastroesophageal reflux, a treatable cause of failure to thrive, aspiration, chronic pneumonia, or apnea. Quantity and quality of food intake should be ascertained. Physical examination and urinalysis, especially for the presence of infections and anomalies, should be performed. Gastrointestinal x rays may be necessary.

Infants up to the age of 1 year to 2 years who vomit should be restricted to very simple feedings, usually clear liquids. These feedings should not be offered more than once or twice. If the vomiting persists, danger of dehydration exists, and the infant should be placed on parenteral fluids.

Diarrhea and vomiting may have similar causes. If the infant has both and is not severely dehydrated, an attempt should be made to feed the child at the same time one treats his diarrhea. This is accomplished by making the diet of the infant as simple as possible by eliminating those foods that had been added most recently to his feeding regimen. Thus, if the child has recently had solid foods, such as meats and vegetables, added to his feeding regimen, these should be eliminated. The least diarrhea-producing foods are breast milk or formula, and fruits with low fiber. If the child still has diarrhea on this simple diet, he should be fed only clear liquids, but these should not be offered for longer than 24 hr. The child is likely to become very irritable if he is given few calories for longer than this time.

If the diarrhea persists in spite of this simplified food intake, the child should be given parenteral fluids to satisfy his water needs. His caloric needs can be met later as the diarrhea ceases. Parenteral fluids consisting of ¼ physiologic salt solution and ¾ 5% glucose in water provide approximately 80% free water. In the presence of severe diarrhea, dehydration, or vomiting, decreased blood pressure may necessitate use of a solution containing half physiologic saline and half 5% glucose in water. Serum electrolytes should be monitored at least daily during the use of IV infusions.

Adding Kaopectate or similar bulk-producing agents to the oral intake can only be recommended if the child is not severely dehydrated when first seen. These agents serve to solidify the stool and make the observer think that the diarrhea is getting better. In addition, they decrease diaper rash and irritation and may absorb certain toxins from the gastrointestinal tract. These agents should not be used in dehydrated infants or in infants with persistent severe diarrhea because they will increase the dehydration. Agents that decrease peristalsis (*e.g.*, paregoric) should not be used in infants with diarrhea, since they may be absorbed and depress the respiration, or they may increase absorption of toxic intestinal contents.

Once a child has been placed on parenteral fluids, realimentation must proceed slowly. Not only may the bowel still be irritable with persistent hyperperistalsis, but it may also have developed decreased enzymes, particularly lactase, so that adding any feeding may be accompanied by recurrence of diarrhea.

The child should be slowly returned to his full feedings. This can be accomplished by first giving clear liquids on the day that the IV fluids are stopped. On the next day one or two feedings of a diluted formula can be offered. On the third day all of the feedings can be dilute formula. On the fourth day the child can return to a full formula, and then daily thereafter each of the foods that he had previously been taking can be returned to his intake. If diarrhea recurs, the physician should return to those feedings that were not associated with diarrhea. It may be necessary in some infants who have had diarrhea for 3 days or longer to introduce lactose-free formulas for several weeks. Infants who have had nonspecific diarrhea for several days develop altered stool flora and may develop vitamin K deficiency. These infants should be given 1 mg to 2 mg vitamin K twice weekly while the diarrhea persists. Complete restriction of fat from the diet may cause diarrhea to persist. If weight gain continues at a normal rate and the stools remain loose and bulky, the child has chronic nonspecific diarrhea, a self-limited disease usually resolving by 4 years of age. Such children should receive a complete diet.

ANEMIA

Anemia, a lower than normal concentration of hemoglobin, red cell volume, or number of red cells per mm^3, is found in children with specific nutritional deficiencies or disorders. The most frequent nutritional causes are deficiencies in the following nutrients:

Iron
Copper
Folic Acid
Vitamin B_{12}, cobalt
Ascorbic acid

Vitamin B_6
Vitamin K
Vitamin E
Protein

Metabolic diseases, such as hypothyroidism, drug toxicity, and allergic states, may cause nutritional deficiencies that may result in anemia. Many children with anemia have multiple deficiencies, all of which must be corrected.

Anemia results in decreased oxygen-carrying capacity of the blood.[4] Children with severe anemia develop tachycardia, heart enlargement, pallor, decreased exercise tolerance, and possibly decreased resistance to infection. Because anemic children are lethargic, they may learn less well than children who are not anemic. Some may be irritable and hyperactive. A physiologic response to the anemia is an increase in red cell 2, 3-diphosphoglycerate (2,3-DPG), which results in more complete transfer of oxygen from red cells to the tissues. With iron deficiency, anemia is manifest by a low hemoglobin concentration, and the red cells are small and hypochromic. Serum iron-binding proteins are elevated, and bone marrow iron is decreased. Hemoglobin levels as low as 11 g or hematocrit levels as low as 33% are considered normal in children.

Microcytic anemias with high serum iron include the thalassemias, the hemoglobinopathies, and sideroblastic anemia. Anemia with chronic infection may be associated with a low serum iron. Anemias of these causes must be distinguished from anemias due to nutritional causes (see Chap. 23).

IRON DEFICIENCY

Iron deficiency is the most frequent cause of anemia in childhood. In some surveys 5% to 25% of children under 6 years have been found to be iron deficient. The newborn infant has about 0.5 g iron, the adult 5.0 g. The premature infant with lower iron stores is more likely to develop iron deficiency. Large intake of cow's milk or iron-poor foods is associated with this common deficiency. In addition, iron deficiency may be a cause of GI blood loss, further aggravating the deficiency.

The infant must absorb about 1 mg of iron/day. Iron-fortified formulas and baby cereals provide absorbable iron and are apparently responsible for a decreasing incidence of iron deficiency. When the infant is old enough to discontinue formula or baby cereals, the foods then introduced should contain absorbable iron.

Treatment consists of decreasing the intake of cow's milk and giving 6 mg elemental iron/kg/day. The iron-deficient infant or child will respond with an increased reticulocyte count and hemoglobin, and this response may be used as a diagnostic test. Medicinal iron may cause diarrhea, constipation, or vomiting. Staining of the teeth has been reported. Chronic excess ingestion of iron results in hemosiderosis with deposition of iron in many tissues. Acute toxicity from ingestion of large amounts of medicinal iron causes GI bleeding, liver failure, and death.

COPPER DEFICIENCY

Copper deficiency anemia resembles iron deficiency in that it is hypochromic and microcytic, with a low serum iron. Copper is a part of ceruloplasmin, the enzyme necessary for the conversion of ferrous to ferric iron, which is the form of iron transported as transferrin. Serum copper and white blood count are low. Serum albumin may be decreased and edema may be present.

Anemia due to copper deficiency is very rare. The usual childhood diet contains about 0.1 mg copper and is sufficient to prevent deficiency. High milk intake, particularly powdered milk, may result in low copper levels. Some children with intestinal diseases, particularly intestinal lymphangiectasia, demonstrate copper deficiency.

Therapeutically, 0.2 mg 0.5% copper sulfate/kg/day given orally results in prompt correction.

LEAD POISONING

Lead poisoning causes hematologic and central nervous system abnormalities in children. One of the earliest signs of lead poisoning is anemia, usually hypochromic and microcytic. It occurs more frequently in those children living in older houses and in those exposed to lead-containing paints or lead fumes.

Most lead poisoning in this country occurs in those children with pica. Such a craving for unusual foods occurs in many malnourished children, but any child may develop a perverted appetite and eat bizarre foods. Most normal children under 3 years put objects in their mouth as part of the normal sucking and mouthing response, and irritable and mentally defective children are especially prone to this habit. Since lead-poisoned children usually have low serum iron, and iron-deficient children are apparently more prone to lead poisoning, it has been suggested that iron-deficient children crave abnormal foods and thus eat lead-containing materials. Diagnosis is made by finding increased blood lead or serum prophyrins and decreased serum aminolevulinic acid dehydrase.

Treatment consists in removing lead from the environment and using chemicals to remove body lead, for example, with ethylene diamine tetra-acetic acid (EDTA). Treatment of the behavioral disorder may be necessary.

FOLIC ACID DEFICIENCY

Folic acid deficiency occurs in some children as a result of decreased intake or absorption and may cause megaloblastic anemia. The megaloblastic cells contain nuclear material resulting from a lack of maturation of red cells. White cells and platelets may be decreased. Serum folate is low, and the urine contains formiminoglutamic acid; serum lactic acid dehydrogenase is elevated. The bone marrow is hypercellular.

Daily requirement of folic acid is 20 µg to 50 µg. Human milk and cow's milk contain sufficient folate for the normal infant, but goat's milk is deficient. Rapid growth, infection, and hemolysis of red cells increase the need for folic acid, and GI diseases causing malabsorption result in folate deficiency. Congenital malabsorption of folate is associated with severe neurologic signs and normal serum vitamin B_{12} levels.

Treatment with 0.5 mg to 1.0 mg folic acid/day results in a rapid hematologic response and should be continued for about 1 month. Toxicity is rare, providing vitamin B_{12} deficiency is not present, but when both deficiencies are present, folic acid produces a hematologic response without correcting the neurologic abnormalities associated with vitamin B_{12} deficiency.

VITAMIN B_{12} DEFICIENCY

Vitamin B_{12} deficiency is rare in children in this country. Vitamin B_{12} is the extrinsic factor and requires the presence of intrinsic factor found in normal gastric mucosa in order to be absorbed. The metabolic functions of vitamin B_{12} in blood formation are closely related to folic acid metabolism, and the type of anemia is indistinguishable from that of folic acid deficiency. In patients with vitamin B_{12} deficiency, vitamin B_{12} is low in the serum and red cells, and urinary excretion of methylmalonic acid is increased. In those with suspected malabsorption of vitamin B_{12}, the Schilling test will indicate lack of intrinsic factor or other causes of malabsorption.

The daily requirement of vitamin B_{12} for the infant is about 0.1 µg, much less than that contained in most infant diets except those of strict vegetarians (vegans). Deficiency occurs in infants whose mothers have pernicious anemia or are taking a diet deficient in vitamin B_{12}. Congenital lack of intrinsic factor causes infantile pernicious anemia even though the gastric mucosa structure and function are normal. Juvenile pernicious anemia is similar to that in adults; children with the juvenile form have gastric atrophy and decreased secretion of gastric acid and pepsin with serum antibodies to intrinsic factor and parietal cells. Endocrinopathies and evidence of immune deficiencies may be present. Both congenital and juvenile pernicious anemia may be inherited as autosomal recessive disorders.

Absorption occurs in the ileum, and children with surgical conditions requiring removal of the ileum or those children infested with the fish tapeworm do not properly absorb vitamin B_{12}. Some bacterial infections, regional enteritis, or congenital malformations may be responsible for malabsorption of vitamin B_{12}.

Transport and utilization of vitamin B_{12} are deficient in the rare autosomal recessive disorder, transcobalamin II deficiency, in which methylmalonate is not increased in the urine (see Chap. 23).

Treatment of vitamin B_{12} deficiency in children is successful with 1 mg vitamin B_{12} IM. This dose should be repeated in 1 month with simultaneous correction of dietary deficiencies. With disorders of transport or absorption, 1 mg/month is given indefinitely.

Orotic aciduria, an autosomal recessive disorder of pyrimidine biosynthesis, results in a megaloblastic anemia similar to that of folate or vitamin B_{12} deficiency. Children with this inborn metabolic error excrete large amounts of orotic acid in the urine and do not respond to folate or vitamin B_{12} administration, but they may improve with dietary supplements of yeast extract containing uridylic and cytidylic acid.

ASCORBIC ACID DEFICIENCY

Ascorbic acid deficiency, rare now in the United States, may cause anemia. In children with scurvy, chronic blood loss results in a microcytic hypochromic anemia, with decreased serum iron, increased iron-binding proteins, and characteristic x-ray changes. Ascorbic acid may also participate in the metabolic activity and absorption of folic acid, and ascorbic acid deficiency may be accompanied by hematologic signs of folic acid deficiency.

The daily requirement of vitamin C in infancy is about 30 mg. Premature infants fed high-protein diets develop increased serum levels of tyrosine and phenylalanine, as well as increased urinary excretion of phenyllactic and phenylacetic acids. These amino acid levels become more nearly normal with increased ascorbic acid intake. Blood levels of tyrosine and phenylalanine remain more nearly normal in those prematurely born infants whose protein intake is 2.5 g/kg/day to 6 g/kg/day, but even in some of these hypertyrosinemia and hyperphenylalanemia occur. The latter may respond to increased vitamin C intake.

Children with infections, severe injuries, such as burns, or those illnesses requiring increased adrenocortical response benefit from increased ascorbic acid intake during the illness.

In children with scurvy, white cell counts and platelet ascorbate are low, and tests for increased capillary fragility are positive. Treatment with 200 mg to 1000 mg ascorbic acid over a period of 3 days to 4 days results in rapid improvement.

VITAMIN B_6 DEFICIENCY

Vitamin B_6 deficiency is a rare cause of microcytic hypochromic anemia in children. Such children may have increased serum iron and increased iron stores in the bone marrow. The diagnosis of vitamin B_6 deficiency or dependency is usually made after the child is found not to be losing blood and is not responsive to oral medicinal iron in adequate doses. Treatment consists of daily supplementation of 10 mg to 100 mg vitamin B_6 orally. Response occurs in several days if the child is deficient in vitamin B_6. Children with vitamin B_6 dependency require daily vitamin B_6 supplements indefinitely.

VITAMIN K DEFICIENCY

Vitamin K deficiency results in anemia secondary to decreased prothrombin and increased bleeding. Prothrombin time is increased, and especially in the neonate serious bleeding into the skin, the head, or the GI tract can result in a severe microcytic hypochromic anemia, so-called hemorrhagic disease of the newborn. Coagulation factors II, VII, IX, and X are decreased in the blood of these infants.

Because sufficient vitamin K is produced by the intestinal flora after the neonatal period, recommended allowance is not established, but 1 mg given at the time of birth prevents hemorrhagic disease. Increased requirements occur in those children receiving diets that change the intestinal flora, in those with diarrhea, or in those receiving antibiotics; 1 mg given IM once weekly suffices. In those with liver disease, vitamin K is not converted to prothrombin. Administration IM of 1 mg to 5 mg vitamin K weekly may decrease the prothrombin time to normal in these children.

VITAMIN E DEFICIENCY

Vitamin E deficiency is rare in term infants, children, or adults. Infants of low birth weight, particularly those fed formulas containing over 20% of the fat as linoleic acid, develop a hemolytic anemia at about 6 weeks to 10 weeks of age. The anemia is associated with an elevated blood reticulocyte count and an increase in circulating platelets. Seborrheic dermatitis and generalized edema have been seen in some of these children. Hemolysis is more common in children receiving formulas that also contain iron; serum tocopherol levels are less than 0.5 mg/dl, and red cells hemolyze in the presence of hydrogen peroxide *in vitro*. This syndrome has not been seen in those receiving very low fat-containing formulas.

Infants with low serum tocopherol respond within 10 days to daily supplementation of α-tocopherol 200 mg until a total dose of 400 mg to 1000 mg is given. Serum tocopherol increases to normal, *in vitro* peroxide hemolysis decreases, platelets and reticulocytes decrease to normal, and seborrhea and edema decrease or disappear. Without treatment, signs and symptoms may disappear spontaneously within 3 weeks to 6 weeks.

MARASMUS AND KWASHIORKOR

Kwashiorkor and marasmus cause multiple signs of malnutrition, including anemia. The anemia may be macrocytic or microcytic, and may be related to specific nutritional factors other than protein or calories. Iron-binding proteins are low in the serum. Partial amelioration of the anemia occurs with specific nutritional additives, such as vitamins or iron. Total correction is not achieved until the general state of the child is improved with protein and calories; intercurrent infections and infestations must also be treated.

Marasmus is the clinical state caused by severe malnutrition in infancy, which results in inanition, starvation, and atrophy of the muscles and subcutaneous tissues. Weight gain is poor, and emaciation is common. The skin is wrinkled and loose: fat is lost from the buttocks and over the body, and finally from the sucking pads of the cheeks. Malnutrition of this extent is rare in the United States but is associated with the high mortality rate of infants and children in the developing countries of Africa, Asia, and Central and South America.

When the deficiency is mainly that of protein and intake of calories is nearly sufficient for the age and size of the child, the children may develop a different appearance. This protein undernutrition state is termed *kwashiorkor*.[16] Worldwide, this is the most common form of malnutrition. Growth retardation becomes most apparent in such children between 1 year to 5 years of age, when the infant is weaned from the breast and the food consumed by the child is high in carbohydrate and very low in protein content and quality.

Gains in height and weight are below those of normal children but are not nearly as deficient as in those with marasmus. The weight deficit is usually greater than the deficit in height. First, second, and third degree protein–calorie malnutrition (PCM) levels are sometimes classified on the 50th percentile of standard height–weight–age charts. Children with heights and weights 75% to 90% of the 50th percentile are said to have first degree PCM; 60% to 75% is second degree, and less than 60% third degree PCM. Fat is mobilized early in deficiency states and adipose tissue diminishes. Physical activity decreases.

The infant becomes irritable and anorexic and loses muscle tone. There is no known tissue storage of protein in contrast to fat, carbohydrate, vitamins, or minerals. Thus, lack of protein in the diet is accompanied by muscle breakdown to provide those amino acids necessary for essential enzymes and hormones. The liver may become enlarged. Immunity is reduced, and multiple infections occur. Edema is common, particularly in those who develop infections and diarrhea. Dermatitis, including dyspigmentation and discoloration, are common. The hair may be sparse, thin, and streaky red. The hair is fragile and its texture coarse. Central nervous system changes, particularly irritability and apathy, are common.

Pancreatic enzymes are deficient. Serum amylase, lipase, cholinesterase, transaminase, and other enzymes are reduced. The serum cholesterol level is low. Anemia is common and may be normocytic, macrocytic, or microcytic. Multiple vitamin and mineral deficiencies usually accompany severe malnutrition.

Laboratory tests of PCM are significant in the more severe degrees of malnutrition. These include decreased serum albumin, decreased blood hemoglobin, decreased serum transferrin, and decreased ratio of essential to nonessential serum amino acids. Hair fragility is increased.

Treatment includes the treatment of the diarrhea, which is common. Electrolyte imbalance is corrected by oral or parenteral infusion. Calories are provided parenterally until the anorexia improves. Mineral imbalances at onset of treatment or those which occur during treatment are corrected as expeditiously as possible. Magnesium deficiency may occur, requiring measurements of this ion as well as the usual serum electrolytes (see Chap. 11). Oral alimentation is begun slowly, noting the tolerance of the infant to oral feedings and the recurrence of diarrhea.

A diet consisting of 10% to 15% of the calories as good quality protein, 35% to 45% as simple carbohydrates, and 40% to 55% fat, supplemented with all vitamins and with one dose of 100,000 IU vitamin A, is recommended. Carbohydrate should not include lactose, since many of these children are lactase deficient. Fat containing medium-chain triglycerides is absorbed better than long-chain fatty acids.[8] Feedings containing larger percentages of protein have been noted to cause enlargement of the liver without hastening recovery from the disease. Infections caused by the decreased body proteins aggravate the malnutrition and must be treated to stop excess protein and calorie losses. Dietary correction hastens recovery in the acute phase and must be supplemented with psychological support, attention to the child's wants and needs, and stimulation and challenge.

Even with recovery, these children do not usually regain normal height and weight, and many may be permanently retarded (see Chap. 11). Extensive studies on mental development related to severe malnutrition appear to indicate that the earlier and more severe the insult, the more likely is permanent retardation. Even when these children are identified late in the course of the disease, intensive realimentation should be attempted before retardation is considered irreversible.[1]

Adverse Reactions to Food

Allergic reactions to foods are expressed by reactions in the GI tract, respiratory tract, skin, central nervous system, and vascular system. The mechanisms of adverse reactions include hereditary enzyme deficiencies and immunologic and psychological factors. The intestinal mucosa contains antibody-forming cells that may cause local reactions. Protein molecules may be absorbed intact through the intestinal wall, especially in the young or following intestinal wall injury, such as follows severe diarrhea. Antibodies formed against these antigens produce a series of reactions resulting in clinical signs and symptoms. This explanation of symptoms is, however, inadequate, since antibodies to some proteins are found in patients who do not develop symptoms when challenged. Likewise, positive skin test reactions to food, and serum immunoglobulin levels of all classes correspond poorly to clinical signs.

Clinical tests for food allergy consist in removing the food and noting prompt improvement of symptoms. This improvement is followed by return of symptoms with reintroduction of the suspect foods.

MILK ALLERGY

In the young infant, adverse reactions occur most frequently to milk, wheat, and egg white, three of the foods introduced early. Very few infants are allergic to human milk. Many signs and symptoms of milk allergy have been described. A diagnosis of milk allergy may be made with supporting evidence limited to poor food intake. Milk allergy has been diagnosed in children whose only symptoms are vomiting or diarrhea owing to overfeeding, irritability owing to improper handling of the infant, or multiple nonrelated causes. Although true milk allergy is less common than diagnosed, a number of different forms of adverse reactions to milk are known.

Milk allergy is associated with bleeding from the GI tract. On feeding the infant small amounts of milk, he becomes anemic with blood loss, which may be gross or microscopic in the stool. When such children are prohibited from ingesting milk, the blood loss ceases. If they are later given small amounts of milk, they may develop anaphylactic shock.

A more insidious and less severe blood loss occurs in infants fed casein-containing foods. These children continuously lose small amounts of blood with excessive milk ingestion. This is less common if the milk is boiled; it is worse if iron deficiency has occurred before the excess casein ingestion.

One syndrome consists of frequent episodes of bronchiolitis, sinusitis, otitis, and rhinorrhea. Children with this acute respiratory syndrome are usually about 4 months to 1 year of age and may appear to have seasonal allergies. Food allergy is rarely suspected as the cause of these symptoms, but when milk is removed from the diet, chest and nasal symptoms disappear.[9]

A syndrome occurs in older children with signs and symptoms suggesting ulcerative colitis or spastic colon. These children may have abdominal pain, diarrhea, and weight loss. Stools may contain excess mucus and fat and may be frequent or infrequent. Constipation may alternate with diarrhea. When milk is removed from the diet, symptoms disappear. This has been related to the lactose in milk because it occurs in children who develop alactasia at about 2 years of age.

As with other food allergies, children allergic to milk may also develop dark circles under the eyes, hyperkinesia, irritability, and lack of attention. They sometimes seem tense and they fatigue easily. These symptoms also disappear after cessation of milk ingestion.

Except for anemia and blood loss in stools (melena), no child should be labeled "allergic to milk" or "milk intolerant" unless the symptoms diappear within 2 weeks to 6 weeks after the cessation of milk ingestion and recur with the reinstitution of milk.

Milk-free formulas with protein derived from soy flour are available (see Table 32-6). Other milk-free formulas are made with meat base. Many of these formulas are lactose-free for those children who do not tolerate lactose or galactose. Though vegetable-constituted formulas contain no carnitine, deficiency states have not been recognized.

TABLE 32-6
Formulas for Special Nutritional Use

Formula	Protein Source	Protein g/100 ml	Fat Source	Fat g/100 ml	Carbohydrate Source	Carbohydrate g/100 ml	Minerals (g/100 ml)
Milk-free formulas, *e.g.* Prosobee*, Isomil†, Nursoy‡ Neo-Mull-Soy§	Soy isolate	1.8–2.5	Vegetable oils	3.0–3.6	Corn syrup or sucrose	6.4–6.8	0.4–0.5
Protein hydrolysate Nutramigen*	Hydrolysed casein	2.2	Vegetable oils	2.6	Sucrose	8.6	.6
Pregestimil*	Hydrolysed casein	2.2	15% MCT	2.6	Starch and glucose	8.6	.6
Very-low-protein formulas‡, *e.g.* S–14 (1.1%),	Cow's milk	1.1	Vegetable	3.7	Lactose	7.1	0.28
S–29 (1.7%),	Dialysed whey	1.7	Vegetable	2.3	Lactose	10.1	0.13
S–44 (1.55%) (For leucine-sensitive hyperglycemia, renal disease, and hypercalcemia)	Dialysed whey	1.55	Vegetable	2.3	Lactose	10.1	0.13

*Mead Johnson
†Ross laboratories
‡Wyeth laboratories
§Syntex

WHEAT ALLERGY

Reactions to wheat and other foods, similar to those described as due to milk, have been reported. These reactions disappear with the removal of the offending substance. One more specific syndrome is commonly associated with wheat ingestion, celiac disease, or sprue. The child with celiac disease is asymptomatic until 6 months to 1 year, at which time he become irritable, refuses to eat or eats little, vomits, fails to gain weight or height, and develops a distended abdomen. Constant whining and crampy abdominal pain, rectal prolapse, constipation, and anemia are seen in those whose symptoms are mild or begin after 2 years of age. Puberty may be delayed. Easy bruising, clubbing of the fingers, and generalized edema may occur. Stools are frequent, foul-smelling, and greasy, and float on water. Tests of fat absorption during these symptoms indicate that little fat is absorbed and that the stools contain excessive fat. If untreated, these children remain irritable and fail to grow. Signs of fat-soluble vitamin deficiencies and tetany develop.

Characteristic changes are demonstrable in the duodenal–jejunal mucosa obtained by peroral biopsy. The mucosa is flattened with elongated crypts, and surface epithelial cells appear damaged. Lactose intolerance may be present, with alactasia demonstrated by enzyme analysis of the mucosa.

Treatment consists in the removal of gluten from the diet. Foods that contain gluten are wheat, barley, rye, and oats. Many baby foods contain vegetable-protein additives, including cereal proteins, and these must be meticulously avoided in children diagnosed as having celiac disease.

Irritability, diarrhea, and abdominal distension decrease within 2 weeks to 6 weeks of exclusion of gluten. Intestinal mucosal biopsy after this time cannot be distinguished from normal. Growth improves and returns to normal after about 2 years. After several years, gluten may be slowly introduced. If symptoms recur, full diet should not be attempted for several years longer.

CYSTIC FIBROSIS

Some signs and symptoms of cystic fibrosis, an autosomal recessively inherited disorder, are similar to those of celiac disease. Cystic fibrosis occurs in approximately 1 in 600 Caucasian live births and may be somewhat less frequent in other races. These children may have diarrhea, steatorrhea, and rectal prolapse, and they fail to thrive. Early in life, they may develop edema and signs of vitamin deficiencies. Other signs are dissimilar from those of celiac disease.

The newborn infant with cystic fibrosis presents with signs of intestinal obstruction and meconium ileus, or he may be born with evidence of intestinal perforation or meconium peritonitis. In contrast to the 6-month-old infant with celiac disease, at a few months of age he appears to have a voracious appetite. He has a happy disposition unless infected. Pulmonary infections (frequently due to *Staphylococcus aureus*), nasal polyps, peripheral edema, chronic cough, and respiratory distress are common. Rickets, eye changes consistent with vitamin A deficiency, and muscle weakness and wasting relate to the severity of the disease. Males are usually sterile.

Diagnosis is made by determining the lack of trypsin and other pancreatic enzymes in the small intestine. Determination of electrolytes in the sweat reveals an elevated concentration of sodium and chloride, over 60 mEq/liter, and is used as an accurate screening test for the disease. At autopsy, secretions of many glands are viscid and the pancreas is fibrotic.

Treatment is complex. For those with intestinal symptoms, a high-calorie diet with hydrolyzed proteins (see Table 32-6), low saturated fat, increased polyunsaturated fats, and pancreatic enzymes orally help control the diarrhea and improve serum albumin levels. Fat-soluble vitamins at two or three times the recommended daily allowances (see Appendix Table A-1) should be given in a water-miscible base. Vitamin E should be included and may lessen muscle weakness. Soybean milks should not be used because of difficult digestion. Medium-chain triglycerides are absorbed better than other fats. Supplementary sodium chloride is needed in hot weather.

Therapy related to the pulmonary complications is difficult and less successful than that related to the GI symptoms. Antibiotics, high humidity, vapor, and physical drainage of the lung are necessary. Patients with good and constant pulmonary care may reach the fourth decade.

ABETALIPOPROTEINEMIA AND ACRODERMATITIS

Abetalipoproteinemia and acrodermatitis are sometimes confused with celiac disease or cystic fibrosis. Abetalipoproteinemia is a rare autosomal recessively inherited disorder with decreased serum levels of fat-transporting proteins. Diarrhea, steatorrhea, acanthocytosis, and very low serum vitamin E levels are associated with failure to thrive in infancy. Later, ataxia, scoliosis, and retinitis pigmentosa further disable the child. Some improvement occurs with low-fat or medium-chain triglyceride-containing diets (see Table 32-6).

Acrodermatitis enteropathica is a disease of infancy characterized by diarrhea and dermatitis of the extremities. Improvement has been noted when infants are fed solely breast milk. Diarrhea is lessened if ingested fat contains a high percentage of linoleic acid or medium-chain triglycerides. Treatment with zinc-containing salts has resulted in improvement; further studies of this treatment are necessary.

LACTOSE INTOLERANCE

Lactose intolerance occurs in three forms:[10] (1) congenital lactose intolerance is rare and is inherited as an autosomal recessive characteristic; (2) acquired lactose intolerance occurs following diarrhea of any cause, including viral gastroenteritis as well as other malabsorption syndromes; and (3) developmental lactose intolerance occurs in 30% to 70% of blacks and Orientals and in about 15% of Caucasians, usually beginning at about 2 years to 3 years of age.

Intolerance is due not to allergy but to the lack of intestinal lactase. When fed lactose-containing foods, the children fail to thrive. Symptoms include vomiting, diarrhea, and abdominal distention. Later symptoms may be limited to abdominal pain and milk diarrhea after drinking milk. Stool pH is below 6 and contains reducing substances, excess fat, and mucus.

Elimination of all lactose-containing foods from the diet (see Table 32-6) improves symptoms. Symptoms may lessen spontaneously with age even though milk ingestion continues.

Sucrase–isomaltase deficiency and glucose–galactose and fructose malabsorption may cause similar symptoms. Elimination of these substances from the diet ameliorates symptoms.

ANOREXIA NERVOSA

Anorexia nervosa is a syndrome of self-starvation more common in adolescent girls than boys. Patients may be obese or may have the self-image that they are obese. They limit their food intake and lose weight but do not stop the limited food intake. In addition to weight loss and failure to eat, adolescent girls may develop amenorrhea. Their appearance must be distinguished from the similar appearance of children with brain tumor or metabolic disease. Children with anorexia nervosa usually have severe psychological problems, though in some, encouragement and psychological support may reverse the process.

Treatment is difficult. Electrolyte imbalance is first corrected, and this may require emergency administration of parenteral fluids. Weight gain following rehydration may lead to false encouragement. Total parenteral nutrition, behavior modification, or intensive psychotherapy may reverse the process (see Chap. 33).

METABOLIC DISEASES

A number of metabolic diseases are best treated by dietary means or are partially treated by changes in the diet. Diabetes is discussed in detail in Chapter 18.

RENAL DISEASE

Children with renal disease must be carefully monitored. Those children with pyelonephritis require extra fluids but maintain their customary diet. They present no nutritional problems unless the disease becomes chronic, when nutritional needs become similar to those of children with degenerative renal disease (see Chap. 34).

Children with the nephrotic syndrome present with edema, hypoalbuminemia, proteinuria, and hypercholesterolemia. The course is variable. In spite of the low serum proteins, a high-protein diet may be followed by anorexia and destruction of tissue proteins. Allowing the child to choose his diet provides calories and may prevent tissue destruction while other measures are taken to ameliorate the underlying disease. In the presence of hypertension sodium chloride intake should be restricted.

Children with degenerative renal disease of any cause are a challenge in management. These children may have growth failure, hypertension, elevated serum urea nitrogen, oliguria, hyposthenuria or isosthenuria, and formed elements and protein in the urine. Nutritional management is directed to the symptoms. Caloric intake is maintained at a high level but short of inducing vomiting or diarrhea. Sodium chloride is restricted in the presence of hypertension. The diet is high in carbohydrate and fat to limit the accumulation of nitrogenous metabolites in the blood. Fluid balance is meticulously maintained to prevent both overhydration and dehydration. Increased phosphate is given if phosphate is being excreted in excess, and a low-phosphate diet with Amphogel or similar phosphate binders is used for those with phosphate retention. Calcium is given to those with hypocalcemia. When associated with vitamin D resistance, 1,25-dihydroxycholecalciferol administration may be helpful.

LIVER DISEASE

Children with chronic liver disease likewise do well on a low-protein diet. In acute liver disease, such as acute viral hepatitis, they should be fed foods that do not cause vomiting. Hepatitis in children generally is a milder disease than that in the adult, and dietary changes are not necessary and are even undesirable. High-protein diets given to such children have resulted in decreased mental responses and neurologic abnormalities.

TABLE 32-7
Approximate Nutritive Composition of Special Dietary Products*

Nutrient	Lofen-alic (MJ)†	PKU–Aid (MS)†	Low-methio-nine Isomil (RL)†	Phenyl-Free (MJ)†	3200–AB (MJ)†	MSUD–Aid (MS)†	MSUD Diet Powder (MJ)†	Methio-naid (MS)†	3200–K (MJ)†	Histi-naid (MS)†	80056 (MJ)†
Calories	460	240	516	406	460	248	476	242	518	240	445
Protein (g)	15	60	12.5	20.3	15	64.4	8.2	63.1	15.8	61.2	0
Fat (g)	18	0	28.1	6.8	18	0	20.1	0	28	0	20.4
CHO (g)	60	0	57.0	66	60	0	63.7	0	51.1	0	65.3
L-AMINO ACIDS (G)											
Essential											
Isoleucine	0.75	2.6	0.56	1.10	0.86	0	0	2.4	0.76	2.5	0
Leucine	1.41	6.1	1.02	1.73	1.76	0	0	32	1.31	3.8	0
Lysine	1.57	6.1	0.77	1.89	1.91	7.1	0.8	6.0	0.98	5.8	0
Methionine	0.45	1.5	0.14	0.63	0.56	1.9	0.25	0.2	0.18	1.6	0
Phenylalanine	0.08	<0.07	0.6	0	0.08	3.8	0.55	4.3	0.86	2.2	0
Threonine	0.77	4.8	0.51	0.94	0.65	3.3	0.55	3.2	0.59	3.1	0
Tryptophan	0.19	0.9	0.12	0.28	0.20	1.2	0.20	0.9	0.18	1.1	0
Valine	1.20	4.6	0.52	1.26	1.38	0	0	3.2	0.80	3.1	0
Histidine	0.39	1.8	0.28	0.47	0.40	2.7	0.25	2.8	0.38	0	0
Nonessential											
Arginine	0.34	3.1	0.83	0.69	0.39	5.1	0.50	4.4	1.08	4.6	0
Alanine	0.64	4.1	0.53	NL	0.76	7.1	0.45	5.6	0.68	5.9	0
Aspartate	1.34	8.1	1.29	5.20	1.60	12.1	1.14	9.5	1.94	10.6	0
Cystine	0.025	1.5	0.15	0.35	0.042	2.1	0.25	3.7	0.107	1.8	0
Glutamate	3.78	9.3	2.48	1.88	4.31	13.3	2.09	11.0	3.12	12.3	0
Glycine	0.35	3.1	0.52	3.35	0.40	3.9	0.60	4.3	0.67	5.9	0
Proline	1.13	3.6	0.6	NL	1.13	2.3	0.90	1.6	0.77	1.9	0
Serine	1.02	4.8	0.68	NL	1.09	2.4	0.60	1.7	0.81	1.9	0
Tyrosine	0.81	6.0	0.40	0.93	<0.04	3.8	0.65	4.3	0.55	4.5	0
Glutamine	NL†	NL	NL	4.75	NL	NL	NL	NL	NL	NL	0

HEART DISEASE

Children with heart disease usually do not require any dietary change and can be managed by the usual pharmacologic treatment for heart disease. However, in those children who develop persistent failure, low-sodium diets are advantageous.

CONGENITAL METABOLIC DISORDERS

Children with certain autosomal recessive disorders of amino acid metabolism have been improved with special diets. Diets are not readily available from natural foods and must be prepared by such techniques as chromatographic separation of the implicated amino acids (see Table 32-7). Children with phenylketonuria, maple syrup urine disease, oxaluria, cystinuria, and diseases of methionine metabolism have been moderately successfully treated. When children with these diagnoses are identified, dietary information from the Academy of Pediatrics or similar agencies should be obtained. A number of vitamin-dependent states have been identified. Such children require true megavitamin therapy (see Table 32-8). Whenever one of these vitamin-dependent states is suspected, specific diagnosis must be made before megavitamin therapy is begun. Not all apparently vitamin-dependent states respond to large doses of vitamins because the underlying enzyme error may involve multiple proteins (see Chap. 25).

HYPERCHOLESTEROLEMIA

Because increased cholesterol levels are considered a risk factor in the development of coronary artery disease, lowering cholesterol by dietary means has been suggested, beginning in childhood. Blood cholesterol can usually be lowered by restricting dietary cholesterol. After examining presently available evidence, the Academy of Pediatrics Committee on Nutrition recommends no such se-

TABLE 32-7
(Continued)

Nutrient	Lofen-alic (MJ)†	PKU–Aid (MS)†	Low-methio-nine Isomil (RL)†	Phenyl-Free (MJ)†	3200–AB (MJ)†	MSUD–Aid (MS)†	MSUD Diet Powder (MJ)†	Methio-naid (MS)†	3200–K (MJ)†	Histi-naid (MS)†	80056 (MJ)†
				VITAMINS							
Vitamin A (IU)	1,151	0	2,200	2,030	1,151	0	1,190	0	1,296	0	1,308
Vitamin D (IU)	288	0	340	406	288	0	297	0	324	0	327
Vitamin E (IU)	7.2	0	12	10	7.2	0	7	0	8.0	0	8
Vitamin C (mg)	37	0	60	53	37	0	39	0	42	0	41
Thiamine (µg)	360	2,000	0.5	609	360	2,000	370	2,000	360	2,000	409
Riboflavin (µg)	430	2,000	0.6	1,015	430	2,000	450	2,000	490	2,000	491
Vitamin B_6 (µg)	290	2,000	0.5	508	290	2,000	300	2,000	290	2,000	327
Vitamin B_{12} (µg)	1.4	20	35	2.5	1.4	20	1.5	20	1.6	20	16.4
Niacin (µg)	5,800	25,000	9	8,122	5,800	25,000	5,900	25,000	6,500	25,000	6,545
Folic acid (µg)	72	400	0.12	102	72	400	74	400	81	400	82
Pantothenic acid (µg)	2,200	20,000	7	3,046	2,200	20,000	2,200	20,000	2,400	20,000	2,454
Choline (mg)	61	0	94	86	61	0	63	0	69	0	69
Biotin (µg)	36	600	0.13	30	36	600	40	600	36	600	41
Vitamin K (µg)	72	0	0.12	102	72	0	74	0	81	0	82
Inositol (mg)	22	0	0	30	22	250	22	100	24	100	25
				MINERALS							
Calcium (mg)	432	2,500	650	609	432	2,500	491	2,500	486	700	491
Phosphorus (mg)	324	1,500	440	457	324	1,500	268	1,500	324	1,500	270
Magnesium (mg)	51	300	40	71	50	300	52	300	49	80	57
Iron (mg)	8.6	25	10	12	8.6	50	9	50	10	4	10
Iodine (µg)	32	150	120	46	32	150	33	150	36	60	37
Copper (µg)	430	2,500	500	609	430	2,500	400	2,500	500	500	491
Manganese (mg)	0.7	3.5	0	1	0.7	3.5	0.7	3.5	0.8	0.5	0.8
Zinc (mg)	2.9	15	4	4.1	2.9	15	3	15	4	0.9	3.3
Sodium (mEq)	9	61	10.4	11	9	61	9.7	61	9	34	2.8
Potassium (mEq)	12	66	10.4	18	12	66	8.6	66	11.4	19	7.9
Chloride (mEq)	9	80	12.7	14	9	80	10.5	80	9	NL	3.5

*Per 100 g of powder. In these formulas, protein = nitrogen in grams × 6.25.

†MJ = Mead Johnson Company; RL = Ross Laboratories; MS = Milner Scientific; NL = not listed.

Adapted from American Academy of Pediatrics, Committee on Nutrition, Special diets for infants with inborn errors of metabolism. Pediatrics 57:783, 1976

vere restriction of cholesterol intake in normal infants and children.[5] Among the considerations is the possible poor development of enzyme systems, such as lecithin cholesterol acyltransferase, necessary for the metabolism of cholesterol.

In those children heterozygous for type II hyperbetalipoproteinemia, early cholesterol restriction may be advantageous. Cholestyramine or similar pharmaceutical agents may be required in addition to dietary restriction of cholesterol. Limited effect is achieved by substituting unsaturated for saturated fatty acids in the diets of these children; lowering total dietary fat has been more effective. Substituting complex carbohydrates and starches for refined sugar may also be effective. It has been suggested that in such children circulating cholesterol does not shut off the production of endogenous cholesterol owing to a congenital lack of feedback mechanism with 3-hydroxy-3-methylglutaryl-CoA reductase.[7] Restriction of dietary cholesterol before the age of 3 years to 4 years should be attempted with caution.

Decrease in dietary fiber, the undigestible part of plants, may be more responsible for the increase of blood cholesterol levels and atherosclerosis than dietary cholesterol. Increase in dietary fiber may aid in lowering serum cholesterol in affected children, but is still hypothetical.

FAILURE TO THRIVE

Failure to thrive physically is an ill-defined term, indicating that the child is below the 3rd percentile of standard growth charts for height, weight, or

TABLE 32-8
Vitamin Dependency States

Disease	Untreated clinical state	Vitamin	Recommended daily dose		Defect
			Normal	Disease	
Darier's disease	Hyperkeratosis follicularis	A	2500 IU	25,000 IU	?
Maple syrup urine disease	Hypotonia, seizures, death	B$_1$	1.4 mg	10 mg	Branched-chain keto acid decarboxylase activity
Hyperpyruvic acidemia Hyperalanemia Hyperlacticacidosis	Ataxia, retardation	B$_1$	1.4 mg	600 mg	Pyruvate decarboxylase activity?
Thiamin-responsive anemia	Megaloblastic anemia	B$_1$	1.4 mg	20 mg	DNA synthesis
Pyruvic kinase deficiency	Hemolysis	Riboflavin	1 mg	10 mg	Pyruvic kinase activity
Cystathioninuria	None?	B$_6$	2 mg	200–400 ml	Cystathionase activity
Homocystinuria	Retardation, thrombi, dislocated lens, osteoporosis	B$_6$	2 mg	25–500 mg	Cystathionine synthetase activity
Pyridoxine-responsive anemia	Microcytic, hypochromic anemia	B$_6$	2 mg	10 mg	δ amino levulinic acid synthesis
Pyridoxine-responsive seizures	Seizures	B$_6$	2 mg	10–25 mg	Glutamic decarboxylase activity
Xanthurenic aciduria	Retardation	B$_6$	2 mg	5–10 mg	Kynureninase activity
Formininotransferase deficiency	Mental deficiency	Folate	50 µg	? 5 mg	
Folic acid reductase deficiency	Megaloblastic anemia	Folate	50 µg	? 5 mg	
Homocystinuria	Retardation	Folate	50 µg	10 mg	Tetrahydrofolate reductase activity
Methylmalonic acidemia	Acidosis, failure to grow, retardation, osteoporosis	B$_{12}$	1 µg	200–1000 µg	B$_{12}$ coenzyme synthesis
Propionic acidemia	Acidosis	Biotin	300 µg	10,000 µg	Propionyl CoA carboxylase activity
B methylcrotonyl glycinuria	Lethargy coma	Biotin	300 µg	10 mg	B methylcrotonyl carboxylase
Chediak–Higashi	Infections	Ascorbate	50 mg	250 mg	Elevated cyclic AMP
Vitamin D dependency (rickets)	Rickets, short stature	D	400 IU	4000 IU	Calcium absorption, phosphate utilization
Familial hypophosphatemic rickets	Rickets, short stature	D	400 IU	50,000–200,000 IU	Absorption of calcium
Hartnup's disease	Ataxia, dermatitis, retardation?	Niacin	10 mg	40–200 mg	Absorption of tryptophan
Glutathione synthetase	Leukocyte activity	E	15 mg	400 mg	Glutathione synthetase deficiency

both. The term encompasses almost all of the illnesses or abnormalities of pediatrics, but the most common cause is lack of calories. Some mothers fail to give their children sufficient calories for psychological reasons, because of ignorance of requirements, or for economic or sociological reasons. Accurate diagnosis is essential for proper management of such children.

First, a good dietary history must be obtained and from this the intake of calories estimated. If the caloric intake seems sufficient or excessive, the informant may be fabricating. If the caloric intake is deficient, the physician must seek causes for the deficiency. Next, an attempt should be made to obtain a sequential growth record. Sudden weight changes are indicative of sudden changes in the metabolic–nutritional state of the child. The heights and weights of the parents and grandparents should be known, since small forebears are more likely to have small progeny. The parental attitude to the child should be observed, since lack of proper affect or good relationship may equal lack of calories in causing failure to thrive.

Except in mild cases it is probably most expeditious to admit the child to a hospital and attempt to feed him. Few laboratory studies should be done initially until the physician obtains an accurate estimate of caloric intake. If the child begins to consume calories and increase his weight, few further studies are necessary. If, however, the child consumes sufficient or excessive calories and does not gain weight, the physician must pursue the diagnosis further, looking particularly for GI losses or hypermetabolic states. Simple tests on the stool for protein, carbohydrate, and fat and on the urine for chronic urinary tract disease should be done. Tests for bone and endocrine diseases, such as hypothyroidism, also should be considered. A good physical examination should be sufficient to rule out diseases in the major systems which can cause failure to thrive, but if all of these tests are within normal limits, the physician must consider some of the rarer causes of failure to thrive, such as disorders of amino acid metabolism and growth hormone deficiencies (see Table 32-9).

OBESITY

Children whose weight is more than 10% greater than the 97th percentile for weight are prone to some complications of the obese. Skin-fold measurements are useful in determining excess fat, but the diagnosis of obesity itself is a judgmental one and includes the prejudices, desires, and evaluation of body image of the child himself, his peers, parents, and other observers (see Chap. 28).

The causes of obesity in children are multiple and are not well understood. When caloric intake is greater than caloric utilization plus waste, the child can respond only with either vomiting and diarrhea or the development of obesity. Infections and sedation, which result in keeping the child at rest, frequently herald the onset of obesity. Early feeding of high-calorie foods during infancy may result in habitual excessive appetite or in the development of fat cells, and increased numbers of fat cells may presage the later development of permanent obesity.[11] Regardless of etiology, obese parents tend to have obese children, and as many as 80% of obese children become obese adults.

Obese infants are prone to respond poorly to res-

TABLE 32-9
Determination of Representative Causes of Failure to Thrive

History
Genetic
  Height of parents and grandparents
Birth weight
  Small for gestational age
Sequential growth record
  Acute or chronic illness
Intake
Losses
  Stool
  Metabolic

Physical Examination
Abnormalities in any system

Suitable History, Physical Examination and Laboratory Tests

Disorder	Tests
Infections	Urinalysis, blood and stool culture, erythrocyte sedimentation rate
Anemias: hemoglobinopathies, hemolysis, deficiency	Complete blood count and smear
Kidney disease	BUN; urine: pH, specific gravity (SG) prot., reducing substance, $FeCl_3$, amino acids, blood pressure
Diabetes	Glucose tolerance
Liver disease	SGOT, alkaline phosphatase, bilirubin
Heart disease	EKG, chest film
Food intolerance	Stool pH, reducing substances, fat, mucus, protein, ova, parasites, bacteria, blood, x-rays of GI tract, proctosigmoidoscopy, jejunal biopsy
Cystic fibrosis	Sweat test, chest film
Endocrine (thyroid, adrenal, pituitary)	Bone age, height age, T_4, serum electrolytes, fasting blood sugar, growth hormone
Immune disorders	Immunoelectrophoresis, CBC, complement, skin tests for hypersensitivity
Other metabolic	Urine as for kidney disease, stool as for food intolerance
Unusual appearance	Buccal smear, chromosomes

TABLE 32-10
Levels of Nutritional Assessment for Infants and Children

Level of Approach*	BIRTH–24 MONTHS History		Clinical evaluation	Laboratory evaluation
	Dietary	*Medical and socioeconomic*		
Minimal	Source of iron Vitamin supplement Milk intake (type and amount)	Birth weight Length of gestation Serious or chronic illness Use of medicines	Body weight and length Gross defects	Hematocrit Hemoglobin
Mid-level	Semiquantitative Iron—cereal, meat, egg yolks, supplement Energy nutrients Micronutrients—calcium, niacin, riboflavin, vitamin C Protein Food intolerances Baby foods processed commercially; home cooked	Family history: diabetes, tuberculosis Maternal: height, prenatal care Infant: immunizations tuberculin test	Head circumference Skin color, pallor, turgor Subcutaneous tissue paucity, excess	RBC morphology Serum iron Total iron-binding capacity Sickle cell testing
In-depth level	Quantitative 24-hr recall Dietary history	Prenatal details Complications of delivery Regular health supervision	Cranial bossing Epiphyseal enlargement Costochondral beading Ecchymoses	Same as above, plus vitamins and appropriate enzyme assays, protein and amino acids, *e.g.* hydroxyproline, should be available
	FOR AGES 2–5 YEARS			
	Determine amount of intake	Probe about pica; Medications	Add height at all levels; Add arm circumference at all levels; Add triceps skinfolds at in–depth level	Add serum lead at midlevel; Add serum micronutrients (*e.g.*, vitamins A, C, folate) at in-depth level
	FOR AGES 6–12 YEARS			
	Probe about snack foods; Determine whether salt intake is excessive	Ask about medications taken; drug abuse	Add blood pressure at midlevel; Add description of changes in tongue, skin, eyes for in-depth level	All of above plus BUN

From Cristakis G (ed): Am J Public Health Supplement, Vol. 63, November, 1973

*It is understood that what is included at a minimal level would also be included or represented at successively more sophisticated levels of approach. However, it may be entirely appropriate to use a minimal level of approach to clinical evaluations and a maximal approach to laboratory evaluations

piratory infections, particularly croup. Obesity can cause serious psychological problems in both the preteen and teenager. Older obese children develop respiratory insufficiency (*e.g.*, the pickwickian syndrome—which includes hypoxemia and lethargy) and also degenerative diseases. Skin infections in skin folds, menstrual irregularities, and impaired glucose tolerance occur in adolescents.

In childhood, obesity is best controlled by advising an increase in activity with little change in the diet. If dietary change is required, it is essential in the young that the diet contain adequate protein, carbohydrate, and fat and that the caloric density and thus the caloric intake be reduced. This can be accomplished most simply by diluting the formula or milk with water or by increasing the intake of low-calorie foods. The practice of feeding obese infants skim milk is not recommended, since skim milk is a very high-protein food that may be associated with an excessively high protein intake. In the older child caloric restriction may be limited to the desired level by eliminating snacks and extra meals. It is desirable to avoid stringent dietary restrictions until after the pubertal growth spurt, since such diets are accompanied by increased protein catabolism, which may interfere with normal growth and hormonal development. Diets similar to those prescribed for adults may be used in the massively obese child.

Evaluation of Nutritional Status

Single tools for evaluation of nutritional status are inexact. However, a combination of careful history, physical examination, and laboratory studies leads to a reasonable evaluation of individuals and can be used in the evaluation of large groups. A convenient outline has been developed by Christakis and colleagues (see Table 32-10).

Such an evaluation includes many of the historic aspects useful in diagnosing the multiple causes of failure to thrive, the development of obesity, and the causes of adverse reactions to food. When obtaining such a record, inference can be drawn of family relationships, the significance of food to the family, and the medical and nutritional care received by the infant or child.

References

1. Chavez A, Martinex C, Yashine T: Nutrition, behavioral development, and mother–child interaction in young rural children. Fed Proc 34:1574–1582, 1975
2. Committee on Nutrition, American Academy of Pediatrics: Childhood diet and coronary heart disease. Pediatrics 49:305, 1972
3. Cornely DA, Barness LA, Gyorgy P: Effect of lactose on nitrogen metabolism and phenol excretion in infants. Pediatrics 51:40–45, 1957
4. Dallman PR: The nutritional anemias. In Nathan DG, Oski FA (eds): Hematology of Infancy and Childhood. Philadelphia, W B Saunders, 1974
5. Fomon SJ: Infant Nutrition, 2nd ed. Philadelphia, W B Saunders, 1974
6. Goldman HT, Goldman JS, Kaufman I, Liebman OB: Late effects of early dietary protein intake on low-birth-weight infants. Pediatrics 85:764, 1974
7. Goldstein JL, Brown MS: Familial hypercholesterolemia: Identification of a defect in the regulation of a 3-hydroxy-3-methyl glutaryl CoA reductase activity associated with overproduction of cholesterol. Proc Natl Acad Sci USA 70:2804–2808, 1973
8. Graham GG, Baertl JM, Cordano A, Morales E: Lactose-free, medium-chain triglyceride formulas in severe malnutrition. Am J Dis Child 126:330–335, 1973
9. Bahna SL, Heiner DC: Cow's milk allergy: Pathogenesis manifestations, diagnosis and management. In Barness (ed): Advances in Pediatrics, Vol 25, p. 1. Chicago, Year Book Medical, 1978
10. Johnson JD, Kretchmer N, Simoons FJ: Lactose malabsorption; its biology and history. In Shulman I (ed): Advances in Pediatrics, 21. Chicago, Year Book Medical, 1974
11. Knittle JL, Ginsberg–Fellmer F: The effect of weight reduction on in vitro adipose tissue lipolysis and cellularity in obese adolescents and adults. Diabetes 21:745, 1972
12. Masirani R: Trace elements and cardiovascular diseases. Bull WHO 40:305–312, 1959
13. Melhorn DK, Gross S: Vitamin E-dependent anemia in the premature infant. II. Effects of large doses of medicinal iron. J Pediatr 79:581, 1971
14. Omans WB, Barness LA, Rose CA et al: Prolonged feeding studies in premature infants. J Pediatr 59:951, 1961
15. Oski FA, Barness LA: Vitamin E deficiency: A previously unrecognized cause of hemolytic anemia in the premature infant. J Pediatr 70:211–220, 1966
16. Payne PR: Safe protein–calorie ration in diets. The relative importance of protein and energy intake as causal factors in malnutrition. Am J Clin Nutr 28:281–286, 1975
17. Synderman SE: The protein and amino acid requirements of the premature infant. In Jonxis JHP, Visser HKA, Troclstra JA (eds): Nutricia Symposium: Metabolic Processes in the Foetus and Newborn Infant. Leiden, Stenfert Korese, 1971
18. Weinberg ED: Nutritional immunity: Host's attempt to withhold iron from microbial invaders. JAMA 231:39, 1975
19. Winick M, Brasel JA, Rosso P: Nutrition and cell growth. In Winick M (ed): Nutrition and Development, p 49. New York, John Wiley, 1972

33
Psychiatry

Morris A. Lipton
Francis J. Kane, Jr.

Historical Perspective

Less than 50 years ago there were more than 200,000 cases of pellagra annually in the United States. Mortality for this illness averaged 33%, and about 10% of the beds in insane asylums throughout the country were occupied by patients with pellagra. In the South, the figure was even higher; from a third to a half of the state hospital beds were so occupied.[64] Of these thousands of cases, some entered the hospital with symptoms of mental illness, a not uncommon finding in pellagra, whereas others developed pellagra, superimposed upon whatever other illness might have caused admission to the hospital, because of poor nutrition within the institution. Pellagra was also common in prisons, orphanages, and other institutions.

Although pellagra had been recognized as an illness in the United States and Europe for more than three centuries, its etiology remained obscure until the classic studies of Goldberger in the 1920s demonstrated that it was not a consequence of infection, intoxication, or genetic taint, but rather a specific nutritional deficiency disease that could be prevented or remedied by yeast, liver, or high-quality protein diets.[70] Goldberger's findings of an animal model, black tongue in dogs, led to the discovery by Elvehjem in 1937 that nicotinic acid (niacin) or nicotinamide was the specific antipellagra vitamin. Within a few years, a national policy of fortifying bread and other cereal products with this water-soluble vitamin was established. This, in conjunction with alterations in the food-growing patterns and dietary customs of rural populations and in

institutions, permitted the eradication of pellagra in the United States and most of Europe. Today, this illness is found very rarely in the United States and then only among debilitated chronic alcoholics, food faddists, or those with Hartnup disease (a rare genetic disorder in the absorption of tryptophan, the amino acid precursor of niacin). However, pellagra remains an endemic problem of great magnitude in parts of Africa, India, and Central America, where extreme poverty makes corn (maize) the staple diet.[64]

The discovery of the cause of pellagra and its subsequent cure and prevention surely must rate among the greatest medical and public health advances. Yet before the cause of pellagra was known, it was for many years considered to be a psychiatric illness because of the high frequency of associated mental and behavioral disturbances. By definition, this means an illness treated by psychiatrists (physicians of the mind). After its etiology was discovered, it was removed from this category, and it is now clearly classified as a nutritional illness. In the same fashion, general paresis, which manifested itself most frequently with symptoms of disordered thinking and feeling, was for many years considered to be a psychiatric illness, but with the discovery of its syphilitic origins and its cure with antibiotics, it too has virtually disappeared and is no longer within the province of responsibility of the psychiatrist.

Psychiatry as a medical discipline deals with illnesses the signs and symptoms of which are manifested in disorders of emotion, thinking, and behavior. Psychiatrists are professionally concerned with disorders of mood, cognition, and behavior, including the affective illnesses (*e.g.,* depression and mania); the cognitive disorders (*e.g.,* mental retardation and organic brain syndromes); personality and behavior disorders, ranging from drug and alcohol abuse to the neuroses; and the psychoses (*e.g.,* schizophrenia), which are called functional because no underlying structural pathology has been discovered. With the exception of some forms of mental retardation and organic brain disease, the etiology of these manifold disorders is not clearly established. Current thinking favors psychological influences as dominant in the genesis of the neuroses and personality disorders. With schizophrenia and the depressive psychoses there is accumulating evidence for a genetic predisposition, but environmental influences that convert the genotype to the phenotype are also invoked. For most psychiatric illnesses it seems likely that univalent causality will not be found. Instead, most recent research points toward the view that there is an interplay between genetics, the antenatal and perinatal physical–chemical environment, and psychological influences in early childhood development, all of which converge to create mental illness.[57]

In this chapter we shall be concerned with nutrition as a branch of biology and shall deal with psychological elements only insofar as they reflect nutritional disorders or interact with the intake of nutrients to alter the mental state.

Strategies of Psychiatric Research

Typically, in studying the biology of mental illness or retardation the research psychiatrist employs two major strategies. One is to seek metabolic defects in individuals or groups of patients who manifest similar spectra of illness. This strategy is based on the model of *inborn errors of metabolism.* The second is based on the premise that when the mechanism of action of effective psychotomimetic or psychotropic drugs is understood, we will be closer to the understanding of the pathophysiology of the illness that they may generate or treat.

On the whole, the search for metabolic abnormalities in mental illness has been disappointing. In mental retardation this strategy has been more fruitful. Tizard has pointed out that, although many inborn errors of metabolism resulting in mental retardation have been found, no known cause can be established for 50% of cases of retardation.[70a] In the "state of the art" today, there are no chemical or physiological laboratory findings that are unequivocally found in most forms of mental illness. Diagnoses are made on the basis of manifest behavior or psychological tests rather than on clin-

ical laboratory findings. Animal models are hardly used with the first strategy because "mental illness" in animals, if it exists, is difficult to define or measure. On the other hand, such models are used extensively in the study of the mode of action of drugs because only with animals can drug effects on the brain be studied directly.

Major advances in the discovery of nutritional disorders have come initially from experimental therapeutics. Foods that would prevent or treat nutritional deficiencies, such as beriberi, scurvy, and pellagra, were discovered. From these, active concentrates were made, and ultimately, vitamins were isolated, chemically characterized, and synthesized. Later, diets specifically lacking in vitamins, essential amino acids, or minerals were created and tested in animals to permit further knowledge of the pathobiology of the deficiency state as well as the metabolic role of the nutrients. Nutritional research has been aided considerably by the discovery of animal models of the deficiency state. It has also depended on the availability of chemical assays or bioassays for vitamins or other nutrients. Unfortunately, neither animal models nor chemical assays are available for the major mental illnesses.

NUTRITIONALLY INDUCED PSYCHIATRIC SYMPTOMS

From nutritional research has come the realization that severe nutritional deficiencies usually manifest themselves in a combination of somatic and psychiatric symptoms and signs. Typically, the psychiatric symptoms associated with vitamin deficiencies do not show a high degree of specificity. Thus, in pellagra, mild and prodromal symptoms may include insomnia, anxiety, vertigo, burning sensations, fatigue, palpitations, numbness, backache, distractibility, and headache. Some students of pellagra noted a breakdown in the personality, with robust men becoming weary, apprehensive, and pessimistic. In more severe cases, patients often became severely melancholic with occasional hallucinations, confusion, disorientation, and loss of memory. Some cases resembling catatonic schizophrenia have been described. In very severe cases, patients became lethargic, stuporous, and comatose. Those advancing to this stage often died. In early cases, "pellagra sine pellagra" may be seen, with psychiatric symptoms appearing without the typical skin lesions or diarrhea. In severe cases the triad of symptoms—diarrhea, dermatitis, dementia—invariably appears. Treatment with niacin is almost always dramatic: the beginning of clinical recovery can be seen in 24 hr and is usually complete within a few weeks.

The psychiatric symptoms of thiamin, riboflavin, or pyridoxine deficiency in adults resemble those of niacin deficiency, but the somatic symptoms differ considerably. Diagnosis of specific deficiency states requires a history, somatic manifestations specific for the vitamin, and laboratory tests for circulating vitamin levels or for the metabolic derangements caused by the deficiency state.[66]

Thus, it is difficult to discriminate between the psychiatric symptoms caused by a clinical deficiency of any single vitamin of the B complex from any other. In part, this may be due to the likelihood that poor nutrition in humans is usually associated with multiple rather than single dietary deficiencies. For example, in clinical pellagra there is often a riboflavin deficiency as well as the niacin deficiency. Similarly, in alcoholism, where so many calories are derived from alcohol that intake of protein and other nutrients is diminished, there are probably combined deficiencies of thiamin and other water-soluble vitamins. More likely, however, the lack of specificity may be attributed to the multiple enzymatic reactions in which the water-soluble vitamins participate as cofactors. For thiamin, there are at least two such reactions; for pyridoxine, there are about 50 reactions. A specific vitamin deficiency would therefore likely involve several metabolic derangements, and these would lead to multiple somatic and psychiatric symptoms.

The wide spectrum of psychiatric symptoms in nutritional deficiencies is probably also associated with the severity and duration of the disorder. Vitamins are usually precursors of coenzymes, and the dissociation constants for a given coenzyme and its many apoenzymes vary considerably. Hence, a mild deficiency would probably not affect all metabolic reactions equally. Furthermore, the metabolic rate of tissues varies with age and endocrine state. Different organs have different metabolic rates and different capacities for recovery or regeneration after injury. Hence, vitamin deficiencies are likely to be more damaging in infants than in adults, and the rapidly growing brain of the child is particularly sensitive. Acute deficiencies treated rapidly can lead to full recovery. Chronic deficiencies or repeated episodes of acute deficiency may lead to permanent brain damage.

In general, there is no substantive evidence that the common major psychiatric illnesses of adults in this country are caused by nutritional deficiencies or that they may be effectively treated by dietary correction. Yet, there is good evidence that inadequate nutrition plays a significant role in the mental retardation and the behavioral disturbances found in children in those nations where the food supply is inadequate. It also plays a role in the rare genetic vitamin-dependency illnesses, where extraordinarily large quantities of specific vitamins are required to prevent and to treat both the somatic and the behavioral disturbances that occur on a "normal" diet.[65] Nutritional inadequacy, especially of vitamins, may also occur following the chronic ingestion of drugs administered by the physician for the treatment of other conditions (see Chap. 19). Each of these will be discussed.

Finally, a group of psychiatrists, who call themselves megavitamin therapists or orthomolecular psychiatrists, advocates the use of huge quantities of vitamins for the treatment of schizophrenia, learning disabilities and hyperkinesis in children, and other mental and physical disorders. The evidence supporting and refuting the use of megavitamins will be critically reviewed.

Protein–Calorie Malnutrition and Mental Retardation

It is estimated that several hundred million people throughout the world suffer from malnutrition. Given continued population growth and the concurrent energy shortages, famine or at least chronic malnutrition will almost certainly worsen in many underdeveloped countries.

Many studies in impoverished societies have shown that severe, prolonged protein–calorie malnutrition is especially devastating to infants and children and that the consequences are prolonged and perhaps irreversible. The results of such studies have been summarized in several excellent monographs derived from international conferences on this subject.[17,66,70a] One exception to these findings is a recent epidemiologic follow-up study of the long-term consequences of a year-long famine in Western Holland during the Nazi occupation of 1944 to 1945.[68] No permanent effects on the physical or mental development of the children born during this period were seen. The Holland study is interesting in its own right, but the results of a brief interlude of malnutrition in an otherwise well-endowed nation cannot be generalized to nations where moderate malnutrition is endemic and where periodic famine is superimposed upon the chronic malnutrition.

Studies of the growth of the human brain and of the effects of malnutrition on the growth and development are more limited than those with animals. Nonetheless, Winick has shown that in the human the number of brain cells increases linearly from gestation until birth, then increases more slowly until about 10 months of age, at which time it virtually stops.[72] Cell size, in contrast to cell number, continues to increase for several years. Myelination occurs rapidly at birth and is still occurring at 2 years of age. The weight of the brain increases rapidly through gestation and the first 2 years of life. Its rate of growth diminishes thereafter, but adult weight is not reached until adolescence.

A few studies have been conducted on the brains of children who have died from malnutrition. The available data show that children dying from marasmus have 15% to 60% fewer brain cells than normal children of comparable age. The 60% reduction is found in infants who weighed less than 5 lb at birth; the 15% reduction is found in children with normal birth weights. It is not certain whether the child with 60% reduction was a premature infant who was more susceptible to malnutrition after birth, or whether this represents a clinical counterpart to the rat that is malnourished during gestation as well as immediately after birth.

Children with kwashiorkor who become malnourished after being taken off the breast in the second or third year of life have a normal number of brain cells, but the size of the cells is diminished.[56]

Behavioral studies of children who survive early severe malnutrition have been reported by several groups of workers. These studies show that such children have profound disturbances in the acquisition of language, in motor skills, in interpersonal relationships, and in adaptive and motivational behavior. Memory defects have also been found.[17]

Most of these studies have been limited to only a few years after recovery from malnutrition. However, an on-going longitudinal study by Cravioto and DeLicardie should ultimately give an answer to the question of whether or not the damaging consequences of early malnutrition are truly irreversible and lead to a vicious cycle in which malnutrition during infancy results in a large pool of poorly functioning people who, because of their poor level of functioning, rear their children under conditions destined to produce a new generation of malnourished people.

ANIMAL STUDIES

The mechanisms by which malnutrition results in structural and functional deficits of the brain have been examined more thoroughly in animals than in humans. In malnourished infant rats there are lower brain weights, fewer neurons, more abnormal neurons, and less DNA, RNA, lipid, cholesterol, phospholipid, and protein. Myelination is retarded, and the pituitaries are smaller, with a diminished concentration of growth hormone. In the rat, DNA synthesis and cell division stop at 17 days to 21 days after birth, but the net protein content (indicating growth in cell size) increases until 99 days. Rats malnourished for the first 17 days of

life show a permanent diminution in the number of brain cells, with different areas of the brain showing greater sensitivity than others. Malnutrition during pregnancy causes an even greater diminution in brain cell number in the offspring, and the brain is apparently sensitized so that additional malnutrition immediately after birth can result in a reduction of cell number by 60%. Rats malnourished after day 21, when brain cell number is no longer increasing, have a diminished cell size, but this is reversible if adequate nutrition is instituted by the 42nd day. Myelination in the rat occurs most rapidly during the 10th to the 21st day. Malnutrition during the first 3 weeks of life causes a deficit in total brain cholesterol and in myelination, which persists for a long period, even when the animals are nutritionally rehabilitated. Acetylcholinesterase activity is persistently elevated after neonatal malnutrition, and norepinephrine and serotonin levels are transiently reduced.[17,70a]

These chemical changes have behavioral correlates. Turkewitz has shown that rats malnourished from infancy show increased spontaneous fighting and increased passive avoidance following foot shock.[71] Adult rats malnourished from infancy show a 50% decrease in biogenic amines following major stress. This suggests a more limited capacity to tolerate stress than is shown by normal adults or by rats malnourished as adults. Rats malnourished during development also show a greater susceptibility than normal to electroconvulsive shock. This is only partially reversed by nutritional rehabilitation. Rats malnourished early in life show a motivational deficit in learning situations and, even when motivation is eliminated as a factor, there remains a deficit in learning tasks involving discrimination. Rats that are the progeny of six to eight generations of malnourishment and that are themselves malnourished show a deficit in learning of tasks that involve discrimination between correct and incorrect stimuli.[66]

The monkey, which is capable of much more complex learning and social interaction than the rat, has been used by Zimmerman and colleagues to study the behavioral consequences of malnutrition.[66] In general, monkeys that are made protein deficient at 4 months of age show less play, less sexual behavior, less grooming, and more aggressive behavior than do animals with adequate protein. Such low-protein monkeys show a striking avoidance of novel stimuli (neophobia), whereas high-protein animals show consistent approach responses. In learning situations, low-protein animals show no deficit in learning set performance or long-term memory, and they are able to perform tasks that do not require detailed attention. On the other hand, they show deficits in tasks requiring attentional or observational behavior. Whether or not this attentional deficit will persist after recovery from malnutrition remains unknown.

Many of the behavioral changes noted in malnourished animals have been shown actually to be a product of both malnourishment and stimulus deprivation. This is particularly striking in ingenious experiments reported by Frankova, who measured exploratory activity in rats.[24] Protein-deficient rats raised with their mothers and litter mates showed about 20% decrement in exploratory activity. They also showed abnormal behavior, including freezing (becoming immobile), trembling, and stereotypy. Rats on a normal diet, that have restricted optical and acoustic stimuli and little contact with the experimenters, show about a 30% decrement in exploratory activity. Rats deprived of both protein and stimuli show a 90% decrement. The effects of both types of deprivation simultaneously are thus more than additive, they are synergistic. The introduction of an "aunt"—a nonpregnant virgin female—into the cages of protein-deprived infant rats elevated their performance to that of normal rats. Such a "mother's helper," though she cannot offer food, tended to normalize the behavior of the rat mother and the pups.

Nutritional and Psychosocial Interaction

Prior to the past decade, research in the field of undernutrition of children focused on the somatic effects of malnourishment. More recently, it has emphasized the effects on mental function. Most studies have shown that survivors of early severe malnutrition differ from normal children in a great variety of functional aspects, ranging from psychomotor behavior to intersensory organization.[17,70a] Deficits have been found in children up to 7 years of age, but the long-term studies required to determine whether these deficits are permanently irreversible have not yet been done. Recent studies of the behavioral effects of early malnutrition have focused on the predisposing ecological conditions, since many of the factors that either cause or accompany malnutrition are themselves capable of retarding mental and behavioral development.

DeLicardie and Cravioto studied the ecological factors that determine which of the children in a cohort of 300 (born in 1 year in a primarily agricultural community in Central America, where literacy is low) developed marasmus or kwashiorkor.[17] In this population, 83% of the children showed no clinical signs of malnutrition, 11.2% showed mild-to-moderate malnutrition, and 5% showed severe malnutrition. Severe malnutrition peaked at 9% after the first year of life, when breastfeeding stopped. To determine the ecological correlates of the severe malnutrition, the authors measured biologic, social, economic, and psychological variables in the environment of those children. No correlations were found with per capita income, family size, sanitary facilities, age of mother, education, literacy, or the mother's personal hygiene. Curiously, mothers who listened to the radio had fewer children with severe malnutrition. On the other hand, positive correlations were found with the microenvironment of the children. Psychologists studying this cohort of children, who were unaware of the nutritional antecedents of the children, found that the degree of psychological stimulation offered at age 6 months to those children who later developed severe malnutrition was significantly lower than that of controls matched by age and birth weight. Similarly, at age 4 years, children who were medically treated and who had recovered from severe malnutrition continued to live in homes where psychosocial stimulation was significantly below that of the control group. Measurement of psychological stimulation in these ecological studies involved the assessment of the following: (1) frequency and stability of adult contact, (2) vocal stimulation, (3) need gratification, (4) emotional climate, (5) avoidance of restriction, (6) breadth of experience, (7) aspects of the physical environment, and (8) available play materials.

The findings of Cravioto and DeLicardie appear to answer the question of why it is that in a relatively homogeneous socioeconomic and cultural macroenvironment, in which many children show mild-to-moderate malnutrition, only a few develop severe malnutrition. These few seem to suffer simultaneously from protein–calorie undernutrition and psychosocial deprivation. The combination seems to be synergistic and leads to devastating developmental consequences. Critical periods in early development exist for adequate nutriton and for the psychological input. Psychosocial deprivation seems to predispose to severe malnutrition those children whose diets are marginal nutritionally. Malnutrition, in turn, diminishes motivation, exploratory behavior, and those complex signals that ordinarily elicit a stimulating and gratifying response from adult parents. A vicious cycle is set up in which the effects of malnutrition synergize with those of environmental deprivation, and the consequences may well lead to irreversible emotional and mental disorders of development. It is interesting that the need for both adequate nourishment and environmental stimulation is not limited to humans but has been demonstrated in every mammalian species that has been studied. Frankova has summarized the work of many investigators who have shown in animal studies that infant stimulation causes increased brain weight and a denser cortex, more rapid myelination, accelerated development of an adult EEG, earlier development of the hypothalamus and pituitary system, and increased exploratory activity in adulthood.[24] Behaviorally, stimulated infants show less emotionality in novel situations and greater tolerance to stress.[17,70a] It is quite remarkable that the effects of infant animal stimulation produce so many positive anatomic, chemical, and behavioral changes that are dramatically opposite to the negative effects produced by malnutrition. There is no reason to believe that similar effects do not occur in humans.

Vitamin Deficiency States

VITAMIN REQUIREMENTS

A variety of methods has traditionally been used to determine the vitamin requirements of a subject. One strategy has been the investigation of large populations in which nutritional deficiency is endemic or smaller populations in which nutritional deficiency is deliberately produced. The quantity of nutrient required to eliminate the signs and symptoms of the deficiency and to maintain health is then considered the recommended dietary allowance (RDA). A second approach is the search for and measurement of abnormal metabolites in the blood and urine known to exist in specific vitamin deficiencies, for example, elevated blood pyruvate in thiamin deficiency. The dose of a specific vitamin required to correct this biochemical abnormality is considered to be the daily requirement. Finally, direct measurement of the vitamin in the blood and urine by chemical or microbiologic means has been employed, and "normal" levels have been established. This strategy involves the use of large populations of healthy subjects of different age, sex, and race in order to obtain normative data.

Recently, a new approach to the measurement of vitamin requirements has been proposed, based on the assumption that enzymes requiring cofactors should be fully saturated with cofactor at all times and that a vitamin deficiency exists if they are unsaturated. With this method, human deficiencies are claimed to be detected and measured by an enzymatic assay based on measuring the degree of saturation by the coenzyme of coenzyme–apoenzyme system. This method employs what has been called the CAS principle.[40]

The assumption that enzymes requiring cofactors should be fully saturated and therefore operating at maximal speed at all times can be questioned. Regulation of enzymatic metabolic reactions is essential for adaptation. Many forms of regulation exist and unsaturation of the enzyme–coenzyme complex may be one of them. Furthermore, the vitamin cofactors act with many apoenzymes, each of which has a different affinity for the cofactor. Saturating the enzyme with the lowest affinity could lead to supersaturation of other enzymes and to undesired reactions. As a case in point, the beneficial effects of L-dopa in parkinsonism can be negated by simultaneously administering gram doses of pyridoxine. This is because the peripheral decarboxylase which converts L-dopa to dopamine in the periphery is ordinarily unsaturated. The additional B_6 saturates it and quickly decarboxylates the L-dopa in the gut and elsewhere in the periphery, thus making it unavailable to the central nervous system where it is needed. Nonetheless, the suggestion that nutritional state can be measured by measuring cofactor-containing enzyme kinetics is intriguing. Its clinical utility remains to be determined.

IATROGENIC-INDUCED VITAMIN DEFICIENCIES

Lasagna has coined the term *disease of medical progress* for those illnesses that come about as a result of the use of pharmacologic agents prescribed by a physician for the treatment of illness. The Boston Drug Surveillance Program has reported the following: (1) 30% of hospitalized medical patients suffer at least one drug-related adverse reaction, affecting up to 3,000,000 patients per year nationally; (2) 3% of all admissions are the result of drug reactions; and (3) deaths in the nation from these causes approximate 29,000/year.[31] Older patients are more at risk for all kinds of illnesses and use a disproportionate number of pharmacologic agents, so they are also at greater risk than other populations for the development of such illness. This section will briefly review the acquired vitamin deficiencies as they occur, usually secondary to the use of pharmacologic agents. These most commonly follow the long-term use of antituberculosis drugs, anticonvulsants, and oral contraceptives. A more comprehensive review of this topic is available.[45] (See also Chap. 19.)

VITAMIN B_6—PYRIDOXINE

The role of this vitamin in neurobiology has recently been reviewed.[19] Adults with proved vitamin B_6 deficiency show a microcytic anemia that fails to respond to iron but improves dramatically following treatment with small doses of the vitamin. Psychological symptoms may include lassitude, weakness, anorexia, depression, and mental confusion. In mild deficiency states the mental symptoms may precede the somatic ones.

Two drugs commonly used in the treatment of tuberculosis can cause vitamin B_6 deficiency. Isoniazid and cycloserine form carboxyl addition compounds with pyridoxal or pyridoxal phosphate and thus inactivate several of the enzymes for which pyridoxal is a coenzyme. Reported complications associated with the use of these drugs usually involve the central nervous system. Neurologic symptoms may include somnolence, headache, tremor, dysarthria, abnormal EEG, and convulsions. Psychiatric symptoms that have been reported include both euphoria and depression, loss of self-control, and acute psychotic episodes in which loss of reality testing is apparent. The administration of vitamin B_6 supplements along with antituberculosis medication is recommended because several reports indicate that neurologic symptoms disappear when the vitamin is given in appropriate quantities.[12] Curiously, the psychiatric symptoms associated with cycloserine administration are less responsive than the neurologic ones. Sodium glutamate administered with pyridoxine has been reported to abolish cycloserine-induced psychoses.[35]

Evidence indicates that estrogens and other steroids compete with pyridoxal phosphate for binding sites, causing a redistribution of the cofactor among apoenzymes. High estrogen levels, which occur during pregnancy or with the use of oral contraceptives, stimulate the activity of hepatic tryptophan oxygenase and thereby might increase the requirements for vitamin B_6. Indeed, deficiency of B_6 has been reported in women taking oral contraceptive agents and in pregnant women, with the deficiency occurring gradually and the most significant decrease paralleling the period of most intensive growth and energy retention of the fetus.[7,60]

Pyridoxal phosphate is an essential cofactor for the decarboxylase involved in the formation of serotonin from tryptophan and of dopamine from dopa. Thus, as a consequence of B_6 deficiency, diminished levels of serotonin and catecholamines might occur. Deficiency of serotonin and the catecholamines has been implicated as a possible cause of depression, and the deficiency of pyridoxine might thereby contribute to the production of depression.[42,52] In therapeutic trials on women who developed depression during pregnancy or while taking oral contraceptives, vitamin B_6 supplementation has been reported to improve mood and to correct the abnormal urinary excretion of tryptophan metabolites.[58,73] Adams and associates found that of 22 depressed women whose symptoms were judged

to be due to the use of oral contraceptive agents, 11 patients exhibited biochemical evidence of a deficiency of pyridoxine.[1] These women responded clinically to the administration of extra B_6, whereas the remaining 11 women, who had normal B_6 levels, did not respond to vitamin supplementation. Based on findings such as these, some investigators recommend the inclusion of supplemental B_6 into oral contraceptive preparations.[59] Oral contraceptives manufactured in Spain at the present time contain 25 mg pyridoxine, and the combination is reported to produce fewer side-effects.[54]

Since vitamin B_6 is a cofactor for about 50 decarboxylase and transaminase enzymes, it is unlikely that only one clinical symptom, that is, depression, would be associated with a pyridoxine deficiency. Consideration must therefore be given to the possibility of functional pyridoxine deficiency being contributory to other types of reported physical and mental side-effects.

VITAMIN B_{12}

Vitamin B_{12} is involved in a wide variety of metabolic processes, including transmethylation reactions and synthesis of amino acids, purines, and pyrimidines. This vitamin is vital for blood formation and the maintenance of neuronal integrity in humans.

A vitamin B_{12} deficiency owing to failure to absorb this vitamin (because of a lack of the gastic intrinsic factor) results in pernicious anemia. Similar absorption failures may result from tropical sprue, ileitis, bowel operations, and some pharmacologic agents.

A number of studies have shown that 25% to 30% of patients with pernicious anemia have either major or minor psychiatric problems.[30] These include depression and apathy, irritability, difficulties in concentration, confusion, and paranoid states. Neurologic symptoms result from demyelination of the dorsal columns and the pyramidal tracts, and constitute a syndrome known as *combined system disease*. As many as 60% of pernicious anemia patients have been found to have abnormal EEG.[14]

Patients with pernicious anemia and low serum B_{12} excrete increased amounts of methylmalonic acid. Treatment with amounts of B_{12} that correct the hematologic abnormality may be inadequate to correct the metabolic abnormality, which disappears slowly with large doses. This may be one reason why mental changes may persist for some time after hematologic remission. Another reason may be that the patchy demyelination that sometimes occurs in the cerebral cortex may be irreversible.

Acquired vitamin B_{12} deficiency may follow the

chronic ingestion of alcohol or may result from folic acid deficiency because folate is required for absorption of B_{12}.[66] A deficiency may also follow the administration of neomycin, para-amino-salicylic acid, or colchicine. There is also an increased requirement for vitamin B_{12} during pregnancy.

The incidence of vitamin B_{12} deficiency in routinely admitted psychiatric patients has been reported to be 2% to 20%. Many of these patients fail to show clinical anemia or megaloblastic bone marrow. Populations especially at risk include elderly patients and any patients receiving tranquilizers, antidepressants, or antituberculosis drugs. Since the chemical assay of vitamin B_{12} blood levels in the preanemic state is neither simple nor routine, patients at risk may be most economically screened by blood smears and observations of cell morphology. Therapeutic trials with large doses of B_{12} may be worthwhile, but results with preanemic psychiatric patients are inconsistent, with both excellent results and failures having been reported.[67]

FOLIC ACID

Folic acid (pteroylglutamic acid) is required in a large number of metabolic reactions in which l-carbon fragments are involved. In deficiency states there is impairment in synthesis of serine from glycine and in the synthesis of purines and pyrimidines needed for DNA synthesis. Folic acid is also involved in transmethylation reactions and is thus required for the synthesis of methionine from homocysteine. Methionine in the form of S-adenosylmethionine is active in the transmethylation of many compounds. Since transmethylation reactions are involved in the metabolic inactivation of norepinephrine, and since aberrant transmethylation has been suggested as a source of endogenous hallucinogens (which might be implicated in schizophrenia), the role of folic acid in the pathogenesis of schizophrenia has received serious attention.[53] Three lines of evidence suggest such a relationship: (1) methionine, at a level of 20 g/day, exacerbates the symptoms of about 20% of stabilized schizophrenics; (2) large doses of folic acid have been reported to act like methionine on schizophrenics; and (3) *in vitro* brain preparations using a folate cofactor have been shown to synthesize dimethyltryptamine and other hallucinogens.

The search for abnormalities in folic acid metabolism in most psychiatric patients has not been rewarding thus far. However, in geriatric studies it has been found that 67% to 80% of admissions to an old age home or to a geriatric mental ward were folate deficient.[38] The symptoms most often seen were apathy, withdrawal, lack of motivation, and depression. Another report suggests that chronic schizophrenics, endogenous depressives, and patients with organic psychoses who are treated with folic acid and vitamin B_{12} in addition to their usual medication have shorter hospital stays and leave the hospital in better condition than do patients treated by conventional methods alone.[45]

Another population at risk is those receiving medication for epilepsy. A number of recent reviews related to the prevalence of folic acid deficiency in patients receiving anticonvulsant medications have implicated phenytoin, but phenobarbital alone produced microcytosis in 34% of one group of patients.[62] Apathy and slowing of the processes were prominent in this population, but Reynolds has reported that most of 26 treated epileptic patients given folic acid supplements improved in drive, alertness, concentration, sociability, and speed of thinking after 1 month to 3 months of treatment.[62]

In a recent study, Hunter, Barnes, and co-workers gave pharmacologic doses of folic acid to 14 healthy volunteers and had to abandon the study after 1 month because of disturbing behavioral effects in most of the subjects.[37] Malaise and irritability were most common. Five subjects became overactive and excitable, several had insomnia, two became depressed, and several had episodes of confusion and difficulty in concentration. Whether or not these symptoms were related to the formation of abnormal metabolites derived from neurotransmitters is not known. Nonetheless, it is interesting that excesses of this vitamin can produce mental symptoms.

VITAMIN DEPENDENCY ILLNESSES

The term *vitamin dependency illness* refers to a group of rare, autosomal recessive genetic illnesses in which the daily requirement for specific vitamins may be 10 to 1000 times the estimated daily requirement of normal subjects. These illnesses are manifest at birth or in early childhood; unless treated with massive doses of the appropriate vitamin, severe mental retardation, convulsions, anemia, heart disease, and similar illnesses occur. If not treated, death will often occur at an early age. These illnesses can be diagnosed by demonstrable abnormalities in amino acid levels or other protein and carbohydrate metabolites in the blood and urine. They have been shown to occur for every one of the water-soluble vitamins with the exceptions of riboflavin, ascorbic acid, and pantothenic acid. We suspect that, sooner or later, dependency illnesses for these vitamins will also be discovered. This topic has been extensively reviewed in the recent literature.[56,65,66]

The first of these illnesses was discovered in 1954, when the sibling of a child who had died from an undiagnosed and untreatable disorder was found to be having convulsions that responded to 3.0 mg pyridoxine daily (10 times the estimated daily requirement for infants).[36] This child was treated too late to prevent mental retardation, but several years later it was demonstrated that early diagnosis and treatment of this condition with large doses of pyridoxine throughout the entire period of childhood is compatible with normal mental development. Later, it was demonstrated that this disorder is genetic in origin, and in 1971 it was shown that reduction of glutamic acid decarboxylase activity occurs in the kidney of a child with pyridoxine-dependent seizure disease. Normal enzyme activity can be restored with the addition of high concentrations of the coenzyme pyridoxal phosphate *in vitro*. Children with this disorder are unable to convert glutamic acid to the inhibitory neurotransmitter, γ-aminobutyric acid (GABA), and this deficiency is apparently responsible for the seizures.

By 1970, 14 vitamin-responsive inherited metabolic diseases had been discovered; by 1974, the number had grown to 25.[65] These genetic illnesses manifest themselves as disorders of many organ systems, and the associated clinical symptomatology may vary from none to death. Of these vitamin-responsive disorders, 14 that involve 6 of the water-soluble vitamins of the B complex have been found to produce neurologic abnormalities. At least 6 vitamin dependency disorders result in medical retardation that is treatable with early detection. One case of childhood schizophrenia responsive to folic acid has been reported.[25]

The nature of the chemical abnormality and the manifest clinical symptoms of each of these illnesses depend not only on the specific vitamin the quantity of which is inadequate when ingested in the usual physiologic dose, but also on the single enzyme and defective metabolic reaction. It will be recalled that each vitamin of the B complex functions as a coenzyme for multiple enzymatic reactions and that the protein apoenzyme determines the specificity of the metabolic reaction associated with the coenzyme (see Chap. 3). Pyridoxine is involved as a coenzyme for more than 50 enzymatic reactions. If any one of the protein apoenzymes is a genetic mutant, that single reaction will be affected. For pyridoxine, for example, if the enzymatic defect is in the glutamic acid decarboxylase, the clinical consequence will be seizures; if it is in the cystathionine synthetase, the consequence will be mental retardation, cerebrovascular accidents, or psychoses; if it is in the kynurinenase, the consequence will be mental retardation. Vitamin dependency illnesses involving thiamin, pyridoxine, vitamin B_{12}, folic acid, and biotin have been demonstrated to involve mental retardation. A single case of homocystinuria presenting with schizophrenic symptoms and responding to large doses of folic acid has been described.[25]

The vitamin dependency illnesses are rare because they are autosomal recessives and therefore express themselves clinically only in the homozygotic state. Diagnosis requires not only the demonstration of clinical symptoms and signs but also an abnormal aminoaciduria or some other distinctive biochemical finding.[65] These illnesses are of interest for several reasons. First, they respond therapeutically to a single specific vitamin in doses 10 to 1000 times the usual estimated daily requirement. Such doses would be pharmacologic in the normal subject, but they are physiologic in the subjects with a vitamin dependency illness. If the metabolic abnormality is detected early in life and adequate quantities of the specific vitamin are given throughout life, the subject can live and grow with no systemic or mental abnormalities. Late detection and treatment may leave the patient with permanent residual neurologic and mental defects. Second, it seems safe to assume that, with improvement in technology, more vitamin-dependent, inherited disorders affecting the central nervous system will be discovered in the near future. Indeed, in principle, there is no reason why similar disorders involving essential minerals might not be discovered. Third, although the incidence of these illnesses is very rare, since they are caused by autosomal recessive genes that become clinically manifest only in the homozygotic state, the incidence of heterozygosity is not nearly so rare. Thus, a homozygotic condition appearing once in 40,000 births would be present in the heterozygotic condition once in 200 births. Since 25 conditions are already known and a rapid rate of discovery of new ones can be anticipated, it seems plausible that a significant portion of the population might be heterozygotic carriers. Techniques for the detection of heterozygotes require a complex technology involving either tissue culture or enzyme assays *in vitro*. Undoubtedly, such techniques will become more readily available, and once this advance is made, it will become possible to determine whether heterozygotes have a normal requirement for nutrients or whether the requirement is intermediate between normal and that of homozygotes for the vitamin dependency illnesses.

Rosenberg comments that with the present state of knowledge vitamin dependency illnesses must be considered in the differential diagnoses of patients with a wide variety of neurologic and mental deficits, because early recognition leads to effective long-term treatment that may prevent lethal or disabling sequelae.[65] This does not imply, however, that all schizophrenic illness or mental retardation will respond to a particular vitamin. Rosenberg feels that a short course of vitamins in large amounts may represent a valuable therapeutic trial in young patients with neurological or psychiatric problems of unknown nature, but he is opposed to the use of vitamins in pharmacologic doses over long periods of time for the treatment of illnesses of unknown etiology and lacking demonstrable laboratory abnormalities.

VITAMIN INSUFFICIENCY ILLNESSES

Falling somewhere between persons with normal vitamin requirements and those with greatly increased requirements owing to a vitamin-dependency illness is a group of patients with so-called *vitamin-insufficiency illness.*[6] This condition is typified by Wernicke–Korsakoff syndrome, an illness with neurologic and psychiatric symptoms that occurs in some alcoholics and that responds to large doses of thiamin. It is interesting that only a very small percentage of severe alcoholics develops the syndrome, despite the inadequate nutrition of most chronic alcoholics. Why is the incidence of the syndrome so low? Blass and Gibson studied four Wernicke–Korsakoff patients and found that they demonstrated a variant of the thiamin-dependent enzyme, transketolase, in which the affinity of the apoenzyme for the cofactor was about one tenth what one would ordinarily find.[6] The authors ran a number of generations of fibroblasts from such patients in tissue culture and found that the affinity of the transketolase apoenzyme for the cofactor did not change; thus, they concluded that the predisposition to Wernicke–Korsakoff illness is genetic. This interesting finding indicates that some individuals can grow and develop normally on an ordinary intake of thiamin, but when they ingest excessive quantities of alcohol, their daily requirement increases about tenfold, a much greater increase than required for the average alcoholic.

Another example of a vitamin insufficiency illness might be the orthopaedic–neurologic disease, carpal tunnel syndrome. Karl Folkers and associates have used enzyme–coenzyme saturation tests to examine the vitamin B_6 status of normal subjects and of patients with carpal tunnel syndrome.[2,20,23,40] The enzymatic system they measured was erythrocyte glutamic-oxaloacetic transaminase (EGOT), which has a pyridoxal phosphate cofactor. In normal, healthy adults 11% to 12% activation of this enzyme occurred when cofactor was added to the *in vitro* system.[40] Another group of healthy subjects, consuming an ordinary diet, averaged 18.5% activation that could be corrected by the administration of 50 mg pyridoxine/day for 3 weeks.[2] From these studies, it appears that many normal diets are inadequate to have a saturation of EGOT and that a deficiency of 10% to 15% generally exists in healthy volunteers.

Following these studies with control subjects, Folkers and co-workers turned their attention to patients with carpal tunnel syndrome, having noted that the erythrocyte apoenzyme of glutamic-oxaloacetic transaminase is not saturated with cofactor in such patients. A group of 11 patients averaged a 26% increase in enzyme activity and were considered to be deficient in pyridoxine.[20] These patients were treated with 100 mg vitamin B_6 tid for 6 weeks to 11 weeks. Not only was the deficiency corrected, but also clinical symptoms markedly diminished.

Folkers and colleagues conducted a longitudinal placebo-controlled study of a single carpal tunnel patient who had a 23% deficiency of B_6 on his normal diet.[23] Following 2 months of 2.0 mg/day pyridoxal phosphate, the recommended dietary allowance, deficiency diminished to 14%, with some improvement in clinical status. Deficiency disappeared after 12 weeks of 100 mg/day of B_6, and there was further clinical improvement to the extent that two independent orthopaedic surgeons deemed surgery of the carpal tunnel to be unnecessary. At this time, placebo was substituted for B_6, and deficiency returned to 12% with a concomitant deterioration in clinical status. Pyridoxine (100 mg/day) was reinstituted, and after 11 weeks deficiency was corrected and the patient was clinically asymptomatic. Another interesting finding from these studies is that administration of 50 mg/day or more of pyridoxine for 5 weeks to 12 weeks led not only to saturation of the available apoenzyme, but apparently to synthesis of new protein, since the basal activity of the enzyme more than doubled.

In all of these studies, doses of pyridoxine ranging from 2 mg/day to 300 mg/day, administered for periods of about 9 weeks to 11 weeks, were required to correct the vitamin B_6 deficiency and to improve the clinical status definitively. The concurrent presence of vitamin B_6 deficiency and the carpal tunnel syndrome, and their correction by pyridoxine supplementation, led these investigators to propose a causal relationship.[20,23] These interesting results require independent replication and confirmation by other investigators at both the basic research and the clinical levels before definitive conclusions can be drawn about their validity and significance.

The concept of vitamin insufficiency illness is new in nutrition. Wernicke–Korsakoff syndrome seems to be genetically determined, perhaps through the mechanism of a heterozygote. It seems likely that other such conditions will be identified in the future. Some megavitamin therapists have suggested that schizophrenia is a vitamin insufficiency illness in which the individual remains mentally healthy on normal quantities of vitamin when ordinarily stressed, but requires massive amounts of vitamins when external or internal stresses that could precipitate psychotic breaks occur. Although this hypothesis has not been disproven, there is no evidence to support it. The lack of dramatic clinical improvement with megavitamins in controlled clinical trials of schizophrenia argues against this hypothesis.[3–5]

Megavitamin and Orthomolecular Therapy in Psychiatry

It is now generally accepted that schizophrenia is a syndrome or a collection of associated symptoms with diverse and complex causes. A genetic diathesis for this condition has been demonstrated from twin and family studies.[49] An interaction of genetics and environment is inferred from these studies on identical twins, which fail to reveal more than 40% concordance for the manifest illness. Although there seems little doubt that there is some biologic defect in schizophrenia, the nature of the biochemical defect is not known. Diminished monoamine oxidase in platelets and dopamine β-hydroxylase in brain have been reported in schizophrenic populations. Aberrant transmethylation with the formation of endogenous hallucinogens has also been proposed.[34,53] It is also generally agreed that the phenothiazines and haloperidol do more than merely attenuate schizophrenic symptoms; rather, they seem to act on the biologic substrates of the psychotic state. The fact that most antipsychotic drugs have dopamine receptor-blocking properties has led to the suggestion that in schizophrenia there is excessive dopaminergic activity.

The nature of the environmental contributions to schizophrenia is also unclear. The pathogenic environment may be toxic or deficient; it may be physical, chemical, or psychosocial. Environmental hazards may be greatest during the antenatal or perinatal period, or they may continue to act throughout childhood and even early adulthood. Research in the area of the etiology of the schizophrenias and in their treatment is very active, but crucial questions remain unanswered.

Almost 20 years ago, when the hypothesis of psychogenesis of schizophrenia was dominant, a biologic hypothesis was formulated that attempted to integrate the psychological, biochemical, and clinical findings in schizophrenia. This hypothesis was among the first to emphasize the biologic nature of schizophrenia and to attempt to characterize the biochemical lesion. From this hypothesis was derived a method of treatment that employed massive doses of vitamin B_3 (niacin) added to other existing forms of treatment, such as electroconvulsive therapy and barbiturates. Over the past 20 years there has been increasing acceptance of pharmacotherapy with the phenothiazines and butyrophenones as crucial, though perhaps not sufficient, in the treatment of this illness. Originators of megavitamin treatment have gradually accepted the new forms of pharmacotherapy, but they always add water-soluble vitamins in huge quantities and claim better results.

Megavitamin therapy is a concept that is loosely defined. Initially, the term dealt with the use of 3 g or more daily of nicotinic acid or nicotinamide for the treatment of schizophrenia. Later, it came to include the use of nicotinamide adenine dinucleotide (NAD), the coenzyme derived from niacin. Over the years, additional water-soluble vitamins (*e.g.,* ascorbic acid, pyridoxine, folic acid, and vitamin B_{12}), minerals, hormones, hypoglycemic and allergy-free diets, and drugs have been added. The name has also been changed; it is now called *orthomolecular therapy.*[49]

The theoretic basis for the use of vitamins in "mega" doses has shifted over the years. The original hypothesis was that aberrant transmethylation caused schizophrenia. Vitamin B_3 was proposed to act as a methyl group acceptor that reduced the formation of endogenous psychotogens (adrenochrome and adrenolutin). In the initial publication 27 years ago, which proposed the hypothesis and treatment, the possibility that schizophrenia was an incipient form of cerebral pellagra was considered to be very remote.[34] Today, the same proponents argue that schizophrenia is a vitamin dependency illness, resulting in cerebral pellagra and requiring exceptionally high quantities of niacin because of a postulated block between the substrate vitamin B_3 and its synthesis into the coenzyme NAD.[32]

In 1968, Pauling published a theoretic paper supporting the possibility that some forms of mental illness might resemble the vitamin dependency illnesses.[55] Treatment was aimed at correcting the molecular defect with appropriate nutrients. This concept was called *orthomolecular psychiatry.* Pauling defined orthomolecular therapy as the "treatment of mental disease by the provision of the optimum molecular environment for the mind, especially the optimum concentration of substances normally present in the human body."[55] Advocates of megavitamin therapy quickly accepted the Pauling concept and changed the name of their treatment approach to orthomolecular psychiatry. They now employ a combination approach that still frequently uses electroconvulsive therapy, the phenothiazines, tranquilizers, and antidepressants but which also adds on very high doses of the water-soluble vitamins as well as some hormones, chelating agents, and special diets.[32] Orthomolecular psychiatrists state that the schizophrenias are a group of illnesses with different biochemical aberrations and that the nutritional needs of each patient must be discovered and appropriate nutrients supplied. However, in marked contrast to the research of the geneticists who continue to discover and treat new vitamin dependency illnesses, orthomolecular psychiatrists say nothing about how the biochemical irregularities are demonstrated or corrected. Furthermore, although in the recognized genetic vitamin dependency illnesses of children, the addition of a specific vitamin alone results in a rapid cure with no other pharmacotherapy being needed, in the common psychiatric conditions for which therapeutic utility is claimed for massive doses of vitamins, additional pharmacologic and somatic treatments are always employed, and these are not orthomolecular.

Orthomolecular psychiatry has been reported to be useful, not only in schizophrenia, but in the treatment of hyperactive children, childhood autism, alcoholism, adverse reactions to psychotomimetic drugs, arthritis, hyperlipidemia, geriatic problems, and even some forms of neuroses and depressions.[32] But the methods and claims of orthomolecular psychiatrists have not been generally accepted by the psychiatric community. One reason has been that no unequivocal biochemical defect has been found either in schizophrenia or in the other psychiatric illnesses for which megavitamin use is proposed. The differences between schizophrenia and the true vitamin dependency illnesses have been emphasized by Rosenberg, a pioneer in the discovery of these latter illnesses.[66] Furthermore, in the past decade, orthomolecular psychiatrists have used questionable diagnostic procedures and have not performed carefully controlled clinical trials. Results of experienced investigators who have conducted carefully controlled double-blind clinical trials to test the megavitamin claims have been negative.[3-5]

Since the claims of therapeutic efficacy became more vigorous over the years, and because the psychiatric profession was castigated for not using these inexpensive forms of treatment, a task force was established by the American Psychiatric Association (APA) to examine critically the evidence for the theory and practice of orthomolecular psychiatry. The APA Task Force found no evidence to support the theory and practice of the orthomolecular psychiatrists.[49] The theory was found to be superficial and inconsistent. For example, a single molecule of nicotinamide cannot simultaneously function as a methyl acceptor and as a precursor for the coenzyme, because once it has been methylated, it cannot be synthesized into the coenzyme. Similarly, the coenzyme cannot be methylated and, hence, cannot be a methyl acceptor. The transmethylation hypothesis and the vitamin dependency hypothesis are therefore incompatible. Yet orthomolecular psychiatrists continue to adhere to both. No evidence could be found to support the contention that adrenochrome is present in the blood or urine of schizophrenics. No evidence could be found to support the view that schizophrenia is associated with an absolute or relative deficiency of niacin. The clinical symptoms of pellagra differ vastly, psychiatrically and somatically, from those of schizophrenia. Successful treatment of pellagra with niacin takes place rapidly, but according to orthomolecular psychiatrists, months or years of treatment with massive doses of the vitamin are required—for therapeutic efficacy of niacin in schizophrenia to become manifest—hence, the need for interim psychotropic drugs.

Nonetheless, since it seemed possible that, despite the lack of evidence to support the theory, the practice might still be beneficial, carefully controlled empirical trials were conducted. The very dramatic claim that the coenzyme NAD made chronic schizophrenics well within a few days could not be replicated by independent groups of investigators.[33,41,50] The claims that niacin addition to conventional procedures enhances the treatment of schizophrenia could not be substantiated by several investigative teams in carefully controlled studies.[3,4] The vitamin in doses of 3 g/day to 6 g/day was found not to diminish the requirement for chlorpromazine or to diminish the duration of hospitalization. The possibility that a small subgroup of schizophrenics might represent a niacin-dependent disease was rendered highly unlikely because, during studies in which several hundred patients were tested, none was found to respond dramatically to niacin.[3,4]

The APA Task Force Report has not remained unchallenged. The advocates of orthomolecular psychiatry have argued that the replications cited in the APA Task Force Report involved antiquated procedures using only niacin, whereas now they use multiple vitamins. They have also argued that they frequently use electroconvulsive therapy along with the vitamins in the types of patients studied by the groups that obtained negative results and that, if this therapy had been used, positive results would have been obtained. However, a recent report found that electroconvulsive therapy is not a crucial variable because patients receiving this treatment along with massive doses of niacin fare no better than those who do not receive the vitamins.

The need for improved treatment of schizophrenia is so great that the authors of the APA Task Force Report reached their negative conclusions reluctantly. They wondered whether the wrong vitamin might have been used in the replication studies. Niacin was selected because it is, historically, the foundation on which all later claims of therapeutic efficacy were made. It was therefore felt that if the initial findings could not be confirmed, the credibility of the orthomolecular psychiatrists would be too low to warrant the expensive and time-consuming trials with other vitamins. Nonetheless, a controlled study testing multiple vitamins in megadoses was conducted at McGill University. Results indicated no significant difference between placebo and multiple megavitamin treatment.[5]

In summary, there is no evidence at present that adult schizophrenics differ from the population at large in their nutritional requirements for niacin. A recent study suggests that the ascorbic acid requirement for schizophrenics does not differ from that of normal persons. The nutritional requirements for the other water-soluble vitamins or trace mineral elements have not been carefully investigated in schizophrenics, but the lack of significant somatic symptoms or biochemical findings in schizophrenia does not favor the suspicion that nutritional requirements for these differ markedly from normal. Although the toxicity of the water-soluble vitamins is not high, ingestion of massive doses of niacin and ascorbic acid over long periods of time has been reported to be damaging. Under similar circumstances, the other water-soluble vitamins may also be damaging. Since there is no evidence of benefit and there is some potential for harm, the treatment of common mental illness with doses of ten to several hundred times the usual daily requirement is not warranted.

MEGAVITAMINS IN AUTISM AND HYPERKINESIS

Although the efficacy of megavitamin therapy is generally unsupported for the many conditions for which proponents have made claims, recent studies suggest beneficial responses in some autistic and hyperkinetic children treated with megadoses of pyridoxine. During preliminary nonblind trials, Rimland identified a subgroup of autistic children whose parents claimed that behavior improved with vitamin B_6, relapsed on withdrawal of the vitamin, and again responded favorably to reinstitution of

the vitamin. Sixteen children from this subgroup participated in a double-blind study of individualized megadoses (75 mg/day to 800 mg/day) of pyridoxine versus placebo.[63] One child, who erroneously was given only the vitamin throughout the trial, was dropped. Of the remaining 15 children, 11 exhibited a small but significant improvement during B_6 versus placebo administration. In open studies Lelord and co-workers administered pyridoxine in megadoses to autistic children and reported dramatic improvement in 10% and some improvement in 30% of the sample.[43] Following B_6 ingestion, the responders exhibited a marked decrease in urinary homovanillic acid, the primary metabolite of dopamine, possibly indicating that these children had a derangement of some metabolic process requiring pyridoxine. The large biochemical improvement with only a small degree of behavioral improvement is disappointing and raises the possibility that irreversible damage occurs with age in untreated children; perhaps at a very young age autistic children could be treated more effectively. Further research with massive doses of vitamin B_6 in autistic children is clearly indicated.

A subpopulation of six hyperkinetic children, whose blood serotonin was found to be low and who had previously responded to methylphenidate, participated in a double-blind trial of 12 mg/kg/day to 25 mg/kg/day pyridoxine.[15] The authors reported that the vitamin both elevated the blood serotonin and caused clinical improvement equivalent to, and perhaps persisting longer than, methylphenidate. Administration of B_6 had no effect upon hyperkinetic children who had normal blood serotonin levels. This preliminary study warrants replication.

THE FEINGOLD DIET FOR HYPERKINESIS

The late Dr. Ben F. Feingold, a pediatrician and allergist from San Francisco, proposed that some children have a central nervous system variation that predisposes them to sensitivity to synthetic food additives, particularly to food colors and the antioxidants butylated hydroxyanisole (BHA) and butylated hydroxytoluene (BHT). In such children, hyperkinetic behavior results from the ingestion of these additives; elimination of food additives from the diet is said to lead to dramatic improvement and even cure. Feingold claimed that between 50% to 70% of hyperkinetic/learning-disabled children placed on a diet devoid of additives will have a complete remission and that 75% of children who have been treated with stimulant medications can discontinue this treatment.[21] The diet is claimed to become effective in several days to several weeks, and the younger the child, the more rapid and complete is the response. Total and permanent adherence to the diet is mandatory, Feingold insisted, because an infringement produces a return of symptoms within about 3 hr which may persist as long as 72 hr. Feingold never conducted controlled, double-blind trials to test his hypothesis, and his claims were based entirely on anecdotal reports and findings from open clinical trials. Nevertheless, the Feingold diet gained considerable popularity among the lay public, and more than 20,000 families of hyperkinetic children adhere to the diet and advocate its use.[51]

Many open studies, in which parents or physicians place children on the additive-free diet and then anecdotally report their results, have been conducted, and these generally support Feingold's claims.[8,16] However, more rigorous, double-blind controlled clinical trials have also been conducted, and these have generally yielded negative results. Based on findings from double-blind studies, it appears that the beneficial results of the diet are largely due to placebo effects.

Because of the difficulty and expense of conducting such trials, only one study has compared the additive-free diet with an ordinary diet containing additives in a controlled blind manner.[27] All of the food for the families participating in the study was provided for the duration of the trial, and neither the investigative team nor the families knew which diet was being consumed. In 36 school-age boys, based on teacher and objective ratings, no significant differences in behavior occurred with diet. With these school-aged children, some parents reported a significant improvement in behavior when the additive-free diet followed the control diet, but they were unable to detect differences when the order of the diets was reversed. With preschool children, parents were better able to detect differences with the additive-free diet compared to the usual diet.

Most of the double-blind studies have been "challenge" trials; that is, children who were reported by their parents to respond to the additive-free diet were blindly "challenged" by the addition of food color additives to the additive-free diet. Harley and colleagues reported that of nine putative diet responders, only one had an adverse reaction to ingestion of 26 mg/day food colors.[28] In a study of 22 children, no positive response to the additive-free diet or deterioration in behavior following active challenge (5 mg/day tartrazine) was detected by teachers, clinicians, or objective ratings.[44] Mothers reported significant improvement with the diet but no detrimental effects with active challenge. Thirteen children from this group were tested further and significant challenge effects were noted only when ratings were done a few hours

after administration of the challenge. Mattes and Gittelman–Klein reported their findings in a single child whose parents had volunteered him because they were certain his responses would unequivocally confirm the efficacy of the Feingold diet.[48] In this child, neither maternal nor teacher ratings revealed a significant difference between active (39 mg/day food color) and placebo challenges, and both the teacher and the child guessed that placebo had been administered throughout the trial. The mother, however, correctly guessed challenge phases in eight out of ten weeks, despite the fact that her objective ratings did not differentiate the periods.

Although the results from double-blind studies have been largely negative, a number of trends are weakly detectable. Younger children may be more sensitive to the effects of additives, and parents (but not objective ratings) have been consistently able to detect improvement in preschool children on the additive-free diet.[27] Transient decrements in attention and concentration have also been reported after challenge with 26 mg to 100 mg food color. Thus, hyperkinetic children who showed no adverse reaction to active challenge in their overall behavior in school or over a day nonetheless showed some decrements in performance in specific laboratory tasks requiring attention and concentration when rated for periods immediately following ingestion of the challenge.[69] Finally, there may be a dose-response curve for food additives just as there is for any toxic substance. These trends raise some doubts that the food additives are completely innocuous. In our opinion, however, existing data do not warrant the removal or severe restriction of these substances from our foods. Further intensive studies of those very few children who seem to react adversely to food dyes, and additional *in vivo* animal research and *in vitro* biochemical research are needed.

Anorexia Nervosa

The metabolic and psychiatric aspects of anorexia nervosa have been reviewed.[9,39] Anorexia nervosa was first defined as a clinical entity by Gull 100 years ago.[9] It is a relatively rare condition about which only a few definitive statements can be made. About 90% of the reported cases occur in adolescent girls, usually within a few years after menarche, and about 10% occur in boys, these being invariably prepubertal. Anorexia nervosa is characterized by a relentless pursuit of thinness that leads to emaciation and occasionally to death. A few of the patients are schizophrenic, but most are very immature, dependent neurotics who are unable to cope with family, social, or sexual pressure except by overeating or by ceasing to eat adequately. Commonly, these patients are exceptionally energetic and active even when severely underweight. They appear to treat food phobically, seeming to fear that if they submit to the temptation of food, they will be unable to moderate their intake. Occasionally this happens, and one finds an alternating bulimia and anorexia.

A dramatic case (observed by M.A.L.) involved a 13-year-old boy who achieved a maximum weight of 230 lb. Teased by his schoolmates, he determined to lose weight. Unable to control his appetite, he would gorge himself and then secretly induce vomiting. When this was discovered by his parents, who attempted to control his food intake, he stopped eating almost entirely and presented at the hospital about 15 months later weighing 85 lb. Initially, in the hospital he cheerfully resumed his pattern of eating publicly and vomiting private.ͺ. When this was prevented, he maneuvered in every conceivable way to avoid eating while giving the appearance that he was enjoying his meals. Medically and endocrinologically, this boy was within normal limits. Psychologically, he was intact except for a substantial conflict with his family, which had always been deeply invested in food. His mother believed that fat babies were the healthiest, but that young men should be vigorous and lean. Typically, he was given huge meals, told to empty his plate, and then criticized for being fat. Treatment involved several months of hospitalization with firm control and clear messages. At one point, tube feeding was necessary; later, he required company while eating and for several hours thereafter to prevent self-induced vomiting. He developed a good relationship with both his physician and nurses and was able to change his self-image to be freer about his choices of food, books, and hobbies. His parents changed in allowing him greater freedom to be himself. When last seen at 16 years of age, he was somewhat overweight but otherwise doing well socially and in school.

This case of anorexia nervosa, though it occurred in a boy, illustrates several of the features of the syndrome. There is a markedly distorted self-image. In girls, breasts and buttocks are abhorred, and they find themselves most attractive when they are emaciated. Years later, when they are well and see a photograph of themselves taken when they were ill, they will be able to recognize their lack of attractiveness, but while they are still sick, they will look at themselves admiringly. Amenorrhea, which is very common, may precede or be concurrent with the weight loss, but it usually follows the weight loss and is welcomed by the patient.

Recent developments in endocrinology have eliminated some misconceptions and illuminated others. For example, the concept that anorexia nervosa resembles Simmonds' disease or panhypopituitarism is incorrect.[39] Although the basal metabolic rate (BMR) is frequently low, direct tests of thyroid function fail to reveal deficient function. Levels of triiodothyronine (T_3), thyroxin (T_4), protein-bound iodine, and butanol-extractable iodine have been found to be within normal limits in severely ill patients. The low BMR is therefore probably an attempt to compensate for the extreme emaciation. At autopsy, the thyroid glands appear normal.[39]

Plasma 17-hydroxycorticosteroids (17-OHCS) are normal, as is the response to adrenocorticotropic hormone, even though 24-hr urinary 17-OHCS are low. Probably, there is decreased catabolism of cortisol. Growth hormone levels tend to be high and do not increase with hypoglycemia. Gonadal function in girls is clearly disturbed, since amenorrhea is universal. Urinary estrogens are low, and this is manifested by atrophic vaginal epithelium. Similarly, in cases coming to autopsy, the gonads are small. The ovarian deficiency is not primary, for if it were, one would find elevated gonadotrophins in response to diminished estrogen, and in anorexia nervosa this is not found. Instead, urinary gonadotrophins are low. Luteinizing hormone (LH) is extremely low, and follicle-stimulating hormone (FSH) is also low in about 50% of patients. Recent studies in which plasma LH is frequently sampled show a plasma LH pattern resembling that of prepubertal girls rather than physically mature women.[39]

Despite this impressive evidence with respect to gonadal activity, selective pituitary malfunction does not seem to be primary. Thus, the administration of hypothalamic luteinizing hormone-releasing factor (LHRF) to five young women patients resulted in elevation of LH and FSH in four of them. This led to the conclusion that the primary difficulty is impaired function in the hypothalamus, which is probably due to disorders of cortical function expressed as psychologic conflict. The clinical impression of disordered hypothalamic function is supported by animal studies, which show glucoreceptors in the hypothalamus that can influence eating behavior.[39]

TREATMENT

There are two major issues in the treatment of anorexia nervosa: (1) nutritional deficiencies and (2) psychiatric disorders. Patients who present with severe cachexia are in a life-threatening situation and must be treated accordingly. No special deficiencies in vitamins, minerals, or protein exist, and hence no special diet is needed. The object is to increase the food intake of such patients to the 2000 Cal/

day to 3000 Cal/day needed in a well-balanced diet. This should be done over a period of weeks. The patients may require gastric tube feeding with liquid semisynthetic diets or even IV feeding, but the latter should be a last resort because of the many hazards involved. Physical restraints or phenothiazines in the doses employed with psychotic patients may be needed to control them during the forced alimentation. Once the patient is over the most critical stage, feeding of solid foods in a high-protein, high-calorie diet should be resumed. Here, the primary problem has been in convincing the patient to take the food. Some success in this has been achieved with authoritative procedures and especially with the techniques of behavior modification.[9] For example, patients are permitted to make or receive phone calls only after eating, or they may be put on enforced bed rest and allowed to get up only after they have achieved a daily specified weight gain.

Once the life-threatening crisis is over, psychological treatment should not focus on the eating problem, but rather on the nature of the interpersonal relationships and stresses that underlie the eating disorder. The family should be treated simultaneously, focusing on the youngster's attempts to individuate herself. An excellent review of the types of treatment that have been useful is offered by Bruch, who points out that unless changes occur in the social and family structure in which the child lives, recurrences are likely.[9] The patient must be encouraged and assisted in increasing her capacity to separate herself psychologically from her family. Although the illness is self-limiting in terms of threatening weight loss, individuals who have not changed psychologically fail to mature and usually end with other severe phobias, compulsions, or character disorders. Psychological treatment over the long run is difficult, but it is the best treatment currently available and in more than half the cases leads to disappearance of both the eating problems and the underlying conflicts, so that an effective and productive life can be achieved.[9]

Diet as Precursor Therapy

The dietary precursors of the neurotransmitters include tryptophan for serotonin (5-hydroxytryptamine, 5-HT), tyrosine for dopamine (DA), and choline for acetylcholine (ACh). Tryptophan is an essential amino acid that cannot be synthesized by any tissue, and it has been found that brain levels of 5-HT are coupled to food consumption.[75] Tyrosine is not essential but its amino acid precursor, phenylalanine, is; phenylalanine is converted to tyrosine largely in the liver. Small quantities of choline can be synthesized, but the large quantities

required for health necessitate dietary intake of choline. The effects of dietary consumption of pharmacologic doses of these amino acids and amines on levels of neurotransmitters are currently being studied.

L-TRYPTOPHAN FOR INSOMNIA

A number of investigators have demonstrated that serotonin and the serotonergic neurons of the raphe system play an important role in the biochemical mechanisms underlying sleep. Because brain serotonin levels appear to be directly dependent on circulating plasma L-tryptophan, the effects of tryptophan on sleep have been investigated.[22] Based on findings in normal subjects and in insomniacs, there is general agreement that L-tryptophan reduces sleep latency and usually reduces waking time. At low doses (1–5 g), these favorable effects on sleep occur without producing distortions of physiologic sleep as measured by EEG recordings. At higher doses (10 g–15 g), alterations in slow-wave sleep and desynchronized sleep occur, but these are less pronounced than changes resulting from the use of hypnotics. L-tryptophan as a remedy for insomnia would have definite advantages over the currently used hypnotic medications and, in 200 subjects and patients prescribed the amino acid, no side-effects other than a few cases of nausea at the highest doses of 10 g to 15 g were reported.[29] On the other hand, this amino acid is not uniformly effective for insomniacs, and its general utility for this purpose has not yet been established. Furthermore, the long-term effects of doses of 5 g/ day to 15 g/day require further investigation.

L-TRYPTOPHAN FOR DEPRESSION

Some depressions appear to be associated with a deficit of brain 5-hydroxytryptamine.[52] The possibility of correcting this deficiency by administering its natural precursor, L-tryptophan, has prompted research in this area. Most of the early studies reported negative results.[10] Recently, some investigators have suggested that the equivocal action of tryptophan could be due to its high rate of catabolism by liver pyrrolase, and that the concomitant administration of a pyrrolase inhibitor would allow tryptophan to reach the brain, where it could form serotonin.[11] Nicotinamide and nicotinic acid are pyrrolase inhibitors that have been used successfully in combination with tryptophan to ameliorate depression.[11] These are preliminary findings, and further research is needed to determine efficacy, dose-response curves, and the types of patients who might benefit from such treatment.

TYROSINE

A very small portion of dietary tyrosine is converted to form the amino acid, L-dopa. L-dopa is decarboxylated to dopamine (DA), which is hydroxylated to norepinephrine (NE), which, in turn, may be methylated to form epinephrine. The process of converting tyrosine to L-dopa is "rate-limiting," and ingestion of large quantities of tyrosine does not result in increased amounts of dopamine or norepinephrine. However, the step from L-dopa to DA is not subject to this control, and it is possible to increase DA by feeding massive amounts of L-dopa.

Parkinson's disease is a chronic neurologic syndrome in which striatal DA is depleted; L-dopa, the immediate precursor of DA, is the most effective treatment for Parkinson's disease. Marketed as levodopa, it has been reported to be effective in as many as 85% of patients with Parkinson's disease.[47]

In addition to improving extrapyramidal symptoms, there are some reports of intellectual improvement in patients treated with L-dopa.[46] These findings have led to the experimental use of L-dopa in patients with senile dementia, but results have been equivocal. A recent report described improvement following L-dopa in two women with senile dementia of Alzheimer's type who exhibited low urinary DA levels.[61] This finding may suggest that there are subgroups among senile patients who may respond to treatment with levodopa.

CHOLINE

Several studies have demonstrated that synthesis of brain acetylcholine (ACh) can be stimulated *in vivo* by elevating tissue concentration of its precursor, choline.[13] This finding has important implications for the efficacy of choline in the treatment of ACh-deficiency conditions. Significant improvement in choreiform movements has been reported in about half or more of patients with tardive dyskinesia who are administered choline.[18,74] Half of a group of patients with Huntington's disease were reported to have transient improvement in speech, balance, and gait, but these patients reverted to their prior disability within 2 weeks, despite continued choline consumption.[26,74] Based on the hypothesis that memory loss and intellectual decline of the aged may be due to impaired functioning of cholinergic neurons, there have also been some suggestions that oral choline might be beneficial in improving memory and intellectual functions in the elderly (see Chaps. 22, 27).[74]

References

1. Adams PW, Rose DP, Folkard J et al: Effect of pyridoxine hydrochloride (vitamin B$_6$) upon depression associated with oral contraception. Lancet 1:897–904, 1973
2. Azuma J, Kishi T, Williams RH et al: Apparent deficiency of vitamin B$_6$ in typical individuals who commonly serve as normal controls. Res Commun Chem Pathol Pharmacol 14:343–348, 1976
3. Ban TA, Lehmann HE: Nicotinic Acid in the Treatment of Schizophrenias. Canadian Mental Health Association Collaborative Study, Progress Report I. Toronto, Canadian Mental Health Association, 1970
4. Ban TA, Lehmann HE: Nicotinic acid in the treatment of schizophrenias. Canadian Mental Health Association Collaborative Study, Progress Report II. Canadian Psychiatric Association J 20:103–112, 1975
5. Ban TA, Lehmann HE, Deutsch M: Negative findings with megavitamins in schizophrenic patients: Preliminary report. Commun Psychopharmacol 1:119–122, 1977
6. Blass JP, Gibson GE: Abnormality of a thiamine-requiring enzyme in patients with Wernicke–Korsakoff syndrome. N Engl J Med 297:1367–1370, 1977
7. Bossé TR, Donald EA: The vitamin B$_6$ requirement in oral contraceptive users. I. Assessment by pyridoxal level and transferase activity in erythrocytes. Am J Clin Nutr 32:1015–1023, 1979
8. Brenner A: A study of the efficacy of the Feingold diet on hyperkinetic children. Clin Pediatr 16:652–656, 1977
9. Bruch H: Eating Disorders, Obesity, Anorexia Nervosa and the Person Within. New York, Basic Books, 1973
10. Carroll BJ: Monoamine precursors in the treatment of depression. Clin Pharmacol Ther 12:743–761, 1971
11. Chouinard G, Young SN, Annable L et al: Tryptophan–nicotinamide combination with depression (letter). Lancet 1:249, 1977
12. Cohen AC: Pyridoxine in the prevention and treatment of convulsions and neurotoxicity due to cycloserine. Ann NY Acad Sci 166:346–349, 1969
13. Cohen EL, Wurtman RJ: Brain acetylcholine: Control by dietary choline. Science 191:561–562, 1976
14. Cohen MM: Nutritional disorders involving the nervous system. In Cohen MM (ed): Biochemistry of Neural Disease, pp 141–159. Hagerstown, MD, Harper & Row, 1975
15. Coleman M, Steinberg G, Tippett J et al: A preliminary study of the effect of pyridoxine administration in a subgroup of hyperkinetic children: A double-blind crossover comparison with methylphenidate. Biol Psychol 14:741–752, 1979
16. Cook PS, Woodhill JM: The Feingold dietary treatment of the hyperkinetic syndrome. Med J Aust 2:85–90, 1976
17. DeLicardie, Cravioto: Behavioral responsiveness of survivors of clinical severe malnutrition to cognitive demands. In Cravioto J, Hambraeus L, Vahlquist B (eds): Early Malnutrition and Mental Development, pp 134–153. Swedish Nutrition Foundation XII. Uppsala, Almqvist & Wiksell, 1973
18. Davis KL, Berger PA, Hollister LE et al: Choline chloride in the treatment of Huntington's disease and tardive dyskinesia: A preliminary report. Psychopharmacol Bull 13:37–38, 1977
19. Ebadi M, Costa E (eds): Role of Vitamin B$_6$ in Neurobiology, Vol. 4. New York, Raven Press, 1972
20. Ellis JM, Kishi T, Azuma J et al: Vitamin B$_6$ deficiency in patients with a clinical syndrome including the carpal

tunnel defect. Biochemical and clinical response to therapy with pyridoxine. Res Commun Chem Pathol Pharmacol 13:743–757, 1976

21. Feingold BF: Why Your Child is Hyperactive. New York, Random House, 1975

22. Fernstrom JD, Wurtman RJ: Brain serotonin content: Physiological dependence on plasma tryptophan levels. Science 173:149–152, 1971

23. Folkers K, Willis J, Watanabe T et al: Biochemical evidence for a deficiency of vitamin B_6 in the carpal tunnel syndrome based on a cross-over clinical study. Proc Natl Acad Sci USA 75:3410–3412, 1978

24. Frankova S: Interaction between early malnutrition and stimulation in animals. In Cravioto J, Hambraeus L, Vahlquist B (eds): Early Malnutrition and Mental Development, pp 202–209. Swedish Nutrition Foundation XII. Uppsala, Amlqvist & Wiksell, 1974

25. Freeman JM, Finkelstein JD, Mudd HS: Folate-responsive homocystinuria and schizophrenia. N Engl J Med 292:491–496, 1975

26. Growden JA, Cohen EL, Wurtman RJ: Huntington's disease: Clinical and chemical effects of choline administration. Ann Neurol 1:418–422, 1977

27. Harley JP, Ray RS, Tomasi L et al: Hyperkinesis and food additives: Testing the Feingold hypothesis. Pediatrics 61:818–828, 1978

28. Harley JP, Matthews CG, Eichman P: Synthetic food colors and hyperactivity in children: A double-blind challenge experiment. Pediatrics 62:975–983, 1978

29. Hartmann E: L-tryptophan: A rational hypnotic with clinical potential. Am J Psychol 134:366–370, 1977

30. Herman M, Most H, Jolliffe N: Psychoses associated with pernicious anemia. Arch Neurol Psych 38:348–361, 1937

31. Hershel J: Drugs—remarkably non-toxic. N Engl J Med 291:824–828, 1974

32. Hoffer A: Orthomolecular treatment of schizophrenia. Canadian Journal of Psychiatric Nursing 14, N. 2:11–14, 1973

33. Hoffer A, Osmond H: Nicotinamide adenine dinucleotide (NAD) as a treatment for schizophrenia. J Psychopharmacol 1:78–95, 1966

34. Hoffer A, Osmond H, Smythies J: Schizophrenia: A new approach. II. Result of a year's research. Journal of Mental Science 100:29–54, 1954

35. Horakova Z, Muratova J, Vitek V et al: An experimental and clinical analysis of cycloserine-amino acid interaction. Activitas Nervosa Superior 7:274–276, 1965

36. Hunt AD, Stokes J, McCrory WW et al: Pyridoxine dependency: Report of a case of intractable convulsions in an infant controlled by pyridoxine. Pediatrics 13:140–145, 1954

37. Hunter R, Barnes J, Oakeley HF et al: Toxicity of folic acid given in pharmacologic doses to healthy volunteers. Lancet 1:61–63, 1970

38. Hurdle ADF, Picton WTC: Folic acid deficiency in elderly patients admitted to hospital. Br Med J 2:202–205, 1966

39. Katz JL: Psychoendocrine considerations in anorexia nervosa. In Sachar EJ (ed): Topics in Psychoendocrinology, pp 121–132. New York, Grune & Stratton, 1975

40. Kishi H, Kishi T, Williams RH et al: Human deficiencies of vitamin B_6. I. Studies on parameters of the assay of the glutamic oxaloacetic transaminase by the CAS principle. Res Commun Chem Pathol Pharmacol 12:557–569, 1975

41. Kline NS, Barclay GL, Cole JO et al: Controlled evaluation of nicotinamide adenine dinucleotide in the treatment of chronic schizophrenia. Br J Psychol 113:731–742, 1967

42. Leklem JE, Brown RR, Rose DP et al: Metabolism of tryptophan and niacin in oral contraceptive users receiving controlled intakes of vitamin B_6. Am J Clin Nutr 28:146–156, 1975

43. Lelord G, Callaway E, Muh JP, et al: Results of urinary HVA dosage in 49 autistic children and 13 mongoloid children with respect to the differential action of vitamin B_6 in each group (trans) In Saletu B, Berner P, Hollister L (eds): Proceedings of Collegium Internationale de Neuropsychopharmacologie (CINP). New York, Pergamon Press, 1978

44. Levy F, Dumbrell S, Hobbes G et al: Hyperkinesis and diet: A double-blind crossover trial with a tartrazine challenge. Med J Aust 1:61–64, 1978

45. Lipton MA, Kane FJ Jr: The use of vitamins as therapeutic agents in psychiatry. In Shader RI (ed): Psychiatric Complications of Medical Drugs, pp 333–368. New York, Raven Press, 1972

46. Loranger AW, Goodell H, Lee JR et al: Levodopa treatment of Parkinson's syndrome. Improved intellectual functioning. Arch Gen Psychiatry 26:163–168, 1972

47. Marsden CD: The need for alternative therapy in Parkinson's disease. In Laake JPWF, Korf J, Wesseling H (eds): Parkinson's Disease: Concepts and Prospects, pp 117–120. Amsterdam, Excerpta Medica, 1977

48. Mattes J, Gittelman–Klein R: A crossover study of artificial food colorings in a hyperkinetic child. Am J Psychol 135:987–988, 1978

49. American Psychiatric Association: Megavitamin and Orthomolecular Therapy in Psychiatry. Task Force Report #7. Washington, DC, American Psychiatric Association, 1973

50. Meltzer H, Shader R, Grinspoon L: The behavioral effects of nicotinamide adenine dinucleotide in chronic schizophrenia. Psychopharmacology 15:144–152, 1969

51. Morrison M: The Feingold diet (letter). Science 199:840, 1978

52. Murphy DL, Campbell I, Costa JL: Current status of the indoleamine hypothesis of affective disorders. In Lipton MA, DiMascio A, Killam KF (eds): Psychopharmacology: A Generation of Progress, pp 1235–1247. New York, Raven Press, 1978

53. Osmond H, Smythies J: Schizophrenia: A new approach. Journal of Mental Sciences 98:309–315, 1952

54. Otte J: Oral contraceptives and depression. Lancet 2:498, 1969

55. Pauling L: Orthomolecular psychiatry. Science 160:254–271, 1968

56. Plum F (ed): Brain Dysfunction in Metabolic Disorders. New York, Raven Press, 1974

57. Pollin W: The pathogenesis of schizophrenia—possible relationships between genetic, biochemical and experiential factors. Arch Gen Psychiatry 27:29–37, 1972

58. Price JM, Thornton MJ, Mueller LM: Tryptophan metabolism in women using steroid hormones for ovulation control. Am J Clin Nutr 20:452–456, 1967

59. Price SA, Toseland PA: Oral contraceptives and depression. Lancet 2:158–159, 1969

60. Reinken L, Dapunt O: Vitamin B_6 nutriture during pregnancy. J Nutr Sci Viminol 48:341–347, 1978

61. Renvoize EB, Jerram T, Clough G: Levodopa in senile dementia (letter). Br Med J 2:504, 1978

62. Reynolds EH, Milner G, Matthews DM et al: Anticonvulsant therapy, megaloblastic haemopoiesis and folic acid metabolism. QJ Med 35:521–537, 1966

63. Rimland B, Callaway E, Dreyfus P: The effect of high doses of vitamin B_6 on autistic children: A double-blind crossover study. Am J Psychiatry 135:472–475, 1978

64. Roe DA: A Plague of Corn—The Social History of Pellagra. Ithaca, Cornell University Press, 1973

65. Scriver CR, Rosenberg LE: Amino Acid Metabolism and Its Disorders. Philadelphia, WB Saunders, 1973

66. Serban G (ed): Nutrition and Mental Functions, pp 33–64; 259–262. New York, Plenum Press, 1975

67. Skaug DE: Vitamin B_{12} deficiency in mental disease. In Walaas O (ed): Molecular Basis of Some Aspects of Mental Activity, pp 475–479. New York, Academic Press, 1967

68. Stein Z, Susser M, Gerhart S et al: The Dutch Hunger Winter of 1944–45. New York, Oxford University Press, 1975

69. Swanson JM, Kinsbourne M: Artificial color and hyperactive behavior. In Knights RM, Bakker D (eds): Treatment of Hyperactive and Learning Disordered Children, pp 131–149. Baltimore, University Park Press, 1980

70. Terris M (ed): Goldberger on Pellagra. Baton Rouge, Louisiana State University Press, 1964

70a.Tizard: Epidemiology of mental retardation. Implications for research on malnutrition. In Carvioto J, Hambraeus L, Vahlquist B (eds): Early Malnutrition and Mental Development, Swedish Nutrition Foundation XII. Uppsala, Almqvist & Wiksell, 1973.

71. Turkewitz G: Learning in chronically protein-deprived rats. In Serban G (ed): Nutrition and Mental Functions, pp 113–120. New York, Plenum Press, 1975

72. Winick M: Malnutrition and the developing brain. In Plum F (ed): Brain Dysfunction in Metabolic Disorders, pp 253–261. New York, Raven Press, 1974

73. Winston F: Oral contraceptives, pyridoxine and depression. Am J Psychiatry 130:1217–1221, 1973

74. Wurtman RJ, Growden JH: Dietary enhancement of CNS neurotransmitters. Hosp Pract 13:71–77, March 1978

75. Young VR, Hussein MA, Murray E et al: Tryptophan intake, spacing of meals, and diurnal fluctuations of plasma tryptophan in man. Am J Clin Nutr 22:1563–1567, 1969

34
Renal Disease

Malcolm A. Holliday

Nutrition therapy is an important aspect of treating patients with renal disease. For the era preceding chronic dialysis and renal transplantation, diet control was the major therapeutic approach to offset symptoms of uremia in patients with progressive renal insufficiency. Addis described the physiologic basis, the clinical application, and the physician–patient relations that underlie this therapy in its best form. His description is a useful guide even today because it is based on the experience of a very rigorous observer and warm physician who could express his observations with grace.[1]

In this chapter, we will describe the physiologic basis for nutrition therapy and strategies used to improve nutritional state and alleviate symptoms of patients with end stage renal disease (ESRD). While nutrition therapy in nephrology today is mainly focused on patients with renal failure, therapy also is useful in hypertension and some renal tubular disorders, such as renal tubular acidosis. Parenteral nutrition therapy is being used in patients with acute renal failure, although its benefit is not well documented. Defined-formula diets, especially those using amino acids or their keto-analogues, are being used with good effect in experimental settings. Continuous ambulatory peritoneal dialysis (CAPD) has added a new perspective to nutrition and metabolism in patients requiring dialysis.

Children with renal insufficiency pose some unique problems.[10] Normal children have both a higher metabolic rate and a higher food requirement per kg body weight, with a correspondingly higher level of renal function than do adults. When renal function declines, the input of metabolic end products from food intake and cell metabolism, normally excreted, remains high, whereas excretory capacity is reduced. Consequently children with ESRD have different and more demanding nutrient and dialysis requirements from those of adults and are more at risk for malnutrition. Children with renal disease also tend to grow poorly, especially in the first few years of life. Retarded growth is related to poor calorie intake and to osteodystrophy. Growth rate improves some with calorie supplementation and with vitamin D therapy but not enough to restore stature to normal. Defined-formula diets using amino acids are being used in experimental studies on children early in life to attempt to improve growth in those years.

Nutrition Therapy

Nutrition therapy in renal insufficiency is based on the concept that normal kidney function allows great latitude in the quantity and composition of the diet because excesses resulting from a varied intake are excreted in urine. Loss of kidney function reduces this latitude. This discretionary excretory function of the kidney is responsive to intake—it allows us to eat "what we want, when we want." In more primitive times, this latitude allowed the hunter–gatherer to gorge or to fast as circumstance dictated. Today it allows us a varied diet on a variable schedule. As function declines, so does tolerance for those variations. The magnitude of the tolerances for several nutrients that are dependent on renal function are illustrated in

Table 34-1.[16] Calories are different from the other nutrients because calorie or energy intake is regulated by appetite in response to energy need. Excesses are miniscule in comparison with other nutrients, and these, of course, are stored, not excreted. Variations between the minimum ($\approx$2300 Cal/day for an adult sedentary male) and maximum ($\approx$6000 Cal/day for a lumberjack) are related to differences in need. However, the level of intake of calories determines, in large degree, the intake of the other nutrients.

The level of intake of these nutrients depends on what is eaten to satisfy energy requirements. The original extraordinary range of tolerance for these nutrients narrows as renal function declines—roughly in proportion to the level of function.

Metabolic alterations that accompany specific impairment of renal function may profoundly affect the need for some nutrients. Renal tubular acidosis alters tolerance for hydrogen ion excretion drastically, and nutrient intake must provide extra alkali. However, with diffuse renal disease, clinical evidence for metabolic nutritional disturbances in adults seldom appears until function is reduced to 30%. In children growth rate may slow with a reduction in function to 50%. The term *renal insufficiency* is appropriate for those states where clinical evidence of impaired renal function appears, that is, where symptoms—including growth failure in children—result from renal disease. Uremia implies symptoms related to nitrogen retention. Uremia develops when clearances are between 5% to 15% of normal in adults and at somewhat higher clearances in children. ESRD is a bureaucratic label that defines patients who require dialysis or renal transplantation.

While excretory function of the kidney is the critical factor affecting nutritional needs, endocrine function of the kidney plays an important role as well. The kidney has at least three endocrine functions, including the synthesis of 1,25-dihydroxyvitamin D_3 (1,25-$(OH)_2D_3$), renin, and erythropoietin. These affect, respectively, calcium and phosphorus metabolism, sodium chloride handling, and red blood cell synthesis. The renin–aldosterone system also affects potassium. Production of 1,25-dihydroxyvitamin D_3 and of erythropoietin is diminished in patients with declining renal mass, and this becomes clinically evident when clearance decreases below 30%. Renin production can remain high even with severe loss of function; other patients become hyporeninemic.

Normal kidney function is permissively important to other metabolic processes. Renal insufficiency alters metabolism in ways that affect nutritional requirements or status; for example, pyridoxine requirement is increased in patients with uremia, and trace mineral requirements often are altered.

The goal of nutrition therapy in renal insufficiency is to provide a diet that meets minimum requirements but does not exceed the limits of tolerance in the patient. In practice, nutrition therapy is limited by uncertainties regarding diet composition, or patient requirements for specific nutrients. Patients also will experience difficulty in adhering to dietary advice. The nutritionist or physician who is giving advice is challenged by the need to construct an appealing diet that limits intake of some nutrients but provides for the greater intake of others. When this challenge is met by the interplay of patients, nutritionists, and physicians,

TABLE 34-1
Minimum and Maximum Daily Intakes of Calories and Six Nutrients, RDA or Average Intake of a Normal Adult Male, and Recommended Amounts for an Adult Male with Uremia

	Minimum	Maximum	Average Intake	Recommended: in Uremia
Calorie (Cal)	2000	6000	2300	2300
Protein (g)	30	300	110	40 (70)‡
Calcium (mg)	400	2000	1000	2000
Phosphorus (mg)	500	4500	1500	800
Sodium (chloride) (mEq)	10	500	200	40
Potassium (mEq)	20	500	100	40
Hydrogen ion (mEq)	−100	300	70	40
Iron (mg)	—	—	10–18†	30–60§
Folacin (μg)	—	—	400*	1000
Pyridoxine (mg)	—	—	2.2*	5–(10)‡

*RDA value.
†RDA: 10 mg for males; 18 mg for females who are menstruating.
‡On hemodialysis.
§If signs of iron deficiency, *i.e.*, low ferratin values are present.

suitable and interesting diets are developed. When this interaction is lacking, the results of nutrition therapy are poor.

Nutrients comprise the macronutrients—protein, fat, and carbohydrate; electrolytes—sodium, potassium, chloride, hydrogen ion, calcium, and phosphorus; and the micronutrients—vitamin and trace minerals.

Recommended dietary allowances (RDA) for normal people at various ages and in different occupations are prepared by the Food and Nutrition Board of the National Academy of Sciences periodically (see Appendix Table A-1). These RDAs may not apply equally well to patients with uremia. However, expressing intakes as a percent of normal RDAs is a useful guide to diet adequacy. Normal values for energy and protein are provided in Table 34-2.

In succeeding sections, we will review metabolism and requirements of several nutrients that are affected in patients with renal disease. The special needs of children are considered.

TABLE 34-2
RDA for Energy and Protein at Different Ages

| | Age (yr) | Energy (Cal/kg/day) | | Protein* (g/kg/day) Male and Female |
		Female	Male	
INFANT	0.5–1	105		2
CHILDREN	1–3	100		1.8
	4–10	85		1.4
	11–14	50	60	1
	15–18	40	45	.85
ADULTS	19–22	40		.80
	23–50	35–40		.80
	>50	35		.80

Taken from Appendix Table A-1. Patients with uremia should be taking at least 80% of RDA for energy.

*Children with uremia should receive between 80%–100% RDA based on present information; adults with uremia should receive 40 g of high-quality protein or 15 g of any protein plus 15 g–20 g essential amino acids or their keto-analogues. Patients on hemodialysis should receive between 100%–150% of RDA based on current information; those on CAPD should receive between 150%–200% of RDA. No data are available on children.

Energy

Energy balance in health embraces two concepts: (1) body composition is normal and (2) energy (calorie) intake and energy expenditure are in a normal range and, over a period of time, are equal. Body composition in this instance refers to body stores of substrate or potential energy,* notably body fat and muscle protein. Strictly speaking there is no store of protein, but, with dietary energy deficiency, muscle contractile protein is consumed. The characteristic features of dietary energy deficiency in terms of change in body composition are a decrease in body fat—skin-fold thickness—and a decrease in muscle mass or work capacity. These features are commonly described as undernutrition or wasting (see Chap. 10).

An adequate energy intake depends on free access to food, and an appetite sensitive to energy need or expenditure, so that intake and expenditure balance while body composition remains normal. Energy expenditure is normal when the individual is free to spend energy and the expenditure is balanced by an equal intake. The range of 2300 Cal/day to 6000 Cal/day in adults is dependent on job and living style. These prosaic definitions cover some subtle complexities. For example, the individual who is chronically undernourished may have

an intake that equals output but work capacity is limited because intake is limited. Adipose tissue and muscle mass are reduced. By contrast, a long-distance runner characteristically has reduced adipose tissue. However, muscle mass, work capacity, and energy expenditure are supranormal and so is energy intake. A patient with muscle disease that limits activity may be in energy balance and have adequate fat stores but may have impaired muscle mass and work capacity for other reasons.

Energy balance in children involves all of these features and, in addition, is essential for normal growth. Small restrictions in energy intake impair growth. Normal growth is an index of energy balance.

Patients with uremia commonly have decreased adipose tissue mass, decreased muscle mass and work capacity, and poor food (calorie) intake. Children grow poorly. Taste perception is impaired in uremic patients. These findings have led to the conclusion that dietary energy deficiency is a common complication in uremia. Its prevalence is not well documented, but several authors using various criteria have found that between one third and two third of patients with ESRD, or those on dialysis, have dietary energy deficiency.[18]

Evaluating energy balance in clinical practice is not easy. Diet records can be used to calculate energy (and other nutrient) intake. Now that a data base for food composition and computer programs are available, this calculation can be done at a reasonable cost.[28] Skin-fold thickness is a suitable

---

*Glycogen is a store of substrate, or potential energy. It is a ready store of carbohydrate that is small and is quickly depleted when a person fasts. Estimating glycogen stores is difficult and not significantly related to assessing the nutritional state relative to energy balance.

method for estimating body fat when the measurement is made by a trained professional (see Chap. 10). Clinically suitable measures of muscle mass and work capacity in these patients are wanting, however. Growth rate in children is an index of adequate energy input.

A dietary intake that falls below 75% of RDA should signal the need for improving energy intake—especially if skin-fold thickness or other clinical signs of muscle wasting are present.[18] Energy intake may be improved by diet counseling to change eating habits, to include high calorie foods, or to add calorie supplements to the diet. Success is more likely when the physician or nutritionist has time to learn the patient's food preferences, style of living, and pattern of eating. We have used two supplements: Polycose (Ross Laboratories, Columbus, Ohio), which is partially hydrolyzed starch that has 10 mEq/Na/100 Cal, and Contralyte (Doyle Chemical Company, Minneapolis, Minnesota), a carbohydrate–fat mix that is free of sodium. These can increase total energy intake by 10% to 30%. Selecting favorite foods, suggesting attractive ways of preparing foods, and eating meals in a pleasant social setting all help to improve intake. We have observed improved growth and normalizing of skin-fold thickness in children given supplements that increased energy intake on average from 75% to 90% of RDA for height. Nutrition therapy to increase intake usually is not needed in patients who have normal skin-fold thickness or whose intake is more than 80% of RDA.

Unfortunately, diets high in carbohydrate increase plasma lipids. Because patients with uremia have hyperlipidemia and a higher rate of early atherosclerosis, the benefits of supplements may incur a cost.[4] One strategy that may prove beneficial is encouraging exercise. Exercise in dialysis patients improves work capacity, lowers plasma lipids, and improves nutritional status.[14]

Uremia is characterized by an exaggerated catabolic response to stress.[17] Fasting in uremic patients is associated with greater losses of nitrogen and higher levels of catabolic hormones. Infection and injury may have greater catabolic responses in uremic patients. Uremic patients can protect themselves by planning more regular schedules for eating and by giving extra attention to nutrition when they have infections.

Obese uremic patients often are "snackers" and are prone to sedentary living; they may benefit from a more planned diet and a more active life.

Low energy intake in children is often associated with poor growth. Increasing energy intake to more than 80% RDA may lead to improved growth but seldom to accelerated growth. It is very important to recognize that children cannot be made to eat.

Skill and patience are necessary on the part of physician, staff, and family in their effort to increase food intake of children. Acceptance by staff of limited successes is important.

Protein

Nitrogen (N) balance in health, like energy balance, embraces the concepts of maintenance of a normal mass of body protein and an intake of amino acid nitrogen sufficient to replace nitrogen lost. The daily requirement for N in the diet is to fill the need for essential and nonessential amino acids. In adult males roughly 7 g of a balanced essential amino acid mix and 15 g to 25 g of nonessential amino acids are needed to replace amino acids catabolized and the nitrogen excreted (see Appendix Table A-1). N is excreted as urea and nonurea nitrogen in the form of uric acid and creatinine. If intake exceeds the minimum requirements, as it usually does, the excess is metabolized almost entirely to urea nitrogen and excreted.

The range of tolerance for protein in normal adults is from 30 g/day to 300 g/day (0.5g/kg/day–5 g/kg/day). The RDA for protein is 0.8 g/kg/day, and the average intake in Western nations is 1.7 g/kg/day, more than twice the RDA and more than 3 times the minimal requirements. The blood urea nitrogen (BUN) concentration of adults and children taking 1.7 g protein/kg/day is in the range of 15 mg/dl to 20 mg/dl, and at 0.5 g/kg/day is in range of 4 mg/dl to 6 mg/dl.

Adults with severe uremia, that is, renal function ≈10% normal, who are on an average diet have a BUN of ≈200 mg/dl. When placed on 0.8 g protein/kg/day, they will decrease BUN to ≈100 mg/dl, and when placed on the very low protein diet (.3 g/kg/day), they will decrease BUN to less than 50 mg/dl. These changes in diet and reduction in BUN are associated with relief of the uremic symptoms. The very low protein intake—0.3 g/kg/day—is below minimum requirements and may be associated with loss of body protein N. Many patients, already malnourished, may find a very low protein diet unpalatable. Patients with moderate uremia are in better N balance when they are given a diet of 35 Cal and 0.6 g protein/kg/day than one providing 0.3 g/kg/day. At least half of the protein should be high biologic value protein, that is, meat, milk, or egg proteins high in essential amino acids.[21]

When patients are given a very low protein diet (less than 0.2 g/kg/day) and are given essential amino acids as supplements, they may improve, gain weight, and retain N. Substituting some keto-analogues for the amino acids and lowering N intake even more lead to further improvement in N balance.[38] The benefits of essential amino acid supplements or of keto-analogue essential amino acid supplements are lost when dietary protein intake is increased to 0.6 g/kg/day.[9]

These observations are at the heart of the controversy over how long diet therapy should be pursued and when dialysis therapy should be initiated in patients with progressive renal insufficiency. Using the strictest diet therapy, patients can be maintained without dialysis when their function is 2% to 5% of normal. Using minimal diet therapy, dialysis is needed when function is 10% to 15% of normal. Proponents of prolonged strict diet therapy feel that patients forestall the restrictions dialysis impose, whereas proponents of early dialysis argue that patients placed on dialysis earlier remain in a better nutritional state.[7,39] Very likely, some patients are better suited for the former and other patients are better suited for the latter. Very restrictive diet therapy using keto-analogues has worked in the hands of Walser.[38] Because diet control is perceived less as therapy by most physicians, and because economic incentives are lacking, there has been less enthusiasm for the strict diet therapy approach of Walser. No controlled studies have been done to ascertain the relative merits of Walser's approach compared with those of early dialysis.

When patients are placed on hemodialysis, protein intake must be increased to 1.0 g/kg/day to 1.2 g/kg/day because there are amino acid losses in the dialysate. The quality of protein is important, and at least half should be high biologic value protein. Patients often elect higher protein intakes. While this may be harmful, careful studies have not been conducted to examine that question.

Patients on CAPD have, in addition to amino acid losses, losses of serum protein in dialysate. They should receive between 1.2 g/kg/day to 1.5 g/kg/day protein, including a generous percentage of high biologic quality protein.[15]

Children who have uremia and require dietary protein restriction presently are recommended to take protein in accordance with the RDA. There are no definitive data on optimal requirements in children. Growth rate has not been linked to protein intake but rather to energy intake. We recommend that children select diets that provide 12% of calories as protein. Energy intakes should exceed 80% RDA for height. Children on dialysis have slightly higher requirements for protein because amino acids are lost by dialysis. Diets providing 15% of total energy as protein appear more appropriate, although it should be noted that studies have not been done to define the requirement of children on dialysis. Children on CAPD who receive a carbohydrate supplement by dialysis and lose protein may need a more protein-rich diet. Preliminary observations of growth and weight gain in children on CAPD do not show significant differences from those on hemodialysis.

Calcium, Phosphorus, and Vitamin D

Calcium (Ca) and phosphorus (P) are the principle elements in bone: more than 99% of body calcium and the major fraction of body phosphorus are in bone. Bone Ca and P are pools from which plasma and cell concentrations can be regulated when intake or excretion is altered. Ca in plasma and in cell membranes regulates many critical biologic functions. Its concentration is closely regulated by a network of controls. P is the currency by which energy is transferred; phosphorylation–dephosphorylation processes are the common means for control of enzyme action. Hence bone Ca and P do more than give bone structure; they provide a pool from which cell Ca and P dynamics can be sustained.

Ca absorption from the gastrointestinal tract is controlled by vitamin D or one of its biologically active analogues, notably $1,25\text{-}(OH)_2D_3$. Ca balance is regulated largely by gastrointestinal function. Renal excretion of Ca is small and relatively consistent; diet has little effect.

The normal dietary requirement for Ca is not well defined, partly because other nutrients affect its absorption (*e.g.*, protein and phosphate, as well as vitamin D). The normal recommendation of the FAO/WHO Committee on Ca requirements for adults is 500 mg/day, whereas the RDA in the United States is 800 mg/day. This discrepancy is due in part to differences in dietary protein and P. The ideal Ca:P ratio is disputed. In growing infants who are forming bone the ideal ratio is 2:1, as is found in human milk. In diets of adults and older children in Western nations the ratio is between 1:1.2 and 1:2, averaging 1:1.6. The major reason for the concern over this variation is the unknown role that Ca intake or the Ca:P ratio plays in osteoporosis in older people. One reason for uncertainty is that changes in dietary Ca have a slow effect on Ca balance. In some cultures dietary intake of 200 mg/day to 400 mg/day appears to suffice.[26]

P is ubiquitous in foods, notably meat, eggs, and milk products, all of which are sources of high biologic quality protein. P is used extensively in food processing. Baked goods, modified proteins, and soft drinks generally contain much added P. Normally more than 50% of ingested P is absorbed and excreted. Renal P excretion is responsive to dietary intake. This control is mediated partly by plasma P concentration, vitamin D, and parathormone.[11]

When patients develop impaired renal function, Ca metabolism and P metabolism are altered, affecting dietary requirements and tolerance of Ca, P, and vitamin D. Ca reabsorption from the gastrointestinal (GI) tract may be decreased with relatively modest reduction in renal function (50%–70%) although both serum levels of 1,25-$(OH)_2D_3$ and hypercalcemic responses to administered 1,25-$(OH)_2D_3$ are normal. Later, when function is less than 30% normal, resistance to the vitamin D effect on Ca absorption develops. As renal insufficiency gives way to ESRD the serum levels of 1,25-$(OH)_2D_3$ become undetectable and Ca absorption is impaired. Hypocalcemia often results, and this will lead to hyperparathyroidism.

By contrast, patients with declining renal function have no difficulty absorbing P but experience progressive loss of excretory capacity. Serum P will rise perceptibly in adults on average P intake (1 g/day–2 g/day) only when renal function decreases below 30% normal.[11] Slatapolsky and Bricker have proposed that regulating P intake early in renal failure will prevent surreptitious elevations in serum P, complexing of serum Ca, and stimulating secretion of parathormone.[35] They reason that this will prevent the hyperparathyroid-induced osteodystrophy. This is one theoretical basis for avoiding excessive P intake in patients with renal insufficiency.[11,35]

Patients who are hypocalcemic should receive Ca supplements of at least 1000 mg Ca daily. Plasma P should be controlled before Ca supplements are given. Indications for giving vitamin D are less clear. Persistent hypocalcemia and x-ray evidence of hyperparathyroid osteodystrophy unresponsive to Ca supplements are clear indications. Treatment should not be initiated until plasma P is below 6 mg/dl. Good results are more likely in patients with pretreatment serum Ca values <10.5 mg/dl and with evidence of hyperparathyroidism.

There is consensus that P intake should be controlled so that plasma phosphate levels remain below 6 mg/dl. There is a strong body of opinion that phosphorus intake should be reduced to levels proportional to the reduction in function in order to prevent hyperparathyroidism and renal injury.[23,35] This opinion prevails even though plasma phosphate levels are seldom elevated in patients until function is less than 30% normal. If normal P intake is accepted as 1.6 g/day, then patients whose function is less than 50% normal would be limited to P intakes of 0.8 g/day—a level that is difficult to achieve unless they accept a low-protein diet. Phosphate-binding gels are effective in lowering plasma phosphate, but patients often find the gels unpalatable. It is common practice to avoid using them until plasma phosphate is elevated.

In children the same goals of therapy are accepted: (1) to maintain plasma phosphate below 6 mg/dl, (2) to maintain plasma Ca between 10 mg/dl and 11 mg/dl, and (3) to follow plasma parathormone and bone mineralization in the effort to prevent or to correct osteodystrophy. The problem is more compelling in children because bones are growing and mineralization should be increasing. It is also more difficult to ascertain what guidelines to use for dietary P control. P intake per kg in children is higher because food intake per kg is higher. Children are at least as prone as adults to find phosphate-binding gels unpalatable. Vitamin D therapy in children may be needed earlier in renal insufficiency because 1,25-$(OH)_2D_3$ levels in children with renal insufficiency are reduced. Vitamin D therapy does promote growth, but, like energy supplements, it does not lead to catch-up growth. Doses of 1,25-$(OH)_2D_3$ are between 0.25 μg/day and 1.0 μg/day. Plasma Ca and P should be followed closely, particularly during the initial phases of treatment. Hypercalcemia and hyperphosphatemia may develop. The intake of either of these, or of 1,25-$(OH)_2D_3$ should then be decreased.

Sodium

Sodium, predominantly as sodium chloride*, is the principal ion governing the volume of extracellular fluid. Sodium balance implies a normal volume and concentration of sodium in extracellular fluid. Intake may be very low or very high, but renal excretion will match it. Control of extracellular fluid volume is carefully regulated by renal function, that is, renal excretion of sodium and chloride.

Recommendations for sodium intake for the normal population present something of an enigma. The minimum intake consistent with sodium balance is 10 mEq/day (250 mg) sodium so long as there are no unusual extrarenal losses, such as GI or skin losses. Some primitive tribes survive on intakes that are this low. Cultures in which intake is less than 40 mEq/day (920 mg) sodium have no hypertension. Disadvantages of this low intake are not documented. The average sodium intake in Western culture is 200 mEq/day (4.6 g) sodium, or 20 times the lowest intake noted above. On this intake roughly 20% of adults develop hypertension. A "low" intake in our culture is 43 mEq/day (1 g) sodium. Tobian has recently summarized the

---

*While sodium intake often is spoken of without mentioning an anion, the most important anion coupled to sodium is chloride. Chloride has unique permeability properties and mechanisms for reabsorption that make sodium and chloride the dominant electrolytes of extracellular fluid. Bicarbonate can fill the role of chloride to a very limited degree, and sodium salts of organic ions lead to bicarbonate generation. Generally, however, sodium intake should be construed as, or preferably documented to be, sodium chloride or salt intake.

evidence linking salt intake to hypertension.[37] The American Academy of Pediatrics, Committee on Nutrition has summarized the evidence on this relationship as it applies to children.[2] A low salt intake approximating 3 g salt/day (50 mEq or 1.2 g sodium) is recommended by many as ideal. Adults with severe hypertension have maintained sodium balance on as little as 2.2 mEq/day (50 mg) sodium. In Japanese communities, people commonly ingest as much as 425 mEq/day (20 g) sodium; in these communities there is a very high prevalence of hypertension. There is considerable evidence that a high salt intake is related to a high prevalence of hypertension in genetically sensitive people.[37]

Sodium depletion effects a decrease in extracellular fluid and circulating blood volume. Sodium excess is expressed as signs of extracellular volume expansion (edema) and circulatory overexpansion (hypervolemia). In nephrosis, edema results from the contracted circulatory volume while total body sodium is expanded.

Infants have an absolute requirement of between 4 mEq/day and 8 mEq/day (100 mg–200 mg) sodium, which is higher than the minimum required by adults. Approximately 2 mEq/day are used for growth. This requirement is met by human milk, with very little excess. Urine sodium in breast-fed infants is quite low.[2,3]

Sodium balance in patients with renal insufficiency is enigmatic. The tolerance for high and low intakes in uremic patients is reduced roughly in proportion to reduction in function. As functional mass decreases and nephrons drop out in patients with progressive renal insufficiency, single nephron filtration rate and fractional excretion of sodium increase.[8] In one study when salt intake in patients with uremia was varied from 3.5 g to 7 g (60 mEq–120 mEq Na/day), the patients tolerated the change by varying the fractional sodium excretion rate so that output matched intake. The fractional excretion rate per nephron was much higher than that seen in normal subjects. However, acute changes outside these limits were not, in these studies, well tolerated.[34] Acute reductions in salt intake lower renal function.[27] While the diseased kidney shows adaptive capacity within the range cited, the normal kidney has a remarkable and rapid ability to respond to changes in sodium intake from as low as 2 mEq/day to as high as 1000 mEq/day and establish sodium balance.

Patients with renal insufficiency have lost the tolerance to marked changes in salt intake. Patients with uremia are sensitive to acute nonrenal losses of sodium and to reductions in salt intake. Some—particularly those with medullary cystic disease—may have unusual requirements of up to 300 mEq/day. We have seen a few patients on normal sodium intakes who were normotensive and had signs of slight loss of skin turgor that responded to prescribed increases in salt intake. The most sensitive indications of a favorable response are a decrease in BUN, an increase in weight, and an improved sense of well-being. Children show improved growth. These patients may respond to successive increments in salt intake with successive reductions in BUN. They should, however, be observed carefully for signs of excess sodium—hypertension, edema, or vascular overload.

Most patients, however, must restrict sodium intake below their accustomed level. For many this means avoiding prepared foods, such as pizza, fried chicken, fried potatoes, and breads, and learning to use homemade substitutes. For patients with renal insufficiency and hypertension, common practice is to pay less attention to dietary sodium restriction and to use diuretic therapy instead. We believe that time spent helping patients to adjust to lower sodium intake is time well spent. Low-salt cooking can be tasty. Indeed, many people rediscover tastes long obscured by a high-salt diet. A second advantage is that patients with progressive renal disease who adapt to a low-salt diet before they require dialysis, start dialysis with fewer adjustments. A low-sodium diet, not diuretic therapy, is the effective way to avoid salt overload in patients on dialysis. It is preferable to ultrafiltration to remove retained fluid and sodium at the time of dialysis. Diets that provide 43 mEq/day to 87 mEq/day (1 g–2 g sodium) are usually satisfactory in controlling blood pressure of anuric adults on dialysis. These require removal of between 0.5 liter to 1.0 liter (8 ml/kg–16 ml/kg) per hemodialysis session when the interval between dialysis is 2 days.

Children can be restricted to 1 mEq/kg/day to 2 mEq/kg/day (25 mg–50 mg) sodium. Normally children eating the same foods as adults ingest more sodium/kg/day than adults because energy intakes per kg are higher. Renal function per kg in normal children also is higher.[10] Children with uremia on a comparable low-sodium diet receive a higher sodium intake per kg than adults on the same diet. Hence, quantitatively it is more difficult to lower sodium intake in children to levels that are achieved in adults. Children on hemodialysis who are anuric and take 1 mEq/kg/day to 2 mEq/kg/day of sodium will require removal of 15 ml to 30 ml fluid per kg per hemodialysis session.

Potassium

Potassium balance implies a normal concentration of potassium in cells and extracellular fluid in the face of an intake within the range usually tolerated. Any normal person meeting usual dietary energy needs from conventional foods will generously exceed the minimum requirement of 20 mEq/day for potassium. Potassium tolerance, like that for sodium, is great. Intakes over 300 mEq/day are common in some cultures, and intakes up to 1000 mEq/day are tolerated. Body potassium can be depleted by diuretic therapy, by frequent laxative use, and by bizarre diets that omit potassium and provide excess sodium. Patients with hyperreninemic hypertension and some with renal tubular acidosis are prone to be potassium deficient because of renal losses of potassium.[13,33] Generally, patients on diuretic therapy do not need potassium supplements; dietary potassium is sufficient. However, patients on diuretic therapy who have hyperreninemic hypertension or are on a high-sodium and low-potassium diet should be followed closely. Patients with renal tubular acidosis and potassium deficiency may need to have part of their alkali therapy given as a potassium salt.[25]

Most patients with progressive renal insufficiency develop a tolerance for potassium intake. As long as function is above 15%, usual dietary potassium intakes are well tolerated. An exception is in patients with aldosterone deficiency and renal insufficiency.[30] These patients, many of whom are diabetic, have moderate renal insufficiency, hyperkalemia, and sometimes renal tubular acidosis. They are not tolerant to usual dietary potassium intakes unless aldosterone replacement therapy is given. Alkali therapy in the form of a sodium salt may be needed when acidosis persists. These patients should have dietary potassium restricted to between 40 mEq/day to 60 mEq/day, or that amount that is compatible with a normal serum potassium.

Patients with uremia, including those on dialysis, also need to limit dietary potassium. Those with uremia must limit intake to excretory capacity. This will be enhanced if acid–base status is kept normal. Those on dialysis accumulate potassium in the interdialytic period, some of which is in extracellular fluid. Since the capacity in such patients to increase the potassium pool without incurring dangerous hyperkalemia is limited, it is important to keep dietary potassium within that limit. During infections, or following stress or severe exercise, hyperkalemia may result from patients becoming catabolic or acidotic. For those patients glucose and alkali therapy may suffice. Some will need a potassium-binding resin (Kayexalate) as well. One gram of Kayexalate removes 1 mEq; the usual dose is 20 g to 30 g in adults and 1 g/kg to 2 g/kg in children.

Acid–Base Balance

Acid–base balance is a term used to imply that body fluid *p*H and buffer capacity remain in a normal range in the face of a considerable range in intake of hydrogen ion or acid. Net acid intake is the sum of hydrogen ion input from diet and metabolism. It may range from a minus value (alkaline input) of 100 mEq/day to one of more than 300 mEq/day. The average for adults is 70 mEq/day. The source of hydrogen ion input is the difference in dietary fixed cation and anion, the metabolic production of fixed acid (phosphate and sulfate), and, when it occurs, the incomplete oxidation of organic anions (*e.g.*, lactate or ketone acids). Bone mineralization releases hydrogen ion; bone demineralization titrates or absorbs it. Relative absorption of cation and anions, particularly Ca and P by the GI tract, also affects net acid intake. For acid–base balance to prevail, net acid loss from body fluids must equal input. Renal acid excretion is largely responsible for effecting this balance. The mechanism of renal acid excretion is complex. It begins with hydrogen ion secretion to reclaim bicarbonate; it continues with hydrogen ion secretion to establish a urine:plasma hydrogen ion gradient of up to 1000:1. In this process phosphate and organic acids are titrated. The secretion of ammonia, a hydrogen ion acceptor, increases the renal capacity to secrete hydrogen ion and reclaim fixed cation. When net intake is alkaline (a negative acid load), bicarbonate reabsorption is depressed until alkali excreted as bicarbonate matches input.

Acidosis is common in patients with renal disease. Two general types exist: renal tubular acidosis (RTA) and the acidosis of uremia. RTA covers a number of diseases that have in common a limitation in renal net acid excretion.[13,25]

Proximal RTA is characterized by a defect in reclamation of bicarbonate from the proximal tubule. A reduction in plasma bicarbonate results; chloride reabsorption and its concentration in plasma increase. When a steady state is established, urine may be acid. Proximal RTA may occur as an isolated disease, but more often it is an expression of diffuse renal injury in which proximal tubule injury is disproportionate. Fanconi's syndrome, particularly that associated with cystinosis, is the most prominent permanent form. In children, poor growth and rickets are common. In the early stages of cystinosis, before glomerular filtration rate (GFR) is reduced, large quantities of alkali—10 mg/kilo/day to 30 mg/kilo/day— as both sodium and potassium salt, are needed to correct the acidosis. These quantities are difficult for patients to take and often interfere with food intake. Thiazide and potassium-sparing diuretics may reduce the alkali needed to restore acid–base balance. In children with cystinosis complete correction is not often achieved. As function declines, it may be possible to restore acid–base balance with lower doses.[12,13,25]

Distal RTA is characterized by a defect in ability

to secrete hydrogen ion in the distal tubule. The disease commonly appears in association with renal injury in adults from many causes. In children it is usually an isolated defect. Its clinical findings are similar to those of proximal RTA, but urine *p*H, even with severe acidosis, remains above 6.0. Nephrocalcinosis develops. In children poor growth and rickets occur as with proximal RTA. Somewhat smaller doses of alkali are needed to restore acid–base balance in distal as opposed to proximal RTA. Between 1 mEq/kg/day to 3 mEq/kg/day of a mixture of sodium and potassium alkaline salts are recommended for adults; between 3 mEq/kg/day to 15 mEq/kg/day are recommended for children.[12] When acid–base balance is restored in children, rickets will heal, "catch-up" growth may occur, and nephrocalcinosis may abate.[24]

Patients with RTA and hyperkalemia either have hypoaldosteronism or a mineralocorticoid-resistant state.[29,30] These patients may require aldosterone replacement therapy and should restrict dietary potassium. In addition, they may require alkali to correct acidosis, and the alkali should be given as a sodium salt.

Patients with acidosis secondary to renal insufficiency may have renal bicarbonate wasting or other features of RTA. They generally have a hyperchloremic acidosis when function is between 20% to 30% of normal.[40] A limitation in the ability to excrete ammonia is the most important factor that impairs net acid excretion and induces acidosis. The ability to excrete ammonia increases in a compensatory way as renal mass declines. This compensatory increase fails to match net acid intake when function declines below 20%.[32]

The acidosis of renal insufficiency can be treated either with dietary alterations to lower net acid intake or with alkali to counter the gap between net acid intake and the capacity for net acid excretion. A low-protein, low-phosphorus diet will lower net acid intake. Giving 30 mEq to 70 mEq (0.5 mEq/kg–1.0 mEq/kg) per day of alkali, usually as a sodium salt, will alleviate the acidosis so long as there is no underlying RTA.

Vitamins

The RDAs for vitamins generally are set well in excess of minimum requirement for the normal population to ensure an adequate intake under most circumstances. These recommended amounts are met with most conventional diets, particularly now that vitamin B enrichment of bread products and vitamin A and D supplementation of milk are common.

However, patients with uremia often are restricted, as noted, in foods that are naturally rich in B vitamins or in foods that are so enriched. For these reasons, probably it is wise to recommend to patients with renal insufficiency who have dietary limitations, especially those with uremia, to take a standard vitamin supplement that provides most of these vitamins in amounts equal to, or slightly greater than, the RDA.[20] Vitamin D has been discussed above; three other vitamins require special comment.

ASCORBIC ACID

The RDA for ascorbic acid has been increased to 60 mg/day based on recent studies of body-pool size and turnover rate. This higher intake ensures reserves for stress and for periods of low intake.[26]

Patients with uremia have dietary restrictions that are likely to lower intake below the RDA, and they sustain losses from dialysis. These patients seem particularly subject to stress of infection or short starvation. For these reasons it is prudent to ensure intakes of at least 60 mg/day, and it may be beneficial to increase this intake to 100 mg/day.

FOLACIN

Folacin losses in normal subjects are estimated to be 40 μg/day. Normal plasma levels are maintained in subjects taking 100 μg/day. The RDA for folacin has been set at 400 μg/day because only half of the naturally occuring folacin is absorbed, and some allowance is made for biologic variation. This amount is provided by conventional diets.

Folacin deficiency is likely to develop in patients with uremia because folacin-rich foods often are restricted because of the potassium content. Prolonged cooking of foods to remove potassium destroys folacin, and folacin is further lost during dialysis. Plasma levels and clinical signs of folate deficiency are reported in patients with uremia.[31] Hyperphosphatemia can inhibit folacin uptake into cells. For these reasons, it is recommended that patients with uremia receive 1 mg of folacin/day in their diet. Those who do not, especially patients on dialysis, should take a supplement of folacin to ensure this intake.[15]

PYRIDOXINE

Pyridoxine is essential as a coenzyme in the pathway of amino acid metabolism leading to protein synthesis. Its deficiency gives rise to changes in plasma amino acid levels, altered immune responses, and hyperlipidemia. Cheilosis, rash, and, in children, convulsions are clinical signs of pyridoxine deficiency (see Chap. 12). The RDA for pyridoxine is 2.2 mg/day.

Pyridoxine metabolism is altered in uremic patients, and signs of pyridoxine deficiency are likely to develop. Biochemical findings suggestive of deficiency are common in patients on dialysis. The abnormal amino acid patterns, altered immune responses, and altered plasma lipid patterns that are seen in patients with uremia may be due to pyridoxine deficiency.[36] In one study, patients on hemodialysis given 300 mg/day pyridoxine showed a return of plasma amino acids toward normal, improvement in response to immune challenge, and an increase in plasma high-density lipoprotein (HDL).[19] These findings are provocative. The doses of pyridoxine used to effect these changes were very high so that the significance of the effect is not clear. Presently, the recommendation is that patients with uremia receive 5 mg/day pyridoxine and those on dialysis receive 10 mg/day.[15]

Trace Elements—Iron and Zinc

Trace elements include iron, zinc, and seven other minerals that are needed in small quantities. Iron and zinc are the most important among these in patients with uremia. Iron requirements for the normal population are greater during rapid growth when iron stores should increase, in women during menstruation when iron is lost, and during pregnancy when iron is stored in the fetus. Iron sources in food include both heme iron that is well absorbed and nonheme iron that is poorly absorbed. These sources provide sufficient iron, except to infants and to women during pregnancy. Infants should receive iron supplements in the second 6 months of life either with iron-enriched formula or infant cereal; women need 30-mg to 60-mg iron supplements daily when they are pregnant (see Chap. 29). Zinc is found in meat and other animal food sources. Zinc deficiency is uncommon in the United States population. About 15 mg of zinc is needed daily.

Anemia is common in patients with uremia, and erythropoietin deficiency may contribute. For most patients the anemia is not due to iron deficiency, and iron supplementation has no value. However, some patients with uremia lose small amounts of blood daily from the GI tract and may become iron deficient. Patients on hemodialysis lose blood during dialysis and may become iron deficient. As with other nutrients, foods that provide iron, particularly heme iron, often are excluded from the diet of patients with uremia. It is important either to monitor patients for laboratory evidence of iron deficiency or to ensure an adequate intake of iron (15 mg/day–30 mg/day) in a suitable bioavailable form. The most dependable assay for iron deficiency in uremia patients is serum ferritin. Values below 80 mg/ml are good evidence of iron deficiency.[5] Iron can be effectively given as an oral supplement.

Zinc intake probably is low in patients with uremia. Zinc deficiency interferes with taste in normal subjects and is a factor causing poor appetite and poor growth in zinc-deficient children (see Chap. 4). Present evidence is not sufficient to recommend routine zinc supplementation in patients with uremia.[22] However, it is quite reasonable in selected patients to provide a supplement in the amount of 10 mg/day to 15 mg/day of elemental zinc given as zinc sulfate and to observe improved taste perception, food intake, or sense of well-being.

Summary

Nutrition therapy in nephrology today has an ill-defined place. There are items that all acknowledge need attention, but our ability to translate that need into effective therapy is hampered. Our understanding of how to help people change ingrained diet practices is inadequate. There are areas in which we see a need for improvement in nutritional status, but we are unsure that a nutritional approach to correction will be effective. This is notably the case in energy balance and calcium–vitamin D metabolism. When there are signs of undernutrition, how do we improve energy intake? If we do, will it work? When there is osteomalacia or hypocalcemia, how do we correct the calcium depletion it represents? How do we prevent it? There are conditions for which we suspect that diet requirements differ significantly from normal, but we lack the knowledge of what the RDA is for uremic patients, and we lack tried and true indices of what path to follow. Pyridoxine and zinc are two such examples. Do we give more to ensure plenty? Is there a risk? What indexes do we monitor?

Further, there is the problem of diet and atherosclerosis. This is an intense problem in patients with renal insufficiency who are progressing to ESRD.[4] Should we seek to limit dietary cholesterol and carbohydrate when energy intake is low? Should we seek to change levels of physical activity to lower plasma lipids?

Given these problems, and the incentives to focus on other aspects of treating uremia, it is not surprising that the place of nutrition in nephrology is unsettled. But being unsettled, it does not follow that either the physician or nutritionist or patient needs to feel paralyzed.

There is general agreement on how to monitor the nutritional–metabolic status of patients with renal insufficiency as they progress to ESRD.[6] We can measure nutrient intake through the use of diet records that can be translated into daily nutrient intake values. A food composition data base developed by Pennington and a computer program are useful.*,28

Table 34-3 summarizes what indexes and laboratory values to follow in relation to several of the nutrients discussed and what changes in their intake may be recommended.

TABLE 34-3
Some Clinical Indexes of Dietary Excesses or Deficiency

ENERGY
Excess: obesity; increased skin-fold thickness
Deficiency: sedentary state; decreased skin-fold thickness; dietary intake of energy <75% RDA

PROTEIN
Excess: high BUN: creatinine ratio (>15) in plasma; history of dietary intake of protein >15% of total calories; improvement in symptoms with a lowering of dietary protein
Deficiency: low plasma albumin; low BUN: creatinine ratio; poor hair growth

CALCIUM
Excess: hypercalcemia
Deficiency: hypocalcemia; high plasma PTH levels; low plasma levels of vitamin D (where available), osteodystrophy

PHOSPHORUS
Excess: hyperphosphatemia; history of intake in excess of 1.2 g/day; high plasma PTH levels; low tubular reabsorption of phosphate
Deficiency: hypophosphatemia; low phosphorus intake; excessive use of phosphate-binding gels

VITAMIN D
Excess: hypercalcemia or hyperphosphatemia in response to vitamin D use
Deficiency: hypocalcemia and osteodystrophy with an adequate calcium intake

SODIUM
Excess: hypertension; edema; pulmonary congestion or heart failure; excessive weight gain between dialyses
Deficiency: fatigue; high BUN: creatinine ratio in plasma; hyponatremia, decrease in BUN in response to adding sodium chloride to the diet

POTASSIUM
Excess: hyperkalemia
Deficiency: hypokalemia

HYDROGEN ION
Excess: low plasma *p*H; low plasma buffer (bicarbonate)
Deficiency: high plasma bicarbonate (may be evidence of K deficiency from diuretic therapy)

*Our computer program may be obtained at cost by writing to Children's Renal Center, U.C.S.F., CA 94143

Having given guidance to what needs to be changed, we can make only a few statements about how to do it. It may be well to drop the term *compliance*. It is authoritarian in tone and counter to the role of a physician who is an adviser. Individuality, culture, economics, convenience, and social pressures are not small forces. We have felt that time spent with patients to help them recognize and contend with these other forces, while we seek to implement changes in diet, is time well spent. A patient or family who can make a change in diet by knowing how to cope with conflicts about individuality, culture, and social pressure is much better served. Trade-offs that can be arrived at openly by adviser and patient provide a much better alternative for effective treatment than strategies to enforce compliance. Some diet changes are more effective when a whole family participates, and the whole family may benefit—or become angry. Lowering dietary salt intake is one example.

Whether dialysis fluid can be used as a conduit for some nutrients rather than a route for loss is being investigated. The use of highly refined diets to forestall dialysis, as proposed by Walser, is a method waiting evaluation.[39] With better delivery systems for these diets, such as indwelling silastic tubes and small portable pumps, the problem of having to eat unpalatable "medical foods" can be bypassed. A new emphasis upon control of dietary input may be in order to improve the support of patients with uremia, including those on dialysis.

References

1. Addis TA: Glomerular Nephritis: Diagnosis and Treatment. New York, Macmillan, 1948
2. American Academy of Pediatrics, Committee on Nutrition: Salt intake and eating patterns of infants and children in relation to blood pressure. Pediatrics 53:115–121, 1974
3. American Academy of Pediatrics, Committee on Nutrition: Commentary on breast-feeding and infant formulas, including proposed standards for formulas. Pediatrics 57:278–285, 1976
4. Bagdade JD, Porte D, Bierman EL: Hypertriglyceridemia: A metabolic consequence of chronic renal failure. N Engl J Med 279:181–185, 1968
5. Bell JD, Kincaid WR, Morgan RG et al: Serum ferritin assay and bone marrow iron stores in patients on maintenance hemodialysis. Kidney Int 17:237–241, 1980
6. Blumenkrantz MJ, Kopple JD, Gutman RD et al: Methods for assessing nutritional status of patients with renal failure. Am J Clin Nutr 33:1567–1586, 1980
7. Bonomini V, Vangelista A, Stefoni S: Early dialysis in renal substitutive programs. Kidney Int 13 (Suppl 8):S112–116, 1978
8. Bricker NS, Fine LG: The "trade-off" hypothesis: Current status. Kidney Int 13 (Suppl 8):S5–8, 1978
9. Burns J, Crisswell E, Ell S et al: Comparison of the effects of keto acid analogues and essential amino acids

on nitrogen homeostasis in uremic patients in moderately protein restricted diets. Am J Clin Nutr 31:1767–1775, 1978

10. Chantler C, Holliday MA: Growth in children with renal disease with particular reference to the effects of caloric malnutrition, a review. Clin Nephrol 1:230–242, 1973

11. Coburn JW, Slatapolsky E: Vitamin D, parathyroid hormone and renal osteodystrophy. In Brenner BM, Rector FC (eds): The Kidney. Philadelphia, WB Saunders, 1981

12. Cogan MG, Rector FC, Seldin DW: Acid–base disorders. In Brenner BM, Rector FC (eds): The Kidney. Philadelphia, WB Saunders, 1981

13. Gennari FJ, Cohen JJ: Renal tubular acidosis. Annu Rev Med 29:521–541, 1978

14. Goldberg AP, Hagberg J, Delmez JA et al: The metabolic and psychological effects of exercise training in hemodialysis patients. Am J Clin Nutr 33:1620–1628, 1980

15. Harvey KB, Blumenkrantz MJ, Levine SE et al: Nutritional assessment and treatment of chronic renal failure. Am J Clin Nutr 33:1586–1597, 1980

16. Holliday MA: Management of the child with renal insufficiency. In Lieberman EL (ed): Clinical Pediatric Nephrology. Philadelphia, JB Lippincott, 1976

17. Holliday MA, Chantler C: Metabolic and nutritional factors in children with renal insufficiency. Kidney Int 14:306–312, 1978

18. Holliday MA, McHenry–Richardson K, Portale A: Nutritional management of chronic renal disease. Med Clin North Am 63:945–961, 1979

19. Kleiner MJ, Tate SS, Sullivan JF et al: Vitamin B_6 deficiency in maintenance of dialysis patients: Metabolic effects of repletion. Am J Clin Nutr 33:1612–1619, 1980

20. Kopple JD: Dietary requirements. In Massery SG, Sellars A (eds): Clinical Aspects of Uremia and Dialysis. Springfield, Ill, Charles C Thomas, 1976

21. Kopple JD, Coburn JW: Metabolic studies of low protein diets in uremia I. Nitrogen and potassium. Medicine 52:583–595, 1973

22. Mahajan SK, Prasad AS, Lambuzon J et al: Improvement of uremic hypogeusia by zinc: A double blind study. Am J Clin Nutr 33:1517–1521, 1980

23. Maschio G, Tessitore N, D'Angelo A et al: Early dietary phosphorus restriction and calcium supplementation in the prevention of renal osteodystrophy. Am J Clin Nutr 33:1546–1554, 1980

24. McSherry E: Acidosis and growth in non-uremic renal disease. Kidney Int 14:349–354, 1978

25. Morris RC: Renal tubular acidosis: Mechanisms classification and implications. N Engl J Med 281:1405–1413, 1969

26. National Research Council, Food and Nutrition Board: Recommended Dietary Allowance, 9th ed. Washington, D.C., National Academy of Sciences, 1980

27. Nickel JF, Lowrance PB, Leiffer E et al: Renal function, electrolyte excretion and body fluids in patients with chronic renal insufficiency before and after sodium deprivation. J Clin Invest 32:68, 1953

28. Pennington JA: Dietary Nutrient Guide. Westport, CT, Avi Publishing, 1976

29. Perez GO, Oster JR, Vaamonde CA: Renal acidosis and renal potassium handling in selective hypoaldosteronism. Am J Med 57:809–816, 1974

30. Schambelan M, Sebastian A, Biglieri EG: Prevalence, pathogenesis, and functional significance of aldosterone deficiency in hyperkalemic patients with chronic renal insufficiency. Kidney Int 17:89–101, 1980

31. Siddiqui J, Freeburger R, Freeman RM: Folic acid, hypersegmented polymorphonuclear leukocytes and the uremic syndrome. Am J Clin Nutr 23:11–16, 1970

32. Simpson DP: Control of hydrogen ion homeostasis and renal acidosis. Medicine 50:503–541, 1971

33. Slaton PE, Biglieri EG: Hypertension and hyperaldosteronism of renal and adrenal origin. Am J Med 38:324, 1965

34. Slatopolsky E, Ekkau IO, Weerts C et al: Studies on the characteristics of the control system governing sodium excretion in uremic man. J Clin Invest 47:521–530, 1968

35. Slatopolsky E, Bricker NS: The role of phosphorus restriction in the prevention of secondary hyperparathyroidism in chronic renal disease. Kidney Int 4:141–145, 1973

36. Stone WJ, Warnock LG, Wagner C: Vitamin B_6 deficiency in uremia. Am J Clin Nutr 28:950–957, 1975

37. Tobian L: The relationship of salt to hypertension. Am J Clin Nutr 32:2739–2748, 1979

38. Walser M: Keto acid therapy in chronic renal failure. Nephron 21: 57–74, 1978

39. Walser M: Conservative management of the uremic patient. In Brenner BM, Rector RC (eds): The Kidney. Philadelphia, WB Saunders, 1981

40. Widmer B, Gerhardt RE, Harrington JT et al: Serum electrolyte and acid–base composition. The influence of graded degrees of chronic renal failure. Arch Intern Med 139:1099–1106, 1979

35
Skin

Robert G. Crounse
Robert A. Briggaman

Recognition of changes in skin, hair, and nails (or in animals, fur and claws) has played a major role in the study of human nutrition. In a few instances (see the sections on copper, zinc, and essential fatty acid deficiencies in this chapter) the outward appearance of animals deficient in a single nutrient has led by analogy to elucidation of the same deficiency in humans whose skin or hair alterations resembled those of the deficient animals. More often, however, cutaneous changes in animals made deficient in a variety of dietary substances are reported simply as scaly skin or paws, rough coats, or hair loss, information that is insufficient to interpret properly or to extrapolate to humans. Although animal deficiencies provide clues to potential signs of human deficiencies, the ultimate unraveling of nutritional events as they affect human skin has been dependent on inadvertant production of individual deficiencies (*e.g.*, essential fatty acid or zinc deficiency during total parenteral nutrition) or purposeful and carefully controlled exclusion from or limitation of a single substance from the diet of volunteers (*e.g.*, manganese, vitamin C, protein). It is only by these "single-substance dietary deletions" that precise interpretation of cutaneous changes can be achieved. Only by these means can new and specific signs be documented and errors perpetuated by the literature be remedied. Angular cheilitis, or *perlèche*, for example, was passed on by authors for years as a relatively specific manifestation of vitamin B_6 deficiency. This explanation was incorrect, as has been shown clearly by the occurrence of cheilitis in zinc deficiency,

folate deficiency, iron deficiency, vitamin C deficiency, as well as other deficiencies.

New "monovalent" nutritional deficiencies have been recognized even since the first edition of this text, and they continue to represent the only sure means of relating specific cutaneous changes to a given substance. The newer information relates especially to trace elements, an aspect of nutrition that is still evolving actively.

The first portion of this chapter will introduce the cutaneous effects of nutritional deficiencies and excesses. (It is now commonly accepted that even essential nutritional substances can have pharmacologic effects when present in larger than physiologic amounts and toxic effects when present in even greater amounts.) The second portion of this chapter will deal with the effect of skin diseases on systemic nutrition and metabolism, a feature of some skin diseases that is often overlooked. The third section will describe briefly a few selected skin disorders in which dietary alterations or additions can play an important therapeutic role.

In all three portions of this chapter, certain basic biologic facts are essential for logical interpretation of the findings. Skin has unique functions that relate to nutritional events. It must provide a tight barrier to the passage of fluids in either direction. This barrier must be flexible, tough, and continuously renewable. Frequently injured, it must have facile reparative properties. It must serve as defense against a host of dangerous and toxic substances or infective microorganisms. It must provide evaporative cooling for body temperature regulation. (Individuals born without sweat glands cannot so regulate.) Finally, it must provide 7-dehydrocholesterol conversion by way of sunlight to cholecalciferol (vitamin D_3), precursor to the hormonally active hydroxycholecalciferol and dihydroxycholecalciferol, prime regulators of calcium metabolism. All of these functions can be affected by nutritional events.

Two cutaneous appendages, hair and nails, are unique in that they synthesize end-products, which are not subject to metabolic turnover. Being both end-product and highly resistant structures produced continuously over long periods of time (nail indefinitely, scalp hair 3–6 years), they are theoretically storage sites for evidence of past nutritional events. A toxic element like lead, for example, may have been cleared from the blood or urine but persists for long periods of time in the metabolically inert hair shaft, having been taken up by the growing hair root and then deposited in the outward growing shaft. Several factors can confuse interpretation of hair trace element or metal content, however. External contamination and analytic error are obvious ones. Decreased rate of growth or even nongrowth are less obvious but equally important, because less uptake, or no uptake, of internal substances will result. Since scalp hair normally has a growing cycle (several years) and a resting cycle (several months), "blind" sampling (*e.g.*, simple clipping) of scalp hair can result in different proportions of growing and resting hairs, which could contain quite different amounts of a given substance. Age and sex differences as well as regional differences have been documented for several elements in hair; correct interpretation of all these variables is best left to expert investigators in the field.

Finally, hair in humans and fur in animals do not generally have similar cycles. In the growing phase, however, both hair and fur are among the most rapidly proliferative and metabolically active tissues in the body, and they are very sensitive to a wide variety of inhibitors or deficiencies. Hair loss is thus a very nonspecific manifestation of metabolic or nutritional insult.

Nutritional Deficiencies and Excesses

Overall, major decrease in food intake, be it due to economically based starvation, unavailability of food in wartime situations, debilitating illness such as cancer, or gross malabsorption, generally results in a combination of signs of deficiency. In severely undernourished young children, dryness, scaling, mosaic fissuring, loss of turgor, an appearance of thinness, laxity, a wizened, aged appearance, and

pallor out of proportion to accompanying anemia are common. In older patients, easy bruising with purpura and ecchymosis are common. Hyperpigmentation is common, especially in light-exposed areas and dorsal surfaces of the feet. Lightening of hair color, diffuse hair loss or thinning, and dystrophic brittle nails may occasionally be accompanied by a paradoxical increase in downy body hair. Poor healing and depressed immunologic reactivity predispose to ulceration and infection.

PROTEIN DEFICIENCY

The prime example of relatively pure protein deficiency in humans is termed *kwashiorkor*. This condition develops predominantly in young children removed from a balanced high-protein source (*i.e.*, mother's milk) and placed on a substitute low-protein diet. The cutaneous changes that result depend on the nature of that new diet and therefore vary somewhat geographically. A cornmeal diet, for example, may result in signs of pellagra. In general, however, the signs of kwashiorkor are readily recognized. Advanced kwashiorkor gives rise to a typical appearance of major skin changes, change in hair color or hair loss, swollen edematous legs, and protuberant abdomen (hepatomegaly), which differs markedly from the appearance of protein–carbohydrate or total caloric starvation (marasmus). The latter does not coincide with weaning and is characterized by emaciation, wasting, wizened facies, scaphoid abdomen, no edema, and relatively little in the way of skin and hair changes (except as described for general caloric deficiency). Cutaneous kwashiorkor has been vividly described using terms such as "enamel-paint" dermatosis, "flaky paint" dermatosis, "crazy-pavement" skin, "mosaic" skin, "elephant" skin, and "dyschromic" skin, and hair changes have been referred to as "achromotrichia," "rabbit fur" hair, and the "flag sign" (color-banded hair). The earliest skin signs are dryness, wrinkling, cracking, scaling, and ichthyosislike changes. The more advanced changes, seen in less than 50% of cases, have led to the fanciful descriptive terms listed above, especially when hyperpigmentation added to areas of epidermal denudation causes alternating dark enamel-paint and red patches ("crazy-pavement" skin). The earliest changes in hair are measurable before clinical hair change is evident, and they include decreased hair root diameter, volume, and DNA or protein content.[12,26] These changes appear to be as sensitive or more sensitive to borderline protein deficiency than commonly employed measures of skin thickness, serum albumin, or transferrin.[26] More advanced protein deprivation causes decreased hair pigment, giving rise to the classic flag sign (*signa de la bandera* in South America), which is loss of darker pigment, and therefore a reddish color, during periods of protein deprivation, with restoration of normal color during periods of better nutrition. The result is a banded appearance of hair that is quite diagnostic when present. Further or more acute progression of protein malnutrition results in hair loss, a not unexpected event given the high metabolic requirements of the actively growing hair roots.

Interestingly, there is some indication that protein malnutrition leads to inhibition of growth or loss of growing (scalp) hairs, while general undernutrition may result in conversion of greater numbers of hairs to the resting stage.[12] These hairs too are lost, a normal physiologic process for resting hairs. Differentiation of resting hairs from growing hairs, even if atrophic, is quite simple and may provide a means of differentiating early total caloric deprivation from predominantly protein deprivation.

There has been extensive verification of the usefulness of changes in hair roots in detecting protein deficiencies in the elderly and in outpatient alcoholics, in distinguishing protein malnutrition from total caloric malnutrition, and in predicting intrauterine growth from maternal hair roots, but not in newborn malnutrition or in malnutrition in school children. Moreover, they are a less sensitive indicator of deficiency than other commonly used parameters such as serum albumin.[8,14,15,66,82,148]

The novelty of the technique as compared to the widely available routine clinical or laboratory measurements will probably relegate hair root analysis to investigational status until a significant advantage in cost, specificity, or sensitivity can be adequately documented.

ESSENTIAL FATTY ACID DEFICIENCY

Three observations have led to recognition of the effects of deficiency of fatty acids on skin. Early experiments with animals raised on diets deficient in fatty acids (*e.g.,* linoleic, linolenic, and arachidonic acids) demonstrated severe scaling of the skin, subsequently shown to be accompanied by greatly increased transepidermal water loss. Biochemical analysis of the skin showed marked depletion of linoleic and arachidonic acids and accumulation of delta-5,8,11, eicosotrienoic acid (converted from oleic acid when linoleic is deficient). This compound is believed to be synthesized to maintain the degree of unsaturation in skin-membrane phospholipids, but is not convertible to prostaglandins, as is arachidonic acid synthesized from linoleic acid.[104] Interestingly, topical prostaglandin E_2 (PGE_2) restores barrier function in essential fatty acid de-

ficient animals, but only in the local areas to which it is applied.

Second, deranged fatty acid metabolism results in a scaly ichthyosiform dermatosis in the inherited metabolic abnormality in humans known as *heredopathia atactica polyneuritiformis,* or *Refsum's disease.* This disorder is characterized by inability to enzymatically degrade phytanic acid, a C_{20} branched-chain fatty acid derived from plants. This compound is incorporated in skin (presumably membrane) phospholipids in place of the normal fatty acids. The result is a hyperproliferative, therefore scaly, reparative response.[28]

Finally, humans made deficient in essential fatty acids from special diets or intravenous alimentation can develop dry, scaly dermatitis and hair loss, confirmed as essential fatty acid deficiency by the presence of increased delta-5,8,11 eicosotrienoic acid in plasma and tissue phospholipids.[106] Intravenous administration of linoleic acid-containing preparations (*e.g.,* Intralipid effects a cure, as does topical application of sunflowerseed oil.[104]

GENERAL CALORIC EXCESS

Consumption of calories in excess of calories used over sufficient time is the cause of obesity, whether of the common adult-onset variety or secondary to other disorders (see Chap. 28). Uncomplicated obesity of sufficient magnitude (redundant body folds, increase in upper leg girth) can result in a variety of dermatologic disorders, especially irritation between body folds called *intertrigo,* sometimes further complicated by secondary bacterial yeast or superficial fungus infections. Such infections are especially common in obesity complicated by diabetes mellitus, and can serve as a portal of entry for bacteria, resulting in thrombophlebitis, septicemia, gangrene, indolent ulceration, and so forth. Eruptive xanthomata may also occur as a manifestation of diabetes.

Acanthosis nigricans (black, thick skin) can occur in uncomplicated obesity, and is characterized by hyperpigmented epidermal roughening and thickening, moist and soft in body fold areas such as axillae or groin and dry and rough when appearing over knuckles, knees, or elbows. Acanthosis nigricans can also occur in the lipodystrophic and insulin-resistant form of diabetes.[71]

Vitamin Deficiencies and Excesses

VITAMIN A

Vitamin A and its derivatives are key substances in modulation of epithelial tissues, a fact known since the early experiments of Fell and Mellanby demonstrated that vitamin A induced mucous metaplasia of various epithelia, including epidermis, in embryonic chick tissue cultures.[34] In hundreds of experiments or clinical trials since then, vitamin A and its congeners or derivatives thereof have been shown to affect normal or abnormal epidermis, hair, or other epithelial structures. As with many vitamins and minerals or trace substances, results vary with chemical compound, dose, route of administration, influence of other nutritional alterations, organ system studied, age, sex, and a host of other factors. In physiologic amounts and normal circumstances, the vitamin A family (retinal, retinoic acid, and so forth) is probably essential for maintenance of normal epithelial differentiation.

Great interest has been generated in the role of the vitamin A group and its synthetic derivatives in causation, prevention, and treatment of epithelial cancer. Vitamin A deficiency in animal systems induces tracheal squamous metaplasia, believed to be a precancerous lesion, and enhances dimethylbenzanthrene (DMBA)-induced oral carcinoma.[54,109] Retinoic acid and its derivatives have preventative and therapeutic effects on animal skin papillomas and carcinomas in DMBA-initiated and croton oil-promoted carcinogenesis and have been used in treatment of keratoses and basal cell epitheliomas in humans.[10,11] Experimental inhibition of animal bladder tumors by 13-*cis*-retinoic acid and of mammary cancer by retinyl methyl ether has been reported.[46,47] Inhibition by vitamin A of induction of ornithine decarboxylase during the $G1$ phase of the cell cycle in synchronous cultures of Chinese hamster ovary cells, with subsequent blockage of DNA synthesis and cell division, relates vitamin A effects to current hypotheses of cellular proliferation and cancer induction.[49]

Dosage and choice of chemical structure and route of administration remain confounding variables. Vitamin A acid, as used to treat acne, causes epidermal hyperplasia, and a possible potentiation of skin tumors induced by ultraviolet light in experimental animals has been reported.[31] Increasing trials of several retinoids in acne and several scaling disorders of humans will probably further elucidate this complex field.

Cutaneous signs of vitamin A deficiency in humans are most commonly reported to be dryness, scaling, gray hyperpigmentation, and follicular hyperkeratosis, traditionally called *phrynoderma*. Although none of these changes is specific, and pure vitamin A deficiency may not exist in humans, experimental induction or occurrence of vitamin A deficiency after small bowel bypass surgery for obesity confirms that follicular hyperkeratosis is an early sign of lack of vitamin A.[64,112,139] Certainly

its occurrence concomitant with night blindness and ultimately keratomalacia signals the likelihood of deficiency.

The clinical spectrum of hypervitaminosis A is well known. Acute toxicity is manifested by sudden increase in intracranial pressure, headache, nausea and vomiting, bulging fontanelles in children, central nervous system impairment, and intense erythema with subsequent scaling of the face and upper trunk. Chronic long-term ingestion, in doses sometimes prescribed for treatment of dermatologic conditions, can result in loss of appetite, dry skin, hepatomegaly, painful extremities with periosteal thickening, anemia, leukopenia, and hair loss. It should be evident by now that "dry skin" is not very helpful in differentiating nutritional deficiencies or excesses—nor is "hair loss" without further specifications of mechanism. Constellations of signs remain helpful, however. An example might be hypervitaminosis A secondary to renal dialysis.[117] Both renal dialysis and hypervitaminosis A can result in dry skin, itching, and hyperpigmentation. Severe alopecia is more likely a sign of the latter and can help to differentiate. However, major weight loss or protein, calorie, or essential fatty acid or zinc deficiency can also cause skin changes and hair loss. Though all nutritional factors must be considered, prolonged administration of therapeutic vitamin A (or food faddism with megavitamin supplements) can result in toxicity and therefore should be monitored carefully.

CAROTENOID PIGMENTS (PROVITAMIN A)

Hypercarotenosis results from prolonged ingestion of large quantities of foods containing carotenoids, such as carrots (see Chap. 3). The condition may also be a result of disturbed carotenoid metabolism, as in diabetes mellitus, hypothyroidism, some hyperlipemias, and anorexia nervosa. The principal manifestation of the disorder is a yellow to orange discoloration of the skin, most prominent on the palms and soles, nasolabial fold, forehead, axillae, and groin. That sclerae and the buccal mucous membrane are spared serves as a distinguishing feature from jaundice. The typical skin pigmentation is usually not prominent until the carotene plasma level is more than 250 μg/100 ml. Skin pigmentation results from secretion of the carotenoids in sweat and sebum and the subsequent reabsorption by the stratum corneum. Hypercarotenosis is not associated with hypervitaminosis A.

Lycopenemia is a condition similar to carotenemia resulting from excessive consumption of foods (*e.g.,* tomatoes) containing lycopene, which is a carotenoid without provitamin A activity. A yellowish orange discoloration of the skin is the only manifestation of this harmless condition.

NIACIN

A deficiency of niacin and its amino acid precursor, tryptophan, results in the clinical syndrome termed *pellagra,* recognized especially because of its cutaneous manifestations. The classic epidemiologic studies of Goldberger in the early 20th century proved that pellagra in the southeastern states of the United States was due to dietary deficiency rather than to an infectious disease as was previously believed. An animal model called *black tongue* in dogs, said to have been brought to Goldberger's attention by a North Carolina veterinarian, led to Elvehjem's identification of niacin as identical with Goldberger's "pellagra-preventative factor." Affected persons in the state of Georgia in the early 1900s occupied one third to one half of the state hospital beds; the reason was the population's dependence upon corn, which is low in both tryptophan and available niacin (much of which is bound and unavailable).[108] Although now rare in the United States by virtue of dietary changes that include niacin-fortified wheat, pellagra still persists in many parts of the world. In one portion of India, dietary dependence on jowar (*Sorghum vulgaris*), despite normal tryptophan amounts and available niacin, results in pellagra (or when fed to dogs, "black tongue"). This is believed to be due to high leucine content, which can inhibit synthesis of niacinamide-adenine dinucleotides, biochemical products of niacin metabolism. High corn consumption alone is not the only cause of pellagra, as is evident from pellagra secondary to other events leading to defects in tryptophan or niacin, including malabsorption, chronic alcoholism, diversions of tryptophan metabolism in disorders such as carcinoid syndrome, Hartnup's disease, and other enzymatic defects in the pathways of tryptophan utilization, and secondary to certain chemotherapeutic agents such as isoniazid, chloramphenicol, 5-fluorouracil, and 6-mercaptopurine.[123] The complexities of these relationships are illustrated by evidence for isoleucine antagonism of the leucine effect and by occurrence of pellagra in an isoniazid-treated (low tryptophan-consuming) vegetarian despite adequate pyridoxine supplementation, a known requirement during isoniazid therapy.[7]

Pellagra begins with a prodromal phase during which the patient feels ill and may complain of a variety of minor symptoms. Overt disease manifests itself with cutaneous changes, gastrointestinal (GI) disturbances, and mental and neurologic alterations. The course of the disease varies greatly. In the progressive cases, more severe neuropsychiatric involvement and a downhill wasting illness follow, terminating in death. A common picture is one of recurrent episodes, usually each spring, with a tendency to worsen with successive occurrences. Sometimes the disease progresses to a fatal termination with the first attack. Also, the disease may resolve completely without specific treatment.

Skin manifestations are important signs of pellagra and occur in virtually all cases. A bright erythema in light-exposed areas is the first evidence of disease. Over a period of weeks, the color deepens to a reddish brown or chocolate hue; desquamation ensues, usually beginning in the center of an area of erythema and progressing toward the periphery. The scale, which may be composed of either fine or large flakes, renders the skin surface rough, hence the name: *pele* (skin) and *agra* (rough). In some cases, induration may accompany the erythema and eventuate in vesiculation and bulla formation, which further evolves into oozing, eroded, crusted, or ulcerated areas (*i.e.,* the wet form of pellagra). Another characteristic skin lesion is the thickened, hyperkeratotic, darkly pigmented plaque, which tends to form fissures in skin creases. Hyperpigmentation, sometimes of marked degree, follows resolution of the active phase of the dermatoses. In general, pellagrous lesions are sharply marginated and symmetrically distributed. Although almost any area of the skin may be affected, there is a striking predilection for light-exposed areas, particularly the face, dorsum of the hands, lower arm, upper chest and neck (Casal's necklace), shins, and extensor surfaces of the feet. Intertriginous sites, such as the groin and medial upper thighs, may exhibit a similar eruption. In these sites, heat and pressure are thought to play a role in the production of lesions. Burning and itching frequently accompany the dermatosis. Burning may sometimes be so violent as to cause the sufferer to plunge into water for relief.

Oral mucous membranes and skin are usually involved concomitantly, but oral changes may precede the skin changes. The tongue is most commonly affected, becoming bright red and presenting a smooth, denuded surface, worse at the tip and along the margins. In more severe involvement, superficial ulceration may occur at the margins and undersurface, accompanied by a yellowish sloughing. Buccal and other oral surfaces may be similarly involved.

The pathogenic mechanism by which niacin deficiency produces the cutaneous lesions is unknown and, indeed, has received little attention. Findley's finding that diphosphopyridine nucleotide (NAD) levels decrease in pellgrous epidermis provides a basis for the idea that the eruption results from disruption of biochemical pathways in skin.[35] Although the skin lesions occur in light-exposed areas, there is confusion in the literature as to whether the patients are photosensitive. Smith and Ruffin were able to induce skin lesions by sunlight exposure in over half of their patients.[120] However, others have had negative results. Findley studied the effect of light on pellagrous Bantu skin and found the cycle of postburn erythema, scaling, and tanning to be more prolonged than in ordinary sunburn.[36] Pellagrous skin lesions may result from failure of the skin to heal normally following physical injury, such as that from light, heat, and pressure. This idea has some support in the previously mentioned prolonged sunburn response. The resemblance of the skin lesions of pellagra to drug- or plant-induced phototoxic reactions is noteworthy. Porphyrins, which may produce photo-induced skin lesions, are elevated in some cases of pellagra; however, this is not a likely explanation for the photosensitivity because porphyrins are not elevated in all patients and show no correlation with the eruption.[108] Porphyrin elevations are usually seen in alcoholic pellagrins and may be related to alcoholism rather than pellagra. Ingestion of plant toxins may predispose some patients to the development of a phototoxic eruption, but this seems unlikely to be the explanation for the eruption in all patients with pellagra.[108]

In addition to its physiologic role as a vitamin, nicotinic acid has been used as a vasodilator and as a cholesterol-lowering agent. Nicotinic acid produces a brisk red flush, especially when administered intravenously. Nicotinamide does not have this effect and should be used in situations where flushing is not desired.

Large doses of nicotinic acid (3 g/day–6 g/day) employed in the therapy of hypercholesterolemia may produce a generalized ichthyosiform eruption associated histologically with marked hyperkeratosis.[110] Relationship to nicotinic acid can be demonstrated by repeated induction and remission of the eruption by alternately administering and withholding the agent.

RIBOFLAVIN

The features of experimental ariboflavinosis (riboflavin deficiency) in humans are angular stomatitis, a seborrheic dermatitislike eruption involving the face, eyelids, and ears, but sparing the scalp, and dermatitis in the groin area.[77] In the clinical setting, a syndrome termed the *oculoorogenital syndrome*, has been ascribed to ariboflavinosis. In addition to the symptoms described under experimental ariboflavinosis, painful magenta-colored tongue and various eye manifestations, including vascularization of the cornea, epithelial keratitis, and nutritional amblyopia, have been reported. None of the individual signs of ariboflavinosis described here are diagnostic because they can all be seen as manifestations of other conditions. However, in the aggregate, they are highly suggestive of riboflavin deficiency.

A therapeutic trial remains the best test of the validity of a clinical diagnosis. Following the administration of a therapeutic dose of 5 mg/day to 15 mg/day riboflavin, symptoms usually disappear within a few days, and lesions resolve over a period of several weeks. A zero or near zero urinary excretion of riboflavin is suggestive of the diagnosis.

PYRIDOXINE (VITAMIN B$_6$)

Several disease states have been related to pyridoxine deficiency in humans, including convulsive disorders, anemia, and peripheral neuropathy associated with isoniazid administration. Cutaneous and mucous-membrane manifestations are a significant part of the pyridoxine deficiency state induced in humans by the administration of the pyridoxine antagonist, 4-desoxypyridoxine.[133] In this study glossitis and a seborrheic dermatitislike eruption on the face, neck, and intertriginous regions are the most commonly encountered findings. Cheilosis, angular stomatitis, conjunctivitis, and a pellagra-like hyperpigmentation of the arms and legs are seen less frequently. All of the above manifestations respond to replacement with pyridoxine but are not influenced by the administration of other B-complex vitamins. Clinical observers in the past have noted a response of angular stomatitis and cheilosis to pyridoxine but not to riboflavin, suggesting that clinically important pyridoxine deficiency does occur. The similarities to riboflavin and niacin deficiencies are noteworthy.

VITAMIN C DEFICIENCY AND SCURVY

Scurvy has long been known to be due to a deficiency of a dietary factor in fresh fruits and vegetables, subsequently identified as L-ascorbic acid. The manifestations of scurvy are mild at the onset but progress in severity as the ascorbic acid depletion persists.[5,59,60] The earliest manifestations of scurvy occur in the skin as follicular hyperkeratoses, which are followed later by perifollicular erythema and hemorrhage, usually on the extremities. Nonfollicular petechiae are also present. As scurvy persists, hemorrhages into the skin become more frequent and more ecchymotic. In addition, they are distributed more widely over the body. Splinter hemorrhages may be seen at the distal ends of the nail beds. "Woody" edema of the legs associated with pain, hemorrhage, and brownish pigmentation may be seen in chronic, long-standing scurvy. This may advance to a scleroderma-like stage.[137] Poor wound healing is noted in new or recent wounds, which become hemorrhagic and tend to break down. Fatigue, muscular pains and aches (particularly in the limbs), swollen and painful joints, peripheral edema, and dyspnea on exertion are characteristic features of both clinical and experimental scurvy. Scorbutic gingivitis begins with redness, swelling, and hemorrhage in the interdental papillae. With progression, the gums become purplish, more swollen, and spongy. Necrosis and free bleeding of the gums may occur. In advanced cases, the teeth are lost. More severe changes are seen in subjects with preexisting gingival disease, and edentulous patients are usually spared.

Infantile scurvy differs in several ways from the picture presented by adult scurvy. Joint, bone, and muscle involvement dominates the clinical presentation. Scorbutic infants exhibit irritability when moved, tenderness of the legs, and pseudoparalysis, but skin hemorrhage is quite infrequent compared to adult scurvy.

Several alterations that are not considered part of clinical scurvy have been observed in experimental scurvy in humans, including the following: (1) exacerbation of acne, (2) Sjögren's syndrome with xerostomia, keratoconjunctivitis sicca, and enlargement of salivary glands, (3) excessive hair loss, and (4) conjunctival telangiectasis and hemorrhage.[5,59,60] Anemia is frequently a feature of clinical scurvy but is not seen in experimentally induced ascorbic acid deficiency.

Senile purpura and sublingual hemorrhages in the elderly are not due to ascorbic acid deficiency, despite the frequent finding of latent scurvy that has been demonstrated biochemically in this age group.

Hemorrhagic phenomena are an essential component of the pathology of scurvy and account for many of the manifestations of the disease, including the skin petechiae and ecchymoses, the muscle pain that results from hemorrhage into muscles, and the joint pain and effusion from hemorrhage into joints.

Recent studies have shed some light on the mechanism by which ascorbic acid deficiency results in the clinical picture of scurvy (see Chap. 3).

BIOTIN

Biotin deficiency in humans was long thought to be associated with an uncommon generalized se-

borrheic dermatitis of infants known as Leiner's disease, a concept supported by reports of low blood and urine biotin levels in affected infants.[125] Enthusiasm over therapeutic trials of biotin were not corroborated by change in biotin levels.[97] Instances of familial Leiner's disease have since been shown to have a defect in opsonization owing to a deficiency of the fifth component of complement, responsive to fresh plasma transfusion.[65,94] The role of biotin is not fully resolved, but may relate to uncertainties in precise diagnosis of seborrheic dermatitislike rash in infants. Good examples of this difficulty are illustrated in recent reports of "skin rashes," blepharitis (a common manifestation of ordinary adult-type seborrheic dermatitis), and alopecia in an infant suffering also from severe hypotonia and lethargy.[18] Despite an initial impression of acrodermatitis enteropathica and low serum zinc level, there was no response to zinc therapy. Urinary screening revealed excessive excretion of 3-hydroxyvaleric acid, subsequently attributed to impaired activity of beta-methylcrotonyl CoA carboxylase, a biotin-dependent enzyme. Administration of oral biotin, 5 mg twice daily, resulted in prompt reversal of both biochemical and clinical abnormalities.

Three other cases of infants with central nervous system dysfunction, alopecia, dermatitis due to Candida with facial, axillary, groin, or distal extremity involvement were believed to be due to biotin-dependent multiple carboxylase deficiency.[25] Immunologic defects, both cellular and humoral, were demonstrated, although they were not identical in the three (unrelated) children.

These metabolic abnormalities are probably the first clear-cut examples of human biotin deficiency, with mechanism not completely known, and show skin abnormalities that might be interpreted as seborrheic. There is no evidence that biotin plays a role in ordinary seborrheic dermatitis. Interestingly, experimental biotin deficiency in humans induced by avidin-rich raw egg-white diets did not result in comparable skin lesions or hair loss, but rather generalized dry skin with greyish pallor and a pale tongue with atrophic lingual papillae, restored to normal with biotin administration.[126]

PERNICIOUS ANEMIA AND OTHER VITAMIN B$_{12}$ DEFICIENCIES

Mucocutaneous manifestations of pernicious anemia are uncommon except for involvement of the tongue, which may be seen in approximately half the patients. The glossitis may be an early symptom occurring even before anemia. The severity of the tongue involvement varies greatly but at its worst can present a painful, beefy red tongue devoid of papillae, occasionally with shallow ulcerations on the surface. The well-known lemon yellow pallor of the skin is a late feature of the pernicious anemia usually associated with severe anemia.

Cutaneous hyperpigmentation has been reported as a sign of vitamin B_{12} deficiency in dark-skinned patients.[4] Pigmentation is usually present on the extremities, especially the fingers and dorsum of the hand, and may be either diffuse or patchy. A peculiar poikilodermatous hyperpigmentation has been reported on the neck, abdomen, groin, and thighs of a Caucasian girl, associated with megaloblastic anemia.[43] Epidermal cells were noted to have unusually large nuclei in the pigmented areas of skin similar to the large nuclei seen in other cells in vitamin B_{12} deficiency. Vitamin B_{12} therapy resulted in clearing of the hyperpigmentation as well as resolution of anemia and nuclear enlargement.

The occurrence of vitamin B_{12} deficiency in the breast-fed infant of a strict vegetarian resulted in increased pigmentation of the dorsal surfaces of hands and feet, especially knuckles, plus ecchymoses over legs and buttocks, along with neurologic abnormalities, a megaloblastic anemia, and a mixed organic and amino aciduria.[56]

FOLIC ACID DEFICIENCY

Folic acid deficiency is known to produce characteristic changes in the bone marrow and other sites of rapid cell proliferation, notably the GI tract. The primary abnormality in folic acid deficiency is inhibition of DNA synthesis. Cutaneous manifestations of folic acid deficiency have been reported.[6] A papulosquamous eruption has also been observed in a patient with prolonged and severe folic acid deficiency.[96] The skin eruption and associated anemia responded to folic acid treatment.

Minerals and Trace Metals

IRON

Iron has important metabolic functions throughout the body in addition to its prime role in the hematopoietic system. Epithelial changes have been observed in iron deficiency. Nail changes are frequently seen and may be an early manifestation, occasionally even before the presence of anemia. The nails are dull, lusterless, and brittle, and tend to break at the free distal edge. The normally convex nail plate flattens and may become concave (koilonychia). The tongue may also be involved, commonly with loss of papillae, but not to the degree seen in pernicious anemia. Fissures may be present at the angles of the mouth. Postcricoid dys-

phagia together with koilonychia, atrophic glossitis, and angular stomatitis constitute the Plummer–Vinson (Paterson–Kelly) syndrome. Whether this syndrome is caused by the iron deficiency or by some associated factors is debatable. Hair growth may also be altered in iron deficiency and occasionally may be seen even before overt anemia occurs.[21,52] Iron deficiency is an uncommon cause of diffuse hair loss in which a low serum iron level and favorable response to iron replacement help to establish the diagnosis. Vulvovaginitis may also complicate iron deficiency. Koilonychia and glossitis may occur even when the total red blood count is normal; determination of hemoglobin will show a low value confirming iron deficiency.

Porphyria cutanea tarda is associated with abnormalities of iron metabolism, which may be important in its pathogenesis. Phlebotomy with attendant iron removal is still a useful form of therapy of porphyria cutanea tarda.

ARSENIC

Arsenic was prescribed frequently in the early part of the 20th century for treatment of several human diseases, including some skin disorders. Arsphenamine was the original "magic bullet" for syphilis. Fowler's solution containing potassium arsenite was used commonly to treat psoriasis, and it is probably still prescribed occasionally in some parts of the world. Of thousands of people who received arsenic as treatment, some developed cutaneous reactions, most commonly small circular keratoses on palms and soles and spotty "raindrop" hyperpigmentation, especially on clothing-covered areas (back, thighs, buttocks). Some of these patients over a period of 10 years to 20 years went on to develop frank invasive epidermal carcinomas in palmar areas, for example; others developed multiple intraepidermal cancers and precancers likened by most investigators to an entity called Bowen's disease.[111,130] These lesions occurred most often on covered areas, and therefore appeared to be of different etiology (presumably arsenic) than the actinic or sunlight-derived keratoses and subsequent epidermal carcinomas in sun-exposed areas.

These observations, the clearly poisonous nature of large, acute doses of arsenic, observations of the cutaneous signs of chronic arsenicism in agricultural workers exposed to arsenic-containing sprays, high statistical correlation in several parts of the world between arsenic content of the drinking water and occurrence of the cutaneous lesions, and some reports of increased internal malignancies in such circumstances have led many to accept arsenic as a prominent carcinogen.[130,136]

Perhaps surprising, then, is the fact that arsenic

has not been shown to be carcinogenic in animal systems despite repeated attempts. This situation, the circumstantial and biostatistical nature of the incriminating data, and occasional observations of either protective effects or even conceivably the essentiality of arsenic have led at least one author to espouse a quite opposite point of view on the putative dangers of arsenic.[40] For the moment, it is only rational that individuals with known exposure to arsenic, particularly if palmar/plantar keratoses and characteristic pigmentary changes are present, be followed carefully by trained observers for the development of cancerous skin lesions.

COPPER

Copper deficiency in humans, either experimentally induced or as the result of relative deficiency during periods of accelerated growth, does not result in observable skin changes. However, it was the apparent similarities of abnormal wool (hair) in sheep deficient in dietary copper to the hair in infants with Menkes' syndrome ("kinky hair," "steely hair" disease) that led to the recognition of biochemical copper deficiency as the underlying defect.[27] Wool or hair from affected individuals contains decreased disulfide cross-linking and increased free cysteine sulfhydryl groups, and the hairs from patients with Menkes' syndrome show increased protein extractibility compatible with less cross-linking.[27,70] Curiously, the "steely" wool in copper-deficient sheep is straighter and less crimped than normal, while in Menkes' syndrome, the hair is abnormally twisted, a condition termed *pili torti.* No specific copper-dependent cross-linking enzyme in hair or wool has been demonstrated, but it has been inferred by the above. Tyrosinase, the enzyme essential for pigment formation, is known to be copper dependent; the hair in Menkes' syndrome is "frosty" in appearance, and general pigmentation is reduced in affected individuals when compared to normal siblings or parents.[20] The precise defect or range of defects in this x-linked disorder is not known. Decreased transport of copper across the intestinal mucosa may not be an adequate explanation, since other tissues can show increased copper storage (including skin fibroblasts in tissue culture, a potential detector system) and intravenous copper replacement may have little effect. It is hoped that prenatal detection might afford opportunity for therapy prior to irreversible damage. The search for pili torti through intrauterine scalp biopsy might aid; pili torti has already been demonstrated in a preterm male with increased skin fibroblast copper uptake.[20] It must be remembered that pili torti may not affect all hairs, and thorough examination is required. Pili torti has been shown to be a marker of x-linked carrier status in females from several affected families.[20]

Hypocupremia has been found in most cases of kwashiorkor and marasmus and, along with zinc deficiency, is suspected by some to contribute to the overall clinical picture.[86] Indeed, the banded depigmentation of published photographs of wool from copper deficient sheep (when refed a normal diet) appear quite similar to the banded hair (flag sign) of human kwashiorkor.

Hypercupremia has been reported repeatedly in psoriasis but not in other dermatoses, although skin tissue levels are not increased in either involved or normal skin.[86] The increased serum copper has been attributed to increased ceruloplasmin, but in some psoriatics, especially those without arthritis, serum ceruloplasmin is said to be normal. It is not possible to further interpret these findings nor the conflicting reports of both high and low serum copper in vitiligo, a common, usually patchy, depigmenting disorder.

NICKEL

Nickel deficiency has not been described in humans. Induced deficiency in chickens, rats, pigs, and goats, however, does result in some cutaneous changes, described respectively as pigmentation and dermatitis of shank skin, rough coat, and parakeratosis.[131] Some suspect that nickel is an essential trace element, but it is so ubiquitous that natural deficiency is exceedingly rare.

The reason for including a discussion of nickel in this chapter is that contact dermatitis due to nickel is one of the most common types of contact dermatitis in the world. There is currently considerable attention being given to ingested nickel as a contributor to the dermatitis, and reports particularly from the Scandinavian countries include evidence for exacerbation of the skin lesions correlated with purposeful ingestion of nickel and remission with placebo, low-nickel diets, or treatment with the nickel chelators, tetraethylthiuram disulfide, or diethyldithiocarbamate.[68] Release of nickel from stainless-steel cooking utensils by acid foods has been implicated in pathogenesis.[16,19,21] Similar reports link nickel ingestion to a chronic vesicular hand dermatitis termed *pompholyx* or *dyshidrotic eczema,* a common disorder of unknown etiology.[90] Studies of serum, urine, sweat, and hair nickel concentrations correlate poorly, however, with the dermatitis. Critical commentary on this literature has been published by Fisher, and major controversies remain on the relationship of average dietary intake to clinical disease.[37,38,67] Since many advances in our knowledge of specific deficiencies in humans have come as the result of experimental or therapeutic deprivation of a given vitamin or element, perhaps observations of individuals made deficient in nickel will yield similar results. One startling observation was an instance of cutaneous leucocytoclastic vasculitis during chelation therapy.[68]

Further evidence that nickel from internal bodily sources can produce cutaneous reactions is found in reports of dermatitis from a nickel-containing coin in the stomach and from nickel-containing metallic prostheses.[76,81]

SELENIUM

The use of selenium salts in treatment of human skin disease is reported to date back to the Napoleonic wars; in modern times selenium disulfide is the apparent active ingredient in commercial preparations commonly used to treat seborrheic scalp disorders. Yet selenium toxicity in animals (and one apparent instance in a human) is manifested by hair loss.[131]

Equally intriguing is evidence that selenium can inhibit chemical carcinogenesis in animal skin as well as in other organs.[113] An inverse relationship between soil selenium or serum selenium levels and human cancer deaths has been reported from many parts of the world, but these reports do not include information on skin cancer.[114]

Selenium has been shown in recent years to be an essential component of the enzyme glutathione peroxidase (see Chap. 4), an enzyme that further metabolizes inorganic and organic peroxides and is believed to convert fatty acid peroxides to hydroxy-fatty acids, thus possibly serving to protect against membrane lipid peroxidation. Levels of both animal and human erythrocyte glutathione peroxidase appear to relate directly to dietary selenium intake. Thus, there is much interest in the essentiality of selenium and its possible role in human disease. Selenium can be measured in human skin, especially epidermis, as can glutathione peroxidase.* Lipid peroxidation products in human skin increase with exposure to ultraviolet light, a known carcinogenic stimulus.[88] It is expected that further research will demonstrate a significant role of selenium in at least some forms of skin disease.

ZINC

It is extremely unlikely that a dermatologist has ever existed who has not prescribed zinc in some form for topical treatment of skin disease. In fact, topical use of zinc was advised well before dermatologists *per se* existed, as recorded in the Ebers papyrus of 3000 B.C.

There may, indeed, be relatively few individuals in the current populations, at least of Western nations, who have not used either a lotion, ointment, or shampoo that contains zinc as a major ingredient. Yet only in recent decades has some degree of rationale for zinc therapy emerged from biochemical and biomedical studies. The nearly 5000-year time lag between empirical use and beginning understanding of the relationship of zinc to functioning of cutaneous tissues may be a record in medical annals. The reason for it is partly technological. Accurate analysis of very small amounts of zinc in biologic tissues has only become possible in recent years. Such microanalytic techniques have been necessary in order to both measure zinc concentrations in tissue under varying circumstances and to establish the essentiality of zinc as a component of a large number of enzymes vital to normal cellular functioning.

It still remained necessary, however, to discover a series of zinc deficiency states in humans before full recognition of the importance of zinc to skin and hair was possible. This recognition occurred by four pathways. One was the role of zinc in wound healing, as championed and reviewed by Pories and colleagues.[101] Another was the insightful elucidation by Moynahan of the inherited recessive disorder acrodermatitis enteropathica as a manifestation of inadequate absorption of zinc.[95] The third was the careful and persistent investigations of Prasad and co-workers and Hambidge and co-workers into acquired chronic zinc deficiencies.[51,102] Finally, inadvertent production of human zinc deficiencies during certain forms of therapeutic intervention, such as penicillamine treatment and total parenteral nutrition (TPN), with reproduction of acrodermatitis enteropathicalike lesions, provided the opportunity to begin to sort out cutaneous effects of zinc deficiency from deficiency of other essential substances.[9,73,124]

The cutaneous signs of zinc deficiency vary with both acuteness and degree of deficiency. It is probably not coincidental that the most severe manifestations occur in patients with acrodermatitis enteropathica and following TPN; both reflect severe zinc lack, a situation no longer likely with TPN since recognition of the syndrome has led to addition of zinc to preparations for intravenous alimentation in virtually all medical centers (see Chap. 13). These signs include facial, periorificial, and acral (distal extremity) eczematous, papulopustular, blistering, and ultimately hemorrhagic skin lesions plus hair loss of progressive severity. Secondary infection with bacteria or yeast is common and may relate to diminished chemotaxis of zinc-deficient

---

*Crounse RG: unpublished data.

leukocytes.[144] The skin lesions are quite resistant to all therapy *except* zinc itself. Remarkably rapid healing (2 days–7 days) is noted with proper replacement of zinc. The "lost" hair does not return so rapidly, which could be interpreted as loss owing to telogen conversion (inducement of resting state of hair roots) rather than to toxicity to anagen (growing) hair roots. Unfortunately, there are no reported investigations of the details of hair loss in these conditions. Two additional facts, however, support the hypothesis of telogen conversion. Mention of greatly decreased hair growth and some reports of normal zinc levels in hairs from affected individuals are best explained by such a mechanism. Alternatively, a significant decrease in rate of hair growth—as in kwashiorkor—could also explain normal concentration of zinc in hair despite low circulating zinc levels.[13] Both explanations illustrate rather dramatically why analysis of hair for metal content may yield useless or paradoxical results without understanding of the biology of hair growth.

Slowly developing, chronic, or less severe zinc deficiency may produce much more subtle cutaneous signs, and may not be reflected in recognized hair loss. The zinc deficiency of childhood dietary deprivation, chronic alcoholism, therapy of other disorders with chelating agents, such as penicillamine and EDTA, chronic gastrointestinal disorders, or protein-losing (and zinc-losing) renal disease may be manifested only by perioral and perinasal scaling or papulopustules, scaling of the scalp, and dry skin generally.[29] Although not always appreciated, perleche, paronychia, and collarette scaling of the palms (the latter especially in reports of zinc-deficiency among Danish beer drinkers) can be signs. The problem of mixed signs of multiple deficiencies is illustrated readily in reports of moderately severe hypozincemia in protein–calorie malnutrition coupled with low vitamin A intake. All three deficiencies can be manifested by both skin and hair signs. In general, follicular hyperkeratosis of vitamin A deficiency, the pigmentary changes, edema, and organomegaly of kwashiorkor, and the less peripherally distributed lesions of essential fatty acid deficiency will help in distinguishing these disease states. The presence of skin ulceration in marasmus and kwashiorkor also correlates significantly with hypozincemia.[44]

The answer to whether or not the common "venous" or "stasis" ulcers of the legs in adults are based at least in part on zinc deficiency, and therefore require zinc to promote healing, may turn out to be relatively simple. After many clinical investigations, a growing concensus seems to indicate that those patients with ulcers *and* hypozincemia benefit from supplemental zinc; those with ulcers and normal serum zinc levels do not benefit.[132] Conflicting results of the efficacy of zinc therapy for acne might reflect similar considerations.[99] Alternatively, there is some indication that the pustular component of acne may be more responsive to zinc therapy than the papular or comedonal elements.[140] Finally, whether for leg ulcers, acne, or a host of other disorders in which zinc treatment is being tried, there is the question of the difference between physiologic/replacement amounts of zinc and pharmacologic doses, as with vitamins or corticosteroids.

Diagnosis of zinc deficiency must rest ultimately upon accurate determination of tissue levels of zinc, plus expansion of our knowledge of the kinetics and distribution of zinc. At this writing, low normal to low serum alkaline phosphatase levels and possible elevated ribonuclease levels may serve as a substitute if accurate zinc determinations are not available. Ideally, both should return to normal with zinc therapy as further evidence of original zinc deficiency.

The pathogenic mechanisms of cutaneous signs of zinc deficiency are not known precisely, but the role of zinc in over 70 enzymatic reactions of all classes provides adequate numbers of hypotheses. Thymidine kinase requirements, for example, might relate readily to tissues with continuous cellular synthesis, such as epidermis and hair. Direct evidence for decreased skin protein incorporation of cysteine in animal models of induced zinc deficiency are especially attractive.[62] Definitive investigations remain for future researchers.

Guidelines for appropriate amounts of zinc replacement therapy are widely available.[141,157] As in all nutrition, it is necessary to indicate that too much zinc may be toxic, and indeed may induce hypocupremia and signs of copper deficiency. It is this area of interactions between elements that will require the most rigorous and extensive research.

Cutaneous Effects on Nutritional and Metabolic Processes

SYSTEMIC NUTRITIONAL AND METABOLIC DISTURBANCES ASSOCIATED WITH SKIN DISEASES

Extensive skin disease can induce clinically significant systemic nutritional and metabolic disturbances. The severe oral mucous membrane bullae and erosions seen in pemphigus vulgaris or severe erythema multiforme (Stevens–Johnson syndrome) present obvious problems in providing for the nutritional needs of the patients. Many severely ill patients with mycosis fungoides or other cutaneous lymphomas, lupus erythematosus, pemphigus, or exfoliative dermatitis have poor appetites, which further complicates their disability through undernutrition. Beyond these more general considerations, skin disorders can induce specific nutritional deficiencies.[118]

PROTEIN AND WATER LOSS

Desquamation of the superficial layers of the stratum corneum is a normal sequence of epidermal activity. Nitrogen loss resulting from desquamated scale under normal conditions has been estimated to be approximately 380 mg/m^2 body surface/day. Skin diseases associated with pronounced scaling, such as exfoliative dermatitis, psoriasis, and lamellar ichthyosis, result in marked nitrogen loss in the exfoliated proteinaceous scale. In severe generalized exfoliation, as much as 20 g to 30 g nitrogen/m^2 may be lost each day. On an adequate protein diet of 1 g nitrogen/kg body weight, normal nitrogen balance is maintained until the scale loss exceeds 17 g/m^2/day, at which point negative nitrogen balance ensues.[39] If negative nitrogen balance persists, as may be the case in chronic exfoliative dermatitis, the consequences are hypoalbuminemia, edema, and loss of muscle mass. Hypoalbuminemia is a common complication of prolonged exfoliative dermatitis, occurring in half or more of the cases.[128] If dietary protein intake is poor, negative nitrogen balance and its sequelae may be expected to occur at a lower rate of scale loss. Roe theorizes that a vicious cycle is established wherein malnutrition leads to dermatitis, as in the case of kwashiorkor or pellagra, and that dermatitis then further complicates the malnutrition by excessive cutaneous protein loss.[107]

Extrarenal water loss (cutaneous insensible water loss plus sweating) normally approximates 400 ml/day at rest in a temperate environment. This may be increased threefold to fivefold or more in extensive exfoliative skin diseases.[39] The water loss is proportional to the extent of the exfoliative process and rapidly decreases as the skin disease resolves. Water loss may be significant in a hot environment and might contribute to dehydration.

METABOLIC ABNORMALITIES ASSOCIATED WITH SKIN DISEASES

Approximately 0.5 mg iron/day is lost through normal epidermal desquamation. Although accurate measurements are not available, it is presumed that severe exfoliative skin disease increases the iron loss, which may lead to iron deficiency. Low serum iron concentration associated with normal or decreased serum iron-binding capacity has been noted in patients with various skin diseases, such as exfoliative dermatitis and psoriasis.[83] Ferrokinetic studies in patients with skin diseases show that a more complicated derangement in iron metabolism may be present, as manifested by variable absorption of ^{59}Fe, rapid disappearance if IV administered ^{59}Fe with a normal or slightly decreased iron turnover, normal red blood cell ^{59}Fe incorporation, and normal marrow iron.[118]

Folic acid deficiency can be demonstrated in patients with extensive dermatoses and psoriasis.[74,129,145] The frequency may be as high as one third of all patients admitted to the hospital for skin disease. Greatly increased turnover of diseased epidermis may increase utilization of folic acid to a degree that a conditioned deficiency results. Malabsorption may also contribute to folic acid deficiency. Occasionally, folic acid deficiency associated with skin diseases may produce overt megaloblastic anemia.

Patients with exfoliative dermatitis may have low blood ascorbic acid levels and may exhibit prolonged saturation times with ascorbic acid, which are thought to result from increased utilization of vitamin C by the diseased skin.

VITAMIN D

Skin plays an essential role in the biogenesis of vitamin D. Under conditions where adequate sunlight is provided to the skin surface, skin produces all the vitamin D that is needed. Only when sunlight is not available does vitamin D become an essential dietary requirement. Human rickets is caused by vitamin D deficiency. The prevalence of rickets today depends on whether artificial vitamin D supplements or sunlight, or both, are provided rather than on what foods are consumed, since most foods contain negligible amounts of vitamin D. The relationship between sunlight and the development of rickets has been recognized for a long time and is supported by the following observations. Rickets is more frequent during the winter months, and its incidence is increased in dark-skinned people and in persons who avoid sunlight exposure to the skin surface (*e.g.,* Moslem women). Both artificial ultraviolet light and natural sunlight irradiation can prevent or cure rickets. The only known precursor of vitamin D in skin, 7-dehydrocholesterol, is found in relatively large amounts within the epidermis where irradiation is thought to occur.

Use of Diet and Specific Nutrients in Dermatologic Therapy

Therapy of nutritional deficiency diseases and their cutaneous manifestations has already been covered in previous sections of this chapter. The response to therapy in deficiency syndromes is usually prompt and complete, as in scurvy or pellagra. In some instances the nutritional deficiency may progress to a stage where irreversible damage is done so that treatment results in incomplete remissions or even failure to respond at all. Early diagnosis and treatment must be stressed in order to avoid these consequences. In several inherited diseases for which specific diet therapy is beneficial, for instance, phenylketonuria or acrodermatitis enteropathica, devastating consequences may result in untreated patients.

In this section, we will be concerned with a variety of skin diseases that are amenable to a greater or lesser degree to therapy employing dietary adjustments or provision of specific nutrients. This type of therapy of skin disease was in vogue in the past, but the pendulum has swung away from stressing dietary factors and specific nutrients in the treatment of dermatologic diseases due to improved understanding of the pathogenesis of many of these diseases and to the availability of more effective therapy.

ACNE VULGARIS

Controversy over both dietary etiology and dietary, vitamin, or trace element therapy of acne has existed for years, and, judging by continued conflicting or contradictory reports, it will persist for some time. Well-documented spontaneous exacerbations and remissions plus a high rate of placebo responses probably account for some of the confusion. Chocolate, greasy foods, soft drinks, and dairy products are believed by many patients and families and some doctors to exacerbate acne (along with emotional stress, sexual activity, indeed most any life experience that is coincident with acne flares). Yet controlled studies, for example, of high versus normal carbohydrate intake or chocolate intake, fail to show consistent effect.[23,42] Large amounts of halides can flare acne or produce an acnelike pustular dermatitis, but iodized salt is said not to be a factor.[58]

Vitamin A used orally in fairly large amounts for treatment of acne apparently has less effect than formerly believed, and can be quite toxic. One report, however, quotes experimental animal evidence of synergism with vitamin E as the basis for combined therapy employing lesser doses of vitamin A than usual in other keratinizing disorders of skin, and suggests such an approach in acne.[2] Curiously, another report cautions that concomitant administration of vitamins A and E results in severe hypervitaminosis A. Caution and measurement would seem to be essential for rational management. Many dermatologists now use topical vitamin A acid (retinoic acid) as an anticomedone

("black" or "white head") preparation.[89] However, possible potentiation of ultraviolet light carcinogenesis is under study.[31] An isomer of vitamin A acid, 13-*cis*-retinoic acid, is being used orally with success in severe acne, but has significant side-effects and is in investigational stages at this writing.[100]

Oral zinc is now being tried widely in treating acne, again with conflicting results. Some report significant improvement when compared to placebo, especially reduction of pustules, while others can detect no significant difference.[57,92,99,140,142] The latter group has found increased plasma zinc levels with placebo as well as with zinc therapy. Of interest are reports of decreased plasma retinol binding protein levels in men with severe acne, but not in women or controls, and even more puzzling, development of acne in several men with experimentally induced zinc deficiency.[3,92] Caution is urged, especially as zinc toxicity is a potential hazard.

DERMATITIS HERPETIFORMIS

Dermatitis herpetiformis (DH) is a chronic, extremely pruritic and therefore often nearly disabling cutaneous disorder characterized by groups of small blisters or papulovesicles. Its pathogenesis is believed to be linked to circulating antigen–antibody complexes of the IgA immunoglobulin class, and it appears to be associated in many individuals with a specific gluten-sensitive enteropathy, although patients with DH seldom have significant clinical signs of gut disease.[72,115] Diets free of wheat proteins (*e.g.*, gluten, gliadin) have been shown to reduce the required therapeutic amounts of sulfapyridine or sulfone therapy most commonly effective in DH, and in some instances maintain a remission.[41,105] One report indicates a return of jejunal mucosa from a villous flattening to a normal appearance, along with a decrease in IgA skin deposits.[53] Antibodies to wheat proteins have been detected in both gluten-sensitive enteropathy and in dermatitis herpetiformis with a frequency significantly higher than controls, thus strengthening the case for gluten hypersensitivity.[63]

ERYTHROPOIETIC PROTOPORPHYRIA

Carotenoid pigments are capable of preventing photosensitivity in light-sensitive variants of several bacteria and plants. In addition, beta carotene prevents photosensitive reactions in mice rendered photosensitive by the administration of large amounts of hematoporphyrin. As a result of these observations, beta carotene was used successfully in the human disease, erythropoietic protoporphyria.[87] This disease is characterized by marked photosensitivity, which is manifested by a burning sensation, edema, crusting, and scarring of light-exposed areas. Preliminary results suggest that some other photosensitive eruptions, including polymorphous light eruption, may also respond to beta-carotene administration. In the effective dose range of 50 mg/day to 75 mg/day beta carotene, cutaneous pigmentation of hypercarotenosis results. Serum vitamin A levels are not elevated; on the contrary, vitamin A blood levels tend to decrease, and these seemingly paradoxical results have not been explained.[80]

INHERITED AND OTHER SCALING DISORDERS AND HAIR ABNORMALITIES

The known modulating effect of vitamin A on epithelial tissues (see vitamin A, this chapter) has led to its therapeutic use (or use of related compounds) in several idiopathic or inherited disorders of abnormal epidermal cellular differentiation. Most notable are pityriasis rubra pilaris, Darier's disease (keratosis follicularis), and several forms of ichthyosis or ichthyosiform dermatoses. Many of these reports are summarized in a symposium proceedings.[85] The side-effects of therapeutic oral doses of retinoic acid (vitamin A acid) or its synthetic stereoisomer 13-*cis*-retinoic acid are similar in general to those of vitamin A; the search for a therapeutically effective, but considerably less toxic, derivative or related compound continues. Similarly, research proceeds to identify a more effective topical regimen with minimal side-effects.

Certain inherited metabolic defects with keratinizing abnormalities are theoretically approachable by dietary manipulation. Refsum's disease is an ichthyosiform dermatosis resulting from inability to degrade exogenous phytanic acid, with subsequent incorporation of phytanic acid in epidermal lipids, including phospholipids, to the exclusion of arachidonic acid.[28,55] The disorder has been reported to respond to a decrease in dietary phytanic acid.[30] A summary of the experience with dietary therapy to date, including initial paradoxical increase in plasma phytanic acid with clinical deterioration, is provided in a recent comprehensive review.[122]

Another example is the response of hypertyrosinemia with palmar and plantar keratoses, keratotic corneal lesions, and mental deficiency (the Richner–Hanhart syndrome) to restriction of dietary phenylalanine and tyrosine.[45,149]

Similarly, low-arginine diets have been used successfully to treat argininosuccinic aciduria, an inherited defect of the enzyme argininosuccinase; the fragile hair abnormality known as trichorrhexis

nodosa found in over half the cases was reported to return to normal and remain so with long-term follow-up.[24,116,143]

PSORIASIS

Psoriasis is a common skin disorder characterized by raised scaly spots or plaques. It may be limited to a few lesions, especially over elbows, knees, and scalp, or it may become quite widespread, sometimes involving the entire body, and it is therefore one cause of generalized exfoliative dermatitis. Its pathogenesis involves greatly accelerated proliferation of epidermal cells, leading to the excessive scaling which, if widespread, can result in significant loss of protein and presumably other constituents of epidermal cells, including vitamins and trace elements.

The increased production and loss of epidermal cells have been thought by some to be worsened by high protein intake, and conversely to be diminished by restriction of dietary protein or total calories. One instance of marked improvement on a low-nitrogen diet and relapse on a high-protein, meat diet was quite convincing.[79] Other reports include failure to observe consistent effects of low-protein or low-calorie diets.[147] These same observers failed to confirm earlier reports of influence of high versus low taurine intake, or a diet high in turkey (once believed to be a low-tryptophan source).[146] Similarly, high-zinc diets, despite reports of low serum zinc levels, failed to significantly improve psoriasis.[135]

The relationship between lipids and psoriasis has been investigated for several decades. A recent study seems to confirm earlier reports of elevated serum cholesterol in psoriasis, although the results are quite variable between men and women, and between different age groups.[48,61] Anecdotal reports by the latter authors of clearing of psoriasis with high-fat (wartime-induced) diets have not been experimentally verified.

The excess proliferation of psoriatic epidermis has led to therapeutic trials of a variety of antimitotic and antimetabolic compounds. The folic acid antagonist methotrexate has been used widely, particularly in severe psoriatics, and dosage forms evolved that minimize toxic potential while maintaining therapeutic benefit. The use of this and other chemotherapeutic agents in psoriasis has been frequently reviewed.[33] An intriguing trial of topical 6-amino-nicotinamide combined with oral niacin in psoriasis implies induced niacin deficiency in the skin with protection from systemic deficiency.[145]

The widespread use of oral lithium compounds, especially in the treatment of bipolar affective psychosis, has resulted in the unexpected production of psoriasis in some patients not apparently otherwise predisposed, or exacerbation of some (but not all) cases of already existing psoriasis.[119] Lithium could theoretically affect psoriasis in several ways, including increased leukocyte numbers, increased leukocyte mobility and phagocytosis, and alterations of cyclic AMP levels.[78]

Finally, experimental observations indicate therapeutic benefit of synthetic vitamin A derivatives, the oral retinoids, in psoriasis. The ability of vitamin A or retinoids to inhibit ornithine decarboxylase, the rate-limiting step in polyamine synthesis, is hypothesized as a potential mechanism, in view of the possible role of polyamines in regulating epidermal (and psoriatic) proliferation.[103,134]

It seems apparent that while gross dietary manipulation may not be of paramount influence upon psoriasis, the role of vitamins, antivitamins, and trace elements may prove to be of significance.

ROSACEA

Rosacea is a common disorder of older persons. It is characterized by facial erythema, telangiectasia, and inflammatory papules and pustules. Dietary indiscretions were previously thought to be important factors in causing rosacea. Tea, coffee, alcoholic beverages, and highly spiced foods do apparently provoke more flushing in rosacea patients than in control subjects.[84] Any of these that specifically produces flushing should be avoided, but the elaborate dietary restrictions of the past are no longer necessary because tetracycline treatment is more effective.

URTICARIA

Foods, including food additives and colorings, are known causes of some cases of hives and angioedema. They are, however, probably less common causes than many people believe. This is especially true in chronic urticaria (*i.e.*, of more than a few weeks duration). True allegic urticaria from foods is even less common, since some "urticariogenic" foods contain direct histamine releasers, which if ingested in sufficient amounts cause short-lived nonallergic hives. Examples include lobsters, shellfish, strawberries, and eggs.[1] Reexposure to the same food in lesser amounts, or to the same food containing less histamine releaser, may not cause hives.

The percentage of cases of urticaria in children attributable to foods ranges in reported series from 44% in one study to 5% or less.[1,17,57] Search for a specific food cause can be rewarding occasionally, but more frequently it is exasperating. If no likely foods are identified immediately by history, a strict, controlled diet may be tried. Although often called *elimination diets*, a more proper term for these controlled diets might be *basal addition* diet. The basal portion might consist of water, green tea, sea salt, whole rice, and one meat rarely eaten (lamb, rabbit, or duck, for example). If the urticaria resolves within a few days (and is not simply obscured by antihistamine therapy) addition of single foods is begun. A single food is one vegetable or fruit, for instance, and not a food mixture like ketchup, salad dressing, or a cake. Urticarial flare with a given food should be repeated at least once for verification.

A series of studies demonstrates a significant number of patients with chronic urticaria who can be shown by provocative testing to react to salicylates, benzoates, and certain food dyes, such as yellow tartrazine (FD + C No. 5).[91,98,138] These compounds are found naturally or as additives in hundreds of food types, as well as in pharmaceutical and oral-hygiene preparations. Cross-reactivity with ordinary aspirin contributes to a fearsome environment to an individual so sensitized. Details of the foodstuffs involved and management tactics can be found in the above references.

References

1. Akers WA, Naverson DN: Diagnosis of chronic urticaria. Int J Dermatol 17:616–626, 1978
2. Ayres S Jr, Mihan R: Acne vulgaris and lipid peroxidation: New concepts in pathogenesis and treatment. Int J Dermatol 17:305–307, 1978
3. Baer MT, King J, Tamura T et al: Acne in zinc deficiency (Letter). Arch Dermatol 114:1093, 1978
4. Baker S, Ignatius M, Johnson S et al: Hyperpigmentation of the skin: A sign of vitamin B_{12} deficiency. Br Med J 1:713–715, 1963
5. Bartley W, Krebs H, O'Brien J: Vitamin C requirements in human adults. London, Medical Research Council Special Report Series No. 280, 1953
6. Bauslag N, Metz J: Pigmentation in megaloblastic anemia associated with pregnancy and lactation. Br Med J 2:737–739, 1969
7. Bender DA, Russell–Jones R: Isoniazid-induced pellagra despite vitamin B_6 supplementation. Lancet 2:1125–1126, 1979
8. Berger HM, King J, Doughty S et al: Nutrition, sex, gestational age, and hair growth in babies. Arch Dis Child 53:290–294, 1978
9. Bernstein B, Leyden JJ: Zinc deficiency and acrodermatitis after intravenous hyperalimentation. Arch Dermatol 114:1070, 1978
10. Bollag W: Prophylaxis of chemically induced epithelial tumors with an aromatic retinoic acid analog (R010-9359). Eur J Cancer Clin Oncol 11:721–724, 1975
11. Bollag W, Ott F: Vitamin A acid in benign and malignant epithelial tumors of the skin. Acta Derm Venereol (Stockh) Suppl 74:163–166, 1975
12. Bradfield RB: Effects of malnutrition on the morphology of hair roots. Montagna W, Parakkal PF (eds): The Structure and Function of Skin, 3rd ed, pp 259–270. New York, Academic Press 1974

13. Bradfield RB, Hambidge KM: Problems with hair zinc as an indicator of body zinc status. Lancet 1:363, 1980

14. Bradfield RB, Lechtig A, Allen L et al: Maternal hair roots in prediction of low birth weight risk. Lancet 2:928–929, 1975

15. Bregar RR, Gordon M, Whitney EN: Hair root diameter measurement as an indicator of protein deficiency in nonhospitalized alcoholics. Am J Clin Nutr 31:230–236, 1978

16. Brun R: Nickel in food: The role of stainless-steel utensils. Contact Dermatitis 5:43–45, 1979

17. Champion R, Roberts S, Carpenter R et al: Urticaria and angioedema. Br J Dermatol 81:588–597, 1969

18. Charles BM, Hosking G, Greene A et al: Biotin-responsive alopecia and developmental regression. Lancet 1:118–120, 1979

19. Christensen OB, Moller H: Release of nickel from cooking utensils. Contact Dermatitis 4:343–346, 1978

20. Collie WR, Goka TJ, Moore CM et al: Hair in Menkes disease: A comprehensive review. In Brown AC, Crounse RG (eds): Hair, Trace Elements and Human Illness. New York, Praeger Scientific Publishers, 1980

21. Comaish S. Metabolic disorders and hair growth. Br J Dermatol 84:83–86, 1971

22. Cordano A: Copper deficiency in clinical medicine. In Hambidge KM, Nicholas BL (eds): Zinc and Copper in Clinical Medicine, pp 119–126. New York, Spectrum Publications, 1978

23. Cornbleet T, Gigli I: Should we limit sugar in acne? Arch Dermatol 83:968–969, 1961

24. Coryell ME, Hall WK, Thevaos TG et al: A family study of a human enzyme defect, arginino–succinic aciduria. Biochem Biophys Res Commun 14:307–312, 1964

25. Cowan MJ, Wara DW, Packman S et al: Multiple biotin-dependent carboxylase deficiencies associated with defects in T-cell and B-cell immunity. Lancet 1:115–118, 1979

26. Crounse RG, Bollet AJ, Owens S: Quantitative tissue assay of human malnutrition using scalp hair roots. Nature 228:465–466, 1970

27. Danks DM, Stevens BJ, Campbell PE et al: Menkes' Kinky hair syndrome. Lancet 1:1100–1103, 1972

28. Davies MG, Reynolds DJ, Marks R et al: The epidermis in Refsum's disease (heredopathia atactica polyneuritiformis). In Marks R, Dykes PJ (eds): The Ichthyoses, pp 51–64. New York, Spectrum Publications, 1978

29. Ecker RI, Schroeter AL: Acrodermatitis and acquired zinc deficiency. Arch Dermatol 114:937–939, 1978

30. Eldjarn L, Try K, Stokke O et al: Dietary effects on serum phytanic acid levels and on clinical manifestations in heredopathia atactica polyneuritiformis. Lancet 1:691, 1966

31. Epstein JH, Grekin DA: Topical retinoic acid (RA) and ultraviolet (UV) carcinogenesis (abstr). J Invest Dermatol 72:272, 1979

32. Evans GE: New aspects of biochemistry and metabolism of copper. In Hambidge KM, Nichols BL, Jr (eds): Zinc and Copper in Clinical Medicine, pp 113–118. New York, Spectrum Publications, 1978

33. Farber EM, Cox AJ: Psoriasis: Proceedings of the Second International Symposium. New York, Yorke Medical Books, 1977

34. Fell HB, Mellanby E: Metaplasia produced in cultures of chick ectoderm by high Vitamin A. J Physiol (London) 119:470–488, 1953

35. Findley G: Epidermal diphosphopyridine nucleotide in normal and pellagrous Bantu subjects. Br J Dermatol 75:249–253, 1963

36. Findley G, Rein L, Mitchell D: Reactions to light on the normal and pellagrous Bantu skin. Br J Dermatol 81:345–351, 1969

37. Fisher AA: Nickel—the ubiquitous contact allergen—possible significance of its presence in food, water, urine, hair and infusion fluids. Cutis 22:542, 1978

38. Fisher AA: Possible role of diet in pompholyx and nickel dermatitis—A critical survey. Cutis 22:412, 1978

39. Freedberg I, Baden H: The metabolic response to exfoliation. J Invest Dermatol 38:277–284, 1962

40. Frost DV: The arsenic problems. In Schrauzer GN (ed): Inorganic and Nutritional Aspects of Cancer, pp 259–279. New York, Plenum Press, 1978

41. Fry L, Riches DJ, Seah PP et al: Clearance of skin lesions in dermatitis herpetiformis after gluten withdrawal. Lancet 1:288–290, 1973

42. Fulton J, Plewig G, Kligman A: Effect of chocolate on acne vulgaris. JAMA 210:2071–2074, 1969

43. Gilliam J, Cox A: Epidermal changes in vitamin B_{12} deficiency. Arch Dermatol 107:231–236, 1973

44. Golden BE, Golden MHN: Plasma zinc and the clinical features of malnutrition. Am J Clin Nutr 32:2490–2494, 1979

45. Goldsmith LA, Kang E, Bienfang DC et al: Tyrosinemia with plantar and palmar keratosis and keratitis. J Pediatr 83:798–805, 1973

46. Grubbs CJ, Moon RC, Sporn MB et al: Inhibition of mammary cancer by retinyl methyl ether. Cancer Res 37:599–602, 1977

47. Grubbs CJ, Moon RC, Squire RA et al: 13-*cis*-retinoic acid: Inhibition of bladder carcinogenesis induced in rats by N-butyl-N (4-hydroxybutyl) nitrosamine. Science 198:743–744, 1977

48. Grutz O, Burger M: Diet Psoriasis als stoffwechsel Problem. Klin Wochenschr 12:373, 1933

49. Haddox MK, Frasier Scott KF, Russell DH: Retinol inhibition of ornithine decarboxylase induction and $^{G}1$ progression in Chinese hamster ovary cells. Cancer Res 39:4930–4938, 1979

50. Halpern S: Chronic hives in children: An analysis of 75 cases. Ann Allergy 23:589, 1965

51. Hambidge KM, Nichols BL (eds): Zinc and Copper in Clinical Medicine. Jamaica, NY, Spectrum Publications, 1978

52. Hard S: Nonanemic iron deficiency as an etiologic factor in diffuse loss of hair of the scalp in women. Acta Dermatol Venereol 43:562–569, 1963

53. Harrington CI, Read NW: Dermatitis herpetiformis: Effect of gluten free diet on skin IgA and jejunal structure and function. Br Med J 1:872–875, 1977

54. Harris CC, Sporn MB, Kaufman DG et al: Histogenesis of squamous metaplasia in the hamster tracheal epithelium caused by vitamin A deficiency or benzo (a) pyreneferric oxide. Journal of The National Cancer Institute 48:743–761, 1972

55. Herndon J, Avigon J, Steinberg D: Refsum's disease: Characterization of the enzyme defect in cell culture. J Clin Invest 48:1017–1032, 1969

56. Higginbottom MC, Sweetman L, Nyhan WL: A syndrome of methylmalonic aciduria, homocystinuria, megaloblastic anemia and neurologic abnormalities in a vitamin B_{12}-deficient breast-fed infant of a strict vegetarian. N Engl J Med 299:317–323, 1978

57. Hillstrom L, Pettersson L, Hellbe L et al: Comparison

of oral ZnSO$_4$ and placebo in acne vulgaris. Br J Dermatol 97:681–688, 1977

58. Hitch J, Greenberg B: Adolescent acne and dietary iodine. Arch Dermatol 84:898–911, 1961
59. Hodges R, Baker E, Hood J et al: Experimental scurvy in man. Am J Clin Nutr 22:535–548, 1969
60. Hodges R, Hood J, Canham J et al: Clinical manifestations of ascorbic acid deficiency in man. Am J Clin Nutr 24:432–443, 1971
61. Howard WR: Psoriasis and serum lipids: A prospective clinical survey. In Farber EM, Cox AJ (eds): Psoriasis: Proceedings of the Second International Symposium, pp 381–382. New York, Yorke Medical Books, 1977
62. Hsu JM: The role of zinc in amino acid metabolism. In Hambidge KM, Nichols BL (eds): Zinc and Copper in Clinical Medicine, pp 25–34. Jamaica, NY, Spectrum Publications, 1978
63. Huff JC, Weston WL, Zirker DK: Wheat protein antibodies in dermatitis herpetiformis. J Invest Dermatol 73:570–574, 1969
64. Hume EM, Krebs H: Vitamin A requirements of human adults: An experimental study of vitamin A deprivation in man. Medical Research Council Special Report Series No. 264, 1949
65. Jacobs JC, Miller ME: Fatal familial Leiner's disease: A deficiency of opsonic activity of serum complement. Pediatrics 49:225–232, 1972
66. Jordan VE: Protein status of the elderly as measured by dietary intake, hair tissue, and serum albumin. Am J Clin Nutr 29:522–528, 1976
67. Jordan WP, King SE: Nickel feeding in nickel-sensitive patients with hand eczema. J Am Acad Dermatol 1:506–508, 1979
68. Kaaber K, Menne T, Tjell JC et al: Antabuse treatment of nickel dermatitis. Chelation—a new principle in the treatment of nickel dermatitis. Contact Dermatitis 5:221–228, 1979
69. Kaaber K, Veien NK, Tjell JC: Low nickel diet in the treatment of patients with chronic nickel dermatitis. Br J Dermatol 98:197–201, 1978
70. Kahler JP, Goldsmith LA: Extractable hair protein in Menkes' syndrome. Pediatrics 92:675, 1978
71. Kahn CR, Flier JS, Bar RS et al: The syndromes of insulin resistance and acanthosis nigricans. N Engl J Med 294:739–745, 1976
72. Katz SI, Strober W: The pathogenesis of dermatitis herpetiformis. J Invest Dermatol 70:63–75, 1978
73. Klingberg WG, Prasad As, Oberleas D: Zinc deficiency following penicillamine therapy. In Prasad AS, Oberleas D (eds): Trace Elements in Human Health and Disease, Vol. 1, pp 51–65. New York, Academic Press, 1976
74. Knowles J, Shuster S, Wells G: Folic acid deficiency in patients with skin disease. Lancet 1:1138–1139, 1963
75. Kusin JA: Vitamin E supplements and absorption of massive doses of vitamin A. Am J Clin Nutr 27:774–776, 1974
76. Lacroix J, Morin CL, Collin P: Nickel dermatitis from a foreign body in the stomach. J Pediatr 95:428–429, 1979
77. Lane M, Alfrey C, Mengel C et al: The rapid induction of human riboflavin deficiency with galactoflavin. J Clin Invest 43:357–373, 1964
78. Lazurus GS, Gilgor RS: Editorial. Psoriasis, polymorphonuclear leukocytes and lithium carbonate—an important clue. Arch Dermatol. 115:1183–1184, 1979

79. Lerner M, Lerner AB: Psoriasis and protein intake. Arch Dermatol 90:217–225, 1974
80. Lewis M: The effect of beta-carotene on serum vitamin A levels in erythropoietic protoporphyria. Aust J Dermatol 13:75–78, 1972
81. Lyell A: Metal allergy and metallic prostheses. Int J Dermatol 18:805–807, 1979
82. Malcolm LA, Balasubramaniam E, Edwards G: Effect of protein supplementation on the hair of chronically malnourished New Guinean schoolchildren. Am J Clin Nutr 26:479–481, 1973
83. Marks J, Shuster S: Iron metabolism in skin disease. Arch Dermatol 98:469–475, 1968
84. Marks R: Concepts in the pathogenesis of rosacea. Br J Dermatol 80:170–177, 1968
85. Marks R, Dykes PJ: The Ichthyoses. New York, Spectrum Publications, 1978
86. Mason KE: A conspectus of research on copper metabolism and requirements of man. J Nutr 109:1981–2066, 1979
87. Mathews–Roth M, Pathak M, Fitzpatrick T et al: Beta-carotene as a photoprotective agent in erythropoietic protoporphyria. N Engl J Med 282:1231–1234, 1970
88. Meffert H, Diezel W, Sonnichsen N: Stable lipid peroxidation products in human skin: Detection, ultraviolet light-induced increase, pathogenic importance. Experientia 32:1397–1398, 1976
89. Melski JW, Arndt KA: Topical therapy for acne—medical intelligence—current concepts. N Engl J Med 301:503–506, 1980
90. Menne T, Kaaber K: Treatment of pompholyx due to nickel allergy with chelating agents. Contact Dermatitis 4:289–290, 1978
91. Michaelsson G, Juhlin L: Urticaria induced by preservatives and dye additives in food and drugs. Br J Dermatol 88:525–532, 1973
92. Michaelsson G, Juhlin L, Valquist A: Effects of oral zinc and vitamin A in acne. Arch Dermatol 113:31–36, 1977
93. Michaelsson G, Valquist A, Juhlin L: Serum zinc and retinol-binding protein in acne. Br J Dermatol 96:283–286, 1977
94. Miller ME, Koblenzer PJ: Leiner's disease and deficiency of C5. J Pediatr 80:879–880, 1979
95. Moynahan EJ: Acrodermatitis enteropathica: A lethal inherited human zinc deficiency disorder (letter to the editor). Lancet 2:399, 1974
96. Nagaraju M, Adamson D, Rogers J: Skin manifestation of folic acid deficiency. Br J Dermatol 84:32–36, 1971
97. Nisenson A: Seborrheic dermatitis of infants: Treatment with biotin injections for the nursing mother. Pediatrics 44:1014–1015, 1969
98. Noid HE, Schulze TW, Winkelmann RK: Diet plan for patients with salicylate-induced urticaria. Arch Dermatol 109:866–869, 1974
99. Orris L, Shalita AR, Sibulkin D et al: Oral zinc therapy in acne. Arch Dermatol 114:1018–1020, 1978
100. Peck GL, Olsen TG, Yoder FW et al: Prolonged remissions of cystic and conglobate acne with 13-*cis*-retinoic acid. N Engl J Med 300:329–333, 1979
101. Pories WJ, Strain WH, Hsu JM et al: Clinical Applications of Zinc Metabolism. Springfield, Ill, Charles C Thomas, 1974
102. Prasad AS, Oberlease D: Trace Elements in Human Health and Disease, Vol 1, Zinc and Copper. New York, Academic Press, 1976
103. Proctor MS, Wilkinson DI, Orenberg EK et al: Lowered

cutaneous urinary levels of polyamines with clinical improvement in treated psoriasis. Arch Dermatol 115:945–949, 1979

104. Prottey C: Essential fatty acids and the skin. Br J Dermatol 94:579–587, 1976
105. Reunala T, Blomquist K, Tarpila S et al: Gluten-free diet in dermatitis herpetiformis. Br J Dermatol 97:473–480, 1977
106. Riella MC, Broviac JW, Wells M et al: Essential fatty acid deficiency in human adults during total parenteral nutrition. Arch Intern Med 83:786–789, 1975
107. Roe D: Nutritional significance of generalized exfoliative dermatoses. NY State J Med 62:3455–3457, 1962
108. Roe D: A Plague of Corn: The Social History of Pellagra. Ithaca, Cornell University Press, 1973
109. Rowe NH, Gorlin RJ: The effect of vitamin A deficiency upon experimental oral carcinogenesis. J Dent Res 38:72–83, 1959
110. Ruiter M, Meyler L: Skin changes after therapeutic administration of nicotinic acid in large doses. Dermatologica 120:139–144, 1960
111. Sanderson KV: Arsenic and skin cancer. In Andrade R, Gumport SL, Popkin GL et al (eds): Cancer of the Skin—Biology, Diagnosis and Management, pp 473–491. Philadelphia, WB Saunders, 1976
112. Sauberlich H, Hodges R, Wallace D et al: Vitamin A metabolism and requirements in the human studied with use of labelled retinol. Vitam Horm 32:251–275, 1974
113. Schamberger RJ: Relationship of selenium to cancer. I. Inhibitory effect of selenium on carcinogenesis. Journal of The National Cancer Institute 44:931–936, 1970
114. Schrauzer GN: Trace elements, nutrition and cancer: Perspectives of prevention. In Schrauzer GN (ed): Inorganic and Nutritional Aspects of Cancer, pp 323–344. New York, Plenum Press, 1978
115. Scott BB, Young S, Rajah SM et al: Coeliac disease and dermatitis herpetiformis: Further studies of their relationship. Gut 17:759–762, 1976
116. Shih VE: Urea cycle disorders and other congenital hyperammonemic syndromes. In Stanbury JB, Wyngaarden JB, Fredrickson DS (eds): The Metabolic Basis of Inherited Disease, pp 362–386. New York, McGraw-Hill, 1978
117. Shmunes E: Hypervitaminosis A in a patient with alopecia receiving renal dialysis. Arch Dermatol 115:882–883, 1979
118. Shuster S: Systemic effects of skin disease. Lancet 1:907–912, 1967
119. Skoven I, Thorman J: Lithium compound treatment and psoriasis. Arch Dermatol 115:1185–1187, 1979
120. Smith D, Ruffin J: Effects of sunlight on clinical manifestations of pellagra. Arch Intern Med 59:631–645, 1937
121. Spruit D, Bongaarts JM, de Jongh GJ: Dithiocarbamate therapy for nickel dermatitis. Contact Dermatitis 4:350–358, 1978
122. Steinberg D: Phytanic acid storage disease: Refsum's syndrome. In Stanburg JB, Wyngaarden JB, Fredrickson DS (eds): The Metabolic Basis of Inherited Disease, pp 689–706. New York, McGraw-Hill, 1978
123. Stratigos JD, Katsambas A: Pellagra: A still existing disease. Br J Dermatol 96:99–106, 1977
124. Strobel CT, Bryne WJ, Abramovits W et al: A zinc-deficiency dermatitis in patients on total parenteral nutrition. Int J Dermatol 17:575–581, 1978
125. Svejcar J, Homolka J: Experimental experiences with biotin in babies. Ann Pediatr 174:175, 1950
126. Sydenstricker VP, Singal SA, Briggs AP et al: Observations on the "egg–white injury" in man and its cure with a biotin concentrate. JAMA 118:1199–1200, 1942
127. Tickner A, Basit A: Vitamin C and exfoliative dermatitis. Br J Dermatol 72:403–408, 1960
128. Tickner A, Basit A: Serum proteins and liver functions in exfoliative dermatitis. Br J Dermatol 72:138–141, 1960
129. Touraine R, Revuz J, Zittoun J et al: Study of folate in psoriasis: Blood levels, intestinal absorption and cutaneous loss. Br J Dermatol 89:335–341, 1973
130. Tseng WP, Chu HM, How SW et al: Prevalence of skin cancer in an endemic area of chronic arsenicism in Taiwan. Journal of The National Cancer Institute 40:453–463, 1968
131. Underwood EJ: Trace Elements in Human and Animal Nutrition. New York, Academic Press, 1977
132. van Rij AM, Pories WJ: Zinc in wound healing. In Nriagu JO (ed): Zinc in the Environment—Part 2: Health Effects, pp 215–236. New York, Wiley & Sons, 1980
133. Vilter R, Mueller J, Glazer H et al: The effect of vitamin B_6 deficiency induced by desoxypyridoxine in human beings. J Lab Clin Med 42:335–357, 1953
134. Voorhees JJ: Editorial. Polyamines and psoriasis. Arch Dermatol 115:943–944, 1979
135. Voorhees JJ, Chakrabati S, Botero F et al: Zinc therapy and distribution of psoriasis. Arch Dermatol 100:669–673, 1969
136. Wagner SL, Maliner JS, Morton WD et al: Skin cancer and arsenical intoxication from well water. Arch Dermatol 115:1205–1207, 1979
137. Walker A: Chronic scurvy. Br J Dermatol 80:625–630, 1968
138. Warin RP, Smith RJ: Challenge test battery in chronic urticaria. Br J Dermatol 94:401–406, 1976
139. Wechsler HL: Vitamin A deficiency following small-bowel bypass surgery for obesity. Arch Dermatol 115:73–75, 1979
140. Weimar VM, Puhl SC, Smith WH et al: $ZnSO_4$ in acne vulgaris. Arch Dermatol 114:1776–1778, 1978
141. Weismann K: Intravenous zinc sulfate therapy in zinc-depleted patients. Dermatologica 159:171–175, 1979
142. Weisman K, Wadskov S, Sonergaard J: Oral zinc sulfate therapy for acne vulgaris. Arch Dermatol Venereol 57:357–360, 1977
143. Westall RG: Treatment of argininosuccinic aciduria. Am J Dis Child 113:160–161, 1967
144. Weston WL, Huff JC, Humbert JR et al: Zinc correction of defective chemotaxis in acrodermatitis enteropathica. Arch Dermatol 113:422–424, 1977
145. Zackheim HS: Topical 6-aminonicotinamide plus oral niacinamide for psoriasis. Arch Dermatol 114:1632–1638, 1978
146. Zackhelm HS, Farber EM: Taurine and psoriasis. J Invest Dermatol 50:227–230, 1968
147. Zackheim HS, Farber EM: Rapid weight reduction and psoriasis. Arch Dermatol 103:136–140, 1971
148. Zain BK, Haquani AH, Qureshi N et al: Studies on the significance of hair root protein and DNA in protein–calorie malnutrition. Am J Clin Nutr 30:1094–1097, 1977
149. Zaleski WA, Hill A, Kusniruk W: Skin lesions in tyrosinosis: Response to dietary treatment. Br J Dermatol 88:335–340, 1973

36
Surgery and Oncology

Bruce V. MacFadyen, Jr.,
Edward M. Copeland, III,
Stanley J. Dudrick

Patients with diseases requiring surgical therapy frequently demonstrate clinical signs of malnutrition more rapidly and acutely than patients with medical diseases. Patients undergoing complicated surgical procedures that necessitate removal of multiple abdominal organs, such as the pancreas, small and large intestine, liver, and the stomach, are especially susceptible to developing malnutrition, which, if present preoperatively, must be corrected using intensive intravenous, oral, or intestinal nutrition techniques. Malnutrition has been defined as a combination of recent weight loss greater than 10% of body weight, serum albumin concentration less than 3 g %, total lymphocyte count less than 1200/mm³, or anergy to a battery of skin test antigens. Significant protein–calorie malnutrition has been demonstrated in 25% to 50% of surgical patients hospitalized for 2 weeks or longer, and these malnourished patients were found to have an increased vulnerability to intercurrent infections.[8] An increased incidence of surgical complications has also been demonstrated in patients whose weight is less than 90% of their ideal body weight. Other patients who are susceptible to nutritional complications include those who have intestinal malabsorption, increased losses of intestinal secretions, pancreatic insufficiency, a long history of drug or alcohol abuse, a prolonged period (2 weeks or longer) of hypocaloric (200 Cal–500 Cal) intravenous feeding, and premature and term infants who require a surgical procedure. Hypermetabolism secondary to fever, infection, multiple trauma, hyperthyroidism, pregnancy, and thermal and electrical burns is also associated with an increased incidence of severe malnutrition.

The catabolic effect on body tissues in patients who are acutely injured consists of two primary manifestations. The first is a local response that depends on the type and extent of the wound and the anatomy and local microcirculation of the injured area. The second response involves an increased output of hormones, which stimulate accentuated utilization of endogenous protein, fat, and carbohydrates. Carbohydrate, in the form of glycogen, is the initial major energy source after which fat and, to a lesser extent, protein become the major energy sources. If the increased postinjury level of catabolism is maintained for 2 weeks or longer, a rapid loss of muscle mass will occur, leading to significant weakness and malaise. Although this catabolic response cannot be significantly altered pharmacologically, the use of intensive nutritional support will minimize the loss of endogenous nutrients, prevent the ravages of malnutrition, and significantly decrease the morbidity and mortality of potentially lethal injuries.

Evaluation of Nutritional State

The importance of recognizing the signs of protein–calorie malnutrition cannot be overemphasized. They include the following: (1) peripheral edema; (2) hair loss, brittle hair, and easy pluckability; (3) muscle wasting; (4) scaly skin and decreased skin turgor; (5) apathy, weakness, and lethargy; (6) abnormal nail growth; (7) moon facies; and (8) hepatomegaly. Abnormal laboratory studies may include decreased serum concentrations of albumin, prealbumin, total protein, retinol-binding protein, and transferrin; a decreased serum carotene level; decreased total lymphocyte count; and decreased phagocytic activity of the white blood cells.[6] The gastrointestinal tract itself is adversely affected and can manifest a decreased thickness of the intestinal wall as well as decreases in the intestinal concentrations of DNA and RNA, decreased protein synthesis, decreases in the concentration and function of absorptive enzymes, and increased gluconeogenic lysosomal enzyme activity.[2] All critically or chronically ill surgical patients should be observed for evidence of these changes because they may be the earliest precursors of nutritional complications, such as progressive weight loss, weakness, impaired wound healing, fistula formation, increased incidence of infection, decreased immunocompetence, diminished response to chemotherapy, and eventually delayed hospital discharge, prolonged convalescence and rehabilitation, and increased medical costs.

Clinical malnutrition is usually classified into two primary categories. The first is the kwashiorkor type, which is primarily related to protein malnutrition manifested by decreased serum albumin and serum transferrin levels, decreased total lymphocyte count, nonreactive skin tests, and obvious loss of somatic protein mass and subcutaneous fat. The second category of malnourished patients includes those who have protein–calorie malnutrition and present with significant decreases in body fat, muscle and visceral protein, along with objective decreases in the weight/height and creatinine/height ratios, in the triceps skin folds, and in arm muscle circumference. Serial objective nutritional assessment is important and includes body weight, nitrogen balance, serum albumin and transferrin levels, total lymphocyte count, and anthropometric measurements. Mullen and colleagues have used regression analysis of nutritional assessment data to categorize the patient's malnourished state and have tried to correlate the nutritional status with surgical morbidity and mortality.[47] However, Shizgal has suggested that anthropometric measurements and serum protein levels are not sufficient for categorization and that body composition studies using radioactive sodium and potassium are far more accurate in relating nutritional status to surgical complications.[57] Because such radioactive tracer studies are not clinically available in most hospitals, the physician must rely on an accurate history and physical examination and serial measurements of serum albumin, total protein, and transferrin levels to assess the patient's nutritional status (see Chap. 10).

Metabolic and Nutritional Changes During Starvation and Injury

Energy is stored in the body in the form of glycogen, protein, and fat. Glycogen is concentrated primarily in the liver and skeletal muscle in combination with water and electrolytes and will yield 1 Cal to 2 Cal of energy/g tissue, in contrast to the anhydrous carbohydrate, which represents one fourth to one fifth muscle weight and has an energy concentration of 4 Cal/g. Amino acids are used in the synthesis of enzymes, plasma, and structural proteins, of cardiac, skeletal, and smooth muscle, and as essential substrates for wound healing. Lipid on the other hand, is stored with water as triglycerides and has a caloric density of 9.4 Cal/g. The total quantity of each nutrient in the body of a normal 70-kg person is shown in Table 36-1.[9] During acute starvation, glycogen is used initially as the energy source, but as starvation progresses, increasing amounts of lipid and protein will be utilized for energy. As was demonstrated by Allen and co-workers, plasma proteins can also be consumed as a source of calories, and it has been observed in prolonged fasting that the synthesis of serum proteins, and particularly albumin, is not rapid enough to compensate for losses, thus necessitating the administration of exogenous amino acids.[4]

In the early fasting state, a 70-kg man can be expected to synthesize approximately 16 g/day of glucose from glycerol, 43 g/day from muscle protein, and an additional 85 g/day from glycogenolysis. Thirty-six grams of glucose can also be produced by recycling glucose through the Cori Cycle and, therefore, the total amount of glucose available for energy is 180 g. The oxidation of fatty acids provides the energy for gluconeogenesis and other body functions except in the brain, where glucose is the primary energy source.

TABLE 36-1
Endogenous Fuel Composition of Normal Humans

Fuel	Kg	Cal
Tissues		
Fat (adipose triglyceride)	15	141,000
Protein (mainly muscle)	6	24,000
Glycogen (muscle)	0.150	600
Glycogen (liver)	0.075	300
Total		165,900
Circulating fuels		
Glucose (extracellular fluids)	0.020	80
Free fatty acids (plasma)	0.0003	3
Triglycerides (plasma)	0.003	30
Total		113

The importance of providing 100 g/day exogenous glucose to the starved patient was first shown by Gamble and co-workers, who demonstrated that this relatively small amount of glucose prevented the breakdown of approximately 50 g endogenous protein, thus decreasing the need for gluconeogenesis and ketogenesis.[31] On the other hand, if protein is not spared, muscle wasting occurs and clinically results in an ineffective cough, pneumonia, impaired wound healing, decreased resistance to infection, and decreased synthesis of enzymes and plasma proteins. Although Blackburn and colleagues demonstrated short-term positive nitrogen balance when amino acids were given without glucose and fat, several other investigators have contested this finding and have emphasized the necessity of concomitant administration of dextrose or lipids as a primary energy source, especially in patients requiring intensive nutritional support for longer than 10 days.

The metabolic effects of accidental or operative trauma and sepsis usually result in (1) hyperglycemia, unless the injury is overwhelmingly fatal; (2) marked fatty acid mobilization and elevation of plasma free fatty acids; (3) significant degradation of muscle protein beyond that needed for energy, in contrast to late starvation when protein is conserved; (4) increased synthesis of urea and the so-called acute phase reactants (haptoglobin, fibrinogen, ceruloplasmin, C-reactive protein, and so forth); and (5) increased extracellular osmolality. Ordinarily, tissue oxygen consumption is not increased during elective operation, but may be increased as much as 25% after multiple fracture, 50% during severe sepsis, and up to 100% following thermal injuries. The initial primary energy source after trauma and during early starvation is glucose, followed by fat. The catabolic hormones, such as catecholamines, glucagon, ACTH, and growth hormone, increase lipid C-AMP and thus increase the activity of the lipolytic enzymes, which hydrolyze triglycerides to free fatty acids and glycerol.

Protein metabolism is also altered following acute injury. Ordinarily, 2 g/day to 3 g/day nitrogen are excreted in the stool and 11 g/day to 17 g/day are excreted in the urine; however, following severe trauma, urinary nitrogen can increase to as much as 30 g/day to 50 g/day. If anuria or oliguria is present, BUN levels may greatly increase shortly after injury, reach a peak during the first week postinjury, and continue for 3 weeks to 7 weeks. On the other hand, a burn patient may lose 50 lb to 75 lb of weight and have large protein losses from the burned surface. It appears from several studies that most of the nitrogen loss is from the muscle and that the integrity of other vital organs is maintained during acute injury at the expense of skeletal muscle.[40,49] This may account for the fact that muscular young men lose more protein than women or debilitated elderly patients. Therefore, it appears that in trauma patients, the excessive muscle protein catabolism far exceeds estimated energy requirements, and the magnitude of the response is directly related to the extent of the injury. However, Duke and co-workers have stated that after severe trauma, the protein contribution to the total calorie requirement rarely exceeds 15%.[25] In addition, it has been observed that the principal amino acids lost during catabolism are leucine, isoleucine, and valine and that the alanine released from muscle is the principle amino acid responsible for regulation of gluconeogenesis in the liver.[27] These amino acids may be increased in the plasma for 2 hr to several weeks after trauma and may contribute to the serum hyperosmolality that is often measured in trauma patients. Following trauma, there is an increase in the acute phase resultant proteins, particularly the C-reactive protein, fibrinogen, and haptaglobin. There is also an increased rate of albumin synthesis and an even greater increase in the degradation of albumin, which is stimulated by the elevated serum cortisol.

The stress of operation or multiple trauma causes the patient to be hypermetabolic. Body-composition studies have indicated that during hypermetabolism, fat and lean body mass contribute approximately 50% of the cellular loss, but fat is the primary calorie source, contributing 80% to 85% of the total calories.[46] The degree of hypermetabolism is determined by the following factors: (1) plasma levels of insulin, growth hormone, glucagon, catecholamines, corticosteroids, and thyroid hormones; (2) cold stress; (3) systemic infection; (4) central nervous system lesions affecting the function of the pituitary gland; and (5) significant tissue injury secondary to the surgical operation, crush injury, long bone fracture, or major full-thickness cutaneous burn.[62] The hormones released by the hypothalamus are regulated by the sympathetic and parasympathetic nervous systems. During acute stress, a sympathetic impulse causes the release of the catabolic hormones, such as catecholamines, glucagon, thyroid hormone, and corticosteroids, which produce glycogenolysis and an increased serum glucose level. On the other hand, parasympathetic stimulation leads to an increase in liver glycogen synthesis and storage and, therefore, the metabolic rate is directly related to the predominance of the anabolic or catabolic hormones. The primary anabolic hormone is insulin, which functions to increase the synthesis of triglycerides and adipose tissue, to oppose the action of catecholamines, ACTH, and glucagon, to increase the amino acid uptake and synthesis in muscle, and to decrease fatty acid and amino acid release from the muscle. The other anabolic hormone is growth hormone, which does not alter the daily nitrogen excretion in fasting subjects but does increase the level of serum insulin. On the other hand, the catabolic hormones increase the rate of nitrogen excretion, increase glycogenolysis in the liver, increase gluconeogenesis by directly opposing the effect of insulin, and have a regulatory effect on circulating amino acids.

Wilmore and co-workers have correlated the metabolic rate and plasma hormone levels in patients with thermal injuries. They demonstrated that as the basal metabolic rate (BMR) increased, there was a concomitant elevation in the urinary excretion of catecholamines. As the BMR decreased, the plasma concentrations of the anabolic hormones increased, and nutrient deposition into tissue occurred. The use of large amounts of oral and intravenous calories and protein did not alter the body's response to stress but rather provided the necessary substrates to counteract the significant nitrogen loss that occurred. Other factors that alter morbidity and mortality in relation to stress include the previous state of nutrition prior to injury, muscle atrophy and inactivity, ambient temperature less than 25°C, and general anesthesia. Therefore, it is extremely important that the patient's nutritional needs are accurately assessed and the necessary nutrients provided in sufficient quantity to produce anabolism, positive nitrogen balance, and weight gain.

Nutritional Alternatives in the Surgical Patient

There are several methods for nutritional support of the surgical patient, and all of these options must provide at least the basic minimum of 1 g/kg/day protein and 30 Cal/kg/day energy in the form of dextrose or fat for the unstressed patients and up to 1.5 g/kg/day to 2 g/kg/day protein and 50 Cal/kg/day to 70 Cal/kg/day nonprotein calories for the hypermetabolic patient. Preferably, nutrients should be supplied by way of the gastrointestinal tract, but at times a surgical patient cannot absorb these nutrients and the intravenous route alone or in combination with the oral route may be the only means by which to promote positive nitrogen balance and weight gain. The therapeutic nutritional options include (1) regular oral diet, (2) nasogastric tube feedings, (3) gastrostomy feedings, (4) jejunostomy feedings, (5) chemically defined (elemental) diets, and (6) total intravenous nutritional support. The effectiveness of oral feedings can be altered by malabsorption, rapid transit time, lack of pancrea-

ticobiliary secretions, deficient mucosal absorptive function, and persistent diarrhea secondary to inflammation of the small and large bowel. Patients with inadequate small intestinal length can have a short bowel syndrome with significant diarrhea and hypergastrinemia that impair nutrient absorption. If these conditions exist, supplemental or complete intravenous hyperalimentation (IVH) feedings may be necessary in order to provide sufficient nutrient intake.

TUBE FEEDINGS

Occasionally, a tumor or radiation injury in the head and neck region or a neurologic or psychological disease may prevent normal swallowing. A #8 or #10 French feeding tube can be inserted through the nose, mouth, hypopharynx, and esophagus and advanced into the stomach or duodenum. Nutrients in the form of a blenderized oral diet, a commercially prepared complete diet, or a chemically defined diet can be administered intermittently or continuously over 24 hours using an infusion pump or gravity flow. The principle advantages of these types of feedings are that the necessity for operative insertion of a gastrostomy or jejunostomy tube is avoided, the nutrients are readily available and inexpensive, and the diets usually are easily digested or absorbed.

When the infusion of these diets is initiated, the concentration should be .25 Cal/ml to .5 Cal/ml, which is increased cautiously to 1 Cal/ml over 3 days to 4 days or more, thus allowing the gastrointestinal tract to adapt gradually to the increasing osmolality, which may vary between 400 mOsm/liter to 100 mOsm/liter. Some of the potential side-effects of these diets include gastric retention, esophageal regurgitation, aspiration pneumonia and asphyxia, pressure necrosis along the nasopharynx, esophagus, and stomach, partial pharyngeal or esophageal obstruction, esophagitis, eustachitis, esophageal stricture, the dumping syndrome, diarrhea, dehydration, and azotemia. However, most of these complications can be avoided if a slow infusion of a dilute feeding is used initially and the patient's head is elevated 45°. If intermittent feedings are used, the initial volume and frequency is usually 200 ml of a .5 Cal/ml diet administered over 45 min every 4 hr to 6 hr and the concentration, volume, and frequency are advanced as tolerated. Supplemental fluids may be given by vein as needed. On the other hand, continuous feedings are best regulated with an infusion pump starting with an initial 24-hr volume of 1200 ml at a concentration of .5 Cal/ml. In general, tube feedings should be used when normal swallowing is impaired and the gastrointestinal tract is functioning normally. This method is safe, relatively easy, economical, effective, and associated with a low incidence of complications if established principles and techniques are observed.

GASTROSTOMY FEEDINGS

Gastrostomy feedings have a similar nutrient composition to nasogastric tube feedings but differ in administration because a surgical procedure is necessary to insert a #20 to #26 French catheter through the anterior abdominal wall directly into the stomach. Primary indications for these feedings include patients who must receive these nutrients for 4 months and longer or patients who are comatose and thus might experience an increased incidence of gastric retention, regurgitation, and subsequent tracheal aspiration. During gastrostomy feedings, the cardioesophageal sphincter minimizes regurgitation, and hence the possibility of aspiration pneumonia is decreased. From the technical standpoint, a permanent gastrostomy is formed by constructing a gastric mucosa-lined tube from the stomach wall and suturing it to the skin. An alternative technique interposes a loop of jejunum between the stomach and skin for nutrient administration and, in general, gastrostomy feedings are effective and their administration is easily accomplished.[32]

Jejunostomy Feedings

When there is gastric outlet or duodenal obstruction and yet the remaining small intestine is functioning normally, jejunostomy feedings are a satisfactory alternative to nasogastric or gastrostomy feedings. These diets can be infused through a #10 to #22 French catheter that is inserted on the antimesenteric border of the proximal jejunum, after which the wall of the jejunum is sutured to the anterior abdominal wall. In the past, leakage of nutrients around the catheter, with associated sepsis, has been reported, but this complication can be minimized with conscientious attention to careful surgical technique. When jejunostomy feedings are no longer required, the tube can be removed and the jejunostomy site will close spontaneously. However, if reinsertion of the jejunostomy tube is desired, another operation is usually required, although occasionally the tube can be reinserted under fluoroscopic control with the use of radiopaque dye to ensure the intraluminal position of the catheter. In the past, a typical jejunostomy feeding regimen provided only 50 g to 80 g protein and 1500 Cal/day to 2000 Cal/day by infusing formulas as outlined in Table 36-2.[56] However, Andrassy and co-workers have advocated infusion of an elemen-

tal diet through a 14-gauge catheter that is inserted into the jejunum on the antimesenteric border and advanced over a long needle through the submucosal space for a few inches before entering into the bowel lumen.[5] This technique produces an S-shaped submucosal catheter tract, which reduces the likelihood of inadvertent catheter withdrawal or leakage. In general, jejunostomy feedings are hyperosmolar and can cause diarrhea, but gradually increasing the volume and concentration of the diet can result in a satisfactory nutrient intake in 90% of patients. During jejunal infusion, proximal reflux of nutrient fluid for distances up to 50 cm may occur, and this should be kept in mind when the site of feeding catheter insertion is chosen. Therefore, it is recommended that these diets should not be given to patients with high intestinal fistulas or to patients in whom total bowel rest is desired.

For adequate enteral nutrient administration, occasionally it may be necessary to create a Roux-en-Y proximal jejunal loop that is secured to the anterior abdominal wall. This mucosa-lined feeding ostomy will permit an easy access for the feeding tube into the bowel lumen while reducing the risk of stricture formation at the entrance site. The primary advantages of this method are that the patient does not have to tolerate a rubber catheter in place at all times and that proximal reflux of nutrient fluid is obviated. In selected cases, feeding jejunostomies can provide all required daily calories, protein, and other essential nutrients at relatively little expense.

CHEMICALLY DEFINED (ELEMENTAL) DIETS

The formulas used in nasogastric and jejunostomy feedings usually are composed of natural foods and often include nutrients that may not be completely digested or absorbed or that are not essential for nutrient replacement. During the past 15 years, the practical and economical production of L-amino acids has been advanced to the point that specific formulations of high biologic value amino acids, together with energy sources such as dextrose or oligosaccharides, are commercially available as chemically defined diets. These formulations also contain electrolytes, minerals, vitamins (except vitamin K), and a small amount of essential fat which, when given in sufficient quantities, will allow normal growth, development, and wound healing to occur (see Table 36-3 and Appendix Table A-38). Their advantages include (1) minimal bulk resulting in ultra-low residue, (2) minimal digestion required prior to absorption, (3) low viscosity allowing infusion through a small catheter, and (4) prolonged positive nitrogen balance and

TABLE 36-2
Jejunostomy Feeding Regimen

	Volume (liters)	Calories (Cal)	Protein (g)
12–18 hr postjejunostomy	0	0	0
1 day: 50 ml 5% dextrose/water/hr × 20	1	200	0
2 day: 100 ml 5% dextrose/water/hr × 20	2	400	0
3 day: 50 ml homogenized milk/hr × 20	1	700	35
4 day: 100 ml homogenized milk/2 hr × 10	1	700	35
5 day: 180 ml homogenized milk/2 hr × 10	1.8	1260	63
6 day: 240 ml homogenized milk/2 hr × 10	2.4	1680	84
Continue same regimen as on 6 day but add an additional half cup of powdered milk to each quart of homogenized milk daily until 1.5 cups/quart homogenized milk daily until 1.5 cups/quart homogenized milk is being used as a feeding formula. Thereafter, give 240 ml of this mixture q 2 × 10 daily. Feedings should begin at 6 A.M. and continue through 12 midnight. Additional water may be given between feedings when indicated.			

Components for mixing:
1. Powdered milk — 1.5 cups
2. Homogenized milk — 1 quart
3. Tween 40 (emulsifying agent) — 1 ml
4. Polyvisol — 0.6 ml
5. Fer-in-sol — 0.6 ml

Adapted from Shires GT, Canizaro PC: Fluid, electrolyte and nutritional management of the surgical patient. In Schwartz SI, Shires GT, Spencer FC, et al: Principles of Surgery, p 65. New York, McGraw–Hill Book Company, 1974

weight gain. However, the osmolarity of these diets ranges from 840 mOsm/liter to 2200 mOsm/liter, and gastric retention or diarrhea will occur if infusion rates are too rapid. Other potential complications such as nausea, vomiting, hyperglycemia, dehydration, fluid overload, and a strongly "organic" taste may necessitate intermittent or continuous infusion by pump through a nasogastric, gastrostomy, or jejunostomy tube. Although these diets may decrease pancreatic, biliary, and gastrointestinal secretions, maximum bowel rest is not achieved because the myoelectric activity in the bowel is only slightly decreased from that observed after a standard oral diet is ingested.

Recently, a chemically defined diet has been formulated using short-chain peptides rather than free amino acids, and with these diets the unpleasant organic flavor can be more easily concealed. However, the efficacy of such diets as protein and calorie sources remains to be determined completely, although they may bridge the nutritional gap in patients whose IVH is being discontinued yet who cannot tolerate a regular diet.

Elemental diets have been advocated for use as an effective bowel preparation for abdominal surgery.[33] Although studies have shown some decreases in the bacterial flora and bulk content of the colon, there has not been any significant alteration in the concentration of the Bacteroides species in the large bowel. Short-term use of this diet preoperatively usually produces diarrhea and potential dehydration, is not an effective nutrient source, and hence its routine use for preoperative bowel preparation is of questionable value.

An elemental diet may be indicated in patients with low intestinal tract fistulas, compensated short bowel syndrome, or inflammatory bowel disease that involves the distal ileum, and in patients who need sufficient oral nutrients but cannot tolerate a regular diet.

INTRAVENOUS HYPERALIMENTATION

When sufficient nutrients cannot be absorbed through the gastrointestinal tract, large quantities of amino acids, dextrose, fat, and other essential nutrients must be given intravenously. This technique, called *intravenous hyperalimentation* (IVH), is a method whereby 2000 to 5000 dextrose calories and 80 g to 200 g amino acids, together with re-

TABLE 36-3
Composition of Current Chemically Defined Diets

	Vivonex 100	Vivonex High Nitrogen	W–T Low Residue Food	Flexical
Carbohydrates (g)	226	210	226	155
	Glucose, glucose oligosaccharides	Glucose oligosaccharides	Dextrin	Sucrose
Nitrogen (g)	3.27	6.67	3	3.5
	Amino acids	Amino acids	Amino acids	Protein hydrolysate and added amino acids
Protein (g)	20.4	41.7	18.8	21.9
Fat (g)	0.74	0.44	0.74	34
	Safflower oil and linoleic acid	Safflower oil	Safflower oil	
Sodium (mEq)	57.6	35.5	55.7	15.7
Potassium (mEq)	29.9	17.9	30	38.9
Calcium (mEq)	22.1	13.3	27.8	26
Magnesium (mEq)	7.11	9.6	18.4	14.6
Iron (mEq)	0.19	0.11	0.34	0.02
Chloride (mEq)	71.2	52.2	85.0	34.3
Osmolarity (mOs/liter)	1175	844	649	805

Adapted from Nutrition Gap, Eaton Laboratories, Norwich, NY: W–T Low Residue Food, Warren–Teed Pharmaceuticals, Inc., Columbus, Ohio; Flexical, Low Residue Elemental Diet, Mead–Johnson Laboratories, Evansville, Indiana

quired vitamins, trace minerals, and electrolytes can be infused intravenously through the superior vena cava over a 24-hr period.[24] (See also Chap. 13.) With this technique, weight gain, normal growth and development, positive nitrogen balance, and wound healing can be achieved along with decreased morbidity and mortality in surgical patients who otherwise would have had complications secondary to malnutrition.

These solutions have an osmolality of 1800 mOsm/liter to 2200 mOsm/liter and, therefore, must be infused into the superior vena cava in order to prevent severe thrombophlebitis which will occur with administration through a peripheral vein. Several techniques for catheter insertion into the superior vena cava have been used. The one preferred by the authors is the infraclavicular approach to the subclavian vein in which a 2-inch-long #14-gauge needle is inserted under the middle third of the clavicle into the subclavian vein. An 8-inch to 10-inch-long #16-gauge polyethylene catheter is advanced through the needle in the subclavian vein into the midportion of the superior vena cava. Other sites of catheter insertion include the internal and external jugular veins, the cephalic vein, and the supraclavicular access to the subclavian vein. Occasionally, the inferior vena cava may be catheterized using a silicone rubber catheter inserted through a branch of the greater saphenous vein in the leg, a method that should be used if there is thrombosis of the superior vena cava. However, this approach is not used routinely

because of the higher incidence of thrombosis and infection. Sterile technique is extremely important during catheter insertion, and dressing and tubing changes should be performed three times each week. Using this procedure, catheters can remain in place safely for periods in excess of 60 days with an infection rate less than 2.2%.[15] In patients who require central venous catheterization for periods less than 60 days, the percutaneously placed polyethylene catheter is used. When IVH is to be used for periods longer than 60 days, however, a surgically implanted silicone rubber catheter is preferred because of the increased longevity and lower incidence of venous thrombosis associated with such catheters.

Although IVH has been discussed in Chapter 13, there are several points regarding its use that must be emphasized. The first consideration is that this technique is safe and is associated with a low incidence of complications. A second point is that complete bowel rest can be achieved with this technique, thus minimizing bowel absorption and decreasing electrical and mechanical activity to a resting potential. This allows gastrointestinal secretions to decrease by 50% to 75% and to reduce significantly intestinal enzyme synthesis.

The Clinical Application of Nutrition in Surgery

Patients with surgical disorders are prime candidates for developing nutritional and metabolic complications. The correction of existing nutritional deficits preoperatively is preferred but occasionally cannot be accomplished because of the acute nature of the surgical problem, and therefore, nutritional support must be limited to the postoperative period. Certain disorders and diseases are particularly associated with development of nutritional deficits. The first group includes patients with partial or complete obstruction of the gastrointestinal tract. Another group includes diseases that alter digestive enzyme secretion or intestinal mucosal absorption. A third group consists of problems which alter the normal metabolism of nutrients, such as renal and liver failure. Clinical problems that stimulate hypermetabolism greatly increase the patient's expenditure and metabolic requirements, and neonates particularly have such a small nutritional reserve that they require immediate nutritional support and repletion. The preferred method of intensive nutritional support is through the gastrointestinal tract whenever possible; however, if sufficient nutrients cannot be supplied in this way, IVH must then be given to provide supplemental or complete nutrition. The use of intensive nutritional support in a few representative clinical problems merits discussion.

GASTROINTESTINAL DISEASE

INFLAMMATORY BOWEL DISEASE

Malnutrition is a frequent sequela to acute and chronic inflammatory bowel disease (IBD), and it has been documented that 65% of these patients weigh 10% to 15% less than their ideal body weights when initially evaluated by their physician. Other clinical signs of malnutrition may include obvious loss of skeletal muscle mass, hypoproteinemia, anemia, edema, weakness, osteomalacia, hypokalemia, and deficiencies of vitamins A, D, E, K, B_{12}, and folic acid. Nutritional problems are usually related to a decreased absorption of carbohydrates, fats, proteins, minerals, and vitamins, to a rapid intestinal transit time, and to an increased secretion of protein into the bowel lumen, which may be 15 times normal during an acute attack. The natural history of IBD includes exacerbations and remissions, and treatment regimens often include short- and long-term courses of corticosteroids, sulfa derivatives, antibiotics, and antimotility drugs, as well as multiple surgical procedures. It is not uncommon for patients to develop partial or complete bowel obstruction, external or internal gastrointestinal fistulas, and short bowel syndrome, all of which accentuate the nutritional complications. Initially, medical treatment is symptomatic and includes Lomotil, Imodium, deodorized tincture of opium, or codeine to slow the intestinal transit time and to solidify the stool.

Corticosteroids can be effective during an acute exacerbation, but they appear to lose their effectiveness on a long-term basis, and their prolonged use is inevitably accompanied by serious nutritional consequences that include negative nitrogen balance, hypoalbuminemia, impaired wound healing, decreased resistance to infection, osteoporosis, hypokalemia, hypocalcemia, and growth retardation in children. Nutriment is preferably given orally using a low-roughage, low-fat, and lactose-free diet or an elemental diet as has been advocated by Rocchio and co-workers.[53] If weight gain and positive nitrogen balance cannot be achieved with oral nutrition, then IVH must be used. The indications for the use of IVH in inflammatory bowel disease include the following: (1) prolonged periods of active disease and associated severe catabolism, (2) nutritional repletion before major surgery, (3) short bowel syndrome, (4) indolent wound healing, (5) alimentary tract fistulas, and (6) adjunctive therapy during an acute exacerbation. IVH enables the gastrointestinal tract to remain at complete rest, which has been shown to decrease intestinal secretion, motility, and inflammatory activity and to improve the healing of the diseased bowel.

The use of IVH and total bowel rest was analyzed in 52 patients with inflammatory bowel disease.[22] Corticosteroids and immunosuppressive drugs were included when deemed advisable, but could usually be reduced or eliminated during the course of IVH therapy (see Table 36-4). One group included 41 patients (78.8%) who had a favorable nutritional response with weight gain and positive nitrogen balance and experienced a clinical remission of their disease. Within this group, 28 patients (53.8%) were restored to a low-residue oral diet within 36.3 days of treatment without exacerbation of the disease. The second subgroup consisted of 13 patients (25%) who required operation for a complication such as intestinal obstruction, fistula, or an abscess. A second major category of patients required operation within 15 days of the beginning of IVH and bowel rest because of extremely virulent and recalcitrant disease, although significant nutritional repletion was accomplished in all patients. This study emphasized the beneficial effect of IVH and total bowel rest in the hospital, but occasionally patients will require prolonged intensive intravenous nutritional support on an outpatient basis. Ambulatory home IVH has been shown to be safe, cost effective, and nutritionally and metabolically beneficial to patients with inflammatory bowel disease.[58]

The exact mechanisms by which IVH and bowel

TABLE 36-4
Intravenous Hyperalimentation in Inflammatory
Bowel Disease

Patients	Results	Duration IVH (days)
GROUP I		
41 (78.8%)	Marked nutritional improvement Clinical remission of disease	
A. 28	Resumed oral diet without exacerbation of disease	36.3
B. 13	Surgery necessary for a complication such as fistula, abscess, or bowel obstruction	26.8
GROUP II		
11 (21.2%)	Marked nutritional improvement Operation for severe activity of primary disease	15

rest allow spontaneous remissions to occur are not known. IVH certainly provides the necessary nutrient substrates for correction of malnutrition, which may improve immunocompetence. Moreover, the lack of food and partially digested foodstuffs in the bowel lumen may greatly reduce the stimulation of any food intolerance or food allergy that might otherwise be present. It is also known that bowel rest decreases not only the caustic intraluminal and pancreatic enzyme secretions but also the intestinal brush border enzyme concentrations, particularly peroxidase, which is derived from leukocytes in the lamina propria.[12,64] The decreased intestinal peroxidase level during bowel rest may indicate a reduction in inflammatory cell infiltration of the bowel wall. In addition, it has also been shown that total bowel rest decreases the myoelectric activity and peristalsis of the bowel, which is ordinarily stimulated by oral and enteral feedings.[45] The decrease in mechanical activity, along with a decrease in the digestive, absorptive, and hormonal activities, is more conducive to healing the inflamed intestine. The combination of IVH and bowel rest is essential to maximize the remission rate and to correct or to prevent primary and nutritional complications of inflammatory bowel disease.

GASTROINTESTINAL TRACT FISTULAS

Patients with gastrointestinal tract fistulas usually develop metabolic and nutritional complications that require intensive nutritional support. In the past, the treatment of gastrointestinal tract fistulas has been associated with a high morbidity and with mortality rates of 40% to 60%.[26] Severe catabolism secondary to malnutrition, sepsis, and renal failure often produces severe complications and death, especially when the patient has not been given intensive nutritional support. Intestinal feedings with an elemental diet can be used in patients with a gastric or colonic fistula, as shown by Rocchio and co-workers.[54] However, most patients are unable to tolerate intestinal nutrients and require the use of IVH.

In 1973, the use of IVH and total bowel rest was reported in a series of 62 patients with 78 gastrointestinal tract fistulas in which prolonged positive nitrogen balance and weight gain occurred with an overall mortality rate of only 6.6%.[44] Moreover, the spontaneous closure rate of both external and internal fistulas was 70.1%. This was the first demonstration that intensive intravenous nutritional support with 80 g to 200 g amino acids and 3000 Cal/day to 5000 Cal/day would significantly improve the mortality rate in this complicated surgical problem. These data have been corroborated by Deitel, who reported a mortality rate of 9.3% in a series of 100 patients in which sufficient intravenous nutrients were supplied, in contrast to a 40% mortality rate in similar patients in whom nutrition was inadequate.[20] His study also showed that duration of hospitalization was twice as long in the patients receiving inadequate nutrition, thus emphasizing the cost-effectiveness of intensive nutritional therapy. Pancreatic and esophageal fistulas have also been reported to respond favorably to a regimen of total bowel rest and IVH, during which spontaneous closure occurred in an average period of 35 days.[23,41]

Patients who have gastrointestinal tract fistulas secondary to active inflammatory bowel disease generally do not experience spontaneous fistula closure unless there is concomitant quiescence of their disease, and it has been documented that IVH and total bowel rest can be successful in decreasing the activity of this disease sufficiently to allow spontaneous fistula closure to occur.[55] Treated with this technique, 75% of a series of 13 patients with 16 fistulas of the small bowel experienced quiescence of their active disease and spontaneous fistula closure within 32 days of starting IVH.[43] However, the closure rate of large bowel fistulas was only 30% during 40 days of IVH. Mullen and colleagues have observed a spontaneous closure rate of 43% in patients with similar problems.[48] Although recurrent fistulas occurred in three patients after IVH therapy alone and in three patients after combination therapy with IVH and surgical closure, they emphasized that the overall morbidity and mortality rates were markedly diminished because sufficient nutrients were provided.

Patients who develop gastrointestinal tract fistulas in the presence of malignant disease can present difficult management problems. The incidence of spontaneous fistula closure is low, especially if the affected bowel has been radiated. When radiation injury to the bowel was not present, Copeland and colleagues noted that 44% of the fistulas spontaneously closed and an additional 28% could be closed surgically.[14] However, the experience with fistulas located in radiated bowel is not as good, and both operative and spontaneous closure rates are very low. Therefore, in these patients, it is recommended that intensive nutritional support be given for 14 days to 21 days preoperatively prior to surgical bypass or resection of the fistula and involved bowel segment. Although nutritional repletion will improve anastomotic healing, recurrent or persistent fistulization may occur in 30% to 40% of patients with cancer.

In the management of all patients with gastrointestinal tract fistulas, certain priorities are necessary to optimize treatment. The first priority is the early institution of IVH, drainage of any abscesses, and external control of fistula drainage. The next priority is delineation of the anatomy of the fistula by radiopaque studies of the gastrointestinal tract, the genitourinary tract, and the fistula tract itself. The patient must remain on an absolutely nothing by mouth (NPO) diet, and nasogastric suction should be instituted in high gastrointestinal tract fistula patients. The use of intravenous cimetidine can also be helpful in reducing fistula output. IVH should be continued for approximately 4 weeks, and if there is no evidence of spontaneous fistula closure, surgical intervention should be considered. If these priorities are followed conscientiously, morbidity and mortality from this devastating problem can be greatly decreased.

SHORT BOWEL SYNDROME

The short bowel syndrome is a clinical problem usually resulting from greater than a 50% resection of the small bowel because of vascular occlusion of the superior or inferior mesenteric arteries or veins, inflammatory bowel disease, multiple gastrointestinal tract fistulas, radiation enteritis, trauma, or malignancy. The complications of this syndrome include significant malabsorption and diarrhea, hypergastrinemia, and severe malnutrition. There are several determining factors that will affect the patient's ultimate nutritional status: (1) the patient's state of nutrition prior to development of the intestinal catastrophe; (2) the underlying disease process; (3) the length, specific segment, and histologic status of the remaining small intestine; and (4) the function of the ileocecal valve. It has been observed that remaining ileum adapts to the functions of the jejunum much better than the jejunum adapts to ileal functions, but the loss of small bowel length is even more critical in pediatric patients, since a resection of 30 cm is associated with an extremely high mortality.

The nutritional and metabolic management of these patients is often complicated and involves a combination of specially tailored oral and intravenous feedings that must be continued for 2 years or longer. During the first month after the short bowel syndrome has developed, it is particularly important to correct fluid and electrolyte abnormalities and to control infection. At this time, nutritional support is primarily by means of IVH, but a low-fat, lactose-free oral diet may be started when the patient is able to tolerate nutrition by mouth. An elemental diet can also be used, although severe diarrhea and taste intolerance may develop. Drugs such as probanthine, Lomotil, codeine, deodorized tincture of opium, and Imodium are necessary to slow intestinal transit; cimetidine must also be given to decrease hyperacidity secondary to hypergastrinemia. Oral food stimulates the release of intestinal chyme and gastrointestinal hormones, which have been implicated in stimulating intestinal cell division and growth. It is important, therefore, to add oral food, even in small amounts, as soon as it is tolerated. In a series of 30 patients with the short bowel syndrome, a combination of IVH and oral nutrition was used during the first 3 months of treatment after which IVH was discontinued in 90% of the patients because they were able to maintain their nutritional status with oral nutrition. However, the patients were extremely susceptible to viral gastroenteritis, and weight loss would occur rapidly, producing malnutrition and cachexia if the patient was not monitored carefully. In this situation, the reinstitution of IVH was usually necessary for 4 weeks until oral nutrition could be restarted without significant diarrhea.

Occasionally some patients will require long-term IVH therapy at home, and this technique and its results have recently been described.[21] The technique is safe and is associated with few complications, it can be life-saving and can allow the patient to return to work and to function normally in society.

PANCREATITIS

In the past, the standard treatment for acute pancreatitis included intravenous fluids, antibiotics, nasogastric suction, and occasionally parasympatholytic drugs. However, total bowel rest and IVH have been shown to minimize pancreatic exocrine function and to induce atrophy of the pancreatic acinar cells.[51] Dudrick and co-workers reported a patient with a pancreatic fistula who had auto-digestion of her anterior abdominal wall when oral feedings were used; but when IVH and total bowel rest were begun, fistula drainage decreased, the skin and wound healed, and the pancreatic fistula spontaneously closed.[23] Subsequent reports have confirmed the efficacy of total bowel rest and IVH in the treatment of pancreatic fistulas.[3,44] A recent study reported a decrease in the overall mortality of patients with acute pancreatitis from 22% to 14% when nutritional repletion with intravenous hyperalimentation was used.[28] Similarly, Goodgame and co-workers retrospectively reviewed their experience with IVH in acute pancreatitis and reported a mortality rate of 22% and noted a decrease in the incidence of such complications as acute respiratory failure and acute renal failure.[34] The averge duration of IVH therapy in these patients was 28 days, although no difference in mortality was observed in patients whose disease was treated for fewer than or more than 30 days. The authors have similarly demonstrated that IVH and total bowel rest in patients with acute pancreatitis will correct or prevent malnutrition coincident or secondary to diminished nutrient intake during treatment for this disease, but the incidence of hemorrhagic pancreatitis is not significantly reduced. The occurrence of hyperglycemia and hypoglycemia is increased during the acute phases of this disease, but these problems can be managed adequately with appropriate adjustments of insulin infusion. Although the elemental diet has been used in patients with acute pancreatitis, it does not rest the pancreas because the volume of pancreatic juice and enzyme concentrations is increased.[11,61] Therefore, it is recommended that total bowel rest and IVH be used in the treatment of acute pancreatitis and pancreatic fistulas in order to minimize metabolic and nutritional complications.

ACUTE RENAL FAILURE

Because of the significant hemodynamic changes that occur in critically ill patients and the increasing use of nephrotoxic drugs, particularly antibiotics, the incidence of acute renal failure has been increasing on surgical services. The overall morbidity and mortality from this complication alone ranges from 30% to 60%, and if a concomitant infection is present, the mortality increases to 90%. Often, malnutrition accompanies acute renal failure and leads to decreased immunocompetence and increased susceptibility to infection. A special oral diet (Giordano–Giovannetti diet) has been formulated to supply primarily the essential amino acids and to limit the total protein intake to 20 g/day to 40 g/day. Since both essential nitrogen and nonessential nitrogen are necessary for body protein synthesis, the exogenous administration of essential amino acids combined with nonessential urea nitrogen could theoretically support tissue synthesis in the presence of appropriate enzymatic activity. In clinical practice, such oral diets are not very effective in promoting positive nitrogen balance and tissue repair, especially in critically ill patients who require very large amounts of nitrogen for tissue synthesis and who often have anorexia, nausea, and vomiting. In order to circumvent this problem, a special intravenous amino acid solution was formulated that is comprised of only the eight essential amino acids. This solution, when combined with concentrated dextrose, has been demonstrated to promote positive nitrogen balance, weight gain, and normal wound healing. In this renal failure formula, 1000 ml of solution provides about 1500 to 2500 dextrose calories and 1 g to 1.5 g essential nitrogen, and is usually infused over 24 hours. Additional nitrogen is added as tolerated if the patient's BUN level does not increase with the initial infusion. Serum phosphate, sulfate, potassium, and BUN concentrations have decreased on this regimen, and the frequency of hemodialysis or peritoneal dialysis is also often decreased.

Able and co-workers reported a decrease in the morbidity and mortality of patients receiving hypertonic dextrose and amino acids compared with patients receiving hypertonic dextrose alone.[1] Recently, a modified renal-failure formula containing essential and nonessential amino acids has been found to be equally effective in some patients, and this formula is listed in Table 36-5. The BUN level may stabilize or even increase with the modified

TABLE 36-5
Intravenous Hyperalimentation Formulas

Normal Formula	Renal Failure Formula	Modified Renal Failure Formula
500 ml 50% dextrose	750 ml–1000 ml 50%–70% dextrose	500 ml–700 ml 50%–70% dextrose
500 ml 8% amino acids (essential and nonessential amino acids)	100 ml–200 ml 5% essential amino acid mixture	250 ml 8% amino acids (essential and nonessential amino acids)
6.4 g nitrogen	1 g–1.5 g essential nitrogen	3.2 g nitrogen
Electrolytes Vitamins	Electrolytes Vitamins	Electrolytes Vitamins

diet and, therefore, the frequency of hemodialysis is not decreased with this regimen.

HEPATIC FAILURE

Malnutrition is a common problem in patients with acute or chronic liver failure. The indiscriminate administration of oral or intravenous amino acids can cause further liver decompensation and encephalopathy, especially if the protein intake exceeds 40 g/day. Although standard oral diets aggravate hepatic encephalopathy, there are several special oral diets that have been formulated to provide an amino acid pattern that promotes tissue synthesis and decreases encephalopathy in some patients. Fischer and co-workers have developed a formula for patients with liver failure that provides higher than usual concentrations of branched-chain amino acids (leucine, isoleucine, valine) and lower than usual concentrations of aromatic amino acids (tyrosine, phenylalamine, methionine).[29] Generally, patients with cirrhosis have high levels of aromatic and low levels of branched-chain amino acids because of increased gluconeogenesis from branched-chain amino acids and decreased peripheral utilization of the aromatic amino acids. With this still experimental parenteral formula, the gastrointestinal tract can be totally bypassed and 50 g to 75 g protein and 2000 to 3000 dextrose calories can be infused every 24 hours. In some clinical studies, a decrease in hepatic encephalopathy and normalization of the serum amino acid pattern has occurred, thus allowing infusion of protein into patients with liver failure in sufficient quantity to produce positive nitrogen balance and tissue synthesis without inducing further liver decompensation.[30]

CANCER

TUMOR GROWTH DYNAMICS

Patients with malignant diseases, particularly tumors of the gastrointestinal tract, will often develop significant weight loss and malnutrition prior to oncologic therapy. Aggressive cancer treatment often increases the degree of malnutrition, and the combination of the effects of aggressive therapy and progressive malnutrition may be a frequent cause of death. The use of intensive nutritional support in such patients will allow weight gain, positive nitrogen balance, and better tolerance of antineoplastic therapy.[17] While studying experimental animals, some investigators have found that protein–calorie malnutrition inhibits or retards the growth of tumors, while Steiger and colleagues and Cameron and co-workers have suggested that intensive nutritional therapy might stimulate tumor growth and DNA synthesis.[10,37,59]

Ota and colleagues addressed this problem by studying the Morris hepatoma implanted into three groups of protein-depleted rats.[50] Group I continued feeding with the protein-free diet; group II was nutritionally restored by a normal protein diet; and group III was given IVH. In the protein-depleted animals, liver protein content was decreased and was repleted to normal by either IVH or a normal oral diet, but the protein content in the tumor remained stable despite variations in protein intake. These investigators concluded that protein–calorie repletion of the malnourished host preferentially benefited the host rather than stimulating tumor growth. Reynolds and co-workers investigated cell replication rates in protein-depleted and nutritionally repleted rats treated with methotrexate, an inhibitor of DNA synthesis.[52] Inhibition of tumor growth was significantly greater in the replenished animals, indicating that DNA replication was greater in these animmals than in those maintained on a protein-free diet.

Stimulation of tumor growth in humans has not been observed clinically in a large series of malnourished cancer patients during periods of nutritional repletion, while intensive nutritional support has been noted to be advantageous to these patients by decreasing morbidity and mortality from intensive cancer therapy. In another study, 20 pediatric patients with metastatic malignancies received chemotherapy and IVH.[60] Thirteen patients responded to chemotherapy, and sepsis occurred in only three patients. The authors drew the following conclusions: (1) IVH did not counteract the effectiveness of chemotherapy in the pediatric patient; (2) IVH did not accelerate tumor growth; and (3) IVH did result in nutritional repletion. Therefore, it appears that intensive nutritional support, either orally or intravenously, is advantageous to the malnourished host during periods of antineoplastic therapy.

CLINICAL APPLICATION OF IVH IN CANCER PATIENTS

The use of IVH as treatment for patients with a wide variety of malignant diseases has been reviewed recently; 406 consecutive patients were evaluated, most of whom received either chemotherapy, radiation therapy, or surgery.[14] Patients were considered malnourished who had lost 10% of their ideal body weight, had a serum albumin level less than 3.4 g %, or had a negative reaction to a battery of recall skin test antigens. Patients who met any two of these three criteria usually were malnourished. Immunodepression associated with oncologic therapy is often secondary to malnutrition and is not necessarily related to a direct suppressor effect on the immune system by a substance released by the cancer cells. The indications for IVH in these patients included chemotherapy (43%), general surgery (24%), head and neck surgery (10%), radiation therapy (10%), fistulas (6%), and supportive care (7%). IVH was infused for an average period of 23.9 days through a total of 428 subclavian vein catheters with an overall catheter-related infection rate of only 2.2%.

IVH was given to 175 patients who received 260 courses of chemotherapy. The average patient gained 5.6 lb and had an evaluable tumor response rate of 27.8%. Those patients who responded to chemotherapy and IVH lived an average time of 8.2 months compared with the nonresponders, who lived an average time of only 1.9 months. Susceptibility to infection should have been increased in 51.5% of the patients who had a leukocyte count less than 2500 cells/mm³ for an average period of 7.7 days; however, the overall catheter-related infection rate was only 1.7%. In addition, chemotherapy complications, such as gastrointestinal irritation, bloody diarrhea, mucositis, and malaise were better tolerated in patients receiving IVH.

The correlation between nutritional status and response to chemotherapy was evaluated in patients with non-oat-cell carcinoma of the lung who were treated with a standard chemotherapeutic protocol.[39] Patients who lost greater than 6% of their ideal body weight prior to treatment and who did not receive IVH had no response to chemotherapy, whereas patients with greater than 6% weight loss who were treated with intensive IVH therapy had a 50% tumor response rate. Patients who lost less than 6% of their body weight prior to chemotherapy and were not, therefore, candidates for IVH had a 75% response to the chemotherapeutic regimen. Issell and co-workers reported a preliminary study in 26 patients with metastatic squamous cell carcinoma of the lung who were treated with *Corynebacterium parvum*, Ifosfamide, and Adriamysin.[36] Thirteen patients received IVH before chemotherapy and were continued on IVH for 31 days during the first course of treatment, whereas the other patients were allowed only oral nutrition. Those patients receiving IVH experienced less nausea and vomiting and had greater improvement in anthropometric measurements than did the non-IVH patients. Four patients in the IVH group and one patient in the non-IVH group responded to chemotherapy. These data support retrospective studies indicating that malnourished patients who are nutritionally replenished prior to or during therapy potentially have a better opportunity for response to chemotherapy than do their malnourished counterparts.[16,39] Therefore, patients who are clinically healthy will respond better to chemotherapy not because of tumor growth stimulation by nutritional repletion but

rather because of a greater ability to tolerate large and prolonged infusions of chemotherapy. If a cancer patient is not malnourished, IVH would not be expected to have any measurable effect on results of antineoplastic therapy.[13]

In a group of 100 general and thoracic surgical patients treated with IVH, 52% underwent major curative resection, whereas 48% had surgical procedures for palliation.[14] IVH was used for average periods of 12.3% days preoperatively and 13.9 days postoperatively, and the operative mortality was only 4%. Increases in serum albumin occurred preoperatively, and the average weight gain was 4.2 lb in contrast to uniform weight loss in all such patients treated without IVH support.

In another group of 39 cancer patients, IVH was given during surgical, radiation, or chemotherapy treatment of their head and neck malignancies. Previous attempts at nutritional correction by means of nasogastric tube feedings had been unsuccessful, and IVH was used to promote nutritional repletion. In this group, the average patient received greater than 2700 Cal/day and 100 g/day of amino acids and gained more than 10 lb. Muscle mass, strength, and tone were restored as well.

Patients receiving radiation therapy were found to respond to intensive nutritional therapy also.[18] In a series of 39 malnourished patients who received IVH as nutritional support during radiation therapy, 95% completed their planned courses of treatment and gained an average of 7.8 lb. Anorexia, nausea, and vomiting disappeared during IVH, and 54% of the patients had greater than 50% reduction in tumor size. Responding patients gained significantly more weight and had greater increases in serum albumin concentrations than did patients whose tumors did not respond to radiation therapy. Prior to the introduction of IVH, these patients would have had their radiation treatment discontinued because of dehydration and malnutrition.

Experience has also been gained in cancer patients with enteric fistulas.[14] These patients were often cachectic at the onset of treatment, but with IVH and total bowel rest, malnutrition was corrected, 44% of the fistulas closed spontaneously, and 28% of the fistulas were successfully closed surgically. However, fistulas arising in areas of radiated bowel did not close spontaneously, and surgical bypass was necessary after 14 days to 21 days of IVH therapy to correct malnutrition. These data emphasize the need for intensive nutritional therapy to decrease the morbidity and mortality from gastrointestinal fistulas that develop in cancer patients.

Immunosuppression during oncologic therapy has been well documented. Jubert and co-workers observed suppression of *in vitro* lymphocyte transformation to mitogens and antigens after major abdominal and thoracic operative procedures.[38] The effect of chemotherapy on the immune response is both dose related and time related, whereas radiation therapy has both an initial and a long-term effect, with persistent lymphopenia having been observed for as long as 10 years following treatment.[19,35] The effect of malnutrition on cell-mediated immunity was evaluated by recall skin test antigens in 65 patients before and during nutritional repletion with IVH.[13] Initially, 46 patients had negative reactions to skin test antigens, but 63% of this group converted skin tests to positive after an average time of 13.6 days of IVH. Tumor response to chemotherapy was greater in those patients whose skin test reactivity was positive. In the radiation therapy group, particularly in those patients with radiation to the mediastinum and pelvis, skin tests often remained negative despite IVH therapy, probably because T-cell-bearing areas, such as the thymus and bone marrow, were within the irradiated field. The immune mechanism is an important host defense against cancer cells, and its optimal function should be maintained. Therefore, intensive nutritional therapy along with chemotherapy, radiation, or surgery should be considered as part of the optimal treatment for the malnourished cancer patient.

Conclusion

It is apparent that patients who have major operations, postoperative complications, and other catabolic conditions require large amounts of high-quality nutrients in order to maintain and to replete body stores. Stress factors must also be minimized or eliminated if the patient is to receive maximal benefit from the nutritional therapy. Preferably, adequate nutrition should be provided orally or through a gastrostomy or nasogastric feeding tube, but if adequate amounts of nutrients are not able to be supplied or absorbed by these methods, patients should receive intensive intravenous nutritional support. The ravages of malnutrition are significant and can lead to increased morbidity and mortality in all patients. Therefore, it is important for all physicians to recognize major nutritional deficits and to correct them aggressively in order to maximize the results of primary treatment and to decrease morbidity and mortality to the lowest possible levels in high-risk patients.

Bibliography

1. Able RM, Shih VE, Abbott W et al: Amino acid metabolism acute renal failure: Influence of intravenous essential L-amino acid hyperalimentation therapy. Ann Surg 180:350, 1974

2. Adams PR, Copeland EM, Dudrick SJ et al: Maintenance of gut mass in bypassed bowel of orally vs. parenterally nourished rats. J Surg Res 24:421, 1978

3. Aguirre A, Fischer JE, Welch CE: The role of surgery and hyperalimentation in therapy of gastrointestinal–cutaneous fistulae. Ann Surg 180:393, 1974

4. Allen JG, Stemmer EA, Head LR: Similar growth rates of littermate puppies maintained on oral protein with those on the same quantity of protein as daily intravenous plasma for 99 days as only protein source. Ann Surg 144:349, 1956

5. Andrassy RJ, Page CP, Feldtman RW: Continual catheter administration of an elemental diet in infants and children. Surgery 82, No. 2:205, 1977

6. Bistrian BR, Blackburn GL, Sherman M et al: Therapeutic index of nutritional depletion in hospitalized patients. Surg Gynecol Obstet 141:512, 1975

7. Blackburn GL, Bistrian BR, Flatt JP et al: Restoration of the visceral component of protein malnutrition during hypocaloric feeding. Clinical Research 23:315A, 1975

8. Butterworth CE, Blackburn GL: Hospital malnutrition. Nutrition Today 10, No. 2:8, 1975

9. Cahill GF Jr: Starvation in man. N Engl J Med 282:668, 1970

10. Cameron IL, Pavlat WA: Stimulation of growth of a transplantable hepatoma in rats by parenteral nutrition. Journal of The National Cancer Institute 56:597, 1976

11. Cassim MM, Allardyce BV: Pancreatic secretion in response to jejunal feeding of an elemental diet. Ann Surg 180:228, 1974

12. Castro GA, Copeland EM, Dudrick SJ et al: Intestinal disaccharidase and peroxidase activities in parenterally nourished rats. J Nutr 105:776, 1975

13. Copeland EM, Daly JM, Ota DM et al: Nutrition, cancer and intravenous hyperalimentation. Cancer 43:2108, 1979

14. Copeland E, Dudrick SJ: Nutritional aspects of cancer. In Hickey RC (ed): Current Problems in Cancer. Chicago, Year Book Medical Publishers, 1976

15. Copeland EM, MacFadyen BV Jr, Dudrick SJ: The use of hyperalimentation in patients with potential sepsis. Surg Gynecol Obstet 138:377, 1974

16. Copeland EM, MacFadyen BV Jr, Lanzotti V et al: Intravenous hyperalimentation as an adjunct to cancer chemotherapy. Am J Surg 129:167, 1975

17. Copeland EM, MacFadyen BV Jr, Lanzotti V et al: The nutritional care of the cancer patient. In Howe CD, Clark RL (ed): Cancer Patient Care at MD Anderson Hospital and Tumor Institute. Chicago, Year Book Medical Publishers, 1976

18. Copeland EM, Souchon EA, MacFadyen BV Jr et al: Intravenous hyperalimentation as an adjunct to radiation therapy. Cancer 39:609, 1977

19. Cosimi AB, Brunstetter FH, Kemmerer WT et al: Cellular immune competence of breast cancer patients receiving radiotherapy. Arch Surg 107:531, 1973

20. Deitel M: Nutritional management of external gastrointestinal fistulas. Can J Surg 19:505, 1976

21. Dudrick SJ, Englert DM, Van Buren CT et al: New concepts of ambulatory home hyperalimentation. JPEN 3, No. 2:72, Mar–Apr 1979

22. Dudrick SJ, MacFadyen BV Jr, Daly JM: Management of inflammatory bowel disease with parenteral hyperalimentation. In Clearfield HR, Denoso VP Jr (eds): Gastrointestinal Emergencies. New York, Grune & Stratton, 1976

23. Dudrick SJ, Wilmore DW, Steiger E et al: Spontaneous closure of traumatic pancreaticoduodenal fistulas with total intravenous nutrition. J Trauma 10:542, 1970
24. Dudrick SJ, Wilmore DW, Vars HM et al: Long-term total parenteral nutrition with growth, development and positive nitrogen balance. Surgery 64:134, 1968
25. Duke JH Jr, Jorgensen SB, Broell JR et al: Contribution of protein to caloric expenditure following injury. Surgery 68:168, 1970
26. Edmunds H Jr, Williams GM, Welsh CE: External fistulas arising in the gastrointestinal tract. Ann Surg 152:445, 1960
27. Felig P, Marliss E, Owen OE et al: Role of substrate in the regulation of hepatic gluconeogenesis in fasting man. Adv Enzyme Regul 7:41, 1969
28. Feller JH, Brown RA, Toussant GPM et al: Changing methods in the treatment of severe pancreatitis. Am J Surg 127:196, 1974
29. Fischer JE, Funovics JM, Aguirre A et al: The role of plasma amino acids in hepatic encephalopathy. Surgery 78:276, 1975
30. Fischer JE, Rosen HM, Ebeid AM et al: The effect of normalization of plasma amino acids on hepatic encephalopathy in man. Surgery 80:77, 1976
31. Gamble JL: Physiological information gained from studies on the life-raft ration. Harvey Lect 42:247, 1947
32. Gibbon JH Jr, Nealon TF, Greco VF: A modification of Glassman's gastrostomy with results in 18 patients. Ann Surg 143:838, 1956
33. Glotzer DJ, Boyle PL, Silen W: Preoperative preparation of the colon with an elemental diet. Surgery 74:703, 1973
34. Goodgame JT, Fischer JF: Parenteral nutrition in the treatment of acute pancreatitis: Effect on complications and mortality. Ann Surg 186:651, 1977
35. Hersh EM, Gutterman JU, Mavligit G et al: Host defence, chemical immunosuppression and the transplant recipient. Relative effects of intermittent vs. continuous immunosuppressive therapy with reference to the objectives of treatment. Transplant Proc 5:1191, 1973
36. Issell BF, Valdivieso M, Zaren HA et al: Protection of chemotherapy toxicities by intravenous hyperalimentation. Cancer Treat Rep 62:1139, 1978
37. Jose DE, Good RA: Quantitative effects of nutritional essential amino acid deficiency upon immune response to tumors in mice. J Exp Med 137:1, 1973
38. Jubert AV, Lee ET, Hersh EM et al: Effects of surgery, anesthesia and intraoperative blood loss on immunocompetence. J Surg Res 15:399, 1973
39. Lanzotti V, Copeland EM, George SL et al: Cancer chemotherapeutic response and intravenous hyperalimentation. Cancer Chemother Reports 59:437, 1975
40. Levenson SM, Howard JM, Rosen IT: Studies of the plasma amino acids and amino conjugates in patients with severe battle wounds. Surg Gynecol Obstet 101:35, 1955
41. Long JM, Steiger E, Dudrick SJ et al: Total parenteral nutrition in the management of esophagocutaneous fistulas. Fed Proc 30:300, 1971
42. MacFadyen BV Jr: Intravenous hyperalimentation in gastrointestinal diseases, In Dudrick SJ (ed): Team Approach to Nutritional Support. East Norwalk, CT, Appleton–Century–Crofts, 1983
43. MacFadyen BV Jr, Dudrick SJ: The management of fistulas in inflammatory bowel disease with parenteral hyperalimentation. In Romieu C, Solassol C, Joyeux H (eds): Proceedings of the International Society of Parenteral Nutrition, p 559. Montpellier, France, 1976
44. MacFadyen BV Jr, Dudrick SJ, Ruberg RL: Management of gastrointestinal fistulas with parenteral hyperalimentation. Surgery 74:100, 1973
45. Moore EP, Copeland EM, Dudrick SJ et al: Effect of an elemental diet on the electrical activity of the small intestine in dogs. J Surg Res 33:205, 1976
46. Moore FD: Metabolic Care of the Surgical patient, p 409. Philadelphia, WB Saunders, 1959
47. Mullen JL, Buzby GP, Waldman MT et al: Prediction of operative morbidity and mortality by preoperative nutritional assessment. Surgical Forum 30:80, 1979
48. Mullen JL, Hargrove WC, Dudrick SJ et al: Ten years experience with intravenous hyperalimentation and inflammatory bowel disease. Ann Surg 187:523, 1978
49. Munro HN, Allison JB (eds): Mammalian Protein Metabolism. New York, Academic Press, 1964
50. Ota DM, Copeland EM, Strobel HW et al: The effect of protein nutrition on host and tumor metabolism. J Surg Res 22:181, 1977
51. Pavlat WA, Rogers W, Cameron IL: Morphometric analysis of pancreatic cancer cells from orally fed and intravenously fed rats. J Surg Res 19:267, 1975
52. Reynolds HM, Daly JM, Rowlands BJ et al: Effects of nutritional repletion on host and tumor response to chemotherapy. Cancer 45:12, 1980
53. Rocchio MA, Cha CJ, Haas KF et al: Use of chemically defined diets in the management of patients with acute inflammatory bowel disease. Am J Surg 127:469, 1974
54. Rocchio MA, Cha CM, Haas KR et al: The use of chemically defined diets in the management of patients with high output gastrointestinal cutaneous fistulas. Am J Surg 127:148, 1974
55. Scofield PF: The natural history and treatment of Crohn's disease. Ann R Coll Surg Engl 36:3, 1965
56. Shires GT, Canizaro PC: Fluid, electrolyte and nutritional management of the surgical patient. In Schwartz SI, Lillehei RC, Shires GT et al (eds): Principles of Surgery, p 65. New York, McGraw–Hill, 1974
57. Shizgal HM: Symposium on nutritional requirements of the surgical patient. 1. Nutrition and body composition. Can J Surg 21:483, 1978
58. Speir AM, Englert D, Dudrick SJ: Thirty man years' experience with ambulatory home hyperalimentation. JPEN 3, No. 6:510, 1979
59. Steiger E, Oram–Smith J, Miller E et al: Effects of nutrition on tumor growth and tolerance to chemotherapy. J Surg Res 18:455, 1975
60. Van Eys J: Nutrition and cancer in children. Cancer 29:40, 1979
61. Voitk A, Brown RA, Echave V et al: Use of an elemental diet in the treatment of complicated pancreatitis. Am J Surg 125:223, 1973
62. Wilmore DW, Long JM, Mason AD et al: Stress in surgical patients as an neurophysiologic reflex response. Surg Gynecol Obstet 132:673, 1976
63. Wilmore DW, Long JM, Mason AD et al: Catecholamines: Mediator of the hypermetabolic response to thermal injury. Ann Surg 180:653, 1974
64. Wolfe BM, Keltner RM, William VL: Intestinal output in regular elemental and intravenous alimentation. Am J Surg 124:803, 1972

Appendix

Contents

627

Recommended Dietary Allowances—Definition and Applications

Recommended Dietary Allowances (RDA) are the levels of intake of essential nutrients considered, in the judgment of the Committee on Dietary Allowances of the Food and Nutrition Board on the basis of available scientific knowledge, to be adequate to meet the known nutritional needs of practically all healthy persons.

RDA are recommendations for the average daily amounts of nutrients that *population groups* should consume over a period of time. RDA should not be confused with requirements for a specific individual. Differences in the nutrient requirements of individuals are ordinarily unknown. Therefore, RDA (except for energy) are estimated to exceed the requirements of most individuals and thereby to ensure that the needs of nearly all in the population are met. Intakes below the recommended allowance for a nutrient are not necessarily inadequate, but the risk of having an inadequate intake increases to the extent that intake is less than the level recommended as safe.

RDA are recommendations established for *healthy* populations. Special needs for nutrients arising from such problems as premature birth, inherited metabolic disorders, infections, chronic diseases, and the use of medications require special dietary and therapeutic measures. These conditions are not covered by the RDA.

RDA are intended to be met by a diet of a wide variety of foods rather than by supplementation or by extensive fortification of single foods. RDA have not been set for all recognized nutrients. (Estimated safe and adequate intakes have been set for some nutrients in this edition.) Therefore, diets should be composed of a *variety* of foods that are acceptable, palatable, and economically attainable by the consumer using the RDA as a guide to assessment of their nutritional adequacy.

ESTIMATION OF RECOMMENDED DIETARY ALLOWANCES

The *ideal* method in developing an allowance would be to determine the average requirement of a healthy and representative segment of each age group for the nutrient under consideration, then to assess statistically the variability among the individuals within the group, and finally to calculate the amount by which the average requirement must be increased to meet the needs of nearly all healthy individuals. Unfortunately, experiments on man are costly, they must often be of long duration, certain types of experiments are not possible for ethical reasons, and, even under the best conditions, only a small number of subjects can be studied in a single experiment. Thus requirement estimates often must be derived from limited information.

In practice, estimates of nutrient requirements are determined by a number of techniques: (1) collection of data on nutrient intake from the food supply of apparently normal, healthy people; (2) review of epidemiological observations when clinical consequences of nutrient deficiencies are found to be correctable by dietary improvement; (3) biochemical measurements that assess degree of tissue saturation or adequacy of molecular function in relation to nutrient intake; (4) nutrient balance studies that measure nutritional status in relation to intake; (5) studies of subjects maintained on diets containing marginally low or deficient levels of a nutrient, followed by correction of the deficit with measured amounts of that nutrient (such studies are undertaken in humans only when the risk is minimal); and (6) in some few instances, extrapolation from animal experiments in which deficiencies have been produced by the exclusion of a single nutrient from the diet. The estimation of precise nutrient requirement by some of these techniques individually may be equivocal. However, with the corroborative evidence arising from application of several reinforcing procedures, the requirements, and hence the allowances, may be stated with greater confidence.

Estimation of the recommended allowances follows essentially four steps:

1. Estimating the average requirement of a population for a given nutrient and the variability of requirement within that population
2. Increasing the average requirement by an amount sufficient to meet the needs of nearly all members of the population
3. Increasing the allowance to account for inefficient utilization by the body of the nutrients as consumed (poor absorption, poor conversion of precursor to active forms, etc.)
4. Using judgment in interpreting and extrapolating allowances when information on requirements is limited

TABLE A-1
Food and Nutrition Board, National Academy of Sciences—National Research Council Recommended Daily Dietary Allowances, Revised 1980

(Designed for the maintenance of good nutrition of practically all healthy people in the USA)

| | Age | Weight | | Height | | Protein | Fat-Soluble Vitamins | | | |
| | | | | | | | Vitamin A | Vitamin D | Vitamin E | Vitamin C |
	yr	kg	lb	cm	in	g	µg RE*	µg†	mg α-TE‡	mg
Infants	0.0–0.5	6	13	60	24	kg × 2.2	420	10	3	35
	0.5–1.0	9	20	71	28	kg × 2.0	400	10	4	35
Children	1–3	13	29	90	35	23	400	10	5	45
	4–6	20	44	112	44	30	500	10	6	45
	7–10	28	62	132	52	34	700	10	7	45
Males	11–14	45	99	157	62	45	1,000	10	8	50
	15–18	66	145	176	69	56	1,000	10	10	60
	19–22	70	154	177	70	56	1,000	7.5	10	60
	23–50	70	154	178	70	56	1,000	5	10	60
	51+	70	154	178	70	56	1,000	5	10	60
Females	11–14	46	101	157	62	46	800	10	8	50
	15–18	55	120	163	64	46	800	10	8	60
	19–22	55	120	163	64	44	800	7.5	8	60
	23–50	55	120	163	64	44	800	5	8	60
	51+	55	120	163	64	44	800	5	8	60
Pregnant						+30	+200	+5	+2	+20
Lactating						+20	+400	+5	+3	+40

From the Committee on Dietetics of the Mayo Clinic: Mayo Clinic Diet Manual, pp 268–269. Philadelphia, WB Saunders, 1981; modified from National Research Council: Recommended Dietary Allowances, 9th ed. Washington, DC, National Academy of Sciences, 1980.

The allowances are intended to provide for individual variations among most normal persons as they live in the United States under usual environmental stresses. Diets should be based on a variety of common foods in order to provide other nutrients for which human requirements have been less well defined.

*Retinol equivalents: 1 retinol equivalent = 1 µg retinol or 6 µg β-carotene.

†As cholecalciferol: 10 µg of cholecalciferol = 400 IU of vitamin D.

‡α-Tocopherol equivalents: 1 mg of d-α-tocopherol = 1 α-TE.

TABLE A-1 (*Continued*)

| | Water-Soluble Vitamins | | | | | | Minerals | | | | | |
Thia-min mg	Ribo-flavin mg	Niacin mg NE§	Vitamin B_6 mg	Fola-cin ¶ μg	Vitamin B_{12} μg	Cal-cium mg	Phos-phorus mg	Mag-nesium mg	Iron mg	Zinc mg	Iodine μg
0.3	0.4	6	0.3	30	0.5#	360	240	50	10	3	40
0.5	0.6	8	0.6	45	1.5	540	360	70	15	5	50
0.7	0.8	9	0.9	100	2.0	800	800	150	15	10	70
0.9	1.0	11	1.3	200	2.5	800	800	200	10	10	90
1.2	1.4	16	1.6	300	3.0	800	800	250	10	10	120
1.4	1.6	18	1.8	400	3.0	1,200	1,200	350	18	15	150
1.4	1.7	18	2.0	400	3.0	1,200	1,200	400	18	15	150
1.5	1.7	19	2.2	400	3.0	800	800	350	10	15	150
1.4	1.6	18	2.2	400	3.0	800	800	350	10	15	150
1.2	1.4	16	2.2	400	3.0	800	800	350	10	15	150
1.1	1.3	15	1.8	400	3.0	1,200	1,200	300	18	15	150
1.1	1.3	14	2.0	400	3.0	1,200	1,200	300	18	15	150
1.1	1.3	14	2.0	400	3.0	800	800	300	18	15	150
1.0	1.2	13	2.0	400	3.0	800	800	300	18	15	150
1.0	1.2	13	2.0	400	3.0	800	800	300	10	15	150
+0.4	+0.3	+2	+0.6	+400	+1.0	+400	+400	+150	**	+5	+25
+0.5	+0.5	+5	+0.5	+100	+1.0	+400	+400	+150	**	+10	+50

§1 NE (niacin equivalent) is equal to 1 mg of niacin or 60 mg of dietary tryptophan.

¶The folacin allowances refer to dietary sources as determined by *Lactobacillus casei* assay after treatment with enzymes (conjugases) to make polyglutamyl forms of the vitamin available to the test organism.

#The Recommended Dietary Allowance for vitamin B_{12} in infants is based on average concentration of the vitamin in human milk. The allowances after weaning are based on energy intake (as recommended by the American Academy of Pediatrics) and consideration of other factors, such as intestinal absorption.

**The increased requirement during pregnancy cannot be met by the iron content of habitual American diets nor by the existing iron stores of many women; therefore the use of 30 to 60-mg of supplemental iron is recommended. Iron needs during lactation are not substantially different from those of nonpregnant women, but continued supplementation of the mother for 2 to 3 months after parturition is advisable to replenish stores depleted by pregnancy.

TABLE A-2
Mean Heights and Weights and Recommended Energy Intake

Category	Age yr	Weight kg	Weight lb	Height cm	Height in	Energy Needs (with range) Cal	Energy Needs (with range) MJ*
Infants	0.0–0.5	6	13	60	24	kg × 115 (95–145)	kg × 0.48
	0.5–1.0	9	20	71	28	kg × 105 (80–135)	kg × 0.44
Children	1–3	13	29	90	3	1300 (900–1800)	5.5
	4–6	20	44	112	44	1700 (1300–2300)	7.1
	7–10	28	62	132	52	2400 (1650–3300)	10.1
Males	11–14	45	99	157	62	2700 (2000–3700)	11.3
	15–18	66	145	176	69	2800 (2100–3900)	11.8
	19–22	70	154	177	70	2900 (2500–3300)	12.2
	23–50	70	154	178	70	2700 (2300–3100)	11.3
	51–75	70	154	178	70	2400 (2000–2800)	10.1
	76+	70	154	178	70	2050 (1650–2450)	8.6
Females	11–14	46	101	157	62	2200 (1500–3000)	9.2
	15–18	55	120	163	64	2100 (1200–3000)	8.8
	19–22	55	120	163	64	2100 (1700–2500)	8.8
	23–50	55	120	163	64	2000 (1600–2400)	8.4
	51–75	55	120	163	64	1800 (1400–2200)	7.6
	76+	55	120	163	64	1600 (1200–2000)	6.7
Pregnancy						+300	
Lactation						+500	

From the Committee on Dietetics of the Mayo Clinic: Mayo Clinic Diet Manual, p 270. Philadelphia, WB Saunders, 1981; modified from National Research Council: Recommended Dietary Allowances, 9th ed. Washington, DC, National Academy of Sciences, 1980.

The energy allowances for the young adults are for men and women doing light work. The allowances for the two older age groups represent mean energy needs over these age spans; they allow for a 2% decrease in basal (resting) metabolic rate per decade and a reduction in activity of 200 Cal/day for men and women between 51 and 75 years, 500 Cal for men over 75 years, and 400 Cal for women over 75 years. The customary range of daily energy output is shown in parentheses for adults and is based on a variation in energy needs of ±400 Cal at any one age; the values emphasize the wide range of energy intakes appropriate for any group of people.

Energy allowances for children through age 18 are based on median energy intakes of children of these ages who participated in longitudinal growth studies. The values in parentheses are 10th and 90th percentiles of energy intake; they indicate the range of energy consumption among children of these ages.
*Megajoule.

Vitamin Supplements*

Under what circumstances is vitamin supplementation appropriate? There is no simple answer, but a general guide is available in the form of the Recommended Dietary Allowances (RDA). However, the RDA are not intended to apply to conditions of stress and illness. The clinician and dietitian must be guided by textbooks and other such sources concerned with the condition at issue.

RECOMMENDED DIETARY ALLOWANCES

The Food and Nutrition Board of the National Academy of Sciences has prepared recommendations for the amounts of a number of vitamins and minerals that should provide for the needs of nearly all normal people living in the United States under usual environmental stresses. These allowances are designed to provide for possible variations in individual needs and in most instances are substantially greater than the minimum amounts needed to prevent symptoms of vitamin deficiency. Thus, a diet supplying less than some of the RDA should not necessarily be considered unsatisfactory or in need of vitamin supplementation.

The RDA should not be confused with the United States Recommended Daily Allowances (USRDA). The latter standards have been derived from the RDA by the Food and Drug Administration as standards for nutrition labeling.

For general vitamin supplementation, there is one generic formulation: Decavitamin USP. This formula consists of the following substances, but the quantity of each component is not specified; only the amount of each vitamin is required to appear on the label: vitamin A (retinol), thiamin (B_1), riboflavin (B_2), pyridoxine (B_6), cyanocobalamin (B_{12}), folic acid, niacin, pantothenate, ascorbic acid (vitamin C), vitamin D (calciferol), and vitamin E (tocopherol). The term *hexavitamin* has been applied to the preparations containing vitamin A, thiamin, riboflavin, niacin, ascorbic acid, and vitamin D.

The responsibility of the clinician is to choose the preparation that will provide the amounts and kinds of vitamins needed for a particular situation.

CLINICAL SETTINGS

For restricted calorie diets below 1,000 Cal to 1,200 Cal, a multivitamin preparation such as a decavitamin or hexavitamin formula with amounts of individual vitamins approximately equal to the

*From the Committee on Dietetics of the Mayo Clinic: Mayo Clinic Diet Manual, pp 272–274. Philadelphia, WB Saunders, 1981.

USRDA may be appropriate. Higher potency or "therapeutic" formulas are not necessary for this purpose.

Patients having malabsorption or maldigestion secondary to pancreatic or intestinal disease may benefit from the regular use of supplemental vitamins. Liquid vitamin preparations may be absorbed better than those in capsule form when rapid transit may interfere with dissolution of the capsule. Measurement of prothrombin activity guides the need for additional vitamin K and the response to this agent. Water-soluble forms of vitamin K, such as menadiol sodium diphosphate (available in 5-mg tablets) and vitamin K_5 (available in 4-mg capsules), used regularly may be effective in states characterized by steatorrhea. Measurements of folate and vitamin B_{12} serum levels may be useful in establishing whether and in what quantities these substances should be given. Folic acid (available in 1-mg tablets) may be given orally in doses of 1 mg to 5 mg daily in malabsorption and, if necessary, may be administered parenterally in doses of 1 mg daily. Vitamin B_{12} is best administered intramuscularly in a dose of 100 µg to 1,000 µg daily until clinical evidences of B_{12} deficiency are corrected; thereafter, 100 µg to 1,000 µg is given at intervals of 2 weeks to 4 weeks.

Emotional stress should not increase vitamin needs, but surgical or traumatic stress possibly increases rates of vitamin losses or degradation. Very little objective information exists on which to base recommendations for vitamin administration in stress, however. The previously well-nourished patient probably experiences no harm if supplementary vitamins are not administered in the first several days after injury or surgery. If regular meals containing the usual complement of vitamins cannot be consumed within a few days, it would be reasonable to provide a decavitamin formula with at least one USRDA, parenterally or orally as circumstances demand.

There does not appear to be any special need for vitamins in old age, but disease and social factors often limit the variety and quality of foods eaten by the elderly. Hence, vitamin supplementation may be needed for the older patient. A diet history may warn of possible vitamin deficiency.

Selected Bibliography

Hine, C Jr: Vitamins: Absorption and malabsorption. Arch Intern Med 138:619–621, 1978

Trace Minerals

The same considerations governing the use of vitamin supplements apply to trace minerals.

TABLE A-3
Estimated Safe and Adequate Daily Dietary Intakes of Additional Selected Vitamins and Minerals

		Vitamins			Trace Elements*						Electrolytes		
	Age yr	Vitamin K μg	Biotin μg	Pantothenic acid mg	Copper mg	Manganese mg	Fluoride mg	Chromium mg	Selenium mg	Molybdenum mg	Sodium mg	Potassium mg	Chloride mg
Infants	0–0.5	12	35	2	0.5–0.7	0.5–0.7	0.1–0.5	0.01–0.04	0.01–0.04	0.03–0.06	115–350	350–925	275–700
	0.5–1	10–20	50	3	0.7–1.0	0.7–1.0	0.2–1.0	0.02–0.06	0.02–0.06	0.04–0.08	250–750	425–1275	400–1200
Children	1–3	15–30	65	3	1.0–1.5	1.0–1.5	0.5–1.5	0.02–0.08	0.02–0.08	0.05–0.1	325–975	550–1650	500–1500
	4–6	20–40	85	3–4	1.5–2.0	1.5–2.0	1.0–2.5	0.03–0.12	0.03–0.12	0.06–0.15	450–1350	775–2325	700–2100
and													
Adolescents	7–10	30–60	120	4–5	2.0–2.5	2.0–3.0	1.5–2.5	0.05–0.2	0.05–0.2	0.10–0.3	600–1800	1000–3000	925–2775
	11+	50–100	100–200	4–7	2.0–3.0	2.5–5.0	1.5–2.5	0.05–0.2	0.05–0.2	0.15–0.5	900–2700	1525–4575	1400–4200
Adults		70–140	100–200	4–7	2.0–3.0	2.5–5.0	1.5–4.0	0.05–0.2	0.05–0.2	0.15–0.5	1100–3300	1875–5625	1700–5100

From the Committee on Dietetics of the Mayo Clinic: Mayo Clinic Diet Manual, p 271. Philadelphia, WB Saunders, 1981; modified from National Research Council: Recommended Dietary Allowances, 9th ed. Washington, DC, National Academy of Sciences, 1980.

Because there is less information on which to base allowances, these figures are not given in the main table of the Recommended Dietary Allowances and are provided here in the form of ranges of recommended intakes.

*Since the toxic levels for many trace elements may be only several times usual intakes, the upper levels for the trace elements given in this table should not be habitually exceeded.

Most of the essential trace minerals are available in adequate amounts in protein-containing foods. Persons who consume adequate amounts of protein are not likely to have trace mineral deficiencies.

Infants and children reared in fluoride-deficient areas and not consuming fluoridated water may require fluoride supplementation. Iodide deficiency is now rare because of the wide use of iodized salt, foods derived from different geographic areas, and some food additives containing iodides.

Iron may be needed for iron-deficient states, but these states are usually the result of blood loss rather than restricted dietary intake. Deficiencies of zinc, manganese, copper, and other trace elements may occur in patients receiving only parenterally administered nutrients. Plasma levels of these substances can be a guide to their administration, but because of the way the substances bind to plasma protein, interpretation of plasma levels in states characterized by protein deficiency is difficult.

TABLE A-4
Recommended Daily Allowances of Vitamins, United States (USRDA; FDA Standard)

	Infants and Children < 4 yr	*Children > 4 yr and Adults*
Vitamin A	2500 IU	5000 IU
Thiamin (B$_1$)	0.7 mg	1.5 mg
Riboflavin (B$_2$)	0.8 mg	1.7 mg
Vitamin B$_6$	0.7 mg	2 mg
Vitamin B$_{12}$	3 μg	6 μg
Folacin (B$_c$)	0.2 mg	0.4 mg
Biotin	0.15 mg	0.3 mg
Niacin	9 mg	20 mg
Pantothenic acid	5 mg	10 mg
Ascorbic acid (C)	40 mg	60 mg
Vitamin D	400 IU	400 IU
Vitamin E	10 IU	30 IU

From White PL: Vitamin preparations: Proper use in medical practice. Postgrad Med 60:204–209, 1976. By permission of McGraw-Hill, Inc.

TABLE A-5
Mayo Clinic Physiologic Values

	(Normal Ranges)

BLOOD OR SERUM VALUES

Ascorbic acid (vitamin C)	0.6–2 mg/dl
Bleeding time–Ivy	1–6 min
Calcium	8.9–10.1 mg/dl
Carotene	48–200 µg/dl
Chloride	100–108 mEq/liter
Copper	0.75–1.45 µg/ml
Erythrocyte count	M, 4.5–6.2 × 10⁶/µl
	F, 4.2–5.4 × 10⁶/µl
Ferritin	M, 20–300 ng/ml
	F, 20–120 ng/ml
Folate (serum)	2–20 ng/ml
Glucose, fasting	70–100 mg/dl
Hematocrit	M, 42%–54%
	F, 38%–46%
Hemoglobin	M, 14–17 g/dl
	F, 12–15 g/dl
Iron	M, 75–175 µg/dl
	F, 65–165 µg/dl
Iron-binding capacity, total	240–430 µg/dl
Iron-binding capacity, % saturation	18%–50%
Lipids	

Lipids, Serum—Upper Limits, 95% (mg/dl)

	Males		Females	
Age	Cholesterol	Triglycerides	Cholesterol	Triglycerides
6	200	86	208	97
8	200	96	208	107
10	200	104	208	113
12	200	114	208	116
14	200	122	208	116
16	200	131	208	115
18	202	138	209	112
20	210	143	210	107
—				
—				
55	291	197	291	133
65	296	199	320	145

Lipids, Lipoproteins Fractions—Upper Limits, 95% Cholesterol, mg/dl

	Males			Females		
Age	VLDL	LDL	HDL	VLDL	LDL	HDL
6–11	20	140	65	20	150	65
12–14	25	140	65	25	150	70
15–19	30	140	65	25	150	70
20–29	45	175	70	35	160	75
30–39	60	190	70	35	170	80
40–49	60	205	70	35	190	80
>50	60	220	70	35	200	80

Triglycerides, mg/dl Upper Limits, 95%

	Males			Females		
Age	VLDL	LDL	HDL	VLDL	LDL	HDL
6–7	60	25	15	60	25	15
8–11	60	25	15	85	25	15
12–14	90	25	15	85	25	15
15–19	105	25	15	85	25	15
20–29	155	30	20	90	30	15
30–39	155	40	20	90	40	15
40–49	155	50	20	90	40	15
>50	155	50	20	90	40	15

TABLE A-5 (*Continued*)

	(*Normal Ranges*)

BLOOD OR SERUM VALUES (*Continued*)

Magnesium	1.7–2.1 mg/dl
Osmolality	275–295 mOsm/kg
Phosphorus	2.5–4.5 mg/dl
Potassium	3.6–4.8 mEq/liter
Protein, total	6.6–7.9 g/dl
Protein electrophoresis	
Albumin	3.05–4.30 g/dl
Alpha-1 globulin	0.13–0.32 g/dl
Alpha-2 globulin	0.60–1.04 g/dl
Beta-globulin	0.72–1.25 g/dl
Gamma-globulin	0.70–1.60 g/dl
Sodium	135–145 mEq/liter
Urea	M, 17–51 mg/dl
	F, 13–45 mg/dl
Uric acid	M, 4.3–8.0 mg/dl
	F, 2.3–6.0 mg/dl
Vitamin A	125–150 IU/dl
Zinc	0.75–1.4 μg/ml

URINE VALUES

Calcium	M, <275 mg/24 hr
	F, <250 mg/24 hr, normal diet
Creatinine clearance	70–135 ml/min/1.73 m² at age 20 (decreased by 6 ml/min/decade)
Osmolality	300–800 mOsm/kg; overhydration <100, dehydration >800
Oxalate	20–60 mg/24 hr
Potassium	30–90 mEq/24 hr
Protein, total	<0.27 g/24 hr
Renal clearance—standard	
Glomerular filtration rate (inulin or iothalamate[125] I)	90–130 ml/min/1.73 m² at age 20 (decreased by 4 ml/min/decade)
Effective renal plasma flow (PAH)	400–700 ml/min/1.73 m² at age 20 (decreased by 17 ml/min/decade)
Filtration fraction	18%–22%
Renal clearance—short	
Glomerular filtration rate (iothalamate[125] I)	90–130 ml/min/1.73 m² at age 20 (decreased by 4 ml/min/decade)
Glomerular filtration rate (creatinine)	See creatinine clearance
Sodium	130–200 mEq/24 hr
Uric acid	<750 mg/24 hr

MISCELLANEOUS VALUES

Basal metabolism rate	−10% to +10%
Stool examination	
Fat, quantitative	2–7 g/24 hr
Nitrogen	1–2 g/24 hr
Vitamin B$_{12}$ absorption (Schilling test)	>9% excretion

From the Committee on Dietetics of the Mayo Clinic: Mayo Clinic Diet Manual, pp 275–277. Philadelphia, WB Saunders, 1981

TABLE A-6
Head Circumference of Boys (Birth–36 Mo)

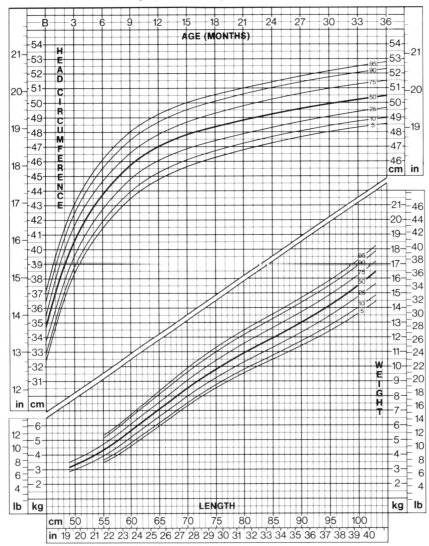

*Adapted from: Hamill PVV, Drizd TA, Johnson CL, Reed RB, Roche AF, Moore
WM: Physical growth: National Center for Health Statistics percentiles. AM J
CLIN NUTR 32:607-629,1979. Data from the Fels Research Institute, Wright
State University School of Medicine, Yellow Springs, Ohio.*

© 1980 ROSS LABORATORIES

TABLE A-7
Physical Growth of Boys (Birth–36 Mo)

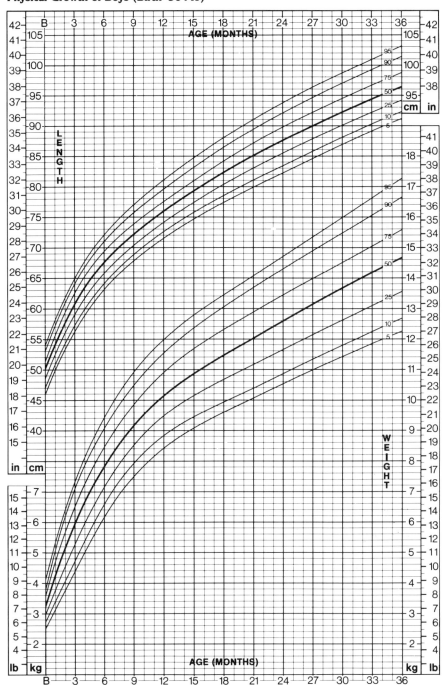

*Adapted from: Hamill PVV, Drizd TA, Johnson CL, Reed RB, Roche AF, Moore
WM: Physical growth: National Center for Health Statistics percentiles. AM J
CLIN NUTR 32:607-629,1979. Data from the Fels Research Institute, Wright
State University School of Medicine, Yellow Springs, Ohio.

© 1980 ROSS LABORATORIES

TABLE A-8
Head Circumference of Girls (Birth–36 Mo)

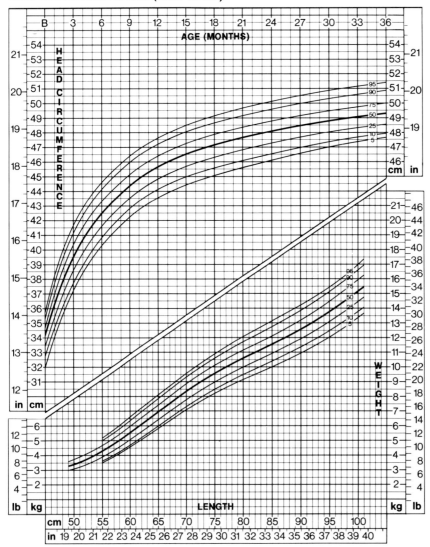

*Adapted from: Hamill PVV, Drizd TA, Johnson CL, Reed RB, Roche AF, Moore
WM: Physical growth: National Center for Health Statistics percentiles. AM J
CLIN NUTR 32:607-629,1979. Data from the Fels Research Institute, Wright
State University School of Medicine, Yellow Springs, Ohio.

© 1980 ROSS LABORATORIES

TABLE A-9
Physical Growth of Girls (Birth–36 Mo)

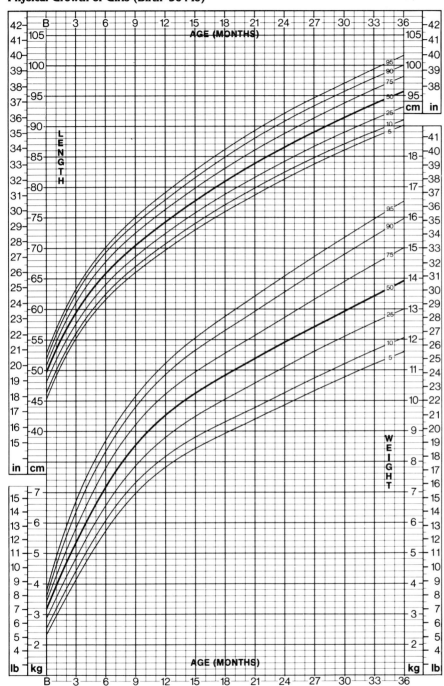

*Adapted from: Hamill PVV, Drizd TA, Johnson CL, Reed RB, Roche AF, Moore
WM: Physical growth: National Center for Health Statistics percentiles. AM J
CLIN NUTR 32:607-629,1979. Data from the Fels Research Institute, Wright
State University School of Medicine, Yellow Springs, Ohio.

© 1980 ROSS LABORATORIES

TABLE A-10
Physical Growth of Boys (2–18 Years)

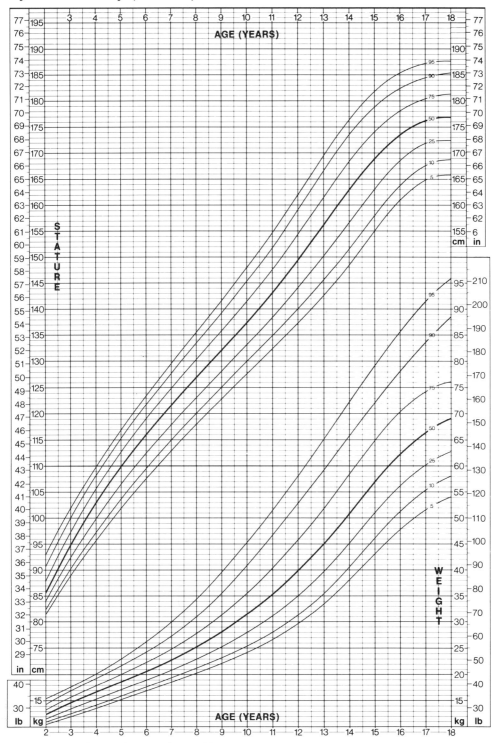

TABLE A-11
Prepubescent Growth of Boys

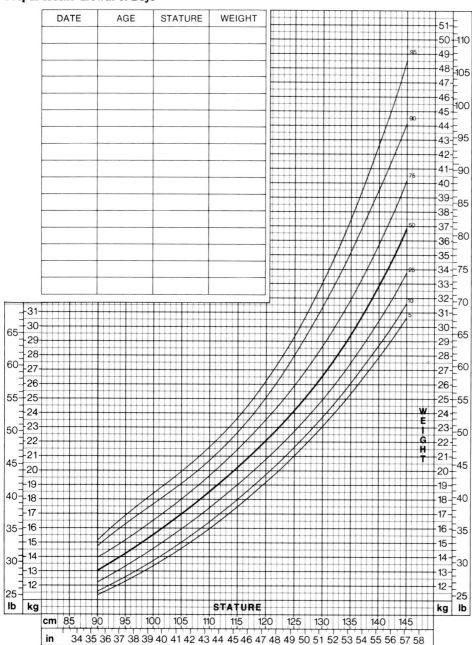

DATE	AGE	STATURE	WEIGHT

*Adapted from: Hamill PVV, Drizd TA, Johnson CL, Reed RB, Roche AF, Moore WM: Physical growth: National Center for Health Statistics percentiles. AM J CLIN NUTR 32:607-629,1979. Data from the National Center for Health Statistics (NCHS) Hyattsville, Maryland.

TABLE A-12
Physical Growth of Girls (2–18 Years)

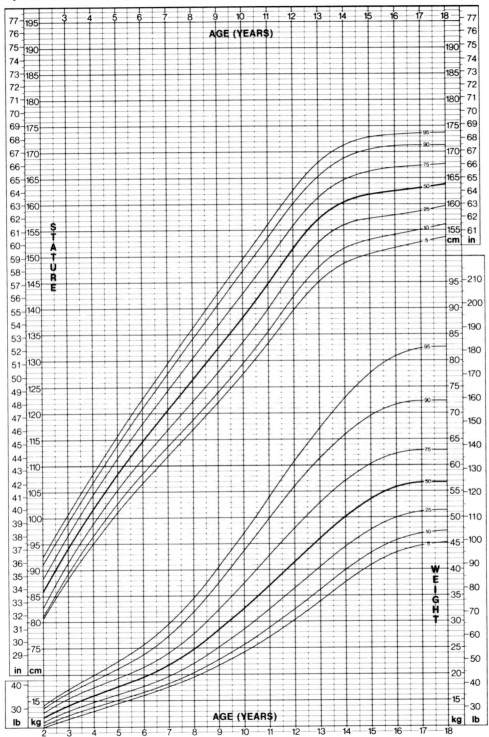

*Adapted from: Hamill PVV, Drizd TA, Johnson CL, Reed RB, Roche AF, Moore
WM: Physical growth: National Center for Health Statistics percentiles. AM J
CLIN NUTR 32:607-629,1979. Data from the National Center for Health
Statistics (NCHS) Hyattsville, Maryland.*

TABLE A-13
Prepubescent Growth of Girls

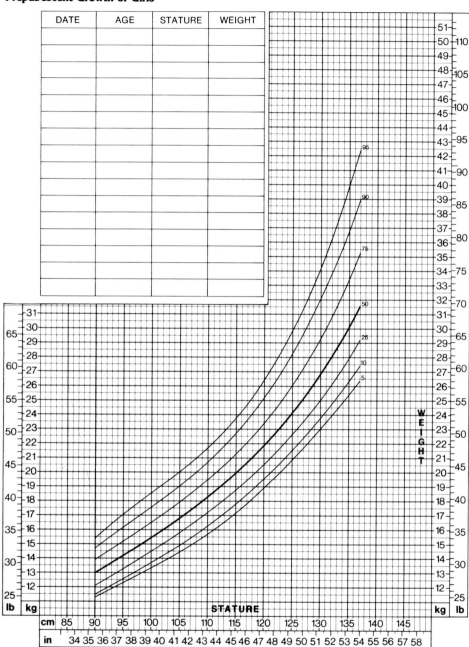

DATE	AGE	STATURE	WEIGHT

*Adapted from: Hamill PVV, Drizd TA, Johnson CL, Reed RB, Roche AF, Moore
WM: Physical growth: National Center for Health Statistics percentiles. AM J
CLIN NUTR 32:607-629,1979. Data from the National Center for Health
Statistics (NCHS) Hyattsville, Maryland.*

TABLE A-14
Average Weights and Selected Percentiles for Each Inch of Height: Men, 18–74 Years, United States, 1971–1974

Height (in)	18–24	25–34	35–44	45–54	55–64	65–74	Height (in)	18–24	25–34	35–44	45–54	55–64	65–74
			Weight in Pounds							Weight in Pounds			
62	175	191	188	194	190	186	69	209	224	224	224	225	216
	165	180	178	183	180	176		199	213	214	213	215	206
	153	167	166	171	167	165		187	200	202	201	202	195
	130	*141*	*143*	*147*	*143*	*143*		*164*	*174*	*179*	*177*	*178*	*173*
	107	115	120	123	119	121		141	148	156	153	154	151
	95	102	108	111	106	110		129	135	144	141	141	140
	85	91	98	100	96	100		119	124	134	130	131	130
63	180	195	193	199	194	190	70	213	229	229	229	230	220
	170	184	183	188	184	180		203	218	212	218	220	210
	158	171	171	176	171	169		191	205	207	206	207	199
	135	*145*	*148*	*152*	*147*	*147*		*168*	*179*	*184*	*182*	*183*	*177*
	112	119	125	128	123	125		145	153	161	158	159	155
	100	106	113	116	110	114		133	140	149	146	146	144
	90	95	103	105	100	104		123	129	139	135	136	134
64	185	200	198	203	200	194	71	218	234	235	234	236	225
	175	189	188	192	190	184		208	223	225	223	226	215
	163	176	176	180	177	173		196	210	213	211	213	204
	140	*150*	*153*	*156*	*153*	*151*		*173*	*184*	*190*	*187*	*189*	*182*
	117	124	130	132	129	129		150	158	167	163	165	160
	105	111	118	120	116	118		138	145	155	151	152	149
	95	100	108	109	106	108		128	134	145	140	142	139
65	190	206	203	207	205	199	72	223	239	239	238	240	229
	180	195	193	196	195	189		213	228	229	227	230	219
	168	182	181	184	182	178		201	215	217	215	217	208
	145	*156*	*158*	*160*	*158*	*156*		*178*	*189*	*194*	*191*	*193*	*186*
	122	130	135	136	134	134		155	163	171	167	169	164
	110	117	123	124	121	123		143	150	159	155	156	153
	100	106	113	113	111	113		133	139	149	144	146	143
66	195	210	208	211	210	203	73	228	244	245	243	244	233
	185	199	198	200	200	193		218	233	235	232	234	223
	173	186	186	188	187	182		206	220	223	220	221	212
	150	*160*	*163*	*164*	*163*	*160*		*183*	*194*	*200*	*196*	*197*	*190*
	127	134	140	140	139	138		160	168	177	172	173	168
	115	121	128	128	126	127		148	155	165	160	160	157
	105	110	118	117	116	117		138	144	155	149	150	147
67	199	215	214	216	215	207	74	233	249	250	247	250	237
	189	204	204	205	205	197		223	238	240	236	240	227
	177	191	192	193	192	186		211	225	228	224	227	216
	154	*165*	*169*	*169*	*168*	*164*		*188*	*199*	*205*	*200*	*203*	*194*
	131	139	146	145	144	142		165	173	182	176	179	172
	119	126	134	133	131	131		153	160	170	164	166	161
	109	115	124	122	121	121		143	149	160	153	156	151
68	204	220	219	220	220	212							
	194	209	209	209	210	202							
	182	196	197	197	197	191							
	159	*170*	*174*	*173*	*173*	*169*							
	136	144	151	149	149	147							
	124	131	139	137	136	136							
	114	120	129	126	126	126							

From the National Center for Health Statistics, Department of Health and Human Services

Examined persons were measured without shoes; clothing weight ranged from 0.20 lb–0.62 lb, which was not deducted from weights shown.

The weight values were computed from the regression equation of weight on height by age. The values above and below the expected mean value represent the $\pm.8416$, ±1.2816, and ±1.6449 standard error of the estimate covering within this range 60%, 80%, and 90% of the population around the mean, respectively. The first range is expected thus to identify 20%, 10%, and 5% percent of the population of the specific height on either side of the range.

Figures in *italics* are the expected means.

TABLE A-15
Average Weights and Selected Percentiles for Each Inch of Height: Women 18–74 Years, United States, 1971–1974

Height (in)	18–24	25–34	35–44	45–54	55–64	65–74	Height (in)	18–24	25–34	35–44	45–54	55–64	65–74
	Weight in Pounds							Weight in Pounds					
57	160	171	183	185	187	178	63	178	192	206	206	208	199
	150	159	170	172	175	167		168	180	193	193	196	188
	138	145	154	157	160	154		156	166	177	178	181	175
	114	*118*	*125*	*129*	*132*	*130*		*132*	*139*	*148*	*150*	*153*	*151*
	90	91	96	101	104	106		108	112	119	122	125	127
	78	77	80	86	89	93		96	93	103	107	110	114
	68	65	67	73	77	82		86	86	90	94	98	103
58	163	174	187	189	191	182	64	181	195	210	210	212	202
	153	162	174	176	179	171		171	183	197	197	200	191
	141	148	158	161	164	158		159	169	181	182	185	178
	117	*121*	*129*	*133*	*136*	*134*		*135*	*142*	*152*	*154*	*157*	*154*
	93	94	100	105	108	110		111	115	123	126	129	130
	81	80	84	90	93	97		90	101	107	110	114	117
	71	68	71	77	81	86		89	89	94	98	102	106
59	166	178	191	192	195	185	65	184	199	214	214	215	206
	156	166	178	179	183	174		174	187	201	201	203	195
	144	152	162	164	168	161		162	173	185	186	188	182
	120	*125*	*133*	*136*	*140*	*137*		*138*	*146*	*156*	*158*	*160*	*158*
	96	98	104	108	112	113		114	119	127	130	132	134
	84	84	88	93	97	100		102	105	111	115	117	121
	74	72	75	80	85	89		92	93	98	102	105	110
60	169	181	195	196	198	188	66	187	203	217	217	219	209
	159	169	182	183	186	177		177	191	204	204	207	198
	147	155	166	168	171	164		165	177	188	189	192	185
	123	*128*	*137*	*140*	*143*	*140*		*141*	*150*	*159*	*161*	*164*	*161*
	99	101	108	112	115	116		117	123	130	133	136	137
	87	87	92	97	100	103		106	109	114	118	121	124
	77	75	79	84	88	92		95	97	101	105	109	113
61	172	185	199	199	202	192	67	190	206	221	221	222	213
	162	173	186	186	190	181		180	194	208	208	210	202
	150	159	170	171	175	168		168	180	192	193	195	189
	126	*132*	*141*	*143*	*147*	*144*		*144*	*153*	*163*	*165*	*167*	*165*
	102	105	112	115	119	120		120	126	134	137	139	141
	90	91	96	100	104	107		108	112	118	122	124	128
	80	79	83	87	92	96		98	100	105	109	112	117
62	175	189	202	203	205	195	68	193	210	225	224	226	217
	165	177	189	190	193	184		183	198	212	211	214	206
	153	163	173	175	178	171		171	184	196	196	199	193
	129	*136*	*144*	*147*	*150*	*147*		*147*	*157*	*167*	*168*	*171*	*169*
	105	109	115	119	122	123		123	130	138	140	143	145
	93	95	99	104	107	110		111	116	122	125	128	132
	83	83	86	91	95	99		101	104	109	112	116	121

From the National Center for Health Statistics, Department of Health and Human Services

Examined persons were measured without shoes; clothing weight ranged from 0.20 to 0.62 pound, which was not deducted from body weight.

The weight values were computed from the regression equation of weight on height by age. The values above and below the expected mean value represent the ±.8416, ±1.2816, and ±1.6449 standard error of the estimate covering within this range 60%, 80%, and 90% of the population around the mean, respectively. The first range is expected thus to identify 20%, 10%, and 5% of the population of the specific height on either side of the range.

Figures in *italics* are the expected means.

TABLE A-16
1983 Metropolitan Height and Weight Tables

		Small	*Medium*	*Large*			*Small*	*Medium*	*Large*
HEIGHT		*Frame*	*Frame*	*Frame*	HEIGHT		*Frame*	*Frame*	*Frame*
FEET	INCHES				FEET	INCHES			
5	2	128–134	131–141	138–150	4	10	102–111	109–121	118–131
5	3	130–136	133–143	140–153	4	11	103–113	111–123	120–134
5	4	132–138	135–145	142–156	5	0	104–115	113–126	122–137
5	5	134–140	137–148	144–160	5	1	106–118	115–129	125–140
5	6	136–142	139–151	146–164	5	2	108–121	118–132	128–143
5	7	138–145	142–154	149–168	5	3	111–124	121–135	131–147
5	8	140–148	145–157	152–172	5	4	114–127	124–138	134–151
5	9	142–151	148–160	155–176	5	5	117–130	127–141	137–155
5	10	144–154	151–163	158–180	5	6	120–133	130–144	140–159
5	11	146–157	154–166	161–184	5	7	123–136	133–147	143–163
6	0	149–160	157–170	164–188	5	8	126–139	136–150	146–167
6	1	152–164	160–174	168–192	5	9	129–142	139–153	149–170
6	2	155–168	164–178	172–197	5	10	132–145	142–156	152–173
6	3	158–172	167–182	176–202	5	11	135–148	145–159	155–176
6	4	162–176	171–187	181–207	6	0	138–151	148–162	158–179

Men	*Women*
Weights at ages 25–59 based on lowest mortality. Weight in pounds according to frame (in indoor clothing weighing 5 lbs, shoes with 1 in heels).	Weights at ages 25–59 based on lowest mortality. Weight in pounds according to frame (in indoor clothing weighing 3 lbs, shoes with 1 in heels).

Source of basic data *1979 Build Study,* Society of Actuaries and Association of Life Insurance Medical Directors of America.
Courtesy of the Metropolitan Life Insurance Company, 1983.

How to Determine Your Body Frame by Elbow Breadth

To make a simple approximation of your frame size, extend your arm and bend the forearm upwards at a 90° angle. Keep the fingers straight and turn the inside of your wrist away from the body. Place the thumb and index finger of your other hand on the two prominent bones on *either side* of your elbow. Measure the space between your fingers against a ruler or a tape measure.* Compare the measurements on the following tables.

These tables list the elbow measurements for medium-framed men and women of various heights. Measurements lower than those listed indicate you have a small frame; higher measurements indicate a large frame.

Men

Height in 1″ heels	Elbow Breadth
5′2″–5′3″	2½″–2⅞″
5′4″–5′7″	2⅝″–2⅞″
5′8″–5′11″	2¾″–3″
6′0″–6′3″	2¾″–3⅛″
6′4″	2⅞″–3¼″

Women

Height in 1″ heels	Elbow Breadth
4′10″–4′11″	2¼″–2½″
5′0″–5′3″	2¼″–2½″
5′4″–5′7″	2⅜″–2⅝″
5′8″–5′11″	2⅜″–2⅝″
6′0″	2½″–2¾″

*For the most accurate measurement, have your physician measure your elbow breadth with a caliper.

TABLE A-17
Subscapular Skin-fold Thickness: Males, 1–17 Years, United States: 1971–1974

Race and Age in Years	Number in Sample	Estimated Population in Thousands	Mean	Standard Deviation	5th	10th	15th	25th	50th	75th	85th	90th	95th
ALL RACES*					*SUBSCAPULAR SKIN FOLD IN MILLIMETERS*								
1	286	1,693	6.2	1.9	4.0	4.0	4.0	5.0	6.0	7.0	8.0	8.5	10.0
2	298	1,747	5.7	2.0	3.0	4.0	4.0	4.5	5.0	6.5	7.0	8.0	10.0
3	308	1,807	5.4	2.0	3.5	4.0	4.0	4.0	5.0	6.0	6.8	7.0	9.5
4	304	1,815	5.1	1.7	3.0	3.5	4.0	4.0	5.0	6.0	6.0	7.0	7.0
5	273	1,563	5.3	2.7	3.0	3.5	4.0	4.0	5.0	6.0	7.0	7.0	8.0
6	179	1,673	5.1	2.4	3.0	3.0	3.5	4.0	4.5	5.0	6.0	7.0	9.0
7	164	1,979	5.5	3.0	3.0	3.0	3.5	4.0	4.5	6.0	7.0	9.0	11.0
8	152	1,861	5.1	2.3	3.0	3.0	3.5	4.0	4.5	6.0	6.0	7.5	9.0
9	169	2,019	7.1	5.1	3.5	3.5	4.0	4.0	5.0	8.0	11.0	14.0	14.0
10	184	2,205	6.8	4.5	3.5	4.0	4.0	4.0	5.5	7.0	10.0	12.0	18.0
11	178	2,177	8.0	6.2	4.0	4.0	4.0	4.5	6.0	8.5	13.0	15.0	19.0
12	200	2,304	8.0	6.0	3.5	4.0	4.5	5.0	6.0	9.0	11.0	14.0	20.5
13	174	1,978	8.8	6.9	3.5	4.0	4.5	5.0	6.5	9.0	13.5	17.0	26.0
14	174	2,030	8.5	6.1	4.0	4.5	5.0	5.0	6.5	9.0	13.0	16.0	20.0
15	171	2,093	9.1	6.5	4.0	5.0	5.0	5.5	7.0	10.0	13.0	15.5	23.0
16	169	2,019	9.8	6.2	5.0	5.5	6.0	6.5	8.0	10.5	13.5	16.5	23.5
17	176	2,095	9.7	5.9	5.0	5.5	6.0	7.0	8.0	10.0	13.0	16.0	23.0
WHITE													
1	211	1,402	6.3	2.0	4.0	4.0	4.0	5.0	6.0	7.0	8.0	8.5	10.0
2	217	1,461	5.6	1.9	3.0	3.5	4.0	4.0	5.0	6.0	7.0	7.5	10.0
3	226	1,536	5.4	2.0	3.5	4.0	4.0	4.0	5.0	6.0	6.5	7.0	10.0
4	229	1,547	5.2	1.8	3.0	4.0	4.0	4.0	5.0	6.0	6.0	7.0	7.0
5	207	1,319	5.3	2.7	3.0	3.5	4.0	4.0	5.0	6.0	7.0	7.0	8.0
6	126	1,343	5.1	2.4	3.0	3.5	3.5	4.0	4.5	5.5	6.0	7.0	10.0
7	125	1,718	5.6	3.1	3.0	3.0	3.5	4.0	5.0	6.0	7.0	8.0	11.5
8	116	1,644	5.1	2.3	3.0	3.0	3.0	4.0	4.5	6.0	6.0	7.5	11.0
9	117	1,636	7.2	4.7	3.5	4.0	4.0	4.0	5.0	8.5	11.5	14.0	14.0
10	148	1,909	6.8	4.5	3.0	4.0	4.0	4.0	5.5	7.0	9.5	12.0	18.0
11	132	1,823	8.2	6.4	3.5	4.0	4.0	4.5	6.0	9.0	14.0	15.0	20.0
12	152	1,970	8.1	5.8	3.5	4.0	4.0	5.0	6.0	9.0	11.5	14.0	21.0
13	129	1,697	9.0	7.1	3.5	4.0	4.0	5.0	6.5	9.0	14.0	17.0	27.0
14	134	1,730	9.0	6.5	4.0	5.0	5.0	5.5	6.5	9.0	14.0	16.0	20.0
15	124	1,728	8.8	6.4	4.0	5.0	5.0	5.5	7.0	9.0	13.0	15.0	22.0
16	128	1,752	9.9	6.4	5.0	5.0	6.0	6.5	8.0	11.0	13.5	17.0	23.5
17	139	1,831	9.7	6.1	5.0	5.5	6.0	6.5	8.0	10.0	13.0	16.0	23.0
BLACK													
1	72	280	6.0	1.6	4.0	4.0	4.0	5.0	6.0	7.0	7.5	8.0	9.0
2	77	267	6.5	2.4	4.0	4.0	4.0	5.0	5.5	7.0	10.0	11.5	11.5
3	72	212	5.3	1.6	3.5	4.0	4.0	4.0	5.0	6.0	6.5	6.5	9.0
4	74	260	4.8	1.2	3.0	3.0	3.5	4.0	5.0	5.1	6.0	6.0	8.0
5	64	226	5.1	2.5	2.5	3.0	3.0	4.0	4.5	5.0	7.0	7.0	8.5
6	52	321	4.9	2.1	3.0	3.0	3.5	4.0	5.0	5.0	5.5	7.0	7.0
7	38	253	5.2	2.4	3.0	3.0	3.0	3.5	4.0	6.0	8.0	10.0	11.0
8	33	203	5.5	2.1	3.5	3.5	4.0	4.0	5.0	6.0	7.5	9.0	9.0
9	52	383	6.6	6.3	3.0	3.0	3.0	4.0	5.0	6.0	8.0	8.0	30.0
10	33	251	6.7	3.8	4.0	4.0	4.0	4.5	5.0	7.0	9.0	12.0	18.5
11	43	313	6.7	4.9	4.0	4.0	4.0	5.0	5.5	6.5	8.0	8.0	12.5
12	47	316	7.4	6.9	4.0	4.0	4.5	4.5	5.0	7.0	7.0	17.0	19.0
13	45	281	7.6	5.9	4.0	4.5	4.5	5.0	6.0	7.0	8.0	18.5	26.0
14	39	282	6.1	2.1	4.0	4.0	5.0	5.0	6.0	7.0	7.0	7.5	12.0
15	43	310	10.6	6.7	4.0	5.0	5.5	7.0	9.0	12.0	12.0	24.0	24.0
16	41	267	8.5	4.2	5.5	5.5	6.5	6.5	7.0	9.0	9.5	10.0	16.0
17	35	235	9.6	5.2	6.0	6.0	6.0	7.0	8.0	10.0	12.0	16.0	16.0

From the National Center for Health Statistics, Department of Health and Human Services.
*Includes data for races that are not shown separately.

TABLE A-18
Subscapular Skin-fold Thickness: Females, 1–17 Years, United States: 1971–1974

Race and Age in Years	Number in Sample	Estimated Population in Thousands	Mean	Standard Deviation	Percentile								
					5th	10th	15th	25th	50th	75th	85th	90th	95th
ALL RACES*					*SUBSCAPULAR SKIN FOLD IN MILLIMETERS*								
1	267	1,620	6.2	1.9	4.0	4.0	4.0	5.0	6.0	8.0	8.0	9.0	9.0
2	272	1,708	6.2	2.4	4.0	4.0	4.0	5.0	6.0	7.0	8.0	9.0	10.0
3	292	1,701	5.8	2.0	4.0	4.0	4.0	4.5	5.5	6.5	7.0	8.0	9.0
4	281	1,599	5.6	1.9	3.5	4.0	4.0	4.5	5.0	6.0	7.0	8.0	9.0
5	314	1,695	6.2	3.3	3.5	4.0	4.0	4.0	5.0	6.5	8.0	9.0	15.0
6	176	1,787	6.0	2.8	3.0	4.0	4.0	4.5	5.5	6.5	7.0	8.0	10.0
7	169	1,754	6.2	3.3	3.0	4.0	4.0	4.5	5.0	7.0	9.0	10.5	11.5
8	152	1,800	7.7	5.5	3.5	4.0	4.0	4.5	5.5	8.0	12.5	14.5	19.5
9	171	2,017	8.5	5.0	4.0	4.0	4.5	5.0	7.0	10.0	13.0	17.0	19.0
10	197	2,173	8.6	5.1	4.0	4.5	5.0	5.5	6.5	10.0	13.0	18.0	20.0
11	166	1,911	10.1	6.4	4.0	5.0	5.0	6.0	8.0	13.0	16.0	19.0	25.5
12	177	1,812	11.1	6.8	5.0	5.0	5.5	6.0	9.5	13.0	16.0	20.0	25.0
13	198	2,175	11.9	7.1	5.0	6.0	6.0	7.0	9.5	15.0	19.0	23.4	26.0
14	184	2,036	13.0	8.0	5.0	6.0	6.5	8.0	10.0	16.0	19.0	24.0	28.0
15	171	2,163	12.2	7.2	6.0	6.5	7.0	7.5	10.0	14.0	18.0	20.0	27.0
16	175	2,145	13.4	7.8	6.0	7.0	7.5	8.0	10.5	15.0	21.0	25.5	29.0
17	157	1,804	15.6	9.4	6.5	7.0	7.5	9.0	12.5	20.0	25.5	27.0	34.1
WHITE													
1	189	1,328	6.3	1.9	3.5	4.0	4.0	5.0	6.0	8.0	8.0	9.0	9.5
2	203	1,434	6.0	2.1	4.0	4.0	4.0	5.0	6.0	7.0	8.0	8.5	10.0
3	211	1,438	5.8	1.9	4.0	4.0	4.0	5.0	5.5	6.5	7.0	8.0	9.0
4	204	1,339	5.7	1.9	3.5	4.0	4.0	4.5	5.0	6.0	7.0	8.0	9.0
5	224	1,416	6.2	3.2	3.5	4.0	4.0	4.5	5.5	6.5	8.0	10.0	15.0
6	125	1,445	6.0	2.7	3.0	3.5	4.0	4.5	6.0	6.5	7.0	8.0	10.0
7	122	1,507	6.2	3.4	3.0	3.5	4.0	4.5	5.0	7.0	8.5	10.0	12.5
8	117	1,507	7.6	5.6	3.5	4.0	4.0	4.5	6.0	8.0	10.0	13.0	21.0
9	129	1,751	8.5	4.7	4.0	4.5	5.0	5.0	7.0	10.0	13.0	16.0	18.0
10	148	1,855	8.8	5.1	4.0	4.5	5.0	5.5	7.0	10.0	13.0	18.0	20.0
11	122	1,569	10.3	6.7	4.0	5.0	5.0	6.0	8.0	13.0	16.5	20.5	25.5
12	128	1,506	11.1	6.4	5.0	5.0	6.0	6.5	9.5	13.5	17.0	20.0	22.0
13	153	1,886	11.6	6.9	5.0	5.5	6.0	7.0	9.0	15.0	19.0	21.0	25.0
14	132	1,731	13.2	8.2	5.0	6.0	6.5	8.0	10.5	16.0	20.0	24.0	30.0
15	125	1,752	12.4	6.9	6.0	7.0	7.0	8.0	10.0	14.5	18.0	20.0	27.0
16	141	1,933	12.9	7.3	6.0	7.0	7.5	8.0	10.0	15.0	20.5	25.0	28.5
17	117	1,549	15.2	9.3	6.0	7.0	7.5	8.0	12.5	18.0	25.0	26.5	34.0
BLACK													
1	73	257	6.1	2.0	4.0	4.0	4.0	5.0	5.5	8.0	8.5	9.0	9.0
2	66	261	6.8	3.3	4.0	4.0	4.5	5.0	6.0	7.5	9.5	12.0	15.5
3	78	245	5.5	2.0	4.0	4.0	4.0	4.5	5.0	6.0	7.0	7.0	8.0
4	73	246	5.2	1.7	3.0	3.5	4.0	4.0	5.0	6.0	6.0	8.0	8.5
5	88	265	5.8	3.5	4.0	4.0	4.0	4.0	5.0	6.0	6.5	7.0	13.0
6	50	336	6.0	3.3	3.0	4.0	4.0	4.5	5.0	7.0	7.5	7.5	10.0
7	46	241	6.4	2.6	3.0	4.0	4.0	5.0	5.5	8.0	11.0	11.0	11.0
8	35	293	8.2	5.2	4.0	4.0	4.0	4.5	5.0	14.0	15.0	16.0	17.5
9	41	247	8.3	6.4	4.0	4.0	4.0	4.5	5.5	7.5	14.5	24.0	24.0
10	48	303	8.1	5.5	4.0	4.0	4.5	5.0	6.0	8.0	12.5	14.3	22.0
11	42	315	9.2	4.5	4.0	5.0	5.0	5.5	8.0	11.0	14.5	14.5	15.5
12	47	284	10.7	8.6	4.5	5.0	5.0	5.5	7.0	11.5	16.0	28.0	31.0
13	44	287	13.9	8.1	6.0	6.0	6.5	8.0	12.0	15.0	26.0	26.0	28.4
14	50	265	12.5	7.3	6.0	6.0	6.5	7.0	10.0	16.5	23.0	23.0	25.0
15	46	411	11.2	8.4	5.5	5.5	6.0	6.5	7.5	10.5	19.0	20.0	33.4
16	33	203	17.8	10.7	6.0	7.0	8.0	10.5	15.0	24.5	31.0	38.0	38.0
17	39	239	16.4	8.4	7.0	7.5	8.0	9.0	12.5	23.5	27.0	28.0	30.0

From the National Center for Health Statistics, Department of Health and Human Services.

*Includes data for races that are not shown separately.

TABLE A-19
Subscapular Skin-fold Thickness: Adult Men, United States, 1971–1974

Race and Age in Years	Number in Sample	Estimated Population in Thousands	Mean	Standard Deviation	Percentile								
					5th	10th	15th	25th	50th	75th	85th	90th	95th
ALL RACES*					*Subscapular Skin Fold in Millimeters*								
	5,261	61,180	15.9	7.7	6.0	7.0	8.0	10.0	14.5	20.0	24.0	26.0	30.5
18–19	260	3,673	12.3	7.1	6.0	6.5	7.0	8.0	10.0	13.0	18.0	23.5	28.5
20–24	513	8,110	13.7	7.4	6.0	7.0	7.0	8.0	12.0	17.0	20.5	24.0	30.0
25–34	804	13,003	15.9	8.1	6.5	7.0	8.0	10.0	14.0	20.0	24.5	26.0	30.5
35–44	664	10,676	16.8	7.2	7.0	8.0	10.0	11.5	16.0	21.0	24.0	26.0	30.5
45–54	765	11,150	17.5	7.9	7.0	8.0	9.0	12.0	16.5	22.0	25.0	29.0	32.0
55–64	598	9,073	16.5	7.5	6.0	7.0	8.5	11.0	15.5	21.0	24.5	27.0	30.0
65–74	1,657	5,496	15.9	7.2	6.0	7.5	9.0	10.5	15.0	20.0	23.0	25.0	30.0
WHITE													
	4,344	54,694	15.9	7.5	6.5	7.5	8.0	10.0	14.5	20.0	24.0	26.0	30.0
18–19	203	3,206	12.5	7.1	6.0	6.5	7.0	8.0	10.0	13.5	18.0	23.5	28.5
20–24	423	7,094	13.8	7.3	6.0	7.0	7.0	8.0	12.0	17.0	21.0	24.0	30.0
25–34	672	11,594	15.8	7.6	7.0	7.5	8.0	10.0	14.0	20.0	25.0	26.0	30.0
35–44	569	9,516	16.6	7.0	7.0	8.5	10.0	11.5	16.0	20.0	24.0	26.0	30.0
45–54	628	10,039	17.6	7.6	7.0	8.0	10.0	12.0	16.5	22.0	25.0	28.5	31.0
55–64	505	8,275	16.5	7.2	6.0	7.0	8.5	11.0	15.5	21.0	24.0	26.5	30.0
65–74	1,344	4,970	15.9	7.0	6.5	8.0	9.0	11.0	15.0	20.0	23.0	25.0	30.0
BLACK													
	847	5,753	16.1	9.9	6.0	6.5	7.0	8.5	14.0	21.9	25.0	28.0	35.0
18–19	52	404	10.9	7.2	4.0	5.5	6.0	7.0	9.0	11.1	15.0	23.5	32.0
20–24	80	866	13.6	8.6	5.5	6.0	7.0	8.0	11.0	17.0	19.0	26.0	30.0
25–34	119	1,232	16.6	11.8	6.0	6.5	7.0	8.0	14.0	21.5	25.0	30.5	42.0
35–44	87	1,005	18.9	8.4	7.0	7.0	8.0	12.0	19.0	24.0	25.5	31.0	33.1
45–54	130	1,057	16.6	9.7	6.0	7.0	7.0	9.0	13.0	22.0	26.0	32.0	35.0
55–64	85	703	17.0	10.5	5.0	5.0	6.5	10.0	14.5	23.0	25.0	28.0	35.0
65–74	294	486	15.2	8.6	6.0	6.0	7.0	8.0	13.0	20.0	23.0	26.0	33.0

From the National Center for Health Statistics, Department of Health and Human Services.
*Includes data for races that are not shown separately.

TABLE A-19a
Subscapular Skin-fold Thickness: Adult Women, United States, 1971–1974

Race and Age in Years	Number in Sample	Estimated Population in Thousands	Mean	Standard Deviation	Percentile								
					5th	10th	15th	25th	50th	75th	85th	90th	95th
ALL RACES*					*Subscapular Skin Fold in Millimeters*								
	8,410	67,837	18.8	10.2	6.5	7.5	8.5	10.5	16.0	25.2	30.0	33.2	38.0
18–19	280	3,679	14.4	7.7	6.5	7.0	7.0	9.0	12.0	19.0	22.0	26.0	30.0
20–24	1,243	9,215	15.4	8.6	6.0	7.0	8.0	9.0	13.0	19.5	23.0	27.0	32.1
25–34	1,896	13,933	17.4	10.1	6.0	7.0	8.0	10.0	14.5	22.5	29.0	32.1	38.0
35–44	1,664	11,593	19.6	10.8	6.5	8.0	9.0	11.0	17.0	26.5	32.0	34.1	39.1
45–54	836	12,163	21.2	10.5	7.0	8.5	10.0	12.0	20.0	28.0	32.5	35.0	40.0
55–64	669	9,976	20.9	10.3	7.0	8.0	9.5	12.5	20.0	28.0	32.0	34.5	38.0
65–74	1,822	7,277	19.5	9.3	7.0	8.0	10.0	12.0	18.0	25.0	30.0	32.5	37.0
WHITE													
	6,757	59,923	18.2	9.8	6.5	7.5	8.0	10.0	16.0	25.0	29.4	32.0	36.5
18–19	208	3,159	14.2	7.4	6.5	7.0	7.0	8.5	12.0	19.0	22.0	26.0	30.0
20–24	956	7,972	15.1	8.5	6.0	7.0	7.5	9.0	13.0	19.0	23.0	27.0	32.0
25–34	1,539	12,161	16.8	9.8	6.0	7.0	8.0	9.5	14.0	21.5	27.5	32.0	37.0
35–44	1,302	10,111	18.8	10.5	6.5	7.5	8.5	10.5	16.0	25.0	30.0	34.0	38.0
45–54	705	10,879	20.4	10.0	7.0	8.5	10.0	12.8	19.0	27.0	31.5	34.0	38.0
55–64	551	9,037	20.2	9.8	6.5	8.0	9.0	12.0	19.0	27.0	31.0	34.0	37.0
65–74	1,496	6,603	19.2	9.1	7.0	8.0	10.0	12.0	18.0	25.0	29.0	32.0	36.0
BLACK													
	1,557	7,302	23.4	12.0	7.0	9.0	10.0	13.0	28.0	31.5	36.1	39.0	44.1
18–19	70	504	14.9	9.4	6.5	7.0	7.5	9.0	12.0	19.0	20.0	26.0	38.0
20–24	259	1,073	17.6	9.3	7.0	8.0	9.0	11.0	15.0	22.5	28.0	30.5	35.1
25–34	335	1,646	21.7	11.3	6.5	8.0	10.0	12.0	20.0	30.0	33.1	36.0	41.0
35–44	334	1,318	26.0	11.0	9.0	10.0	12.0	17.0	26.5	34.0	38.0	40.1	42.4
45–54	126	1,237	28.5	12.0	10.5	11.5	14.0	17.5	30.0	37.1	40.0	43.1	46.0
55–64	115	871	27.5	13.4	7.5	9.5	12.0	19.0	27.0	35.5	40.0	47.0	55.0
65–74	318	652	22.8	10.5	6.0	8.0	10.0	14.0	24.0	31.0	34.0	35.5	39.0

From the National Center for Health Statistics, Department of Health and Human Services.

*Includes data for races that are not shown separately.

TABLE A-20
Triceps Skin-fold Thickness: Males, 1–17 Years, United States: 1971–1974

Race and Age in Years	Number in Sample	Estimated Population in Thousands	Mean	Standard Deviation	Percentile 5th	10th	15th	25th	50th	75th	85th	90th	95th
ALL RACES*					*Triceps Skin Fold in Millimeters*								
1	286	1,693	10.4	3.1	6.0	7.0	7.5	8.0	10.0	12.0	14.0	15.0	16.0
2	298	1,747	10.0	2.7	6.0	6.5	7.0	8.0	10.0	12.0	12.5	13.5	15.0
3	308	1,807	9.9	2.7	6.5	7.0	7.0	8.0	10.0	11.0	12.5	13.1	14.5
4	304	1,815	9.4	2.5	5.0	6.5	7.0	8.0	9.0	11.0	12.0	12.5	14.0
5	273	1,563	9.5	3.3	5.0	6.0	7.0	7.0	9.0	11.0	12.5	13.5	15.0
6	179	1,673	8.6	3.0	5.0	5.5	6.0	6.5	8.0	10.0	12.0	12.0	14.0
7	164	1,979	8.9	3.5	4.0	5.0	6.0	6.5	8.0	10.0	12.0	13.0	15.5
8	152	1,861	9.0	3.3	5.0	5.5	6.0	6.5	8.0	10.0	12.0	13.0	16.0
9	169	2,019	10.6	4.8	5.0	6.0	6.5	7.0	9.0	14.0	17.0	17.0	19.0
10	184	2,205	10.9	4.4	5.5	6.0	6.0	8.0	10.0	13.5	15.0	17.0	19.5
11	178	2,177	11.9	6.4	5.0	6.0	6.0	7.5	10.0	14.5	18.0	20.0	24.0
12	200	2,304	11.9	6.3	4.5	6.0	6.5	8.0	10.5	13.5	16.5	20.0	27.0
13	174	1,978	11.2	6.6	5.0	5.0	5.5	7.0	10.0	13.0	19.0	22.0	25.0
14	174	2,030	10.3	6.2	4.0	5.0	5.5	6.5	8.0	12.0	16.5	19.0	22.5
15	171	2,093	10.0	6.1	4.0	5.0	5.0	6.0	8.0	11.5	15.0	19.0	23.5
16	169	2,019	9.7	5.2	4.0	5.0	5.0	6.0	8.0	12.0	14.0	17.0	22.0
17	176	2,095	9.2	5.4	4.0	5.0	5.0	6.0	7.5	11.0	12.5	15.0	19.0
WHITE													
1	211	1,402	10.7	3.0	7.0	7.0	7.5	8.0	10.0	12.0	14.0	15.0	16.5
2	217	1,461	9.9	2.6	6.0	6.5	7.0	8.0	10.0	12.0	12.5	13.0	14.7
3	226	1,536	9.9	2.6	6.5	7.0	7.0	8.0	10.0	11.0	12.5	13.5	14.5
4	229	1,547	9.6	2.4	6.0	7.0	7.0	8.0	10.0	11.0	12.0	12.5	14.0
5	207	1,319	9.8	3.2	6.0	6.5	7.0	7.5	9.0	11.0	12.5	13.5	15.0
6	126	1,343	8.9	3.1	5.5	5.6	6.0	7.0	9.0	10.0	12.0	12.5	14.0
7	125	1,718	9.1	3.5	5.0	6.0	6.0	7.0	8.0	10.5	12.0	13.5	17.0
8	116	1,644	9.1	3.3	5.0	5.5	6.0	7.0	8.5	10.5	12.0	13.0	16.0
9	117	1,636	11.1	4.8	5.5	6.5	6.5	7.5	10.0	14.0	17.0	17.0	19.0
10	148	1,909	11.1	4.2	5.5	6.0	7.0	8.0	10.0	14.0	15.5	17.0	19.5
11	132	1,823	12.5	6.5	6.0	6.0	7.0	8.0	10.0	15.0	19.0	20.5	24.5
12	152	1,970	12.4	6.1	6.0	6.0	7.0	8.5	11.0	14.0	18.0	21.0	27.0
13	129	1,697	11.7	6.7	5.0	5.0	6.0	7.0	10.0	14.0	19.0	22.0	25.5
14	134	1,730	10.9	6.4	4.0	5.0	6.0	7.0	9.0	13.0	18.0	20.0	24.0
15	124	1,728	10.2	6.1	4.0	5.0	6.0	6.0	8.0	12.0	15.0	19.0	24.0
16	128	1,752	10.1	5.2	4.0	5.0	5.0	6.5	9.0	12.5	15.0	17.0	22.0
17	139	1,831	9.3	5.4	4.5	5.0	5.5	6.0	7.5	11.0	13.0	15.0	19.0
BLACK													
1	72	280	9.4	3.4	4.5	6.0	7.0	8.0	8.0	11.0	12.0	13.0	15.0
2	77	267	10.1	3.2	4.5	6.0	6.5	8.0	10.0	12.0	14.0	15.0	15.0
3	72	212	9.1	2.6	6.0	6.5	6.5	7.0	9.0	10.5	12.0	12.0	13.0
4	74	260	8.0	2.6	5.0	5.0	5.0	6.5	7.0	9.0	10.0	10.5	15.0
5	64	226	7.7	3.4	4.5	5.0	5.0	5.0	7.0	9.0	10.0	12.0	15.5
6	52	321	7.1	1.8	4.0	4.0	5.0	6.0	7.0	8.0	9.0	9.0	9.0
7	38	253	7.5	3.2	4.0	4.0	4.0	5.0	6.5	9.0	11.5	13.0	15.0
8	33	203	7.8	3.4	4.0	5.0	5.0	6.0	6.5	10.0	11.0	11.0	12.5
9	52	383	8.2	3.9	3.5	4.0	4.5	6.0	7.0	8.0	12.0	13.0	18.0
10	33	251	9.1	5.3	5.0	5.0	6.0	6.0	7.5	10.0	13.0	15.0	20.0
11	43	313	8.0	5.0	4.0	4.0	5.0	5.0	6.0	8.5	11.0	12.0	15.0
12	47	316	9.4	7.0	4.0	4.0	4.5	6.0	7.5	10.7	11.0	15.0	24.0
13	45	281	8.2	4.4	4.0	5.0	5.0	5.0	7.0	8.5	11.0	19.0	19.0
14	39	282	6.6	2.6	3.5	3.5	3.5	5.0	6.5	7.0	8.0	9.0	12.0
15	43	310	8.9	6.1	4.0	4.5	5.0	5.0	6.5	9.0	10.0	21.0	21.0
16	41	267	7.2	4.8	4.0	4.0	4.0	5.0	6.0	7.5	8.0	11.0	15.0
17	35	235	8.7	5.8	3.5	3.5	5.0	5.0	7.0	10.5	12.0	12.0	23.2

From the National Center for Health Statistics, Department of Health and Human Services
*Includes data for races that are not shown separately.

TABLE A-21
Triceps Skin-fold Thickness: Females, 1–17 Years, United States: 1971–1974

Race and Age in Years	Number in Sample	Estimated Population in Thousands	Mean	Standard Deviation	Percentile								
					5th	10th	15th	25th	50th	75th	85th	90th	95th
ALL RACES*					*Triceps Skin Fold in Millimeters*								
1	267	1,620	10.1	2.8	6.0	6.5	7.0	8.0	10.0	12.0	13.0	14.0	15.0
2	272	1,708	10.5	2.5	7.0	7.5	8.0	9.0	10.0	12.0	13.5	14.0	15.0
3	292	1,701	10.9	2.7	6.0	7.0	8.0	9.0	11.0	12.5	13.5	14.0	15.0
4	281	1,599	10.5	2.7	7.0	7.5	8.0	8.0	10.0	12.0	13.0	14.0	15.0
5	314	1,695	10.5	3.8	6.0	7.0	7.0	8.0	10.0	12.0	13.0	15.0	17.5
6	176	1,787	10.3	3.3	6.0	6.5	7.0	8.0	10.0	12.0	13.0	13.5	15.0
7	169	1,754	10.8	4.2	4.0	6.0	7.0	8.0	10.5	12.0	15.0	16.0	18.0
8	152	1,800	12.3	4.8	6.5	8.0	8.0	9.0	11.0	15.0	17.0	18.0	22.5
9	171	2,017	13.2	4.8	7.0	7.5	8.0	10.0	12.5	16.0	18.0	20.0	22.0
10	197	2,173	13.1	5.0	7.0	8.0	8.0	9.5	12.0	15.5	19.0	20.0	23.0
11	166	1,911	14.5	6.2	7.0	8.0	8.5	10.0	13.0	18.0	20.5	23.5	28.5
12	177	1,812	15.0	5.9	7.5	8.0	9.0	10.5	14.0	18.5	20.0	23.0	27.0
13	198	2,175	16.2	6.8	7.0	8.0	10.0	11.5	15.0	20.0	24.0	25.0	30.0
14	184	2,036	17.5	7.3	8.5	9.5	10.0	13.0	16.0	21.0	24.0	27.0	33.0
15	171	2,163	17.0	7.0	8.0	10.0	11.0	12.0	16.0	20.5	23.0	25.0	28.5
16	175	2,145	18.2	6.7	10.0	10.5	12.0	13.5	17.0	21.0	24.0	26.0	32.5
17	157	1,804	19.6	8.1	10.0	11.5	12.0	13.0	19.0	24.0	26.5	29.5	35.0
WHITE													
1	189	1,328	10.2	2.8	6.0	7.0	7.0	8.0	10.0	12.0	13.0	13.5	15.5
2	203	1,434	10.6	2.6	7.0	7.5	8.0	9.0	10.0	12.0	13.5	14.0	15.0
3	211	1,438	11.1	2.6	7.0	8.0	8.5	9.0	11.0	13.0	13.5	14.0	15.0
4	204	1,339	10.8	2.6	7.5	8.0	8.0	9.0	10.5	12.0	13.0	14.5	16.0
5	224	1,416	10.7	3.7	6.0	7.0	8.0	8.5	10.0	12.0	13.0	15.0	17.5
6	125	1,445	10.6	3.3	6.5	7.0	7.5	8.0	10.5	12.0	13.0	14.0	16.0
7	122	1,507	10.9	4.2	4.0	6.0	7.0	8.0	11.0	12.0	15.0	15.5	17.5
8	117	1,507	12.4	4.7	7.0	8.0	8.0	9.0	11.5	15.0	16.5	18.0	22.0
9	129	1,751	13.6	4.6	7.5	8.0	9.0	10.0	13.0	16.0	18.0	20.0	22.0
10	148	1,855	13.4	4.8	7.5	8.0	8.5	10.0	12.5	15.5	19.0	20.0	23.0
11	122	1,569	14.9	6.1	8.0	8.5	9.0	10.0	13.0	17.5	20.5	24.5	28.5
12	128	1,506	15.2	5.6	8.0	9.0	10.0	11.0	14.0	18.5	20.0	23.0	26.0
13	153	1,886	16.2	6.8	7.0	8.0	10.0	11.5	15.0	20.0	24.0	25.0	28.5
14	132	1,731	17.8	7.3	9.0	9.5	10.5	13.0	16.7	21.0	24.0	28.5	33.0
15	125	1,752	17.7	6.7	9.0	10.5	11.0	13.0	17.0	21.0	24.0	25.0	28.5
16	141	1,933	18.2	6.6	10.0	10.5	12.5	14.0	17.0	21.0	24.0	26.0	32.1
17	117	1,549	19.8	8.0	10.0	12.0	12.5	13.5	19.0	24.0	26.5	29.5	35.0
BLACK													
1	73	257	10.0	3.0	5.5	5.5	7.0	8.0	10.0	12.0	13.0	14.0	15.0
2	66	261	10.0	2.3	7.0	8.0	8.0	8.0	10.0	11.0	12.0	14.0	15.5
3	78	245	9.7	2.9	6.0	7.0	7.0	8.0	10.0	11.0	12.0	13.0	14.0
4	73	246	8.8	2.7	5.0	6.0	7.0	7.0	8.0	10.5	12.0	13.0	14.0
5	88	265	9.4	3.9	5.0	5.0	6.5	7.0	8.0	10.0	12.0	13.5	17.0
6	50	336	9.0	3.1	5.5	6.0	6.0	8.0	8.0	10.0	11.5	12.0	13.0
7	46	241	10.1	4.0	5.0	6.0	7.0	7.5	9.0	11.0	17.5	18.0	18.0
8	35	293	11.5	5.1	5.0	6.5	7.0	8.0	10.0	13.5	18.0	18.0	23.0
9	41	247	10.2	5.1	5.5	6.0	6.0	6.5	8.0	12.0	18.0	18.0	20.0
10	48	303	11.7	5.6	6.5	6.5	7.0	7.5	10.0	16.0	18.0	19.0	24.0
11	42	315	12.7	6.4	4.0	5.0	6.5	7.5	10.0	18.0	22.0	23.0	23.0
12	47	284	13.6	7.6	5.5	6.0	6.0	7.5	12.0	17.0	22.0	25.0	30.0
13	44	287	16.1	7.0	7.0	8.5	10.0	11.0	14.0	18.0	24.0	24.0	33.5
14	50	265	15.9	6.7	8.0	8.0	9.0	10.5	14.0	20.5	24.0	24.5	24.5
15	46	411	14.0	7.6	6.5	6.5	8.0	10.0	12.5	16.0	16.5	20.0	32.8
16	33	203	18.9	8.0	8.0	8.0	10.0	12.0	19.0	24.0	24.5	33.0	33.1
17	39	239	16.9	6.6	7.5	9.0	11.0	12.0	14.5	20.0	24.0	28.0	31.0

From the National Center for Health Statistics, Department of Health and Human Services.
*Includes data for races that are not shown separately.

TABLE A-22
Triceps Skin-fold Thickness: Adult Men, United States, 1971–1974

Race and Age in Years	Number in Sample	Estimated Population in Thousands	Mean	Standard Deviation	Percentile								
					5th	10th	15th	25th	50th	75th	85th	90th	95th
ALL RACES*					*Triceps Skin Fold in Millimeters*								
	5,261	61,180	12.0	5.9	4.5	6.0	6.5	8.0	11.0	15.0	18.0	20.0	23.0
18–19	260	3,673	11.0	6.1	4.5	5.0	6.0	7.0	8.5	15.0	18.0	19.5	23.5
20–24	513	8,110	11.2	6.2	4.0	5.0	6.0	7.0	10.0	14.0	17.5	20.0	23.0
25–34	804	13,003	12.6	6.4	4.5	5.5	6.0	8.0	12.0	16.0	18.5	21.5	24.0
35–44	664	10,676	12.4	5.5	5.0	6.0	7.0	8.5	12.0	15.5	17.5	20.0	23.0
45–54	765	11,150	12.4	5.9	5.0	6.0	7.0	8.0	11.0	15.0	18.0	20.0	25.5
55–64	598	9,073	11.6	5.2	5.0	6.0	6.5	8.0	11.0	14.0	16.5	18.0	21.5
65–74	1,657	5,496	11.8	5.5	4.5	5.5	6.5	8.0	11.0	15.0	17.0	19.0	22.0
WHITE													
	4,344	54,694	12.2	5.8	5.0	6.0	6.5	8.0	11.0	15.0	18.0	20.0	23.0
18–19	203	3,206	11.3	5.9	5.0	5.5	6.0	7.0	9.0	15.0	18.0	20.0	23.0
20–24	423	7,094	11.5	6.0	4.0	5.0	6.0	7.0	10.0	15.0	18.0	21.0	23.0
25–34	672	11,594	12.7	6.2	5.0	6.0	6.5	8.0	12.0	16.0	18.5	21.0	24.0
35–44	569	9,516	12.6	5.4	5.0	6.0	7.0	9.0	12.0	15.5	17.5	20.0	23.0
45–54	628	10,039	12.6	5.9	5.5	6.5	7.0	8.5	11.0	15.0	18.0	20.0	26.0
55–64	505	8,275	11.7	5.0	5.0	6.0	7.0	8.0	11.0	14.0	16.5	18.0	21.0
65–74	1,344	4,970	12.0	5.4	5.0	6.0	7.0	8.0	11.0	15.0	17.0	19.0	22.0
BLACK													
	847	5,753	10.6	7.0	3.5	4.0	4.5	6.0	8.5	13.0	16.0	20.0	23.0
18–19	52	404	8.9	6.7	2.0	4.0	5.0	5.1	7.0	8.0	12.0	21.0	24.0
20–24	80	866	10.0	7.9	3.0	4.0	4.0	6.0	8.0	11.0	13.0	18.0	24.0
25–34	119	1,232	11.8	8.4	4.0	4.0	4.0	5.0	10.0	15.0	20.0	22.0	23.0
35–44	87	1,005	11.3	6.5	4.0	4.5	5.0	7.0	10.0	14.0	17.0	18.4	22.0
45–54	130	1,057	10.0	5.1	4.0	4.0	5.0	6.0	10.0	12.5	14.0	16.0	20.0
55–64	85	703	10.7	7.2	3.0	4.0	4.5	5.0	8.0	14.0	20.0	22.0	26.0
65–74	294	486	9.7	5.4	4.0	4.5	5.0	6.0	9.0	12.0	14.0	15.0	19.5

From the National Center for Health Statistics, Department of Health and Human Services.
*Includes data for races that are not shown separately.

TABLE A-22a
Triceps Skin-fold Thickness: Adult Women, United States, 1971–1974

Race and Age in Years	Number in Sample	Estimated Population in Thousands	Mean	Standard Deviation	Percentile								
					5th	10th	15th	25th	50th	75th	85th	90th	95th
ALL RACES*					*Triceps Skin Fold in Millimeters*								
	8,410	67,837	23.0	8.4	11.0	13.0	14.0	17.0	22.0	28.0	32.0	34.0	37.5
18–19	280	3,679	18.6	6.8	9.0	11.0	12.0	14.0	17.5	22.0	24.0	27.0	32.0
20–24	1,243	9,215	19.7	7.8	10.0	11.0	12.0	14.0	18.0	24.0	27.9	30.5	34.5
25–34	1,896	13,933	21.9	8.2	10.5	12.0	13.5	16.0	21.0	26.5	30.5	33.5	37.0
35–44	1,664	11,593	24.0	8.4	12.0	14.0	16.0	18.0	23.0	29.5	32.5	35.5	39.0
45–54	836	12,163	25.4	8.3	13.0	15.0	17.0	20.0	25.0	30.0	34.0	36.0	40.0
55–64	669	9,976	24.9	8.5	11.0	14.0	16.0	19.0	25.0	30.5	33.0	35.0	39.0
65–74	1,822	7,277	23.3	7.5	11.5	14.0	16.0	18.0	23.0	28.0	31.0	33.0	36.0
WHITE													
	6,757	59,923	22.9	8.1	11.0	13.0	14.5	17.0	22.0	28.0	31.0	34.0	37.0
18–19	208	3,159	18.9	6.6	9.5	12.0	13.0	14.5	18.0	22.5	24.0	26.5	33.5
20–24	956	7,972	19.8	7.7	10.0	11.0	12.0	14.0	19.0	24.0	27.9	30.5	34.0
25–34	1,539	12,161	21.8	8.0	11.0	12.5	14.0	16.0	20.5	26.0	30.0	33.0	36.5
35–44	1,302	10,111	23.7	8.3	12.0	14.0	15.9	18.0	22.5	29.0	32.0	35.1	38.5
45–54	705	10,879	25.3	8.1	13.0	15.0	17.0	20.0	25.0	30.0	33.5	35.5	39.5
55–64	551	9,037	24.6	7.9	11.5	14.5	16.0	19.0	24.0	30.0	33.0	34.1	38.0
65–74	1,496	6,603	23.3	7.3	12.0	14.0	16.0	18.0	23.0	28.0	31.0	33.0	35.5
BLACK													
	1,557	7,302	23.7	10.3	9.0	11.0	12.0	15.5	23.0	30.5	34.0	36.6	41.0
18–19	70	504	16.2	7.3	8.0	9.0	9.0	11.5	14.0	20.0	25.0	29.0	32.0
20–24	259	1,073	19.3	8.7	9.0	10.0	11.5	12.5	17.0	24.5	28.6	32.0	36.0
25–34	335	1,646	22.5	9.6	8.5	10.0	12.0	14.0	22.0	30.0	32.6	34.1	40.0
35–44	334	1,318	25.8	9.2	11.5	13.0	16.0	20.0	25.5	32.0	35.0	36.5	41.0
45–54	126	1,237	26.8	9.8	12.0	14.0	17.0	20.0	26.0	34.0	37.1	40.0	42.2
55–64	115	871	28.2	12.9	10.0	11.0	13.0	19.0	28.0	34.0	40.0	45.0	51.5
65–74	318	652	23.8	9.0	7.5	11.5	15.0	17.5	24.0	30.0	32.2	35.5	40.0

From the National Center for Health Statistics, Department of Health and Human Services.

*Includes data for races that are not shown separately.

TABLE A-23
The Indispensable Nutrients of Human Nutrition

A. *Water*

B. *Chemical elements:*
   Major: Na, K, Cl, Ca, P, Mg, S
   Minor: Fe, Zn, Cu, Mn
   Trace: I, F, Mb, Se, Co, Cr

C. *Amino acids:*
   Leucine, isoleucine, valine, lysine, methionine (spared by cystine), phenylalanine (spared by tyrosine), threonine, tryptophan

   arginine and histidine (conditional on growth in infants and, in adults, for N equilibrium in long-term total parenteral nutrition)

D. *Vitamins:*
   A, D (spared by exposure to sunlight), E, K, ascorbic acid, folacin, niacin (spared by tryptophan), pyridoxine, riboflavin, thiamin, vitamin B_{12}, biotin, pantothenic acid

E. *Essential polyunsaturated fatty acids:*
   Linoleic acid (spared by linolenic and arachidonic acids)

TABLE A-24
Fatty Acid and Cholesterol Content of Foods

Food	Amount	Total Fat (g)	Fatty Acids, g* Saturated	Fatty Acids, g* Polyunsaturated	Cholesterol (mg)
Meat, lean (≤ 3 g fat/oz)	1 oz				
Beef		2.6	0.9	0.1	25
Lamb		2.9	1.2	0.1	28
Pork		2.8	0.8	0.3	25
Veal		3.1	1.3	0.2	28
Poultry (without skin)	1 oz				
Chicken					
Light		1	trace	trace	22
Dark		2.7	0.7	0.5	25
Turkey					
Light		0.7	trace	trace	22
Dark		1.5	0.4	0.3	28
Others: duck, goose, pheasant		2.3	0.5	0.2	25
Finfish	1 oz				
≤ 5% fat		0.5	trace	trace	18
Bass, cod, halibut, haddock, skipjack tuna, sole, red snapper, pike perch					
5–10% fat		2	trace	race	18
Trout; drained anchovy, salmon, albacore, and sardines; mackerel; Atlantic herring					
≥ 12% fat		3.8	0.6	0.6	27
Pacific herring					
Shellfish	1 oz				
< 2% fat		0.5		0.2	15
Abalone, clams, mussels, oysters, scallops					
Crab, lobster		0.5		0.2	26
Shrimp		0.4		0.2	42
Caviar		4.2			84
Organ meats	1 oz				
Heart		1.6	0.5	0.2	77
Liver					
Beef, veal		1.1	0.4	0.2	122
Chicken		1.2	0.5	0.3	208
Brains		2.4	0.6	0.3	560
Sweetbreads		6.5	2.7	0.3	130
Kidney		3.4	1.3	0.5	225
Tongue		4.7	1.6	0.6	25
Giblets		0.9	0.3	0.2	60
Gizzard		0.9	0.3	0.2	55
Meat, medium–fat (≤ 5 g fat/oz): cooked, separable lean	1 oz				
Beef		4.3	1.8	0.2	25
Pork		4	1.3	0.4	25
Meat, high–fat (≥ 10 g fat/oz)	1 oz				
Beef		9	3.7	0.3	26
Pork		8.6	3.3	1.0	25
Lamb (untrimmed)		8.2	3.8	0.5	27
Veal (untrimmed)		7	2.6	0.4	28
Cold cuts		7.6	2.7	0.9	25
Sausage		12.4	4.5	1.5	25
Bacon: cooked, 50% fat	1 slice	3.4	1.3	0.4	3

TABLE A-24
Fatty Acid and Cholesterol Content of Foods (*Continued*)

Food	Amount	Total Fat (g)	Fatty Acids, g*		Cholesterol (mg)
			Saturated	Polyunsaturated	
Dairy products					
Milk	1 cup				
Skim (< 1% fat)		0.2	0.1		4
Buttermilk		0.2	0.1		4
1%		2.4	1.4	trace	7
2%		4.8	2.9	0.2	14
Whole		8.4	5.3	0.3	32
Chocolate					
Skim		5.5	2.2	0.1	16
Whole		8.2	5.2	0.3	32
Yogurt	1 cup				
Part skim milk		2	1.3	0.1	11
Whole milk		8.2	5.3	2.4	32
Processed milk	1 oz				
Condensed		2.4	1.5	0.1	10
Evaporated		2.4	1.4	trace	9
Cottage cheese	1/4 cup (2 oz)				
1%		0.5	0.3	trace	2
2%		1	0.6	trace	3
Regular		2.3	1.4	0.7	7
Cheese	1 oz				
< 1% fat		0.3	0.2	trace	2
Dietetic					
< 10% fat		2.2	1.4	0.1	9
Imitation processed cheese spread					
< 20% fat		4.6	2.9	0.1	18
Farmer, mozzarella (part skim), ricotta					
< 30% fat		7.4	4.7	0.2	27
Pasteurized processed cheese, foods and spreads, Bel Paese, Camembert, Edam, feta, Gouda, Limburger, mozzarella (low-moisture), Neufchâtel, Parmesan, Samsoe, Swiss					
> 30% fat		9.2	5.6	0.3	29
Blue, Brick, cheddar, colby, cream, Muenster, Port du Salut					
Polyunsaturated cheese		6.4	0.8	3.7	1
Cream	1 oz				
Half-and-half		3.3	2.0	0.9	12
Light (sweet or sour)		5.8	3.6	0.2	18
Heavy		10.6	6.6	0.4	38
Whipped (aerosol)		6.5	4.1	0.3	24
Dairy desserts	3 1/2 oz				
Ice milk		5.1	3.2	0.2	14
Ice cream					
Regular		10.6	6.6	0.4	40
Rich		16	10	0.6	57
Ice cream sandwich		8.2	4.7	0.5	40
Butterfat	1 tsp				
Butter		4	2.5	0.2	12
Butter oil		5	3.1	0.2	14
Eggs					
Whole	1				
Small (≤ 40 g)		4.5	1.4	0.5	192
Medium (≤ 44 g)		5	1.5	0.6	222
Large (≤ 50 g)		5.7	1.7	0.6	252
Extra large (≤ 57 g)		6.4	1.9	0.7	281
Yolk	100g	33.5	10.1	3.8	1480

TABLE A-24 (*Continued*)

| Food | Amount | Total Fat (g) | Fatty Acids, g* | | Cholesterol (mg) |
			Saturated	Polyunsaturated	
Fats and oils					
Margarine	1 tsp				
Vegetable (P/S ratio†)					
> 3: *e.g.*, soft safflower		4	0.5	2.3	
2.6–3: *e.g.*, stick safflower		4	0.6	1.7	
2–2.5: *e.g.*, soft corn		4	0.7	1.8	
1.6–1.9: *e.g.*, stick corn		4	0.8	1.3	
1–1.5: *e.g.*, liquid soybean		4	0.9	1.3	
0.5–0.9: *e.g.*, partially hydrogenated oil		4	0.8	0.5	
< 0.5: *e.g.*, hydrogenated oil		4	0.8	0.5	
Vegetable–animal		4	1.7	0.3	4
Animal fats					
Beef	1 tsp				
Tallow		5	2.4	0.2	5
Lard		5	2	0.6	5
Chicken					
Fat	1 tsp	5	1.6	0.8	4
Skin, 35% fat	5g	1.8	0.5	0.5	6
Salt pork, raw	1 oz	23.8	8.5	2.7	19
Mutton	5g	5	2.2	0.4	4
Vegetable oils	1 tsp				
Safflower		5	0.5	3.7	
Sunflower		5	0.5	3.2	
Soybean					
Nonhydrogenated		5	0.8	2.9	
Part hydrogenated		5	0.7	2	
Wheat germ		5	0.9	3	
Corn		5	0.6	2.9	
Sesame		5	0.8	2	
Cottonseed		5	1.3	2.5	
Peanut		5	0.9	1.2	
Olive		5	0.7	0.4	
Palm		5	2.4	0.5	
Cocoa butter		5	3	0.2	
Coconut		5	4.3	0.1	
Soybean lecithin		5	0.8	2.4	
Processed vegetable oils	1 tsp				
Oil blends					
90% sunflower and 10% cottonseed		5	0.6	3.1	
90% soybean and 10% cottonseed		5	0.8	2.8	
50% cottonseed and 50% soybean		5	1.2	2.7	
10% olive and 90% other vegetable		5	0.7	1.8	
Shortenings					
All vegetable		5	1.6	1	
Vegetable–animal		5	2.1	0.5	3
Dressings					
Mayonnaise		4	0.6	2.3	4
Mayonnaise-type		2.1	0.3	1.1	2.5
Salad					
All creamy: *e.g.*, French, garlic		2	0.3	1.1	
Creamy with egg or mayonnaise or both: *e.g.*, tartar sauce, Thousand Island		2.5	0.4	1.3	3
Clear: *e.g.*, French, Italian		3	0.5	1.7	
Sandwich spread		2.5	0.3	1.5	2.6
Meat substitutes					
Meat loaf	1 oz	2.5	0.4	1.4	
Sausage, piece					
Link	23 g	4.3	1	1.6	

TABLE A-24
Fatty Acid and Cholesterol Content of Foods (*Continued*)

Food	Amount	Total Fat (g)	Saturated	Polyunsaturated	Cholesterol (mg)
			Fatty Acids, g*		
Patty	38 g	7.2	1.5	2.6	
Ham, slice	1 oz	2.4	0.4	0.8	
Frankfurter	1 oz	5.5	0.8	2.9	
Textured vegetable protein	1 oz	2	0.3	1.1	
Nuts	1/2 oz				
Peanuts					
Runner		7.6	1.3	2.1	
Virginia		7.1	1.2	1.8	
Spanish		7.4	1.4	2.4	
Unspecified		7.3	1.3	2	
Almonds		8.1	0.6	1.5	
Brazil nuts		10.2	2.6	3.8	
Cashews		6.8	1.4	1.1	
Chestnuts		0.4	trace	0.2	
Filberts		9.7	0.7	1	
Macadamia nuts		11.3	1.5	0.2	
Pecans		10.6	0.9	2.7	
Pistachios		8.1	1.1	1.1	
Walnuts					
English		9.6	1	6.1	
Black		8.9	0.7	4.9	
Peanut butter	2 tbsp				
Hydrogenated		14.4	2.9	4.2	
Unhydrogenated		13.8	2.5	4.1	
Avocado, 50 g	1/4	8.2	1.2	0.9	
Coconut: shredded, sweetened	1 tbsp	5.3	4.7	1	
Olives	1/2 oz				
Green		3.6	0.5	0.3	
Black		3.9	0.5	0.3	
Cereal products					
Bread, all varieties	1 slice	0.8	0.2	0.3	
Bagel, small	1/2				
Plain		2	0.3	0.9	
Egg		2	0.3	0.9	28
English muffin	1/2	0.9	0.2	trace	
Roll	1	0.8	0.2	0.3	
Bun, frankfurter or hamburger	1/2	1.5	0.6	0.2	
Cereals					
Dry	3/4 cup	trace	trace	trace	
Cooked	1/2 cup	trace	trace	trace	
Pasta	1/2 cup				
Plain		trace			
Egg		2	0.2	0.2	31
Wheat germ	1/4 cup	2.5	0.5	1.6	
Crackers	5				
Low-fat (< 12%)					
Saltines		< 1	< 0.7	0.2	
High-fat (> 12%)					
Ritz		3.2	1.3	0.4	3
Prepared foods					
Biscuit	1 oz	2	‡	‡	
Corn bread, small	1 oz	2.8	‡	‡	

TABLE A-24 (*Continued*)

Food	Amount	Total Fat (g)	Fatty Acids, g* Saturated	Fatty Acids, g* Polyunsaturated	Cholesterol (mg)
Muffin, small	1 oz	2.1	‡	‡	
Potatoes, fried	1 oz	5	‡	‡	
Potato chips	1 oz	11	‡	‡	
Pancake, 4 in round	1 oz	2	‡	‡	
Waffle, 4 1/2 in sq	1 1/2 oz	5	‡	‡	

From the Committee on Dietetics of the Mayo Clinic: Mayo Clinic Diet Manual, pp 284–289. Philadelphia, WB Saunders, 1981.

*Polyunsaturated fats include all unsaturated fats with two or more double bonds. Monounsaturated fats (one double bond) are not listed in the table because they do not affect serum lipids and are not used in calculating the ratio of polyunsaturated to saturated fat (P/S ratio).

†Check label for content of saturates, polyunsaturates, and cholesterol.

‡Fatty acid content depends on type of fat used in preparation.

Selected Bibliography

Comprehensive evaluation of fatty acids in foods (series), J Am Diet Assoc

    I. Dairy products (Posati L P, Kinsella J E, Watt B K). 66:482–488, 1975
    II. Beef products (Anderson B A, Kinsella J E, Watt B K). 67:35–41, 1975
    III. Eggs and egg products (Posati L P, Kinsella J E, Watt B K). 67:111–115, 1975
    IV. Nuts, peanuts, and soups (Fristrom G A, Stewart B C, Weihrauch J L, et al). 67:351–355, 1975
    V. Unhydrogenated fats and oils (Brignoli C A, Kinsella J E, Weihrauch J L). 68:224–229, 1976
    VI Cereal products (Weihrauch J L, Kinsella J E, Watt B K). 68:335–340, 1976
    VII. Pork products (Anderson B A). 69:44–49, 1976
    VIII. Finfish (Exler J, Weihrauch J L). 69:243–248, 1976
    IX. Fowl (Fristrom G A, Weihrauch J L). 69:517–522, 1976
    X. Lamb and veal (Anderson B A, Fristrom G A, Weihrauch J L). 70:53–58, 1977
    XI. Leguminous seeds (Exler J, Avena R M, Weihrauch J L). 71:412–415, 1977
    XII. Shellfish (Exler J, Weihrauch J L). 71:518–521, 1977

Adams CF: Nutritive Value of American Foods in Common Units. Agriculture Handbook No. 456. Washington DC, United States Department of Agriculture, 1975

Feeley RM, Criner PE, Watt BK: Cholesterol content of foods, J Am Diet Assoc 61:134–149, 1972

Nazir DJ, Moorecroft BJ, Mishkel MA: Fatty acid composition of margarines. Am J Clin Nutr 29:331–339, 1976.

TABLE A-25
Sodium and Potassium Content of Foods

Food	Amount	Sodium, mEq	Potassium, mEq
Meat and meat substitutes			
Bacon	1 strip	2	trace
Beef potpie, commercial	1	38	5
Beef stew, canned	1 cup	43	10
Casserole, commercial	1 cup	39	11
Cheese, cheddar type	1 oz	9	1
Cheese, processed American	1 oz	15	1
Cheese, processed spread	1 oz	21	2
Chili, canned	1 cup	23	6
Chow mein	1/2 cup	12.5	4
Cold cuts	1 oz	16	2
Corned beef	1 oz	23	1
Dried beef	1 oz	56	2
Fish sticks	1 oz	3	2.5
Frankfurter	1	24	3
Ham	1 oz	14	3
Kosher meat	1 oz	4	2
Peanut butter, regular	2 tbsp	8	5
Peanuts, salted	3/4 cup	18	17
Pizza	1/4 of 16 oz	29	3
Salmon, regular, canned	1/4 cup	7	3
Sardines	1 oz	11	4.5
Sausage, link	2	16.5	3
Sausage, patty	1 oz	12.5	2
Soup, canned, undiluted	1/2 cup	37	3
Spaghetti sauce, canned	1/2 cup	18	4
Tuna, regular, canned	1/4 cup	10	2
TV dinner	10–12 oz	47	*
Fats			
Gravy	2 tbsp	10	*
Olives	3	31	0.5
Salad dressing	1 tbsp	8	1
Milk			
Buttermilk	1 cup	14	8
Starches			
Crackers, saltines	5	7	0.5
Crackers, snack	6	10	0.5
Popcorn, salted	1 cup	15	
Potato chips	1 oz	14	10
Potatoes, packaged	1/2 cup	22	10
Pretzels, round, ring	6–15	14	0.5
Pretzels, very thin	60	28	0.5
Vegetables			
Frozen combination vegetables with sauce	1/3 cup	13	5
Sauerkraut	1/2 cup	33	4
Tomato juice, canned	1/2 cup	9	23
Tomato paste	1 tbsp	3	4
Tomato sauce	1/2 cup	36	11
Desserts			
Cake, commercial	1 piece	6	2
Cookies, commercial	1	3	1
Ice cream	1 cup	4	6
Pie, commercial	1/6 of 9-in pie	20	4
Pudding, commercial	1/2 cup	6	4

TABLE A-25 (*Continued*)

Food	Amount	Sodium, mEq	Potassium, mEq
Miscellaneous			
Baking powder	1 tsp	14	
Baking soda	1 tsp	59	
Barbecue sauce	1 tbsp	10	1
Bouillon	1 cube	52	trace
Catsup, mustard	1 tbsp	8	1
Cheese sauce, packaged	1/4 cup	29	trace
Cocoa mixes	1 tbsp	1.6	2.5
Coconut	2 tbsp	0.1	3
Meat and vegetable sauces, packaged	1/4 cup	13	1
Monosodium glutamate	1 tsp	33	
Pickles, dill	1 large	62	5
Pickles, dill	1 small	19	1.5
Salt	1 tsp	92	trace
Salt substitutes	1 tsp		50–65
Soft water	1 liter	5–8	
Soy sauce	1 tsp	16	

From the Committee on Dietetics of the Mayo Clinic: Mayo Clinic Diet Manual, pp 290, 291. Philadelphia, WB Saunders, 1981

*Data not available

Selected Bibliography

Adams CF: Nutritive Value of American Foods in Common Units. Agriculture Handbook No 456. Washington, DC, United States Department of Agriculture, 1975

Kraus B: The Dictionary of Sodium, Fats, and Cholesterol. New York, Grosset & Dunlap, 1974

Church CF, Church HN (eds): Bowes and Church's Food Values of Portions Commonly Used, 12th ed. Philadelphia, JB Lippincott, 1975

TABLE A-26
Calcium and Phosphorus Content of Foods

Food	Amount	Calcium, mg	Phosphorus, mg
Meat, fish, poultry			
Beef	1 oz	3	56
Pork	1 oz	3	70
Chicken	1 oz	4	74
Liver	1 oz	4	137
Fish, average	1 oz	12	76
Tuna	1/4 cup	2	95
Sardines, canned, with bones	1 oz	86	101
Salmon, canned, with bones	1 oz	74	98
Luncheon meat	1 oz	3	53
Bacon, strip	1–5 g	1	11
Meat substitutes			
Eggs	1	28	90
Dried beans, average, cooked	1/2 cup	44	144
Lentils, cooked	1/2 cup	25	119
Peanuts and peanut butter	1 tbsp	11	60
Milk	1 cup		
Whole milk		290	227
2% milk		297	232
Skim milk		302	247
Buttermilk		285	219
Chocolate milk		280	251
Hot cocoa		298	270

TABLE A-26
Calcium and Phosphorus Content of Foods (*Continued*)

Food	Amount	Calcium, mg	Phosphorus, mg
Other dairy products			
Yogurt, plain, low-fat	8 oz	415	326
Cheddar cheese	1 oz	204	145
Swiss cheese	1 oz	272	171
Processed American cheese	1 oz	174	211
Cottage cheese, creamed	1/4 cup	31	69
Half-and-half	2 tbsp	32	28
Vanilla ice cream	1/2 cup	88	67
Sherbet	1/2 cup	51	37
Cereal and grain products			
Bread, white	1 slice	21	24
Bread, whole wheat	1 slice	23	52
Bread products made from white flour			
Biscuit	2-in diameter	42	61
Doughnut, cake	1 average	13	61
Doughnut, raised	1 average	11	23
Pancake	4-in diameter	45	63
Sweet roll	1 average	35	57
Waffle	5-in diameter	85	130
Cereal, refined	1/2 cup cooked; 3/4 cup dry	35	57
Cereal, whole grain	1/2 cup cooked; 3/4 cup dry	14	109
Crackers, saltines	5 2-in squares	2	15
Crackers, graham	2 2 1/2 in squares	6	21
Macaroni; spaghetti; noodles	1/2 cup cooked	8	47
Rice	1/2 cup cooked	7	21
Vegetables	100 g (approx) 1/2 cup cooked		
Artichokes		51	69
Asparagus		21	50
Bean sprouts		17	48
Broccoli		88	62
Brussels sprouts		32	72
Cabbage		44	20
Corn		4	48
Cress		61	48
Greens			
Beet greens		99	25
Collards		152	39
Dandelion greens		140	42
Kale		134	46
Mustard greens		183	50
Spinach		98	30
Swiss chard		73	24
Turnip greens		184	37
Leeks		52	50
Lima beans		47	121
Mushrooms		6	116
Okra		92	41
Parsnips		45	62
Peas		20	66
Potatoes, white		9	65
Rutabagas		59	31
Winter squash		28	48
Other vegetables, average		25	26

TABLE A-26 (*Continued*)

Food	Amount	Calcium, mg	Phosphorus, mg
Fruit			
Blackberries	5/8 cup	32	19
Orange	1 small	41	20
Raspberries	2/3 cup	30	22
Rhubarb	3/8 cup	78	15
Tangerine	1 large	40	18
Fresh fruit, average	1/2 cup or 1 medium	16	20
Canned fruit, average	1/2 cup	10	12
Fruit juice	1/2 cup	10	13
Fats and oils			
Butter or margarine	1 tsp	1	1
Nondairy cream substitute, nondairy powder	1 tsp	trace	8
French dressing	1 tbsp	2	2
Gravy	1 tbsp		2
Mayonnaise	1 tsp	1	1
Sweets			
Candy, sugar	1/2 oz		
Candy, milk chocolate	1/2 oz	26	28
Honey	1 tbsp	4	3
Jelly	1 tbsp	2	2
Sugar, white	1 tbsp		
Sugar, brown	1 tbsp	9	6
Syrup, maple	1 tbsp	33	3
Desserts			
Assorted cookies	1 2-in	7	32
Cake, white	2 in by 3 in by 2 in	34	46
Pie, cream	1/8 of 9-in pie	62	88
Pie, fruit	1/8 of 9-in pie	23	30
Snack foods			
Popcorn	1 cup	2	39
Potato chips	5	3	15
Beverages			
Beer	8 oz	10	62
Carbonated beverages			
Colas, average	8 oz	7	42
Ginger ale, average	8 oz	3	
Coffee	6 oz	5	5
Tea	6 oz	5	4

From the Committee on Dietetics of the Mayo Clinic: Mayo Clinic Diet Manual, pp 292–294. Philadelphia, WB Saunders, 1981

Selected Bibliography

Adams CF: Nutritive Value of American Foods in Common Units. Agriculture Handbook No. 456. Washington, DC, United States Department of Agriculture, 1975

Church, CF, Church HN (eds): Bowes and Church's Food Values of Portions Commonly Used, 12th ed. Philadelphia, JB Lippincott, 1975

United States Agriculture Research Service, Consumer Food Economics Institute: Composition of Foods: Dairy and Egg Products; Raw, Processed, Prepared. Agriculture Handbook No 8-1. Washington DC, United States Department of Agriculture, 1976

TABLE A-27
Conversion of Milligrams to Milliequivalents

To convert milligrams (mg) to milliequivalents (mEq):

$$\frac{\text{Milligrams}}{\text{Atomic weight}} \times \text{Valence} = \text{Milliequivalents}$$

Mineral Element	Chemical Symbol	Atomic Weight	Valence
Chlorine	Cl	35.4	1
Potassium	K	39	1
Sodium	Na	23	1
Calcium	Ca	40	2
Magnesium	Mg	24.3	2
Sulfur	S	32	
Sulfate	SO_4	96	2

To convert specific weight of sodium to sodium chloride:

Milligrams of sodium $\times$ 2.54 = Milligrams of sodium chloride

To convert specific weight of sodium chloride to sodium:

Milligrams of sodium chloride $\times$ 0.393 = Milligrams of sodium

Sodium Milligrams	Sodium Milliequivalents	Sodium Chloride Grams
500	21.8	1.3
1000	43.5	2.5
1500	75.3	3.8
2000	87	5

From the Committee on Dietetics of the Mayo Clinic: Mayo Clinic Diet Manual, p 304. Philadelphia, WB Saunders, 1981

TABLE A-28
Acid–Base Reaction of Foods

POTENTIALLY ACID OR ACID–ASH FOODS:

Meat	Meat; fish; fowl; shellfish; eggs; all types of cheese; peanut butter; peanuts
Fat	Bacon; nuts (Brazil nuts, filberts, walnuts)
Starch	All types of bread (especially whole wheat), cereals, and crackers; macaroni; spaghetti; noodles; rice
Vegetable	Corn; lentils
Fruit	Cranberries; plums; prunes
Dessert	Plain cakes; cookies

POTENTIALLY BASIC OR ALKALINE–ASH FOODS:

Milk	Milk and milk products; cream; buttermilk
Fat	Nuts (almonds, chestnuts, coconut)
Vegetable	All types (except corn, lentils), especially beets, beet greens, Swiss chard, dandelion greens, kale, mustard greens, spinach, turnip greens
Fruit	All types (except cranberries, prunes, plums)
Sweets	Molasses

NEUTRAL FOODS:

Fats	Butter; margarine; cooking fats; oils
Sweets	Plain candies; sugar; syrup; honey
Starch	Arrowroot; corn; tapioca
Beverages	Coffee; tea

From the Committee on Dietetics of the Mayo Clinic: Mayo Clinic Diet Manual, p 124. Philadelphia, WB Saunders, 1981

TABLE A-29
Crude Fiber Content of Selected Foods

	Grams Per Serving			
	< 0.2	0.2 to 1 (avg, 0.6)	1 to 2 (avg, 1.5)	> 2
Fruit (1/2 cup or 1 medium)	Juice	Applesauce Apricots Banana Cantaloupe Cherries Fruit cocktail Grapefruit Grapes Honeydew melon Nectarine Orange Peaches Pears without skin Pineapple Plums Raisins Strawberries Watermelon	Apples with skin Avocado Blueberries Dates Figs Pears with skin Prunes Raspberries	Blackberries
Vegetables (1/2 cup)	Juice	Asparagus Bean sprouts Beets Cabbage Carrots Cauliflower Celery Collards Corn Cucumber Dandelion greens Eggplant Green pepper Kale Kohlrabi Lettuce Mushrooms Mustard greens Okra Onions Potatoes Radishes Sauerkraut Spinach Split peas String beans: green, yellow Summer squash Sweet potatoes Tomatoes Turnip greens Turnips	Baked beans Beet greens Black beans Broccoli Brussels sprouts Chick-peas Kidney beans Lentils Lima beans Parsnips Peas Pinto beans Pumpkin Rutabaga Winter squash	Artichoke
Bread* (1 slice)	Cracked wheat French Rye White	Pumpernickel Raisin Whole wheat		

TABLE A-29
Crude Fiber Content of Selected Foods (*Continued*)

	Grams Per Serving			
	< 0.2	0.2 to 1 (avg, 0.6)	1 to 2 (avg, 1.5)	> 2
Cereals, cooked (1/2 cup)	Cream of Rice Cream of Wheat Farina Maltex	Oatmeal Wheatena		
Cereals, ready-to-eat (1 oz = 1/4 to 1 1/4 cup)	Puffed corn Puffed rice	Cornflakes Granola Raisin bran Shredded wheat Wheat flakes Wheat germ	Bran flakes	100% bran cereals
Crackers (20 g = 2 to 4 crackers)	Saltines Soda crackers	Graham crackers Rye wafers Whole wheat crackers		
Snack foods	Popcorn (1 cup) Pretzels (10 medium)	Corn chips (10 medium) Potato chips (10 medium)		
Other starches (1/2 cup)	Grits Macaroni Noodles Spaghetti White rice	Barley Brown rice		
Flours (1 cup)	Wheat, cake or pastry	Cornmeal, degermed Rye, light Wheat, all purpose	Cornmeal, whole, ground	Whole rye Whole wheat
Nuts and seeds (1/4 cup)		Almonds Cashews Peanuts Pecans Pumpkin seeds Walnuts	Brazil nuts Coconut Roasted soybeans Sunflower seeds	

From the Committee on Dietetics of the Mayo Clinic: Mayo Clinic Diet Manual, pp 140, 141. Philadelphia, WB Saunders, 1981; based on data from Watt BK, Merrill AL: Composition of Foods: Raw, Processed, Prepared. Agriculture Handbook No. 8. Washington, DC, United States Department of Agriculture, United States Agricultural Research Service, 1963. These are the most recent and nearly complete data available.

*Several so-called high-fiber breads are on the market. Generally, they contain added cellulose and have a crude fiber content of 1.5–2 g, whereas whole wheat bread contains approximately 0.4 g crude fiber per slice.

TABLE A-30
Components of Dietary Fiber

Fraction	*Principal Constituents*
ACCEPTED BY MOST INVESTIGATORS	
Celluloses ⎫ crude fiber	Cell wall polysaccharides, unbranched glucose polymers
Lignins ⎬	Non-carbohydrate cell wall material, phenylpropane polymers
Hemicelluloses	Cell wall polysaccharides derived from various pentoses and hexoses
Pectins	Cell wall galacturonic acid polymers with pentose and hexose side chains
ADDITIONAL SUBSTANCES ACCEPTED BY SOME INVESTIGATORS	
Gums	Non-cell wall, complex polysaccharides containing glucuronic and galacturonic acids, xylose, arabinose, mannose
Mucilages	Non-cell wall, complex polysaccharides some of which are also storage polysaccharides (*e.g*, guar)
Algal polysaccharides	Highly complex polymers
RECENTLY SUGGESTED ADDITIONS	
Indigestible storage polysaccharides	
Indigestible plant protein	
Fungal chitins	
Associated indigestible minerals, waxes, other substances	

From Talbot JM: Role of dietery fiber in diverticular disease and colon cancer. Fed Proc 40:2338, 1981

TABLE A-31
Nutritive Value of Desserts and Snack Foods

Food	Amount	Protein g	Fat g	Carbohydrate g	Calories
Bread					
Coffee cake	4 1/2 in diameter	3	5	26	160
Sweet roll	1 average	5	4	30	175
Cake	1 piece				
Chocolate, iced	2 in by 3 in by 2 in	2	5	33	185
Pound cake	3 in by 3 in by 1/2 in	3	9	27	200
White, iced	2 in by 3 in by 2 in	2	5	30	175
Candy	About 1 oz				
Bar candy, chocolate covered	1 oz	3	8	20	165
Butterscotch	6 pieces		3	24	125
Caramels	3 medium	1	3	22	120
Chocolate					
Creams	2 average	1	4	18	110
Fudge	1 1/4-in sq	1	3	24	127
Mints	3 small	1	4	23	130
Hard candy	6 squares			30	120
Peanut brittle	2 1/2-in sq	2	4	18	115
Cookies	1				
Assorted	2-in diameter	1	4	14	95
Brownies	2-in square	2	10	15	160
Doughnuts	1				
Cake, plain		2	6	16	125
Yeast-leavened, plain		2	8	11	125
Pudding	1/2 cup				
Chocolate		3	5	26	160
Custard		3	4	23	140
Vanilla		4	4	16	115
Pie	1/6 of 9-in pie				
Chiffon		7	13	45	325
Cream		7	15	60	400
Custard		9	15	35	310
Fruit		4	15	60	390
Soup	1 cup				
Bean		6	2	26	145
Beef		6	4	12	110
Cream		7	12	18	210
Vegetable		4	2	14	90

From the Committee on Dietetics of the Mayo Clinic: Mayo Clinic Diet Manual, p 295. Philadelphia, WB Saunders, 1981

Selected Bibliography

Adams CF: Nutritive Value of American Foods in Common Units. Agriculture Handbook No. 456. Washington, D C, United States Department of Agriculture, 1975

Church CF, Church HN (eds): Bowes and Church's Food Values of Portions Commonly Used, 12th ed. Philadelphia, JB Lippincott, 1975

TABLE A-32
Nutritive Value of Alcoholic and Carbonated Beverages

Beverage	Amount	Calories	Carbohydrate, g	Alcohol,* g
Alcoholic beverages				
Beer	8 oz	100	9	9
Brandy	Brandy glass	75		11
Gin; rum; vodka; whiskey	1 jigger			
80 proof		70		10
90 proof		80		11
100 proof		90		13
Liqueurs, average	Cordial glass	65	6	7
Wines	3 1/2 oz			
Champagne		75	3	10
Muscatel		160	14	15
Sauterne		85	4	10
Table wine		85		10
Vermouth, French		105	1	15
Vermouth, Italian		165	12	18
Carbonated beverages	1 cup			
Carbonated waters				
(sweetened quinine soda)		75	19	
Colas		95	24	
Ginger ale		75	19	
Root beer		100	25	
Soda, cream or fruit-flavored		105	26	

From the Committee on Dietetics of the Mayo Clinic: Mayo Clinic Diet Manual, p 296. Philadelphia, WB Saunders, 1981
*Alcohol calculated as 7 Cal/g

Caloric Value of Alcoholic Beverages

The caloric contribution of an alcoholic beverage can be estimated by multiplying the number of ounces by the proof and then again by the factor 0.08. For beers and wines, calories can be estimated by multiplying ounces by percentage of alcohol and then by the factor 1.6.

Selected Bibliography

Adams CF: Nutritive Value of American Foods in Common Units. Agriculture Handbook No. 456. Washington, DC, United States Department of Agriculture, 1975
Church CF, Church HN (eds): Bowes and Church's Food Values of Portions Commonly Used, 12th ed. Philadelphia, JB Lippincott, 1975
Gastineau CF: Alcohol and calories. Mayo Clin Proc 51:88, 1976

TABLE A-33
Caffeine Content of Selected Beverages

Beverage	Caffeine, mg/5-oz cup
Coffee, percolated	110
Coffee, drip	146
Instant coffee	66
Decaffeinated coffee	3
Tea, black	28–46
Tea, green	20–35
Instant tea	20–58
Cocoa beverages	4
Some carbonated beverages	
(usually colas)	32–65*

Adapted from the Committee on Dietetics of the Mayo Clinic: Mayo Clinic Diet Manual, p 297. Philadelphia, WB Saunders, 1981

*Per 12-oz can

Selected Bibliography

Bunker ML, McWilliams M: Caffeine content of common beverages J Am Diet Assoc 74:28–32, 1979
Graham DM: Caffeine—its identity, dietary sources, intake and biological effects. Nutr Rev 36:97–102, 1978
Zoumas BL, Kreiser WR, Martin RA: Theobromine and caffeine content of chocolate products. J Food Sci 45:314–316, 1980

TABLE A-34
Composition of Pediatric Formulas

Product	Description and use	Cal/oz	Renal solute load	Osmolarity mOsm/kg	Carbohydrate source	Fat source	Nitrogen source
Advance (Ross)		16	182	230	Lactose and corn syrup solids	Soy and corn oil	Cow's milk, soy isolate
Enfamil (Mead Johnson)	Infant formula for routine feeding	20	110	262	Lactose	80% soy oil, 20% coconut oil	Cow's milk protein
Enfamil Premature Formula (Mead Johnson)	Low birth weight	24	220	264	Glucose polymers, lactose	MCT, corn oil, coconut oil	Whey, skim milk (60% lactalbumin, 40% whey)
Isomil (Ross)	Cow's milk protein intolerance	20	126	228	Corn syrup solids and sucrose	Coconut, soy oils	Soy isolate
Lofenalac (Mead Johnson)	Proved phenylketonuria	20	130	407	Corn syrup solids, tapioca starch	Corn oil	Hydrolyzed casein
Lytren (Mead Johnson)	Oral fluid and electrolyte therapy	10	80	267	Glucose, corn syrup solids	None	None
MBF (Meat-Based Formula); (Gerber)	Galactosemia; cow's milk protein allergy	20	176	NA	Sucrose, tapioca starch	Animal fat, sesame oil	Beef hearts
Milk, cow's	Not recommended for routine infant feeding until 6–12 months of age	20	232	260	Lactose	Butterfat	Cow's milk
Milk, skim		11	242	290	Lactose	Butterfat	Cow's milk
Milk, cow's, 2% low-fat		18	289	350	Lactose	Butterfat	Cow's milk
Milk, human	Routine infant feeding	22	79	273	Lactose	Human milk	Human milk (60% lactalbumin, 40% casein)
Nursoy (Wyeth)	Cow's milk protein allergy	20	131	NA	Corn syrup solids, sucrose	Oleo; coconut, safflower, and soybean oils	Soy protein isolate
Nutramigen (Mead Johnson)	Protein hydrolysate formula; protein allergy or intolerance; malabsorption, celiac disease, galactosemia, diarrhea	20	130	397	Sucrose, tapioca starch	Corn oil	Casein hydrolysate
Oral Electrolyte Solution (Wyeth)	Oral fluid and electrolyte therapy	10	80	517	Glucose	None	None
Pedialyte (Ross)	Oral fluid and electrolyte therapy	6	80	376	Glucose	None	None

TABLE A-34 (*Continued*)

												Ca	P	
						Composition/liter								
Protein		Fat		CHO		Na		K						
g	Cal	g	cal	g	cal	mg	mEq	mg	mEq			(mg)	(mg)	Comments
28	20	20	34	62	46	450	20	1100	28			800	500	
15	9	37	50	70	41	276	12	690	18			540	460	Also available with iron, 13.6 mg/L
24	12	41	44	89	44	317	14	896	23			950	476	1.7 mg vitamin E/g linoleic acid; iron, 1.3 mg/liter
20	12	36	48	68	40	300	13	710	18			700	500	
22	13	27	35	88	52	313	14	677	16			625	470	Phenylalanine, 113 mg/liter; incomplete; requires careful management of phenylalanine levels
0	0	0	0	79	100	690	30	875	25			160	155	Nutritionally incomplete
27	16	32	48	60	36	171	7	360	9			937	625	Additional carbohydrates required
36	21	36	49	50	30	515	22	1490	38			1220	960	Requires supplementation with iron
38	40	1	2	54	58	540	24	1510	39			1260	990	Not recommended for infants
44	26	21	31	64	41	1850	48	1850	48			1520	1190	Recommended after age 2 in familial hyperlipidemias
11	6	45	55	72	390	160	7	510	13			340	140	Represents the standard against which artificial formulas are compared; nutritionally complete
23	13	36	50	68	37	201	9	741	19			634	444	
22	13	26	35	88	52	313	14	677	16			625	470	
0	0	0	0	75	100	690	30	780	20			140	155	Nutritionally incomplete
0	0	0	0	50	100	690	30	780	20			900	0	Nutritionally incomplete

TABLE A-34
Composition of Pediatric Formulas (*Continued*)

Product	Description and use	Cal/oz	Renal solute load	Osmolarity mOsm/kg	Carbohydrate source	Fat source	Nitrogen source
Pregestimil (Mead Johnson)	Malabsorption, cow's milk protein allergy or intolerance, diarrhea, celiac disease, cystic fibrosis	20	130	449	Glucose, tapioca starch, corn syrup solids	MCT oil, corn oil	Casein hydrolysate
Probana (Mead Johnson)	Celiac syndrome, systic fibrosis	20	250	531	Banana powder, glucose	Corn oil, butterfat	Casein hydrolysate, milk protein
ProSobee (Mead Johnson)	Infant formula for routine feeding in cow's milk protein allergy or intolerance, lactose intolerance, diarrhea galactosemia	20	150	233	Sucrose, corn syrup solids (glucose and complex glucose forms)	Soybean oil	Soy protein isolate
S-14 (Wyeth)	For infants with leucine-sensitive hypoglycemia	20	73	NA	Lactose	Oleo; coconut, safflower, soybean oil	Cow's milk
S-29 (Wyeth)	Low renal solute load; for heart failure, renal disease, diabetes insipidus	20	77	NA	Lactose	Oleo; coconut, safflower, soybean oil	Demineralized whey
S-44 (Wyeth)	Low renal solute load; for infants with severe hypercalcemia	20	77	NA	Lactose	Oleo; coconut, safflower, soybean oil	Demineralized whey
Similac (Ross)	Routine infant feeding	20	108	262	Lactose	Coconut, soy oils	Cow's milk protein
Similac 24 LBW (Ross)	Premature infants	24	154	256	Lactose and corn syrup solids	MCT, coconut, soy oils	Cow's milk
Similac PM 60/40 (Ross)	Premature infants	20	92	239	Lactose	Coconut, corn oil	Cow's milk and whey (60% lactalbumin, 40% casein)
SMA (Wyeth)	Routine infant feeding	20	91	271	Lactose	Oleo; coconut, safflower, soy oil	Cow's milk and whey (60% lactalbumin, 40% casein)

TABLE A-34 (*Continued*)

						Composition/liter						
Protein		Fat		CHO		Na		K		Ca	P	
g	Cal	g	cal	g	cal	mg	mEq	mg	mEq	(mg)	(mg)	Comments
22	13	28	35	88	52	313	14	677	16	625	470	Initial feeding of 333 Cal/liter recommended
42	24	22	29	79	47	600	26	1200	34	1155	893	
25	15	34	15	68	40	416	18	730	19	780	520	Nutritionally complete
11	6	37	53	71	41	158	7	476	12	423	317	Low but apparently adequate levels of leucine
17	10	23	33	101	57	10	<1	317	8	138	169	Mineral content inadequate for growth and development
17	10	23	33	101	57	10	<1	317	8	138	169	Same as S-29 but without added vitamins
16	9	36	48	72	48	250	11	780	20	510	390	Also available in 24- and 27-Cal/oz concentrations: also available with iron, 12 mg/liter
22	11	45	47	85	42	370	16	1000	26	730	560	
16	9	38	50	69	41	160	7	580	15	400	200	
15	9	36	48	72	43	150	6	560	14	440	550	Also available in 13-, 24-, and 27-Cal/oz concentrations; only available with iron, 13.6 mg/liter

From Weinsier R, Butterworth CE Jr: Handbook of Clinical Nutrition, pp 86–89. St Louis, CV Mosby, 1981

TABLE A-35
Intravenous Fat Emulsions

Product:	Intralipid	Liposyn
Manufacturer:	Cutter	Abbott
Concentration:	10%	10%
Fat source: *Component fatty acids:*	Soybean oil (10%) Linoleic (54%) Oleic (26%) Palmitic (9%) Linolenic (8%)	Safflower oil (10%) Linoleic (77%) Oleic (13%) Palmitic (9%) Stearic (2.5%)
Other additives:	Egg yolk phospholipid (1.2%) Glycerin (2.25%) Water	Egg yolk phospholipid (1.2%) Glycerin (2.5%) Water
Cal/ml:	1.1	1.1
Osmolarity (mOsm/liter):	280	300
Fat particle size(μ):	0.5	0.4

TABLE A-36
Recommended Intravenous Vitamin Allowances, with Vitamin Contents of Commercial Preparations

	Recommended daily allowance (per kg body weight)		*MVI (Multivitamin infusion) concentrate (2.5 ml)*	*Berocca-C (2 ml)*	*Folbesyn (2 ml)*	*Betalin Complex F.C. (2 ml)*	*Solu-B-Forte (1 ml)*
	Newborns and Infants	*Adults*					
Thiamin (mg)	0.05	0.02	25	10	10	12.5	25
Riboflavin (mg)	0.1	0.03	5	10	10	3	5
Niacin (mg)	1	0.2	50	80	75	50	125
Pyridoxine (mg)	0.1	0.03	7.5	20	5	5	5
Vitamin B_{12} (μg)	0.2	0.03	—	—	15	—	—
Folate (μg)	20	3	—	—	3,000	—	—
Pantothenate (mg)	1	0.2	12.5	20	10	2.5	50
Biotin (μg)	30	5	—	200	—	—	—
Ascorbate (mg)	3	0.5	250	100	300	75	100
Vitamin A (μg)	100	10	1,500	—	—	—	—
D_3 Cholecalciferol (μg)	2.5	0.04	12.5	—	—	—	—
Vitamin E (mg)	3	1.5	2.5	—	—	—	—
Vitamin K (μg)	50	2	—	—	—	—	—

From Butterworth C E Jr, Weinsier R: Handbook of Clinical Nutrition, pp 96, 97. St. Louis, C V Mosby, 1981; based on data from Wretlind A: Nutr Metab 14(Suppl):1, 1972

TABLE A-37
Approximate Daily Adult and Pediatric Requirements for Minerals During Complete Parenteral Alimentation

Mineral	*Child*	*Adult*
Sodium	3–5 mEq/kg	60+ mEq
Potassium	2–5 mEq/kg	60+ mEq
Calcium	1–4 mEq/kg	10–15 mEq
Phosphate	0.7–3 mmol/kg	20–50 mmol
Magnesium	0.3–2 mEq/kg	8–20 mEq

From Butterworth C E Jr, Weinsier R: Handbook of Clinical Nutrition, p 98. St. Louis, C V Mosby, 1981

Table A-38
Guidelines for Essential Trace Elements for Daily Parenteral Use

Element	Child (Stable)	Adult		
		Stable	Acutely Catabolic	With Gastrointestinal Losses
Zinc	100–300 μg/kg*	2.5–4. mg	4.5–6 mg	Add 12 mg/liter small bowel fluid loss; 17 mg/liter
Copper	20 μg/kg	0.5–1.5 mg	NA†	diarrheal fluid
Chromium	0.14–0.2 μg/kg	10–15 μg	NA	NA
Manganese	2–10 μg/kg	0.15–0.8 mg	NA	20 μg
Iodine	5 μg/kg	50–100 μg	NA	NA
				NA

From Department of Foods and Nutrition Advisory Group: Guidelines for essential trace element preparations for parenteral use, JAMA 241:2051–2054, 1979. Copyright 1979, American Medical Association.

*300 μg/kg recommended for premature infant 1,500–3,000 g weight; 100 μg/kg recommended for full-term infant and until age 5 years; thereafter, adult guidelines apply.

†NA, no information available.

TABLE A-39
Weights and Measures

	Weights	Approximate equivalents of metric
1 ounce (oz)	= 28.35 g	30 g
1 pound (lb)	= 453.6 g	
1 stone	= 6.35 kg	
1 gram (g)	= 0.0353 oz	
1 kilogram (kg)	= 2.205 lb	2.2 lb
	Fluid measures	
1 fluid ounce (fl oz)	= 28.41 ml	30 ml
1 pint	= 568.2 ml	600 ml
1 (English) gallon	= 4.546 liter	
	= 1.2 USA gallons	
1 teaspoonful	= 1/8 fl oz	4 ml
1 dessertspoonful	= 1/4 fl oz	8 ml
1 tablespoonful	= 1/2 fl oz	15 ml
1 milliliter (ml)	= 0.0352 fl oz	
1 liter	= 1.760 pints	2 pints
	Measures of length	
1 inch (in)	= 2.54 cm	
1 foot	= 30.48 cm	30 cm
1 mile	= 1.609 km	
1 centimeter (cm)	= 0.394 in	
1 kilometer (km)	= 0.6214 mile	

From Davidson S, Passmore R, Brock JF: Human Nutrition, 5th ed, p 566. Edinburgh, Churchill Livingstone, 1973

TABLE A-40
Conversion Factors for Weights and Measures

To change	To	Multiply by
Inches	Centimeters	2.54
Feet	Meters	.305
Miles	Kilometers	1.609
Meters	Inches	39.37
Kilometers	Miles	.621
Fluid ounces	Cubic centimeters	29.57
Quarts	Liters	.946
Cubic centimeters	Fluid ounces	.034
Liters	Quarts	1.057
Grains	Milligrams	64.799
Ounces (av.)	Grams	28.35
Pounds (av.)	Kilograms	.454
Ounces (troy)	Grams	31.103
Pounds (troy)	Kilograms	.373
Grams	Grains	15.432
Kilograms	Pounds	2.205
Kilocalories	KiloJoules	4.184
Kilocalories	MegaJoules	.004

From Bogert LJ, Briggs GM, Calloway DH: Nutrition and Physical Fitness, 9th ed, p 576. Philadelphia, WB Saunders, 1973

Appendix

TABLE A-41
Equivalent Weights and Measures

	Milligram	Gram	Kilogram	Grain	Ounce	Pound
Weight equivalents						
1 microgram (μg)	.001	.000001				
1 milligram (mg)	1.	.001		.0154		
1 gram (g)	1000.	1.	.001	15.4	0.35	.0022
1 kilogram (kg)	1,000,000.	1000.	1.	15,400.	35.2	2.2
1 grain (gr)	64.8	.065		1.		
1 ounce (oz)		28.3		437.5	1.	.063
1 pound (lb)		453.6	.454		16.0	1.

	Cubic millimeter	Cubic centimeter	Liter	Fluid ounce	Pint	Quart
Volume equivalents						
1 cubic millimeter (mm³)	1.	.001				
1 cubic centimeter (cc)	1000.	1.	.001			
1 liter (l)	1,000,000.	1000.	1.	33.8	2.1	1.05
1 fluid ounce		30.(29.57)	.03	1.		
1 pint (pt)		473.	.473	16.	1.	
1 quart (qt)		946.	.946	32.	2.	1.

	Millimeter	Centimeter	Meter	Inch	Foot	Yard
Linear equivalents						
1 millimeter (mm)	1.	.1	.001	.039	.00325	.0011
1 centimeter (cm)	10.	1.		.39	.0325	.011
1 meter (m)	1000.	100.	1.	39.37	3.25	1.08
1 inch (in.)	25.4	2.54	.025	1.	.083	.028
1 foot (ft)	304.8	30.48	.305	12.	1.	.33
1 yard (yd)	914.4	91.44	.914	36.	3.	1.

From Cooper LF, Barber EM, Mitchell HS, Rymbergen HJ: Nutrition in Health and Disease, 12th ed, p 712. Philadelphia, JB Lippincott, 1953

Index

Index

An *f* following a page number represents a figure; a *t* indicates tabular material.